**American Academy of Pediatrics**

# Signs & Symptoms IN PEDIATRICS

**Editors**
Henry M. Adam, MD, FAAP
Jane Meschan Foy, MD, FAAP



American Academy of Pediatrics
DEDICATED TO THE HEALTH OF ALL CHILDREN™

**American Academy of Pediatrics Publishing Staff**

*Director, Department of Publishing:* Mark Grimes
*Director, Division of Professional and Consumer Publishing:* Jeff Mahony
*Senior Product Development Editor:* Chris Wiberg
*Editorial Assistant:* Carrie Peters
*Director, Division of Editorial and Production Services:* Sandi King, MS
*Manager, Publishing and Production Services:* Theresa Wiener
*Manager, Art Direction and Production:* Peg Mulcahy
*Manager, Editorial Services:* Jason Crase
*Director, Department of Marketing and Sales:* Mary Lou White
*Brand Manager, Clinical and Professional Publications:* Linda Smessaert

Published by the American Academy of Pediatrics
141 Northwest Point Blvd, Elk Grove Village, IL 60007-1019
847/434-4000
Fax: 847/434-8000
www.aap.org

Library of Congress Control Number: 2013949735

ISBN: 978-1-58110-850-7
eBook: 978-1-58110-855-2
MA0703

This book has been developed by the American Academy of Pediatrics. The authors, editors, and contributors are expert authorities in the field of pediatrics. No commercial involvement of any kind has been solicited or accepted in the development of this publication.

The recommendations in this publication do not indicate an exclusive course of treatment or serve as a standard of medical care. Variations, taking into account individual circumstances, may be appropriate.

Every effort has been made to ensure that the drug selection and dosage set forth in this text are in accordance with the current recommendations and practice at the time of publication. It is the responsibility of the health care provider to check the package insert of each drug for any change in indications and dosage and for added warnings and precautions.

The mention of product names in this publication is for informational purposes only and does not imply endorsement by the American Academy of Pediatrics.

The American Academy of Pediatrics is not responsible for the content of the resources mentioned in this publication. Web site addresses are as current as possible but may change at any time.

The publishers have made every effort to trace the copyright holders for borrowed material. If they have inadvertently overlooked any, they will be pleased to make the necessary arrangements at the first opportunity.



Printed in the United States of America

9-349/0215
1 2 3 4 5 6 7 8 9 10

# Editors

**Henry M. Adam, MD, FAAP**
Bronx, New York

**Jane Meschan Foy, MD, FAAP**
Professor of Pediatrics
Wake Forest University School of Medicine
Winston-Salem, North Carolina

# Tools Editors

**Rebecca Baum, MD, FAAP**
Department of Pediatrics
The Ohio State University
Nationwide Children's Hospital
Columbus, Ohio

**Kelly J. Kelleher, MD, MPH, FAAP**
Professor of Pediatrics, Psychiatry, and Public Health
The Ohio State University
Nationwide Children's Hospital
Columbus, Ohio

# Contributors

**Jeffrey R. Avner, MD, FAAP**
Professor of Clinical Pediatrics
Codirector, Medical Student Education in Pediatrics
Albert Einstein College of Medicine
Chief, Pediatric Emergency Medicine
The Children's Hospital at Montefiore
Bronx, New York
**32:** *Gastrointestinal Hemorrhage*

**Sarah Bagley, MD**
Addiction Medicine Fellow
Boston University Medical Center
Boston, Massachusetts
**75:** *Substance Use: Initial Approach in Primary Care*

**Nancy K. Barnett, MD, FAAP**
Dermatology of Cape Cod
Falmouth, Massachusetts
Affiliate, Tufts Medical Center
Department of Dermatology
Boston, Massachusetts
**3:** *Alopecia and Hair Shaft Anomalies*
**43:** *Hyperhidrosis*
**61:** *Pruritus*

**Rebecca Baum, MD, FAAP**
Department of Pediatrics
The Ohio State University
Nationwide Children's Hospital
Columbus, Ohio
**54:** *Medically Unexplained Symptoms*

**Peter F. Belamarich, MD, FAAP**
Director, Division of General Pediatrics
The Children's Hospital at Montefiore
Associate Professor of Clinical Pediatrics
Albert Einstein College of Medicine
Bronx, New York
**1:** *Abdominal Distention*
**11:** *Constipation*

**John P. Bent, MD**
Director, Pediatric Otolaryngology-Head and Neck Surgery
Professor, Albert Einstein College of Medicine
The Children's Hospital at Montefiore
Bronx, New York
**74:** *Stridor*

**Robert J. Bidwell, MD**
Associate Clinical Professor of Pediatrics
University of Hawai`i John A. Burns School of Medicine
Honolulu, Hawai`i
**33:** *Gender Expression and Identity Issues*

**Diane E. Bloomfield, MD, FAAP**
Department of Pediatrics
The Children's Hospital at Montefiore
Bronx, New York
**84:** *Weight Loss*

**Joel S. Brenner, MD, MPH, FAAP**
Director, Sports Medicine and Adolescent Medicine
Children's Hospital of The King's Daughters
Associate Professor of Pediatrics
Eastern Virginia Medical School
Norfolk, Virginia
**8:** *Back Pain*

**Michael G. Burke, MD, MBA, FHM, FAAP**
Department of Pediatrics
Johns Hopkins University School of Medicine
Saint Agnes Hospital
Baltimore, Maryland
**24:** *Extremity Pain*

**John Campo, MD**
Professor and Chair
Ohio State University Wexner Medical Center
Department of Psychiatry and Behavioral Health
Columbus, Ohio
**54:** *Medically Unexplained Symptoms*

**Jayanthi Chandar, MD**
Associate Professor of Clinical Pediatrics
University of Miami Miller School of Medicine
Medical Director, Pediatric Kidney Transplant Program
Miami Transplant Institute
Miami, Florida
**40:** *High Blood Pressure*

**Marcela Del Rio, MD**
Department of Pediatrics
Montefiore Medical Center
Bronx, New York
**37:** *Hematuria*

**Linda M. Dinerman, MD, PC**
Adolescent and Young Adult Medicine
Private Practice
Huntsville, Alabama
**18:** *Dysmenorrhea*
**82:** *Vaginal Discharge*

**Elaine A. Dinolfo, MD, MS, FAAP**
Assistant Clinical Professor of Pediatrics
Columbia University College of Physicians and Surgeons
Attending Physician, Department of Pediatrics
Harlem Hospital Center
New York, New York
**84:** *Weight Loss*

**Mary Iftner Dobbins, MD, FAAP**
Department of Family and Community Medicine
Southern Illinois University School of Medicine
Carbondale, Illinois
**27:** *Family Dysfunction*

**Sarah Edwards, DO**
Assistant Professor
Director of Training, Child and Adolescent Psychiatry Fellowship
Medical Director of Child and Adolescent Psychiatry Hospital Services
Division of Child and Adolescent Psychiatry
University of Maryland School of Medicine
Baltimore, Maryland
**69:** *Self-stimulating Behaviors*

**Mohammad F. El-Baba, MD**
Division Chief, Pediatric Gastroenterology
Fellowship Program Director
Children's Hospital of Michigan
Wayne State University
Detroit, Michigan
**19:** *Dysphagia*

**Lisa Figueiredo, MD**
Division of Pediatric Hematology/Oncology
The Children's Hospital at Montefiore
Bronx, New York
**58:** *Petechiae and Purpura*

**Barbara L. Frankowski, MD, MPH, FAAP**
Department of Primary Care Pediatrics
University of Vermont Children's Hospital
Burlington, Vermont
**49:** *Learning Difficulty*

**Mariam Gangat, MD**
Department of Pediatrics
Division of Pediatric Endocrinology
Rutgers Robert Wood Johnson Medical School
New Brunswick, New Jersey
**41:** *Hirsutism, Hypertrichosis, and Precocious Sexual Hair Development*

**Jack Gladstein, MD**
Professor of Pediatrics and Neurology
University of Maryland School of Medicine
Baltimore, Maryland
**34:** *Headache*

**Mary Margaret Gleason, MD, FAAP**
Associate Professor
Child Psychiatry and Pediatrics
Tulane University School of Medicine
New Orleans, Louisiana
**76:** *Symptoms of Emotional Disturbance in Young Children*

**Beatrice Goilav, MD**
Assistant Professor of Pediatrics
Director, Pediatric Nephrology Training Program
Division of Pediatric Nephrology
The Children's Hospital at Montefiore
Albert Einstein College of Medicine
Bronx, New York
**21:** *Dysuria*

**David L. Goldman, MD**
Associate Professor of Pediatrics
Assistant Professor of Microbiology
The Children's Hospital at Montefiore
Albert Einstein College of Medicine
Bronx, New York
**64:** *Recurrent Infections*

**Waseem Hafeez, MBBS, FAAP**
Associate Professor of Clinical Pediatrics
Albert Einstein College of Medicine
Attending Physician
Division of Pediatric Emergency Medicine
The Children's Hospital at Montefiore
Bronx, New York
**46:** *Irritability and Fussiness*

**Caroline Breese Hall, MD**†
**52:** *Lymphadenopathy*

**David C. Hanson, MD**
Assistant Professor
Divison of General Pediatrics
Department of Pediatrics
University of Minnesota Masonic Children's Hospital
Minneapolis, Minnesota
**24:** *Extremity Pain*

**J. Peter Harris, MD**
Professor Emeritus
Department of Pediatrics
University of Rochester Medical Center
Rochester, New York
**9:** *Cardiac Arrhythmias*

**Nancy Heath, PhD**
Department of Educational and Counselling Psychology
McGill University
Montreal, Quebec
**68:** *Self-harm*

**Sebastian Heersink, MD, FACS**
Eye Center South
Dothan, Alabama
**65:** *Red Eye/Pink Eye*

**Norman T. Ilowite, MD**
Professor of Pediatrics
Albert Einstein College of Medicine
Department of Pediatrics
Division of Rheumatology
The Children's Hospital at Montefiore
Bronx, New York
**50:** *Limp*

**Ginger Janow, MD**
Department of Pediatrics
Division of Rheumatology
Joseph M. Sanzari Children's Hospital
Hackensack, New Jersey
**50:** *Limp*

†Deceased.

**Alain Joffe, MD, MPH, FAAP**
Director, Student Health and Wellness Center
Johns Hopkins University
Associate Professor of Pediatrics
Johns Hopkins University School of Medicine
Baltimore, Maryland
**4:** *Amenorrhea*
**81:** *Vaginal Bleeding*
**82:** *Vaginal Discharge*

**Paul Kaplowitz, MD, PhD, FAAP**
Division of Endocrinology
Children's National Medical Center
George Washington University School of Medicine and Health Sciences
Washington, DC
**70:** *Short Stature*

**Frederick J. Kaskel, MD, PhD**
Professor and Vice Chair of Pediatrics
Albert Einstein College of Medicine
Director, Division and Training Program in Pediatric Nephrology
The Children's Hospital at Montefiore
Bronx, New York
**21:** *Dysuria*

**Diana King, MD, FAAP**
Assistant Professor of Clinical Pediatrics
Albert Einstein College of Medicine
Attending Physician
Division of Pediatric Emergency Medicine
Children's Hospital at Montefiore
The Bronx, New York
**46:** *Irritability and Fussiness*

**Robert A. King, MD**
Professor of Child Psychiatry
Yale Child Study Center
Yale University School of Medicine
New Haven, Connecticut
**79:** *Tics*

**Genna W. Klein, MD**
Division of Pediatric Endocrinology
Joseph M. Sanzari Children's Hospital
Hackensack University Medical Center
Hackensack, New Jersey
**41:** *Hirsutism, Hypertrichosis, and Precocious Sexual Hair Development*

**Robert K. Kritzler, MD**
Deputy Chief Medical Officer
Johns Hopkins HealthCare LLC
Assistant Professor, Johns Hopkins University
Glen Burnie, Maryland
**62:** *Puberty: Normal and Abnormal*

**Daniel Krowchuk, MD, FAAP**
Department of Pediatrics
Wake Forest School of Medicine
Winston-Salem, North Carolina
**63:** *Rash*

**Erik Langenau, DO, MS, FACOP, FAAP**
Department of Learning Technologies
Philadelphia College of Osteopathic Medicine
Philadelphia, Pennsylvania
**57:** *Odor (Unusual Urine and Body)*

**Judith B. Lavrich, MD**
Associate Surgeon
Department of Pediatric Ophthalmology and Ocular Genetics
Wills Eye Hospital
Clinical Instructor
Sidney Kimmel Medical College
Thomas Jefferson University
Philadelphia, Pennsylvania
**65:** *Red Eye/Pink Eye*

**Adam S. Levy, MD**
Associate Professor of Clinical Pediatrics
The Children's Hospital at Montefiore
Albert Einstein College of Medicine
Bronx, New York
**5:** *Anemia and Pallor*
**58:** *Petechiae and Purpura*

**Paul A. Levy, MD, FACMG, FAAP**
Attending Geneticist
Assistant Professor of Pediatrics and Pathology
The Children's Hospital at Montefiore
Bronx, New York
**22:** *Edema*

**Sharon Levy, MD, MPH, FAAP**
Director, Adolescent Substance Abuse Program
Boston Children's Hospital
Assistant Professor of Pediatrics
Harvard Medical School
Boston, Massachusetts
**75:** *Substance Use: Initial Approach in Primary Care*

**Samuel M. Libber, MD, FAAP**
Department of Pediatrics
Johns Hopkins University School of Medicine
Baltimore, Maryland
**59:** *Polyuria*

**Steven E. Lipshultz, MD, FAHA, FAAP**
Schotanus Professor of Pediatrics and Chair
Carman and Ann Adams Department of Pediatrics
Wayne State University School of Medicine
Pediatrician-in-Chief
Children's Hospital of Michigan
President, University Pediatricians
Detroit, Michigan
**40:** *High Blood Pressure*

**Anthony M. Loizides, MD**
Assistant Professor of Pediatrics
Albert Einstein College of Medicine
Attending Physician

Division of Pediatric Gastroenterology and Nutrition
The Children's Hospital at Montefiore
Bronx, New York
**2:** *Abdominal Pain*

**Dominique Long, MD**
Division of Pediatric Endocrinology
Department of Pediatrics
Johns Hopkins Children's Center
Baltimore, Maryland
**62:** *Puberty: Normal and Abnormal*

**Michael G. Marcus, MD**
Vice Chair, Pediatric Ambulatory Network
Director, Division of Pulmonary Medicine and Pediatric Allergy and Immunology
Maimonides Infants and Children's Hospital
Brooklyn, New York
**12:** *Cough*

**Ronald V. Marino, DO, MPH, FAAP**
Professor of Pediatrics
Stony Brook University Medical School
College of Osteopathic Medicine at the New York Institute of Technology
Associate Chairman, Department of Pediatrics
Winthrop University Hospital
Mineola, New York
Pediatric Residency Director
Good Samaritan Hospital Medical Center
West Islip, New York
**66:** *School Absenteeism and School Refusal*

**Robert W. Marion, MD**
Chief, Division of Genetics
Professor of Pediatrics and Obstetrics and Gynecology and Women's Health
The Children's Hospital at Montefiore
Albert Einstein College of Medicine
Bronx, New York
**25:** *Facial Dysmorphism*

**Bethany Marston, MD**
Department of Pediatrics and Medicine
University of Rochester
Rochester, New York
**48:** *Joint Pain*

**Anne May, MD, FAAP**
Assistant Professor of Clinical Pediatrics
The Ohio State University
Nationwide Children's Hospital
Columbus, Ohio
**71:** *Sleep Disturbances (Nonspecific)*

**Jay H. Mayefsky, MD, MPH, FAAP**
Professor of Pediatrics and Family and Preventive Medicine
Rosalind Franklin University of Medicine and Science
Associate Medical Director
School Based Health Centers
Heartland Health Centers
Chicago, Illinois
**20:** *Dyspnea*

**Alicia K. McFarren, MD, FAAP**
Department of Pediatric Hematology, Oncology, and Blood and Marrow Transplantation
Children's Hospital Los Angeles
Los Angeles, California
**5:** *Anemia and Pallor*

**Nancy McGreal, MD**
Assistant Professor of Medicine and Pediatrics
Divisions of Adult and Pediatric Gastroenterology
Duke University Medical Center
Durham, North Carolina
**51:** *Loss of Appetite*
**83:** *Vomiting*

**Sarah E. Messiah, PhD, MPH**
Research Associate Professor
Perinatal/Pediatric Epidemiologist
University of Miami Miller School of Medicine
Department of Pediatrics
Division of Pediatric Clinical Research
Batchelor Children's Research Institute
Miami, Florida
**40:** *High Blood Pressure*

**Ryan S. Miller, MD**
Division of Pediatric Endocrinology
Department of Pediatrics
Johns Hopkins University School of Medicine
Baltimore, Maryland
**59:** *Polyuria*

**Timothy R. Moore, PhD, LP, BCBA-D**
Clinical Director
Minnesota Life Bridge
Cambridge, Minnesota
**68:** *Self-harm*

**Joshua P. Needleman, MD, FAAP**
Pediatric Pulmonary Medicine
Maimonides Medical Center
Brooklyn, New York
**85:** *Wheezing*

**Katherine Atienza Orellana, DO**
Pediatric Gastroenterology
Valley Medical Group
Ramsey, New Jersey
**2:** *Abdominal Pain*

**Philip Overby, MD, DABPN**
Department of Pediatrics and Neurology
New York Medical College
Valhalla, NY
**7:** *Ataxia*

**Philip O. Ozuah, MD, PhD, FAAP**
Professor of Pediatrics
Professor of Epidemiology and Population Health
Albert Einstein College of Medicine
President
Montefiore Health System
Bronx, New York
**28:** *Fatigue and Weakness*
**39:** *Hepatomegaly*
**73:** *Splenomegaly*
**80:** *Torticollis*

**Lane S. Palmer, MD, FACS, FAAP**
Division of Pediatric Urology
Cohen Children's Medical Center of New York
Hofstra North Shore-LIJ School of Medicine
Long Island, New York
**67:** *Scrotal Swelling and Pain*

**Debra H. Pan, MD**
Assistant Professor of Pediatrics
Albert Einstein College of Medicine
Attending Physician
Division of Pediatric Gastroenterology and Nutrition
The Children's Hospital at Montefiore
Bronx, New York
**47:** *Jaundice*

**Sanjay R. Parikh, MD, FACS**
Division of Pediatric Otolaryngology
Seattle Children's Hospital
Associate Professor
Department of Otolaryngology–Head and Neck Surgery
University of Washington
Seattle, Washington
**42:** *Hoarseness*

**Leslie Plotnick, MD**
Professor of Pediatrics, Department of Pediatrics
Johns Hopkins Medical Institutions
Baltimore, Maryland
**59:** *Polyuria*
**62:** *Puberty: Normal and Abnormal*

**Gregory E. Prazar, MD, FAAP**
Elliot Pediatric Specialists
New Hampshire Hospital for Children
Manchester, New Hampshire
**78:** *Temper Tantrums and Breath-holding Spells*

**Oscar H. Purugganan, MD, MPH**
Assistant Professor of Pediatrics
Department of Pediatrics
NewYork Presbyterian/Columbia University Medical Center
New York, New York
**53:** *Macrocephaly*
**55:** *Microcephaly*

**Andrew D. Racine, MD, PhD, FAAP**
Senior Vice President and Chief Medical Officer
Montefiore Medical Center
Executive Director, Montefiore Medical Group
Bronx, New York
**26:** *Failure to Thrive: Pediatric Undernutrition*

**Prema Ramaswamy, MD**
Director, Division of Pediatric Cardiology
Maimonides Infants and Children's Hospital of Brooklyn
Brooklyn, New York
**77:** *Syncope*

**Kimberly J. Reidy, MD**
Assistant Professor
Department of Pediatric Nephrology
The Children's Hospital at Montefiore
Albert Einstein College of Medicine
Bronx, New York
**37:** *Hematuria*

**Marina Reznik, MD, MS**
Associate Professor of Pediatrics
Department of Pediatrics
The Children's Hospital at Montefiore
Albert Einstein College of Medicine
Bronx, New York
**28:** *Fatigue and Weakness*
**39:** *Hepatomegaly*
**73:** *Splenomegaly*

**Yolanda Rivas, MD**
Assistant Professor of Pediatrics
Albert Einstein College of Medicine
Attending Physician
Division of Pediatric Gastroenterology and Nutrition
The Children's Hospital at Montefiore
Bronx, New York
**47:** *Jaundice*

**Ruby F. Rivera, MD, FAAP**
Department of Pediatrics
Albert Einstein College of Medicine
The Children's Hospital at Montefiore
Bronx, New York
**17:** *Dizziness and Vertigo*

**Sarah M. Roddy, MD, FAAP**
Associate Professor of Pediatrics and Neurology
Associate Dean of Admissions
Loma Linda University School of Medicine
Loma Linda University Children's Hospital
Loma Linda, California
**56:** *Nonconvulsive Periodic Disorders*

**Maris Rosenberg, MD, FAAP**
Children's Evaluation and Rehabilitation Center
Department of Pediatrics
Albert Einstein College of Medicine
The Children's Hospital at Montefiore
Bronx, New York
**72:** *Speech and Language Concerns*

**Ann Rothpletz, PhD, CCC-A**
Program in Audiology
Department of Surgery
University of Louisville
**35:** *Hearing Loss*

**Joy Samanich, MD**
Department of Pediatrics
Division of Genetics
The Children's Hospital at Montefiore
Bronx, New York
**25:** *Facial Dysmorphism*

**Richard M. Sarles, MD**
Retired Professor of Psychiatry and Pediatrics
University of Maryland School of Medicine
Baltimore, Maryland
**69:** *Self-stimulating Behaviors*

**Miriam Schechter, MD, FAAP**
Assistant Professor of Pediatrics
Albert Einstein College of Medicine
Department of Pediatrics
The Children's Hospital at Montefiore
Bronx, New York
**23:** *Epistaxis*

**Scott A. Schroeder, MD, FCCP**
Department of Pediatrics
The Floating Hospital for Children at Tufts Medical Center
Boston, Massachusetts
**10:** *Chest Pain*
**38:** *Hemoptysis*

**George B. Segel, MD**
Professor of Medicine
Emeritus Professor of Pediatrics
Wilmot Cancer Center
University of Rochester School of Medicine and Dentistry
Rochester, New York
**52:** *Lymphadenopathy*

**Catherine R. Sellinger, MD, FAAP**
Assistant Professor of Clinical Pediatrics
Albert Einstein College of Medicine
Associate Director, Division of Pediatric Emergency Medicine
Department of Pediatrics
The Children's Hospital at Montefiore
Bronx, New York
**17:** *Dizziness and Vertigo*

**David M. Siegel, MD, MPH, FAAP**
Edward H. Townsend Chief of Pediatrics
Rochester General Hospital
Professor of Pediatrics and Medicine
Chief, Division of Pediatric Rheumatology and Immunology
Division of Adolescent Medicine
University of Rochester School of Medicine and Dentistry
Bronx, New York
**48:** *Joint Pain*

**Pamela S. Singer, MD**
Assistant Professor
Division of Pediatric Nephrology
Department of Pediatrics
Cohen Children's Medical Center
New Hyde Park, New York
**60:** *Proteinuria*

**Catherine C. Skae, MD**
Vice President for Graduate Medical Education
Montefiore Medical Center
Associate Dean for Graduate Medical Education
Albert Einstein College of Medicine
Bronx, New York
**80:** *Torticollis*

**Douglas P. Sladen, PhD, CCC-A**
Mayo Clinic
Rochester, Minnesota
**35:** *Hearing Loss*

**David V. Smith, MD, FAAP**
Assistant Professor of Pediatrics
Department of Pediatrics
Children's Hospital of The King's Daughters
Norfolk, Virginia
**8:** *Back Pain*

**Alfred J. Spiro, MD, FAAP**
Professor of Neurology and Pediatrics
Albert Einstein College of Medicine
Attending in Neurology and Pediatrics
Montefiore Medical Center
Bronx, New York
**44:** *Hypotonia*

**Mark L. Splaingard, MD, FAAP**
Nationwide Children's Hospital
Professor of Pediatrics
The Ohio State University School of Medicine
Columbus, Ohio
**71:** *Sleep Disturbances (Nonspecific)*

**David M. Stevens, MD, FAAP**
Assistant Professor
Department of Pediatrics
The Children's Hospital at Montefiore
Albert Einstein College of Medicine
Bronx, New York
**23:** *Epistaxis*

**Frank Symons, PhD**
Department of Educational Psychology
University of Minnesota
Minneapolis, Minnesota
**68:** *Self-harm*

**Nancy Tarshis, MA, MS, CCC-SLP**
Supervisor of Speech and Language Services
Children's Evaluation and Rehabilitation Center
Albert Einstein College of Medicine
Bronx, New York
**72:** *Speech and Language Concerns*

**Anne Marie Tharpe, PhD**
Professor and Chair
Department of Hearing and Speech Sciences
Associate Director
Vanderbilt Bill Wilkerson Center
Vanderbilt University School of Medicine
Nashville, Tennessee
**35:** *Hearing Loss*

**John F. Thompson, MD**
Professor of Pediatrics
Albert Einstein College of Medicine
Director, Division of Pediatric Gastroenterology and Nutrition
The Children's Hospital at Montefiore
Bronx, New York
**2:** *Abdominal Pain*

**Jessica R. Toste, PhD**
Assistant Professor
Department of Special Education
The University of Texas at Austin
Austin, Texas
**68:** *Self-harm*

**Christine Tracy, MD, FACC**
The Heart Center
Akron Children's Hospital
Akron, Ohio
**36:** *Heart Murmurs*

**Maria Trent, MD, MPH, FAAP**
Associate Professor of Pediatrics
Division of General Pediatrics and Adolescent Medicine
Johns Hopkins University School of Medicine
Baltimore, Maryland
**4:** *Amenorrhea*
**81:** *Vaginal Bleeding*

**Martin H. Ulshen, MD**
Clinical Professor
Pediatric Gastroenterology
University of North Carolina School of Medicine
Chapel Hill, North Carolina
Professor Emeritus
Pediatric Gastroenterology
Duke University School of Medicine
Durham, North Carolina
**15:** *Diarrhea and Steatorrhea*
**51:** *Loss of Appetite*
**83:** *Vomiting*

**H. Michael Ushay, MD, PhD, FAAP**
Medical Director PCCU
Professor of Clinical Pediatrics
Department of Pediatrics
Division of Critical Care
The Children's Hospital at Montefiore
Bronx, New York
**13:** *Cyanosis*

**Élise W. van der Jagt, MD, MPH, FAAP, SFHM**
Professor of Pediatrics and Critical Care
Department of Pediatrics
Golisano Children's Hospital
University of Rochester School of Medicine and Dentistry
Rochester, New York
**29:** *Fever*
**30:** *Fever of Unknown Origin*

**Sandra Vicari, PhD, LCPC**
Southern Illinois University School of Medicine
Springfield, Illinois
**27:** *Family Dysfunction*

**Alfin G. Vicencio, MD**
Chief, Division of Pediatric Pulmonology
Associate Professor of Pediatrics
Mount Sinai School of Medicine
Kravis Children's Hospital
New York, New York
**74:** *Stridor*
**85:** *Wheezing*

**Christine A. Walsh, MD, FAAP, FACC**
Department of Pediatrics
The Children's Hospital at Montefiore
Bronx, New York
**36:** *Heart Murmurs*

**Geoffrey A. Weinberg, MD, FIDSA, FAAP**
Professor of Pediatrics and Director, Pediatric HIV Program
University of Rochester School of Medicine and Dentistry
Golisano Children's Hospital at University of Rochester Medical Center
Rochester, New York
**52:** *Lymphadenopathy*

**Benjamin Weintraub, MD, FAAP**
Marblehead Pediatrics
Marblehead, Massachusetts
**31:** *Foot and Leg Problems*

**Lawrence S. Wissow, MD, MPH**
Professor, Department of Health, Behavior, and Society
Johns Hopkins Bloomberg School of Public Health
Baltimore, Maryland
**6:** *Anxiety*
**14:** *Depression*
**16:** *Disruptive Behavior and Aggression*
**45:** *Inattention and Impulsivity*

**Robert P. Woroniecki, MD, MS**
Chief, Division of Pediatric Nephrology and Hypertension
Associate Professor of Clinical Pediatrics
SUNY, School of Medicine
Stony Brook Children's Hospital
Stony Brook, New York
**60:** *Proteinuria*

**Gaston Zilleruelo, MD**
Professor of Pediatrics
Director, Division of Pediatric Nephrology
Fellowship Training Program Director
Department of Pediatrics
University of Miami Miller School of Medicine
Miami, Florida
**40:** *High Blood Pressure*

# American Academy of Pediatrics Reviewers

Committee on Adolescence
Committee on Child Abuse and Neglect
Committee on Child Health Financing
Committee on Drugs
Committee on Genetics
Committee on Medical Liability and Risk Management
Committee on Native American Child Health
Committee on Pediatric Emergency Medicine
Committee on Practice and Ambulatory Medicine
Committee on Psychosocial Aspects of Child and Family Health
Committee on Substance Abuse
Council on Children With Disabilities & Autism Subcommittee
Council on Communications and Media
Council on Early Childhood
Council on Environmental Health
Council on Foster Care, Adoption, and Kinship Care
Council on School Health
Section on Adolescent Health
Section on Allergy and Immunology
Section on Cardiology and Cardiac Surgery
Section on Child Abuse and Neglect
Section on Clinical Pharmacology and Therapeutics
Section on Developmental and Behavioral Pediatrics
Section on Gastroenterology, Hepatology, and Nutrition
Section on Hematology/Oncology
Section on Infectious Diseases
Section on Lesbian, Gay, Bisexual, and Transgender Health and Wellness (Provisional)
Section on Nephrology
Section on Neurology
Section on Oral Health
Section on Pediatric Pulmonology and Sleep Medicine
Section on Rheumatology
Section on Urology
Task Force on Early Hearing Detection and Intervention

# Contents

**Preface,** xxiii

1 **Abdominal Distention,** 1
*Peter F. Belamarich, MD*

2 **Abdominal Pain,** 13
*Anthony M. Loizides, MD*
*Katherine Atienza Orellana, DO*
*John F. Thompson, MD*

3 **Alopecia and Hair Shaft Anomalies,** 27
*Nancy K. Barnett, MD*

4 **Amenorrhea,** 39
*Maria Trent, MD, MPH*
*Alain Joffe, MD, MPH*

5 **Anemia and Pallor,** 47
*Alicia K. McFarren, MD*
*Adam S. Levy, MD*

6 **Anxiety,** 63
*Lawrence S. Wissow, MD, MPH*

7 **Ataxia,** 77
*Philip Overby, MD*

8 **Back Pain,** 85
*Joel S. Brenner, MD, MPH*
*David V. Smith, MD*

9 **Cardiac Arrhythmias,** 97
*J. Peter Harris, MD*

10 **Chest Pain,** 111
*Scott A. Schroeder, MD*

11 **Constipation,** 119
*Peter F. Belamarich, MD*

12 **Cough,** 135
*Michael G. Marcus, MD*

13 **Cyanosis,** 145
*H. Michael Ushay, MD, PhD*

14 **Depression,** 161
*Lawrence S. Wissow, MD, MPH*

15 **Diarrhea and Steatorrhea,** 173
*Martin H. Ulshen, MD*

**16 Disruptive Behavior and Aggression,** 203
*Lawrence S. Wissow, MD, MPH*

**17 Dizziness and Vertigo,** 215
*Ruby F. Rivera, MD*
*Catherine R. Sellinger, MD*

**18 Dysmenorrhea,** 221
*Linda M. Dinerman, MD, PC*

**19 Dysphagia,** 227
*Mohammad F. El-Baba, MD*

**20 Dyspnea,** 235
*Jay H. Mayefsky, MD, MPH*

**21 Dysuria,** 247
*Beatrice Goilav, MD*
*Frederick J. Kaskel, MD, PhD*

**22 Edema,** 255
*Paul A. Levy, MD*

**23 Epistaxis,** 263
*Miriam Schechter, MD*
*David M. Stevens, MD*

**24 Extremity Pain,** 275
*Michael G. Burke, MD, MBA*
*David C. Hanson, MD*

**25 Facial Dysmorphism,** 287
*Robert W. Marion, MD*
*Joy Samanich, MD*

**26 Failure to Thrive: Pediatric Undernutrition,** 301
*Andrew D. Racine, MD, PhD*

**27 Family Dysfunction,** 317
*Mary Iftner Dobbins, MD*
*Sandra Vicari, PhD, LCPC*

**28 Fatigue and Weakness,** 329
*Philip O. Ozuah, MD, PhD*
*Marina Reznik, MD, MS*

**29 Fever,** 343
*Élise W. van der Jagt, MD, MPH*

**30 Fever of Unknown Origin,** 361
*Élise W. van der Jagt, MD, MPH*

**31 Foot and Leg Problems,** 371
*Benjamin Weintraub, MD*

**32 Gastrointestinal Hemorrhage,** 395
*Jeffrey R. Avner, MD*

33 **Gender Expression and Identity Issues,** 409
*Robert J. Bidwell, MD*

34 **Headache,** 443
*Jack Gladstein, MD*

35 **Hearing Loss,** 451
*Anne Marie Tharpe, PhD*
*Douglas P. Sladen, PhD*
*Ann Rothpletz, PhD*

36 **Heart Murmurs,** 459
*Christine Tracy, MD*
*Christine A. Walsh, MD*

37 **Hematuria,** 471
*Kimberly J. Reidy, MD*
*Marcela Del Rio, MD*

38 **Hemoptysis,** 479
*Scott A. Schroeder, MD*

39 **Hepatomegaly,** 489
*Philip O. Ozuah, MD, PhD*
*Marina Reznik, MD, MS*

40 **High Blood Pressure,** 497
*Jayanthi Chandar, MD*
*Sarah E. Messiah, PhD, MPH*
*Gaston Zilleruelo, MD*
*Steven E. Lipshultz, MD*

41 **Hirsutism, Hypertrichosis, and Precocious Sexual Hair Development,** 523
*Genna W. Klein, MD*
*Mariam Gangat, MD*

42 **Hoarseness,** 539
*Sanjay R. Parikh, MD*

43 **Hyperhidrosis,** 549
*Nancy K. Barnett, MD*

44 **Hypotonia,** 551
*Alfred J. Spiro, MD*

45 **Inattention and Impulsivity,** 559
*Lawrence S. Wissow, MD, MPH*

46 **Irritability and Fussiness,** 569
*Diana King, MD*
*Waseem Hafeez, MBBS*

47 **Jaundice,** 581
*Debra H. Pan, MD*
*Yolanda Rivas, MD*

**48 Joint Pain,** 597
*David M. Siegel, MD, MPH*
*Bethany Marston, MD*

**49 Learning Difficulty,** 607
*Barbara L. Frankowski, MD, MPH*

**50 Limp,** 619
*Ginger Janow, MD*
*Norman T. Ilowite, MD*

**51 Loss of Appetite,** 633
*Nancy McGreal, MD*
*Martin H. Ulshen, MD*

**52 Lymphadenopathy,** 637
*Geoffrey A. Weinberg, MD*
*George B. Segel, MD*
*Caroline Breese Hall, MD*

**53 Macrocephaly,** 649
*Oscar H. Purugganan, MD, MPH*

**54 Medically Unexplained Symptoms,** 657
*Rebecca Baum, MD*
*John Campo, MD*

**55 Microcephaly,** 665
*Oscar H. Purugganan, MD, MPH*

**56 Nonconvulsive Periodic Disorders,** 673
*Sarah M. Roddy, MD*

**57 Odor (Unusual Urine and Body),** 679
*Erik Langenau, DO, MS*

**58 Petechiae and Purpura,** 691
*Lisa Figueiredo, MD*
*Adam S. Levy, MD*

**59 Polyuria,** 699
*Ryan S. Miller, MD*
*Samuel M. Libber, MD*
*Leslie Plotnick, MD*

**60 Proteinuria,** 709
*Robert P. Woroniecki, MD, MS*
*Pamela S. Singer, MD*

**61 Pruritus,** 719
*Nancy K. Barnett, MD*

**62 Puberty: Normal and Abnormal,** 723
*Robert K. Kritzler, MD*
*Dominique Long, MD*
*Leslie Plotnick, MD*

**63 Rash,** 733
*Daniel Krowchuk, MD*

**64 Recurrent Infections,** 747
*David L. Goldman, MD*

**65 Red Eye/Pink Eye,** 759
*Judith B. Lavrich, MD*
*Sebastian Heersink, MD*

**66 School Absenteeism and School Refusal,** 775
*Ronald V. Marino, DO, MPH*

**67 Scrotal Swelling and Pain,** 785
*Lane S. Palmer, MD*

**68 Self-harm,** 799
*Nancy Heath, PhD*
*Jessica R. Toste, PhD*
*Timothy R. Moore, PhD*
*Frank Symons, PhD*

**69 Self-stimulating Behaviors,** 811
*Richard M. Sarles, MD*
*Sarah Edwards, DO*

**70 Short Stature,** 819
*Paul Kaplowitz, MD, PhD*

**71 Sleep Disturbances (Nonspecific),** 827
*Mark L. Splaingard, MD*
*Anne May, MD*

**72 Speech and Language Concerns,** 859
*Maris Rosenberg, MD*
*Nancy Tarshis, MA, MS*

**73 Splenomegaly,** 869
*Marina Reznik, MD, MS*
*Philip O. Ozuah, MD, PhD*

**74 Stridor,** 877
*Alfin G. Vicencio, MD*
*John P. Bent, MD*

**75 Substance Use: Initial Approach in Primary Care,** 887
*Sharon Levy, MD, MPH*
*Sarah Bagley, MD*

**76 Symptoms of Emotional Disturbance in Young Children,** 901
*Mary Margaret Gleason, MD*

**77 Syncope,** 919
*Prema Ramaswamy, MD*

**78 Temper Tantrums and Breath-holding Spells,** 929
*Gregory E. Prazar, MD*

**79 Tics,** 935
*Robert A. King, MD*

**80 Torticollis,** 947
*Philip O. Ozuah, MD, PhD*
*Catherine C. Skae, MD*

**81 Vaginal Bleeding,** 953
*Maria Trent, MD, MPH*
*Alain Joffe, MD, MPH*

**82 Vaginal Discharge,** 963
*Linda M. Dinerman, MD, PC*
*Alain Joffe, MD, MPH*

**83 Vomiting,** 971
*Martin H. Ulshen, MD*
*Nancy McGreal, MD*

**84 Weight Loss,** 979
*Diane E. Bloomfield, MD*
*Elaine A. Dinolfo, MD, MS*

**85 Wheezing,** 987
*Alfin G. Vicencio, MD*
*Joshua P. Needleman, MD*

**Index,** 997

# Preface

Traditionally, medical textbooks have been organized by areas of specialty: infectious diseases, cardiology, pulmonary medicine, and so on. This organizational strategy allows us convenient access to information on diseases we have the need to learn more about. For the practicing physician, however, this presentation has its limits; it is more useful when we know the diagnosis than when we are faced with making one. Very few parents or children come to us with a chief complaint of nephrosis, for instance, or of psoriasis. Rather, what we hear is that "My son's feet and face are swollen," "My daughter has a rash," or even "My child has been struggling in school."

*Signs and Symptoms in Pediatrics* is our effort to address the need of the pediatrician and other primary care physicians for information organized to reflect the way practice really happens. Here you have access to a concise yet thorough discussion of each sign or symptom that may be the chief complaint you are asked to address. Each chapter begins with contextual information on areas like pathophysiology and epidemiology and provides a guide to the history, physical examination, and laboratory and imaging studies that generate an appropriate differential diagnosis. Next are approaches to initial management and suggestions about when to refer or admit.

You will notice too as you look over the table of contents that we take seriously the responsibility of caring for children's mental health as an integral part of pediatric practice. Mental health symptoms may augur the emergence of a mental health problem or impair a child's functioning even in the absence of a diagnosable disorder, and they often complicate acute and chronic medical conditions. They may drive a child's use of health services and affect adherence to treatment. For these reasons, symptoms of emotional disturbance have chapters alongside syncope and disruptive behavior gets the same attention as dizziness.

Not only are our authors expert physicians themselves, but each chapter has been critiqued by members of the pertinent American Academy of Pediatrics (AAP) sections, committees, and councils, providing an additional layer of expertise and supporting our effort to make this reference evidence-based and as reliable as possible. Most also include a listing of helpful Tools for Practice, curated in partnership with Drs Rebecca Baum and Kelly Kelleher, as well as a bibliography of the most relevant AAP policy. We hope you will find this book a robust and easily accessible tool in our shared mission of caring for the health of all children.

Henry M. Adam, MD, FAAP
Jane Meschan Foy, MD, FAAP

# Chapter 1

# Abdominal Distention

*Peter F. Belamarich, MD*

Abdominal distention can be a challenging clinical problem. There are no statistical definitions of distention available to pediatricians; therefore, determining what is likely to be pathological distention takes experience that includes many examinations of children of various ages in illness and in health.

Establishing the precise cause of abdominal distention in childhood from the history and physical examination alone can be also be difficult. The number of possible diagnoses is very large, and the most likely diagnoses vary greatly with the age of the child. Furthermore, not all distention is pathological. Healthy infants may have variable degrees of abdominal distention caused by aerophagia, and healthy toddlers may have a potbelly resulting from a combination of lumbar lordosis and relative hypotonia of the abdominal rectus muscles. The nonpathological distention often seen in infants and toddlers may exceed the mild distention seen with an intraabdominal malignancy. Therefore, a careful systematic approach should be used whenever concerns about abdominal distention are raised. The assessment of distention invites us to combine a systematic diagnostic thinking process and the art of physical diagnosis to minimize tests, radiation, discomfort, and expense.

## ▶ APPROACH TO THE CHILD WITH ABDOMINAL DISTENTION

### *History*

The history should establish the tempo of the obstruction, the presence or absence of gastrointestinal (GI) symptoms, pain, and constitutional symptoms.

Symptoms of GI obstruction (vomiting, pain, constipation, delayed passage of meconium at birth) or malabsorption (failure to thrive, diarrhea or greasy, bulky, malodorous stools) should be sought.

Although pain is present in most cases, an episode of acutely painful distention is a surgical emergency until proved otherwise. Painless distention raises the question of ascites, progressive organomegaly, tumors, and cysts, as well as abdominal hypotonia.

The presence of fever, weight loss, failure to thrive, anorexia, fatigue, irritability, or bone pain should be sought because these symptoms may suggest a malignancy; however, their absence does not exclude one.

See Table 1-1 for a list of symptoms that suggest specific causes of distention.

Medication use, including herbal and alternative therapies, should be reviewed, with particular attention to laxative dependence as a clue to Hirschsprung disease or another organic cause of constipation and to the use of agents that can cause GI ileus and constipation.

**Table 1-1**
**Symptoms That Suggest Causes of Abdominal Distention**

| SYMPTOM | CAUSE |
|---|---|
| Fever | Peritonitis |
| Diffuse severe pain | Obstruction, peritonitis, pancreatitis |
| Constitutional symptoms–weight loss | Malignancy |
| Perception of a mass | Malignancy |
| Bilious or pernicious vomiting | GI obstruction, ruptured ectopic pregnancy |
| Progressive, asymptomatic distention | Malignancy, ascites |
| Malodorous stools | Malabsorption |
| Amenhorrhea | Imperforate hymen |
| Weakness | Rickets |

Travel history should be covered to explore the possibility of geographically specific causes of distention, such as ascariasis, which in many parts of the world is a common cause of GI obstruction.

Given the vast differential diagnosis, the past medical history should be comprehensive. Conditions that predispose children to an intraabdominal malignancy include the WAGR syndrome (*W*ilms tumor, *a*niridia, *g*enitourinary abnormalities, and mental *r*etardation) and Denys-Drash syndrome, which are associated with increased risk for Wilms tumor, and Beckwith-Wiedemann syndrome, which puts affected children at increased risk for Wilms tumor, hepatoblastoma, and adrenal carcinoma. Children with trisomies, DNA fragility syndromes, and immunodeficient states are at risk for lymphoma and leukemia. A history of abdominal surgery suggests the possibility of intestinal adhesions causing obstruction. Behavioral and psychiatric disorders should raise the question of a bezoar.

The family history should include questions about cystic fibrosis (meconium ileus), polycystic kidney disease, metabolic diseases, and whether any history exists of fetal demise or early neonatal death that might indicate an unrecognized metabolic disease, some of which produce hepatomegaly, splenomegaly, and congenital ascites.

In newborns, additional clues may be found in the pregnancy history: oligohydramnios suggests distal urinary obstruction, whereas polyhydramnios is seen with upper GI obstruction.

For infants and toddlers with otherwise asymptomatic distention, a diet history may suggest that the child is at risk for rickets. One must be careful to differentiate a parent's concern about the potbelly appearance of a toddler from more ominous reports of progressive or marked distention or the perception of a mass.

In female adolescents, the possibility of a pregnancy mandates that a confidential history of sexual activity be obtained. A history of amenorrhea despite advanced puberty raises the question of imperforate hymen with hematocolpos.

### *Physical Examination*

The value of an unhurried, calm, reassuring, and gentle approach to the anxious younger child with an abdominal problem cannot be overstated. Having the child's parents model the examination, using the child's doll or toy to demonstrate what will happen, is key to achieving this. To this end, sometimes the examination table must be forgone in favor of lying the child down across the parent's lap. The abdominal examination of an unwilling, anxious child who is struggling and crying is uniformly unsatisfying and nondiagnostic.

The profile of the abdomen should be inspected with the child in a supine position, noting whether the distention is generalized (maximum at the umbilicus) or localized. Box 1-1 presents commonly encountered causes for focal abdominal distention and common masses. The pattern and prominence of the abdominal veins should be noted. Prominent superficial veins on the abdomen may indicate portal hypertension or obstruction to the systemic venous return. The abdomen should be auscultated for hyperactive bowel sounds (malabsorption, acute obstruction), rushes (incomplete obstruction), and absence of sounds (paralytic ileus), as well as for bruits (vascular malformation).

Percussion can be used to differentiate diffuse from the more focal epigastric tympani and to identify shifting dullness in older children.

Gentle palpation should begin from the lower quadrants and progress upward so that the inferior edge of the liver and spleen are appreciated (massive hepatomegaly may be missed if the liver is compressible and the liver's edge is near the child's pelvis). The abdomen should be assessed for focal or generalized tenderness. Involuntary guarding noted on gentle palpation is a sensitive sign of peritoneal inflammation; assessment of rebound tenderness in young children is vulnerable to false-positive results.

**BOX 1-1**

## *Causes of Focal Abdominal Distention or Mass*

**EPIGASTRIUM**

- Duodenal atresia
- Pyloric stenosis
- Malrotation
- Gastric duplication
- Bezoar

**FLANK**

- Wilms tumor
- Hydronephrosis
- Multicystic kidney
- Polycystic kidney
- Neuroblastoma
- Renal vein thrombosis
- Adrenal hemorrhage

**RIGHT UPPER QUADRANT**

- Choledochal cyst
- Hepatomegaly
- Hepatic tumors
- Hydrops of the gallbladder

**LEFT UPPER QUADRANT**

- Splenomegaly
- Splenic cyst

**RIGHT LOWER QUADRANT**

- Ovarian mass
- Intussusception
- Appendiceal abscess
- Crohn disease
- Fecal mass

**LEFT LOWER QUADRANT**

- Ovarian mass
- Fecal mass

**HYPOGASTRIUM**

- Hydrometrocolpos
- Hematocolpos
- Fecal mass
- Presacral teratoma
- Obstructed bladder
- Urachal cyst

When an abdominal mass is appreciated, the examiner should note its location and whether it is painful, is mobile (intraabdominal) or nonmobile (retroperitoneal, malignant), moves with respiration (liver and spleen), is cystic or solid or malleable (fecal masses), is smooth or nodular, and whether it crosses the midline (often seen with neuroblastoma). Ballottement—"throwing" the kidney anteriorly with a finger in the costovertebral angle while palpating the surface of the abdomen with the other hand—can help elicit masses in the flank that cannot be appreciated with simple palpation.

Although rectal examination is often avoided, properly done it can add considerable information to the evaluation of children who have constipation, anal stenosis, Hirschsprung disease, and pelvic masses.

Infants who have ascites have bilateral bulging flanks in the supine position; in older children, the examiner may be able to elicit shifting dullness by percussion or appreciate a fluid wave. An acquired umbilical hernia may indicate massive ascites.

In female patients, a genital examination is necessary to exclude imperforate hymen with hydrometrocolpos or, in adolescents, hematocolpos and pregnancy. In both sexes, lower genitourinary tract malformation raises the question of upper genitourinary tract malformation.

Examination of the inguinal region and the scrotum in males for an inguinal hernia is always warranted with gaseous distention or symptoms of obstruction. Scrotal edema may accompany ascites caused by hypoalbuminemia.

Finally, an assessment of muscular tone and a search for the signs of rickets are warranted in all children whose distention remains unexplained.

## ▶ DIFFERENTIAL DIAGNOSIS

The differential diagnosis can be narrowed further based on whether the child has a tympanitic abdomen or prominent GI symptoms, a palpable mass, organomegaly, ascites, or hypotonia of the abdominal wall (Table 1-2). Causes of hepatomegaly and splenomegaly are reviewed separately in Chapters 39 and 73, respectively.

Life-threatening causes of abdominal distention are presented in Box 1-2.

### *Tympanitic Abdomen in Newborns and Neonates*

Tympanitic abdominal distention may occur in healthy infants, in infants who have systemic conditions, and in newborns who have congenital causes of intestinal obstruction.

Some healthy infants experience transient mild distention because of air swallowing with crying or feeding. This distention is variable, greatest after feeding or fussing, and absent at other times. Vomiting is absent, and the stooling pattern and physical examination are normal.

In the ill newborn, many systemic conditions cause a paralytic intestinal ileus characterized by quiet, nontender abdominal distention: sepsis, pneumonia, birth asphyxia, hypothyroidism, and electrolyte imbalance. In premature infants, necrotizing enterocolitis (NEC) should be considered.

Congenital causes of proximal GI obstruction causing distention in newborns include intestinal atresias, annular pancreas, and abnormalities of intestinal rotation and fixation. The most common proximal GI obstruction is duodenal atresia,[1] characterized by polyhydramnios in 50% of patients and the onset of bilious vomiting in the first hours of life in conjunction with focal epigastric distention (Figure 1-1). Upright plain radiographs

**Table 1-2**
**Differential Diagnosis of Abdominal Distention Based on Physical Examination Findings**

| PHYSICAL SIGN | POSSIBLE CAUSES |
|---|---|
| Tympanitic abdomen | GI ileus<br>GI obstruction<br>Peritonitis<br>Malabsorption<br>Aerophagia<br>Pneumoperitoneum |
| Palpable mass | Renal tumor or hydronephrosis<br>Adrenal, sympathetic chain tumor<br>Hepatomegaly or hepatic tumor<br>GI duplication<br>Mesenteric, omental cyst<br>Ovarian cyst or tumor, hematocolpos<br>Splenic or lymphatic enlargement or tumor |
| Ascites | Hypoalbuminemia from nephrosis, protein-losing enteropathy<br>Hepatic cirrhosis, liver failure<br>Heart failure<br>Urinary ascites from a ruptured urinary tract<br>Chylous ascites—congential, traumatic, postoperative |
| Abdominal wall hypotonia | Generalized hypotonia<br>Rickets<br>Hypothyroidism |
| Signs of peritonitis | GI perforation<br>Bacterial peritonitis<br>Chemical peritonitis–leak of bile or pancreatic fluid |

**BOX 1-2**

***Life-Threatening Causes of Abdominal Distention***

- Sepsis
- Peritonitis (GI perforation, infected ascites, primary bacterial, chemical)
- Intraabdominal bleeding
- Liver, spleen, or GI laceration or hematoma
- Severe pancreatitis
- Splenic sequestration crisis
- Acute renal failure
- Acute liver failure
- Ruptured ectopic pregnancy
- Severe electrolyte disturbances or toxicological etiologies leading to ileus

are diagnostic of duodenal obstruction when they demonstrate the double-bubble sign. Because malrotation is present in up to 19% of patients who have intrinsic duodenal obstruction, a barium enema should establish normal intestinal rotation in infants whose surgery is deferred.

Upper abdominal distention is a common, although not universal, finding in newborns and infants who have symptomatic intestinal malrotation,[2] most of whom have bilious

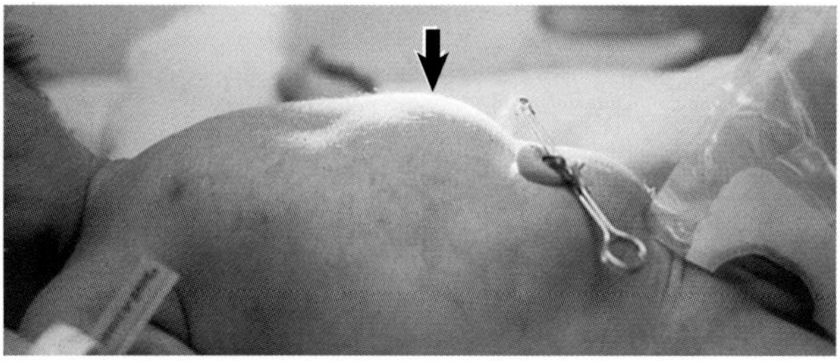

**Figure 1-1**
Newborn infant with duodenal atresia and upper abdominal distention.

vomiting in the first 4 weeks of life. Plain radiographs may demonstrate a distended stomach or duodenal distention with a paucity of gas distally, or the radiographs may appear normal. Therefore, clinical suspicion even in the face of a normal plain radiograph warrants an upper GI series.

Congenital causes of lower intestinal obstruction include distal intestinal atresias, meconium ileus, Hirschsprung disease, small left colon syndrome, and anorectal malformations. Newborns who have lower intestinal obstruction typically develop generalized tympanitic distention over the course of 24 to 48 hours, with bilious vomiting and failure to pass meconium. Although an imperforate anus or an incarcerated hernia will be apparent on physical examination, differentiation of the remaining causes of lower intestinal obstruction involves radiographic evaluation.

Marked tympanitic abdominal distention can be a manifestation of pneumoperitoneum, which is demonstrated by upright and cross-table lateral abdominal radiographs revealing free air within the peritoneum. When pneumoperitoneum is associated with peritonitis, intestinal perforation is likely, and the causes include NEC, volvulus, an intestinal obstruction causing perforation, appendicitis, and spontaneous perforations. In infants on a respirator, pneumoperitoneum may occur without peritonitis as a complication of pneumomediastinum.

## *Tympanitic Abdomen Beyond the Neonatal Period*

Beyond the neonatal period, the causes of a tympanitic abdomen include intestinal ileus, mechanical obstruction, pneumoperitoneum, and malabsorption.

Children with paralytic ileus have a clinical picture similar to that seen with distal mechanical bowel obstruction; however, bowel sounds are diminished or absent, and plain radiographs demonstrate air throughout the GI tract. Common precipitants include abdominal surgery, peritonitis, trauma, shock, sepsis, hypokalemia, and anesthesia, as well as numerous medications.

GI obstruction causing a tympanitic abdomen beyond the neonatal period can be either a late presentation of a congenital problem or an acquired condition, including an intraluminal obstruction such as pyloric stenosis, intussusception, a bezoar, meconium ileus equivalent, intestinal polyps, ascariasis, or an intrinsic tumor. Extraluminal obstructions include postoperative adhesions, an appendiceal abscess, a Meckel diverticulum, and extrinsic compression by abdominal or pelvic masses.

Tympanitic distention occurs in conjunction with the fat malabsorption syndromes, cystic fibrosis, and celiac disease. These conditions are characterized by steatorrhea and variable degrees of malnutrition and suboptimal growth. Although idiopathic constipation is extremely common throughout childhood and impaction can cause abdominal distention (Figure 1-2), marked distention or recurrent distention should not be attributed to functional constipation (see Chapter 11, Constipation).

## Abdominal Masses in Newborns and Neonates

Two-thirds of abdominal masses in neonates originate from the kidney or the urinary tract.[3] Renal masses are retroperitoneal, nonmobile, and appreciated either in the flank or on deep abdominal palpation. Cystic masses predominate and have a slightly compressible quality. A multicystic kidney is the single most common neonatal flank mass. It can be appreciated on physical examination as a soft mass with a slightly irregular contour. The next most frequently encountered renal mass is caused by hydronephrosis. A smooth unilateral flank mass in an otherwise well newborn is usually from a ureteropelvic junction obstruction. Posterior urethral valves, a common cause of bilateral hydronephrosis and hydroureters in male infants, may present as bilateral flank masses or a palpable bladder. Newborns who have autosomal recessive polycystic kidney disease may have palpable bilateral firm flank masses, oliguria, hematuria, and hypertension. The most common renal tumor encountered in newborns is a mesoblastic nephroma, a tumor that can cause massive unilateral nephromegaly.

Renal vein thrombosis is a rare but important cause of a smooth flank mass and hematuria, which develop concurrently in an ill newborn after an episode of asphyxia, sepsis, or dehydration or in an infant whose mother has diabetes.

Of the remaining one third of neonatal abdominal masses that arise outside the urinary tract, neuroblastoma, GI duplications, hydrometrocolpos, and ovarian cysts account for a large proportion.[3]

When a newborn has a palpable flank mass after a traumatic or breech delivery, the possibility of an adrenal hemorrhage should be considered, as should hepatic and splenic hematomas.

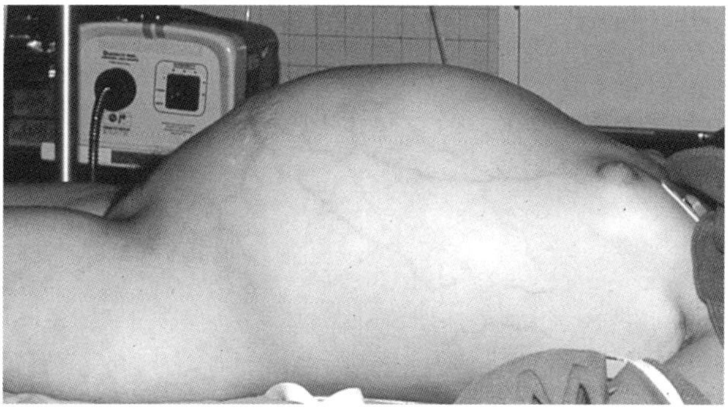

**Figure 1-2**
Thirteen-year-old girl with severe fecal impaction.

Female newborns may have a lower abdominal or pelvic mass from hydrometrocolpos. An imperforate hymen will be evident on the genital examination as a bulging round membrane within the introitus. A rectal examination can be diagnostic for the presence of a dilated vagina in higher obstructions.

Although rare, a significant number of benign epithelial cysts may arise in the neonatal period, including choledochal cysts (right upper quadrant), splenic cysts (left upper quadrant), mesenteric cysts (midabdominal, mobile in the transverse plane), and urachal cysts (hypogastrium). Retroperitoneal cysts include abdominal lymphangiomas and pancreatic cysts.

### Abdominal Masses Beyond the Neonatal Period

The differential diagnosis of masses in infants and older children includes late presentations of congenital masses, malignancies, fecal masses, bezoars, and pancreatic pseudocysts. Of the congenital masses, GI duplications, mesenteric cysts, and choledochal cysts may enlarge slowly and become apparent in later infancy or childhood. Similarly, an adolescent who has an imperforate hymen or vaginal septum may not become symptomatic with hematocolpos until the onset of cyclical uterine bleeding.

The abdomen is the site of origin of Wilms tumor, hepatic tumors, ovarian tumors, about 70% of neuroblastomas, and 30% of non-Hodgkin lymphomas. Neuroblastoma, Wilms tumor, and hepatoblastoma may produce an asymptomatic abdominal distention or mass that is noted by the parent during bathing or dressing the child or by the physician on routine physical examination. Wilms tumor tends to occur in older infants and toddlers, with a peak incidence in 2- to 5-year-old children (Figure 1-3). Hepatoblastoma, the most common primary hepatic malignancy in childhood, is also overwhelmingly discovered as an asymptomatic abdominal mass, with a median age at diagnosis of 12 months. In the second decade, tumors detected as an abdominal mass are predominantly ovarian (Figure 1-4) or non-Hodgkin lymphoma.

Fecal masses are extremely common in childhood and adolescence and may be found in the right lower quadrant (when a redundant sigmoid colon loops to the right), in the hypogastrium, or in the left lower quadrant. They are mobile, nontender, and malleable. Reexamination after laxative therapy should confirm that the masses are no longer present.

Bezoars, which are intragastric concretions of indigestible material, can cause a large array of GI complications, including upper abdominal discomfort and a large mass. Most commonly, they result from the ingestion of hair.

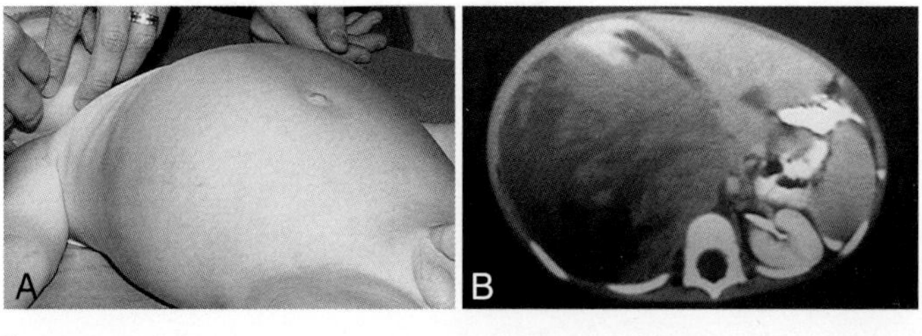


**Figure 1-3**
**A,** Abdominal distention from a right-sided Wilms tumor. **B,** Computed tomographic scan of tumor.

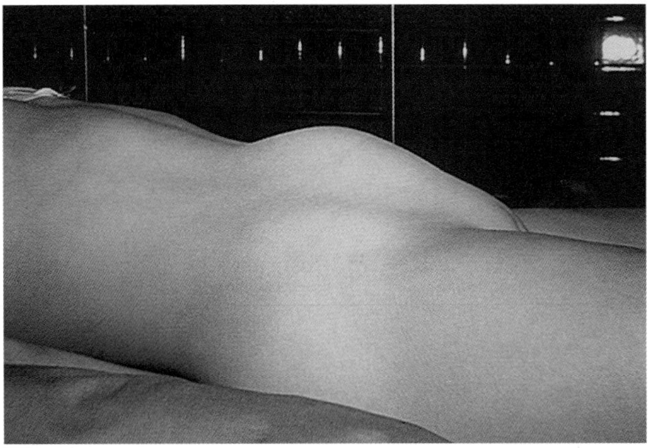

**Figure 1-4**
Lower abdominal distention caused by ovarian teratoma.

## Ascites

The newborn with ascites has a distended, nontympanitic abdomen with bulging and dullness in the flanks, findings that may be mimicked by a massively dilated bladder, a severely hydronephrotic kidney, or a large ovarian cyst. In the newborn, ascites results most often from a perforation within an obstructed urinary tract; in boys, posterior urethral valves are a common precipitant.[4]

Beyond the neonatal period, ascites occurs most commonly as a consequence of nephrotic syndrome. It is also commonly seen in chronic liver disease with cirrhosis and portal hypertension, and in congestive heart failure.

Chylous ascites is a rare condition that occurs when lymphatic fluid leaks directly into the peritoneum because of a malformation or perforation of the intestinal lymphatics. The diagnosis is made by paracentesis.

## Abdominal Wall Hypotonia

Abdominal distention is frequently encountered in healthy infants and may also be seen in infants with a variety of neuromuscular conditions that produce generalized hypotonia. Hypothyroidism and rickets can cause abdominal distention to develop insidiously.

## Radiographic Approach

Although the history and physical examination sometimes provide the diagnosis, many children who have abdominal distention require radiographic imaging. The choice of initial imaging modality is dictated by clinical suspicion, primary findings on physical examination, and locally available resources and expertise.

Given that a single abdominal computed tomography (CT) scan can deliver the same radiation dose as 250 chest radiographs, the judicious and informed use of CT scanning for the evaluation of children with abdominal distention is encouraged.

Therefore, consulting with the radiologist is helpful. Some general guidelines for choosing an initial radiologic study are presented in Figure 1-5.

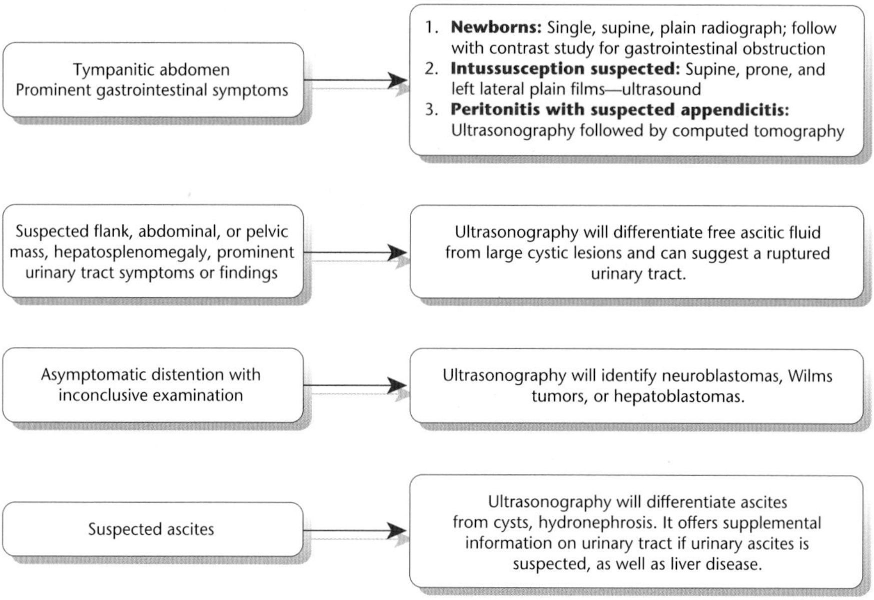


**Figure 1-5**
Initial radiographic approach to abdominal distention in infants and children.

*The author wishes to thank Kenneth Kenigsberg, MD, for providing the photographs used in this chapter.*

## When to Admit

Abdominal distention in the presence of:
- Refractory vomiting, dehydration
- Peritonitis
- Toxic or septic appearance
- Moderate or severe pain that is undiagnosed or not well controlled
- Mass suspicious for malignancy
- Urgently needed surgical or radiologic procedures

### *TOOLS FOR PRACTICE*

#### Medical Decision Support

- *Evaluation and treatment of constipation in infants and children: recommendations of the North American Society for Pediatric Gastroenterology, Hepatology and Nutrition* (guideline), North American Society for Pediatric Gastroenterology, Hepatology and Nutrition (www.naspghan.org/user-assets/Documents/pdf/PositionPapers/constipation.guideline.2006.pdf)
- *North American Society for Pediatric Gastroenterology, Hepatology and Nutrition* (Web site), (www.naspghan.org)

## *AAP POLICY STATEMENTS*

American Academy of Pediatrics Subcommittee on Chronic Abdominal Pain. Chronic abdominal pain in children. *Pediatrics.* 2005;115(3):812–815 (pediatrics.aappublications.org/content/115/3/812.full)

American Academy of Pediatrics Subcommittee on Chronic Abdominal Pain. Chronic abdominal pain in children. *Pediatrics.* 2005;115(3):e370–e381 (pediatrics.aappublications.org/content/115/3/e370.full)

Brody AS, Frush DP, Huda W, Brent RL; American Academy of Pediatrics Section on Radiology. Radiation risk to children from computed tomography. *Pediatrics.* 2007;120(3):677–682 (pediatrics.aappublications.org/content/120/3/677.full)

## *REFERENCES*

1. Escobar MA, Ladd AP, Grosfeld JL, et al. Duodenal atresia and stenosis: long-term follow-up over 30 years. *J Pediatr Surg.* 2004;39:867–871
2. Torres MA, Ziegler MM. Malrotation of the intestine. *World J Surg.* 1993;17(3):326–331
3. McVicar M, Margouleff D, Chandra M. Diagnosis and imaging of the fetal and neonatal abdominal mass: an integrated approach. *Adv Pediatr.* 1991;38:135–149
4. Griscom NT, Colodny AH, Rosenberg HK, et al. Diagnostic aspects of neonatal ascites: report of 27 cases. *Am J Roentgenol.* 1977;128:961–969
5. Avner JR. Abdominal distention. In: Fleisher G, Ludwig S, eds. *Textbook of Pediatric Emergency Medicine.* 6th ed. Philadelphia, PA: Lippincott Williams & Wilkins; 2010
6. Worth L. Molecular and cellular biology of cancer. In: Berman RE, Kliegman RM, Jensen HB, eds. *Nelson Textbook of Pediatrics.* 17th ed. Philadelphia, PA: WB Saunders; 2004

# Chapter 2

# Abdominal Pain

*Anthony M. Loizides, MD; Katherine Atienza Orellana, DO; John F. Thompson, MD*

Abdominal pain is one of the most common symptoms in children and adolescents and is estimated to account for approximately 5% of unscheduled office visits.[1] Acute abdominal pain may require medical or surgical intervention to prevent disability or even death. The precise number of children who experience acute abdominal pain is unknown, but acute appendicitis is the most common abdominal emergency in the pediatric population, with an estimated 81,000 appendectomies performed in the United States annually.[2] More commonly, abdominal pain is a recurrent symptom not associated with physical disability or mortality.[3]

Abdominal pain is determined by several different factors, including the provocation itself, the type of receptor involved, the organization of the neural pathways from the site of injury to the central nervous system, and complex communication between transmission, understanding, and reaction to pain. Abdominal pain is transmitted through distinct types of afferent nerve fibers. These result in the perception of 3 different types of abdominal pain: visceral, parietal, and referred pain.

The principal mechanical signal to which visceral nociceptors are sensitive is stretch, and visceral pain is transmitted by nonmyelinated nerves that are found in muscle, mesentery, peritoneum, and viscera. Pain from abdominal viscera tends to be burning, dull, diffuse, crampy, poorly localized, more gradual in onset, and long in duration. Abdominal organs convey sensation to both sides of the spinal cord; therefore, visceral pain is usually perceived to be in the midline. The area involved may be contingent on the organ affected. For example, lower esophageal, gastric, and duodenal pain tends to be felt in the epigastrium. Small intestinal distention may be periumbilical or in the hypogastrium. Colonic pain may be felt in the lower abdomen. Innervation of most viscera is multisegmental, and because there are fewer nerve endings in the viscera than in more sensitive organs such as the skin, visceral pain is not well localized. Secondary effects such as sweating, restlessness, nausea, vomiting, perspiration, and pallor often accompany visceral pain. The patient may shift position in an attempt to relieve the distress.

Parietal pain is mediated by myelinated nerve receptors that are distributed principally to skin and muscle. These pain receptors respond to tearing or inflammation. Pain is perceived as sharp, sudden, and well-localized such as that which follows an acute injury. Parietal pain occurring from injurious stimulation of the parietal peritoneum is more powerful and more precisely localized than visceral pain. In acute appendicitis, early vague periumbilical visceral pain is followed by the localized parietal pain at McBurney point that is produced by inflammatory involvement of the parietal peritoneum. Parietal pain is typically heightened by movement. Reflexive responses, such as abdominal rigidity and involuntary guarding, are facilitated by spinal reflex arcs that contain parietal pain pathways.[4]

Referred pain results from the interplay between visceral and parietal pain. It is felt in regions distant from the diseased organ and results when visceral and somatic neurons from different areas meet at second-order neurons in the same spinal segment as nerve fibers from cutaneous dermatomes. Examples of this type of pain include referred right scapular pain secondary to acute cholecystitis and mid-back pain from acute pancreatitis.

Functional abdominal pain (FAP), the most common cause of chronic abdominal pain in the pediatric population, was first characterized by Apley and Naish as pain that occurs at least 3 times over a period of 3 or more months severely enough to affect daily activities in children older than 3 years.[5] The prevalence of FAP is estimated to be between 0.3% and 19%, although in large studies the prevalence is far lower, 0.3% to 8%.[6] One reason for the broad range may be the lack of uniformity of criteria for making the diagnosis of FAP: its definitions may be too broad and may include other functional gastrointestinal disorders, such as functional dyspepsia.[6]

A multidimensional measurement of FAP has been created,[7] which, according to the Rome III criteria, must include episodic or continuous abdominal pain, insufficient criteria for other functional gastrointestinal disorders, and absence of an inflammatory, anatomic, metabolic, or neoplastic process that explains the subject's symptoms. The experience of the pain must occur once a week for at least 2 months. Regardless, no consensus exists on an exact definition. Some trends have been noted, such as a higher prevalence of FAP in girls. The highest prevalence occurs in children between 4 and 6 years of age and in early adolescence. Studies have also demonstrated associations between FAP and the child's family dynamics (eg, children living in a single-parent household are more likely to experience chronic abdominal pain[8]), psychological comorbidity such as anxiety,[9] and socioeconomic environment (eg, children living in low-income, low-educated–worker families are more likely to experience pain).[10]

Criteria have been established to categorize FAP. Initially, the Rome I criteria, later updated as Rome II, improved the definition of functional gastrointestinal disorders. Although this classification system can help categorize patients so that appropriate treatment options can be considered, not all children can be clearly placed in these categories. Some authorities have argued against using the classification in children,[11] with one major reason being that the most common location of FAP is periumbilical pain, which is not in the Rome II criteria. Twenty-seven percent of children with abdominal pain do not meet Rome II criteria overall.[12]

Pediatric gastroenterologists have identified and developed similar criteria for childhood functional disorders, including FAP.[13] These criteria—the Rome III Criteria for Functional Bowel Disorders Associated With Abdominal Pain or Discomfort in Children—are based on symptom classification. Four classes were identified, including functional dyspepsia, irritable bowel syndrome, childhood functional abdominal pain as defined above (with a subgroup of children having childhood functional abdominal pain syndrome), and abdominal migraine. The usefulness of the Rome III criteria still needs to be established.[14]

As difficult as characterizing different types of FAP is assessing the effectiveness of various treatments. Significant inconsistencies exist in the methodologic approaches currently used to assess pain.[15] The influence of age and developmental maturation, individual differences (eg, temperament, coping patterns), family interactions, and community and cultural contexts may influence the expression of FAP, and these areas have not been addressed in the assessment of pain. To attend to some of these issues, a multidimensional analytic approach has been developed to assess the primary outcome in clinical trials.[7]

In light of suboptimal classification and assessment tools, a symptom-based differential diagnosis with an emphasis on identifying the warning signals for organic disease is currently the most useful approach to patient care. Pediatricians and other physicians must recognize that chronic abdominal pain can lead to significant dysfunction and disability, with school absences, repeated visits to health care professionals, and secondary psychological problems if assessment and initiation of treatment are either ignored or delayed.[16]

## ▶ DIFFERENTIAL DIAGNOSIS

The differential diagnosis of acute abdominal pain can be subdivided into 3 broad categories: conditions that require immediate surgical intervention (Box 2-1), conditions that may be managed medically at first but may require surgical involvement (Box 2-2), and conditions that can be managed medically (Box 2-3).[17] The differential diagnosis of acute abdominal pain based on age is provided in Box 2-4. The differential diagnosis of chronic or recurrent

BOX 2-1

### *Differential Diagnosis of Acute Surgical Abdomen*

- Closed loop intestinal obstruction
- Volvulus (gastric, midgut, sigmoid)
- Incarcerated hernia (inguinal, internal, external)
- High-grade bowel obstruction
- Nonreducible intussusception
- Malrotation with Ladd bands
- Ovarian torsion
- Testicular torsion
- Acute appendicitis
- Perforated viscus with diffuse peritonitis or toxicity
- Ruptured tumor
- Ectopic pregnancy

BOX 2-2

### *Differential Diagnosis of Acute Abdominal Pain That May Require a Combined Surgical and Medical Approach*

- Partial small bowel obstruction
- Postsurgical adhesions
- Crohn disease
- Lymphoma
- Periappendiceal abscess
- Abdominal abscess
- Cholecystitis
- Gallbladder hydrops
- Pancreatitis
- Pancreatic pseudocyst
- Toxic megacolon or typhlitis

BOX 2-3

## *Differential Diagnosis of Acute Abdominal Pain That May Require Medical Management*

- Upper respiratory infection, pharyngitis
- Viral gastroenteritis (mesenteric adenitis)
- Pneumonia
- Partial bowel obstruction
- Paralytic ileus
- Fecal impaction
- Meconium ileus equivalent in cystic fibrosis
- Bacterial enterocolitis
- Acute gastritis or peptic ulcer
- Acute constipation
- Flare of functional abdominal pain
- Acute hepatitis
- Perihepatitis (Fitz-Hugh–Curtis syndrome)
- Inflammatory bowel disease (Crohn disease and ulcerative colitis)
- Henoch-Schönlein purpura
- Hemolytic uremic syndrome
- Collagen vascular disease
- Hereditary angioedema
- Pyelonephritis
- Renal calculi
- Pelvic inflammatory disease
- Sickle cell crisis
- Diabetic ketoacidosis
- Dysmenorrhea
- Mittelschmerz
- Poisoning
- Porphyria
- Intestinal gas pain

BOX 2-4

## *Main Causes of Acute Abdominal Pain by Age*

**NEONATE**

- Necrotizing enterocolitis
- Spontaneous gastric perforation
- Hirschsprung disease
- Meconium ileus
- Intestinal atresia or stenosis
- Peritonitis owing to gastroschisis or ruptured omphalocele
- Traumatic perforation of viscus (difficult birth)

**INFANT (<2 YEARS)**

- Colic (<3 months)
- Acute gastroenteritis or viral syndrome
- Traumatic perforation of viscus (child abuse)
- Intussusception
- Incarcerated hernia
- Volvulus (malrotation)
- Sickling syndromes

**SCHOOL AGE (2–13 YEARS)**

- Acute gastroenteritis or viral syndrome
- Urinary tract infection
- Appendicitis
- Trauma
- Constipation
- Pneumonia
- Sickling syndromes

**ADOLESCENT**

- Acute gastroenteritis or viral syndrome
- Urinary tract infection
- Appendicitis
- Trauma
- Constipation
- Pelvic inflammatory disease
- Pneumonia
- Mittelschmerz

abdominal pain include those functional entities defined in the Rome III criteria as well as nonfunctional entities as shown in Box 2-5.

Entities that may require combined surgical and medical management are primarily associated with the gastrointestinal lumen as well as its associated organs (see Box 2-2) and can include postsurgical complications such as abdominal abscess or pancreatitis.

The concept of *referred pain* is especially relevant when discussing acute abdominal pain in children. A complete history may provide crucial information that suggests the abdominal pain may originate outside the abdomen. For example, a 3-year-old who has pneumonia may have inflammatory irritation of the diaphragm, resulting in acute abdominal pain as the presenting complaint. In addition, perihepatitis (Fitz-Hugh–Curtis syndrome) can produce acute abdominal pain, and the physician should be sensitive to an adolescent girl's possible reluctance to spontaneously disclose a history of sexual intercourse. The differential diagnoses of medical entities, including those that are extraabdominal or systemic, are listed in Box 2-3.

Box 2-4 lists some of the major diagnostic considerations for acute abdominal pain in children by age.[17] Although diagnostic considerations overlap for each age group, the child's age and physiologic development can help the physician focus the differential diagnosis. For example, Hirschsprung disease should be considered more likely in an infant in the first weeks of life; Mittelschmerz should most certainly be in the differential diagnosis for an adolescent girl.

**BOX 2-5**

## *Main Causes of Chronic Abdominal Pain by System*

**GI TRACT**

- Gastroesophageal reflux disease
- *Helicobacter pylori* gastritis
- Peptic ulcer
- Esophagitis
- Lactose intolerance
- Celiac disease
- Parasitic infection (*Giardia, Blastocystis hominis*)
- Inflammatory bowel disease
- Meckel diverticulum
- Malrotation with intermittent volvulus
- Chronic appendicitis
- Constipation

**GALLBLADDER, LIVER, AND PANCREAS**

- Cholelithiasis
- Choledochal cyst
- Hepatitis
- Liver abscess
- Recurrent pancreatitis

**GENITOURINARY TRACT**

- Hydronephrosis
- Urinary tract infection
- Urolithiasis
- Dysmenorrhea
- Pelvic inflammatory disease
- Mittelschmerz

**MISCELLANEOUS**

- Familial Mediterranean fever
- Malignancies
- Sickle cell crisis
- Lead poisoning
- Vasculitis (especially Henoch-Schönlein purpura)
- Angioneurotic edema
- Acute intermittent porphyria

The cause of chronic abdominal pain in an adolescent female merits particular attention as it may be gynecologic, resulting from dysmenorrhea, endometriosis, pelvic inflammatory disease, or ovarian abnormalities.[18] Dysmenorrhea is common among adolescent females: up to 90% report symptoms when surveyed, but only 40% have told their physician about the pain. Dysmenorrhea is categorized into primary and secondary dysmenorrhea, depending on whether there is underlying pelvic pathology. Symptoms usually begin 6 to 12 months after menarche. Patients complain of lower abdominal pain that is crampy, spasmodic, stabbing, or dull. The pain typically occurs during menstruation but can begin a day or 2 before the onset of menses. Other symptoms can include nausea, vomiting, and diarrhea (see Chapter 18, Dysmenorrhea). Adolescents with endometriosis can present with cyclic abdominal pain, nausea, diarrhea, and constipation in addition to typical symptoms of dysmenorrhea. The pain may be severe enough for patients to miss school, visit their pediatrician, or go to an emergency department for medical care. Sexually active adolescents can have lower abdominal pain from pelvic inflammatory disease and may even have fever and vomiting depending on the severity of the infection. Ovarian abnormalities that may cause pain include ovarian cysts, ruptured ovarian cysts, ovarian torsion, and Mittelschmerz.

Constipation is a frequent cause of abdominal pain and should be considered when a child presents with chronic abdominal pain. Three percent of general pediatric outpatient visits and 25% of pediatric gastroenterology consultations are related to possible dysfunction of defecation.[19] The stool history may be unreliable, and an abdominal radiograph may not be helpful,[20] but serious consideration should be given to empirical treatment with a stool softener (see Chapter 11, Constipation).

## ▶ EVALUATION

### *History*

The approach to the evaluation of abdominal pain begins with a complete history and a thorough physical examination. The findings should direct the use of selected laboratory studies that are based on a reasonable differential diagnosis and will permit a clear therapeutic strategy to be created. Figure 2-1 summarizes the evaluation of the child or adolescent who has abdominal pain.[21,22] The history alone accounts for most of the data the physician uses in making a diagnosis.

A systematic history should elicit information about the location, onset, and severity of the pain, alleviating and precipitating factors, and associated symptoms. The timing of the onset and changes in the intensity, location, and quality of pain over time are essential factors in determining its cause. For children or adolescents who have recurring abdominal pain, information about the timing of the onset of the pain in relation to other events (eg, mealtime, school days), as well as the duration of each episode and the frequency of recurrence, is helpful. The effect of abdominal pain on school, work, sleep, and mood should be assessed. Additional information about family (inherited disorders, concurrent illnesses, chronic pain disorders), medical history (prior surgery, chronic medication, faltering growth), and environmental or behavioral factors (recent changes in family or school, travel, unusual food) should also be obtained. In adolescents, additional history should include menstrual history in females, sexual history, drug and alcohol use, and screening for depression. The timing of abdominal pain in relation to menses must be considered.

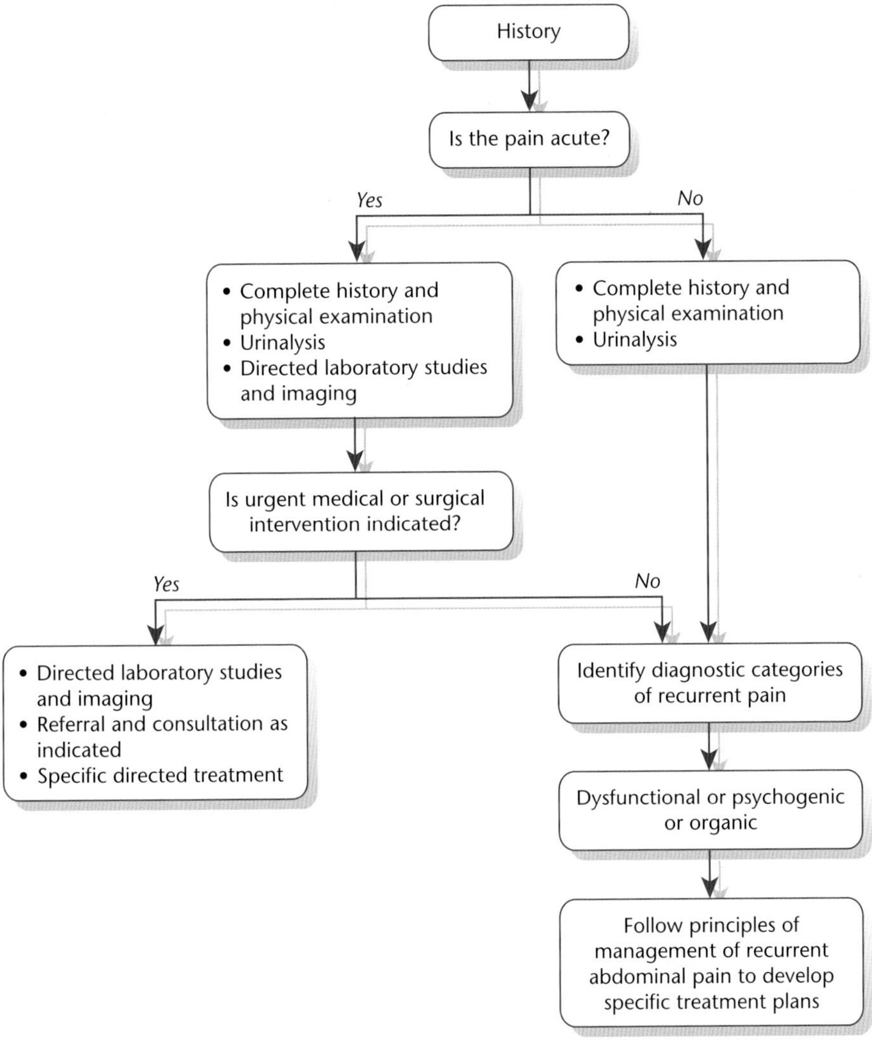


**Figure 2-1**
Evaluation of child or adolescent who has abdominal pain.

One must keep in mind that pain frequency, severity, location, presence or absence of associated symptoms, and effects on lifestyle cannot be used to distinguish between an organic or a functional cause for chronic abdominal pain. Nonetheless, children with FAP are more likely than children without FAP to have headache, joint pain, anorexia, vomiting, nausea, excessive gas, and altered bowel symptoms. The presence of alarming symptoms or signs suggests a higher probability or prevalence of organic disease and may justify performing diagnostic tests and referring the child to a subspecialist. Alarm symptoms or signs include, but are not limited to, involuntary weight loss, deceleration of linear growth, gastrointestinal blood loss, significant vomiting, chronic severe diarrhea, persistent right upper or right lower quadrant pain, unexplained fever, and family history of inflammatory bowel disease (see When to Refer).[23] No single test can diagnose FAP. In patients with FAP a component of pain can be visceral hyperanalgesia,[24] which provides a physiologic explanation of symptoms in children who have distinct functional gastrointestinal disorders.

The physician should help the family understand the importance of the history during the assessment. Both the parents and the patient should be interviewed. Patients must feel comfortable in discussing their own symptoms and concerns, even if these are different from those expressed by the parents. Confidentiality should be addressed with the adolescent patient when the parent is not present. Obtaining a history from the patient without the parents is therefore often useful; similarly, the parents may want to relate some of their concerns without the child being present. Important diagnostic information can be missed if the pediatrician does not give the child and parents the opportunity to provide separate histories.

In addition to the presence of specific symptoms and positive history, negative aspects of the history can provide important information to narrow the differential diagnosis. For example, the absence of dysuria in an older child or adolescent would make the diagnosis of urinary tract infection unlikely.

### Physical Examination

Specific findings on the physical examination of children with FAP have rarely been described. The presence of tenderness on abdominal palpation has been reported to be characteristic of children with recurrent episodes of abdominal pain without evidence of organic disease,[25] but most children's physical examination will be normal. A normal examination and the absence of alarm signals point toward a functional diagnosis for abdominal pain. A complete physical examination, however, including a careful external examination of the urethral orifice and vaginal orifice as well as a rectal examination, should always be part of an initial assessment of abdominal pain. The history of the presenting symptoms will alert the pediatrician to consider more specific aspects of the physical examination.

### Laboratory Evaluation

Laboratory and diagnostic studies performed without any medical indications are generally not helpful and may actually hinder the therapeutic suggestions made by the pediatrician in FAP. The common pitfall of overtesting occurs when the physician responds to the parents' initial request to rule everything out by performing a battery of laboratory or radiographic studies.[26] Maintaining a systematic approach to FAP will not only minimize the use of expensive, unnecessary laboratory studies but will also decrease recurrent emergency visits and, most important, prevent a delay in beginning effective treatment.

Dysfunctional and psychogenic causes account for most diagnoses of FAP, with organic causes identified in only approximately 5% to 8% of cases. However, diagnostic testing is indicated when alarm signals or abnormal physical findings suggest the possibility of an organic disorder. Tests to consider are listed in Box 2-6. When the history and physical examination indicate a dysfunctional or psychogenic cause, urinalysis could suffice as the initial laboratory study, but suggested screening laboratory tests are listed in the table below.

Laboratory and other diagnostic studies such as urinalysis (particularly in female patients of childbearing age), stool, or genital tract cultures; serum chemistries or erythrocyte sedimentation rate; radiographic studies (eg, barium swallow, upper or lower gastrointestinal series, gallbladder series); and abdominal or pelvic ultrasound or computed tomographic

BOX 2-6

## *Suggested Screening Laboratory Tests*

**ALL PATIENTS**

- Complete blood count with differential
- Erythrocyte sedimentation rate
- Comprehensive metabolic panel
- Stool hemoccult

**DIARRHEA**

- Stool ova and parasite
- *Giardia* enzyme-linked immunosorbent assay
- *Clostridium difficile* toxin or PCR
- Celiac panel
- Lactose or fructose breath test
- Dyspepsia
- *Helicobacter pylori* stool antigen testing

scans should be directed to evaluate specific concerns identified in the history and physical examination. For example, when pancreatitis is suspected, laboratory investigations should include amylase and lipase. When indicated, abdominal and pelvic ultrasound provides a safe, noninvasive way to assess bowel and pelvic organ structures and help clarify the need for urgent surgical intervention (eg, intussusception, ovarian torsion, kidney abscess). In general, the physician should consider the least invasive procedures first, keeping in mind the cost of special studies in terms of pain, discomfort, and time.

Common laboratory tests (complete blood cell count, erythrocyte sedimentation rate, comprehensive metabolic panel, urinalysis, stool parasite analysis)[27] are not helpful in distinguishing between organic and functional abdominal pain. The coexistence of abdominal pain and an abnormal test result does not necessarily indicate a cause-and-effect relationship. For example, eliminating dietary lactose as the treatment for patients with demonstrable lactose malabsorption does not necessarily result in the resolution of abdominal pain. Children found to have *Helicobacter pylori* infection are not more likely to have abdominal pain than children without *H pylori*.[23]

### *Imaging Studies*

Ultrasound of the abdomen or pelvis is not useful in the absence of alarm symptoms. When atypical symptoms are present, such as jaundice,[23] urinary symptoms, back or flank pain, vomiting, or abnormal findings at physical examination, abdominal and pelvic ultrasound is more likely than not to detect an abnormality. Endoscopy with biopsy in the absence of alarm symptoms similarly fails to reveal organic disease.[23] Insufficient evidence exists to suggest that the use of esophageal pH monitoring in the absence of alarm symptoms results in finding organic disease.[23] In patients who experience recurrent vomiting, an upper gastrointestinal series should be considered to define potential anatomic abnormalities such as gastric outlet disorder or malrotation. The choice of radiologic test should be guided by the differential diagnosis generated by the history and the physical examination.

## ▶ TREATMENT

The treatment of abdominal pain that results from an organic process should be pursued according to accepted practice guidelines for that condition. The treatment of FAP should be approached as a biopsychosocial phenomenon. FAP is still real pain. However, the response to pain can be subjective and understood through life experience. The treatment may therefore be a combination of psychotherapy, pharmacology, dietary, or alternative medicine techniques. It must always begin with educating the child and parent about the cause of the pain and the treatment plan. This approach not only improves the adherence to the treatment plan but also has been shown to affect the outcome. Treatment response may be influenced by whether the parents perceive the pain to have an organic cause.[28] Similarly, children of parents who are open to a psychiatric consultation are more likely than not to report less pain.[28]

## ▶ MANAGEMENT

A discussion of FAP as a real entity that is a product of an alteration in the brain-gut axis makes understanding the cause of the pain easier for parents. A good analogy is that of a migraine: no specific test exists to confirm the diagnosis, but stress and other inciting events may trigger a headache. When explained this way, parents may be better able to understand that the current thinking of autonomic dysfunction and visceral hypersensitivity as causes of the child's recurrent FAP does not mean that the pain is purely in the child's head or solely the effect of an undiagnosed physical ailment. Equally important is to inform the parents that the goal of therapy is not so much to arrive at a diagnosis, but rather to be able to have the child resume the lifestyle that preceded the onset of the abdominal pain, including school attendance, sleep patterns, and appetite.

### *Psychosocial Treatment*

Several different psychological strategies have been tried in a variety of conditions associated with functional pain, including treatment aimed at individuals or parent–child couples in one-to-one contacts with a therapist, group-based interventions, or a mixture of individual and group treatment. Psychological treatments, principally relaxation and cognitive-behavioral therapy, are effective in reducing the severity and frequency of chronic headache in children and adolescents. However, no evidence has been found for the effectiveness of psychological therapies in attenuating pain in conditions other than headache.[29,30]

Cognitive-behavioral therapy that combines operant elements and stress management may provide an effective treatment for FAP, however.[31] Cognitive-behavioral therapy results in short-term improvement, with more than one-half of patients experiencing freedom from pain.[32,33] The child's coping skills and the parent's caregiving strategies predict the effectiveness of treatment.[34] Disengagement and involuntary engagement are correlated with increased anxiety, depression, and somatic symptoms. Anxiety as a comorbidity has also been associated with FAP,[35] and therefore psychological therapy may be used as a strategy in treating FAP.

Alternative medical techniques for the treatment of functional gastrointestinal disorders, including FAP of childhood, are becoming more common.[36] Specific mind-body techniques include various breathing techniques, guided imagery, progressive muscle relaxation, biofeedback, hypnosis, cognitive-behavioral training, and music therapy. Of those techniques, guided imagery, relaxation, biofeedback, and hypnosis have shown the most promise in treating FAP of childhood. Reported improvement in the pain, fewer school absences, better engagement in social activities, and fewer visits to the physician's office may result from guided imagery and progressive relaxation techniques taught over approximately 4 office visits.[37] Such techniques are easy to learn and teach and are office friendly, even with children.

### *Medication*

Many drugs have been used in the attempt to treat FAP in childhood, including famotidine, pizotifen, and peppermint oil.[38] Peppermint oil in the form of a pH-dependent, enteric-coated capsule has been shown in evidence-based studies to be helpful in alleviating abdominal pain. Other commonly used medications are anticholinergics, antiemetics, antidepressants, and simethicone, but they have not yet been adequately studied. Citalopram, a selective serotonin reuptake inhibitor, has been used to treat FAP, with improvement of abdominal pain, anxiety, depression, and functional impairment.[35] Amitriptyline has also been shown to reduce pain, depressive symptoms, and somatization in children with FAP and irritable bowel syndrome.[39]

Probiotics have been used to treat alterations in gut flora in ulcerative colitis and antibiotic-associated diarrhea, but there is little evidence to support their use in FAP. Only one study has shown that the probiotic VSL#3 improves abdominal pain as well as bloating, gassiness, discomfort, and quality of life in patients with irritable bowel symptoms. Other studies suggest that Lactobacillus GG does not relieve abdominal pain but can decrease its frequency and reduce bloating.[40]

### *Dietary Interventions*

Dietary manipulation has been used to treat the pain in functional disorders. Common dietary interventions include a high-fiber diet, avoidance of lactose, an oligoantigenic diet, and a low-oxalate diet in abdominal migraine.[41] A high-fiber diet may be helpful primarily in constipated children, to substitute for nutrient-poor, high-fat, and high-calorie diets. Avoidance of high-fructose corn syrup and glucose-based drinks and of sugar-free gum and candy may improve symptoms. Sorbitol, the sugar substitute in gum and candy, can cause bloating, cramping, abdominal pain, and diarrhea. Dietary manipulation is easily understood by parents and children and can empower the family.

## ▶ CONCLUSION

The causes of abdominal pain range from acute, life-threatening disease to chronic, functional conditions. Regardless of the cause, the consequences of abdominal pain can be far reaching and can affect not only the emotional and psychological well-being of the child but also the social and economic dynamics of the family. The need to diagnose and treat emergent conditions quickly must be balanced with unnecessary testing when a functional cause seems likely. In the case of functional conditions, a caring approach that educates and reassures the patient and parents is essential for good adherence and an effective therapeutic relationship.

### When to Refer

- Involuntary weight loss
- Deceleration of linear growth
- Gastrointestinal blood loss

- Significant vomiting
- Chronic severe diarrhea
- Persistent right upper or right lower quadrant pain
- Unexplained fever
- Family history of inflammatory bowel disease
- Extraintestinal symptoms
- History of psychiatric disorder
- Abnormal test results
- Anemia or low mean corpuscular volume
- Peripheral eosinophilia
- Increased erythrocyte sedimentation rate
- Increased transaminases
- Increased blood urea nitrogen or creatinine
- Hypoalbuminemia
- Low complement-4 protein

## When to Admit

Hospitalization is seldom indicated for patients with FAP; in fact, some studies suggest that placing patients with FAP in the hospital may lead to worse outcome. Some patients do experience relief of symptoms during hospitalization. However, no data suggest that the natural history of the pain is affected. Hospitalization does not help the fundamental goals of environmental modification and will likely reinforce pain behavior. Hospitalization is required in the following circumstances:

- Surgical or medical emergency as determined by diagnostic or therapeutic intervention
- Inability to tolerate enteral nutrition
- Inability to maintain hydration
- Diagnosis that requires observation to evaluate the progress or natural history of the illness

### TOOLS FOR PRACTICE

#### Engaging the Patient and Family

- *Abdominal Pain* (Web page), American Academy of Pediatrics (www.healthychildren.org/English/tips-tools/Symptom-Checker/Pages/Abdominal-Pain.aspx)
- *Abdominal Pain in Children* (fact sheet), American Academy of Pediatrics (www.healthychildren.org/English/health-issues/conditions/abdominal/Pages/Abdominal-Pain-in-Children.aspx)
- *Abdominal Pain in Infants* (fact sheet), American Academy of Pediatrics (www.healthychildren.org/English/health-issues/conditions/abdominal/Pages/Abdominal-Pains-in-Infants.aspx)

#### Medical Decision Support

- *Pediatric Nutrition Handbook,* 7th ed (book), American Academy of Pediatrics (shop.aap.org)

### AAP POLICY STATEMENT

American Academy of Pediatrics Subcommittee on Chronic Abdominal Pain. Chronic abdominal pain in children. *Pediatrics.* 2005;115(3):812–815 (pediatrics.aappublications.org/content/115/3/812.full)

## REFERENCES


1. Scholer SJ, Pituch K, Orr DP, Dittus RS. Clinical outcomes of children with acute abdominal pain. *Pediatrics.* 1996;98:680–685
2. Gasior AC, St Peter SD, Knott EM, Hall M, Ostlie DJ, Snyder CL. National trends in approach and outcomes with appendicitis in children. *J Pediatr Surg.* 2012;47(12):2264–2267
3. Caty MG, Azizkhan RG. Acute surgical conditions of the abdomen. *Pediatr Ann.* 1994;23:192–201
4. Sengupta JN, Gebhardt GF. Gastrointestinal afferent fibers and sensation. In: Johnson LR, ed. *Physiology of the Gastrointestinal Tract.* New York: Raven Press; 1994:483
5. Apley JNN. Recurrent abdominal pains: a field survey of 1000 school children. *Arch Dis Child.* 1957;33:165–170
6. Chitkara DK, Rawat DJ, Talley NJ. The epidemiology of childhood recurrent abdominal pain in Western countries: a systematic review. *Am J Gastroenterol.* 2005;100:1868–1875
7. Malaty HM, Abudayyeh S, O'Malley KJ. Development of a multidimensional measure for recurrent abdominal pain in children: population-based studies in three settings. *Pediatrics.* 2005;115:e210–e215
8. Bode G, Brenner H, Adler G, Rothenbacher D. Recurrent abdominal pain in children: evidence from a population-based study that social and familial factors play a major role but not *Helicobacter pylori* infection. *J Psychosom Res.* 2003;54:417–421
9. Hyams JS, Burke G, Davis PM, Rzepski B, Andrulonis PA. Abdominal pain and irritable bowel syndrome in adolescents: a community-based study. *J Pediatr.* 1996;129:220–226
10. Grøholt EK, Stigum H, Nordhagen R, Köhler L. Recurrent pain in children, socio-economic factors and accumulation in families. *Eur J Epidemiol.* 2003;18:965–975
11. Christensen MF. Rome II classification—the final delimitation of functional abdominal pains in children? *J Pediatr Gastroenterol Nutr.* 2004;39:303–304
12. Walker LS, Lipani TA, Greene JW, et al. Recurrent abdominal pain: symptom subtypes based on the Rome II Criteria for pediatric functional gastrointestinal disorders. *J Pediatr Gastroenterol Nutr.* 2004;38:187–191
13. Rasquin-Weber A, Hyman PE, Cucchiara S, et al. Childhood functional gastrointestinal disorders. *Gut.* 1999;45(Suppl 2):II60–II68
14. Chogle A, Dhroove G, Sztainberg M, Di Lorenzo C, Saps M. How reliable are the Rome III criteria for the assessment of functional gastrointestinal disorders in children? *Am J Gastroenterol.* 2010;105: 2697–2701
15. Ball TM, Weydert JA. Methodological challenges to treatment trials for recurrent abdominal pain in children. *Arch Pediatr Adolesc Med.* 2003;157:1121–1127
16. Stone RTBG. Recurrent abdominal pain in childhood. *Pediatrics.* 1970;45:732
17. Boyle JT. Pediatric gastrointestinal disease. In: Walker WA, ed. *Pathophysiology, Diagnosis, Management.* 4th ed. Hamilton, Ontario, Canada: BC Decker; 2004
18. Song AH, Advincula AP. Adolescent chronic pelvic pain. *J Pediatr Adolesc Gynecol.* 2005;18:371–377
19. Constipation Guideline Committee of the North American Society for Pediatric Gastroenterology, Hepatology and Nutrition. Evaluation and treatment of constipation in infants and children: recommendations of the North American Society for Pediatric Gastroenterology, Hepatology and Nutrition. *J Pediatr Gastroenterol Nutr.* 2006;43:e1–e13
20. Pensabene L, Buonomo C, Fishman L, Chitkara D, Nurko S. Lack of utility of abdominal x-rays in the evaluation of children with constipation: comparison of different scoring methods. *J Pediatr Gastroenterol Nutr.* 2010;51:155–159
21. Green M. Diagnosis and treatment: psychogenic, recurrent, abdominal pain. *Pediatrics.* 1967;40:84–89
22. Poole SR, Schmitt BD, Mauro RD. Recurrent pain syndromes in children: a streamlined approach. *Contemp Pediatr.* 1995;12:47–50, 52, 58
23. Di Lorenzo C, Colletti RB, Lehmann HP, et al. Chronic abdominal pain in children: a technical report of the American Academy of Pediatrics and the North American Society for Pediatric Gastroenterology, Hepatology and Nutrition. *J Pediatr Gastroenterol Nutr.* 2005;40:249–261

24. Di Lorenzo C, Youssef NN, Sigurdsson L, et al. Visceral hyperalgesia in children with functional abdominal pain. *J Pediatr.* 2001;139:838–843
25. Alfvén G. The pressure pain threshold (PPT) of certain muscles in children suffering from recurrent abdominal pain of non-organic origin. An algometric study. *Acta Paediatr.* 1993;82:481–483
26. Coleman WL, Levine MD. Recurrent abdominal pain: the cost of the aches and the aches of the cost. *Pediatr Rev.* 1986;8:143–151
27. Bhisitkul DM, Listernick R, Shkolnik A, et al. Clinical application of ultrasonography in the diagnosis of intussusception. *J Pediatr.* 1992;121:182–186
28. Crushell E, Rowland M, Doherty M, et al. Importance of parental conceptual model of illness in severe recurrent abdominal pain. *Pediatrics.* 2003;112:1368–1372
29. Eccleston C, Yorke L, Morley S, Williams AC, Mastroyannopoulou K. Psychological therapies for the management of chronic and recurrent pain in children and adolescents. *Cochrane Database Syst Rev.* 2003;(1):CD003968
30. Huertas-Ceballos A, Macarthur C, Logan S. Psychosocial interventions for recurrent abdominal pain (RAP) in childhood (protocol for the Cochrane Review). In: *The Cochrane Library.* Issue 3, Chichester, UK: John Wiley & Sons; 2004
31. Blanchard EB, Scharff L. Psychosocial aspects of assessment and treatment of irritable bowel syndrome in adults and recurrent abdominal pain in children. *J Consult Clin Psychol.* 2002;70:725–738
32. Sanders MR, Rebgetz M, Morrison M, et al. Cognitive-behavioral treatment of recurrent nonspecific abdominal pain in children: an analysis of generalization, maintenance, and side effects. *J Consult Clin Psychol.* 1989;57:294–300
33. Sanders MR, Shepherd RW, Cleghorn G, Woolford H. The treatment of recurrent abdominal pain in children: a controlled comparison of cognitive-behavioral family intervention and standard pediatric care. *J Consult Clin Psychol.* 1994;62:306–314
34. Thomsen AH, Compas BE, Colletti RB, et al. Parent reports of coping and stress responses in children with recurrent abdominal pain. *J Pediatr Psychol.* 2002;27:215–226
35. Dorn LD, Campo JC, Thato S, et al. Psychological comorbidity and stress reactivity in children and adolescents with recurrent abdominal pain and anxiety disorders. *J Am Acad Child Adolesc Psychiatry.* 2003;42:66–75
36. Gerik SM. Pain management in children: developmental considerations and mind-body therapies. *South Med J.* 2005;98:295–302
37. Youssef NN, Rosh JR, Loughran M, et al. Treatment of functional abdominal pain in childhood with cognitive behavioral strategies. *J Pediatr Gastroenterol Nutr.* 2004;39:192–196
38. Weydert JA, Ball TM, Davis MF. Systematic review of treatments for recurrent abdominal pain. *Pediatrics.* 2003;111:e1–e11
39. Saps M, Youssef N, Miranda A, et al. Multicenter, randomized, placebo-controlled trial of amitriptyline in children with functional gastrointestinal disorders. *Gastroenterology.* 2009;137:1261–1269
40. Guandalini S, Magazzù G, Chiaro A, et al. VSL#3 improves symptoms in children with irritable bowel syndrome: a multicenter, randomized, placebo-controlled, double-blind, crossover study. *J Pediatr Gastroenterol Nutr.* 2010;51:24–30
41. Huertas-Ceballos A, Macarthur C, Logan S. Dietary interventions for recurrent abdominal pain (RAP) in childhood (protocol for the Cochrane Review). In: *The Cochrane Library.* Issue 3, Chichester, UK: John Wiley & Sons; 2004

# Chapter 3

# Alopecia and Hair Shaft Anomalies

*Nancy K. Barnett, MD*

Hair matters. It does not serve an essential function, inasmuch as people can live without it. Nevertheless, the symbolism over the ages, from Samson to John Lennon, and the emotional investment people have in their hair make any of its abnormalities a matter of concern. This anxiety is particularly so with alopecia: loss of hair is a disturbing event.

## ▶ INTRODUCTION

A sequence of events makes up the life of a single hair, from active growth over 2 to 6 years, a busy period known as the *anagen phase,* to passivity, a resting period of about 3 months, known as the *telogen phase.* As many as 15% of scalp hairs may be in the telogen phase at any specific time. These hairs are soon lost in the constant turnover of scalp hair, a continuous shedding that is hardly apparent to a casual observer. Surprisingly, about 50% of the hair must be shed for loss to be noticeable. Normally, up to 100 hairs are lost from the scalp daily, and 200 are lost with shampooing.[1]

Hair loss may increase to as much as 60% during a period known as a *telogen effluvium.* During such a period, the situation is similar to that of animals, which shed seasonally. In humans, this change in the normal anagen-to-telogen ratio may occur after a period of stress, such as a prolonged fever, a pregnancy, or a severe illness. It may occur in either gender and results in a diffuse, nonpatterned and nonscarring loss of hair. The diagnosis of telogen effluvium can be confirmed simply by plucking a group of hairs and examining them microscopically (see Evaluation, later in this chapter). Notably, plucking these hairs does not hurt because they are in the resting phase, with the number of resting hairs increased well beyond the usual 10% to 15%.

Excessive hair loss is a matter deserving careful attention. A precise, pointed history and physical examination are necessary. Determining whether an alopecia is scarring or nonscarring is important. The pediatrician must not limit the examination simply to the site of hair loss. The whole body and all its hair-bearing parts must be observed and hairs themselves examined microscopically. Under the light microscope, the normality of the individual hair and the ratio of anagen to telogen hairs can be judged. The pediatrician may need to consult with a dermatologist.

Lanugo, the first hair made by hair follicles in utero, feels silky and covers the entire body of the fetus. It is most often shed in utero, to be replaced by hair that begins to grow on the scalp in the third trimester, continues to grow after birth, and is lost a few months after birth in a normal process that results in temporary near-baldness. In many instances, parents are concerned with the thinning or with a more markedly localized area of loss, usually over the occiput, once thought to be the result of the pressure of the head as the infant lies in the crib. Finally, however, the lost early hair is gradually replaced by new hair, which has more of a "feel" to it; thicker, usually darker, and more stable, it grows longer before loss and does not shed quite so readily.

The constant ebb and flow of growth and shedding and the extreme activity of the hair follicle put it at great risk when exposed to antimetabolites and mitotic inhibitors. When a child loses scalp hair rather suddenly, the physician should be concerned with the possibility of a toxic event. Children treated with antimetabolites for a malignancy suffer hair loss because of the damage done by the drugs during the anagen phase, resulting in an anagen effluvium. Occasionally, similar hair loss is caused by accidental poisoning, as with rat poison that contains thallium or coumarin. In most instances, over a period of several months, new hairs will replace lost hairs, unless the exposure to the toxic element is chronic.

The prognosis for the return of hair depends in large part on elimination of the toxic stimulus and on whether the loss is accompanied by scarring. Loss with scarring (eg, from iatrogenic scalp injury during delivery or from a burn) is permanent. Additionally, hair will not grow at the site of most nevi and hemangiomas. In children, alopecia of both known and unknown causes usually occurs without scarring, as in alopecia areata (spotty loss of scalp hair); alopecia totalis (loss of all scalp hair); alopecia universalis (loss of all scalp and body hair); drug-induced, postfebrile, and postpartum alopecias; and alopecias associated with an endocrinopathy (hypothyroidism, hyperthyroidism, or hypoparathyroidism) or a nutritional deficiency (vitamins A, B, and C, or kwashiorkor).

When scarring is present, as with a kerion associated with tinea capitis, keloid formation, or discoid lupus erythematosus, little hope exists for hair recovery.

## ▶ EVALUATION

Appropriate diagnosis requires microscopic differentiation of the hair and its root in both the anagen and the telogen stages. Anagen hairs have fat, healthy follicle bulbs and an attached emerging long terminal hair, whereas telogen hairs have a small bulb and an attached hair resulting in a club-shaped appearance. Deformities of the hair shaft can be seen, particularly with aminoacidopathies and in a variety of rare syndromes, including Menkes kinky hair syndrome. The physician can differentiate microscopically monilethrix (usually an inherited, autosomal dominant disorder in which the diameter of the hair shaft varies) from pili torti (a disorder in which the hair is twisted on its long axis).

## ▶ DIFFERENTIAL DIAGNOSIS

A variety of congenital and hereditary disorders can produce hair loss, either total or less obvious with thinning (Table 3-1). True congenital alopecia is rare and may be inherited as an isolated autosomal recessive trait or as one feature of a significant hereditary disorder. Hairs may be thin or poorly anchored to the scalp or have a variety of shaft abnormalities. The pediatrician must look for signs of ectodermal dysplasia, and thus consider radiographic exploration for skeletal defects (as with cartilage-hair hypoplasia, congenital ectodermal dysplasia, or orofaciodigital syndrome), as well as for evidence of inherited metabolic or endocrine disorders such as phenylketonuria, homocystinuria, and congenital hypothyroidism.

**TABLE 3-1**
**Distinguishing Characteristics of Alopecia**

| CONDITION | PATTERN OF LOSS | PULLED-HAIR CHARACTERISTICS AS EXHIBITED WITH LIGHT MICROSCOPY |
|---|---|---|
| **NONSCARRING WITH HAIR SHAFT ABNORMALITIES** | | |
| Trichorrhexis nodosa | Fragile, short hair with grayish-white nodules | Nodes along hair shaft similar to interlocking broom or brush ends |
| Monilethrix | Fragile, short, stubble-like growth | Variable shaft thickness gives beaded appearance with internodal breakage |
| Pili torti | Fragile, short, light-colored hair appears spangled as a result of light reflection | Irregularly spaced twists along the shaft appear flattened |
| **NONSCARRING WITHOUT HAIR SHAFT ABNORMALITIES** | | |
| Alopecia areata | Sharply demarcated, round, nearly bald patches appearing suddenly | Exclamation-point hairs from periphery of patches with poorly pigmented shaft and tapered attenuated bulb |
| Androgenetic alopecia | Thinned scalp hair in common male baldness pattern or diffuse thinning with retained frontal hair in the female | Increased telogen-to-anagen ratio<br>Biopsy shows miniaturized anagen bulbs |
| Trichotillomania | Irregularly shaped areas of thinned stubble of varying lengths | Normal cuticle, shaft, and anagen bulb of varying lengths |
| Traumatic alopecia | Bizarre patterns conforming to site and method of injury (eg, head trauma, braiding) | Normal cuticle, shaft, and anagen bulb of varied lengths |
| Telogen effluvium | Diffuse thinning with easy epilation from all areas of scalp | More than 25% of pulled hairs are telogen club hairs with no pigment |
| Anagen effluvium | Significant thinning | Tapered anagen bulbs |
| Loose anagen syndrome | Slight diffuse or patchy thinning | Anagen hairs have misshapen pigmented bulbs with ruffled cuticle |
| **POTENTIALLY SCARRING WITHOUT HAIR SHAFT ABNORMALITIES** | | |
| Tinea capitis and kerion | Varied, ranging from round, minimally inflamed alopecic area with slight seborrheic scale to the boggy, tender, often pustular, severely inflamed kerion | Potassium hydroxide preparation of broken hairs (black-dot hairs) reveals clusters of chains of arthrospores around or in hair shaft and bulb |
| Lupus erythematous | Discoid, well-demarcated erythematous plaques with scale, plugging of follicles, and atrophy or thinning as a result of broken, fragile hair with acute flares (lupus hair) | Not applicable if scarred<br>Short, broken (frayed) anagen hairs |

Children with serious chromosomal defects (eg, de Lange syndrome or trisomy 13 syndrome) usually provide a surfeit of signs and symptoms beyond simple loss of hair.

## *Hair Shaft Anomalies*

Anomalies of the hair usually result in a stubbly growth of broken hair rather than true alopecia. Ectodermal defects, brittle fingernails, or perhaps cataracts and tooth anomalies may accompany hair shaft anomalies. Fragile hair with resultant breakage (trichorrhexis) and stubble can be seen in a variety of rare conditions. Trichorrhexis nodosa is a familial condition in which the hair is fragile without other associated findings. Children with argininosuccinic aciduria, a rare inborn error of metabolism, have stubbly hair and show evidence of severe intellectual disability in the first year of life.

The texture of hair may be helpful in finding the source of difficulty. In an infant who has hypothyroidism, the hair may be coarse, brittle, and without luster; with progeria and cartilage-hair hypoplasia syndrome, it may be fine and even silky. In all these circumstances, the hair may break off, and apparent baldness increases. Whenever the hair is abnormal, it becomes weakened, fragile, and fractured, and it may be lost or unevenly shortened, often resulting in a stubbly, ragged alopecia. Given that a variety of abnormalities (congenital, traumatic, or endocrine) can lead to such fragility and loss, referral to a dermatologist is appropriate so that a specific diagnosis can be pursued.

### Loose Anagen Syndrome

Loose anagen syndrome is characterized by hairs that are quite easily and painlessly pulled from the scalp.[2] Generally, but not always, affected children are blond female preschoolers between 2 and 5 years of age.[2] Their hair appears sparse. The individual hairs are not fragile. On examination, they have misshapen anagen bulbs with a cuffed cuticle and no external root sheath. Hairs are not firmly anchored because of an inner root sheath defect.

Typically, the child's hair is said to be slow growing, seldom requiring cutting. The hair over the occiput often is matted and sticky. The condition may wane with time, although adult-onset cases have been reported.[3] The hair grows thicker and longer, and its pigmentation increases. Nonetheless, even in adulthood, it may pull out easily and painlessly. A hereditary factor may be involved, but most cases are sporadic. The diagnosis can be made from the history and examination, the painless *pull test* (when hair is growing normally, it usually hurts to pull it), and light microscopy to view the recovered hairs. Management is limited to reassurance.

### Trichorrhexis Nodosa

Trichorrhexis nodosa is a common abnormality of the hair shaft that becomes obvious under the light microscope, where the *nodes* resemble the effect observed when the ends of 2 brushes are pushed together. Most often congenital, trichorrhexis nodosa results in breakage of hair and short stubble over the scalp; it may also be a genetic predisposition in some black patients, who experience hair breakage over large areas of the scalp and whose hair will not grow beyond a relatively short length. Trichorrhexis nodosa is usually accompanied by a history of hair straightening or repeated vigorous brushing and combing. Avoiding this kind of steady abuse and using a more gentle cosmetic approach can result in some gradual improvement. White and Asian individuals can experience the same difficulty, probably without congenital or familial relationship, and the breakage occurs most often at the distal end of the hair. White specks marking the nodes may appear after some physical and chemical injuries. Here again, a gentle approach and elimination of any noxious exposure are appropriate.

### Monilethrix

Monilethrix (beaded hair syndrome) is a condition in which scalp hairs have regularly spaced differences in their circumference, suggesting a chain of beads. The cause is unknown but probably genetic, and no treatment is known. Although some degree of recovery may occur spontaneously, particularly after puberty or during pregnancy, this period is a long time to wait, inasmuch as hair breakage becomes obvious during infancy. Variable expressivity was noted in 3 kindreds in whom monilethrix was mapped to the type II keratin gene cluster at chromosome 12q13.[4] Occasionally, associated problems (cataracts, brittle nails, faulty teeth) are suggestive of a more widespread ectodermal defect.

### Pili Torti

Pili torti simply means *twisted hair,* which indeed is the way this hair appears under the microscope. The color is "off," and the hair is coarse and lusterless. It is as though straight and curly hair were competing for a place in the same strand. In cross-section, a straight hair appears round, and a curly hair appears oval. In pili torti, both configurations may be seen in a single strand, an abnormality that can be an important clue to Menkes kinky hair syndrome, an X-linked disease characterized by low serum copper, progressive cerebral degeneration with hypotonia and often with seizures, arterial degeneration, and osteoporotic bones.

## Alopecia Areata

Alopecia areata, most often seen as an acute problem, results in a sudden and total loss of hair in sharply circumscribed, round areas, often several centimeters in diameter, usually on the scalp, but possibly anywhere on the body where hair is found (Figure 3-1). Hairs at the periphery of an area are plucked easily and may be particularly colorless and thin. *Exclamation-point hairs* (broken hairs with a narrow bulb) may appear throughout the patch, which is sometimes salmon colored as a manifestation of the presumed inflammation seen histologically around the hair follicle. The fingernails may be pitted, possibly indicating a more extensive ectodermal problem.

Just a few patches of loss may be found, or a total absence of body hair (alopecia universalis) may occur, including eyebrows and eyelashes. The more extensive the loss and the younger the child, the less likelihood there is of a full recovery. The prognosis is best when the loss is less widespread and only 1 or 2 patches are present. Although the cause is unknown, some suggestion has been made of a T-cell–mediated autoimmune process against the anagen hair follicle, explaining recent interest in T-cell "biologics" as therapy, but thus far they have not been helpful. Occasionally, autoimmune antibodies are identified in patients who have alopecia areata when no other clinical evidence exists of autoimmune disease. An increased incidence of alopecia areata also occurs in persons who have acute autoimmune thyroid disease and vitiligo. The association with multiple genes[5] suggests a susceptibility to alopecia areata, which manifests with various environmental factors.

About one-third of patients who have alopecia areata will regrow hair spontaneously in 6 months; for another one-third, hair will regrow within 5 years. For the remaining one-third, treatment is needed to stimulate hair growth.

Cortisone creams applied topically have been used with some success. In the older, more cooperative child, direct injection of corticosteroid into the scalp or eyebrow hair follicles can be effective, but the process is painful. The primary care pediatrician should seriously question the appropriateness of this procedure, carefully assessing the effect of the disease and of the treatment on the child, and should refer the patient to a dermatologist for consideration

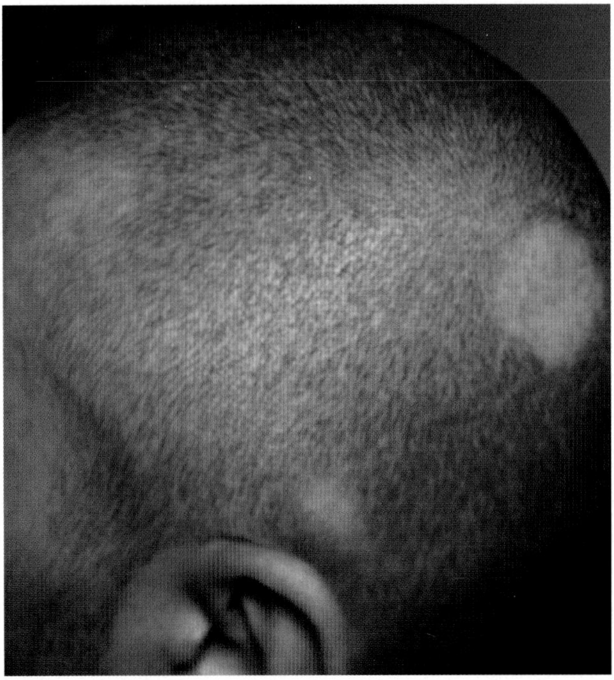

**Figure 3-1**
This 30-year-old man developed slow, expanding hair loss on the scalp 1 month earlier. Although a potassium hydroxide preparation was supposedly positive, he did not improve on topical ciclopirox shampoo and oral itraconazole. At a subsequent visit 1 month later, several new patches were noted, and the diagnosis was changed to alopecia areata. *(Reprinted with permission from DermAtlas.org. Courtesy of Manoj Ram, MD.)*

of this intervention. Excimer laser has shown some success even in children as young as 6 years of age with patchy alopecia areata.[6]

Large areas (>50% scalp hair loss) that require steroid infiltration present obvious difficulty. Oral steroid therapy has the risk for serious complications but is occasionally used. Minoxidil 5% solution can be used twice daily as an adjunct to topical steroids for small, stubborn areas of alopecia. Latanoprost, a prostaglandin analog used to treat glaucoma, was noted by chance to promote the growth of eyelashes and is now commercially available; it and several newer agonists have had mixed results thus far in attempts to treat eyebrow and eyelash alopecia areata.[7] There is no guarantee that if hair regrows in response to therapy it will persist, especially once treatment is stopped.

For extensive alopecia, some irritants (dinitrochlorobenzene immunotherapy and tars such as short-contact anthralin) and psoralen with ultraviolet A light (known as *PUVA therapy*) have been used. These agents should be used only in children older than 12 years and only by a knowledgeable dermatologist in controlled circumstances.

An oddity of alopecia areata is that when hair does regrow, it may initially be white. Eventually color returns, and casual observers cannot identify the formerly affected area.

The efficacy of treatment is difficult to assess because of the waxing-and-waning nature of alopecia areata. The National Alopecia Areata Foundation (www.naaf.org) offers education and support to families, and sponsors an annual children's camp. In counseling patients and their families, primary care pediatricians should remind them that the disease is nonscarring and that there is always the potential for full regrowth. Also, it is hoped that further elucidation of the genetics of alopecia areata will lead to more targeted therapies in the future.

### *Telogen Effluvium*

Telogen effluvium, the diffuse loss of hair in the telogen phase of growth, may be difficult to distinguish from diffuse alopecia areata. Actually the most common form of hair loss in children, telogen effluvium is what occurs in most infants at 6 to 8 weeks of age, probably as a result of the stress of birth, and it is the type of hair loss that can follow the stress of a febrile illness, surgery, or trauma. Presumably, the stress causes a synchronization of the hair follicles so that many of them reach the telogen phase simultaneously, reversing the normal 4:1 ratio of anagen to telogen. This is evident on the hair pull/pluck test, when the hairs of diffuse alopecia areata appear as dystrophic anagen rather than telogen hairs. Telogen effluvium is generally reversible.

### *Androgenetic Alopecia*

Androgenetic alopecia is a genetically determined loss of hair that begins most often with a receding hairline and some thinning over the vertex. It occurs most often in men but can happen to women. The fullest expression is most common in the mature adult, but pediatricians are confronted with the problem in 15% of adolescents older than 14 years. Hairs from affected follicles do not epilate easily on pulling, but they are shorter and finer as a result of normal pubertal androgen increase. No therapy is reliably effective, although topical minoxidil twice daily and hair transplant micrografts may help some individuals. Finasteride can be tried after 18 years of age with male patients but is contraindicated in female patients because of the possibility of genital defects in exposed male fetuses if a pregnancy occurs.

### *Trichotillomania*

Some children have a compulsive need to pull out their hair or even their eyebrows or eyelashes. Although not always of emotional significance, trichotillomania may provide a major clue to an underlying psychosocial problem. The hair loss often appears in large, patchy, ill-defined patterns. The family structure and the interaction with siblings and parents and with friends at home and at school should be explored in an effort to find stressors. Consulting a psychiatrist should also be considered. The primary care pediatrician can paint the attacked areas with petroleum jelly in an attempt to frustrate the habit; however, without attention to the possibility of an underlying emotional issue, this approach is quite obviously temporary. Both imipramine and fluoxetine have been used successfully to control trichotillomania in some children.[8]

The hair lost is that which is most accessible to the probing hand. In some cases, enough is pulled to simulate alopecia areata (Figure 3-2). The patient who eats hair may accumulate it in the stomach and create a trichobezoar (hairball), which may ultimately lead to acute intestinal obstruction or, most often, to the complaint of abdominal pain. A trichobezoar may be palpable as an abdominal mass and is demonstrable on a radiograph. Referral for either endoscopic or surgical removal is indicated.

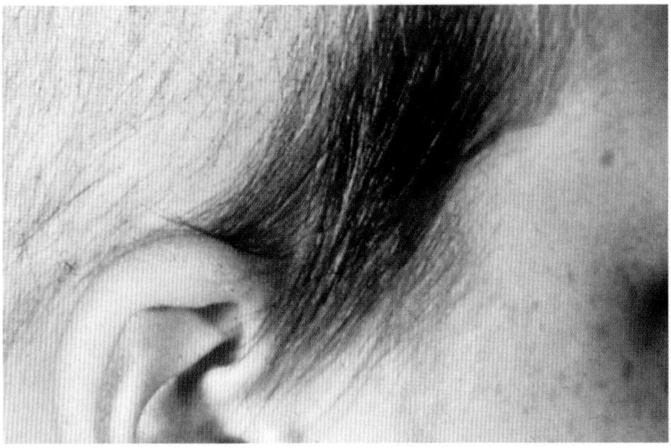

**Figure 3-2**
Trichotillomania in a 7-year-old boy.

### *Traumatic Alopecia*

Hair is fragile. It should be handled gently and without physical or chemical assault. In children, hair is probably best left alone, except for simple washing, combing, and cutting.

Constant teasing or straightening with heat or chemicals may seriously damage hair. Some hairstyles, particularly with barrettes, ponytails, braids, or cornrows, cause constant and prolonged traction, especially along the hairline. The hair may then fall out, accompanied by redness and inflammation, even with pustular involvement of the follicles. Generally, simply discontinuing the stress will help. In childhood, the hair will almost always return, although the regrowth can be slow. Injured hair follicles, whether from trichotillomania or simple traction, do not heal quickly, often taking 3 months or longer to return to an anagen phase.

### *Tinea Capitis*

Whenever a child has patches of alopecia or stubbly hair growth, even in the absence of crusting, scaling, redness, or other inflammatory signs, the physician should consider the possibility of tinea capitis, along with seborrheic dermatitis, atopic dermatitis, or psoriasis (Figure 3-3). Certainly, seborrhea and atopy are more common in children than fungal scalp infection; but particularly when alopecia is accompanied by local adenopathy, tinea capitis should be in the differential diagnosis.[9] Obviously, if crusting, scaling, or redness is present, then the likelihood of alopecia areata is diminished because inflammation is not a symptom of that condition. In any event, the practitioner should perform a mycologic examination, looking particularly for the usual fungus, *Trichophyton tonsurans.* Clinically, the lesions tend to be more elevated than in other forms of tinea and may be characterized by black dots. In rare cases, the endothrix fungi *Microsporum canis* and *Microsporum audouinii* can invade the hair shaft and cause breakage and stubble. *M canis* tends to cause much more inflammation than does *M audouinii.* Endothrix fungal infections, but not *T tonsurans,* can produce a greenish fluorescence under Wood light in a darkened room.

On occasion, particularly with *M canis* or after treatment with an irritant, the affected area may become secondarily infected and seriously inflamed, requiring treatment with an antibiotic. Kerion, a delayed hypersensitivity reaction to the fungus, may develop, and if it is unchecked, the resultant scarring interferes with the regrowth of hair (Figure 3-4). Early diagnosis and treatment are therefore helpful.

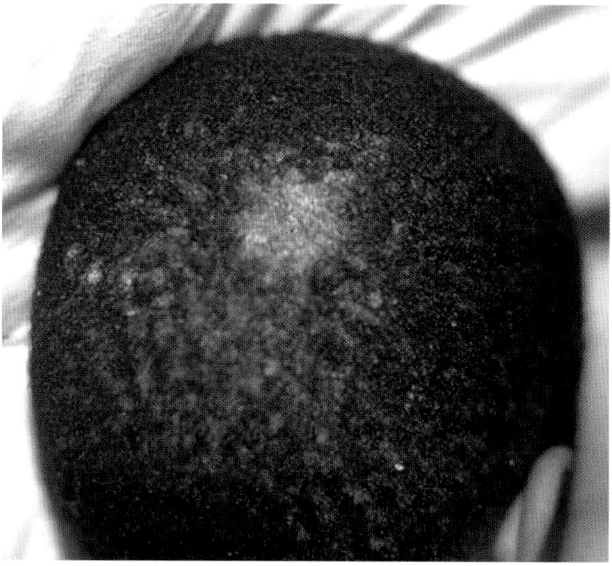

**Figure 3-3**
A young boy admitted for asthma therapy was incidentally noted to have a scalp lesion. The scaling and focal alopecia suggested the diagnosis of tinea capitis. The child was successfully treated with griseofulvin.

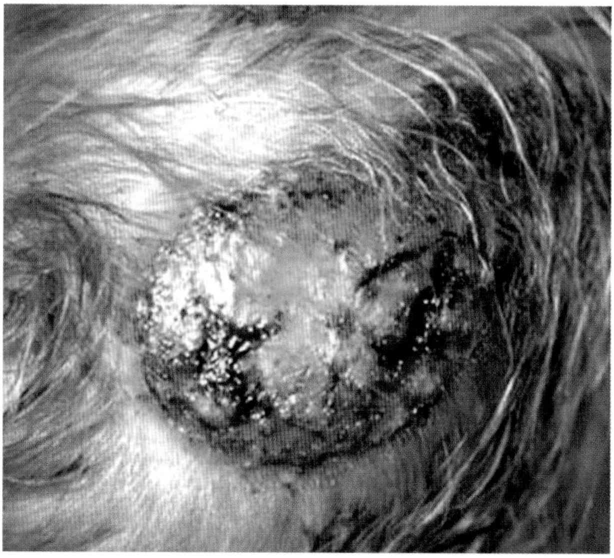

**Figure 3-4**
A 2½-year-old boy with a kerion caused by chronic, progressive tinea capitis.

Topical antifungal agents do not provide adequate treatment because the fungus is deep in the follicle. Oral griseofulvin had been the standard of care, but the usual course of 2 to 3 months of therapy may present difficulties with adherence in a young child. Several newer agents have the appeal of offering a shorter course, despite their expense. The fungicidal drug terbinafine seems effective for tinea capitis when given for 6 weeks and is currently approved for children 4 years and older for this use by the US Food and Drug Administration; neither itraconazole nor fluconazole is approved, but they may be similarly safe for short courses in children.[10] These agents certainly provide alternatives if griseofulvin therapy fails or is not tolerated, but they have not proved effective for *Microsporum* tinea capitis. Liquid itraconazole has been associated with diarrhea in children and with pancreatic adenocarcinoma in laboratory animals and should be avoided.[11] Liver function should be tested if antifungal medications are used for longer than 12 weeks and at the start of therapy if any suggestion of preexisting liver disease exists. Oral prednisone tapered over 10 days may help rapidly decrease the tenderness and inflammation of a kerion and prevent a widespread id reaction. (For medication dosage information, consult the American Academy of Pediatrics *Red Book*.)

## Acrodermatitis Enteropathica

Acrodermatitis enteropathica, an autosomal-recessive disorder characterized by abnormal zinc absorption, has several important cutaneous manifestations, simulating, at times, psoriasis, epidermolysis bullosa, pyoderma, or candidiasis. Zinc deficiency can result in abdominal pain and diarrhea, as well as a wispy alopecia and dystrophic development of the fingernails, suggesting widespread ectodermal involvement. Oral zinc sulfate is the treatment of choice.

## Discoid and Systemic Lupus Erythematosus

Discoid lupus erythematosus can be disfiguring to the scalp and, with scarring, can cause a permanent loss of hair (Figure 3-5). Early treatment with topical or intralesional steroids may prevent scarring. Systemic lupus erythematosus can also cause alopecia, and the scalp

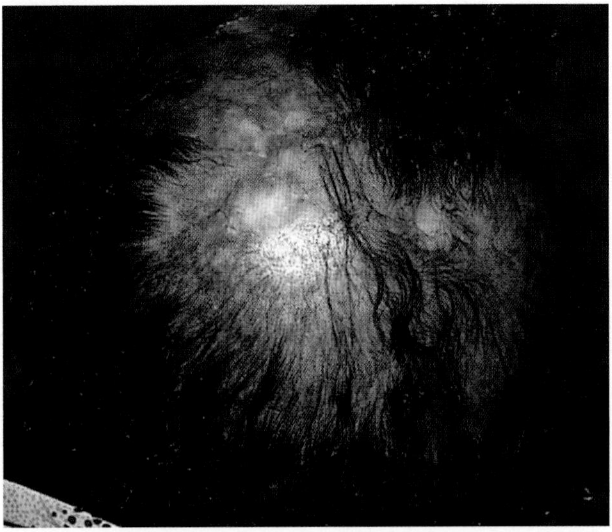

**Figure 3-5**
This 43-year-old woman had an 11-year history of slowly progressive red scaly plaques with central scarring and hair loss in sun-exposed areas. A biopsy showed changes typical of discoid lupus. She was otherwise well and complained of itching of her feet where she had new lesions. She also had some asymptomatic erosions on the tongue and buccal mucosa. *(Reprinted with permission from DermAtlas.org. Courtesy of Kosman Sadek Zikry, MD.)*

itself can be erythematous; however, the loss of hair is generally temporary and does not involve the scarring characteristic of discoid disease.

## ▶ MANAGEMENT

Treatment for alopecia depends, of course, on the cause. Physicians are accustomed to seeing children who are being treated with antimetabolites wearing baseball caps or bandannas to hide their full or partial baldness from anagen arrest. A noticeable loss of hair from any cause may be disturbing to both patient and parent; therefore, the suggestion that the child wear a baseball cap or other concealing adornment may be appropriate. Even a hairpiece can be designed for a child. These steps serve in the interim while physicians attempt potentially helpful treatments or wait expectantly in circumstances in which their role is diagnostic and supportive. The possibility that hair will not fully regrow must be considered when loss follows high fever (telogen effluvium) or chronic toxicity (anagen effluvium); is accompanied by scarring; or occurs in the areas of nevi, aplasia cutis, or persistent hemangiomas. The pediatrician must talk this through with the child who is old enough and with the parents as well, exploring the emotional reaction and discomfort and, if recovery of hair is questionable, working with them to achieve an emotional balance consistent with reality and to adopt suitable coping mechanisms. In most instances, this goal is achievable, and the pediatrician should not back away from trying. The physician, sometimes frustrated by the lack of a practical, successful management regimen, should not forget the value of a willing, listening ear. Plastic surgery expertise should be sought for consideration of hair transplants and scalp reduction (for scarred areas) when possible.

### When to Refer

- Rapid, diffuse hair loss
- Chronic, progressive, localized, or diffuse hair loss without regrowth
- Scarring alopecia
- Inability to grow hair as a result of breakage, loss, or abnormal texture of hair
- Appearance of scalp mass or plaque affecting localized hair loss

### *TOOLS FOR PRACTICE*

#### Engaging Patient and Family

- *National Alopecia Areata Foundation* (Web site), (www.naaf.org)
- *Teens—Alopecia Areata Fact Sheet* (fact sheet), National Alopecia Areata Foundation (www.naaf.org/ kids/teen-facts.asp)
- Locks of Love (Web site), (www.locksoflove.org)

#### Medical Decision Support

- *Pediatric Dermatology: A Quick Reference Guide* (book), American Academy of Pediatrics (shop.aap.org)

### *REFERENCES*


1. Price VH. Androgenetic alopecia in adolescents. *Cutis.* 2003;71(2):115–121
2. Price VH, Gummer CL. Loose anagen syndrome. *J Am Acad Dermatol.* 1989;20(2 Pt 1):249–256
3. Tosti A, Peluso AM, Misciali C, et al. Loose anagen hair. *Arch Dermatol.* 1997;133(9):1089–1093

4. Birch-Machin AM, Healy E, Turner R, et al. Mapping of monilethrix to the type II keratin gene cluster at chromosome 12q13 in three new families, including one with variable expressivity. *Br J Dermatol.* 1997;137:339–343
5. Petukhova L, Duvic M, Hordinsky M, et al. Genome-wide association study in alopecia areata implicates both innate and adaptive immunity. *Nature.* 2010;466(7302):113–117
6. Al-Mutairi N. 308-nm excimer laser for the treatment of alopecia areata in children. *Pediatr Dermatol.* 2009;26(5):547–550
7. Faghihi G, Andalib F, Asilian A. The efficacy of latanoprost in the treatment of alopecia areata of eyelashes and eyebrows. *Eur J Dermatol.* 2009;19(6):586–587
8. Sheikha SH, Wagner KD, Wagner RF Jr. Fluoxetine treatment of trichotillomania and depression in a prepubertal child. *Cutis.* 1993;51(1):50–52
9. Williams JV, Eichenfield LF, Burke BL, Barnes-Eley M, Friedlander SF. Prevalence of scalp scaling in prepubertal children. *Pediatrics.* 2005;115(1):e1–e6
10. Gupta AK, Solomon RS, Adam P. Itraconazole oral solution for the treatment of tinea capitis. *Br J Dermatol.* 1998;139(1):104–106
11. Roberts BJ, Friedlander SF. Tinea capitis: a treatment update. *Pediatr Ann.* 2005;34(3):191–200

# Chapter 4

# Amenorrhea

*Maria Trent, MD, MPH; Alain Joffe, MD, MPH*

Amenorrhea is a common clinical complaint; its frequency varies based on the gynecologic age of the young woman (the number of months or years elapsed since menarche). For example, in a study of high school adolescent girls, the rates of girls who missed 3 consecutive menstrual periods in a single year were 12.5% in the first year after menarche and 5.4% after 7 postmenarchal years.[1] Traditionally, amenorrhea has been classified as being either primary or secondary. Primary amenorrhea is defined as the failure to initiate menstruation, whereas secondary amenorrhea refers to cessation of menses in an adolescent who has previously menstruated. Although some value can be found in knowing whether the absence of menses results from a disruption or lack of initiation, this distinction is of limited clinical utility because many diseases and clinical states cause both primary and secondary amenorrhea.

The mean age of menarche among girls in the United States has decreased slightly in recent years. In 1973, the average age of menarche was 12.76 years among participants in the National Health Examination Survey (NHES). Recent analyses using the combination of the NHES and National Health and Nutrition Examination Surveys (NHANES) have documented that the current average age of menarche in the United States is 12.54 years, with some variation by race or ethnicity.[2] Further analyses from the NHANES data demonstrated that 90% of girls will have menstruated by age 13.75 years and that fewer than 10% menstruate before 11 years of age.[3]

Amenorrhea is a symptom, not a disease, and has a variety of causes. The differential diagnosis for the patient with amenorrhea includes maturational (constitutional) factors, disorders of the central nervous system (CNS), adrenal and ovarian disease, congenital abnormalities of the reproductive tract (primary amenorrhea), thyroid disease, nutritional disorders, systemic illness, and pregnancy. Therefore, a thoughtful, systematic approach to the patient who has a menstrual disorder usually identifies the cause. The major causes of amenorrhea are listed in Box 4-1.

Menstruation usually begins about 2 years after breast budding; however, the interval between these events can be as short as 6 months or as long as 4 years. Given this broad range of individual variation in the onset of puberty and menarche, the physician first must assess pubertal status, noting breast and pubic hair development. An evaluation is warranted if

1. No signs of secondary sexual development are present by 14 years of age. In this instance, the evaluation should include an assessment for delayed puberty. (See Chapter 62, Puberty: Normal and Abnormal.)
2. Menarche has not occurred by 16 years of age even if the patient has experienced development of secondary sexual characteristics and growth has been normal.

BOX 4-1

## *Major Causes of Amenorrhea in Adolescent Girls by Organ System*

**CENTRAL NERVOUS SYSTEM**

- Familial-physiologic delay
- Systemic illness
- Developmental defects (eg, Kallmann syndrome)
- Laurence-Moon-Bardet-Biedl syndrome
- Prader-Willi syndrome
- Infiltrative disease
- Head trauma
- Sheehan syndrome (postpartum necrosis)
- Primary empty sella syndrome
- Irradiation
- Surgery
- Depression
- Drugs (eg, hormonal contraception, cocaine, phenothiazines)
- Psychological stressors
- Eating disorders (eg, anorexia nervosa)
- High-level athletic training with low weight for height (eg, female athlete triad)
- Psychosocial stress
- Central nervous system tumor (eg, prolactinoma)

**THYROID**

- Hyperthyroidism
- Hypothyroidism

**ADRENAL**

- Addison disease
- Cushing syndrome
- Late-onset congenital adrenal hyperplasia (21-hydroxylase deficiency)
- Tumor

**OVARIES**

- Gonadal dysgenesis
- Premature ovarian failure
- Radiation or chemotherapy
- Ovarian removal or destruction
- Polycystic ovary syndrome
- Tumor

**UTERUS**

- Pregnancy
- Uterine synechiae
- Congenital abnormalities (müllerian agenesis, androgen insensitivity)

**VAGINA, CERVIX, HYMEN**

- Agenesis
- Imperforate hymen
- Transverse septum

3. Menarche has not occurred and the patient has been at Tanner stage 5 for at least 1 year or has had breast development for 4 years.
4. Three consecutive menstrual cycles are absent in a patient with signs of an eating disorder.
5. The patient has previously menstruated but has had amenorrhea for more than 6 months.
6. The patient has not had menses and has symptoms or stigmata of another disease process such as Turner syndrome.
7. The patient has had menstrual cycles, has missed one period, and has had unprotected sexual intercourse in the interim. In this instance, the patient should be evaluated for pregnancy.

Gynecologic age is important when evaluating an adolescent who seems to have secondary amenorrhea. After the onset of menarche, many teenagers will menstruate sporadically; regular monthly cycles often are not established until 1 to 2 years after menarche.[4] Clearly, the abrupt cessation of menstruation in a teenager who has established regular cycles is of greater concern than the absence of menses for 3 to 4 months in a teenager who has a gynecologic age of 6 months to 1 year. The point at which the physician elects to pursue an evaluation depends on the anxiety of the patient and her family, the possibility of pregnancy, and the likelihood that a potentially serious disease is responsible for the amenorrhea. For a general approach to the evaluation of amenorrhea, see Figure 4-1.

## ▶ HISTORY

The history and physical examination are critical elements in the diagnostic approach. Although the adolescent should always be interviewed alone during the visit, many adolescent girls may have difficulty with the details of their own medical and family medical histories, making maternal involvement during the visit extremely useful. Mothers are able to provide detailed medical histories for their daughters from infancy to the present, the details of their own menstrual and medical histories, and usually that of first-degree female relatives. Finally, mothers are often acutely aware of behavioral factors within the home, such as a daughter's menstrual patterns, symptoms associated with menstrual cycles, consumption of pads or tampons, dietary and exercise patterns, stressors on the family and children, and the subtle development of physical features such as weight gain, acne, or hirsutism. Detailed discussions of personal lifestyle factors such as sexual activity should be conducted without the parent present. Use of the HEADDSS assessment (*h*ome situation, *e*ducational status of the patient, *a*ctivities, *d*iet, *d*rug use, *s*uicidality or depression, and *s*exuality or sexual behavior) facilitates this portion of the interview.

The hypothalamic-pituitary-ovarian axis of the adolescent is more sensitive to physical and psychological stress than is that of the adult woman. Stress, emotional upset, fever accompanying viral illness, and changes in weight or environment (eg, going away to college) all can induce amenorrhea. Comments about weight or body image may be a clue to anorexia nervosa. The history also should include questions about drug or medication use, including any forms of hormonal contraception that the patient may be using. Most women who develop amenorrhea while using combined estrogen-progesterone contraceptive methods resume menstruation within 6 months of discontinuing their use. Pregnancy should be the primary consideration in patients who have a history of sexual intercourse. Unfortunately, denial of sexual activity does not exclude pregnancy, inasmuch as many teenagers are reluctant to admit to something they believe will be met with condemnation from adults. Sudden cessation of menstruation is more likely to indicate pregnancy or stress as a cause, whereas a gradual cessation suggests polycystic ovary disease or premature ovarian failure. A history of uterine surgery or abortion raises the possibility of uterine synechiae. Given that many women are involved in sports, questions about exercise patterns or participation in athletics (frequency, duration, intensity) are essential. The physician must be sure to seek clues to any of the endocrine abnormalities (eg, galactorrhea), a history of past CNS insults (eg, meningitis), or symptoms of an intracranial tumor. The age at which the patient's mother and sisters first menstruated is also helpful information because such a pattern may be familial.[2] Finally, chronic diseases such as inflammatory bowel disease or renal failure may be subtle in their early presentation; hence, questions aimed at uncovering these illnesses must be included in the review of systems.

## ▶ PHYSICAL EXAMINATION

Plotting of previous growth data (both height and weight) is essential. A short girl who has amenorrhea should prompt a search for the other physical characteristics of Turner

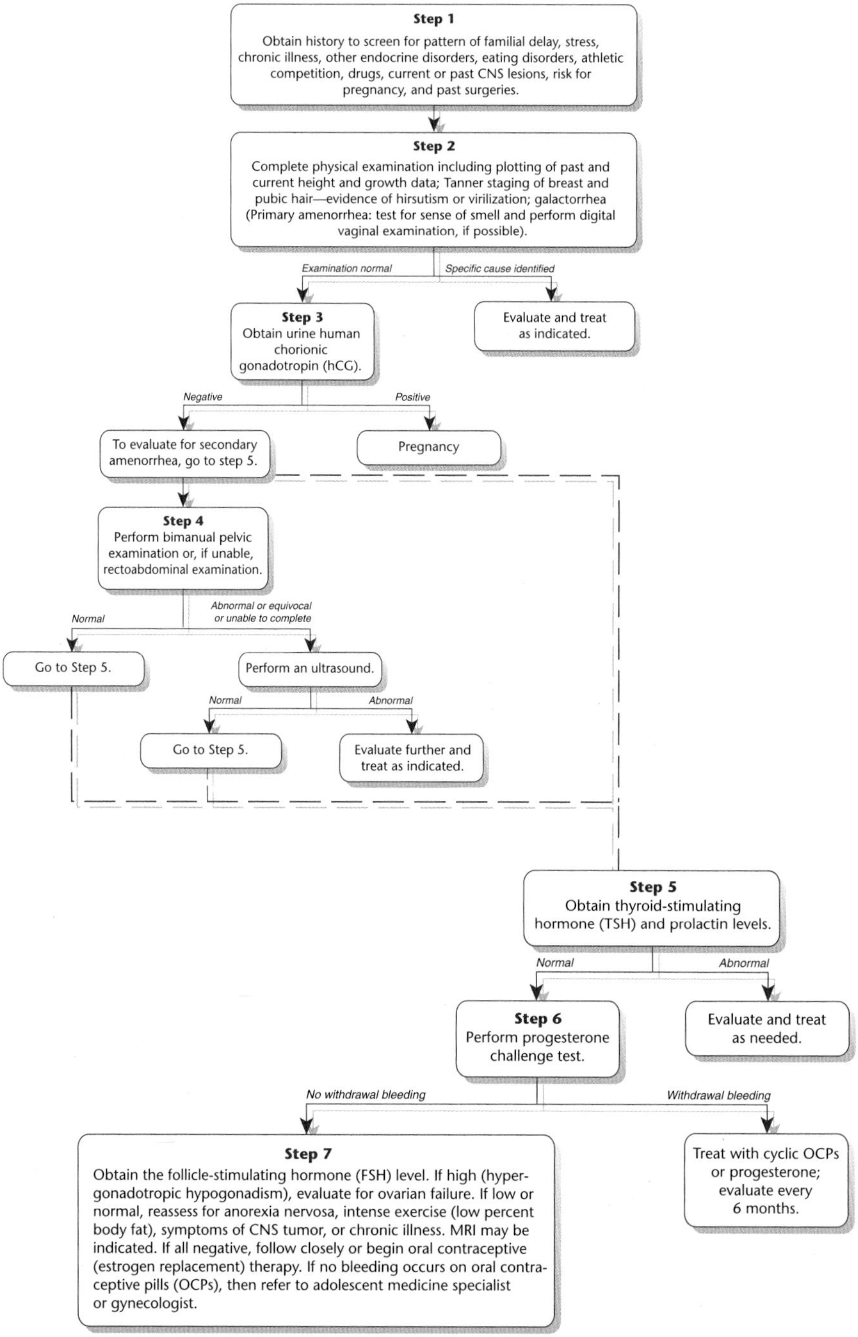


**Figure 4-1**
Evaluation of patients who have amenorrhea in whom secondary sex characteristics are present.

syndrome.[1] Diagnostic criteria for anorexia nervosa include loss of weight or failure to gain the weight expected with pubertal development. A complete physical examination, which in most cases will include a pelvic examination, should be performed.[5] Obesity or excessive thinness can result in amenorrhea. Abnormalities of the visual field, smell, or other cranial nerve function; papilledema; or disturbances of reflexes suggest a CNS tumor. Hirsutism, a receding hairline, excessive acne, moon facies, striae, enlarged thyroid, or buffalo hump suggests an endocrine disorder. A webbed neck, short stature, or widely spaced nipples suggest Turner syndrome. Nipple discharge may indicate elevated prolactin levels, and lack of or scant pubic hair in a girl who has Tanner stages 3 to 4 breast development suggests androgen insensitivity syndrome.

A pelvic examination is essential to ensure the presence of normal internal and external female genitalia. An imperforate hymen or transverse vaginal septum prevents menstrual blood from escaping. If the hymenal opening is patent, then the examination should proceed to determine the presence of a normal vagina, cervix, and uterus. If the hymenal opening is very small, then the cervix and uterus can be palpated by means of a bimanual rectoabdominal examination. The size of the clitoris should be noted because clitoromegaly indicates the presence of excess androgens (eg, partial 21-hydroxylase deficiency). In the few cases in which a pelvic or rectoabdominal examination cannot be performed to determine the presence or absence of a uterus, an ultrasound may be necessary.

Although a pink vaginal mucosa indicates the presence of some degree of estrogenization, the patient's estrogen status can be assessed using a progesterone challenge, vaginal maturation index, or measurement of serum estradiol levels. The progesterone challenge is particularly useful because a positive result indicates an estrogen-primed uterus. The progesterone challenge is conducted by administering 10 mg of medroxyprogesterone acetate for 5 to 10 days. Any spotting or bleeding in the week afterward is considered a positive test. Some experts in the field recommend measuring follicle-stimulating hormone (FSH) levels before performing a progesterone challenge because some women who have hypergonadotropic amenorrhea will have a withdrawal bleed.[6] A vaginal maturation index is performed by collecting cells from the upper lateral sidewall of the vaginal wall using a moistened cotton-tipped applicator, rolled on a glass slide, and fixed using the same technique in Papanicolaou smear preparation. Cytologic assessment will determine the number of parabasal, superficial, and intermediate cells present. Samples can be scored using Meisel's modified scoring system to interpret results in terms of estrogen and pubertal status.[7]

## ▶ LABORATORY TESTS

For the girl with primary amenorrhea who has an unremarkable history, review of systems, and general physical examination, and no evidence of vaginal outlet obstruction, the next step is to determine, either by pelvic examination, ultrasound, or both, whether a uterus is present. If not, then karyotyping and serum testosterone levels should be determined to screen for müllerian agenesis or androgen insensitivity syndrome. If a uterus is present, then an evaluation comparable to that for secondary amenorrhea should be pursued.

Patients with primary or secondary amenorrhea who have a history of sexual activity should first be screened for pregnancy using a urine pregnancy test. If negative, then initial laboratory evaluation includes FSH, prolactin, and thyroid-stimulating hormone. Low or normal FSH levels are usually associated with physiologic delay, hypothalamic and pituitary causes of amenorrhea, and chronic illnesses. Elevated levels of FSH indicate ovarian failure. Follow-up testing in patients with elevated FSH levels should include karyotyping and screening for autoimmune endocrinopathies. Patients with amenorrhea and clinical evidence of androgen excess most likely have polycystic ovary syndrome (PCOS)[8] or, less commonly, late-onset congenital adrenal hyperplasia (21-hydroxylase deficiency). Additional useful laboratory tests to assess for PCOS and other disorders associated with androgen excess include serum testosterone (total and free) and dehydroepiandrosterone (DHEA) and its sulfate (DHEA-S). Measurement of the first morning 17-hydroxyprogesterone levels is also indicated for patients with elevations in DHEA-S to further assess for late-onset congenital adrenal hyperplasia. If the patient has evidence of virilization (eg, clitoromegaly), or if the androgens are elevated in the tumor range, then adrenal and ovarian imaging are indicated, depending on the source of androgens. Isolated elevations of testosterone are suggestive of ovarian origin, whereas DHEA-S is suggestive of adrenal origin. (See also Chapter 41, Hirsutism, Hypertrichosis, and Precocious Sexual Hair Development.)

Imaging is indicated for other specific presentations of amenorrhea. Pelvic sonography is indicated if abnormalities are noted on bimanual examination or if bimanual examination is not possible. Magnetic resonance imaging of the pelvis is indicated for patients with possible congenital abnormalities. Dual-energy radiograph absorptiometry bone density evaluations should be obtained in girls with hypoestrogenic amenorrhea, given the association with low bone mineral density.[9] Hypoestrogenic amenorrhea is commonly seen in patients with restrictive eating disorders, athletic amenorrhea, and ovarian failure.[10–13]

## ▶ MANAGEMENT

Definitive recommendations for treatment of secondary amenorrhea depend on the underlying cause. When adolescent girls initiate puberty late, but progression through puberty seems normal and the findings of a thorough history and physical examination are also normal, the patient can be reassured that she should anticipate menarche 2 to 3 years after the initiation of puberty. This probability is particularly true when family history suggests late menarche in first-degree female relatives. Regularly scheduled follow-up visits until menarche occurs are warranted. Any halt in development or absence of menarche by age 16 years merits an evaluation.

In patients with secondary amenorrhea and normal estrogen levels, medroxyprogesterone 5 to 10 mg for 12 to 14 days can be used every 1 to 3 months to stimulate withdrawal bleeding. For sexually active patients and patients with PCOS, treatment with combined contraceptives is indicated. Patients with PCOS may also benefit from additional medications to address underlying metabolic abnormalities or clinical findings associated with androgen excess (hirsutism and acne). In patients with low levels of estrogen, normalizing weight for height is important by addressing disordered eating and intensity of athletic training.

Although many pediatric practices provide gynecologic care, patients who cannot receive a thorough gynecologic assessment in the pediatrician's office should be referred to an adolescent medicine specialist or pediatric gynecologist for evaluation. Adolescent medicine physicians may be particularly well suited to address other developmental or endocrinologic issues that may also be present. Patients who have evidence of complicated endocrine disease; evidence of a CNS, adrenal, or androgen tumor; genetic disorder; eating disorder; or structural abnormality should also be referred to the appropriate specialty team for further evaluation and management.

## When to Refer

- The amenorrhea appears secondary to a chronic illness that the pediatrician is unable to manage
- The pediatrician feels uncomfortable performing a pelvic examination
- Long-term hormonal therapy is required
- The patient has an eating disorder
- Evidence exists of anatomic or chromosomal abnormality
- Evidence exists of a complicated endocrine disorder
- Evidence exists of a CNS, adrenal, or ovarian tumor
- The patient is pregnant and the pediatrician is unwilling or unable to provide comprehensive options counseling or referral for all options[14]

### *REFERENCES*


1. Johnson J, Whitaker AH. Adolescent smoking, weight changes, and binge-purge behavior: associations with secondary amenorrhea. *Am J Public Health*. 1992;82(1):47–54
2. Anderson SE, Dallal GE, Must A. Relative weight and race influence average age at menarche: results from two nationally representative surveys of US girls studied 25 years apart. *Pediatrics*. 2003; 111(4 Pt 1):844–850
3. Chumlea LC, Schubert CM, Roche AF, et al. Age at menarche and racial comparisons in US girls. *Pediatrics*. 2003;111:110–113
4. World Health Organization multicenter study on menstrual and ovulatory patterns in adolescent girls. I. A multicenter cross-sectional study of menarche. World Health Organization Task Force on Adolescent Reproductive Health. *J Adolesc Health Care*. 1986;7:229–235
5. Braverman PK, Breech L; American Academy of Pediatrics Committee on Adolescence. Gynecologic examination for adolescents in the pediatric office setting. *Pediatrics*. 2010;126(3):583–590
6. Rebar RW, Connolly HV. Clinical features of young women with hypergonadotropic amenorrhea. *Fertil Steril*. 1990;53:804–810
7. Meisels A. Computed cytohormonal findings in 3,307 healthy women. *Acta Cytol*. 1965;9:328–333
8. Rotterdam ESHRE/ASRM-Sponsored PCOS consensus workshop group. Revised 2003 consensus on diagnostic criteria and long-term health risks related to polycystic ovary syndrome (PCOS). *Hum Reprod*. 2004;19:41–47
9. White CM, Hergenroeder AC, Klish WJ. Bone mineral density in 15- to 21-year-old eumenorrheic and amenorrheic subjects. *Am J Dis Child*. 1992;146:31–35
10. Golden NH, Jacobson MS, Schebendach J, et al. Resumption of menses in anorexia nervosa. *Arch Pediatr Adolesc Med*. 1997;151:16–21
11. Yeager KK, Agostini R, Nattiv A, Drinkwater B. The female athlete triad: disordered eating, amenorrhea, osteoporosis. *Med Sci Sports Exerc*. 1993;25:775–777
12. Hetland ML, Haarbo J, Christiansen C, Larsen T. Running induces menstrual disturbances but bone mass is unaffected, except in amenorreheic women. *Am J Med*. 1993;95:553–558
13. Gidwani GP. Amenorrhea in the athlete. *Adolesc Med*. 1999;10:275–290
14. American Academy of Pediatrics Committee on Bioethics. Physician refusal to provide information or treatment on the basis of claims of conscience. *Pediatrics*. 2009;124:1689–1693

# Chapter 5

# Anemia and Pallor

*Alicia K. McFarren, MD; Adam S. Levy, MD*

## ▶ INTRODUCTION

Anemia is a laboratory finding reflecting a decrease in red blood cell (RBC) mass below an age-appropriate normative value. Anemia may be associated with pallor, but it is more likely a silent symptom and detected only on routine screening studies. Pallor and anemia are not diagnoses; rather, they are signs and symptoms of an underlying disease process requiring a thorough evaluation by the primary care physician.

## ▶ DEFINITIONS AND CLINICAL MANIFESTATIONS

### Pallor

Pallor, derived from the Latin *pallere,* meaning "to be pale," is a clinical sign associated with a variety of systemic illnesses resulting in a decrease in the amount of oxygenated hemoglobin visible through the superficial and translucent layers of the skin and mucosa. Accurate assessment of pallor may be hindered by fluorescent lighting, dark skin color, jaundice, or cyanosis. Although a common finding in children with moderate to severe anemia, pallor does not necessarily indicate a low hemoglobin level. Sepsis may cause pallor resulting from a decrease in peripheral perfusion. Vasoconstriction from exposure to cold or febrile illnesses may also lead to pallor. Disorders that lead to an accumulation of fluid in the interstitium such as heart failure, hypoproteinemia, or myxedema can also result in pallor.

### Anemia

Anemia can be defined as a reduction in RBC number, RBC mass (hematocrit), or hemoglobin concentration.[1] For each value, the lower limit of the normal range is defined as 2 standard deviations from the mean for age and gender (Table 5-1). Normal ranges for hemoglobin and hematocrit vary with age and gender. Racial differences exist as well. Black children on average have normal hemoglobin values that are approximately 0.5 g/dL lower than white and Asian children.[2]

## ▶ CLASSIFICATION AND DIFFERENTIAL DIAGNOSIS

Anemias can be systematically evaluated based on RBC size (mean corpuscular volume [MCV]). Normal MCV values vary with age, but microcytic anemias generally have an MCV less than 70 fL, normocytic anemias have an MCV of 72 to 90 fL, and macrocytic anemias have an MCV of greater than 90 fL. Subclassification of anemias as microcytic, normocytic, and macrocytic will greatly reduce the differential diagnosis and limit the number

**Table 5-1**
**Mean Values for Hemoglobin, Hematocrit, and Mean Corpuscular Volume**

| AGE | HEMOGLOBIN (g/dL) | HEMATOCRIT (%) | MCV (fL) |
|---|---|---|---|
| Cord blood | 15.3 | 49 | 112 |
| 1 day | 19.0 | 61 | 119 |
| 1 wk | 17.9 | 56 | 118 |
| 1 mo | 17.3 | 54 | 112 |
| 2 mo | 10.7 | 33 | 100 |
| 3 mo | 11.3 | 33 | 88 |
| 6 mo–2 yr | 12.5 | 37 | 77 |
| 2–4 yr | 12.5 | 38 | 79 |
| 5–7 yr | 13 | 39 | 81 |
| 8–11 yr | 13.5 | 40 | 83 |
| 12- to 14-year-old girls | 13.5 | 41 | 85 |
| 12- to 14-year-old boys | 14 | 43 | 84 |
| 15- to 17-year-old girls | 14 | 41 | 87 |
| 15- to 17-year-old boys | 15 | 46 | 86 |

Modified from Nathan DG, Orkin SH. A diagnostic approach to the anemic patient. In: *Nathan and Oski's Hematology of Infancy and Childhood*. 5th ed. Philadelphia, PA: WB Saunders; 1998. Copyright © 1998, Elsevier, with permission.

of laboratory tests needed to attain the diagnosis. Figures 5-1 and 5-2 contain guidelines for a diagnostic approach to children and newborns with anemia. Box 5-1 lists the differential diagnoses of specific pathologic RBC features.

## *Microcytic Anemia*

The differential diagnosis of a microcytic anemia is listed in Table 5-2, and the main causes are reviewed in detail here.

### Iron Deficiency

Iron deficiency is the most common cause of anemia in the United States.[3] Iron deficiency may be attributed to poor iron intake, poor iron absorption, or blood loss. Full-term neonates are born with sufficient iron stores to last for the first 6 months of life. Iron deficiency is rare during this period. The incidence of iron deficiency anemia peaks at age 12 to 24 months and then again in adolescence. The peak in childhood corresponds to the transition of children from human milk or iron-containing formulas to whole milk. Iron deficiency in adolescents is typically related to a poor dietary intake of iron, as well significant blood and iron loss in adolescent girls with menstrual bleeding.

In children of all ages, occult blood loss must be considered as a source for iron loss leading to deficiency. Blood loss may be acute, chronic, or intermittent. A thorough history should be obtained to rule out melena, hematochezia, tarry stools, and bloody or coffee-ground emesis. Stool guaiac tests for occult blood should be performed at several different times

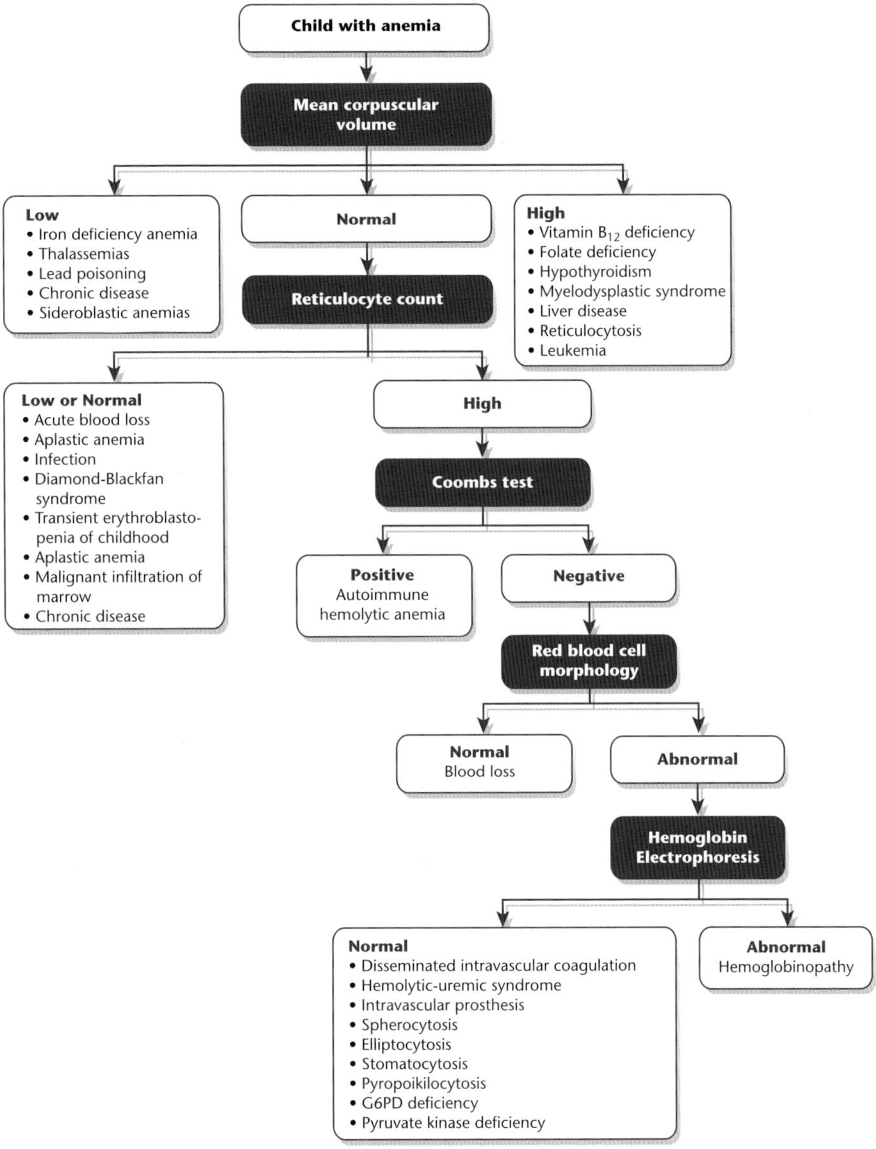


**Figure 5-1**

Diagnostic approach to anemia in childhood based on red blood cell mean corpuscular volume. *G6PD,* glucose-6-phosphate dehydrogenase. *(Derived from Nathan DC, Oski F.* Hematology of Infancy and Childhood. *3rd ed. Philadelphia, PA: WB Saunders; 1987.)*

to capture any intermittent bleeding. Common causes of gastrointestinal bleeding include gastric and duodenal ulcers, Meckel diverticulum, polyps, hemorrhoids, and gastritis. Signs and symptoms of inflammatory bowel disease should also be considered in the history and physical examination. Patients with iron deficiency anemia have symptoms similar to those in other forms of anemia, including pica as a craving for ice.

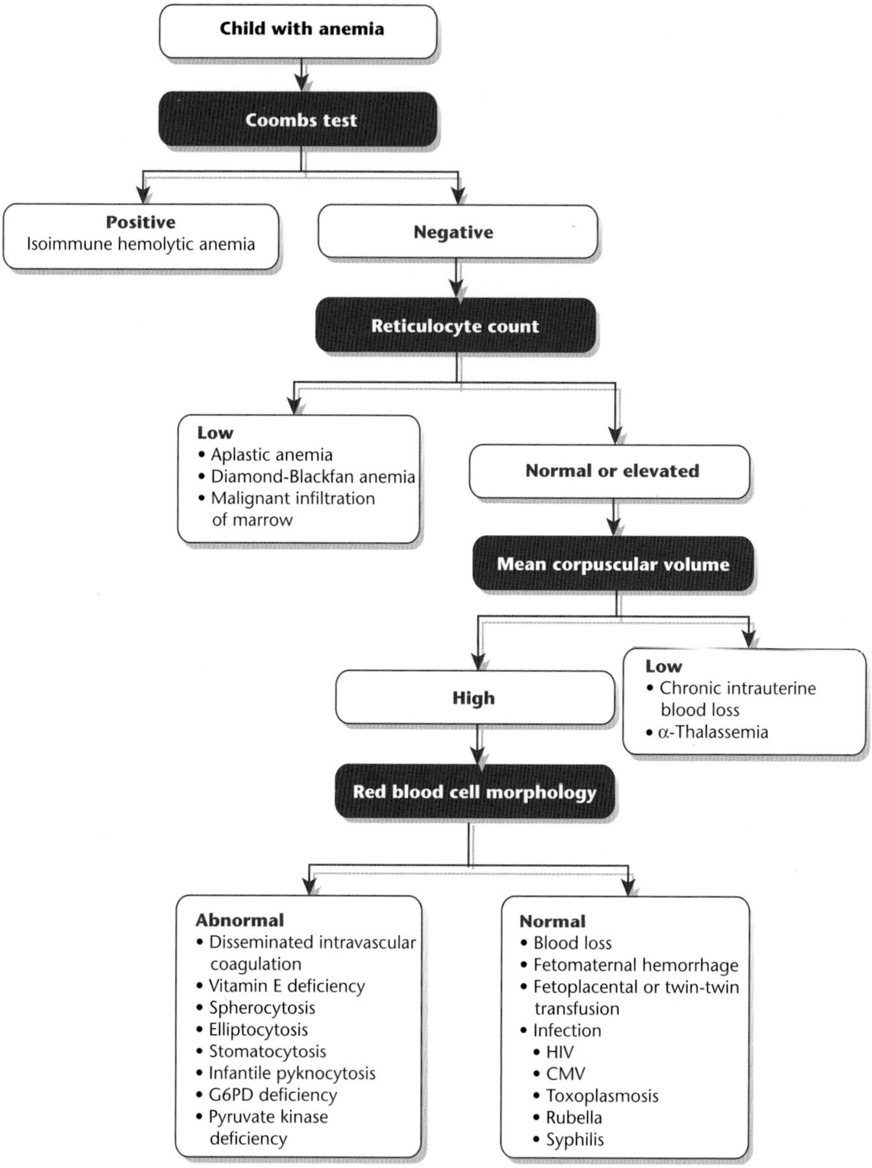


**Figure 5-2**
Diagnostic approach to anemia in the newborn. *CMV,* cytomegalovirus; *G6PD,* glucose-6-phosphate dehydrogenase; *HIV,* human immunodeficiency virus. *(Derived from Nathan DC, Oski F.* Hematology of Infancy and Childhood. *3rd ed. Philadelphia, PA: WB Saunders; 1987.)*

When iron deficiency is sufficient to cause anemia, other abnormalities may be seen on routine laboratory testing. In addition to being microcytic, the RBCs will be hypochromic, with target cells and elliptocyte forms visible on the peripheral blood smear. These features and a low reticulocyte count are sufficient to make the diagnosis of iron deficiency anemia. In many instances, further testing is not necessary but may be helpful in some settings.

BOX 5-1

## *Differential Diagnosis of Specific Pathologic Red Blood Cell Features*[a]

### TARGET CELLS

(Surface-to-volume ratio increased)
- Thalassemia
- Hemoglobinopathies
- Hemoglobin E disease
- Hyposplenism or postsplenectomy
- Hepatic disease
- Severe iron deficiency anemia
- Abetaproteinemia
- Lecithin or cholesterol acyltransferase deficiency

### SPHEROCYTES

(Hyperdense cells with a decrease in surface-to-volume ratio and an increased mean corpuscular hemoglobin concentration)
- Hereditary spherocytosis
- Hemolytic anemia (autoimmune, ABO incompatibility, water dilution)
- Microangiopathic hemolytic anemia
- Hemoglobin SS disease
- Hypersplenism
- Burns
- After RBC transfusions
- Pyruvate kinase deficiency

### ACANTHOCYTES (SPUR CELLS)

(Cells with 10–15 spicules that are typically irregular in length, spacing, and width; cells usually smaller than normal RBCs)
- Disseminated intravascular coagulation
- Microangiopathic hemolytic anemia
- Hyposplenism or postsplenectomy
- Hepatic disease
- Hypothyroidism
- Vitamin E deficiency
- Abetalipoproteinemia
- Malabsorption

### ECHINOCYTES (BURR CELLS)

(Cells with 10–30 spicules that are typically of comparable size and distributed evenly)
- Dehydration
- Renal disease
- Hepatic disease
- Pyruvate kinase deficiency
- Peptic ulcer disease
- After RBC transfusion

### PYKNOCYTES

(Hyperchromic RBCs with a decreased volume and distorted shape)
- Similar to acanthocytes and echinocytes

### BLISTER CELLS

(Contain a clear area in RBCs that contains no hemoglobin)
- Hemoglobin SS disease
- G6PD deficiency
- Pulmonary emboli

### BASOPHILIC STIPPLING

(Retention of RNA resulting in fine blue inclusions in the cytoplasm)
- Iron deficiency anemia
- Lead poisoning
- Hemolytic anemias
- Pyrimidine 5'-nucleotidase deficiency

### ELLIPTOCYTES

(Elliptical-shaped cells)
- Hereditary elliptocytosis
- Iron deficiency anemia
- Thalassemia
- Hemoglobin SS disease
- Sepsis
- Megaloblastic anemia
- Malaria
- Leukoerythroblastic reaction

### TEARDROP CELLS

(Microcytic and hypochromic cells that are in the shape of a teardrop)
- Normal finding in newborns
- Thalassemia
- Myeloproliferative diseases
- Leukoerythroblastic reaction

### SCHISTOCYTES

(RBC fragments that result from trauma)
- Disseminated intravascular coagulation
- Hemolytic anemia and microangiopathic hemolytic anemia
- Kasabach-Merritt syndrome
- Purpura fulminans
- Hemolytic-uremic syndrome
- Uremia, glomerular nephritis, acute tubular necrosis

*Continued*

BOX 5-1

## *Differential Diagnosis of Specific Pathologic Red Blood Cell Features—cont'd*

- Cirrhosis of the liver
- Malignant hypertension
- Thrombosis
- Thrombotic thrombocytopenia purpura
- Amyloidosis
- Chronic relapsing schistocytic hemolytic anemia
- Burns
- Connective tissue disorders

**STOMATOCYTE**

(Area of central pallor is more slit-like than round)

- Present in small numbers in normal individuals
- Stomatocytosis (hereditary)
- Thalassemia

**NUCLEATED RED BLOOD CELLS**

(Normal on a peripheral blood smear in the first week of life only)

- Normal newborns
- Significant bone marrow stimulation
- Congenital infections
- Hyposplenism or postsplenectomy
- Leukoerythroblastic reaction, particularly with severe infections and leukemias or metastatic tumors in the bone marrow
- Megaloblastic anemia
- Dyserythropoietic anemias

[a]Frequently, normal blood smears will contain abnormal-appearing RBCs that are simply an artifact of trauma during the blood draw or ex vivo processing of the blood.

*G6PD,* glucose-6-phosphate dehydrogenase; *RBC,* red blood cell.

Modified from Nathan DG, Orkin SH. A diagnostic approach to the anemic patient. In: *Nathan and Oski's Hematology of Infancy and Childhood.* 5th ed. Philadelphia, PA: WB Saunders; 1998.

**Table 5-2**
**Classification of Anemia in Childhood**

| MICROCYTIC | NORMOCYTIC | MACROCYTIC |
|---|---|---|
| Iron deficiency anemia | Infection | Megaloblastic anemias from $B_{12}$ or folate deficiency |
| Lead poisoning | Acute blood loss | Reticulocytosis |
| Copper deficiency | Renal disease | Postsplenectomy |
| Malnutrition | Connective tissue disorder | Myelodysplastic syndrome |
| Chronic disease | Hepatic disease | Aplastic anemia |
| Thalassemia | Hemolysis | Fanconi anemia |
| Hemoglobin E trait | Hypersplenism | Diamond-Blackfan syndrome |
| Sideroblastic anemia | Malignancy | Pearson syndrome |
| Atransferrinemia | Aplastic anemia | Dyskeratosis congenita |
| Inborn errors of metabolism | Dyserythropoietic anemia | Paroxysmal nocturnal hemoglobinuria |
| | Drugs | Down syndrome |
| | | Hypothyroidism |
| | | Hepatic disease, jaundice |
| | | Drugs (eg, phenytoin, methotrexate) |

Serum iron and ferritin levels are low, whereas the total iron-binding capacity is elevated. Many children also have an elevated platelet count.

When a primary care physician is treating a child with hypochromic, microcytic anemia found on a routine screening blood cell count, and a history of poor iron intake or excessive milk intake is elicited, a reasonable approach would be to give a trial of supplemental iron

(6 mg/kg of elemental iron per day divided into 2 or more doses) rather than to draw additional blood for biochemical analysis. The reticulocyte count should increase within 5 to 7 days once therapy is initiated. Assuming the dietary deficiency is corrected, supplemental iron should continue for 2 to 3 months after the hemoglobin concentration has normalized to replenish iron stores fully. For patients with a hypochromic microcytic anemia who do not seem to be at risk based on diet alone, and for those who do not respond to supplemental iron, additional testing is required. Iron deficiency, although common, is still abnormal, and the etiology of the deficiency should be clearly defined.

## Thalassemias

The thalassemias are a heterogenous group of disorders of hemoglobin production. The α-thalassemias have deficient production of the α chain, and the β-thalassemias have deficient production of the β chain. In either case, the excess of one chain relative to the other results in precipitation and destruction of the RBCs.

**β-THALASSEMIA.** Thalassemia minor (or thalassemia trait) is common among black patients and results from a mutation of 1 of the 2 genes on chromosome 11 encoding for the β-chain. When only 1 gene is affected, a mild decrease in β-chain production occurs, resulting in a mild anemia. Patients with thalassemia trait frequently have a hypochromic, microcytic anemia found on a routine complete blood count, similar to patients with iron deficiency anemia. Target cells are also common to both diseases. However, patients with thalassemia trait usually have an increase in the number of RBCs, whereas patients with iron deficiency commonly have a decrease in RBC number. A hemoglobin electrophoresis may also be helpful in diagnosing thalassemia trait. Both the hemoglobin F and hemoglobin $A_2$ levels are commonly elevated. Although treatment is not necessary, diagnosing thalassemia trait is important so that appropriate genetic counseling may be offered to patients and families.[4]

**THALASSEMIA MAJOR.** Thalassemia major (Cooley anemia) results from defects in both β-globin genes and manifests as a severe hemolytic anemia. Marked compensatory erythropoiesis causing expansion of the medullary space results in a prominence of the cheeks and frontal bossing.[4] Long-term transfusion therapy is required for these patients, and immediate referral to a hematologist is necessary.

**α-THALASSEMIA.** Each chromosome 16 contains 2 identical genes (4 genes total) for the α chain. Abnormalities in these genes, most commonly seen in blacks and Asians, result in α-thalassemia.[5] When 1 gene is affected, the patient will be asymptomatic, with little or no abnormality on routine testing. α-Thalassemia trait is the result of a mutation in 2 genes. Patients with α-thalassemia trait are also asymptomatic. They have laboratory findings similar to patients with α-thalassemia trait or iron deficiency (microcytic, hypochromic) anemia. However, unlike α-thalassemia trait, the anemia is usually less severe, and the hemoglobin electrophoresis is normal. The diagnosis is based on the findings of a microcytic, hypochromic mild anemia in patients of Asian or black descent with a normal electrophoresis and no evidence of iron deficiency. Molecular genetic testing of *HBA1* and *HBA2* detects deletions in about 90% and point mutations in about 10% of affected individuals.[6] For purposes of genetic counseling, the typical Asian genotype, with both abnormal genes on the same chromosome, is of more concern than the usual genotype in black patients, with 1 abnormal gene on each chromosome 16. When 3 of the 4 genes are affected, hemoglobin H disease is the result. Patients with hemoglobin H disease may be asymptomatic but on laboratory testing show a moderate to severe anemia (hemoglobin, 7–10 g/dL). The anemia is microcytic and hypochromic, with RBC fragments visible on review of the peripheral blood smear. A hemoglobin electrophoresis shows 5% to 30% hemoglobin H (hemoglobin consisting of 4 β chains). In the newborn period, hemoglobin Barts may be detected, which consist of 4 gamma chains. With mutations in all 4 genes, no normal hemoglobin is made, and unless the diagnosis is made prenatally to allow for intrauterine transfusions, the fetus will die with hydrops fetalis.[4]

## Lead Poisoning

Any measurable lead in the plasma is abnormal, but clinically significant lead poisoning occurs at lead levels higher than 10 mcg/dL, and levels higher than 5 mcg/dL deserve attention. In most instances, lead poisoning is diagnosed on routine screening tests.[7] The anemia in lead poisoning is microcytic and hypochromic, similar to iron deficiency. However, intense basophilic stippling of the RBCs may also be observed. Lead inhibits the insertion of iron into the protoporphyrin ring, thus inactivating heme synthesis and leading to an accumulation of free erythrocyte protoporphyrin, the levels of which can be elevated in both iron deficiency and lead poisoning.

## Chronic Inflammation

Chronic illness may be associated with anemia, likely the result both of decreased production and shortened RBC survival. Iron flow from the reticuloendothelial cells to the erythroblasts may also be diminished, resulting in a hypochromic, microcytic anemia. Anemia of chronic disease can be associated with malignancies, autoimmune diseases, renal failure, and chronic infections. Frequently, RBCs in chronic disease are normocytic and normochromic, but microcytic and hypochromic anemias are seen as well. The hemoglobin typically is in the range of 7 to 10 g/dL with a normal to low reticulocyte count.

### *Sideroblastic Anemias*

The sideroblastic anemias, caused by the retention of iron in the mitochondria of immature erythrocytes, are rare forms of anemia in childhood. Acquired sideroblastic anemia is a disease primarily of adulthood, whereas inherited forms of the disease occur in childhood.

### *Normocytic Anemia*

Normocytic anemia is defined as a decreased circulating RBC mass with an MCV in the appropriate range for age.[1] As noted previously, the distinction of age-appropriate normative values is well established and important to consider lest the physician misinterpret a child's results and pursue an unnecessary evaluation (see Table 5-1).

The differential diagnosis of normocytic anemia (see Table 5-2) is broad and can be divided into primary hematologic disorders or systemic disorders with secondary anemia. Primary hematologic causes of normocytic anemia include early iron deficiency anemia, aplastic anemia and other bone marrow failure syndromes, and hemolytic anemias (most commonly sickle cell disease). Systemic disorders with secondary normocytic anemia include anemia of chronic disease, systemic infection, acute blood loss, renal failure, and other disorders.[8] The physician can also classify normocytic anemia as a disorder of decreased RBC production or increased RBC destruction.[9] Whichever way is chosen to develop a diagnostic algorithm, approaching the diagnosis of anemia in a structured way that can consistently consider the broad range of diagnostic possibilities is useful.

## Primary Hematologic Causes of Normocytic Anemia

For many patients, the diagnosis of anemia is made on routine screening. Iron deficiency anemia is the most common cause of nutritional anemia in childhood discovered by routine screening. Although the classic indices for iron deficiency anemia include a low MCV and a high red cell distribution width, early iron deficiency anemia may appear as a normocytic anemia. A reticulocyte count will be lower than expected for a patient with anemia because RBC production will be decreased. Iron studies should corroborate the diagnosis of iron deficiency anemia, but a trial of supplemental iron should be both diagnostic and therapeutic.

Aplastic anemia and bone marrow failure syndromes can result in normocytic anemia as a result of decreased RBC production.[10] Examples include congenital or acquired aplastic anemia, transient erythroblastopenia of childhood,[11,12] pure red cell aplasia (Diamond-Blackfan anemia), and viral infections (eg, parvovirus, Epstein-Barr virus).[13]

Bone marrow infiltration from a malignant process (either leukemia or metastatic solid tumors) can result in decreased RBC production and cause a normocytic anemia. Again, the reticulocyte count will be lower than expected for the degree of anemia. Abnormalities in the white blood cell count and platelet count may also be noted. Immature cells may be noted on review of a peripheral blood smear. Evidence of hemolysis and increased RBC turnover should be absent.

Hemolytic anemias result from RBC membrane defects (eg, hereditary spherocytosis, elliptocytosis),[4] enzyme defects (eg, glucose-6-phosphate dehydrogenase [G6PD] deficiency, pyruvate kinase deficiency),[14] hemoglobin defects (eg, sickle cell disease, thalassemias), and autoimmune hemolytic anemias. In general, the hemolytic anemias are characterized by an elevated reticulocyte count and evidence of increased RBC destruction (elevated serum bilirubin level). A patient with a personal or a family history of early cholecystectomy or intermittent jaundice may suggest a familial hemolytic anemia. Obtaining the complete blood count results of immediate family members may help confirm the diagnosis. Although routine newborn screening will identify patients with sickle cell disease born in the United States, children born in areas without routine screening may well have their sickle cell disease diagnosed later in life.[15]

Rarely, normocytic anemia may result from a combination of a microcytic anemia (iron deficiency) and a macrocytic anemia (folate deficiency). The MCV is a mean and, as such, 2 populations of RBCs may average out to a normal MCV.

## Systemic Causes of Normocytic Anemia

Acute blood loss will result in a normocytic anemia. Patients with chronic blood loss (eg, gastrointestinal bleeding) will likely become iron deficient and develop a microcytic anemia. However, in the early stage of the process, the patient will have normocytic RBCs. Testing the stool for occult blood is indicated in the evaluation.

Anemia of chronic disease is a poorly understood but well-recognized cause of normocytic anemia in children and adults. Anemia of chronic disease can be associated with a variety of illnesses, including rheumatologic conditions, systemic infections, endocrine dysfunction, liver failure, lung disease, and renal disease.[9,16,17]

## Evaluation of Normocytic Anemia

In general, normocytic anemias that are nonresponsive to supplemental iron and not clearly associated with a systemic illness warrant referral to a pediatric hematologist. A reticulocyte count and review of the peripheral blood smear are indicated for every child with normocytic anemia referred to a hematologist. The smear may help identify morphologic features to aid in the diagnosis (eg, spherocytosis, sickle cells) or reveal evidence of hemolysis (schistocytes, RBC fragments).

The percentage reticulocyte count must be considered within the context of the patient's hemoglobin level and hematocrit. A high percentage reticulocyte count is expected in a child who can mount an appropriate response to anemia. An apparently normal reticulocyte percentage (1.1%–3.5%) in a child with severe anemia is actually relatively lower than it should be to compensate for the anemia. For this reason, the reticulocyte index is a useful calculation: the reticulocyte count multiplied by the ratio represented by the patient's hematocrit divided by the normal hematocrit.[10]

A relatively low reticulocyte count (<1%) suggests decreased RBC production. The primary care physician must then consider aplastic anemia, malignancy, transient erythroblastopenia of childhood, and other causes of bone marrow suppression. A bone marrow aspirate and biopsy are rarely indicated but must be considered to rule out malignancy, especially when more than a single blood cell line is abnormal.

An elevated reticulocyte count suggests that the bone marrow is compensating for blood loss either from hemolysis or from hemorrhage. Causes of blood loss must be considered. Patients with an elevated reticulocyte count and an elevated bilirubin level likely have ongoing hemolysis. A positive Coombs test (direct antiglobulin test) suggests an autoimmune hemolytic anemia. Without evidence of an autoimmune process, hemoglobinopathies (sickle cell disease and variants and thalassemias) must be evaluated by hemoglobin electrophoresis.

Other specialized assays may define specific RBC disorders that result in hemolysis. G6PD deficiency, which is X-linked, is the most common enzyme defect in males. Many variants have been found, and the assay may be falsely negative in patients with a high reticulocyte count immediately after a hemolytic crisis. Families need to be educated regarding the triggers for hemolysis in G6PD deficiency, including a variety of medications, infections, exposure to mothballs, and, for some variants, fava beans (favism). A positive osmotic fragility test helps confirm the diagnosis of hereditary spherocytosis and should be considered in patients with RBC morphology consistent with the diagnosis.[18]

### *Macrocytic Anemias*

Macrocytic anemias in childhood are extremely rare and are typically the result of deficiencies in folate or vitamin $B_{12}$.[1] Folate deficiency can be associated with inborn errors of metabolism, poor dietary intake, increased utilization in patients with hemolytic anemias, malabsorption, and drugs that inhibit folate metabolism (methotrexate). Vitamin $B_{12}$ deficiency may be caused by inborn errors of metabolism, poor dietary intake, and malabsorption. In cases of significant deficiencies, these anemias can be quite severe, with an MCV between 100 and 140 fL. In addition to normochromic macrocytic RBCs, hypersegmented neutrophils may be visible on the peripheral blood smear. Serum folate and $B_{12}$ levels may help confirm the diagnosis, but the underlying cause of the vitamin deficiency must be determined.

A macrocytic anemia in a child is always concerning for an underlying disorder in bone marrow production. Myelodysplasia, early aplasia, and leukemia may all manifest as macrocytosis with or without anemia. In the absence of a clear $B_{12}$ or folate deficiency, a referral to a hematologist is warranted for assessment of macrocytosis to rule out myelodysplasia or malignancy.

### Anemia of the Newborn

The differential diagnosis of anemia in a newborn is distinctly different from that in older children. Peripartum hemorrhage and maternal factors, such as alloantibodies, are important in deciphering neonatal anemias. Iron deficiency in the newborn period is quite rare. Anemias with similar origins may also be displayed differently in infants and children.

Table 5-1 lists the normal hematologic parameters for infants and children. Hematologic parameters in children evolve over the first couple of months of life. Typically, a normal hemoglobin level in a term newborn is approximately 19 g/dL. The hemoglobin concentration falls gradually to a nadir of 10 to 11 g/dL by 8 to 12 weeks of age. This nadir, termed *physiologic anemia of the newborn,* is more pronounced in preterm infants with nadirs as low as 7 to 8 g/dL. Despite the low nadir, transfusions are necessary only if the anemia is uncompensated, although early supplementation with iron is usually indicated.[1]

When considering the differential diagnosis of anemia in newborns, classifying the cause of the anemia into 1 of 3 broad groups is helpful: (1) blood loss, (2) hemolysis, or (3) decreased production.[19,20] Blood loss may occur at any time during a pregnancy. Common causes include fetomaternal transfusion, twin-to-twin transfusion, placental abruption, placenta previa, and internal hemorrhage (eg, intraventricular hemorrhage, cephalohematoma, caput succedaneum). The Betke-Kleihauer test detects the presence of fetal RBCs in the mother. Fetal cells can be detected in the circulation of 50% of pregnancies; however, rarely is the hemorrhage significant enough to cause anemia in the newborn. Mothers who are blood type O with infants who are not type O may have a false-negative Betke-Kleihauer test result.

At least 15% of monochorionic twins develop significant twin-to-twin transfusions, with differences in hemoglobin concentrations of 5 g/dL or more. At birth, the donor twin typically is smaller and may have pallor, oligohydramnios, and even shock. Polycythemia, polyhydramnios, and congestive heart failure may be present at birth in the recipient twin.[21]

The clinical manifestation of neonatal anemia from blood loss is dependent on the severity and rapidity of the blood loss. Infants with chronic blood loss throughout pregnancy may have pallor and microcytic, hypochromic anemia but appear otherwise well and hemodynamically stable. Infants with acute blood loss may have pallor, tachypnea, tachycardia, hypotension, and decreased tone. A normocytic, normochromic anemia with a reticulocytosis is detectable soon after birth.[19,20]

The most common cause of hemolytic anemia in the newborn is isoimmune hemolytic anemia caused by an incompatibility in maternal and fetal RBC antigens, including Rh, ABO, and minor blood groups. Mothers who are Rh negative may become immunized against the Rh antigen when pregnant with an Rh-positive fetus. During subsequent pregnancies, if the fetus is Rh positive, then maternal anti-Rh antibodies will readily cross the placenta and destroy the Rh-positive RBCs in the fetus. In utero and perinatal hemolysis may be rapid and severe, resulting in life-threatening hemolysis and hyperbilirubinemia.

However, with the prenatal administration of Rh immune globulin to Rh-negative mothers, life-threatening Rh incompatibility is rare today. In cases of hemolytic anemia from ABO or minor blood group antigen incompatibility, the mechanism of immunization and hemolysis is similar to Rh incompatibility, but the hemolysis is rarely severe.[1] Hemolytic anemia in the newborn may also occur as a result of maternal drug use and neonatal infections, including bacterial sepsis, cytomegalovirus, toxoplasmosis, herpes, and rubella. Microangiopathic hemolysis may occur in infants with thrombi, disseminated intravascular coagulation, and Kasabach-Merritt syndrome (multiple cavernous hemangiomas).

Hemolysis from hemoglobinopathies rarely causes symptomatic anemia in newborns. Anemia from β chain defects (eg, sickle cell disease, β-thalassemias) may not appear until later in infancy when the hemoglobin concentration is more dependent on β-chain production. α-Thalassemia major will manifest as erythroblastosis fetalis in the newborn period. RBC membrane and enzyme defects may be apparent at birth but more commonly appear later in the newborn period.

RBC production deficiencies are rare in the newborn period and are typically the result of infection or drugs. Diamond-Blackfan anemia is a rare congenital pure RBC precursor aplasia. However, affected patients are typically not anemic until 3 to 12 months of age. Congenital leukemias and osteopetrosis may also result in deficient RBC production but are also typically associated with disorders in the other cell lines and are extremely rare.

## ▶ EVALUATION

Anemia is frequently identified in the first or second year of life and in adolescence on routine screening performed by primary care physicians. By using information obtained from a thorough history and physical examination, as well as results of routine laboratory studies, most causes of anemia can be accurately diagnosed in the primary care physician's office. Diseases leading to anemia and pallor in infants and children are listed in Table 5-2, Figure 5-1, and Figure 5-2.

### *History*

Many children with anemia are asymptomatic and have their condition diagnosed only on routine screening evaluations. Nonetheless, a thorough history may help identify patients most at risk for developing anemia, as well as help identify the cause of an existing anemia. Demographic factors such as age, gender, and ethnicity will identify risk groups for specific types of anemia. Toddlers and adolescent girls account for most cases of iron deficiency anemia. Blacks are at greatest risk for sickle cell anemia, whereas the thalassemias occur primarily in patients of Mediterranean and Southeast Asian descent. A diet history is crucial in identifying children most likely to develop iron deficiency anemia. Sulfa drugs can produce a hemolytic anemia in patients with G6PD deficiency. Many common acute bacterial and viral infections may result in a mild anemia from decreased RBC production or increased RBC destruction, or both. Anemias resulting from such infections are typically short-lived but are commonly the cause of abnormalities identified on routine screening. Acute or chronic blood loss (or both) should be considered in all patients with anemia. Common sites of blood loss in otherwise asymptomatic patients include the gastrointestinal tract for all patients and the genitourinary tract for female patients. Anemia may be the benign manifestation of an underlying systemic disease such as autoimmune disorders and may be associated with signs of systemic illness (fevers, weight loss, among other signs). Finally, a family history may help guide the workup for a patient with anemia. In addition to a family history of hemoglobinopathies, a history of jaundice during systemic illnesses, cholecystectomy at a young age, or splenectomy may suggest a hereditary hemolytic anemia. Historical factors worthy of note in evaluating an anemic patient are listed in Table 5-3.

### *Physical Examination*

Infants and toddlers may experience fatigue, irritability, pallor, increased periods of sleep, poor feeding, and failure to thrive. Older children and adolescents may experience fatigue, pallor, exercise intolerance, dizziness, headaches, shortness of breath, or palpitations. However, most mild to moderate anemias in childhood are asymptomatic because they develop slowly over time, and patients are usually well compensated. In fact, seeing a child for a routine physical examination only to find out later that routine laboratory studies reveal anemia is not uncommon.

Pallor is the classic physical examination finding suggestive of anemia but is rare in mild anemias and frequently only seen reliably with hemoglobin concentrations less than

**Table 5-3**
**Pertinent Historical Factors in the Diagnosis of Childhood Anemia**

| | |
|---|---|
| Age | Nutritional anemias are rare in infancy in term infants but are more common in infants born preterm, as well as in school-aged children and adolescents. Significant anemia diagnosed in the first 6 months of life in a term infant is most likely a congenital anemia. |
| Gender | G6PD is an X-linked disorder. |
| Race and ethnicity | Hemoglobin S and C are more common among patients of African descent. $\alpha$-Thalassemias are most common in patients of African or Asian ancestry. $\beta$-Thalassemia syndromes are more common in patients from the Mediterranean. |
| Nutrition | Sources of iron, folate, $B_{12}$, and vitamin E should be documented. A history of pica suggests iron deficiency. |
| Medications | Phenytoin and methotrexate can induce a megaloblastic anemia. Oxidants can induce hemolytic anemias. |
| Family history | Document a history of anemia, jaundice, gallstones, cholecystitis, splenomegaly, splenectomy, or hemolytic crisis, which may suggest an inherited hemolytic anemia. |
| Infection | Infections may induce hemolysis or red blood cell hypoplasia or aplasia (parvovirus B19), whereas hepatitis may induce aplastic anemia. |
| Gastrointestinal | The gastrointestinal tract is a common source of blood loss. Nutritional deficiencies may result from malabsorption syndromes. |

*G6PD,* glucose-6-phosphate dehydrogenase.
Modified from Nathan DG, Orkin SH. A diagnostic approach to the anemic patient. In: *Nathan and Oski's Hematology of Infancy and Childhood*. 5th Ed. Philadelphia, PA: WB Saunders; 1998. Copyright © 1998, Elsevier, with permission.

8 g/dL. Pallor may be more easily identified in the nail beds, mucosa, conjunctiva, and palmar creases than in a cursory examination of the skin. Splenomegaly, scleral icterus, and jaundice in the setting of anemia are highly suggestive of a hemolytic process. In chronic hemolytic anemia such as thalassemia, frontal bossing and maxillary prominence are indicative of the marrow expansion necessary to keep pace with ongoing hemolysis. Leukemia or lymphoma may manifest as an anemia associated with focal lymphadenopathy and hepatosplenomegaly. Regardless of the cause of the anemia, a mild to moderate decrease in RBC mass may result in a pulmonary valve flow murmur, whereas more severe anemias may be associated with signs and symptoms of congestive heart failure. Compensated anemia usually refers to anemia associated with sufficient cardiovascular compensation to preserve normal oxygen delivery to tissues. Patients in whom the anemia develops or persists over a long period may have hemoglobin concentrations less than 6 g/dL but no signs or symptoms of anemia other than pallor. Cardiac stroke volume is increased, allowing patients to maintain normal oxygen delivery to tissues with normal or near-normal heart rates. Patients who lose blood more rapidly, from hemolysis or hemorrhage, may not have time for compensatory mechanisms to maintain tissue perfusion and oxygenation. Tachycardia is an early sign, followed by orthostasis, headache, dizziness, and hypotension, all of which are reasons to hospitalize a patient with anemia.

### *Laboratory Findings*

In addition to a determination of the hemoglobin level and hematocrit, which may be done exclusively in some practice settings, RBC morphology and reticulocyte count should be assessed. Anemias may be classified by RBC size as determined by the MCV and by RBC production as determined by the reticulocyte count. An elevated reticulocyte count implies bone marrow compensation for chronic blood loss or hemolysis, whereas a low reticulocyte count may suggest impaired RBC production or acute blood loss. Although not necessary in the initial diagnosis of all patients with anemia, iron studies may be performed and erythrocyte sedimentation rate, serum bilirubin, and serum lactate dehydrogenase levels may be assessed easily in most practice settings and may provide clues to the cause of the anemia. The mean corpuscular hemoglobin (MCH) and mean corpuscular hemoglobin concentration (MCHC) are generally of minimal value in the classification and diagnosis of an anemia. Changes in the MCH typically parallel changes in the MCV. The MCHC is a measure of RBC hydration status. Higher MCHC values (>35/dL) are seen in dehydrated red cells associated with spherocytosis, and low MCHC values may be seen in iron deficiency.

## ▶ TREATMENT

Treatment of a compensated anemia will be dictated by the cause of the anemia. Patients with uncompensated anemia should be admitted to the hospital for observation and possible transfusion. Effective treatment of the anemia is best accomplished by treating the underlying disorder. A substantial number of patients with a microcytic anemia or a normocytic anemia have early iron deficiency anemia, and a course of supplemental iron is appropriate. However, for patients with anemia that is nonresponsive to nutritional supplements and not clearly related to a systemic illness, referral to a pediatric hematologist is warranted. Referral to a pediatric oncologist is also warranted for management of most macrocytic anemias that are not related to nutritional deficiencies. Specific treatment will be predicated on the underlying hematologic disorder.

## When to Refer

- Hemoglobin level less than 8 g/dL or hematocrit less than 25%
- Anemia of unknown origin
- Anemia is associated with disorder in white blood cells or platelets
- Diagnosis of hemoglobinopathy or RBC membrane defect is suspected or confirmed

## When to Admit

- Profound anemia (hemoglobin level <5)
- Uncompensated anemia or anemia associated with a rapidly dropping hemoglobin level
- Anemia in an ill child

## *TOOLS FOR PRACTICE*

### Engaging Patient and Family

- *Anemia and Your Young Child* (handout), American Academy of Pediatrics (patiented.solutions.aap.org)
- *Iron and Iron Deficiency* (fact sheet), Centers for Disease Control and Prevention (www.cdc.gov/nccdphp/dnpa/nutrition/nutrition_for_everyone/iron_deficiency/index.htm)

### Medical Decision Support

- *Pediatric Nutrition Handbook,* 7th ed (book), American Academy of Pediatrics (shop.aap.org), pp 403–417

## *REFERENCES*


1. Nathan DG, Orkin SH. A diagnostic approach to the anemic patient. In: *Nathan and Oski's Hematology of Infancy and Childhood.* 5th ed. Philadelphia, PA: WB Saunders; 1998
2. d'Onfrio G, Chirillo R, Zini G, et al. Simultaneous measurement of reticulocyte and red blood cell indices in healthy subjects and patients with microcytic and macrocytic anemia. *Blood.* 1995;85:818–823
3. Dallman PR, Yip R, Johnson C. Prevalence and causes of anemia in the United States. *Am J Clin Nutr.* 1984;49:437–445
4. Weatherall DJ, Clegg JB. *The Thalassemia Syndromes.* 3rd ed. Oxford, UK: Blackwell Scientific Publications; 1981
5. Higgs DR, Vickers MA, Wilkie AO, et al. A review of the molecular genetics of the human alpha-globin gene cluster. *Blood.* 1989;73:1081–1104
6. Galanello R, Cao A. Gene test review. Alpha-thalassemia. *Genet Med.* 2011;13:83–88
7. Piomelli S, Seaman C, Zullow D, Curran A, Davidow B. Threshold for lead damage to heme synthesis in urban children. *Proc Natl Acad Sci U S A.* 1982;79:3335–3339
8. Lanzkowsky P. Classification and diagnosis of anemia during childhood. In: *Manual of Pediatric Hematology and Oncology.* 4th ed. Burlington, MA: Elsevier Academic Press; 2005
9. Brill JR, Baumgardner DJ. Normocytic anemia. *Am Fam Physician.* 2000;62:2255–2264
10. Perkins SL. Pediatric red cell disorders and pure red cell aplasia. *Am J Clin Pathol.* 2004;122 (Suppl):S70–S86
11. Mupanomunda OK, Alter BP. Transient erythroblastopenia of childhood (TEC) presenting as leuko-erythroblastic anemia. *J Pediatr Hematol Oncol.* 1997;19:165–167

12. Gerrits GP, van Oostrom CG, de Vaan GA, Bakkeren JA. Transient erythroblastopenia of childhood. A review of 22 cases. *Eur J Pediatr*. 1984;142:266–270
13. Irwin JJ, Kirchner JT. Anemia in children. *Am Fam Physician*. 2001;64:1379–1386
14. Prchal JT, Gregg XT. Red cell enzymes. *Hematology Am Soc Hematol Educ Program*. 2005;19–23
15. Carreiro-Lewandowski E. Newborn screening: an overview. *Clin Lab Sci*. 2002;15:229–238
16. Abshire TC. The anemia of inflammation. A common cause of childhood anemia. *Pediatr Clin North Am*. 1996;43(3):623–637
17. Christensen RD, Hunter DD, Goodell H, Rothstein G. Evaluation of the mechanism causing anemia in infants with bronchopulmonary dysplasia. *J Pediatr*. 1992;120:593–598
18. Deters A, Kulozik AE. Hemolytic anemia. In: Sills RH, ed. *Practical Algorithms in Pediatric Hematology and Oncology*. Basel, Switzerland: S. Kargar AG; 2003
19. Lubin B, Vichinsky E. Anemia in the newborn period. *Pediatr Ann*. 1979;8:416–434
20. Oski FA, Naiman JL. *Hematologic Problems of the Newborn*. 3rd ed. Philadelphia, PA: WB Saunders; 1982
21. Blickstein I. The twin-twin transfusion syndrome. *Obstet Gynecol*. 1990;76:714–722

# Chapter 6

# Anxiety

*Lawrence S. Wissow, MD, MPH*

## ▶ INTRODUCTION

Symptoms of anxiety affect many children, including a large number whose symptoms do not rise to the level of a disorder. At some stages and in some circumstances, a certain level of anxiety is developmentally appropriate (eg, stranger anxiety in late infancy or anxiety in anticipation of a painful medical procedure). However, from 6% to 20% of youth will meet diagnostic criteria for an anxiety disorder at some time during childhood,[1] with approximately half experiencing impairment of daily functioning.[2] Anxiety disorders (generalized anxiety disorder, panic disorder, separation anxiety disorder, agoraphobia, social phobia, post-traumatic stress disorder [PTSD], obsessive-compulsive disorder [OCD], specific phobias; see Table 6-1) are among the most common mental health disorders in children and adolescents.[2] Anxiety disorders often occur concomitantly with chronic medical conditions—affecting children's use of medical resources through frequent emergency department visits and hospitalizations[3]—and with other psychiatric disorders, especially depression.[4] Anxious children often have an anxious or a depressed parent.

The guidance in this chapter applies to the care of children presenting with symptoms of anxiety in pediatric clinical settings. Though, as noted above, there are several distinct forms of anxiety disorders, they often co-occur, sharing core symptoms and approaches to initial treatment. Thus the pediatrician may want to start building competence in this area by learning about anxiety problems in general before trying to further differentiate the various disorders.

The following guidance is based on the work of the World Health Organization, whose recommendations may be updated annually. The most up-to-date information can be found at www.who.int.

## ▶ FINDINGS SUGGESTING ANXIETY

Symptoms of anxiety vary by age. Children may experience developmentally normal fears; they may have fears that are exaggerated or persistent beyond norms for their age; and they may have fears and associated reactions or panic attacks that impair their functioning at school, at home, or with peers. Box 6-1 provides a summary of the symptoms and clinical findings that suggest anxiety. These may be elicited from either parents or youth. Parents and youth often disagree on the severity of anxiety symptoms; however, agreement is much better if the discussion is about whether there are symptoms at all, regardless of

**Table 6-1**
**General Overview of Anxiety and Anxiety-Related Disorders**

| TYPE | DESCRIPTION |
|---|---|
| **ANXIETY** | |
| Generalized anxiety disorder | Excessive anxiety and worry about a number of events or activities. Children tend to worry excessively about their competence or the quality of their performance at school or in sporting events. |
| Panic disorder | Recurrent, unexpected, abrupt surge of intense fear or discomfort that reaches a peak within minutes and includes symptoms such as sweating, trembling, palpitations, and dizziness. |
| Separation anxiety disorder | Developmentally inappropriate and excessive fear or anxiety concerning separation from those to whom the individual is attached. |
| Agoraphobia | Marked fear or anxiety in using public transportation, being in open or enclosed spaces, standing in line or being in a crowd, or being outside of the home alone. |
| Social phobia | Marked fear or anxiety about 1 or more social situations in which the individual is exposed to possible scrutiny by others. In children, the anxiety must occur in peer settings and not just during interactions with adults. |
| Specific phobias | Marked fear or anxiety about a specific object or situation (eg, insects, heights, storms, needles, airplanes, loud sounds, costumed characters). In children, the fear or anxiety may be expressed by crying, tantrums, freezing, or clinging. |
| **OBSESSIVE-COMPULSIVE DISORDERS** | |
| Obsessive-compulsive disorder (OCD) | Presence of obsessions or compulsions. Obsessions are recurrent and persistent thoughts, urges, or images that are experienced as intrusive and unwanted. Compulsions are repetitive behaviors or mental acts that an individual is driven to perform, often in response to an obsession or rigidly applied rules. |
| **TRAUMA- AND STRESSOR-RELATED DISORDERS** | |
| Post-traumatic stress disorder (PTSD) | Development of characteristic symptoms following exposure to actual or threatened death, serious injury, or sexual violence. |

Derived from American Psychiatric Association. *Diagnostic and Statistical Manual of Mental Disorders.* 5th ed. Arlington, VA: American Psychiatric Association; 2013.

severity or effect on function. Agreement at this level may facilitate further discussion of how to approach the problem.

## ▶ TOOLS TO ASSIST WITH IDENTIFICATION

Because many children do not spontaneously disclose their symptoms, standardized psychosocial screening instruments may be used to identify children with symptoms of anxiety. Several instruments have versions to collect information directly from the youth or from parents or teachers. Table 6-2 provides an overview of general psychosocial screening tools available in the public domain, along with results suggesting that anxiety may be present. Use of additional instruments, such as the Spence Children's Anxiety Scale or Screen for Child Anxiety Related Disorders 2 (SCARED), can help to confirm findings of the initial screening; and use of a functional assessment tool, such as the Strengths & Difficulties Questionnaires (SDQ) or Columbia Impairment Scale (CIS), will assist in determining whether the child is significantly impaired by the symptoms. Use of a tool to assess the effect

**BOX 6-1**

## *Symptoms and Clinical Findings Suggesting Anxiety*

- Normal fears (eg, strangers, dark, separation, new social situations, unfamiliar animals or objects, public speaking) are exaggerated or persistent.
- Fears are keeping child from developmentally appropriate experiences (eg, school refusal, extreme shyness or clinging, refusal to sleep alone).
- Tantrum, tearfulness, acting-out behavior, or another display of distress occurs when child is asked to engage in feared activity.
- Child worries about harm coming to self or loved ones or fears something bad is going to happen.
- Behavior changes following a traumatic experience, such as abuse, witness to violence, loss of a loved one, or medical trauma, as follows:
  - **Infants and toddlers:** Crying, clinging, change in sleep or eating habits, regression to earlier behavior (eg, bed-wetting, thumb-sucking), repetitive play or talk
  - **3- to 5-year-olds:** Separation fears, clinging, tantrums, fighting, crying, withdrawal, regression to earlier behavior (eg, bed-wetting, thumb-sucking), sleep difficulty
  - **6- to 9-year-olds:** Anger, fighting, bullying, irritability, fluctuating moods, fear of separation or of being alone, fear that traumatic events will recur, withdrawal, regression to earlier behavior, physical complaints (eg, stomachaches, headaches), school problems (eg, avoidance, academic difficulty, difficulty concentrating)
  - **10- to 12-year-olds:** Crying, aggression, irritability, bullying, resentment, sadness, social withdrawal, fears that traumatic events will recur, suppressed emotions or avoidance of situations or discussions that evoke memories of the traumatic event, sleep disturbance, concern about physical health of self or others, academic problems or decline related to lack of attention
  - **13- to 18-year-olds:** Numbing, reexperiencing, avoidance of feelings (or situations or discussions that evoke memories of the traumatic event), resentment, loss of trust or optimism about future, depression, withdrawal, mood swings, irritability, anxiety, anger, exaggerated euphoria, acting out, substance use, fear of similar events, appetite and sleep changes, physical complaints, academic decline, school refusal
- Somatic features accompany worries: palpitations, stomachaches, headaches, breathlessness, difficulty getting to sleep, nausea, feeling wobbly ("jelly legs"), butterflies.
- *Panic attacks* occur in response to feared objects or situations, or happen spontaneously. These are unexpected and repeated periods of intense fear, dread, or discomfort along with symptoms such as racing heartbeat, shortness of breath, dizziness, light-headedness, feeling smothered, trembling, sense of unreality, or fear of dying, losing control, or losing one's mind. Panic attacks often develop without warning and last minutes to hours.

of the child's problem on other members of the family may also be helpful; the Caregiver Strain Questionnaire (CGSQ) is an example.

It is important to differentiate the use of these tools as screening instruments at routine visits from their use to refine concerns that have already been raised. When used as screening tools, they tend to have relatively low sensitivity and positive predictive value. That is, positive results need further discussion to understand the meaning of the result, and negative results may not be reassuring if the parent or youth are truly concerned. When used to follow up on existing concerns, results still need discussion with families, but are more likely be a fair indicator of the nature and severity of the child's problems.

**Table 6-2**
**General Psychosocial Screening/Results Suggesting Anxiety**

| SCREENING INSTRUMENT | SCORE SUGGESTING ANXIETY |
|---|---|
| Pediatric Symptom Checklist (PSC)-35 | • Total score ≥24 for children 5 years and younger.<br>• ≥28 for those 6–16 years.<br>• ≥30 for those 17 years and older.<br>AND<br>• Further discussion of items related to anxiety confirms a concern in that area. |
| PSC-17 | • Internalizing subscale is ≥5.<br>AND<br>• Further discussion of items related to anxiety confirms a concern in that area. |
| Strengths & Difficulties Questionnaire (SDQ) | • Total symptom score of >19.<br>• Emotional symptom score of 7–10 (see instructions at www.sdqinfo.com).<br>• Impact scale score of 1 (medium impairment) or ≥2 (high impairment).<br>AND<br>• Further discussion of items related to anxiety confirms a concern in that area. |

## ▶ ASSESSMENT

Assessment begins by differentiating the child's symptoms from normal behavior. Some children have a temperament that is, from the outset, marked by having more difficulty with change and wariness of new situations or individuals. Recognizing that these are longstanding traits can help parents promote active coping skills and avoid misinterpreting the child's behavior as oppositional. Anxiety is a universal experience, and it can occur predictably at partcular stages of life or in particular situations. When anxiety persists outside of these stages and situations, or when its severity is disruptive, further assessment and treatment may be warranted. Some stages in which particular anxieties may normally emerge include the following:

- **8 to 9 months:** Peak of stranger anxiety.
- **Toddlers and early school age:** Development of separation anxiety (fear of new people, places, or being away from trusted caregivers), usually ends by age 2 to 3 years. Depending on their temperament, toddlers and young children may have greater or lesser tolerance of changes to routine or expectations or of novel experiences (which can include new clothing, foods). Fears of the dark (or of unseen monsters) are common and exacerbated by other stresses and exposure to frightening media.
- **5 to 8 years:** During this period, many children experience an increase in worry about harm to parents or attachment figures. Worries may be triggered by illness or death in family members, by the child's own illness, or by world events.
- **School-aged children of any age:** Many children experience anxiety and distress at the time of high-stakes testing, as well as initial reluctance to socialize in new situations.
- **Adolescence:** Previously resolved anxiety issues often occur again in early adolescence, sometimes associated with concerns about appearance, new social situations, and school performance.

Children with anxiety disorders have fear and distress that interferes with functioning in response to everyday situations. Verbal older children and adolescents are usually able to describe their fears ("worries" may be a more understandable concept), but evaluating reports of younger children's anxiety may be challenging, especially if the parent giving information is also anxious; therefore, it is important to communicate directly with children about these symptoms and to observe or get the child's report of physiologic symptoms (eg, increased heart rate, shortness of breath, numbness, tingling). Sometimes children will display anxiety through repetitive play that acts out their concerns—crashing toy cars or having violent or tragic things happen to dolls—or through drawings that they make in response to simple requests to "draw something." Bad behavior can also be a masked presentation of anxiety. Children and youth at any age may become irritable or oppositional in the face of situations—imminent or anticipated—that they fear. Depression or bereavement may mimic or co-occur with anxiety, so at least some exploration of other emotional symptoms and of current stressors is always warranted. When children and youth of any age are anxious, it is always important to ask about stressors in the family environment—serious illness (including anxiety and depression) in a family member, economic problems, or marital discord.

Anxiety, like depression, also may occur in multiple family members. When children are found to be anxious, it is not unusual to find that one or more close family members are anxious as well. Helping parents manage their own anxiety can be very important, especially, as discussed in the following text, when trying to use modelling as a form of treatment. Table 6-3 provides a summary of these conditions.

Children with anxiety sometimes have panic attacks, which are episodes of autonomic arousal that occur suddenly, often (but not always) cued by thoughts of a feared situation. People experiencing panic attacks usually report sudden onset of shortness of breath, palpitations, trembling, diaphoresis, and often a feeling of faintness, dread, or impending doom. The attacks usually subside by themselves over the course of several minutes, but it is not unusual, especially among teenagers, for some of the symptoms to be prolonged and result in a call for emergency medical assistance. Differentiating panic attacks from hypoglycemia, asthma exacerbations, or cardiac conditions may in itself help with their treatment; often they will improve as other aspects of anxiety are treated. As noted in the following text, they can sometimes be suppressed with medication if their frequency is causing disability, which can facilitate treatment of the underlying anxiety problem.

Treatment for anxiety generally involves identifying the specific situations in which it is triggered and helping individuals learn how to reduce anxious feelings when they occur and gradually become tolerant of the triggers to the point where anxious responses are either no longer evoked or remain manageable. Treatment is usually tailored to the specific triggering situation, often through carefully supported increasing exposure to the trigger coupled with practice of a variety of cognitive, somatic, and social coping strategies. Treatment of OCD and PTSD involves these same treatment elements, but differs in that the etiology of the disorders takes on a role in treatment (whereas in the treatment of other anxiety disorders there is less emphasis on how the problem began and more on how to get it to remit). For OCD, the fact that obsessions and compulsions develop without particular triggers (though they can be worsened by other stresses) plays an important role in children's and family's

**Table 6-3**
**Conditions That May Mimic or Co-occur With Anxiety**

| CONDITION | RATIONAL |
|---|---|
| Learning problems or disabilities | If symptoms of anxiety are associated with problems of school attendance or performance, the child may be experiencing academic difficulties. (See Chapter 49, Learning Difficulty, for more information.) |
| Somatic complaints | Anxious children may present with a variety of somatic complaints (eg, gastrointestinal symptoms, headaches, chest pain). These may elicit medical workups if they are not recognized. Conversely, acute or chronic medical conditions or pain syndromes may cause anxiety. |
| Depression | This can be very difficult to distinguish from anxiety. Depression coexists in half or more of anxious children. Marked sleep disturbance, disturbed appetite, low mood, or tearfulness in the absence of direct anxiety provocation could indicate that a child is depressed. |
| Bereavement | Most children will experience the death of a family member or friend sometime in their childhood. Other losses may also trigger grief responses—separation or divorce of parents, relocation, change of school, deployment of a parent in military service, breakup with a girlfriend or boyfriend, or remarriage of a parent. Such losses are traumatic. They may result in feelings of insecurity and anxiety immediately following the loss or exacerbate existing anxiety. Furthermore, they may make the child more susceptible to impaired functioning at the time of subsequent losses. |
| Autism spectrum disorders including pervasive developmental disorder and Asperger syndrome | Children who have these difficulties also have problems with social relatedness (eg, poor eye contact, preference for solitary activities), language (often stilted), and range of interest (persistent and intense interest in a particular activity or subject). They often will have very rigid expectations for routine or parent promises and become anxious or angry if these expectations are not met. |
| Exposure to adverse childhood experiences (ACE) | Children who have experienced or witnessed trauma, violence, a natural disaster, separation from a parent, parental divorce or separation, parental substance use, neglect, or physical, emotional, or sexual abuse are at high risk of developing emotional difficulties such as adjustment disorder or PTSD. Determination of the temporal relationship between the trauma and onset of anxiety symptoms is essential. Denial of trauma symptoms does not mean trauma did not occur; questions about ACE should be repeated as a trusting relationship is established. |
| Psychosis | Symptoms associated with psychosis, such as hallucinations or delusions, may occur in children with PTSD. They may also occur infrequently with adolescent onset of bipolar disorder and are features of schizophrenia, which may also have its onset in adolescence. The teen may manifest fear without disclosing the hallucinations or delusions. |
| Physical illness | Medical issues that can mimic or provoke anxiety symptoms include thyroid disease, hypoglycemia, side effects of medications (eg, bronchodilators), and endocrine tumors (pheochromocytoma). Drug or alcohol withdrawal is a consideration for teens (the latter potentially a medical emergency). |
| Selective mutism | Consider this if a child who has had normal language development suddenly stops talking in certain situations (most often in school and to adults outside the home). This can be confused with children making a language transition (eg, a child raised speaking Spanish who is suddenly placed in an English-speaking class.) |

understanding of the condition. For PTSD, linking what may be nonspecific symptoms to a particular past trauma can be an important part of treatment.

- **Consider OCD in the presence of marked rituals or compulsive behaviors.** Most children have phases of ritualized behavior that usually can be distinguished from OCD by the degree of distress caused if a ritual is interrupted. Individuals with OCD usually report—or after discussion will admit—that the symptoms have a major effect on how they plan their activities or interact with others, and that attempts to stop the thoughts or actions have been difficult to carry out or even contemplate. School-aged children and adolescents will often—once the symptoms can be openly discussed—admit being aware that there is something objectively out of proportion about their concerns, even though they remain difficult to resist. The most common concerns center on contamination—fears of touching things that may be dirty, or the need to repetitively wash or bathe. Other common difficulties are the need to check that something has been done (usually related to security—doors locked, stove turned off) or a need to have one's personal possessions in a particular order or place.
- **Consider PTSD if the onset of anxiety was preceded by an extremely distressing experience,** such as witnessing violence, losing a loved one, undergoing medical trauma, or experiencing sexual or physical abuse. Parents may be unaware of exposures to trauma, such as bullying at school or in the community, and there may be major traumas in the family (eg, serious illness in a parent, pending divorce) that are similarly not discussed or disclosed; consequently, clinicians may need to interview children and parents separately to elicit a complete history. It is important to note that the triggering circumstances need only be traumatic in the eye of the child. Most antecedents have in common situations in which the child felt that there was risk to her life, or that of someone close to her. The 3 hallmark symptoms of anxiety in the wake of trauma are *re-experiencing* (often repetitive play in young children), *avoidance* of memories or situations that recall the trauma, and *hypervigilance* (eg, increased worry about safety, startling or anxiousness at unexpected sounds or events). Avoidance can also take the form of changing the subject or acting inappropriately when subjects related to trauma are brought up in conversation. Children most at risk for developing PTSD following trauma or loss are those with preexisting mental health conditions, those whose caregivers are experiencing emotional difficulties, those facing preexisting or consequent family life stressors, such as divorce or loss of job, those with previous loss or trauma experiences, those repeatedly exposed to media coverage of traumatic events, and those with a limited support network.[4] Clinicians can provide the child with a safe and comfortable environment to express her feelings and allow the child to control the interview, taking breaks or discontinuing as needed. Even children with limited symptoms of PTSD after a trauma can benefit from treatment.

## ▶ PLAN OF CARE FOR CHILDREN WITH ANXIETY

The care of a child experiencing anxiety can begin in the primary care setting from the time symptoms are recognized, even if the child's symptoms do not rise to the level of a disorder and regardless of whether referral to a mental health specialist is ultimately part of the care plan. Both children and parents may, by temperament, be more or less socially outgoing and more or less open to new or unexpected experiences. Helping parents appreciate their own areas of comfort and discomfort, and how these may differ from those of their child, can be a first step toward treatment. Regardless of parent or child temperament, parents can be helped to learn ways to help their child gain better emotional regulation.

## Engage Child and Family in Care

Without engagement, most families will not seek or persist in care. The process may require multiple primary care visits.[5]

Reinforce strengths of the child and family (eg, good relationships with at least 1 parent or important adult, prosocial peers, concerned or caring family, help-seeking, connection to positive organizations) as a method of engagement, and identify any barriers to addressing the problem (eg, stigma, family conflict, resistance to treatment). Use "common factors" techniques[6] to build trust and optimism, reach agreement on incremental next steps, develop a plan of care, and collaboratively determine the role of the primary care physician. Regardless of other roles, the primary care physician can encourage a positive view of treatment on the part of the child and family.

Remember that it is in many ways normal for people with anxiety problems to initially resist their treatment. This is because most people cope with anxiety through avoidance, and initiating treatment means that one has to start thinking about the situations that trigger the anxious feelings.

## Provide Psychoeducation

Tell the family a little bit about anxiety; much of the material discussed previously in this chapter could be useful. Emphasize that anxiety is a normal human emotion, that anxiety problems are very common, and that they can be addressed. For some children and families, it can be helpful to talk about variations in temperament or personal style that make some people more or less anxious in new situations or more or less responsive to threats. Again, acknowledge that these are traits we are born with and not to be ashamed of. The clinician can also say that anxiety has nothing to do with bravery or accomplishment, noting that many famous performers and athletes experience serious degrees of "stage fright" and yet, with support and encouragement, have become very successful (usually by working hard to prepare themselves). It can be helpful to point out that one can very much enjoy and be good at things but still experience anxiety when having to do them in front of others or in particularly high-stakes circumstances.

## Encourage Healthy Habits

Encourage exercise, outdoor play, balanced and consistent diet, sleep (critically important to mental health), special time with parents, frequent acknowledgment of the child's strengths, and open communication with a trusted adult about worries. Children, particularly younger ones, should be shielded from certain types of media, such as the news, when there are violent or disturbing images or stories. Likewise, TV shows, even some cartoons, may contribute to a child's feeling anxious. For preteens and teens, media messages about body image and social media may contribute to or exacerbate anxiety.

## Reduce Stress

Consider the child's social environment (eg, family social history, parental depression screening, results of any family assessment tools administered, reports from child care or school). Questions to raise might include the following:

- *Is an external problem causing the child to be anxious* (eg, bullying at school, academic difficulties, disruption at home)? Take steps to address the problem.

- *Is the child exposed to frightening electronic media?* Sometimes this results from unsupervised access to television or Internet content, but it may also occur during shared family activities (eg, movies, TV, video games) when parents or other family members underestimate or fail to recognize how frightened the child has become. Limiting these exposures, and providing reassuring explanations if they occur, can be an important part of reducing anxiety, especially among younger children.
- *Is the child's worry about a parent's welfare legitimate because of a serious illness, domestic violence, or parent impairment?* Address environmental issues, enlisting the help of school personnel or social services as appropriate to the situation.
- *Is the parent anxious or depressed or impaired because of substance abuse? Has the parent experienced trauma or loss?* Anxious children very often have an anxious or a depressed parent. Advise parents to minimize their own displays of fear or worry when the child is present. A referral to adult mental health services might also be appropriate.

## Offer Initial Intervention(s) to Address the Anxiety Symptoms

The strategies described in the following text are common elements of evidence-based psychosocial interventions for anxiety disorders. They are applicable to the care of children with mild or emerging anxiety symptoms and to those with impairing symptoms that do not rise to the level of a disorder. They can also be used as initial primary care management of children with anxiety disorders and while readying children for referral or awaiting access to specialty care. Medications can be helpful, especially to speed suppresion of panic and OCD symptoms or when very time-limited and severe stressors need to be faced, but, in the absence of psychosocial treatments, symptoms may recur as the medications are discontinued. Interpreting the results of a medication trial can also be problematic, because the severity of anxiety problems is often cyclic. Families may seek care as symptoms are peaking. If medication is started at this point, it often cannot be determined if the condition improved on its own or responded to medication. Thus, starting with a carefully administered psychosocial treatment plan may be a reasonable first step until the severity and natural history of the anxiety concerns are better understood.

*Guide parents in managing the child's fears.* Help the parents to identify their child's fear(s) and reach consensus with the child and family on the goal of reducing symptoms and on a way to do it. This could include teaching the child and parent cognitive behavioral strategies to improve coping skills at times when the child feels anxious. Examples of these skills include deep breathing, muscle relaxation, positive self-talk, thought stopping, and thinking of a safe place. The child and family may also benefit from reading material or a Web course, as appropriate to their literacy level.

*Gradually increase exposure.* One of the best validated approaches to anxiety and phobias is to gradually increase the child's exposure to feared objects or experiences. The eventual goal is to master rather than avoid feared things. To do this, the parent might start out with brief exposure to the feared object or activity and gradually lengthen the exposure. First, help the child imagine or talk about the feared object or activity or look at pictures; then learn to tolerate a short exposure with support from the parent; proceed to tolerate a longer exposure in a group or with the parent or another coach; and, finally, tolerate the feared activity alone (when that is appropriate) but with a chance to get help if needed. During these trials, parents need to stay as calm and confident as possible; if they become distressed, it will be a cue for the child to become distressed.

*Manage school phobia.* For some children who are vulnerable to anxiety, it is necessary to return the child promptly to the anxiety-producing situation. School phobia is an example. For the child who is afraid at school or resists going to school, rule out bullying, trauma, learning difficulties, and medical conditions that may be contributing to stress and fear. Also, the primary care physician can partner with school personnel to manage the child's return to school and gently, but firmly, insist that the child attend school, in addition to providing positive feedback and calm support. If absence becomes prolonged or parents are reluctant to support the child's return, referral to a mental health specialist will be necessary.

If anxiety is secondary to environmental stress, support the parents' efforts to protect the child, buffer stress, and help the child master his anxiety. Help the child to rename the fear (ie, "annoying worry") and assist the child to become the boss of the worry. It is also helpful to reward brave behavior (see Table 6-4).

*Attend to overall parenting style.* Children can become anxious if parents are inconsistent about rules and expectations. Determine whether there are catastrophic consequences for failure ("I know Dad will get angry if I bring home a bad grade...."). Explore the child's sense of responsibility for the family's stresses ("I know that the only reason Mom and Dad work hard is so I can go to a better school, so I'm afraid that if don't do well....").

*Treat panic attacks.* Early treatment, including psychosocial and psychopharmacologic therapy, is useful and may prevent progression to agoraphobia and other problems such as depression and substance abuse.[7] When children are aware of the triggers for their attacks, developing alternative responses to those triggers can diminish the frequency of attacks. When attacks appear without apparent triggers, referral for pharmacologic treatment may be most effective.

Links for further information regarding the treatment of anxiety symptoms are provided in Tools for Practice at the end of this chapter.

## Provide Resources

Helpful handouts and publications are included in Tools for Practice: Engaging Patient and Family at the end of this chapter. Provide the family with contact numbers and resources in case of emergency.

**Table 6-4**
**Tips for Reward System**

| REWARD SYSTEMS FOR BRAVE BEHAVIOR | GUIDELINES FOR USE |
|---|---|
| Small rewards | Include positive feedback. |
| Star charts | • Focus on only 1 or 2 behaviors at a time.<br>• Have 1 star chart per behavior.<br>• Negotiate rules for the star chart (eg, sleeping in own bed for 1 night = 1 star; 4 stars = trip to the pool).<br>• Ignore mistakes and failures; do not even mark them on the star chart.<br>• Continue awarding stars when they are earned. |

## Monitor the Child's Progress Toward Therapeutic Goals

Child care, preschool, or school reports can be helpful in monitoring progress. Screening instruments that gather information from multiple reporters (youth, parent, teacher), such as the SDQ, can be helpful in monitoring progress with symptoms and functioning.

It is important for the primary care physician to work with the family to understand that it is not uncommon for treatment to be successful for a period of time and then seem to lose effectiveness. This can happen when there are new stresses or demands, or when, after a period of success, there has been a letup on treatment. If troubleshooting existing treatment and ways of dealing with new stresses does not help get function back to baseline, new treatments or new diagnoses need to be considered. In particular, as school demands increase, learning issues may need to be considered even if they were not seen as contributing problems in the past.

## Involve Specialist(s)

Involve specialist(s) if the child does not respond to initial interventions or if the following clinical circumstances exist:

- Child has severe functional impairments at school, at home, or with peers—for example, if anxiety threatens to interfere with academic progress or other developmentally important goals.
- Multiple symptoms of anxiety occur in many domains of life (eg, fearful of new situations, reluctant to do things in public, trouble separating, worries a lot).
- The child or parent is very distressed by the symptom(s).
- There are co-occurring behavior problems. (The combination of shyness, anxiety, and behavior problems is thought to be particularly risky for future behavior problems of a more serious nature.)
- The anxiety was preceded by serious trauma or symptoms suggesting PTSD.
- The child seems to have panic disorder or OCD, both of which require specialized treatment.
- The anxiety occurs in a child with an autism spectrum disorder. Anxiety about both normal childhood issues (weather, animals), as well as the orderliness and predictability of daily routines, is relatively common among higher functioning children who display autism spectrum symptoms, including stereotyped interests and poor social perceptions and skills.

*When specialty care is needed, ensure that it is evidence-informed and assist the family in accessing it.* A variety of evidence-based and evidence-informed psychosocial interventions, and some pharmacologic interventions, are available for the treatment of anxiety disorders in children and adolescents. Ideally, those referred for care in the mental health specialty system would have access to the safest and most effective treatments. Table 6-5 provides a summary of these interventions. Youth referred for mental health specialty care complete the referral process only 61% of the time, and a significantly smaller number persist in care.[8] Approaches to improving the referral process include making sure that the family is ready for this step in care, has some idea of what the specialty care will involve, and understands what the primary care physician's ongoing role may be. If the specialty appointment is not likely to occur shortly, the physician can work with them on a plan to manage the problem as well as possible in the meantime.

**Table 6-5**
**Psychosocial and Psychopharmacologic Treatments for Anxiety (as of November 2014)[a]**

| | PSYCHOSOCIAL TREATMENTS | |
|---|---|---|
| **CLUSTER AREA** | **LEVEL 1 (BEST SUPPORT)** | **LEVEL 2 (GOOD SUPPORT)** |
| Anxious or avoidant behaviors[b] | • Cognitive behavior therapy (CBT)<br>• CBT and medication<br>• CBT with parents (includes parent and child, focusing on the child's concerns)<br>• Education<br>• Exposure<br>• Modeling | • Assertiveness training<br>• Attention<br>• CBT for child and parent (child and parent receive CBT separately, focusing on each of their concerns)<br>• Cultural storytelling<br>• Family psychoeducation<br>• Hypnosis<br>• Relaxation<br>• Stress inoculation |
| Traumatic stress[b] | • CBT<br>• CBT with parents (includes the parent as well as the child, focusing on the child's concerns) | • Exposure<br>• Eye movement desensitization and reprocessing |
| **US FOOD AND DRUG ADMINISTRATION–APPROVED PSYCHOPHARMACOLOGIC INTERVENTIONS[c]** | | |
| **DIAGNOSTIC AREA** | **PSYCHOPHARMACOLOGIC INTERVENTION** | |
| Anxiety disorders | Currently (as of November 2014), the only psychopharmacologic interventions approved by the US Food and Drug Administration are selective serotonin reuptake inhibitors (SSRIs) (sertraline, fluvoxamine) and clomipramine for the treatment of obsessive-compulsive disorder (OCD). Currently, no psychopharmacologic interventions have been approved for other anxiety disorders, although a number of randomly controlled clinical trials suggest their efficacy and safety. | |

[a]For AAP policy, please visit pediatrics.aappublications.org/site/aappolicy.
[b]Excerpted from PracticeWise Evidence-Based Child and Adolescent Psychosocial Interventions. Reprinted with permission from PracticeWise. For updates and an explanation of PracticeWise determination of evidence level, please visit www.aap.org/mentalhealth.
[c]For up-to-date information about Food and Drug Administration (FDA)-approved interventions, go to www.fda.gov/ScienceResearch/SpecialTopics/PediatricTherapeuticsResearch/default.htm.

Note that not all evidence-based interventions may be available in every community. If a particular intervention is not available, this becomes an opportunity to collaborate with others in the community to advocate on behalf of children. Increasingly, states offer both telepsychiatry services and consultation/referral support "warmlines" that help physicians provide initial treatment and locate resources. The availability of the latter form of help is tracked at www.nncpap.org.

*Reach agreement on respective roles in the child's care.* If the child is referred to mental health specialty care for an anxiety disorder, the physician may be responsible for initiating medication or adjusting doses; monitoring response to treatment; monitoring adverse effects; engaging and encouraging the child and family's positive view of treatment; and coordinating care provided by parents, school, medical home, and specialists. In fact, the child may improve just knowing that the physician is involved and interested. Resources available to help clinicians in these roles are provided in Tools for Practice: Medical Decision Support.

### ACKNOWLEDGMENT

The author and editor wish to acknowledge the contributions of Linda Paul, MPH, manager of the AAP Mental Health Leadership Work Group.

### TOOLS FOR PRACTICE

#### Engaging Patient and Family

- *How to Ease Your Child's Separation Anxiety* (fact sheet), American Academy of Pediatrics (www.healthychildren.org/English/ages-stages/toddler/Pages/Soothing-Your-Childs-Separation-Anxiety.aspx)
- *Tips for Parenting the Anxious Child* (handout), American Academy of Pediatrics (www.brightfutures.org/mentalhealth/pdf/families/mc/tips.pdf)
- *Helping Your Anxious Child: A Step-by-Step Guide for Parents,* 2nd ed (book), New Harbinger Publications
- *Feelings Need Check-ups Too* (toolkit), American Academy of Pediatrics (www.aap.org/en-us/advocacy-and-policy/aap-health-initiatives/Children-and-Disasters/Pages/Feelings-Need-Checkups-Too-Toolkit.aspx)

#### Medical Decision Support

- *Pediatric Symptom Checklist* (screen), Massachusetts General Hospital (www.massgeneral.org/psychiatry/services/psc_home.aspx)
- *Strengths & Difficulties Questionnaires* (screen), Youth in Mind, Ltd (www.sdqinfo.com)
- *Spence Children's Anxiety Scale* (scale), Susan H. Spence, PhD (www.scaswebsite.com)
- *Screen for Child Anxiety Related Disorders* (screen), University of Pittsburgh (child version: www.psychiatry.pitt.edu/sites/default/files/Documents/assessments/SCARED%20Child.pdf; parent version: www.psychiatry.pitt.edu/sites/default/files/Documents/assessments/SCARED%20Parent.pdf)

### REFERENCES

1. Connolly SD, Bernstein GA; Work Group on Quality Issues. Practice parameter for the assessment and treatment of children and adolescents with anxiety disorders. *J Am Acad Child Adolesc Psychiatry.* 2007;46:267–283
2. Merikangas KR. Vulnerability factors for anxiety disorders in children and adolescents. *Child Adolesc Psychiatr Clin N Am.* 2005;14:649–679, vii
3. Bernal P. Hidden morbidity in pediatric primary care. *Pediatr Ann.* 2003;32:413–418; quiz 421–422
4. Williamson DE, Forbes EE, Dahl RE, Ryan ND. A genetic epidemiologic perspective on comorbidity of depression and anxiety. *Child Adolesc Psychiatr Clin N Am.* 2005;14:707–726, viii
5. Foy JM; American Academy of Pediatrics Task Force on Mental Health. Enhancing pediatric mental health care: algorithms for primary care. *Pediatrics.* 2010;125(Suppl 3):S109–S125
6. The Anxious Child. American Academy of Child and Adolescent Psychiatry, Facts for Families Web site. http://www.aacap.org/cs/root/facts_for_families/the_anxious_child. No. 47. Updated November 2004. Accessed November 26, 2014
7. Kemper KJ, Wissow L, Foy JM, Shore SE. *Core Communication Skills for Primary Clinicians.* Wake Forest School of Medicine. nwahec.org/45737. Accessed January 9, 2015
8. Chisolm DJ, Klima J, Gardner W, Kelleher KJ. Adolescent behavioral risk screening and use of health services. *Adm Policy Ment Health.* 2009;36:374–380

# Chapter 7

# Ataxia

*Philip Overby, MD*

Ataxia derives from the Greek—*a* (without), *taxia* (order) and means a "lack of order." Broadly, ataxia encompasses disorders in which there is an absence of coordinated movements, often involving gait. Although ataxia can certainly be chronic, as a presenting symptom in pediatrics it is almost always acute. For the treating physician, the list of its potential causes can be daunting (see Box 7-1), in part because ataxia can be caused by dysfunction at any level of the motor system from brain to muscle. Diagnostically, the goal is to localize the ataxia to the level of dysfunction.

## ▶ EVALUATION

### *History*

Practically, the initial approach to the child with acute ataxia should focus on the serious causes of ataxia. Once these have been excluded clinically, more common as well as treatable causes can be considered. Life-threatening conditions fall into 4 broad categories: infection or inflammation, neoplasm, stroke, and ingestion. Although the initial history should be directed foremost at identifying serious causes of acute ataxia, in most cases, the causes of acute ataxia are self-limited and benign.[1] One retrospective study of 40 pediatric cases found that 80% could be attributed to acute cerebellitis, toxic ingestion, and Guillain-Barré syndrome (GBS).[2] Note that although it certainly is a common cause of acute ataxia in children, ingestion in this discussion is included among the more serious causes because missing the diagnosis can be life threatening.

The history should explore evidence of recent or current infection: fever, rash, respiratory symptoms, or vomiting. Questions about possible toxic exposures in the home, such as medications, alcohol, or illicit drugs, are essential. The possibility of trauma, observed or unobserved, should be explored with all caregivers and children who might be aware of it.

Associated symptoms can further guide the history. Although acute cerebellitis is characterized by preservation of alertness, a change in mental status is concerning and can signal a systemic process. Considerations include toxic ingestion, infection, or mechanical compression of the brainstem by a tumor or abscess. Headaches, recurrent vomiting, visual loss or diplopia, and worsening of symptoms when supine can be signs of elevated intracranial pressure (ICP) from hydrocephalus in the setting of posterior fossa masses. It should be noted, however, that these findings can be late or even intermittent, and their absence does not exclude elevated ICP.

Recent and abrupt onset of symptoms is more suggestive of a vascular, toxic, or infectious cause. Tumors and immune-mediated processes are typically more subacute in their

BOX 7-1

## *Causes of Acute Ataxia in Childhood*

**Infectious/immune-mediated cerebellar disorders**
- Acute cerebellar ataxia[a]
- Acute demyelinating encephalomyelitis[a]
- Systemic infections
- Brainstem encephalitis
- Multiple sclerosis

**Mass lesions**
- Tumors
- Vascular lesions
- Abscesses

**Hydrocephalus**

**Trauma**
- Cerebellar contusion or hemorrhage
- Posterior fossa hematoma
- Postconcussion syndrome
- Vertebrobasilar dissection

**Stroke**
- Vertebrobasilar dissection or thromboembolism
- Cerebellar hemorrhage

**Paraneoplastic disorders**
- Opsoclonus-myoclonus syndrome

**Sensory ataxia**
- Guillain-Barré syndrome
- Miller-Fisher syndrome

**Paretic ataxia**
- Upper motoneuron
- Lesions of frontal lobe, corticospinal pathways
- Lower motoneuron
- Spinal cord: transverse myelitis, vascular lesions, cord compression
- Peripheral nerve: Guillain-Barré syndrome, Miller Fisher syndrome, tick paralysis

**Other neurologic disorders**
- Inborn errors of metabolism (see Box 7-2)[a]
- Basilar migraine, benign paroxysmal vertigo
- Nonconvulsive seizures
- Central pontine myelinolysis
- Wernicke encephalopathy

**Functional ataxia**

[a]Most common.
From Ryan MM, Engle EC. Topical review: acute ataxia in childhood. *J Child Neurol.* 2003;18:309–316, with permission from SAGE Publications.

progression. The exception is tumors that hemorrhage. If a patient with a known brain tumor has an acute change in mental status, or acute ataxia, he or she should be evaluated for hemorrhage acutely with a head CT. If hemorrhage is present, neurosurgery should be contacted immediately. Prior similar episodes are suggestive of chronic conditions such as migraine, or even seizures. Recurrent episodes are also potentially suggestive of metabolic processes (see Box 7-2).[3]

### Physical Examination

Life-threatening causes of acute ataxia typically originate in the central nervous system. They tend to involve the posterior fossa or brainstem. In particular, symptoms are referable to 3 sources: cranial nerves, the pyramidal tracts, and the cerebellum. Moreover, the involvement of brainstem and cerebellar structures typically results in abnormalities both on history and physical examination. As such, a normal neurologic examination, carefully performed, is a pertinent negative.

The physical examination begins with vital signs. Fever suggests infection. Autonomic changes can be seen in the setting of acute stroke, elevated ICP, or peripheral processes such as GBS.[4] The examination can be challenging because the child may be uncooperative. Given this, the examination should move from the least to the most invasive. General observations (Does the child appear ill or uncomfortable? Is she agitated or careful not to move?) are

BOX 7-2

## *Causes of Episodic or Intermittent Ataxia in Childhood*

**Recurrence of acute cerebellar ataxia**[a]

**Migraine or migraine equivalents**
- Basilar migraine[a]
- Benign paroxysmal vertigo
- Benign paroxysmal torticollis of infancy
- Alternating hemiplegia of childhood

**Metabolic disorders**
- Mitochondrial disorders
  - Pyruvate decarboxylase deficiency
  - Pyruvate dehydrogenase deficiency
  - Leigh disease
- Amino acidopathies
  - Maple syrup urine disease, intermittent form Hartnup disease
  - γ-Glutamylcysteine synthetase deficiency
- Urea cycle disorders
  - Carbamoyl phosphate synthetase type 1 deficiency
  - Ornithine transcarbamylase deficiency
  - Citrullinemia
  - Arginosuccinic aciduria
- Organic acidopathies
  - Holocarboxylase deficiency
  - Biotinidase deficiency
  - Isovaleric acidemia
- Carnitine acetyltransferase deficiency

**Recurrent genetic ataxias**
- Episodic ataxia type 1 (paroxysmal ataxia with myokymia)
- Episodic ataxia type 2 (acetazolamide responsive)
- Episodic ataxia types 3 and 4
- Episodic ataxia with paroxysmal dystonia
- CAPOS syndrome (cerebellar ataxia, areflexia, pes cavus, optic atrophy, sensorineural hearing loss)

**Nonconvulsive seizures**

**Drug ingestion**[a]

**Paroxysmal tonic upgaze of childhood**

**Cogan syndrome**

[a]Most common.
From Ryan MM, Engle EC. Topical review: acute ataxia in childhood. *J Child Neurol.* 2003;18:309–316, with permission from SAGE Publications.

valuable. The somatic examination should explore for evidence of meningismus: neck stiffness as well as photophobia and discomfort with movement. Next, attention should be given to the child's mental status. Behavioral changes, decreased alertness, inattention, or dysarthria can all be clues to elevated ICP, brainstem compression, or cranial neuropathies that may affect eye movements. If possible, fundi should be inspected for papilledema. The presence or absence of associated findings to suggest elevated ICP, such as restriction of upward gaze or lateral eye movements, should also be noted.

Cerebellar hemisphere dysfunction is often associated with a wide-based gait. Attempts to stand with feet close together can result in swaying from side to side with eyes open or closed. Unilateral weakness or pyramidal tract dysfunction manifests as asymmetries in arm or leg use. Subtle gait difficulties can be elicited with tandem walking. Sensory ataxia can be elicited by asking the child to stand still with feet together and eyes closed, the "Romberg test," which examines the dorsal columns. A positive test is one in which swaying or a frank fall occurs.

## Differential Diagnosis—Serious Disorders

### Acute Stroke

In the absence of trauma, hemorrhagic stroke (intracerebral hemorrhage, or ICH) in children most commonly results from an arteriovenous malformation (AVM). Emergent neurologic and neurosurgical evaluation is critical. Associated symptoms of ICH include headache, seizure, or visual loss. Decompression of a posterior fossa hemorrhage can be life saving. Hemorrhagic stroke will be apparent on head computed tomography. Ischemic stroke of the posterior circulation is rare in children but can be seen in the setting of vertebral dissection—often from trauma.

## Acute Disseminated Encephalomyelitis

Acute disseminated encephalomyelitis (ADEM) is an acute demyelinating event that is typically most severe at onset. It is an immune-mediated encephalitis often occurring in the context of viral or postviral infections.[5] The white matter of the brain and spinal cord are preferentially affected. Typically, ADEM follows a prodrome of fever, vomiting, headache, and malaise. The neurologic features are broad[5]: unilateral or bilateral pyramidal signs (60%–95%), acute hemiplegia (76%), ataxia (18%–65%), cranial nerve palsies (22%–45%), visual loss from optic neuritis (7%–23%), seizures (13%–35%), and spinal cord involvement (24%).[6] Ultimate outcome does not seem to be affected by immunologic therapy, which can, however, hasten recovery.

## Tumor

Childhood brain tumors occur most frequently in the posterior fossa. The most common tumors are medulloblastoma, brainstem glioma, ependymoma, and cystic astrocytoma. There are 3 potential areas of involvement: cranial nerves, pyramidal tracts, and the cerebellum. Although symptoms may be reported to have developed over the course of days, a careful history typically reveals subtle signs of weakness and coordination difficulties lasting weeks to months. Signs from obstruction of cerebrospinal fluid (CSF) flow are common, and children younger than 2 years typically present with increasing head circumference. In older children, symptoms such as headaches and ataxia are more common. The average time from symptom onset to diagnosis is 7 months.[7] Although less common than brain tumors, spinal tumors can also present with ataxia. Depending on the spinal level, signs of weakness or sensory loss referable to the lower or upper extremities with preservation of reflexes will be present. In addition, paraneoplastic presentation of tumors (eg, opsoclonus–myoclonus syndrome) at times need to be considered in the differential diagnosis of ataxia.

## Cerebellitis

Acute cerebellitis, also known as acute cerebellar ataxia, is a common, typically benign infectious or parainfectious phenomenon.[8] It typically occurs in preschool- and school-aged children. Generally, the acute ataxia is most prominent on awakening and improves over the course of hours to days. Rarely, however, fulminant cerebellitis occurs. Unlike its more benign form, fulminant cerebellitis progresses from its onset to the development of encephalopathy, with hydrocephalus caused by obstruction of the fourth ventricle. Outcomes can be favorable with aggressive management.[9]

## Trauma

Life-threatening conditions to consider in the setting of trauma are hemorrhagic stroke and ischemic stroke from vertebrobasilar artery dissection. In the absence of more diffuse injury causing associated encephalopathy, it is unusual for trauma to present with isolated ataxia. The important exception to this rule is vertebral artery dissection, which represents 7% to 20% of pediatric ischemic strokes.[10] The vertebral arteries supply the posterior circulation. Presenting signs and symptoms are referable to the posterior fossa: ataxia, vertigo, vomiting, diplopia, and head and neck pain. Although these symptoms are common and nonspecific, 88% of patients in a 2005 review had focal neurologic deficits.[9] Fifty percent of children in the same study had a history of trauma.

### Toxic Ingestion

Ingestion of a toxin represents a major cause of ataxia in children, accounting for up to 32.5% of cases.[2] Ingestion associated with ataxia includes antihistamines, alcohol, anticonvulsants (especially phenytoin and carbamazepine), piperazine, diphenylhydantoin, barbiturates, carbon monoxide, organic solvents, and bromides.[11] Accidental ingestion occurs in young children. Adolescents can also present after ingestion in attempts to self-harm. Symptoms of ingestion can be nonspecific. Indeed, when symptoms do not fit well into a clinical syndrome, ingestion should become a concern. When considering toxic ingestion, it is also important to evaluate for other evidence of metabolic aberrations, such as hypoglycemia, hyponatremia, and hyperammonemia.

## *Common Causes of Ataxia*

### Sensory or Motor Ataxia Caused by Guillain-Barré Syndrome

Studies of the incidence of GBS in children younger than 16 years old, most of which have been performed in Europe and North America, suggest rates between 0.4 and 1.4 per 100,000.[12] Although the typical presentation of symmetrical weakness is well known, an acute progressive ataxia is another presentation of GBS seen particularly in young children. Important early clues include distal paresthesias or numbness. Younger children may present with prominent symptoms of leg pain, agitation, or vomiting, and meningeal signs may be present on examination.[4] Reflexes are depressed or absent. Lumbar puncture typically demonstrates dissociation between cells and protein, with elevated protein and borderline-to-normal WBC counts. The CSF may be normal on initial presentation.

Three disorders need to be considered in the setting of suspected GBS. First, transverse myelitis (TM) can also present with limb weakness, back pain, and depressed reflexes. Sustained sphincter dysfunction and a sensory level distinguish TM from GBS. Second, tick paralysis can also present with pure motor weakness and absent reflexes.[13] Particularly in the late spring or summer if careful inspection reveals a tick, its removal is typically curative. Oculomotor paralysis can be a clue and can appear similar to the Miller Fisher variant of GBS, characterized by ataxia, oculomotor palsies, and absent deep tendon reflexes. Finally, brainstem encephalitis can also mimic the Miller Fisher variant of GBS.[14]

### Acute Cerebellar Ataxia

Acute cerebellar ataxia (ACA) occurs most commonly in children younger than 5 years old but can occur at any age.[15] It has been associated with a variety of infections but is usually the result of postinfectious demyelination rather than direct infection. The presentation is characterized by maximal deficits at onset, and often on awakening. Pancerebellar dysfunction can result in truncal ataxia, with the consequent inability to sit or stand without assistance. Head titubation, nystagmus, and dysmetria are sometimes present. Mental status is normal. Full recovery is typical but can take as long as 3 to 6 months.[14] There is no evidence that immune therapy such as steroids alters the outcome of ACA.

## Migraine

Vertigo as the primary or sole manifestation of migraine occurs with very young children and teenaged girls.[16] Children younger than 4 years can have the abrupt onset of unsteadiness lasting seconds to minutes. More commonly, adolescents describe repeated bouts of isolated vertigo, or headache and vertigo. In both cases, there is usually a family history of migraine and a propensity to motion sickness in the context of a normal neurologic examination.

## Labyrinthitis

The clinical symptoms of labyrinthitis are superficially similar to ACA: acute onset of ataxia and nystagmus. However, children with acute labyrinthitis generally appear more ill, have prominent vomiting, and hold themselves still to minimize exacerbation of symptoms. This condition frequently occurs in clusters of exposed individuals, most frequently in spring and early summer, supporting an infectious (likely viral) cause.[17] In particular, the vestibular nerve is inflamed.

### *Laboratory Evaluation*

A thorough history and physical examination often make laboratory testing unnecessary. At a minimum, however, urine toxicology should be considered. If there is a high clinical suspicion, blood and urine samples should be held with the intention of sending targeted analysis following consultation with poison control.[2,11]

Lumbar puncture should be considered in the setting of suspected infectious or inflammatory processes. Normal white blood cell count or a mild pleocytosis is typical in ACA. More significant pleocytosis or low glucose raises the concern for bacterial meningitis or encephalitis, and an expanded evaluation for viral (especially herpes simplex virus) and bacterial causes is warranted.

### *Imaging*

Imaging of the brain is indicated in the presence of a focal neurologic examination, or with the inability to perform a reliable neurologic examination in the presence of illness or sedation. Imaging in the absence of these indications is low yield. Acutely, head CT is effective for evaluating for hemorrhage or hydrocephalus. However, magnetic resonance imaging of the brain both spares the child radiation and provides more sensitive visualization of the brain parenchyma. Additional studies with contrast are indicated if there is concern for infection and inflammation or tumor. Imaging of the vasculature with magnetic resonance angiography or magnetic resonance venographyis useful when stroke is a consideration. Neurologic consultation should typically be obtained before ordering imaging to optimize the study, and before considering conventional cerebral angiography or computed tomographic angiography.

# ▶ MANAGEMENT

## Treatment Approach

Treatment is directed at the underlying diagnosis. Initial attention to vital signs in the ill child is crucial. Posterior fossa hemorrhage requires urgent neurosurgical consultation. Ischemic stroke requires neurologic consultation and admission to a pediatric critical care unit for further management. In the case of ADEM, immune modulating therapy such as steroids, intravenous immunoglobulin (IVIG), or plasma exchange (PLEX) can be considered: treatment can hasten recovery, but does not appear to alter ultimate outcome.[5] A 2004 study of vestibular neuritis in adults found that vestibular function was improved in patients treated with methylprednisolone but not valacyclovir.[18]

Infectious processes, such as cerebellar abscess or brainstem encephalitis, are treated initially with broad antimicrobial therapy (including ampicillin for *Listeria* in the case of brainstem encephalitis) as well as antiviral therapy (acyclovir for herpes simplex virus) until the causative agent is identified. Brain tumors require neurologic, oncologic, and neurosurgical consultation.

GBS requires admission for monitoring of vital signs and respiratory function. Respiratory function can worsen from presentation, and initial monitoring in the PICU for 24 to 48 hours should be considered. Treatment with IVIG or PLEX speeds recovery, and IVIG is favored because it is less invasive.[19] IVIG should not be used in patients who are immunogloblin A deficient.

## Ongoing Care

Long-term treatment is not typically required for the common causes of pediatric acute ataxia. However, follow-up 2 to 4 weeks after discharge to monitor recovery is reasonable. Prognosis and management are linked to diagnosis. If persistent or permanent dysfunction results, physical therapy and adaptive devices should be coordinated. Aside from ingestion, few of the causes of ataxia are preventable. In most cases, the outcome is a good one.[1,2] In patients requiring admission, early recognition leading to early admission and treatment may improve outcomes.

### TOOLS FOR PRACTICE

#### Medical Decision Support

- *Intravenous Immunoglobulin for Gullain-Barré Syndrome* (article), *Cochrane Database of Systematic Reviews,* Issue 16, Article No CD002063, 2010

### REFERENCES


1. Ryan MM, Engle EC. Acute ataxia in childhood. *J Child Neurol.* 2003;18:309–316
2. Gieron-Korthals MA, Westberry KR, Emmanuel PJ. Acute childhood ataxia: 10-year experience. *J Child Neurol.* 1994;9:381–384
3. García-Cazorla A, Wolf NI, Serrano M, et al. Inborn errors of metabolism and motor disturbances in children. *J Inherit Metab Dis.* 2009;32:618–629
4. Jones HR. Guillain-Barré syndrome: perspectives with infants and children. *Semin Pediatr Neurol.* 2000;7:91–102
5. Rust RS. Multiple sclerosis, acute disseminated encephalomyelitis, and related conditions. *Semin Pediatr Neurol.* 2000;7:66–90
6. Tenembaum S, Chitnis T, Ness J, Hahn JS, International Pediatric MS Study Group. Acute disseminated encephalomyelitis. *Neurology.* 2007;68:S23–S36

7. Mehta V, Chapman A, McNeely PD, Walling S, Howes WJ. Latency between symptom onset and diagnosis of pediatric brain tumors: an Eastern Canadian geographic study. *Neurosurgery.* 2002;51:365–372
8. Sawaishi Y, Takada G. Acute cerebellitis. *Cerebellum.* 2002;1:223–228
9. de Ribaupierre S, Meagher-Villemure K, Villemure JG, et al. The role of posterior fossa decompression in acute cerebellitis. *Childs Nerv Syst.* 2005;21:970–974
10. Rafay MF, Armstrong D, Deveber G, et al. Craniocervical arterial dissection in children: clinical and radiographic presentation and outcome. *J Child Neurol.* 2006;21:8–16
11. Riordan M, Rylance G, Berry K. Poisoning in children 1: general management. *Arch Dis Child.* 2002;87:392–396
12. McGrogan A, Madle GC, Seaman HE, de Vries CS. The epidemiology of Guillain-Barré syndrome worldwide. A systematic literature review. *Neuroepidemiology.* 2008;32:150–163
13. Li Z, Turner RP. Pediatric tick paralysis: discussion of two cases and literature review. *Pediatr Neurol.* 2004;31:304–307
14. Odaka Mm Yuki N, Yamada M, et al. Bickerstaff's brainstem encephalitis: clinical features of 62 cases and a subgroup associated with Guillain-Barré syndrome. *Brain.* 2003;126:2279–2290
15. Connolly AM, Dodson WE, Prensky AL, Rust RS. Course and outcome of acute cerebellar ataxia. *Ann Neurol.* 1994;35:673–679
16. Weisleder P, Fife TD. Dizziness and headache: a common association in children and adolescents. *J Child Neurol.* 2001;16:727–730
17. Baloh RW. Clinical practice. Vestibular neuritis. *N Engl J Med.* 2003;348:1027–1032
18. Strupp M, Zingler VC, Arbusow, et al. Methylprednisolone, valacyclovir, or the combination for vestibular neuritis. *N Engl J Med.* 2004;351:354–361
19. Rabie M, Nevo Y. Childhood acute and chronic immune-mediated polyradiculoneuropathies. *Eur J Paediatr Neurol.* 2009;13:209–218

# Chapter 8

# Back Pain

*Joel S. Brenner, MD, MPH; David V. Smith, MD*

## ▶ DEFINITION

The back encompasses the region from the upper thoracic vertebra (T1) and shoulder girdle to the sacrum and surrounding musculature. The patient who complains of pain in this region may have difficulty localizing the source of the pain and describe it simply as deep pain, or the patient may localize pain to a specific muscle group or vertebral body. Allowing patients to define in their own words the nature, location, and duration of the pain is an important first step in arriving at a clinical diagnosis. If parents, coaches, or peers are available during the interview, they can be valuable to confirm or elaborate on the patient's symptoms. One should keep in mind that young children and adolescents may minimize pain out of imagined fears of diagnostic or therapeutic procedures. Functional disability such as interference with sports, play, or school may prompt more urgent diagnostic evaluation and treatment.

## ▶ EPIDEMIOLOGY

Population-based data on back pain in children are limited, and estimates of prevalence vary considerably depending on sample size and method used. At the least, most studies have consistently shown that the prevalence of back pain increases with age. In non-clinical populations, the prevalence is less than 10% in preteens, progressing to nearly 50% of 18- to 20-year-olds reporting at least one episode of low-back pain.[1] Clearly, most people who experience such pain do not seek medical care. In preadolescent children, back pain is not only unusual but also likely to indicate serious underlying illness when severe or persistent enough to prompt a medical visit.[2] One 6-year study in a tertiary orthopedic setting found that back pain constituted fewer than 2% of referrals in children ages 15 years or younger, but that roughly 50% of these children had serious underlying diseases.[3] From early adolescence onward, back pain becomes more common as a presenting complaint but is more likely to be a benign condition related to acute injury or repetitive stress. The physician presented with a child or adolescent complaining of back pain should use a careful history and physical examination to guide any further laboratory or radiologic evaluation. Overall, they should be aware of the relatively higher risk for serious underlying disease in younger children, even without specific physical findings.

## ▶ DIFFERENTIAL DIAGNOSIS

### Infants

From infancy through the third or fourth year of life, the patient is not capable of localizing or complaining of pain in the back. Unexplained fever or toxicity, along with refusal to walk or stand, may be the presenting signs of diskitis.[4,5] Other pathologies localized to the back to consider include leukemia, lymphoma, pyelonephritis, vaso-occlusive crisis, or vertebral osteomyelitis in a child who has sickle cell disease, or accidental or nonaccidental trauma.

### Children

As children mature and become more capable of communicating and localizing symptoms, a specific history of the duration, quality, associated symptoms, and radiation of back pain becomes possible. Back pain before adolescence remains an uncommon presenting complaint and should prompt thorough evaluation. Only after a thorough diagnostic evaluation should the physician consider the diagnosis of muscular or ligamentous strain as a cause of back pain in younger children. The differential diagnosis of back pain in this age group is broad and includes acute leukemia, lymphoma, and primary vertebral tumors, such as Ewing sarcoma, aneurysmal bone cyst, benign osteoblastoma, and osteoid osteomas.[4] Other etiologies include diskitis, an unusual if not rare condition that is most common in children younger than 10 years (mean age, about 6 years). Diskitis is an inflammatory process presumed to be a bacterial infection in the intervertebral disk space. Vertebral osteomyelitis usually affects school-aged children and teenagers and presents as severe back pain and systemic symptoms. A family history of rheumatoid disease should prompt consideration of ankylosing spondylitis. In the presence of sickle cell disease, a vaso-occlusive crisis is a strong consideration. Back pain on walking may be the only sign of a tethered cord.[4] An underlying leg-length discrepancy of any cause may result in chronic or recurrent low-back pain from musculoligamentous strain.

### Adolescents

Classifying the causes of back pain in adolescents as acute or chronic is helpful (Table 8-1). In adolescent patients, a diagnostic consideration of acute back pain caused by muscular or ligamentous strain is reasonable. Other causes of acute back pain include lumbar disk disease, apophyseal ring fractures, vertebral osteomyelitis, epidural abscess, and sciatica caused by piriformis syndrome. The adolescent who has chronic pain (>3 weeks) may still have a strain, but stronger consideration should be given at this point to spondylolysis or spondylolisthesis, which are the most common identifiable causes of low-back pain in this age group.[2] The most frequent cause of spondylolysis is a stress fracture of the pars interarticularis (posterior arch) of the spine, thought to be acquired through repetitive extension loading. Athletes who participate in gymnastics, dance, cheerleading, football, and diving are at highest risk. For example, ballet dancers, as a group, as well as football players (offensive lineman), have great flexibility but may be predisposed to lumbar lordosis by postural demands and relatively weak core musculature, possibly making them prone to spondylolysis and disk disease.[6] Individuals with benign hypermobility syndromes may also be at risk. Less commonly, spondylolysis can be an asymptomatic congenital deformity. Spondylolisthesis is the anterior movement of one vertebral body on top of another, usually L5 on S1, as a result of bilateral spondylolysis.

**Table 8-1**
**Differential Diagnosis of Back Pain**

| INFANTS | CHILDREN | ADOLESCENTS |
|---|---|---|
| Diskitis | Diskitis | **Acute** |
| Leukemia, lymphoma | Tethered cord | Muscle, ligament strain |
| Vaso-occlusive crisis | Osteomyelitis | Lumbar disk disease |
| Osteomyelitis | Ankylosing spondylitis | Apophyseal ring fractures |
| Trauma | Vaso-occlusive crisis | Sciatica |
| | Leukemia, lymphoma | Piriformis syndrome |
| | Ewing sarcoma | Osteomyelitis |
| | Osteoid osteoma | Epidural abscess |
| | Spinal tuberculosis | Spinal tuberculosis |
| | | **Chronic** |
| | | Spondylolysis |
| | | Spondylolisthesis |
| | | Scheuermann kyphosis |
| | | Facet, vertebral dysfunction |
| | | Sacroiliac dysfunction |
| | | Lumbar disk disease |
| | | Spinal stenosis |
| | | Spondyloarthropathy |
| | | Tumor or malignancy |
| | | Soft tissue strain |
| | | Functional (nonorganic) |

Chronic low-back pain, especially in adolescent athletes or others who have cumulative trauma, may indicate lumbar disk disease. Other chronic causes of back pain in this age group include Scheuermann kyphosis, facet or vertebral dysfunction, sacroiliac dysfunction, spinal stenosis, the spondyloarthropathies (ie, ankylosing spondylitis, psoriatic arthritis, Reiter syndrome, arthritis of inflammatory bowel disease that with the exception of psoriatic arthritis can be classified as enthesitis-related juvenile idiopathic arthritis), and tumor or malignancy. Chronic back pain can also be a disorder of the soft tissues of the back, postulated to be caused by a combination of repetitive strain, genetic predisposition, and environmental factors. Assessing for discrepancy in leg lengths and for tight hamstrings is advisable because both alter the dynamic stress put on the muscles and ligaments of the low back. Modifiable contributing factors may include prolonged seated posture, forward bending of the spine while sitting at a desk for long periods, or carrying an excessively heavy backpack (>10%–20% of body weight).[7-9]

## ▶ PSYCHOSOCIAL CONSIDERATIONS

Although malingering or the use of pain symptoms for secondary gain may be relatively common in adults, it should not be a strong consideration in the diagnosis of back pain in children or adolescents. Back pain is not as common a somatoform symptom among adolescents as is headache, abdominal pain, or chest pain. If a thorough diagnostic evaluation of chronic back pain in an adolescent is unrevealing and the usual management involving exercise and stretching is not beneficial, then a psychosocial or nonorganic cause should be considered. The Waddell test, a series of 5 questions, may be used to help determine whether significant psychological stress is associated with chronic low-back pain.[10]

If 3 or more of the following 5 criteria are present, then the test is considered positive:

1. Inappropriate tenderness that is superficial or widespread
2. Pain on pressing the top of the head or on passive rotation of shoulders and pelvis
3. Distraction signs such as inconsistent performance between straight-leg raising in the seated and the supine positions
4. Strength and sensory loss patterns that do not fit with accepted neuroanatomy
5. Overreaction during the physical examination[10]

## ▶ EVALUATION

### *Infants, Children, and Adolescents*

The age of the patient is a critical factor in the diagnostic evaluation, with the extent and urgency of evaluation usually being greater for preadolescent patients.[11,12] The duration of symptoms is an additional factor because chronic pain, even in adolescent patients, is uncommon and may indicate structural or serious underlying disease. The evaluation of acute or chronic back pain should always include motor, sensory, and reflex examination to help differentiate any nerve root involvement (Figure 8-1).

Chronic pain should prompt a diagnostic evaluation possibly to include rectal examination for sphincter tone loss, radiographs of the spine (anteroposterior, lateral, and oblique views), uric acid, lactate dehydrogenase, white blood count, sedimentation rate, C-reactive

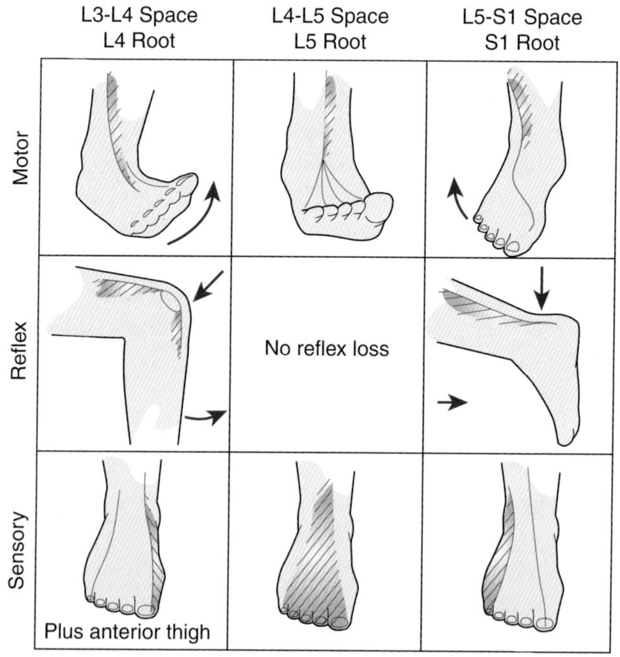


**Figure 8-1**
Sensory, motor, reflex grid. *(From Lewis RC.* Primary Care Orthopedics. *New York: Churchill Livingstone; 1988, with permission from Elsevier.)*

protein, and urinalysis and urine culture. Infants, young children, or adolescents who have fever and back pain must be considered as having an infectious, inflammatory, or neoplastic process until proved otherwise. Diagnoses that should be considered include diskitis, vertebral osteomyelitis, ankylosing spondylitis, pyelonephritis, vaso-occlusive crisis in a patient who has sickle cell anemia, acute lymphoblastic leukemia, Ewing sarcoma, and Hodgkin lymphoma.[4,11] Spinal tuberculosis (Pott disease) is rare but should be considered when back pain is accompanied by low-grade fever.[12]

A child with diskitis is typically uncomfortable in an upright posture, may refuse to walk, or may have pain when bending forward. Even in the absence of fever, a child who refuses to walk, particularly a preschooler, should be evaluated promptly for diskitis. Typically, diskitis is associated with an elevated erythrocyte sedimentation rate and a high white blood cell count; plain radiographs of the spine may show narrowing of the disk space. In a recent review, 76% of children with diskitis had changes evident on plain radiographs; however, plain radiographs are often negative in the first 2 to 3 weeks of the disease. If a second imaging test is needed, magnetic resonance imaging (MRI) is generally thought to be sensitive in identifying diskitis.[4,5]

Weight loss, bone pain in other locations, bruising, organomegaly, or adenopathy should prompt aggressive diagnostic evaluation for malignancies such as leukemia, lymphoma, or sarcomas. Especially in the presence of fever or other systemic signs and symptoms, acute leukemia and lymphoma are serious concerns and must be ruled out.

A child with nocturnal back pain, even if relieved by nonprescription analgesics, should be evaluated for osteoid osteoma or osteoblastoma with a bone scan if plain radiographs are normal.[2,4] Primary vertebral tumors almost always are visible on plain radiographs, but computed tomography (CT) or MRI may be needed.

Fever accompanied by back pain should prompt an aggressive diagnostic evaluation and orthopedic surgery consultation because aspiration and culture to evaluate for possible vertebral osteomyelitis should be considered.[2] Dysuria, urinary urgency, or urinary frequency, especially if accompanied by fever, warrants consideration of pyelonephritis.

Idiopathic scoliosis usually does not cause back pain in children.[12] Scoliosis with pain should raise concern about an alternative cause, including malignancy in the region of the spine or a benign osteoid osteoma.

## Adolescents

Muscular or ligamentous strain begins to become common during adolescence. The typical presentation is low-back pain of 3 weeks' or less duration, with or without recollection of an acute injury, that is exacerbated by postural changes or specific movements. Associated signs and symptoms such as neurologic deficits of the lower extremities; limited straight-leg raising; sciatic pain; bowel, bladder, or sexual dysfunction; fever; weight loss; adenopathy; urinary urgency or frequency; scoliosis; or marfanoid habitus should be absent.[3] The pain is exacerbated by lifting, stooping, and exercising. Radiologic studies are not needed if muscular or ligamentous strain is thought to exist. However, very localized tenderness in the spine after an injury (eg, motor vehicle crash, athletic trauma) warrants radiologic evaluation for compression fracture.[4] Plain radiographs (anteroposterior and lateral) should be ordered initially.

Low-back pain associated with excessive lordotic curvature, especially in an athlete subjected to repetitive extension loading (eg, gymnasts, football linemen), may indicate spondylolysis or spondylolisthesis. Spondylolysis may be unilateral or bilateral and is most common at L5. Symptoms of spondylolysis are not usually acute; it more commonly exhibits as a gradual worsening of back pain on extension, usually in an athlete during the growth spurt or after intense training. Pain can be reproduced reliably by having the patient hyperextend the back while standing on one leg (the stork test) (Figure 8-2).[2] The sensitivity of the stork test is modest, however, and a negative stork test should not be relied on to rule out an active spondylolysis.[15] The patient usually has no pain with flexion, rotation, or lateral bending of the back. Hamstring tightness is a common associated finding.[14] Plain radiographs of the lumbar spine should be ordered (anteroposterior, lateral, oblique views). The *Scotty dog with a collar* is visualized on the oblique radiographs (Figure 8-3). Normal plain radiographs alone do not rule out spondylolysis. One study reported that oblique views detected only 32% of spondylolyses detected on CT.[16] A single-photon emission computed tomography (SPECT) scan should be ordered if the diagnosis is highly suggested. A positive plain radiograph with a negative SPECT scan is indicative of a nonmetabolically active spondylolysis that may not be the cause of the patient's back pain. Back pain on extension with normal plain radiographs and SPECT scan is usually from facet or vertebral dysfunction.

Spondylolisthesis may be accompanied on physical examination not only by excess lumbar lordosis but also by the sensation of a shelf at the base of the lordotic curvature, where the lower of the 2 affected vertebrae has held its position while the upper vertebral body

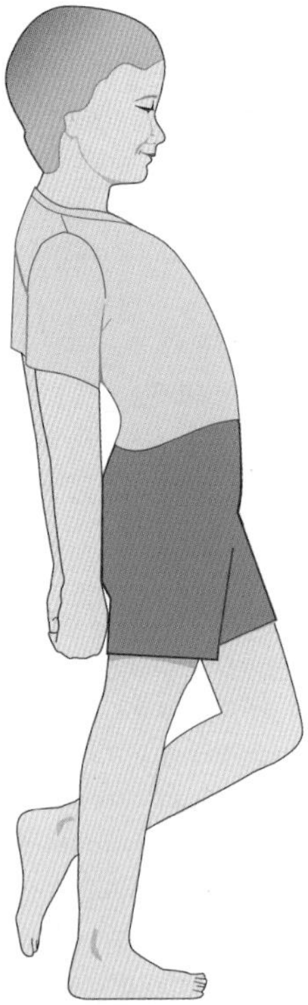

**Figure 8-2**
One-leg hyperextension test (stork test).

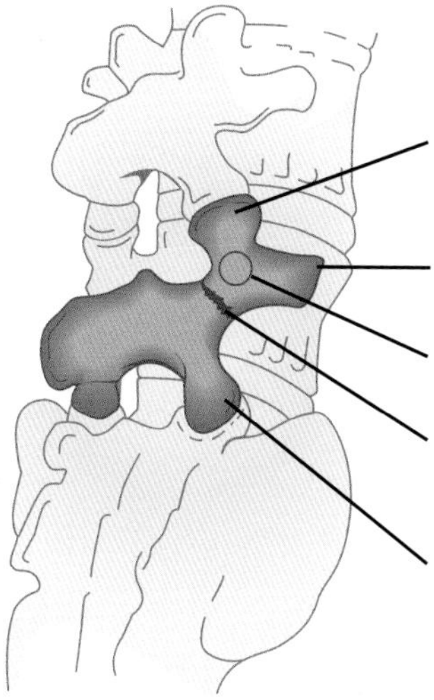


**Figure 8-3**
Scotty dog with a collar. *(From Smith JA, Hu SS. Management of spondylolysis and spondylolisthesis in the pediatric and adolescent population.* Orthop Clin North Am. *1999;30(3):487–499, ix, with permission from Elsevier.)*

slipped forward. The anterior slippage is diagnosed and staged for treatment purposes on the lateral plain radiographs. In rare cases, radiographs will reveal congenital absence of a lumbosacral articular process.[17]

Accompanying neurologic symptoms, including radicular pain down the leg, numbness or tingling, bowel or bladder problems, erectile dysfunction, or loss of sphincter tone on rectal examination, may indicate lumbar disk herniation or other nerve compression and should prompt an urgent evaluation and referral.[4,11] Symptoms are typically worsened by mechanical strain, as with lifting or coughing.[4] A positive straight-leg raise test or a *slump test* (Figure 8-4) is highly suggestive of nerve root compression.[14] Using cervical flexion to accentuate the patient's symptoms during straight-leg raising may add to the test's sensitivity. Any reproduction of the patient's usual symptoms during testing before 60 degrees of hip flexion, or marked asymmetry in symptoms, should be considered a positive test.[18,19] Pain after 60 degrees or limited to the posterior thigh is more likely caused by hamstring tightness.

A spondyloarthropathy should be suspected when there is limited lumbar flexion (modified Schober test), tenderness at entheses (particularly the Achilles-calcaneal enthesis, the origin or insertion of the plantar fascia, or the base of the fifth metatarsal), pain in the sacroiliac (SI) area with *f*lexion-*ab*duction and *e*xternal *r*otation (an abnormal FABER test), or tenderness over the SI joints. MRI with gadolinium of the SI joints and ultrasonography of the entheses can confirm local inflammation. The presence of HLA-B27 antigen is not diagnostic because it is present in 10% to 30% of individuals of European ancestry.

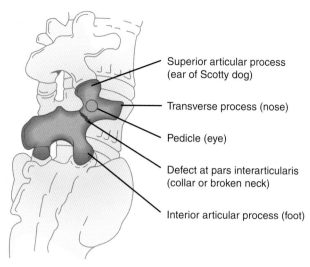

Scheuermann disease, or butterflyer's back, typically exhibits in an adolescent, particularly a competitive swimmer, with thoracic back pain after exercise or late in the day. Patients have rigid thoracic kyphosis on examination and pain worsened by forward flexion.[2,4,20] It must

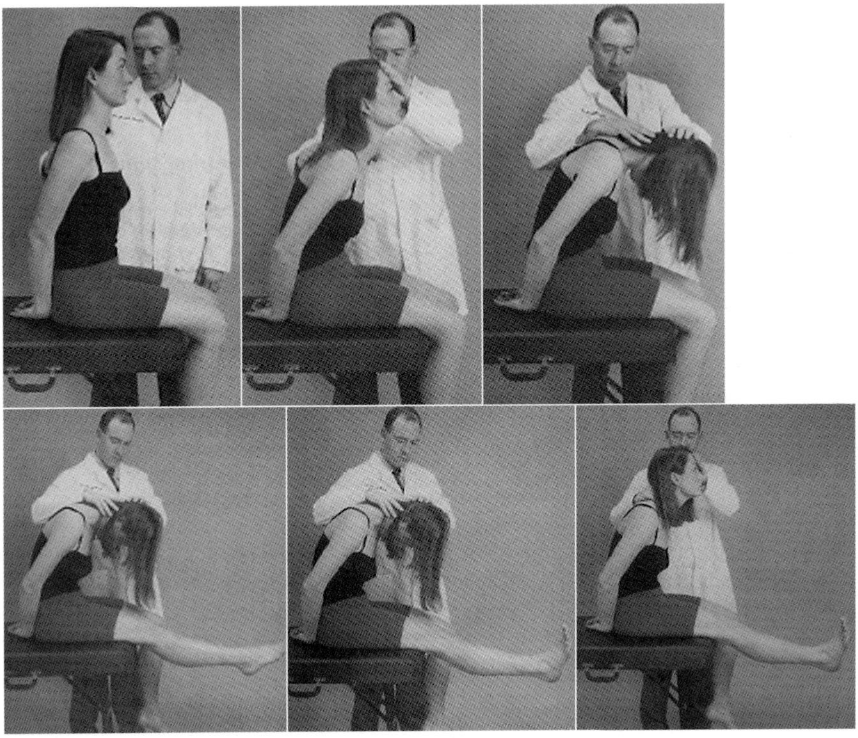

**Figure 8-4**
Slump test. *(From Reider B.* The Orthopedic Physical Examination. *Philadelphia, PA: WB Saunders; 1999, with permission.)*

be differentiated from postural kyphosis, which is commonly seen in adolescents. Postural kyphosis is a flexible kyphosis that disappears on forward flexion and conscious postural straightening. Scheuermann disease is confirmed by anterior wedging of 5 degrees or greater in 3 or more contiguous vertebrae shown on lateral plain spine radiographs.[20] Oblique radiographs also should be obtained because spondylolysis is associated with Scheuermann disease.[21]

Stigmata of Marfan syndrome include joint hyperextensibility, pectus excavatum, pes planus, dislocated lenses, hernias, arachnodactyly, and scoliosis. The scoliosis may result from a dural ectasia or widening of the subarachnoid space in the lumbar area, which has been associated with low-back pain in adolescents and young adults.[22] Patients who have Marfan syndrome are also at increased risk for spondylolysis.[12]

## ▶ MANAGEMENT

Pain that is acute and lasting fewer than 3 weeks, especially with a history of musculoskeletal injury, may be managed expectantly in many cases, whereas more chronic pain in a child or adolescent demands further investigation.[11,12] When back pain results from an underlying disorder, treatment of the pain itself should be undertaken in addition to treatment of the primary condition.

### Infants

Treatment for diskitis is variable, depending on its cause. Most experts recommend parenteral followed by oral antibiotic administration, if evidence of bacterial infection exists, and relative rest to promote pain control.[23,24] Staphylococcal infection is the most common cause of vertebral osteomyelitis and should be treated with antibiotics, rest, and a prompt orthopedic surgery consultation.[2]

### Children

Treatment for diskitis and osteomyelitis in children is the same as that for infants. Management of patients with ankylosing spondylitis is best coordinated by a pediatric rheumatologist, who will often use anti-inflammatory medications with physical and occupational therapy. Treatment of vaso-occlusive crisis entails pain management, hydration, and physical therapy. Leukemia, lymphoma, and Ewing sarcoma should be managed by a pediatric oncologist. Pain from osteoid osteoma is typically relieved with nonsteroidal anti-inflammatory agents, and patients should be referred to a pediatric orthopedic surgeon for possible excision or ablation.[26,27]

### Adolescents

When the adolescent exhibits back pain acutely after an injury that is thought to be a muscular or ligamentous strain, the PRICEMMMS mnemonic (*p*rotection, *r*elative rest, *i*ce, *c*ompression, *e*levation, *m*edication, *m*otion, *m*odalities, *s*trength) should be used. Bed rest, which has been shown to delay recovery, should be discouraged.[28] Continuous-frequency ultrasound and massage are often helpful. Pain-free activity may be resumed gradually, and low-back and hamstring flexibility, as well as the strengthening of the core musculature (abdominal area, hip, and back) with an exercise ball, Yoga, or Pilates exercises, should be emphasized.

Evidence indicates that full sit-ups with the feet fixed and the knees bent, by using hip flexors rather than abdominal muscles, increase intervertebral disk pressure and should be discouraged. The goal of abdominal muscle strengthening is to reduce pelvic tilt and its accompanying tendency toward lordosis and low-back strain. Because decreased strength and endurance of spinal extensor muscles is associated with low-back pain, extensor exercises such as raising the torso and head off the floor or exercise ball while lying prone are recommended. These same exercises, and stretching after warming the muscles by gentle exercise or moist heat, are recommended for chronic low-back pain of muscular origin. Proper posture should also be taught, and backpack weights should not exceed 10% to 20% of the person's body weight.[7-9] Acupuncture may be a useful adjunct for chronic back pain. If a leg-length discrepancy is discovered, a heel lift as well as physical therapy to reduce any accompanying flexion contractures at the knee and hip and genu valgus could be of benefit.

The treatment of spondylolysis is controversial and may best be managed by a pediatric sports medicine specialist or orthopedic surgeon. All regimens include the initial cessation of extension-loading activities while providing symptomatic relief and physical therapy that promotes abdominal strengthening and hamstring stretching (the Williams program). Thoracolumbar bracing to prevent extension has been shown to be helpful in some studies; however, others showed no difference in outcomes with or without the use of a brace.[29] Some experts advocate restricting extension activities without a brace.[30-32] When bracing is implemented, it can be used for up to 6 months or until the patient is pain free with extension. Bone stimulators have been used as adjunctive therapy.[33]

Treatment of the spondyloparthropathic conditions involves anti-inflammatory and immunomodulatory therapies along with physical therapy, and the patient should be referred to a pediatric rheumatologist. Treatment for Scheuermann disease is usually conservative, including physical therapy with strengthening and stretching exercises, avoiding painful activities, and analgesic medication if needed.[20] Thoracolumbar bracing and surgery may be indicated if kyphosis is more than 60 degrees.[2,20] Patients should be referred to an orthopedic surgeon (pediatric or spinal) for failure of conservative management, intractable pain, or progression of the kyphotic deformity.

Referral to a mental health professional may not be necessary for functional or nonorganic back pain. If the family has a high degree of trust with the physician, then a sensitive evaluation of family and social factors may be an effective first step. In these cases, the physician should not assume that the pain is feigned but rather consider it as a very real physical symptom rooted in psychological or emotional distress. At the very least, chronic pain and its accompanying disability can, of itself, lead to psychological distress, which should be addressed openly by the physician.

## When to Refer

- Abnormality of posture or gait
- Neurologic findings
- Persistent pain in a preteen
- Pain unrelated to activity or on awakening from sleep
- Functional disability (decreased play or sports activity)
- Diagnosis and evaluation are outside of the primary care physician's scope of expertise

## When to Admit

- Whenever a prompt and thorough outpatient diagnostic assessment cannot be completed for a child who has back pain and associated fever or neurologic findings

## TOOLS FOR PRACTICE

### Engaging Patient and Family

- *Backpack Safety* (fact sheet), American Academy of Pediatrics (www.healthychildren.org/English/safety-prevention/at-play/Pages/Backpack-Safety.aspx)
- *Sports Shorts: Lower Back Pain in Athletes* (fact sheet), American Academy of Pediatrics (www.healthychildren.org/English/health-issues/injuries-emergencies/sports-injuries/Pages/Lower-Back-Pain-in-Athletes.aspx)

### Medical Decision Support

- *Care of the Young Athlete*, 2nd ed (book), American Academy of Pediatrics (shop.aap.org)
- *Essentials of Musculoskeletal Care*, 3rd ed (book), American Academy of Orthopaedic Surgeons and American Academy of Pediatrics (shop.aap.org)

## AAP POLICY STATEMENT

American Academy of Pediatrics Committee on Psychosocial Aspects of Child and Family Health, Task Force on Pain in Infants, Children, and Adolescents. The assessment and management of acute pain in infants, children, and adolescents. *Pediatrics.* 2001;108:793–797 (pediatrics.aappublications.org/content/108/3/793.full)

## REFERENCES


1. Leboeuf-Yde C, Kyvik KO. At what age does low back pain become a common problem? A study of 29,424 individuals aged 12–41 years. *Spine (Phila Pa 1976).* 1998;23(2):228–234
2. Hollingsworth P. Back pain in children. *Bri J Rheumatol.* 1996;35(10):1022–1028
3. Turner PG, Green JH, Galasko CS. Back pain in childhood. *Spine (Phila Pa 1976).* 1989;14(8):812–814
4. Payne WK, Ogilvie JW. Back pain in children and adolescents. *Pediatr Clin North Am.* 1996;43(4): 899–917
5. Staheli LT. Pain of musculoskeletal origin in children. *Curr Opin Rheumatol.* 1992;4(5):748–752
6. Bryan N, Smith BM. Back school programs. The ballet dancer. *Occup Med.* 1992;7(1):67–75
7. Mackenzie W, Sampath J, Kruse R, Sheir-Neiss GJ. Backpacks in children. *Clin Orthop Rel Res.* 2003;409:78–84
8. Negrini S, Carabalona R, Sibilla P. Backpack as a daily load for schoolchildren. *Lancet.* 1999;354(9194):1974
9. Brackley HM, Stevenson JM. Are children's backpack weight limits enough? A critical review of the relevant literature. *Spine (Phila Pa 1976).* 2004;29(19):2184–2190
10. Wadell G, McCulloch JA, Kummel E, Venner RM. Nonorganic physical signs in low back pain. *Spine (Phila Pa 1976).* 1980;5(2):117–125
11. Dyment PG. Low back pain in adolescents. *Pediatr Ann.* 1991;20(4):170, 173–178
12. Sponseller P. Evaluating the child with back pain. *Am Fam Physician.* 1996;54(6):1933–1941
13. Fernandez M, Carrol CL, Baker CJ. Discitis and vertebral osteomyelitis in children: an 18-year review. *Pediatrics.* 2000;105(6):1299–1304
14. Reider B. *The Orthopaedic Physical Examination.* Philadelphia, PA: WB Saunders; 2004
15. Masci L, Pike J, Malara F, et al. Use of the one-legged hyperextension test and magnetic resonance imaging in the diagnosis of active spondylolysis. *Br J Sports Med.* 2006;40(11):940–946
16. McCleary MD, Congeni JA. Current concepts in the diagnosis and treatment of spondylolysis in young athletes. *Curr Sports Med Rep.* 2007;6(1):62–66
17. Ikeda K, Nakayama Y, Ishii S. Congenital absence of lumbosacral articular process: report of three cases. *J Spin Dis.* 1992;5(2):232–236
18. Farrell JP, Drye CD. Back school programs. The young patient. *Occup Med.* 1992;7(1):55–66
19. Epstein JA, Epstein NE, Marc J, Rosenthal AD, Lavine LS. Lumbar intervertebral disk herniation in teenage children: recognition and management of associated anomalies. *Spine (Phila Pa 1976).* 1984;9(4):427–432
20. Lowe TG. Scheuermann's disease. *Orthop Clin North Am.* 1999;30(3):475–487
21. Ogilvie JW, Sherman J. Spondylolysis in Scheuermann's disease. *Spine (Phila Pa 1976).* 1987;12(3):251–253
22. Schlesinger EB. The significance of genetic contributions and markers in disorders of spinal structure. *Neurosurgery.* 1990;26(6):944–951
23. Ring D, Johnston CE, Wenger DR. Pyogenic infectious spondylitis in children: the convergence of discitis and vertebral osteomyelitis. *J Pediatr Orthop.* 1995;15(5):652–660
24. Cushing AH. Diskitis in children. *Clin Infect Dis.* 1993;17(1):1–6
25. Cassidy J, Petty R, Laxer R, et al. *Textbook of Pediatric Rheumatology.* 6th ed. Philadelphia, PA: Elsevier Saunders; 2010
26. Lindner N, Ozaki T, Roedl R, et al. Percutaneous radiofrequency ablation in osteoid osteoma. *J Bone Joint Surg Br.* 2001;83(3):391–396
27. Wenger D, Rang M. *The Art and Practice of Children's Orthopaedics.* New York, NY: Raven Press; 1993
28. Malmivaara A, Häkkinen U, Aro T, et al. The treatment of acute low back pain—bed rest, exercises, or ordinary activity? *N Engl J Med.* 1995;332(6):351–355

29. Klein G, Mehlman CT, McCarty M. Nonoperative treatment of spondylolysis and grade I spondylolisthesis in children and young adults: a meta-analysis of observational studies. *J Pediatr Orthop.* 2009;29(2):146–156
30. Anderson K, Sarwark JF, Conway JJ, Logue ES, Schafer MF. Quantitative assessment with SPECT imaging of stress injuries of the pars interarticularis and response to bracing. *J Pediatr Orthop.* 2000;20(1):28–33
31. Steiner ME, Micheli LJ. Treatment of symptomatic spondylolysis and spondylolisthesis with the modified Boston brace. *Spine (Phila Pa 1976).* 1985;10(10):937–943
32. Smith JA, Hu SS. Management of spondylolysis and spondylolisthesis in the pediatric and adolescent population. *Orthop Clin North Am.* 1999;30(3):487–499
33. Stasinopoulos D. Treatment of spondylolysis with external electrical stimulation in young athletes: a critical literature review. *Br J Sports Med.* 2004;38(3):352–354

# Chapter 9

# Cardiac Arrhythmias

*J. Peter Harris, MD*

Arrhythmias in young people are common and may occur as a result of normal rhythm variations, premature beats, atrial or ventricular tachyarrhythmias, or conduction defects. They can occur at any age, and their clinical implications range from benign to lethal. Newer diagnostic modalities such as event recorders to capture infrequent episodes have enhanced our ability to detect arrhythmias. Empirical therapy without arrhythmia identification does not meet the current standard of practice. A 12-lead electrocardiogram (ECG) should always be obtained when an arrhythmia is suspected, because electrophysiologic alterations may be quite subtle and not always identified on a rhythm strip. A thorough family history is required, with particular emphasis on sudden and premature death, syncope, seizures, and recurrent arrhythmias.

Infants with arrhythmias may have nonspecific signs and symptoms such as fatigue, malaise, poor feeding, nausea, and pallor. Older children tend to exhibit more specific symptoms such as palpitations (the disquieting awareness of the person's own heartbeat), lightheadedness, syncope, visceral chest pain, and dyspnea.

Premature beats and supraventricular tachyarrhythmias in infancy may be noted incidentally on a visit for other reasons, but, more commonly, infants with supraventricular tachycardia (SVT) present with signs and symptoms of congestive heart failure: tachypnea, dyspnea, truncal diaphoresis, diminished pulses, pallor, hepatomegaly, and poor feeding. Older children and adolescents are able to verbalize discomfort, including palpitations, chest pain, dyspnea, and nausea, with various forms of SVT. Ventricular tachyarrhythmias often compromise cardiac output to a greater degree than SVT and have more overt signs of congestive failure, chest pain, syncope, dyspnea, and palpitations. Myocardial dysfunction is usually related to increased oxygen demand owing to the tachycardia, inadequate time for ventricular filling, ischemia from insufficient time for diastolic coronary perfusion, and loss of atrioventricular synchrony. Infants and children with moderate or severe bradycardia from advanced second-degree and complete heart block also display signs and symptoms of inadequate cardiac output, including fatigue, reduced exercise capacity, pallor, presyncope, and syncope.

## ▶ APPROACH TO ARRHYTHMIAS

As a part of the systematic approach to ECG interpretation, the cardiac rhythm should be analyzed in an organized fashion. The answers to the following 4 questions will define most arrhythmias:

1. Is the rhythm fast or slow?
2. Is the rhythm regular or irregular?

**Table 9-1**
**Bradycardia by Age and State**

| AGE | HEART RATE |
|---|---|
| **SURFACE ELECTROCARDIOGRAM** | |
| Neonates and infants | <100 beat/min, awake |
| Children to 3 years | <100 beats/min |
| Children 3–9 years | <60 beats/min |
| Adolescents 9–16 years | <50 beats/min |
| Adolescents >16 years | <40 beats/min |
| **AMBULATORY (HOLTER) MONITORING** | |
| Neonates and infants | <60 beats/min, sleeping; 80 beats/min, awake, quiet |
| Children 2–6 years | <60 beats/min |
| Children 7–11 years | <45 beats/min |
| Adolescents >11 years | <40 beats/min |
| Athletes | <30 beats/min |

3. Are the QRS complexes narrow or wide?
4. What is the relationship between the P waves and the QRS complexes?

## ▶ NORMAL RHYTHM VARIATIONS

Recognizing normal rhythm variations allays patient and parental anxiety and avoids unnecessary investigations and interventions. For instance, sinus arrhythmia (phasic respiratory variations of sinus rate with inspiratory acceleration and expiratory slowing) is common in childhood; so too is wandering atrial pacemaker, usually noted with slower heart rates and characterized by different P-wave morphologies. These rhythm variations are related to alterations in vagal tone.

A wide range of heart rates is present in the young. Sinus tachycardia has been documented at rates of 230 to 250 beats per minute during infancy, but a rate in excess of 200 beats per minute in a teenager who is not involved in maximal exertion would be abnormal. Sinus bradycardia is a sinus rate below what is expected for a patient's age. A sinus rate below 100 beats per minute in an awake neonate would be abnormal, but during sleep, rates down to 80 beats per minute are commonly observed on ECG monitoring. Brief dips into the 60- to 80-beats-per-minute range are also observed in sleeping neonates during normal, vagally induced episodes of junctional rhythm that arise from either the atrioventricular node or the bundle of His and that are characterized by a narrow QRS without a preceding P wave. A highly conditioned adolescent endurance athlete may have a resting heart rate of 40 beats per minute or less. Table 9-1 provides guidelines for the diagnosis of sinus bradycardia on the surface ECG and during ambulatory monitoring.

## ▶ PREMATURE BEATS

Premature beats are common, but usually benign, arrhythmias and may arise in the atria, the atrioventricular junction, or the ventricles. By definition, premature beats are early and thus are distinguished from escape or late beats occurring when higher pacemaker cells fail to produce an impulse at the expected interval. Two premature beats in a row constitute a couplet. If every second or third beat is a premature impulse, then a bigeminal or trigeminal rhythm is present.

## Atrial Premature Contractions

Atrial premature contractions (APCs) are characterized by premature P waves with an axis and morphology that are different from the sinus P waves. If an APC occurs when one of the bundle branches is refractory, then the premature beat will be conducted down the other bundle branch, resulting in an aberrant APC with a QRS morphology wider and different from sinus QRS complexes (Figure 9-1). If both bundle branches are refractory, then the APC will not be conducted to the ventricles (blocked APC) but may reset the sinus node with a resultant pause greater than the previous RR interval. If every other beat is a blocked APC (blocked atrial bigeminy) in a newborn infant who is dependent on an adequate heart rate for normal cardiac output, then slowing of the heart rate sufficient to alter feeding and arousal time may be present. T waves are usually smoothly inscribed, and consistent sharp deflections in the T waves may represent P waves (Figure 9-2). APCs usually occur with normally conducted QRS complexes; but if wide beats are also noted, then the apparently prolonged QRS beats are likely to be aberrant APCs because premature atrial and ventricular contractions rarely occur together, especially in the newborn period.

The incidence of APCs is 50% to 75% in children on Holter monitoring. Most are benign and require no therapy; however, there are occasional associations with myocarditis, atrial stretch, sympathomimetic or other stimulant drugs, intracardiac catheters, and electrolyte disturbances. They are most often without an obvious incitant and are usually not

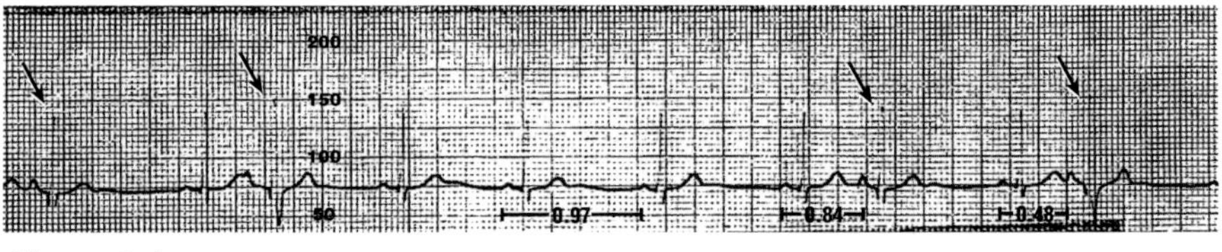


**Figure 9–1**
Atrial premature contractions (arrows) with normal and aberrated conduction.

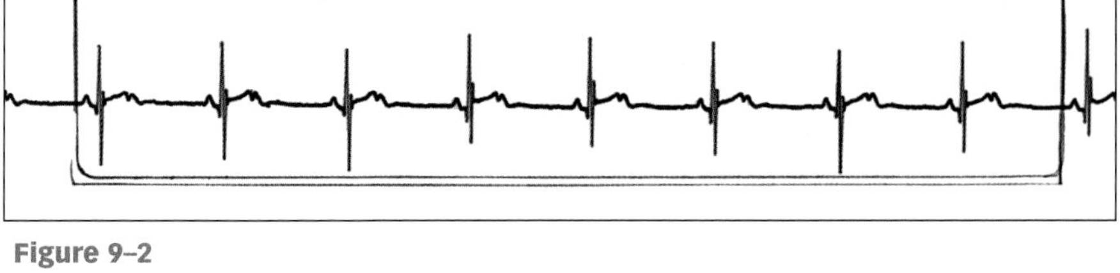

**Figure 9–2**
Every other beat is a blocked atrial premature contraction (blocked atrial bigeminy) represented by a consistent sharp deflection in the T waves.

recognized by the child or adolescent. If suppressive therapy is required, then either digoxin or propranolol is suitable.

### Premature Ventricular Contractions

Premature ventricular contractions (PVCs) are less common than APCs but may be present on Holter monitoring in up to 25% of healthy infants, children, and adolescents. PVCs are characterized by a QRS morphology that is different from sinus QRS beats, occur before the next expected sinus beat, and are not preceded by a premature P wave. The QRS duration may be only slightly prolonged. Uniform PVCs have similar morphology to one another, and multiform PVCs have diverse morphology. The designations *unifocal* and *multifocal* are no longer used, because the form of PVCs is now known not to correlate reliably with focus of origin. If a PVC occurs late, at the beginning of the next expected sinus beat, then it will produce a hybrid or fusion beat derived, in part, from the normal conduction pathways and, in part, from the PVC. Fusion beats have a morphology that is intermediate between the sinus QRS and PVC.

Although most PVCs are observed in healthy children and adolescents, PVCs can occur in patients with underlying heart disease, such as myocarditis, hypertrophic and dilated cardiomyopathies, and ventricular dysfunction in congenital cardiac malformations. The new appearance of PVCs in the setting of a febrile illness should raise the question of myocarditis. Other causes include sympathomimetic and street stimulant drugs, electrolyte imbalances, and intraventricular catheters. A 12-lead ECG should always be obtained to assess the premature beat morphology and to look for chamber enlargement but also to calculate the corrected QT interval.

$$QTc = \frac{QT\ interval\ (seconds)}{\sqrt{Preceding\ RR\ interval\ (seconds)}}$$

PVCs are considered benign if no evidence of heart disease exists, the QTc is normal (≤0.44 second), the family history is not adverse (no sudden premature deaths or cardiac arrests, important arrhythmias, or cardiomyopathies), and the PVCs are uniform in appearance and are either suppressed or not aggravated with exercise. Conversely, the presence of any of these risk factors should prompt referral for further investigation. Because underlying heart disease may be subtle, an echocardiogram to assess cardiac structure and function is usually obtained in referred patients.

Benign PVCs do not require treatment or curtailment of exercise, even if a bigeminal rhythm is present. However, if frequent benign PVCs persist, then cardiology surveillance should be arranged to detect the unusual situation of arrhythmia-induced ventricular dilation or dysfunction, especially if the ectopy burden constitutes more than 5% of the total beats on a 24-hour ambulatory electrocardiogram.[1] PVCs that are not clearly benign require the expertise of a pediatric cardiologist to determine whether there is a need for therapy. Ventricular couplets are assessed in the same manner, but triplets represent ventricular tachycardia and are discussed later in this chapter.

## ▶ SUPRAVENTRICULAR TACHYCARDIA

Supraventricular tachycardia (SVT) is common in the young, affecting as many as 1 in 250 children. More than 90% of pediatric SVT is reentrant in nature, involving 2 distinct

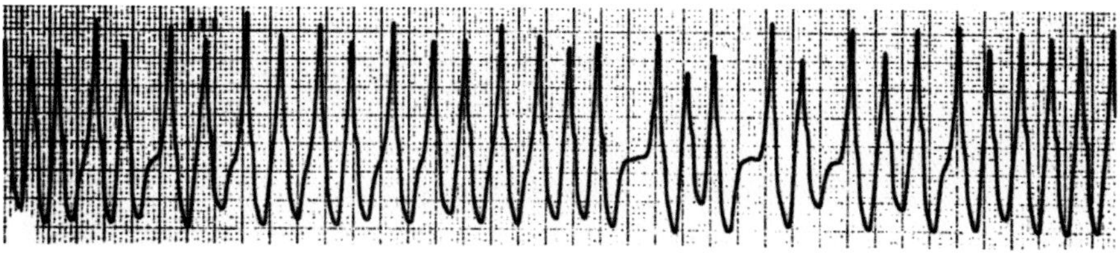

**Figure 9–3**
Antegrade conduction over an accessory pathway during atrial fibrillation in a 15-year-old boy with syncope. The short RR intervals represent rapid conduction over the accessory connection and a risk for ventricular fibrillation.

atrioventricular pathways with differing conduction characteristics and unidirectional block in one pathway. An APC may initiate SVT by entering the unblocked pathway, activating the ventricle, and then re-entering the atrium retrograde through the blocked pathway, completing the re-entrant circuit. Most re-entrant SVT in infants and children results from an accessory pathway, but the incidence of atrioventricular nodal reentry increases during adolescence with further development of the atrioventricular node. Wolff-Parkinson-White (WPW) syndrome is present if the ECG demonstrates prograde conduction through the accessory pathway in sinus rhythm as a short PR interval, delta wave, and wide QRS. The prevalence of WPW syndrome in the general population is 0.15%, but in many affected individuals, no SVT occurs. Patients with asymptomatic WPW syndrome carry a small (0.05%–0.5% per year) but definite risk for sudden death related to rapid antegrade conduction down the accessory pathway if atrial fibrillation occurs (see Figure 9-3).

WPW syndrome (with tachycardia) may be inherited in an autosomal-dominant fashion, and for these individuals the risk for sudden death is substantially increased. Automatic atrial tachycardias account for less than 10% of SVTs in children and tend to be incessant with a variable rate dependent on autonomic tone.

About 50% of patients with SVT present with tachycardia during the first 4 months of life, and 60% of this group will have recurrences, particularly if WPW syndrome is present. Although potentially still inducible at an electrophysiologic study, more than 90% will be free of clinical episodes of tachycardia at 1 year of age. However, as many as one-third of children who have a history of SVT in early infancy and clinical resolution by 1 year of age may have a recurrence at a mean age of 8 years. SVT presenting for the first time in a child 5 years or older implies a likelihood of recurrent episodes of tachycardia as high as 75% to 80%.[2] SVT is usually initiated by an APC or sinus tachycardia in early infancy, but in childhood and adolescence, PVCs and sinus pauses with junctional escape beats are additional initiators. Most children with SVT have a structurally normal heart, but if WPW syndrome is present, there is a somewhat higher incidence of cardiac defects such as hypertrophic cardiomyopathy, Ebstein malformation, or levotransposition of the great vessels.

## ▶ PRESENTATION OF SVT

During infancy, SVT may be detected incidentally on a routine examination; more commonly, however, young infants exhibit varying degrees of congestive heart failure related to the rate and duration of tachycardia and the presence of associated heart disease. As a general rule, 25% of infants develop congestive heart failure after tachycardia for 24 hours, and 50% have heart failure after SVT for 48 hours. Often, a history of poor feeding and pallor over several days is present, culminating in respiratory distress. Children older than 5 years are usually able to communicate their distress soon after the onset of SVT—hence the relative rarity of congestive heart failure caused by SVT in older children. The duration of SVT in children and adolescents ranges from a few seconds to several hours. Palpitations are the only symptom in some children; others have lightheadedness, chest discomfort, pallor, diaphoresis, and nausea. SVT-induced syncope is rare. In infancy, the heart rate with SVT may range from 230 to 300 beats per minute but is usually between 260 and 280 beats per minute, in contrast to older patients who typically have rates between 180 and 240 beats per minute. The QRS complexes are usually narrow but may be transiently wide at initiation as a consequence of aberrancy (Figure 9-4). A 12-lead ECG may reveal sharp deflections in the T waves, representing retrograde conduction from the ventricles to the atria through an accessory pathway (Figure 9-5).

## ▶ MANAGEMENT OF SVT

If cardiogenic shock is present with SVT, then direct current synchronized cardioversion should be performed; otherwise, adenosine can be administered through an intravenous bolus of 100 mcg/kg, followed by a second doubled dose if the first dose is ineffective. Adenosine always should be administered with ECG monitoring to detect the rare conversion to a more malignant arrhythmia. If adenosine is ineffective, or if SVT quickly recurs, cardiology consultation is advised. In this circumstance, an infusion of procainamide can be administered to infants and young children after appropriate loading, with a subsequent

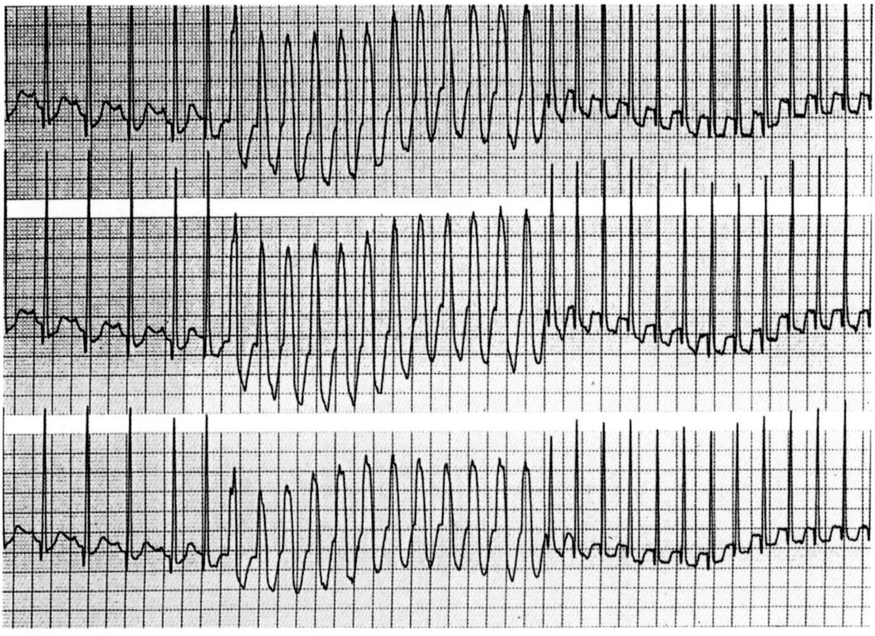

**Figure 9–4**

Transient aberrant conduction at the onset of supraventricular tachycardia during an exercise test in a 14-year-old adolescent. The QRS duration then returns to normal.

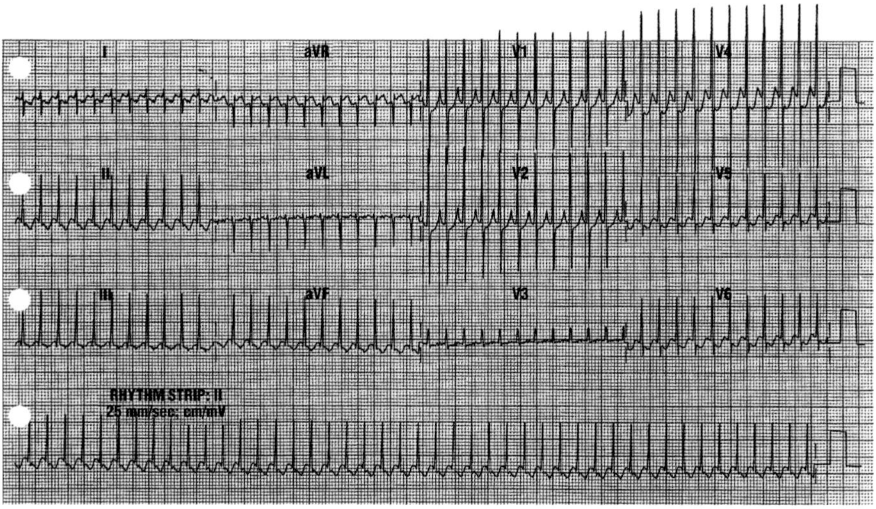


**Figure 9–5**

Twelve-lead electrocardiogram (ECG) of supraventricular tachycardia in a 2-week-old infant. Consistent sharp deflections in the T waves are present in lead III, indicating retrograde atrial activation via an accessory pathway. A repeat ECG after conversion to sinus rhythm did not reveal any pre-excitation; therefore, a concealed accessory pathway is present. Note also the ST depression in the lateral precordial leads, indicating an element of myocardial ischemia.

repeat trial of adenosine. Alternatively, amiodarone (5 mg/kg) may be administered intravenously over 20 to 60 minutes, followed by a repeat bolus if conversion is not achieved with the first dose. In general, in children younger than 1 year, intravenous verapamil and propranolol are contraindicated.

After conversion to a sinus rhythm is achieved, a 12-lead ECG should be repeated to look for evidence of pre-excitation. If WPW syndrome is present, suppressive therapy with propranolol is appropriate. Digoxin and verapamil should be avoided in children with WPW because either medication may shorten the antegrade refractory period of the accessory pathway, allowing more rapid conduction to the ventricles, a potentially fatal scenario if atrial fibrillation develops. If pre-excitation is not present, either digoxin or propranolol has been used with success to prevent recurrences. Many cardiologists currently avoid the use of digoxin because of concerns about unproven efficacy and its potential for toxicity. Beta blockers are not universally effective either and may aggravate congestive heart failure, sick sinus syndrome, or bronchospasm. Other possible medical therapies include flecainide, sotalol, or amiodarone, all of which require hospitalization for drug initiation because of possible proarrhythmic effect. Infants who have SVT are usually treated for 6 to 12 months and then observed in view of the risk for later recurrence. Because of the higher risk for complications, including the prospect that the resultant myocardial scar may grow with the patient and become a subsequent nidus for malignant and often drug-refractory arrhythmias, ablations are not commonly recommended in the first 2 years of life. If surgery for a cardiac defect is contemplated and episodes of SVT have occurred, then preoperative assessment and ablation should be considered to reduce arrhythmia-related postoperative morbidity and mortality.

Depending on the frequency and ease of conversion of episodes, older children and adolescents have 3 therapeutic choices:

1. No therapy other than self-conversion through a supine Valsalva maneuver or headstand
2. Drug therapy, although the duration, adherence issues, and cost of this approach need to be addressed with the family
3. Radiofrequency ablation, currently at least 90% successful but with a chance of a later recurrence

Automatic ectopic tachycardias in childhood are often incessant and relatively drug resistant, with the eventual possible outcome of a tachycardia-induced cardiomyopathy if conversion is not achieved. However, spontaneous resolution may occur, especially in patients younger than 3 years.[3]

## ▶ ATRIAL FLUTTER

Atrial flutter, a primary atrial re-entrant tachycardia, is seen in a bimodal distribution in newborns and in older children, the latter usually with cardiomyopathies and after repair of complex congenital heart malformations.

In the newborn, the characteristic rapid sawtooth pattern with inverted P waves in the inferior limb leads is found with an atrial rate typically between 350 and 500 beats per minute and variable, commonly 2:1, atrioventricular block, resulting in a mean ventricular rate typically about 200 beats per minute.[4] If the onset is in utero, then hydrops fetalis may develop. After birth, congestive heart failure tends to be less severe than in SVT. Structural cardiac problems are uncommon. Spontaneous conversion may occur within a few hours of birth. Although most require electrical cardioversion, chronic pharmacotherapy is usually unnecessary because recurrences are rare.

Although the typical form of atrial flutter may be seen in older children and adolescents, more common in this age group is a different variety called intra-atrial re-entrant tachycardia (IART), characterized by a slower atrial rate and distinct P waves separated by isoelectric periods. IART is usually seen after repair of complex congenital cardiac lesions (Figure 9-6).[5] Management is often difficult, but if conversion to and maintenance of a sinus rhythm cannot be achieved, morbidity is substantial, with a 4- to 5-fold increase in the risk for sudden death.[6] If an inappropriately rapid heart rate of 100 to 140 beats per minute is noted in an older child after repair of congenital heart defect, a 12-lead ECG should be obtained to look for IART, even if the surgical repair is in the remote past.

## ▶ ATRIAL FIBRILLATION

Atrial fibrillation, an irregular tachycardia with variable atrioventricular conduction, is much less common than the other forms of SVT and is seen in older patients with structural heart disease, cardiomyopathies, and alcohol binges. However, the incidence of idiopathic and paroxysmal atrial fibrillation in adolescence may be underestimated. If pre-excitation (WPW syndrome) is present and the accessory pathway is capable of rapid antegrade conduction, atrial fibrillation may conduct quickly to the ventricles, with a resultant decrease in cardiac output, syncope, and the potential for ventricular fibrillation and sudden death (see Figure 9-3).

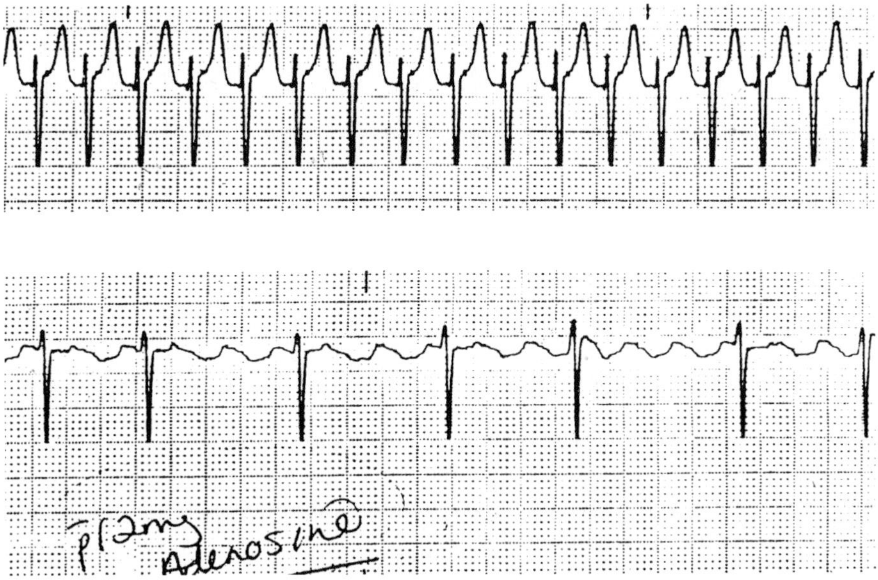

**Figure 9–6**
Intra-atrial re-entry tachycardia before and immediately after adenosine treatment in a 12-year-old boy after a Mustard repair of transposition of the great arteries in infancy. Adenosine produces high-grade AV block revealing but not converting the underlying IART.

## ▶ VENTRICULAR TACHYCARDIA

Ventricular tachycardia (VT) is defined as 3 or more repetitive excitations arising from the ventricles with a rate more than 120 beats per minute or 25% faster than the sinus rate. The QRS complexes are different from the sinus QRS complexes and are typically wide, except in young infants in whom minimal QRS prolongation (0.08–0.09 second) may be seen. VT may be extremely rapid, up to 500 beats per minute, and slightly irregular because of intermittent sinus capture beats. The differential diagnosis includes SVT with persistent aberrancy (see Figure 9-4) and SVT with antegrade conduction across an accessory pathway (see Figure 9-3), both of which are relatively uncommon. Safety dictates that all wide QRS tachycardias be considered VT until proved otherwise. The presence of similar but isolated PVCs and fusion beats in sinus rhythm assists in establishing the diagnosis, but VT is confirmed by the presence of atrioventricular dissociation (Figure 9-7).

VT in the newborn and young infant is rare, and when it is drug resistant and incessant, a ventricular tumor may be present. Mitochondrial fatty acid β-oxidation disorders can also cause VT in neonates.[7] Predisposing factors in older children and adolescents include myocarditis, repaired and unrepaired congenital cardiac lesions, cardiomyopathies, long QT syndrome, catecholamine- or exercise-induced VT, marked electrolyte imbalances, and use of street drugs (eg, cocaine). In general, VT is a marker for myocardial disease.[8]

Acute management depends on the patient's clinical status, which is determined by the rate and duration of VT and the presence of structural cardiac lesions or prior myocardial dysfunction. Hemodynamic compromise dictates electrical cardioversion with 1 to 2 watt-seconds/kg. If reasonable clinical stability is present, then intravenous amiodarone, procainamide, magnesium, or lidocaine can be administered.

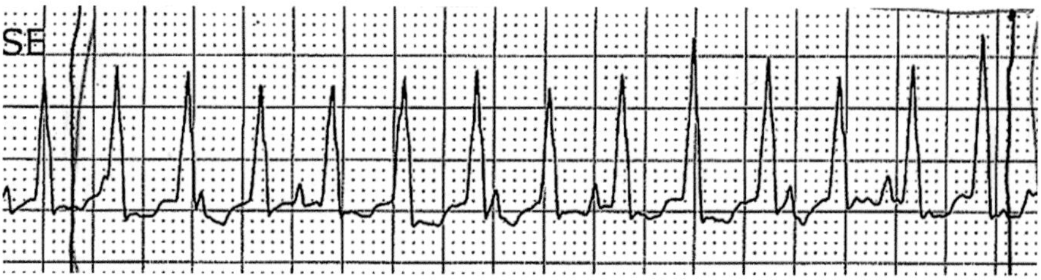


**Figure 9–7**
Ventricular tachycardia: wide QRS tachycardia with atrioventricular dissociation.

Chronic suppressive therapy is predicated on the risk for recurrence, the morbidity and mortality of the type of VT, and the risk-to-benefit ratio of treatment. Beta blockers, sotalol, and amiodarone are commonly used to prevent VT recurrences. Other treatments include implantation of an automatic cardioverter-defibrillator and VT ablation. In contrast to classic VT, accelerated ventricular rhythm is characterized by a rate of 120 beats per minute, or less than 25% faster than the basic sinus rate. Accelerated ventricular rhythm is benign when it occurs in an otherwise normal heart.

## ▶ CONDUCTION ABNORMALITIES

First-degree atrioventricular block is a prolongation of the PR interval beyond the upper limit of normal for age, with all impulses conducted. It may be seen in patients who have congenital cardiac malformations (especially atrioventricular septal defects), electrolyte disorders, rheumatic fever, myocarditis, and congenital muscular disorders. Patients receiving antiarrhythmic agents frequently exhibit first-degree atrioventricular block, which is usually benign in most settings.

Mobitz type I second-degree atrioventricular block, also known as *Wenckebach block*, is a progressive prolongation of the PR interval until a dropped ventricular beat (non-conducted P wave) occurs. It is a normal finding in healthy children during sleep and in highly conditioned athletes at rest, circumstances that are associated with a predominance of vagal tone. In general, this entity, when it occurs without exertional symptoms or syncope, is benign.

On the other hand, Mobitz type II second-degree atrioventricular block is characterized by intermittent loss of atrioventricular conduction without preceding lengthening of the PR interval. Because the site of Mobitz type II block is more distally located in the bundle of His (in contrast to type I, in which the site of block is in the atrioventricular node), there is greater risk for progression to complete atrioventricular block. The presence of type II block implies an abnormal conduction system with greater risk for associated symptoms and threatening complications, so referral to a cardiologist is appropriate for ongoing medical surveillance and evaluation for potential pacemaker implantation.

Complete atrioventricular block (CAVB), in which no atrial impulses are conducted to the ventricles, occurs in 1 of 10,000 to 20,000 live-born infants and may be acquired or congenital. Acquired block is usually a consequence of conduction system injury at the time of repair of congenital cardiac malformations but can also be seen in myocarditis, including Lyme disease, and with ingestion of beta blockers, clonidine, opioids, and sedatives. About 50% of newborns who have complete congenital atrioventricular block (CCAVB)

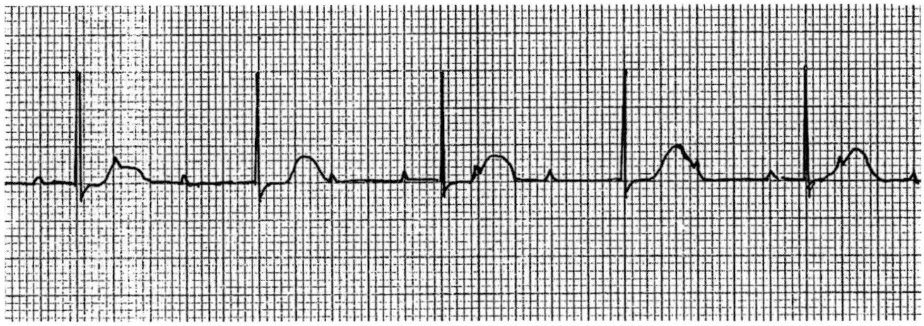

**Figure 9–8**
Complete congenital atrioventricular block in a newborn infant whose mother has Sjögren syndrome. The atrial rate is 150 beat/min, and the ventricular rate is 60 beats/min. The QRS duration is normal.

have underlying complex congenital heart malformations, particularly levotransposition of the great vessels and complex atrioventricular septal defects. Even with permanent pacing, the mortality rate of CCAVB in the setting of structural heart disease is high (>75%). The other 50% of neonates with CCAVB have immune-mediated block associated with the passage in utero of immunoglobulin G SS-A/Ro and SS-B/La antibodies from the mother who has overt or occult autoimmune disease. When the fetus is exposed to these maternal antibodies, particularly to high levels (≥100 U/mL) of maternal anti-Ro antibodies between 15 and 24 weeks of gestation, there may be fibrotic replacement of atrioventricular nodal tissue with consequent second-degree block or CAVB (Figure 9-8).[9] Fewer than 5% of infants born to mothers who have autoimmune disease develop CCAVB.[10] Infants without CCAVB born to anti-Ro/SS-A–positive mothers with autoimmune disease may have QT prolongation and sinus bradycardia.[11] If a mother bears a child who has CCAVB, the risk in future pregnancies is 15%.[12] An immune-mediated myocarditis may also occur in fetuses exposed to maternal anti-Ro and anti-La antibodies, with possible development of a postnatal dilated cardiomyopathy (endocardial fibroelastosis).

Risk factors for fetal, neonatal, or late death with CCAVB include fetal hydrops, premature birth, the presence of complex structural heart disease, a prolonged QT interval seen in up to 25% of affected patients, congestive heart failure, ventricular ectopy, atrioventricular valve insufficiency, and a low or decreasing ventricular rate (55 beats per minute or less in a neonate).[13] In view of the risk for mortality, early pacemaker implantation is advised if any of these risk factors or signs of an inadequate cardiac output is present. An infusion of isoproterenol can be administered, if necessary, to increase the heart rate while awaiting pacemaker therapy but should not delay implantation. In patients who do not require pacemaker implantation in early infancy, pacing usually becomes necessary in adolescence.

## ▶ SUDDEN CARDIAC DEATH

Sudden cardiac death, a rare but devastating event in the young, strikes approximately 1 in 100,000 children and teenagers, with the highest incidence in mid-adolescence. In decreasing order of frequency, predisposing factors include the following:

1. Repaired complex congenital heart malformations
2. Cardiomyopathies
3. Myocarditis

4. Congenital coronary artery anomalies (especially origin of the left main coronary artery from the right sinus of Valsalva)
5. Primary arrhythmias such as long QT syndrome (LQTS), WPW syndrome, and catecholamine-sensitive polymorphic VT

LQTS is a familial, clinically and genetically heterogeneous ion channel cardiac disorder that prolongs repolarization and may cause syncope, seizures, and sudden death as a consequence of polymorphic VT (torsades de pointes). The autosomal-dominant Romano-Ward subcategory, which accounts for 95% of patients with LQTS, is related to a heterozygotic mutation on chromosomes 11, 7, 3, 4, or 21. The remaining 5% are characterized by homozygotic mutations on chromosome 11 leading to the autosomal-recessive Jervell and Lange-Nielsen (JLN) syndrome, which is characterized by marked prolongation of the corrected QT intervals and congenital deafness.[14] Patients with JLN syndrome have a greater degree of QTc prolongation and a substantially higher incidence of sudden death compared with patients with the much more common Romano-Ward variant.[15] Potassium-channel function is affected by mutations on chromosomes 11, 7, 4, and 21, whereas the sodium channel is perturbed as a consequence of mutations on chromosome 3.

The incidence of LQTS is estimated at 1 in 2,500 individuals, with no gender predisposition, but the incidence may be underestimated because of incomplete genetic ascertainment. The annual mortality rate after onset of symptoms in untreated young patients is 1% to 5%, with a nearly 10% risk for sudden death as the initial symptom. The cumulative probability of a cardiac event (predominantly syncope) occurring in patients who are genotyped LQT1, 2, and 3 by 15 years of age ranges between 10% for patients with LQT3 and 69% for those with LQT1.[16] LQTS has been identified as a rare cause of the sudden infant death syndrome. The highest risk for sudden death occurs in patients with a history of syncope and a QTc of more than 500 milliseconds.[17] Syncope, atypical seizures, or cardiac arrest usually occur during exertion or emotional stress, except for long QT3 subtype events, in which symptoms predominantly occur at rest. Other than bradycardia, the physical examination is usually normal. LQTS is defined by a corrected QT interval in excess of 460 milliseconds, with a borderline QTc defined by an interval of 440 to 460 milliseconds. In general, the longer the QTc, the greater the risk for polymorphic VT. The differential diagnosis of QTc prolongation also includes electrolyte abnormalities such as hypokalemia, hypocalcemia, and hypomagnesemia. Myocardial ischemia or injury, acute central nervous system events, and cardiomyopathies may be associated with mild QTc prolongation. Cisapride, imipramine, pentamidine, and intravenous erythromycin may also prolong the QT interval. Management of LQTS includes beta-blocker therapy, restriction from competitive sports, avoidance of sympathomimetics and drugs capable of prolonging the QTc, and avoidance and rapid correction of electrolyte abnormalities. More invasive management is often necessary, including pacing, left stellate ganglionectomy, and implantation of an internal cardiac defibrillator. Gene-specific therapy with potassium channel opening agents and sodium channel blockers is on the horizon.

Beyond infancy, 25% of sudden cardiac deaths in the young occur during exercise; most occurrences are electrical in nature, with ventricular fibrillation as the final common pathway. Athletic risk may be stratified by asking 2 critical questions in pre-sports clearance evaluations: (1) Has the patient ever passed out, had visceral chest pain, or experienced symptomatic palpitations during strenuous exercise? (2) Has any family member died suddenly and unexpectedly before the age of 35 years? An affirmative answer to either question should prompt a referral to a cardiologist before participation in competitive sports. For any child or adolescent who collapses suddenly with no discernible cardiac output, rapid resuscitation including early defibrillation is mandated. Automatic external defibrillators that are available in some school systems have already begun to decrease the incidence of sudden cardiac death in the young.

## When to Refer

- Arrhythmias associated with presyncope, syncope, chest pain, or a sense of doom
- Arrhythmias associated with repaired or unrepaired congenital heart disease or cardiomyopathies
- Family history of premature (<35 years) sudden cardiac death
- Persistent or repetitive bradycardias or tachycardias
- Premature ventricular beats that increase with exercise
- Asymptomatic WPW syndrome

## When to Admit

- Arrhythmias associated with congestive heart failure, syncope, or low cardiac output
- Symptomatic high-grade atrioventricular block
- Difficult-to-control SVT, atrial flutter
- VT
- Heart disease with syncope, aborted sudden death

## TOOLS FOR PRACTICE

### Engaging Patient and Family

- *Irregular Heartbeat (Arrhythmia)* (fact sheet), American Academy of Pediatrics (www.healthychildren.org/English/health-issues/conditions/heart/Pages/Irregular-Heartbeat-Arrhythmia.aspx)
- *Sudden Cardiac Death* (fact sheet), American Academy of Pediatrics (www.healthychildren.org/English/health-issues/injuries-emergencies/sports-injuries/Pages/Sudden-Cardiac-Death.aspx)

### Medical Decision Support

- *Preparticipation Physical Evaluation*, 4th ed (book), American Academy of Pediatrics (shop.aap.org)
- *Preparticipation Physical Evaluation Forms* (questionnaire), American Academy of Pediatrics (shop.aap.org)
- *Watch, Learn and Live (Arrhythmias)* (interactive media), American Heart Association (watchlearnlive.heart.org/CVML_Player.php?moduleSelect=arrhyt)

## AAP POLICY STATEMENTS

American Academy of Pediatrics, American Heart Association, American College of Cardiology Foundation. ACC/AHA/AAP recommendations for training in pediatric cardiology. *Pediatrics*. 2005; 116(6):1574–1575. Reaffirmed December 2008 (pediatrics.aappublications.org/content/116/6/1574.full)

American Academy of Pediatrics Committee on Sports Medicine and Fitness. Medical conditions affecting sports participation. *Pediatrics*. 2008;121:841–848. Reaffirmed May 2011 (pediatrics.aappublications.org/content/121/4/841.full)

American Academy of Pediatrics Section on Cardiology and Cardiac Surgery. Guidelines for pediatric cardiovascular centers. *Pediatrics.* 2002;109(3):544–549. Reaffirmed October 2007 (pediatrics.aappublications.org/content/109/3/544.full)

## REFERENCES


1. Yarlagadda RK, Iwai S, Stein KM, et al. Reversal of cardiomyopathy in patients with repetitive monomorphic ventricular ectopy originating from the right ventricular outflow tract. *Circulation.* 2005;112(8):1092–1097
2. Perry JC, Garson A. Supraventricular tachycardia due to Wolff-Parkinson-White syndrome in children: early disappearance and late recurrence. *J Am Coll Cardiol.* 1990;16(5):1215–1220
3. Salerno JC, Kertesz NJ, Friedman RA, Fenrich AL Jr. Clinical course of atrial ectopic tachycardia is age-dependent: results and treatment in children $<3$ or $\geq 3$ years of age. *J Am Coll Cardiol.* 2004;43(3):438–444
4. Texter KM, Kertesz NJ, Friedman RA, Fenrich AL Jr. Atrial flutter in infants. *J Am Coll Cardiol.* 2006;48(5):1040–1046
5. Cecchin F, Johnsrude CL, Perry JC, Friedman RA. Effect of age and surgical technique on symptomatic arrhythmias after the Fontan procedure. *Am J Cardiol.* 1995;76(5):386–391
6. Garson A, Bink-Boelkens M, Hesslein PS, et al. Atrial flutter in the young: a collaborative study of 380 cases. *J Am Coll Cardiol.* 1985;6(4):871–878
7. Bonnet D, Martin D, De Lonlay P, et al. Arrhythmias and conduction defects as presenting symptoms of fatty acid oxidation disorders in children. *Circulation.* 1999;100(22):2248–2253
8. Alexander ME, Berul CI. Ventricular arrhythmias: when to worry. *Pediatr Cardiol.* 2000;21(6):532–541
9. Jaeggi E, Laskin C, Hamilton R, Knigdom J, Silverman E. The importance of the level of maternal anti-Ro/SSA antibodies as a prognostic marker of the development of cardiac neonatal lupus erythematosus a prospective study of 186 antibody-exposed fetuses and infants. *J Am Coll Cardiol.* 2010;55(24):2778–2284
10. Brucato A, Frassi M, Franceschini F, et al. Risk of congenital complete heart block in newborns of mothers with anti-Ro/SSA antibodies detected by counterimmunoelectrophoresis: a prospective study of 100 women. *Arthritis Rheum.* 2001;44(8):1832–1835
11. Cimaz R, Stramba-Badiale M, Brucato A, et al. QT interval prolongation in asymptomatic anti-SSA/Ro-positive infants without congenital heart block. *Arthritis Rheum.* 2000;43(5):1049–1053
12. Buyon JP, Hiebert R, Copel J, et al. Autoimmune-associated congenital heart block: demographics, mortality, morbidity and recurrence rates obtained from a national neonatal registry. *Am J Cardiol.* 1998;31(7):1658–1666
13. Lopes LM, Tavares GM, Damiano AP, et al. Perinatal outcome of fetal atrioventricular block. *Circulation.* 2008;118(12):1268–1275
14. Weintraub RG, Gow RM, Wilkinson JL. The congenital long QT syndromes in childhood. *J Am Coll Cardiol.* 1990;16(3):674–680
15. Komsuoğlu B, Göldeli O, Kulan K, et al. The Jervell and Lange-Nielsen syndrome. *Int J Cardiol.* 1994;47(2):189–192
16. Zareba W, Moss AJ, Schwartz PJ, et al. Influence of genotype on the clinical course of the long-QT syndrome. International Long-QT Syndrome Registry Research Group. *N Engl J Med.* 1998;339(14):960–965
17. Goldenberg I, Moss AJ, Peterson DR, et al. Risk factors for aborted cardiac arrest and sudden cardiac death in children with the congenital long-QT syndrome. *Circulation.* 2008;117(17):2184–2191

# Chapter 10

# Chest Pain

*Scott A. Schroeder, MD*

Although chest pain from cardiac disease in children is extremely rare, few symptoms result in more fear and anxiety in children and their parents. Undiagnosed cardiac disease causes chest pain in less than 5% of patients, and if children with preexisting heart disease are excluded, then cardiac abnormalities are found in less than 1% of patients. Although chest pain from cardiac disease occurs in a few children, much of the pediatrician's evaluation and teaching will be focused on convincing families that the heart is normal. If the care of a child with chest pain is managed inappropriately, then grief, anxiety, restriction of activities, and distrust by the family may result. However, a thorough history and physical examination will usually uncover the cause of the chest pain and will almost always allow the physician to state emphatically that the chest pain in this case is certainly not from heart disease.

## ▶ DIFFERENTIAL DIAGNOSIS

Of children and adolescents with chest pain, by far the largest number have musculoskeletal chest wall trauma or other conditions identified as the source of the pain. Pulmonary diseases—pneumonia, asthma, pneumothorax, and cough itself—account for approximately one-fifth of cases, and the rest are the result of hyperventilation or psychiatric causes, gastrointestinal disorders, and, finally, cardiac disease.[1-6] Approximately 15% of cases remain idiopathic. However, most studies on the causes of chest pain in children originate in pediatric emergency departments and pediatric cardiology clinics, and therefore these studies have not rigorously looked for the presence of esophageal disorders or reactive airway disease, both of which have been shown to be common in children with idiopathic chest pain.[7-9]

## ▶ PATHOPHYSIOLOGIC FEATURES OF CHEST PAIN

Because numerous organ systems are within the thorax, and because of the confusing overlap of sensory inputs from the various tissues in the chest, a systematic approach to the thorax is essential to determine the source of the child's pain. Pain from the chest wall and the supporting musculoskeletal structures is transmitted from these inflamed or irritated tissues to the central nervous system through the primary sensory afferents that terminate in the dorsal root ganglia. Spinal neurons then transmit the sensation from the inflamed chest wall tissues to the brain, where it is perceived as a sharp, localized pain. This feature is why chest wall pain (eg, from costochondritis or trauma) is sharp, localized, and easily reproduced on palpation.

Spinal neurons that receive input from the organs within the thorax also receive sensory input from the thoracic dermatomes. This overlap of sensory input leads to the phenomenon of *referred pain,* which often makes the evaluation of chest pain challenging. Diffuse, poorly localized chest pain can originate from any of the organs within the thorax. Inflammation of the structures that pass through the mediastinum results in pain over dermatomes T1 to T4, from the retroclavicular to the retrosternal regions. Pain over dermatomes T5 to T8, especially in the xiphoid area, suggests lower chest wall or diaphragmatic irritation or even intra-abdominal disease. Because both the intercostal nerves and the phrenic nerve innervate the diaphragm, peripheral diaphragmatic irritation causes pain in the lower anterior chest or epigastric regions, and central diaphragmatic inflammation results in ipsilateral shoulder pain because of its innervation by the phrenic nerve. The pericardium, positioned on the central diaphragm, has pleural connections and is innervated by the phrenic, vagus, and recurrent laryngeal nerves. Therefore, when the pericardium is inflamed or infected, sharp substernal pain can occur. The pain of pericarditis may be limited to the sternal and precordial areas; however, if the left lobe of the diaphragm is irritated, then pain will be referred to the ipsilateral shoulder or neck. Pleural pain results from distention or inflammation of the pleura that can occur during the course of pneumonia, pneumothorax, or empyema. Pain from pleural inflammation is aggravated by respiratory movements. The pain is characterized as well localized and sharp, exaggerated by coughing or deep inspiration. The pain associated with a pneumothorax can be pleuritic in nature, or it can be referred to the ipsilateral shoulder. Pleurodynia is a specific cause of pleuritic chest pain heralded by fever and associated with coxsackievirus B; an idea of its intensity comes from its apt nickname as "the devil's grip."

The pain associated with esophageal disorders can seem indistinguishable from that associated with myocardial ischemia because the sensory afferents from the esophagus are through the cardiac and esophageal plexi as well as the sympathetic trunk. Within the lungs, sensory input exists only from the larger airways and parietal pleura; thus, the pain arising from pulmonary parenchymal disease results from inflammation of or traction on contiguous structures.

## ▶ EVALUATION

### *History*

Because pathognomonic findings are rare on physical examination in the evaluation of a child with chest pain, a detailed history will help focus the differential diagnosis, develop a logical intervention, and allow the child and family to voice their concerns. A meticulous history should address the nature of the pain as well as the child's response to the pain. If possible, children should describe the pain in their own words, and they should be asked what they think is causing the pain. Along with a description of the location, duration, radiation, and quality of the pain, the pediatrician should elicit any associated signs and symptoms, as well as any aggravating and alleviating factors, and attempt to uncover the family history and dynamics. To many adolescents, chest pain is synonymous with heart disease; therefore, this issue should be addressed, and if no cardiac cause is discovered, then the physician should unequivocally state to the adolescent and the family that the heart is normal.

Pain that occurs with exercise points toward either a cardiac or a respiratory cause. If the pain awakens the child from sleep, then the cause might be respiratory, cardiac, musculoskeletal, or gastroesophageal, but it is never psychological. When the pain is poorly localized or is associated with recurrent somatic complaints or family or school stress, and when a family history of chest pain can be found, a psychogenic source of the pain is likely. Conversely, deep, poorly localized pain that radiates to the neck or shoulders is characteristic of visceral pain. Superficial sharp pain that is exacerbated by lifting or movements of the torso suggests musculoskeletal pain.

Peripheral pain that increases with inspiratory efforts originates from pleural inflammation. Questions regarding trauma to the chest wall should always be asked, and even if the trauma occurred 1 to 3 months before the pain, it should not be discounted because the pain might represent a posttraumatic pericardial effusion. Sharp pain that decreases when the child leans forward is characteristic of pericardial inflammation. Children with a family history of Marfan or Turner syndromes, as well as those with a history of Kawasaki disease or congenital heart disease, warrant referral to a pediatric cardiologist.

Even if the history is highly suggestive of the cause for the chest pain, the pediatrician should be careful and thorough because the potential exists for 2 different causes of the pain. Children with asthma can also have gastroesophageal reflux. Children with sickle cell disease who develop acute chest syndrome may have chest pain as a result of medication-induced gastritis, vaso-occlusive crisis, or asthma.

## Laboratory Evaluation

Laboratory tests are usually not helpful in establishing a specific diagnosis; therefore, a thorough history and physical examination should guide the physician in ordering tests. In most cases, chest radiographs and electrocardiographs will only confirm what is suspected clinically. If a child has a fever, acute onset of chest pain, and an abnormal cardiac examination suggestive of pericarditis, then a chest radiograph and electrocardiogram are indicated. If a child has fever, tachypnea, chest pain, and decreased breath sounds over a segment of the lungs, then a chest radiograph is appropriate to determine whether a pneumothorax, a pneumonia, a pleural effusion, or other pulmonary disease is present. If the pain occurs with exercise, then exercise testing or spirometry may help uncover underlying asthma or exercise-induced bronchospasm. One cause of idiopathic chest pain may be an esophageal disorder.[7] Signs and symptoms of children with chest pain who warrant hospitalization or specialty evaluation are listed in Box 10-1.

**BOX 10-1**

### *Signs and Symptoms That Accompany Chest Pain and Warrant Referral or Hospitalization*

**SIGNS**

- Syncope
- Fevers, chills, weight loss, malaise, anorexia
- History of Kawasaki disease, Turner syndrome, Marfan syndrome, sickle cell disease, or cystic fibrosis
- Recent elective abortion, calf pain, oral contraceptive use
- Family history of hypertrophic obstructive cardiomyopathy or unexplained syncope
- Pica
- Foreign body aspiration
- Conversion disorder

**SYMPTOMS**

- Cyanosis, toxic appearance, or respiratory distress
- Murmur that increases with Valsalva maneuver
- Pleural or pericardial friction rub
- Pulsus paradoxus
- Cardiac clicks, thrills, gallop, or third heart sound
- Chest pain with exercise
- Palpitation or tachycardia

## ▶ SPECIFIC CAUSES OF CHEST PAIN IN CHILDREN

### *Musculoskeletal and Chest Wall Conditions*

After a determination has been made that the child is in no distress, inspection of the thorax will determine the presence of bruising, swelling over joints, splinting, signs of trauma, or an abnormal breathing pattern. Palpation and percussion are extremely important to localize and reproduce the pain because disturbances in the chest wall are the most common diagnoses in children with chest pain. Each rib cartilage should be palpated with only one finger or with the child's finger because palpation with 2 or more digits may cause splinting and will not recreate the pain. Reproduction of point tenderness at the origin of the spontaneous pain is the strongest evidence favoring the diagnosis of chest wall disease. Pain from the thoracic cage that can be elicited by movements of the torso or by flexion of the arms is highly suggestive of a musculoskeletal chest wall injury. The pain of costochondritis causes tenderness over the affected costochondral or costosternal junctions and can occur at rest or with movement. Adolescents with gynecomastia or breast pain may experience chest pain that is easily discernible on inspection and palpation of the developing breast tissue. No laboratory testing is needed if any of the these conditions is identified as a cause of the chest pain. Table 10-1 lists common, uncommon, and rare causes of chest pain and their associated signs and symptoms.

### *Pulmonary Conditions*

Children with asthma may have chest pain from excessive coughing and overuse of their intercostal muscles. Having pain alone as a manifestation of asthma is unusual for a child; usually, nocturnal cough, adventitial breath sounds, abnormal pulmonary function tests, or other signs of atopic diseases can exist.

A variety of other diseases of the airways, pleurae, and parenchyma can cause substernal or pleuritic chest pain. Pneumonia, asthma, exercise-induced bronchospasm, pleural effusions, and air in the pleural space can cause pain, but the chest pain is never the sole sign of the underlying disease process. A child with a parapneumonic effusion will classically have fever, tachypnea, tachycardia, a pleural friction rub or crackles (or both) on auscultation, and dullness to percussion in addition to the pleuritic chest pain that intensifies with inspiration.

Exercise-induced chest pain or chest tightness that resolves with the cessation of the exercise or the administration of bronchodilators may be a manifestation of cardiac disease but is more commonly related to exercise-induced bronchospasm. Exercise testing, cold air challenge, or a therapeutic trial of bronchodilators can confirm the diagnosis of exercise-induced or cold air–induced bronchospasm. Treatment with bronchodilators will help these children participate in sports and allow them to lead normal, active lives.

Spontaneous pneumothorax can occur in teenagers with chronic illnesses such as cystic fibrosis, asthma, and Marfan syndrome, but it can also occur in healthy teenagers. A child with cystic fibrosis who experiences chest pain should be assumed to have a pneumothorax until proven otherwise. Dyspnea, shoulder pain, and tachypnea are often observed in addition to the chest pain in a typically tall, thin adolescent who develops a spontaneous pneumothorax.

### *Gastrointestinal Conditions*

Acid reflux to the esophagus can mimic the pain of angina and can cause both acute and chronic chest pain. Pain that originates from the esophagus or stomach is described as an

**Table 10-1**
**Common, Uncommon, and Rare Causes of Chest Pain and Associated Signs and Symptoms**

| CAUSE OF CHEST PAIN | SIGNS AND SYMPTOMS |
|---|---|
| **MUSCULOSKELETAL** | |
| Costochondritis (common) | Localized, superficial, reproducible pain over rib cartilage |
| Exercise, overuse, muscle strain (common) | Reproducible pain with use of involved muscle group |
| Protracted coughing or vomiting (common) | Intercostal muscle tenderness |
| Trauma | Localized pain; pain with movement of involved areas |
| Stitch (common) | Sharp, crampy costal pain that occurs with running |
| Precordial catch (uncommon) | Transient, stabbing pain at left sternal border; relieved by forced inspiration |
| **PULMONARY** | |
| Asthma (common) | Associated with cough, shortness of breath, wheezing, abnormal pulmonary function tests; relief with inhaled anti-inflammatory drugs or bronchodilators |
| Exercise-induced bronchospasm (common) | Abnormal exercise tests; improvement with bronchodilators |
| Pneumonia (common) | Crackles, fever, cough |
| Pleural effusion (uncommon) | Pleural rub, fever, decreased breath sounds |
| Pneumothorax (uncommon) | Sudden pain, referred shoulder pain, dyspnea, hyperresonance and/or absent or reduced breath sounds on affected side |
| Pulmonary embolus (rare) | Contraceptive use or recent abortion, pleuritic pain |
| **GASTROINTESTINAL** | |
| Esophagitis (common) | Retrosternal pain; relief with antacids |
| Gastroesophageal reflux (common) | Retrosternal burning pain; worse after eating and when reclining; relief with antacids |
| **CARDIAC** | |
| Hypertrophic cardiomyopathy (rare) | Syncope, family history, systolic ejection murmur |
| Pericarditis (rare) | Associated fever with acute onset of pain; pain increases with movement; narrow pulse pressure, distant heart sounds; alleviated by leaning forward |
| Myocarditis (rare) | Precedent viral illness, anorexia, shortness of breath, third heart sound or gallop, cardiomegaly |
| **NONORGANIC** | |
| Psychogenic (common) | Normal physical examination, trouble sleeping, family or school problems, life stresses, family history of chest pain, other somatic complaints |
| Hyperventilation (common) | Associated light-headedness, paresthesias, underlying anxiety |

uncomfortable, gnawing substernal burning sensation. The pain can last for hours, and it intensifies after meals and on reclining. Any inflammation of the esophagus, abnormalities of peristalsis, esophageal foreign body, or trauma can cause chest pain. The most common gastrointestinal cause of chest pain is esophagitis. However, because the clinical presentation of esophagitis can be nonspecific, children with idiopathic chest pain may benefit from a trial of antacids or $H_2$-receptor antagonists before embarking on an exhaustive evaluation.

### Cardiac Conditions

The least likely but most worrisome causes of chest pain in children are cardiac disorders that cause myocardial ischemia. Cardiac disease in children rarely produces isolated chest pain and is always associated with other findings at evaluation. Sudden death from cardiac disease in children is caused by a small subgroup of disorders: abnormalities of the myocardium or coronary vessels, specific congenital heart lesions, arrhythmias, and conduction disorders.[10] Signs and symptoms that identify children with these disorders and warrant cardiology evaluation include exertional nonrespiratory dyspnea, syncope, and palpitations. A pediatric cardiologist should also see children with chest pain and a family history of sudden death.

A child with chest pain from myocarditis or pericarditis usually appears ill, with fever, dyspnea, changes in the pain associated with the respiratory cycle, and abnormal auscultatory findings. In most instances, the echoviruses, especially coxsackievirus B, are identified as the culprit responsible for myocarditis. Pericarditis can result from either an infectious agent or an autoimmune process.

Aortic stenosis and idiopathic hypertrophic cardiomyopathy, which are the most important lesions that cause left ventricular outflow obstruction, can cause chest pain as a result of the heart's inability to increase the cardiac output with exercise. These disorders cause syncope and chest pain with exertion. Mild aortic stenosis does not cause chest pain.

Chest pain may be, but is not usually, the primary complaint of children with arrhythmias unless they perceive the palpitations as painful. More commonly, older children complain of light-headedness or dizziness along with the palpitations. The arrhythmia can usually be detected on auscultation and confirmed by resting electrocardiogram. If the palpitations or chest pain occur infrequently or are not associated with exercise, then referral to a pediatric cardiologist is indicated for Holter monitoring.

Although mitral valve prolapse (MVP) is commonly thought to cause chest pain in adolescents, most children with MVP are asymptomatic. Chest pain has been found to be no more common in teenagers with MVP than it is in those without MVP.[11]

Findings on auscultation that point to a cardiac source of pain include clicks, rubs, and systolic murmurs. A murmur can be worrisome if it increases in intensity with the Valsalva maneuver or any other procedure that expands the degree of left ventricular outlet obstruction. A third heart sound or gallop is heard in myocarditis and congestive heart failure. Pleural friction rubs, wheezes, tachypnea, and crackles suggest a pulmonary cause. Conversely, hyperventilation associated with light-headedness, paresthesias, dizziness, and a high level of stress or anxiety suggests a hyperventilation syndrome.

### Idiopathic Causes

Especially among adolescents, as many as 39% of patients complaining of chest pain will not have a readily identifiable cause.[3,4] Children with chronic chest pain, no history of respiratory or cardiac disease, and a normal physical examination are unlikely to have a serious cause for their pain. For teenagers, a careful explanation of the pathophysiologic features in concrete terms is a fundamental part of their therapeutic regimen. Several studies of children with idiopathic chest pain have shown that most of them have no further pain 1 to 2 years after their initial evaluation.[12]

### Psychogenic Chest Pain

A child with a long history of chest pain, other recurrent somatic problems, school or sleep problems, a family history of chest pain, or any combination of these factors may have a psychogenic cause for the pain. If a psychogenic cause is entertained, then the diagnosis should not be made by exclusion of organic disease; rather, the diagnosis should be based on positive psychiatric evidence. As with any somatic illness, if the family or the child is able to articulate a relationship between the chest pain and stress or emotional upheaval, then the diagnosis will be easier for them to comprehend and accept.[13] Emotional causes for chest pain seem to be more common in adolescents than in children younger than 12 years.[1] Hyperventilation can be associated with the chest wall syndrome but is more commonly seen in teenagers with underlying anxiety. The diagnosis is usually made by history alone because the child may need to hyperventilate for 20 minutes to reproduce the pain.

Almost all children with hyperventilation syndrome have associated paresthesias, carpopedal spasm, and light-headedness. For a child with an acute episode of hyperventilation, the treatment is to have the child breathe into a paper bag to relieve the hypocapnia. Resolution of the chronic problem is based on techniques to allow the children to understand the nature of their anxiety and allow them to regain control of their emotional state. The treatment of other forms of psychogenic chest pain should be focused on the family's comprehension of the cause of the pain and reassurance that no long-term sequelae exist, all while acknowledging that the pain is real. For children with more significant psychiatric problems, referral to a psychiatrist may be necessary.

## When to Admit

Rarely will a child with chest pain need to be hospitalized because, for the most part, chest pain is usually benign, self-limited, and not associated with severe intrathoracic illness. Box 10-1 provides guidance for when to refer and when to admit. However, children with the following should be hospitalized:

- Myocarditis
- Pericarditis
- Empyema
- Pneumothorax
- Significant thoracic trauma
- Acute chest syndrome
- Esophageal foreign bodies
- Coronary artery anomalies or other cardiac lesions
- Myocardial ischemia
- Chest pain and palpitations
- Cyanosis
- Distress

## REFERENCES


1. Selbst SM, Ruddy RM, Clark BJ, Henretig FM, Santulli T Jr. Pediatric chest pain: a prospective study. *Pediatrics.* 1988;82:319–323
2. Rowe BH, Dulberg CS, Peterson RG, Vlad P, Li MM. Characteristics of children presenting with chest pain to a pediatric emergency department. *CMAJ.* 1990;143:388–394
3. Pantell RH, Goodman BW. Adolescent chest pain: a prospective study. *Pediatrics.* 1983;71:881–887
4. Driscoll DJ, Glicklich LB, Gallen WJ. Chest pain in children: a prospective study. *Pediatrics.* 1976;57:648–651
5. Massin MM, Bourguignont A, Coremans C, et al. Chest pain in pediatric patients presenting to an emergency department or to a cardiac clinic. *Clin Pediatr.* 2004;43:231–239
6. Fyfe DA, Moodie DS. Chest pain in pediatric patients presenting to a cardiac clinic. *Clin Pediatr.* 1984;23(6):321–324
7. Glassman MS, Medow MS, Berezin S, Newman LJ. Spectrum of esophageal disorders in children with chest pain. *Dig Dis Sci.* 1992;37:663–666
8. Weins L, Sabath R, Ewing L. Chest pain in otherwise healthy children and adolescents is frequently caused by exercise-induced asthma. *Pediatrics.* 1992;90:350–353
9. Thull-Freedman J. Of 3700 children thought to have non-cardiac chest pain at initial paediatric cardiology clinic evaluation, none suffered cardiac death over a median of 4 years follow-up. *Evid Based Med.* 2012;17:190–191
10. Liberthson RR. Sudden death from cardiac causes in children and young adults. *N Engl J Med.* 1996;334:1039–1044
11. Savage DD, Garrison RJ, Devereux RB. Mitral valve prolapse in the general population. 1. Epidemiologic features: the Framingham Study. *Am Heart J.* 1983;106:571–576
12. Rowland T, Richards M. The natural history of idiopathic chest pain in children: a follow-up study. *Clin Pediatr (Phila).* 1986;25:612–614
13. Green M. *Sources of Pain.* Philadelphia, PA: WB Saunders; 1983

# Chapter 11

# Constipation

*Peter F. Belamarich, MD*

The term *constipation*, which denotes both a symptom and a chronic condition, refers to the infrequent elimination of large or hard stools that may cause pain on defecation. In childhood, constipation that is not caused by another condition is known as idiopathic or functional constipation. Given that constipation encompasses both objective and subjective complaints that vary by age, it has defied a comprehensive standard definition. Several consensus groups have developed definitions of constipation; however, none of these definitions seems entirely satisfactory to all.[1] One expert consensus definition of constipation is presented in Box 11-1.

Constipation is a common symptom among children in the industrialized world. In parental surveys, 16% to 37% of toddlers are reported to suffer from it.[2] Functional constipation presents a challenge to the pediatrician, as suggested by the observation that the evaluation and treatment of constipation occupies 25% of all referrals to pediatric gastroenterologic services, although these children rarely require an invasive procedure.[3] To pediatricians caring for chronically constipated children, treatment failure raises the question of Hirschsprung disease. Among referral populations, more than 90% of childhood constipation is functional; ultimately, 50% to 90% of these children are cured.[4]

The approach to constipated children used by gastroenterologists is well within the scope of the primary care pediatric practice. The focus of this chapter is on identifying and treating children who have functional constipation. An evidence-based guideline, endorsed by the American Academy of Pediatrics, has been published on evaluating and treating constipation.[5]

## ▶ PATHOPHYSIOLOGIC MECHANISM OF FUNCTIONAL CONSTIPATION

### *Normal Colonic Function*

The role of the colon is to reclaim water from the liquid ileal effluent. This task is accomplished, in part, by a motility pattern that includes focal circular contractions, which impede the progress of the luminal contents while solutes and water are absorbed. Subsequently, forward progress of the relatively dehydrated fecal stream is achieved by coordinated contractile waves, which propel the bolus of stool to the next colonic segment and ultimately to the rectum. The final elimination of stool is controlled by defecation, a coordinated sequence of neuromuscular events with both reflexive and conscious components. Control of defecation, continence, is a critically important social achievement in early childhood. At rest, continence is maintained by the involuntary resting tonic contraction of the smooth

BOX 11-1

## *Definition of Constipation*

Constipation is a symptom defined by the occurrence of any of the following, independent of stool frequency:

- Passage of hard, scybalous, pebble-like, or cylindrical cracked stools
- Straining or painful defecation
- Passage of large stools that may clog the toilet
- Stool frequency less than 3 per week, unless the child is breastfed

Adapted from Hyams J, Colletti R, Faure C, et al. Functional gastrointestinal disorders: Working Group Report of the First World Congress of Pediatric Gastroenterology, Hepatology, and Nutrition. *J Pediatr Gastroenterol Nutr.* 2002;35 (Suppl 2):S110.

muscle cuff of the internal anal sphincter and by the posterior turn of the anal canal in relation to the anterior angulation of the rectal vault. This angle is modulated by the puborectalis sling muscle, which loops posteriorly around the anorectal junction and is anchored anteriorly on the pubic bone.

When stool arrives in the rectal ampulla, causing distention of the rectal walls, a reflexive relaxation of the internal anal sphincter occurs, which lowers the pressure of the anal canal and allows the stool bolus to descend to the anal canal, a phenomenon known as the rectoanal inhibitory reflex. Control of defecation then occurs by the voluntary (and learned) deliberate contraction of the striated muscle of the external sphincter and puborectalis sling muscles, which increase the pressure in the anal canal and make the exiting angle more acute. Conversely, a Valsalva maneuver, in combination with relaxation of the external anal sphincter and the puborectalis sling, permits defecation to proceed. Normal stool frequency decreases from about 4 stools per day in infancy to 1.2 stools per day at 4 years old.[6]

### *Factors in Functional Constipation*

The pathophysiologic basis of functional constipation is not clear. It may be the final common pathway for a number of underlying distinct conditions:[7] a disorder of the dynamics of defecation; a problem with rectal sensation; or a disorder of colonic transit, leading to impacted, overly desiccated stool in the colon. Functional constipation can also arise solely from a behavioral aversion to or learned problems with the process of defecation.

Stool withholding, the act of voluntarily deferring defecation to avoid pain, significantly contributes to the chronicity of constipation in childhood independently of the primary cause.

### *Stool Withholding*

In practical terms, several commonly recognized clinical scenarios can result in constipation, including painful anal fissures, perianal streptococcal cellulitis, traumatic toilet-training experiences, and transient periods of dehydration, illness, or immobility. Stool withholding likely figures prominently in the perpetuation of constipation when pain or an aversive experience is the primary insult. Withholding behavior in the toddler or child is strongly self-reinforcing. The child is avoiding painful bowel movements, which makes the stool harder and more painful to pass. Parents who focus with great concern on the withholding crisis, often believing that the child is valiantly trying to defecate rather than to withhold, also reinforce stool withholding unwittingly. Toddlers love the worried attention of their parents! The lack of privacy commonly found in some school lavatories can engender withholding by older children. Anorectal manometric studies have documented abnormalities in the dynamics of defecation in a large series of chronically constipated children, the most common being a paradoxic contraction of the external anal sphincter and the puborectalis sling in response to the rectoanal inhibitory reflex.

This commonly identified abnormality is known variously as rectoanal pelvic floor dyssynergia, abnormal defecation dynamics, and anismus.[8] Most experts consider dyssynergia a learned phenomenon. For a large proportion of chronically constipated children, painful defecation and withholding antedate the clinical presentation of constipation by 1 to 5 years.[9] In a significant subset of children who experience persistent constipation, withholding becomes entrenched and particularly difficult to unlearn. In fact, initial enthusiasm over manometrically based biofeedback training was based on its potential to help patients identify and unlearn this withholding behavior. However, controlled studies have not documented greater improvements in the outcome for patients who have undergone biofeedback training than for those given a standard treatment regimen.[8]

### Sensory Abnormalities

Another common manometric abnormality found in chronically constipated children is known as megarectum. As the name implies, the rectum is dilated with a chronic impaction, a finding associated with an increase in the sensory threshold to minimal rectal distention, as well as an increase in the minimal volume required to initiate the urge to defecate. These sensory abnormalities persist for several years in some patients after successful treatment, suggesting that ongoing sensory abnormalities contribute to relapses and perhaps to the initial pathogenesis of constipation in some children.

### Slow Transit

Constipation from abnormally slow transit of the fecal stream through the colon occurs predominantly in young women but can occur in children.[10] Whether slowed colonic transit is the primary problem or is secondary to distal difficulties with defecation is unclear. Slow-transit constipation in children is not easily differentiated clinically from normal-transit constipation. A unique therapeutic approach to slow-transit constipation has not emerged.

### Dietary Factors

Whether dietary factors alone cause constipation is unclear. In infancy, human milk is highly protective. Despite broad agreement that dietary fiber has an important role in promoting a regular bowel habit, very little literature and no prospective studies support this belief. A case-control study has documented decreased fiber intake as a risk factor for childhood constipation; however, substantial overlap exists in the fiber intake between cases and controls.[11] Nonetheless, many physicians have remarked that, in infancy, the transition from human milk or formula to whole cow's milk, or periods of excess protein intake such as occur in toddlers with excessive whole cow's milk consumption, are associated with constipation.

The tenacious and harmful myth that iron-containing formula causes constipation has been disproved many times.

## ▶ DIFFERENTIAL DIAGNOSIS

The differential diagnosis of chronic childhood constipation includes many conditions (Box 11-2). Despite the large number of possible diagnoses, at least 90% of affected children have functional constipation.

Frequently, the foremost consideration in the differential diagnosis of chronic constipation is Hirschsprung disease. The most common basis for this concern is treatment failure, an appropriate concern in early infancy when functional constipation is unusual and easily treatable. However, treatment failure in the toddler and the school-aged child more often reflects the complexity and duration of intervention required to treat functional constipation adequately than a missed diagnosis of Hirschsprung disease. Fortunately, several findings in the history are useful in the process of ruling out Hirschsprung disease. Perhaps most useful is that almost all children with functional constipation withhold stool in response to the rectoanal inhibitory reflex, whereas this reflex is absent with Hirschsprung disease. Simply stated, stool withholding behaviors are a historical finding that almost always rule

BOX 11-2

### *Differential Diagnosis of Constipation in Childhood*

**FUNCTIONAL CONSTIPATION**

- Disorders of intestinal neuromuscular function

**ANAL AND RECTAL DISORDERS**

- Anal fissure
- Anterior ectopic anus
- Anal stenosis
- Anorectal malformations
- Rectal duplication
- Anal trauma (abuse)
- Pelvic tumor (presacral teratoma, ganglioneuroma, ovarian cyst, hematocolpos)

**NEUROLOGIC—NEUROMUSCULAR**

- Hirschsprung disease
- Pseudoobstruction syndromes
- Spinal cord lesions
- Spinal dysrhaphism, including spina bifida
- Cerebral palsy
- Neuromuscular diseases with hypotonia

**METABOLIC AND ENDOCRINE**

- Hypothyroidism
- Diabetes insipidus
- Hypercalcemia
- Hypokalemia

**MEDICATION AND TOXIN RELATED**

- Antihistamines
- Anticholinergics
- Anticonvulsants
- Opioids
- Bismuth, aluminum hydroxide
- Tricyclic antidepressants
- Iron preparations (not iron-fortified formulas)
- Plumbism
- Infant botulism

**MISCELLANEOUS**

- Celiac disease
- Cystic fibrosis
- Cow milk allergy
- Scleroderma
- Systemic lupus erythematosus

out Hirschsprung disease. Conversely, Hirschsprung disease should be considered in any child with refractory constipation who has had any of the following:

1. Failure to pass meconium in the first 24 hours of life.
2. Onset of constipation before 3 months of age.
3. Symptoms of intestinal obstruction at any time (distention, emesis).
4. Lifelong dependence on laxatives, enemas, or mechanical manipulation to initiate defecation.
5. History of enterocolitis in early infancy (sometimes misdiagnosed as gastroenteritis).
6. Constipation in children with syndromes associated with Hirschsprung disease (eg, trisomy 21, Waardenburg-Shah, congenital central hypoventilation).
7. Failure to thrive or growth faltering. See Table 11-1 for a summary of features that distinguish Hirschsprung disease from functional constipation.

Other conditions that specifically affect the neuromuscular function of the colon include the pseudoobstruction syndromes, which are characterized by intermittent episodes of functional intestinal obstruction. Furthermore, a large percentage of children who have generalized neuromuscular disabilities (eg, cerebral palsy, muscular dystrophy, generalized hypotonia) have refractory constipation that is frequently multifactorial and difficult to treat.

Anorectal disorders producing constipation include anal fissures, anal stenosis, anterior ectopic anus, and extrinsic masses that partially obstruct the rectum. Fissures may induce a self-perpetuating cycle of withholding and worsening of constipation that causes reinjury. Congenital anal stenosis is characterized by straining during the production of small-caliber stools; it is frequently diagnosed during infancy. The anal canal is noted to be narrow and not distensible during digital examination. Occasionally, chronic constipation is caused by a subtle anorectal malformation known as anterior ectopic anus,[12] in which the anal orifice

**Table 11-1**
**Comparison of Hirschsprung Disease to Functional Constipation**

| CHARACTERISTIC | HIRSCHSPRUNG DISEASE | FUNCTIONAL CONSTIPATION |
|---|---|---|
| Prevalence | ~1 in 6,000 births | 1.5% of 7-year-old boys |
| Failure to pass meconium <24 hr | 58%–94% | ~5% |
| Constipation in first 3 mo | 90% | Rare |
| Symptoms or signs of obstruction | Common | Absent |
| Abdominal distention | Common | Mild or absent |
| Stool size | Narrow, ribbon-like | Intermittent large-caliber stools |
| General appearance | Chronically ill | Well |
| Stool-withholding behavior | Rare | Extremely common |
| Soiling | Unusual | Common |
| Stool in ampulla | Unusual | Common |
| Plain radiographs | Empty rectum | Dilated enlarged rectum |
| Rectal manometry | Rectoanal reflex absent | Rectoanal reflex present |
| Typical barium enema | Distal spasm, proximal dilatation | Diffusely dilated colon and rectum |

is misplaced anteriorly so that the stool bolus must turn anteriorly at the perineum to exit. The parents may report seeing a perineal bulge when the infant attempts to defecate. Surgical reconstruction may be necessary in children who fail to improve with medical therapy. In rare cases, constipation is a manifestation of an intermittent or partial extrinsic obstruction of the rectum by a rectal duplication cyst or by a pelvic mass such as a neuroblastoma, presacral teratoma, or ovarian tumor.

Spinal cord lesions affecting the second, third, and fourth sacral nerves are associated with both sensory and motor deficits affecting defecation. Trauma to the sacral cord, intraspinal and extraspinal tumors, and congenital malformations that can alter the spinal cord function should be suspected when constipation is accompanied by abnormalities in bladder function or gait, or when there are visible abnormalities or palpable findings over the lumbosacral spine, including hair tufts, dimples, pigmentary abnormalities, or a deviated gluteal cleft.

Metabolic and endocrine disorders associated with constipation include hypothyroidism, hypercalcemia, diabetes insipidus, hypokalemia, and plumbism. These conditions generally do not manifest with chronic constipation as a sole symptom.

Both cystic fibrosis and celiac disease can cause constipation. Physicians should be alert to these possibilities in children with poor growth in weight or height, recurrent respiratory complaints, anemia, or hypoproteinemia.

Many medications and toxins are reported to cause constipation (see Box 11-2).

Recently, 2 reports have linked constipation to cow milk protein allergy.[13,14] In a study of a referral population of 65 children who had treatment-resistant chronic constipation, 44 had a positive therapeutic response to the substitution of soy milk for cow milk. Questions remain, however, about the generalizability of these findings to the primary care setting.

Box 11-3 presents a diagnostic approach for children thought to have an organic cause of their constipation.

**BOX 11-3**

## *Studies in Children With Constipation*

- For growth failure, failure to thrive, short stature
  - Thyroid function tests
  - Celiac panel
  - Sweat test
  - Hirschsprung disease
- For delayed passage of meconium
  - Anorectal manometry
  - Rectal suction biopsy
  - Unprepared contrast enema
  - Sweat test
- For hair tufts, lipomas or hemangiomas overlying the lumbosacral spine and for abnormalities of gait, urination, absence of anal wink or cremaster reflex
  - Consider imaging the lumbosacral spinal cord (ultrasound, magnetic resonance imaging)
- For refractory constipation
  - Thyroid function tests
  - Serum calcium
  - Potassium
  - Lead
  - Celiac panel
  - Sweat test

Routine studies of children who are thought to have functional constipation are not recommended.

## ▶ COMMON PRESENTATIONS OF FUNCTIONAL CONSTIPATION

### Infancy

Particularly in the first 6 months of life, parental notions of what constitutes constipation may be incorrect. Breastfed infants may have a mushy stool as infrequently as once a week. In the otherwise healthy infant, this situation does not deserve the label constipation and requires no intervention. In general, stool consistency rather than frequency is the critical determinant of constipation in the infant. Parents also worry about infants who strain or grunt excessively (often turning deep red) in the course of producing a soft stool of normal caliber. Manometric studies have documented the presence of a functioning rectoanal inhibitory reflex at birth, and infants exhibiting this behavior are likely attempting, unsuccessfully, to coordinate the voluntary with the involuntary components of defecation.

The truly constipated infant, who does require treatment, typically displays a pattern of straining associated with either the production of a desiccated plug of stool followed by loose stool or by the production of a consistently desiccated stool that has a pebbly consistency.

### Toddlers

Although parents of toddlers are usually aware of when their child is constipated, they frequently do not recognize stool withholding. During the act of withholding, the child may hide quietly, clinging to an inanimate object, while squeezing the buttocks together. Numerous variations of stool-withholding behavior exist, including crouching, dancing or walking on tiptoes, and crying out in anticipation of the pain. Not infrequently, these episodes are misinterpreted by the parents as valiant attempts to defecate, and they generate great concern. Eliciting a history of stool withholding is critical for both diagnostic and therapeutic purposes.

### Childhood

Once the child has attained privacy in the bathroom, parents are not likely to be involved in the toilet routine, and constipation becomes occult. The child often goes to the bathroom with a regular or increased frequency but during defecation passes only a small, hard piece of desiccated stool. Not infrequently, the child emerges from the bathroom not terribly bothered. The parent inquires, "Did you go?" The child answers, "Yes." Thus both parties are happy. This stooling pattern, known as incomplete evacuation, is common in school-age children and is punctuated episodically by the passage of massive bowel movements. Many children do not seem very bothered by their constipation and are brought in by their parents not for the constipation itself but rather for associated phenomena, such as soiling, recurrent abdominal pain, blood streaks seen on the stool, excessive flatus, or anorexia. Finally, pelvic floor dyssynergia seen in children with stool withholding can affect urinary voiding dynamics, predisposing some to enuresis or urinary tract infection. Box 11-4 lists features that support the diagnosis of functional constipation.

## ▶ EVALUATION

Functional constipation frequently can be diagnosed by history, physical examination, and therapeutic response to a comprehensive treatment regimen. The history should incorporate

BOX 11-4

## *Findings That Support the Diagnosis of Functional Constipation*

- Onset after infancy
- Presence of stool-withholding behavior
- Absence of red flags
- Episodic passage of large-caliber stools

the frequency, consistency, and caliber of the stools that the child passes, as well as the age of the child at the onset of constipation. The newborn history should specifically establish whether the child passed meconium in the first day of life. A history of the child's toilet-training experience and whether traumatic toileting experiences occurred is critical in toddlers and preschool-aged children. The diet history can establish whether the onset of constipation occurred concurrently with the transition to cow milk or with periods of high protein intake (excessive cow whole milk consumption).

Common complications of constipation should be assessed: fissures, bleeding, abdominal pain, anorexia, enuresis, and urinary tract infection. A history of distention and vomiting is explored because they are not caused by functional constipation. Eliciting a history suggesting stool withholding is critical because it strongly supports the diagnosis of functional constipation and should be addressed in the therapeutic plan. Details of prior evaluations and treatments should be explored, including over-the-counter medicines, home remedies, alternative therapies, and culturally specific therapies that can be incorporated in the treatment plan, if they pose no harm.

Specific questions should address the differential diagnosis. Symptoms of Hirschsprung disease, as well as endocrine, metabolic, and neurologic disease, should be sought. The possibility of an occult spinal process affecting the sacral nerves can be addressed by inquiring about any changes in the urinary voiding pattern (urinary stream or urinary continence) or in the child's gait. The family history covers heritable conditions in the differential diagnosis and a family history of functional constipation, which has been shown to have a heritable component. A developmental history may also be important.

On physical examination, the child's growth parameters, including recent growth velocity, should be normal. The child should appear well and not wasted or malnourished. The abdomen should not be distended, and the examination should establish the presence or absence of a fecal impaction in the lower quadrants or in the hypogastric area. The external examination of the perineal area is performed to establish normal placement of the anal orifice and to look for evidence of soiling, fissures, skin tags, and a normal anal wink in response to touch.

When a rectal examination can be done with the child's cooperation, it should be part of the evaluation. In most children who have functional constipation, desiccated stool is found in the rectal vault on rectal examination. For older children who have long-standing constipation and a megarectum, chronic rectal distention may efface the internal sphincter along the rectal wall, making the anal canal feel foreshortened. Children who soil from chronic constipation with a megarectum have only a sensory disorder; thus, the tone of the internal sphincter should be normal. The examiner should be alert during the digital examination for the rare situation in which an extrinsic mass is compressing the rectum. A patulous anus is indicative of a neurologic lesion or of sexual abuse involving the anus. Especially in infants, an empty rectum on digital examination raises the possibility of Hirschsprung disease, particularly in conjunction with an explosive gush of stool on withdrawal or a hard, impacted mass palpated in the pelvis or lower abdomen. Impactions in infancy are unusual and may indicate Hirschsprung disease. In the older child who has functional constipation, an empty rectum may be found occasionally if the child has just defecated. Nonetheless, the possibility of Hirschsprung disease should be considered carefully.

The evaluation should continue with an examination of the spine, looking for a dimple, hair tuft, or palpable vertebral deformity (signs of spina bifida occulta), and from this evaluation to a thorough neurologic examination that explicitly assesses the tone, strength, symmetry, and reflexes of the lower extremities and to an analysis of the patient's gait.

Routine laboratory tests are not indicated in evaluating for functional constipation.[5] In addition, a recent systematic review has shown that plain abdominal radiographs do not have significant diagnostic value.[15] Nonetheless, plain radiographs of the abdomen can be used selectively for confirmation that an abdominal mass appreciated on physical examination is indeed a fecal impaction.

Children thought to have Hirschsprung disease should be discussed with a consulting surgeon and radiologist to decide on the choice of initial diagnostic testing, keeping in mind that rectal biopsy is the gold standard. Box 11-5 presents red flags in constipation.

## ▶ TREATMENT

Treatment of constipation involves laxatives, parental education, diet, and behavioral modification. Consideration must be given to the age of the patient and the duration of symptoms. Whereas transient constipation of several days' duration typically can be managed with 1 to a few days of laxative use and dietary change, most patients who have functional constipation are affected for weeks to months before coming to attention and require a phased approach and months of treatment. Successful treatment of functional constipation in older children may even require 1 to 2 years of laxative therapy. Ultimately, the goals of treatment are to establish a pattern of soft bowel movements at a regular frequency (at least 3 per week), to wean the child from pharmacotherapy, and to have the child and family manage the problem on their own with diet and behavioral modification.

**BOX 11-5**

### *Red Flags in Childhood Constipation*

- Failure to thrive, weight loss, poor growth
- Vomiting
- Abdominal distention
- Persistent anal fissures, perianal disease
- Persistent blood in stool or guaiac-positive stool
- Delayed passage of meconium
- Weak urinary stream, diurnal enuresis

### Treatment of Infants

Before they are introduced to infant food, constipated infants can be treated by the addition to the diet of undigestible, osmotically active carbohydrates: either dark corn syrup or malt soup extract can be added to the formula in a dose of 2 to 6 teaspoons divided in several bottles per day. Once juice and infant food are introduced, apple or prune juice and fruits can be added to the diet. Infant glycerin suppositories can be used at the beginning of therapy to remove a desiccated rectal plug but should not be the mainstay of therapy because infants can become behaviorally conditioned to depend on rectal stimulation to initiate defecation. Infants should not receive mineral oil because of the risk for pneumonia from aspiration. Externally visible anal fissures should be treated with petroleum jelly. Two studies have established the efficacy of polyethylene glycol (PEG) in infants.[16,17] Infants whose constipation is refractory to these measures should be referred to a pediatric gastroenterologist.

### Treatment in Toddlers and Older Children

The treatment of established constipation is divided into 3 phases: (1) education and disimpaction, (2) maintenance, and (3) weaning. This method has been adopted widely by pediatric gastroenterologists and advocated in published guidelines.[5]

#### Education

The treatment of constipation begins with parental education regarding the pathogenesis of constipation. Particular focus is given to the concept that, once established, constipation frequently engenders withholding, which is self-perpetuating. Toddlers, in particular, require several months of laxative treatment that produces soft stools before they abandon this behavior. Parents should be instructed to ignore stool withholding events as they would a temper tantrum. At times when the child is not withholding, parents should talk directly to toddlers and engage them in the therapeutic program: "I want you to push the poo-poo out of your body; don't hold it in. That's how you will get better, and it will stop hurting!"

Physicians should address the widely held misconceptions that long-term laxative use in childhood is not safe or engenders laxative dependence. This fear, compounded by a general reluctance to medicate children for what is widely perceived as a transient problem, almost always leads to premature discontinuation of therapy. In fact, innumerable studies have established that nonstimulant laxatives such as mineral oil, milk of magnesia, PEG, and lactulose do not result in dependence. On the other hand, experts discourage the prolonged use of stimulant laxatives (Senna, Bisacodyl),[5,18] but the limited use of Senna, an anthraquinone-stimulant laxative, is acceptable.

#### Disimpaction

Treatment begins with disimpaction in the toddler or child who has had months to years of symptoms or an impaction on examination. For children attending school, disimpaction treatment (Table 11-2) should be deferred until the weekend; in the interim, the child can be treated with mineral oil to lubricate the impacted stool. Enemas once a day for 3 to 6 days are simple and effective and, with some important caveats, are safe. Dose guidelines should be followed, and the child should be brought to medical attention in the rare event of failure to stool following an enema. Sodium phosphate enemas are contraindicated in children who weigh less than 10 kg, in those who have any cardiac or renal impairment or electrolyte disorders, and in those who may have any form of intestinal obstruction.[19] In 4- to 11-year-old children, a comparison of daily oral PEG for 6 days versus daily enemas for 6 days showed equal efficacy in resolving fecal impactions. The choice of enemas versus the oral route should be made with the child and family's input.[20]

The goal of disimpaction is to remove all the hard-formed stools throughout the colon. A follow-up telephone call after 2 to 3 days can ascertain whether the child is still passing hard stools. Any questions about whether the disimpaction phase of treatment is complete should prompt a revisit for an abdominal and rectal examination or an abdominal radiograph. Last, children who have extremely hard or treatment-resistant impactions can be admitted for nasogastric administration of a PEG solution or surgical disimpaction. Failure to achieve a thorough disimpaction, a common therapeutic mistake, undermines successful treatment because laxatives given in maintenance doses do not penetrate or remove the impaction. For the same reason, fiber is withheld during the disimpaction phase of treatment.

## Maintenance

The maintenance phase of treatment follows disimpaction and should incorporate laxative use and dietary and behavioral advice. Maintenance doses of laxatives are listed in Table 11-2. Telephone follow-up within 2 to 3 days of starting therapy is essential so that the laxative can be titrated to a dose that induces a daily soft bowel movement. Results

**Table 11-2**
**Regimens for Older Toddlers and Children Who Have Chronic Constipation[a]**

| LAXATIVE DOSAGES | |
|---|---|
| **DISIMPACTION** | |
| Enema | |
| Hypertonic sodium phosphate[a,b] | 3 mL/kg/dose, once daily via rectum for 3–6 days, maximum 135 mL |
| Mineral oil | 30–60 mL, once daily via rectum for 1–6 days |
| Oral | |
| Polyethylene glycol, electrolyte free | 1.5 g/kg/day, maximum 100 g for 3–6 days |
| Mineral oil | 30 mL/year of age to maximum 8 oz twice daily for 3 days |
| Polyethylene glycol with electrolytes | 10–40 mL/kg/hr, via nasogastric tube (maximum 2 L/hr) until stool effluent clear |
| **MAINTENANCE** | |
| Polyethylene glycol, electrolyte free powder | 0.8–1.5 g/kg/day |
| Mineral oil | 1–3 mL/kg/day |
| Milk of magnesia | 1–3 mL/kg/day |
| Lactulose 10 g/15 mL | 1–2 mL/kg/day |
| Senna syrup 218 mg/5 mL[b] | 10–20 mg/kg/dose po qhs |

[a]Not recommended for children younger than 2 years of age.
[b]See maximum doses in the *Physicians' Desk Reference*.

of a Cochrane review support both PEG and mineral oil as superior to other agents for the treatment of constipation.[21] If mineral oil is used, then it should not be prescribed to children younger than 2 years or to children who are at risk for pulmonary aspiration.[22] PEG has gained wide use for the treatment of functional constipation. PEG, an osmotic laxative, is a polymer of ethylene glycol that is not absorbed or fermented by colonic bacteria. One appeal of PEG is that it is a fairly tasteless, water-soluble powder that can be disguised when mixed into a child's drink. Pediatric studies of PEG have established clinical tolerance, effective dose, and the absence of unanticipated or serious adverse effects in small groups of study subjects.[23,24]

A recent systematic review of nonpharmacologic therapies for childhood constipation concluded that apart from an increase in fiber intake, other therapies such as an increase in fluid intake, the addition of probiotics/prebiotics to the diet, an increase in physical activity, and yoga are not studied to the point at which they can be offered as evidence-based recommendations.[25] These therapies deserve further study because they may be beneficial and are associated with little harm. The addition of dietary fiber is a widely advocated adjunct to the treatment of childhood constipation, and a recent randomized controlled trial has shown benefits of a fiber supplement when prescribed with a laxative.[26] Alternatively, dietary changes that increase the child's fiber intake can be made and include the introduction of whole-grain breads and cereals and increasing the child's fruit and vegetable intake.

Simple behavioral advice has been a mainstay of treatment recommendations. For toddlers, the focus is on replacing stool-withholding behavior with deliberate attempts to defecate. Toilet-training efforts are deferred until the child stops withholding. For older children, a behavioral modification program of sitting on the toilet for 5 to 10 minutes after meals to capitalize on the gastrocolic reflex is recommended, with success rewarded by the use of a star-chart system: the child should be rewarded for the targeted behavior (sitting). The physician is responsible for titrating the laxative dose to achieve the desired effect (a soft bowel movement every day), which requires an active partnership with the child and parents, who need to report to the physician frequently. Referral to a child behavior specialist or psychiatrist is warranted when toileting is the focus of a power struggle or when a significant mental health problem complicates the treatment regimen.

## Weaning From Maintenance Therapy

Weaning, as opposed to abrupt cessation, of laxative therapy is the next phase of treatment. Successful weaning can occur following 6 to 12 weeks of maintenance treatment in some toddlers but may not be possible for 6 to 12 months in older children. Typically, the daily laxative dose is decreased to 75%, 50%, and 25% of the initial dose over successive months, or the full dose is given every second day for 6 to 8 weeks and then every third day for another 6 to 8 weeks. Efforts to increase the child's fiber intake and to comply with the behavioral program are redoubled during weaning. Older school-aged children are encouraged to practice self-monitoring of the frequency and adequacy of their bowel movements, and a rescue plan for an enema, a suppository, or a dose of stimulant laxative must be in place for a transient relapse (no stool for longer than 3 days) that may occur during weaning. The inability to wean from laxatives after 12 months of therapy is not uncommon in functional constipation but may reasonably justify referral to a pediatric gastroenterologist. Box 11-6 presents common reasons for treatment failure of functional constipation.

BOX 11-6

## *Common Reasons for Treatment Failure of Functional Constipation*

- Reliance on dietary advice alone
- Inadequate disimpaction
- Failure to escalate laxative dose to achieve 1 to 2 soft stools per day
- Failure to address widely held notion that laxatives are addictive, leading to premature discontinuation
- Relying on dietary fiber alone

Remaining optimistic and involved at this point is important because improvement beyond 12 months of therapy is well documented.[4,27,28]

## When to Refer

- Abnormal studies
- Findings that are inconsistent with functional constipation (growth failure, distention, vomiting, bleeding)
- Significant behavioral, emotional, and parenting problems complicating treatment
- Refractory to comprehensive treatment regimen

## When to Admit

- Constipation associated with obstruction or enterocolitis
- Failure of disimpaction as an outpatient

### *TOOLS FOR PRACTICE*

#### Engaging Patient and Family

- *Constipation and Your Child* (handout), American Academy of Pediatrics (patiented.solutions.aap.org)
- *Constipation* (Web page), American Academy of Pediatrics (www.healthychildren.org/English/health-issues/conditions/abdominal/Pages/Constipation.aspx)
- *Everyone Poops* (book), Kane/Miller Book Publishers
- *Guide to Toilet Training* (book), American Academy of Pediatrics (shop.aap.org)
- *Toilet Training* (Web page), American Academy of Pediatrics (www.healthychildren.org/English/ages-stages/toddler/toilet-training/Pages/default.aspx)
- *Toilet Training* (handout), American Academy of Pediatrics (patiented.solutions.aap.org)

#### Medical Decision Support

- *Constipation in Infants and Children: Evaluation and Treatment* (guideline), *Journal of Pediatric Gastroenterology and Nutrition,* Vol 43, Issue 3, 2006

### *AAP POLICY STATEMENTS*

American Academy of Pediatrics Subcommittee on Chronic Abdominal Pain. Chronic abdominal pain in children. *Pediatrics.* 2005;115(3):e370–e381 (pediatrics.aappublications.org/content/115/3/e370.full)

American Academy of Pediatrics Subcommittee on Chronic Abdominal Pain. Chronic abdominal pain in children. *Pediatrics.* 2005;115(3):812–815 (pediatrics.aappublications.org/content/115/3/812.full)

## REFERENCES


1. Maffei HVL, Moreira FL, Oliveira WM Jr, et al. Defining constipation in childhood and adolescence: from Rome, via Boston, to Paris and…? *J Pediatr Gastroenterol Nutr.* 2005;41:485–486
2. Issenman RM, Hewson S, Pirhonen D, Taylor W, Tirosh A. Are chronic digestive complaints the result of abnormal dietary patterns? Diet and digestive complaints in children at 22 and 40 months of age. *Am J Dis Child.* 1987;141:679–682
3. Taitz LS, Wales JK, Urwin OM, Molnar D. Factors associated with outcome in management of defecation disorders. *Arch Dis Child.* 1986;61:472–477
4. Loening-Baucke V. Chronic constipation in children. *Gastroenterology.* 1993;105:1557–1564
5. Baker SS, Liptak GS, Colletti RB, et al. Constipation in infants and children: evaluation and treatment. A medical position statement of the North American Society for Pediatric Gastroenterology and Nutrition. *J Pediatr Gastroenterol Nutr.* 1999;29:612–626
6. Palit S, Lunniss PJ, Scott SM. The physiology of human defecation. *Dig Dis Sci.* 2012;57:1445–1464
7. Croffie JM, Fitzgerald JF. Idiopathic constipation. In: Walker WA, Goulet OJ, Kleinman RE, et al, eds. *Pediatric Gastrointestinal Disease.* 4th ed. St. Louis, MO: Mosby; 2003
8. Loening-Baucke V. Biofeedback training in children with functional constipation. A critical review. *Dig Dis Sci.* 1996;41:65–71
9. Partin JC, Hamill SK, Fischel JE, et al. Painful defecation and fecal soiling in children. *Pediatrics.* 1992;103:1007–1009
10. Benninga MA, Büller HA, Tytgat GN, et al. Colonic transit time in constipated children: does pediatric slow-transit constipation exist? *J Pediatr Gastroenterol Nutr.* 1996;23:241–251
11. Morrais MB, Vitolo MR, Aguirre AC, et al. Measurement of low dietary fiber intake as a risk factor for chronic constipation. *J Pediatr Gastroenterol Nutr.* 1999;29:132–135
12. Leape LL, Ramenofsky ML. Anterior ectopic anus: a common cause of constipation in children. *J Pediatr Surg.* 1978;13:627–630
13. Iacono G, Cavataio F, Montalto G, et al. Intolerance of cow's milk and chronic constipation in children. *N Engl J Med.* 1998;339:1100–1104
14. Daher S, Sol D, Nuspitz CK, et al. Cow's milk protein intolerance and chronic constipation in children. *Pediatr Allergy Immunol.* 2000;12:399–342
15. Reuchlin-Vroklage LM, Bierma-Zeinstra S, Benninga MA, Berger MY. Diagnostic value of abdominal radiography in constipated children: a systematic review. *Arch Pediatr Adolesc Med.* 2005;159:671–678
16. Michail S, Gendy E, Preud'Homme D, Mezoff A. Polyethylene glycol for constipation in children younger than eighteen months old. *J Pediatr Gastroenterol Nutr.* 2004;39:197–199
17. Loening-Baucke V, Krishna R, Pashankar DS. Polyethylene glycol 3350 without electrolytes for the treatment of functional constipation in infants and toddlers. *J Pediatr Gastroenterol Nutr.* 2004;39: 536–539
18. Benninga MA, Voskuijl WP, Taminiau JA. Childhood constipation: is there new light in the tunnel? *J Pediatr Gastroenterol Nutr.* 2004;39:448–464
19. Harrington L, Schuh S. Complications of Fleet enema administration and suggested guidelines for use in the pediatric emergency department. *Pediatr Emerg Care.* 1997;13:225–226
20. Bekkali NL, van den Berg MM, Dijkgraaf MG, et al. Rectal fecal impaction treatment in childhood constipation: enemas versus high doses oral PEG. *Pediatrics.* 2009;124:e1108–e1115
21. Gordon M, Naidoo k, Akobeng AK, Thomas AG. Osmotic and stimulant laxatives for the management of childhood constipation. *Cochrane Database Syst Rev.* 2012;7:CD009118
22. Hari R, Baudla R, Davis SH, et al. Lipoid pneumonia: a silent complication of mineral oil aspiration. *Pediatrics.* 1999;103:e19

23. Youssef NN, Peters JM, Henderson W, et al. Dose response of PEG 3350 for the treatment of childhood fecal impaction. *J Pediatr.* 2002;141:410–414
24. Bell EA, Wall GC. Pediatric constipation therapy using guidelines and polyethylene glycol 3350. *Ann Pharmacother.* 2004;38:686–693
25. Tabbers MM, Boluyt N, Berger MY, Benninga MA. Nonpharmacologic treatments for childhood constipation: systematic review. *Pediatrics.* 2011;128:753–761
26. Loening-Baucke V, Miele E, Staiano A. Fiber (glucomannan) is beneficial in the treatment of childhood constipation. *Pediatrics.* 2004;113:259–264
27. Pijpers MA, Bongers ME, Benninga MA, Berger MY. Functional constipation in children: a systematic review on prognosis and predictive factors. *J Pediatr Gastroenterol Nutr.* 2010;50:256–268
28. Nolan T, Debelle G, Oberklaid F, Coffey C. Randomised trial of laxatives in treatment of childhood encopresis. *Lancet.* 1991;338:523–527
29. Dupont C, Leluyer B, Maamri N, et al. Double-blind randomized evaluation of clinical and biological tolerance of polyethylene glycol 4000 versus lactulose in constipated children. *J Pediatr Gastroenterol Nutr.* 2005;41:625–633
30. Erickson BA, Austin C, Cooper CS, et al. Polyethylene glycol 3350 for constipation in children with dysfunctional elimination. *J Urol.* 2003;107:1518–1520
31. Hyams J, Colletti R, Faure C, et al. Functional gastrointestinal disorders: Working Group Report of the First World Congress of Pediatric Gastroenterology, Hepatology, and Nutrition. *J Pediatr Gastroenterol Nutr.* 2002;35(Suppl 2):S110–S117
32. Liangthanasarn P, Nemet D, Sufi R, Nussbaum E. Therapy for pulmonary aspiration of a polyethylene glycol solution. *J Pediatr Gastroenterol Nutr.* 2003;37:192–194
33. McClung HJ, Boyne LJ, Linsheid T, et al. Is combination therapy for encopresis nutritionally safe? *Pediatrics.* 1993;91:591–594

# Chapter 12

# Cough

*Michael G. Marcus, MD*

## ▶ INTRODUCTION

Cough is among the most common complaints of children. Although generally resulting from acute viral infections and therefore self-limited, cough may be the harbinger of a more serious problem. Because cough can be exceedingly disruptive to the child and family, it can lead to significant anxiety for all involved parties. Allaying this anxiety through appropriate diagnosis and management is of prime importance to the primary care physician.

## ▶ PATHOPHYSIOLOGIC FEATURES

Cough can be described as a forceful exhalation. Its primary purpose is to facilitate the removal of inhaled irritants and secretions from the airway. The cough reflex can be triggered by stimulation of the cough receptors located at all levels of the respiratory tract, beginning at the sinus level and extending caudally throughout the respiratory tree and ending at the terminal bronchi. It also includes the auricular branch of the vagus nerve (Arnold nerve), which carries afferent impulses from the concha of the ear and posterior portion of the external auditory canal. Impulses from these cough receptors travel through the cranial nerve afferent pathway to the medullary cough center. The reflexive efferent response of this activation causes the coordinated activity of glottic closure and diaphragmatic, chest wall, abdominal, and pelvic floor contraction, resulting in cough.[1]

The cough sequence can be divided into 3 classic phases. The first phase, termed the inspiratory phase, results in a deep inspiration ending in glottic closure. During the short second phase, termed the compressive phase, intrathoracic pressure increases as a result of coordinated contraction of the expiratory muscles. With the expiratory third phase, the glottis opens rapidly, leading to the sudden, sometimes explosive, release of the pent-up intrathoracic air (ie, cough). Coupled with this third phase, secretions and irritants are expelled from the airway. Incomplete or inefficient removal of these materials will result in recurrence of the cough sequence, as will ongoing irritation or inflammation.

## ▶ CLASSIFICATION

Many classification schemes for cough have been developed over the years, and each has its benefits and limitations.[2] Ultimately, any useful classification scheme must help in planning an efficient and successful evaluation and management plan. When classifying cough, 2 basic questions need to be addressed. First is whether the cough is acute or chronic

(>4 weeks' duration), with chronic cough likely requiring a more extensive evaluation plan. The second question is whether the cough is triggered by upper, lower, or combined airway pathology (although the effect of the upper airway on the etiology of cough is somewhat controversial), and whether it is specific or nonspecific. This is not always apparent, especially in younger children, but is critical to determine to minimize unnecessary testing, treatment, or both.

## ▶ DIFFERENTIAL DIAGNOSIS

In considering a functional differential diagnosis, the physician should try to answer the above 2 questions on the initial assessment. In this regard, the character of the cough can sometimes be helpful, with *croupy, throaty,* and *honking (foghorn)* coughs being more likely to originate in the upper airway. However, young children with asthma (clearly a disease of the lower airways) may initially exhibit a croupy cough, presumably from the physiologic narrowing of the subglottic space in children younger than 4 years.

At the other extreme, although a productive cough with expectoration of sputum is classically associated with lower airway inflammation (eg, pneumonia, asthma), children with severe chronic sinusitis (a disease of the upper airway) will often cough and expectorate or swallow thick sputum, which may at times even be tinged with blood. Therefore, cough character, although helpful, should not limit the differential diagnosis. A variety of qualities attributed to cough character have been described that can be useful starting points in the evaluation of cough, including paroxysmal for pertussis; staccato for *Chlamydia* infection; barking for laryngotracheal infection; throat clearing for postnasal secretions; and honking for habit cough syndrome.[3] History and pattern of illness progression are crucial for putting these cough qualities into perspective. For example, cough that occurs only during the daytime, increases with attention, and does not limit or change with physical activity is more likely habit cough syndrome. However, such a cough can also indicate tracheal pathology if it does not possess all of these characteristics. In contrast, if the cough clearly increases with activity and limits the child from participating in desired physical activities, then asthma is a likely diagnosis. Night cough is frequently seen with asthma; however, when nasal symptoms are present it could also suggest allergy or sinusitis (or both) as triggers; cough during feeding suggests swallowing dysfunction or tracheoesophageal fistula with aspiration; and cough after feeding with spitting up, retching, or arching of the back suggests gastroesophageal (GE) reflux.[4]

Age of onset is also an important feature in planning a workup. Chronic or recurrent cough that begins in early infancy, especially in children younger than 3 months, suggests a congenital or anatomic origin and clearly requires a more aggressive evaluation. These children are also at risk for protracted bacterial bronchitis, although the effect of this entity is still being delineated. Similarly, an aggressive approach should be considered when cough begins relatively suddenly, especially in toddlers, since this might suggest foreign-body aspiration. In both of these scenarios visualization of the airway using bronchoscopy should be considered early in the evaluation process. Cough beginning at more than 6 months of age may suggest airways hyperreactivity, and a therapeutic trial of treatment with a beta-2 agonist may be a reasonable first step. Cough beginning relatively suddenly in adolescents, especially at times of psychosocial stress, might indicate a psychogenic origin.[5–7]

Classifying cough in this way, using key historical information, can provide a useful starting point in developing a differential diagnosis. Studies have shown that an organized approach to the assessment and management of cough can greatly improve diagnostic and treatment success.[8,9]

## ▶ EVALUATION

### History

#### Personal and Family History

The history from a patient complaining of cough should begin with an accurate description of the cough, with a focus on the pattern and progression of symptoms. The duration of cough; the frequency of discrete cough episodes; quiet periods between cough (daily cough vs days or weeks between cough episodes); and the quality, timing, and triggers of the cough are all important pieces of information to help make an accurate diagnosis. Associated fever suggests a respiratory tract infection; cough worsening with exercise suggests asthma; and night cough in the absence of any other daytime symptomatology may suggest a postnasal drip, as with allergy or sinusitis. Past history is also important. Previous episodes, especially with a recurrent pattern of spring and fall seasonal variation, may suggest allergy, and chronic cough with poor weight gain suggests a more severe systemic illness such as cystic fibrosis or an immune deficiency. Family history can be especially helpful with more chronic symptoms. A family history of allergies, atopy or asthma makes these diagnoses far more likely in the child with chronic or recurrent cough, given that a history of asthma or atopy in first-degree relatives confers a 2- to 4-fold increase in risk of asthma in the child.[10] Similarly, a family history of early childhood death related to infection makes an immune deficiency more likely.

#### Neonatal History

Neonatal history is similarly important because preterm infants are more likely than full-term infants to have persistent airways hyperreactivity, laryngotracheomalacia, and GE reflux. Infants with poor Apgar scores, perinatal hypoxia, or a difficult postnatal course may have central nervous system sequelae and therefore have suck or swallow dysfunction, increasing the risk of aspiration. Finally, associated congenital abnormalities (eg, diaphragmatic hernia) may result in pulmonary hypoplasia, leading to chronic respiratory dysfunction and recurrent pneumonia.

#### Environmental History

Environmental history is also important in determining the source of cough. Children who live in households with smokers have significantly more respiratory infections and asthma symptoms than children not exposed to secondhand smoke. Exposure to molds from household water leaks, decaying garbage, vegetation or ineffective cleaning of bathroom tile; dust mites from mattresses, pillows, stuffed animals, or forced air heating systems; and roaches, mice, and household pets all increase the risk of allergy and asthma symptoms.[11] Exposure to other children through school, child care, babysitters, or school-aged siblings all make recurrent respiratory tract infections far more common. Even thirdhand smoke, residual chemicals from tobacco use which remain on surfaces such as walls, clothing, and even hair, may play a role in chronic cough.

## Physical Examination

The physical examination plays a critical role in pinpointing the trigger for the cough and identifying signs of a more serious underlying or chronic condition. A nasal speculum examination can help determine the color and quality of the nasal mucosa, as well as the presence or absence of nasal secretions. Inflamed nasal mucosa, coupled with thick secretions, suggests rhinitis; when the symptoms have been prolonged, sinusitis can be considered. Associated maxillary, ethmoid or frontal sinus tenderness and pharyngeal drip with a cobblestone appearance (lymphoid hyperplasia) further support the diagnosis of sinusitis.[12] Halitosis may also be present. In contrast, pale, boggy, swollen nasal mucosa makes allergic rhinitis more likely. Associated atopic symptoms, such as eczema, further support this diagnosis. Other features of the pharyngeal examination can also be helpful. Chronic pharyngeal inflammation, in the absence of other signs of acute infection, suggests GE reflux. Oral mucosal ulcerations or thrush suggests an immune deficiency. When pertussis is a consideration, cough paroxysms triggered by a tongue depressor support the diagnosis. Signs of an acute infectious process, such as fever, adenopathy, pharyngitis, or rash, are important to appreciate but do not necessarily rule out a predisposing condition, especially when the pattern of illness suggests chronicity or frequent recurrence. A thorough assessment of other body systems is important in judging whether a more global workup is necessary. Growth failure, poor developmental milestone achievement, clubbing, heart murmurs, hepatosplenomegaly, and chronic lymphadenopathy are all potential clues to a more severe underlying process.

A thorough examination of the respiratory system is critical in making an accurate diagnosis. Stridor and inspiratory rhonchi or wheeze suggest upper and large central airway disease, whereas rales, expiratory rhonchi, and wheeze are indicative of lower or distal airway inflammation. Similarly, a change in the quality of air exchange can be an early finding in asthma and other diseases of airways obstruction.[13,14]

An accurate lower airway examination depends on the cooperation of the patient. Wheeze and distal airway sounds can be masked by a patient's vocalization or crying. Similarly, force of airflow insufficient to uncover milder changes may mask both inspiratory and expiratory findings in infants and children who do not take deep breaths on command. Every effort should be made to place the child at ease during the examination. Game playing, such as blowing on a feather or blowing up a balloon, can be helpful. In younger children and infants, the examiner can mimic a forced expiratory maneuver by firmly but gently compressing the anteroposterior chest wall inward once the child has begun voluntary exhalation. This approach will frequently uncover milder degrees of wheezing previously not appreciated with passive breathing. The examiner should allow the child to begin exhalation passively before performing this maneuver to ensure that the glottis is relaxed and the procedure proceeds safely and effectively.

## Laboratory Evaluation

### Hematologic Tests

Acute cough rarely needs extensive laboratory assessment. A detailed history and physical examination are usually sufficient to reach an accurate presumptive diagnosis, and response to empiric therapy will confirm this assessment. In cases where this approach does not lead to a resolution of symptoms, or when the cough is either recurrent or chronic, an organized approach using a standardized algorithm has proven to be very helpful in identifying the cause and optimizing treatment, thereby shortening the duration of cough. A complete blood cell count (CBC) with differential may help distinguish a bacterial from a viral cause if infection is suspected. However, localized infections such as sinusitis are not always accompanied by an elevated white blood cell count with a shift to the left. The total eosinophil count on the CBC may be an important clue to atopy. Similarly, an elevated IgE level or positive nasal smear for eosinophils would further corroborate the diagnosis of allergy and suggest the possibility of asthma. Although increased polymorphonuclear leukocytes on a nasal smear may suggest rhinosinusitis, the result is difficult to quantify, and the test may be misleading. Ultimately, if sinusitis is suspected, empiric therapy should be initiated based on history and physical examination, and response to therapy should be monitored.[12,15] Advanced imaging techniques (computed tomography) can be considered in complicated cases.

## Gastroesophageal Tests

When aspiration or GE reflux (although the effect of GE reflux as a trigger for cough has not been clearly proven) is a consideration, a barium swallow (modified for aspiration and standard for GE reflux) may be useful. Although barium swallow is of limited use in diagnosing GE reflux (approximately 40% false negative), looking for anatomic causes related to esophageal abnormalities such as partial obstruction, tracheoesophageal fistulae, and vascular rings, is important in infants. Monitoring with a pH probe is the gold standard for diagnosing GE reflux; however, many experts suggest a period of empiric therapy if reflux is suggested by history and physical examination findings, with the pH probe being reserved for patients in whom primary empiric treatment fails.[16–18]

## Pulmonary Function Tests

Early use of pulmonary function testing can be very helpful in making the distinction between upper and lower airways disease and differentiating obstructive from restrictive changes. Children must be old enough to exhale fully and inhale forcefully on command, and the test should be reproducible to ensure accuracy and reliability of results.[19]

Flattening of the inspiratory portion of the flow-volume loop suggest upper airway obstruction, whereas changes in the ratio of the forced expiratory volume in the first 1 second to the forced vital capacity of the lungs ($FEV_1$/FVC) or the forced midexpiratory flow rate over the middle half of the FVC (FEF 25%–75%) indicate airways obstruction consistent with distal disease. Reversibility of these changes (20% improvement) with a β-2 agonist confirms the diagnosis of asthma and leads to effective therapy.

In younger children, 3 to 6 years old, impulse oscillometry may be used to assess airways resistance and response to bronchodilators. This can be helpful in children too young to perform formal spirometry. Infant pulmonary function testing can be used in even younger ages; however, the results are less reliable and require a high level of expertise to be performed accurately.

## Other Tests

Chest radiograph is important when cough is chronic and no clear diagnosis is evident on first assessment. Other tests, such as the sweat test, tuberculin skin test, immunologic studies, and alpha-1 antitrypsin levels (although these patients characteristically present with lung disease in the third or fourth decade of life), can all be useful in the proper clinical setting. Bronchoscopy can be useful to diagnose abnormalities of both the upper and lower airways and should be considered in patients with chronic symptoms not responsive to empiric treatment. It is especially helpful in confirming the diagnosis of protracted purulent bronchitis and directing appropriate antimicrobial therapy.[20] Furthermore, it is the test of choice when a foreign body or chronic aspiration are considered likely. In cases in which an upper airways origin is likely, flexible bronchoscopy (vs laryngoscopy) is still preferred to make the definitive diagnosis since lesions below the vocal cords up to the thoracic inlet can still be the cause of upper airway symptomatology.[21,22]

## ▶ TREATMENT

Once the history and physical examination have led to an initial assessment, the fact that cough is a symptom of an underlying condition should be discussed with the patient and family. Treatment of the underlying disorder (if necessary) should always be the prime focus.[23–26] Empiric therapy, based on primary assessment, can be a reasonable starting point. Judicious use of laboratory testing, as previously discussed, can be helpful in confirming the diagnosis and allaying parental anxiety. Furthermore, in some conditions, cough is an important component of the body's natural response to the primary illness, and suppressing the cough in the absence of effective therapy of the primary disorder may actually worsen the problem.

Treatment of the underlying disorders causing cough is discussed in other sections of this book; this chapter is limited to a review of medications used to treat cough itself. The decision to use a cough medicine as an adjunct to the treatment of the primary disease is left to the primary care physician and family. When cough is limiting or otherwise debilitating the patient, symptomatic treatment may be attempted; however numerous studies question whether over-the-counter cough preparations offer any significant clinical benefit.[27–30] In addition these cough and cold medications should not be given to children younger than 4 years because serious and potentially life-threatening side effects can occur from their use.[31,32] Finally, several studies have shown that honey may be beneficial in children older than 2 years of age.[33,34]

### *Expectorants*

Expectorants such as guaifenesin (formerly known as glyceryl guaiacolate) may be used in an attempt to make secretions more fluid and reduce sputum thickness, however the effectiveness of this treatment has been called into question.[35] This therapeutic approach may be useful when drainage of secretions is important, as with sinusitis. Because expectorants work by increasing the fluid content of secretions, water is probably the most effective expectorant. Saline nose sprays can make secretions more fluid and easily cleared by the patient and systemic hydration, but not overhydration, should always be optimized. Despite widespread use, expectorants have not been shown to decrease cough in children. Other older expectorants, such as potassium iodide and ammonium chloride, are no longer prescribed to children because of their adverse effects when used at effective doses.

## Mucolytic Agents

Acetylcysteine was previously used as a mucolytic agent to help liquefy thick secretions, especially in diseases such as cystic fibrosis; however, its propensity for inducing airway reactivity and inflammation has lately made it less popular.[36,37]

## Cough Suppressants

Cough suppressants, which can be divided into peripheral and centrally acting agents, can be effective in transiently decreasing cough severity and frequency. Peripheral agents include demulcents (eg, throat lozenges), which soothe the throat, and topical anesthetics, which can be sprayed or swallowed. Topical agents block the cough receptors, but their effects are short-lived because oral secretions rapidly wash them away. Centrally acting cough suppressants, including both narcotic and nonnarcotic medications, suppress the cough reflex at the brain stem level. The narcotic agent most commonly used in children is codeine. Although it has been shown to be effective in adults, studies on its safety and efficacy in children are lacking. Furthermore, data from adults should not be extrapolated to children, particularly those younger than 2 years, because the metabolic pathway for clearance of codeine is immature in infants. In older children, codeine should still be avoided and only used in extreme cases and with very clear instructions because of the unpredictable and potentially dangerous variation of its metabolism in the pediatric population. Other agents, such as hydrocodone, have no demonstrated advantage and pose a greater risk of dependency. Dextromethorphan (the dextro-isomer of codeine) is the most commonly used nonnarcotic antitussive; and despite data from adults, evidence of efficacy for children is lacking.

## Decongestants

Decongestants such as pseudoephedrine can be used either topically or systemically to decrease nasal mucosal swelling. Decongestants can also facilitate sinus drainage by decreasing sinus ostia obstruction, and may work well in combination with expectorants to optimize treatment of chronic sinusitis. Care should be taken in the use of these agents because they have been shown to lead to tachyarrhythmias in individuals who use them in excess. In addition, these agents have not been studied in children and should be avoided in children younger than 2 years. Multiple reviews of the data from children between 2 and 6 years old also show lack of efficacy combined with a risk of side effects in this age group. It is therefore recommended that these agents not be used in children younger than 6 years.

## Antihistamines

Antihistamines, which can be helpful in the treatment of cough triggered by allergy, have minimal effect when cough is the result of viral or bacterial infection and may actually be detrimental because they can increase the thickness of secretions. First-generation $H_1$-receptor antagonists may decrease nasal drip by exerting an anticholinergic effect. Additionally, diphenhydramine may have a modest direct effect on the medullary cough center. The clinical benefits of these agents are unclear.[38]

## When to Refer

- Cough persists despite adequate therapy of primary disease
- Cough thought to be from hyperreactive airways is not easily reversible with β-2 agonist
- Cough recurs more frequently than every 6 to 8 weeks
- Cough associated with failure to thrive
- Cough associated with other systemic illness

## When to Admit

- Patient has respiratory distress
- Infant is unable to feed
- Cough is associated with bacterial pneumonia not responsive to oral antibiotic trial

### *TOOLS FOR PRACTICE*

**Engaging Patient and Family**

- *Cover Your Cough* (flyers and posters), Centers for Disease Control and Prevention (www.cdc.gov/flu/protect/covercough.htm)

**Medical Decision Support**

- *Managing Cough as a Defense Mechanism and as a Symptom: A Consensus Panel Report of the American College of Chest Physicians* (article), *Chest*, Vol 142, Issue 2, 1998 (journal.publications.chestnet.org/article.aspx?articleid=1073794)
- *A Cough Algorithm for Chronic Cough in Children: A Multicenter, Randomized Controlled Study* (article), *Pediatrics*, Vol 131, Issue 5, 2013 (pediatrics.aappublications.org/content/131/5/e1576)

### *AAP POLICY STATEMENTS*

American Academy of Pediatrics Committee on Drugs. Use of codeine- and dextromethorphan-containing cough remedies in children. *Pediatrics.* 1997;99(6):918–920. Reaffirmed October 2006 (pediatrics.aappublications.org/content/99/6/918.full)

Wald ER, Applegate KE, Bordley C, et al. Clinical practice guidelines for the diagnosis and management of acute bacterial sinusitis in children aged 1 to 18 years. *Pediatrics.* 2013;132(1):e262–e280 (pediatrics.aappublications.org/content/132/1/e262.full)

### *REFERENCES*

1. Chang AB, Phelan PD, Sawyer SM, Robertson CF. Airway hyperresponsiveness and cough-receptor sensitivity in children with recurrent cough. *Am J Respir Crit Care Med.* 1997;155:1935–1939
2. Irwin RJ, Cloutier F, Gold H, et al. Managing cough as a defense mechanism and as a symptom: a consensus panel report of the American College of Chest Physicians. *Chest.* 1998;114(2):133S–181S
3. Chang AB, Gaffney JT, Eastburn MM, et al. Cough quality in children: a comparison of subjective vs. bronchoscopic findings. *Respir Res.* 2005;6:3
4. Callahan CW. Etiology of chronic cough in a population of children referred to a pediatric pulmonologist. *J Am Board Fam Pract.* 1996;51:630–631
5. Chang AB, Powell CV. Non-specific cough in children: diagnosis and treatment. *Hosp Med.* 1998;59:680–684
6. Doull IJ, Williams AA, Freezer NJ, Holgate ST. Descriptive study of cough, wheeze and school absence in childhood. *Thorax.* 1996;51:630–631
7. Brooke AM, Lambert PC, Burton PR, et al. Recurrent cough: natural history and significance in infancy and early childhood. *Pulmonology.* 1998;26:256–261

8. Chang AB, Glomb WB. Guidelines for evaluating chronic cough in pediatrics: ACCP evidence-based clinical practice guidelines. *Chest.* 2006;129:260S–283S
9. Chang AB, Robertson CF, Van Asperen PP, et al. A multicenter study on chronic cough in children: burden and etiologies based on a standardized management pathway. *Chest.* 2012;142:943–950
10. Burke W, Fesinmeyer M, Reed K, Hampson L, Carlsten C. Family history as a predictor of asthma risk. *Am J Prev Med.* 2003;24:160–169
11. Wilson NW, Robinson NP, Hogan MB. Cockroach and other inhalant allergies in infantile asthma. *Ann Allergy Asthma Immunol.* 1999;83:27–30
12. Steel RW. Rhinosinusitis in children. *Curr Allergy Asthma Rep.* 2006;6:508–512
13. Faniran AO, Peat JK, Woolcock AJ. Persistent cough: is it asthma? *Arch Dis Child.* 1998;79:411–414
14. Wright AL, Holberg CJ, Morgan WJ, et al. Recurrent cough in childhood and its relation to asthma. *Am J Respir Crit Care Med.* 1996;153:1259–1265
15. Wald ER, Applegate KE, Bordley C, et al. Clinical practice guidelines for the diagnosis and management of acute bacterial sinusitis in children aged 1 to 18 years. *Pediatrics.* 2013;132(1):e262–e280
16. Chawla S, Seth D, Mahajan P, et al. Gastroesophageal reflux disorder: a review for primary care providers. *Clin Pediatr.* 2006;45:7–13
17. Sontag SJ. The spectrum of pulmonary symptoms due to gastroesophageal reflux. *Thorac Surg Clin.* 2005;15:353–368
18. Callahan CW. Primary tracheomalacia and gastroesophageal reflux in infants with cough. *Clin Pediatr.* 1998;37:725–731
19. Zanconato S, Meneghelli G, Braga R, Zacchello F, Baraldi E. Office spirometry in primary care pediatrics: a pilot study. *Pediatrics.* 2005;116:e792–e797
20. Zgherea D, Pagala S, Mendiratta M, et al. Bronchoscopic findings in children with chronic wet cough. *Pediatrics.* 2012;129:e364–e369
21. Nicolai T. Pediatric bronchoscopy. *Pediatr Pulmonol.* 2001;31:150–164
22. Saito J, Harris WT, Gelfond J, et al. Physiologic, bronchoscopic, and bronchoalveolar lavage fluid findings in young children with recurrent wheeze and cough. *Pediatr Pulmonol.* 2006;41:709–719
23. Chang AB, Phelan PD, Carlin JB, Sawyer SM, Robertson CF. A randomised, placebo controlled trial of inhaled salbutamol and beclomethasone for recurrent cough. *Arch Dis Child.* 1998;79:6–11
24. Cochrane D. Diagnosing and treating chesty infants: a short trial of inhaled corticosteroids is probably the best approach. *BMJ.* 1998;316:1546–1547
25. O'Brien KL, Dowell SF, Schwartz B, et al. Cough illness/bronchitis: principles of judicious use of antimicrobial agents. *Pediatrics.* 1998;101:178–181
26. Chang AB, Lasserson TJ, Kiljander TO, et al. Systematic review and meta-analysis of randomised controlled trials of gastro-oesophageal reflux interventions for chronic cough associated with gastro-oesophageal reflux. *BMJ.* 2006;332:11–17
27. Chang CC, Cheng AC, Chang AB. Over-the-counter (OTC) medications to reduce cough as an adjunct to antibiotics for acute pneumonia in children and adults. *Cochrane Database Syst Rev.* 2012;2:CD006088
28. Paul IM. Therapeutic options for acute cough due to upper respiratory infections in children. *Lung.* 2012;190:41–44
29. Smith SM, Schroeder K, Fahey T. Over-the-counter (OTC) medications for acute cough in children and adults in ambulatory settings. *Cochrane Database Syst Rev.* 2012;8:CD001831
30. Vassilev ZP, Kabadi S, Villa R. Safety and efficacy of over-the-counter cough and cold medicines for use in children. *Expert Opin Drug Saf.* 2010;9:233–242
31. Shehab N, Schaefer MK, Kegler SR, Budnitz DS. Adverse events from cough and cold medications after a market withdrawal of products labeled for infants. *Pediatrics.* 2010;126:1100–1107
32. Rimsza ME, Newberry S. Unexpected infant deaths associated with use of cough and cold medications. *Pediatrics.* 2008;122:e318–e322
33. Cohen HA, Rozen J, Kristal H, et al. Effect of honey on nocturnal cough and sleep quality: a double-blind, randomized, placebo-controlled study. *Pediatrics.* 2012;130:465–471

34. Oduwole O, Meremikwu MM, Oyo-Ita A, Udoh EE. Honey for acute cough in children. *Cochrane Database Syst Rev.* 2012;3:CD007094
35. Schroeder K, Fahey T. Over-the-counter medications for acute cough in children and adults in ambulatory settings. *Cochrane Database Syst Rev.* 2004;4:CD001831
36. Duijvestijn YC, Brand PL. Systematic review of N-acetylcysteine in cystic fibrosis. *Acta Paediatr.* 1999;88:38–41
37. Duijvestijn YC, Gerritsen J, Brand PL. [Acetylcysteine in children with lung disorders prescribed by one third of family physicians: no support in the literature] (Dutch). *Ned Tijdschr Geneesk.* 1997;141:826–830
38. Arroll B. Non-antibiotic treatments for upper-respiratory tract infections (common cold). *Respir Med.* 2005;99:1477–1484

# Chapter 13

# Cyanosis

*H. Michael Ushay, MD, PhD*

## ▶ INTRODUCTION

Cyanosis is a bluish purple appearance of the skin or mucous membranes usually caused by an increased concentration of deoxygenated (unsaturated or reduced) hemoglobin (Hgb). While occasionally a benign finding, as in a healthy newborn with acrocyanosis or when observed in the lips and fingers of a child who has been in the cold ocean, acute cyanosis often indicates a significant reduction in oxygen concentration and may signify a life-threatening event. The presence or history of cyanosis requires careful evaluation.

Cyanosis occurs in all ages and may be the result of congenital or acquired disorders of the respiratory or cardiovascular systems. In the neonatal period, persistent pulmonary hypertension of the newborn (PPHN) and congenital heart disease are common causes of cyanosis, while respiratory disorders are the most common cause of life-threatening cyanosis in older children.[1]

Observed most easily in the nail beds, the lips, mucous membranes of the mouth, the ears, the conjunctivae, and the tip of the nose, cyanosis is especially visible in buccal mucosa and beneath the tongue. At these locations, capillary beds are close to the surface and arterial and venous blood are seen together. Cyanosis can be present peripherally, centrally on the head and trunk, and also differentially with only lower parts of the body affected. The location where cyanosis is observed can help in determining the cause.

Cyanosis is made worse by vasoconstriction, so a patient should be examined in a warm environment. The perception of cyanosis depends on the quality of ambient lighting and by an examiner's ability to perceive subtle shades of blue.

To most observers, cyanosis becomes visible when the concentration of deoxygenated Hgb approaches 3 to 5 g/dL,[2] but some reports suggest that the threshold for detecting cyanosis may be as low as 1.5 g/dL.[3] The appearance of cyanosis is related to the absolute concentration of deoxygenated Hgb rather than to a specific oxyhemoglobin saturation ($SaO_2$). Cyanosis in a patient with a Hgb concentration of 15 g/dL will be apparent at an arterial $SaO_2$ somewhere between 70% and 80%: 5 g/dL of Hgb is desaturated at 70% arterial saturation, and 3 g/dL is desaturated at 80% saturation. The higher the patient's Hgb concentration, the more readily cyanosis becomes evident. For example, 5 g/dL represents one-half of the Hgb in a child with 10 g/dL but only one-third in a patient with 15 g/dL of Hgb. Thus, as Hgb concentration falls, cyanosis becomes apparent only at lower oxyhemoglobin saturations. Because Hgb concentration varies in both healthy and ill children and throughout life, cyanosis appears at different degrees of desaturation in different children and at different times.

Whereas patients becoming progressively more anemic do not manifest cyanosis until their oxygen saturations have fallen substantially, a patient who is polycythemic with a Hgb concentration of 20 g/dL, for example, might manifest cyanosis when 92% saturated (1.5 g/dL desaturated Hgb) and certainly when 75% saturated (5 g/dL desaturated Hgb). It is important to remember that in an anemic patient, a severe degree of oxygen desaturation can occur without cyanosis. Although cyanosis is always a concern, the absence of cyanosis is not necessarily reassuring in a patient with respiratory distress.

The arterial Hgb oxygen saturation measured with a pulse oximeter is referred to as $SpO_2$ to distinguish it from a saturation measurement obtained from an arterial blood gas (ABG), which is referred to as $SaO_2$. $SpO_2$ and $SaO_2$ are often used interchangeably and are usually almost identical in the absence of significant amounts of carbon monoxide, methemoglobinemia, elevated bilirubin levels, or very poor perfusion.[4] A pulse oximeter measures $SaO_2$ directly and permits the recognition of decreasing degrees of $SaO_2$ before cyanosis becomes visible. Screening newborns using pulse oximetry detects degrees of Hgb desaturation indicative of congenital heart disease that may not be obvious on examination.[5]

In an ABG sampling, the pH, $PCO_2$, $PO_2$, and $SaO_2$ are determined in addition to other values. Depending on the type of ABG analyzer, the $SaO_2$ is measured directly in a process called co-oximetry or is calculated based on the pH, $PCO_2$, $PO_2$, and oxyhemoglobin dissociation curve.[6]

## ▶ CENTRAL AND PERIPHERAL CYANOSIS

Cyanosis is described as being *central* or *peripheral* in origin. Central cyanosis occurs when the origin of desaturation is either an oxygenation defect of the lungs or the result of addition of venous blood to arterial blood from shunts or mixing lesions in the heart. In central cyanosis, the arterial blood leaving the heart is desaturated. Peripheral cyanosis occurs when blood leaves the heart and lungs fully saturated, but, from either excessive tissue oxygen extraction or sluggish blood flow in tissue beds (including some, such as the nail beds or lips, that are visible), the venous blood becomes desaturated to the extent that cyanosis becomes evident. Whether cyanosis is central or peripheral is a function of the physiologic dysfunction rather than where the cyanosis is evident on physical examination.

*Acrocyanosis* refers to bluish color in the hands and feet and around the mouth (circumoral cyanosis). The mucus membranes generally remain pink. A form of peripheral cyanosis that usually reflects benign vasomotor changes in the affected extremities, acrocyanosis does not indicate pathology unless cardiac output is extremely low, resulting in severe venous desaturation from increased oxygen extraction.

In the newborn, acrocyanosis is a striking example of cyanosis arising from intense peripheral vasoconstriction and variable perfusion in the extremities compared with the central circulation.[7,8] It is seen in well babies and resolves within the first few days of life.

Acrocyanosis may also occur in infants when they cry, regurgitate, vomit, cough, or hold their breath. This finding is often very alarming to the caregiver who witnesses the event, and it requires careful questioning and observation to differentiate it from serious underlying pathology (eg, seizure, apneic episode, cardiac arrhythmia, congenital heart defect). The child with acrocyanosis typically does not have major changes in mental status during the event and appears well on physical examination.

Moderate cold exposure slows the transit time of blood through capillary beds and allows for increased unloading of oxygen from the blood to the tissues in infants and young children, leading to cyanosis, especially in the lips and perioral region. This form of acrocyanosis rapidly resolves with warming of the patient.

## ▶ OXYGEN CONTENT, DELIVERY, AND TRANSPORT

Because deoxygenated Hgb has a dark blue to purplish color, the higher the concentration of desaturated Hgb, the bluer the blood and the more cyanotic the patient appears. Hgb desaturation and hence cyanosis result from disorders of oxygen uptake, transport, and utilization.

In an intact postnatal circulation, venous blood with a saturation of approximately 75% travels via the pulmonary artery to the pulmonary capillary bed where it becomes fully saturated upon exposure to oxygen from the alveolus across the alveolar capillary membrane. Fully oxygenated blood returns to the left atrium via the pulmonary veins and from there moves through the left ventricle to the aorta.

Oxygen in the blood is either bound to Hgb or dissolved in plasma. The amount bound to Hgb is reflected by the oxyhemoglobin saturation, and the amount dissolved in plasma is measured by the $PaO_2$. The role of oxyhemoglobin saturation on the oxygen content of blood is described by the equation

$$CaO_2 = [Hgb] \times SaO_2 \times 1.36 \text{ mL/g} + 0.003 \times PaO_2$$

where $CaO_2$ is the oxygen content, [Hgb] is the concentration of hemoglobin in g/dL, $SaO_2$ is the oxyhemoglobin saturation, 1.36 mL/g is the binding capacity for oxygen in mL/g of Hgb, and $PaO_2$ is the tension of dissolved (unbound) oxygen in the plasma. Approximately 97% of the oxygen in blood is bound to Hgb, leaving only a small amount unbound and dissolved in blood. Delivery of oxygen to the tissues is a function of the flow of blood produced by the systemic ventricle of the heart (cardiac output) and the oxygen content of the blood.

In a normal circulation, beyond the neonatal period, arterial blood with an oxyhemoglobin saturation of 95% to 98% flows to capillary beds throughout the body, where in the course of traversing the tissue beds approximately 25% of the Hgb-bound oxygen molecules are offloaded to the tissues. This is known as oxygen consumption or utilization. The end-capillary oxyhemoglobin saturation is, on average, about 25% less than at entrance to a capillary bed. Some tissues will extract more oxygen and some may extract less. The 25% difference in oxygen content between arterial and venous blood is relatively conserved as long as cardiac output is adequate to meet tissue oxygen demands. In tissue beds with reduced cardiac output (blood flow), a higher proportion of oxygen is drawn from Hgb, resulting in greater than 25% extraction.[6]

Hypoxemia is the term used to describe decreased oxygen tension ($PaO_2$) and saturation ($SaO_2$) of arterial blood. Hypoxia is the state that occurs when inadequate oxygen is delivered to tissues with resultant decreased function and a transition to anaerobic respiration.[9]

With oxygenated arterial blood appearing red and deoxygenated venous blood usually appearing dark red or bluish, the color of a capillary bed becomes a function of the relative amounts of arterial and venous blood present in the bed. The more deoxygenated

Hgb present, the bluer (cyanosed) the capillary bed appears to be. When cardiac output to a tissue falls below normal, more than 25% of oxygen may be extracted from each Hgb molecule to meet the metabolic requirements of the tissue. This increased off-loading will result in a decrease in oxyhemoglobin saturation for the end capillary blood and an increase in the arterial to venous oxygen content difference, thus making cyanosis more prominent. As the oxyhemoglobin saturation of the end capillary blood decreases, cyanosis becomes obvious.

In cirucmstances in which the Hgb of the arterial blood entering a capillary bed is not fully saturated with oxygen, venous blood leaving the capillary bed will be desaturated to an even greater degree and the capillary beds will look even more cyanotic. For example, if arterial blood enters a capillary bed with an oxyhemoglobin saturation of 85%, the resultant venous blood may have an oxyhemoglobin saturation of 60% after the off-loading of 25% of oxygen molecules. Thus, the blood in the capillary bed will look cyanotic. The preservation of an arterial to venous oxygen content difference of approximately 25% is used as a surrogate indicator of adequate cardiac output and tissue oxygen delivery. In the presence of adequate cardiac output and an appropriate Hgb concentration, adequate tissue oxygen delivery can occur even in the presence of significantly desaturated or cyanotic arterial blood.

## ▶ PULMONARY MECHANISMS OF CYANOSIS

The Hgb desaturation of central cyanosis can result from pathology of the airways, lungs, heart, or Hgb itself. Normally, Hgb is close to 100% saturated with oxygen when it leaves the alveolar capillary unit and slightly less than 100% when it leaves the left ventricle—there is a normal, very small amount of venous blood shunted to the blood entering the left side of the heart from the lungs. With pulmonary disease, a disturbance of alveolar gas exchange may result in desaturated blood entering the pulmonary veins and left atrium. The desaturation of pulmonary venous blood is a key factor distinguishing desaturation caused by pulmonary disease from desaturation caused by congenital heart disease. In congenital heart disease, pulmonary venous blood is usually fully saturated even when systemic saturations may be very low. Five pathophysiologic mechanisms explain why blood does not become fully oxygenated as it travels through the pulmonary alveolar capillary beds. These 5 mechanisms of hypoxemia are mismatching of alveolar ventilation to perfusion, intrapulmonary shunt, hypoventilation, diffusion block, and breathing hypoxic gas mixtures.[10]

In patients with parenchymal lung disease such as pneumonia, ventilation-perfusion (V/Q) mismatch is the most important mechanism for hypoxemia. For blood to become fully oxygenated, the flow of blood to an alveolar-capillary unit must match the ventilation in the unit. V/Q mismatching occurs when the relationship of alveolar ventilation to capillary bed perfusion is not appropriately balanced. The matching of ventilation to perfusion is along a continuum. At 1 extreme are alveolar capillary units that are ventilated but not perfused; these are described as having dead space ventilation ($V/Q = \infty$). At the other extreme are lung units that are perfused but not ventilated ($V/Q = 0$); these are described as intrapulmonary shunt, occurring when blood travels through the lungs from the right side of the heart to the left without being exposed to aerated alveoli. Between the 2 extremes is a continuous range of V/Q ratios that, overall, result in a normal ABG. In lung diseases such as acute respiratory distress syndrome, pneumonia, bronchiolitis, pulmonary edema, and asthma, most hypoxemia is the result of V/Q mismatching with only a small component from intrapulmonary shunt.

Hypoventilation occurs in patients with neurologic, traumatic, pharmacologic, or chemical suppression of respiratory drive, as well as with suffocation. A patient who develops apnea or acute upper airway obstruction caused by a foreign body will become profoundly hypoxemic and very rapidly become cyanotic. Cyanosis associated with viral laryngotracheobronchitis (croup) or pertussis (whooping cough) are examples of hypoventilation-induced hypoxemia. Any acquired or congenital abnormality of the airway that obstructs airflow can potentially cause significant hypoventilation and result in hypoxemia to the extent that cyanosis becomes apparent.

Breathing hypoxic gas mixtures occurs when victims are trapped in a hypoxic environment such as a closed-space fire or when exposed to high concentrations of gases such as methane and helium that are not in themselves toxic but induce hypoxia by displacing breathable oxygen. Another example of breathing hypoxic gas is the effect of altitude on barometric pressure. At higher altitudes, the barometric pressure, and hence the amount of oxygen available to breathe, is lower: arterial $PaO_2$ and $SaO_2$ thus fall in proportion to the decrease in barometric pressure.

Diffusion block occurs when the interstitial space between the pulmonary capillary and the alveolus becomes so thickened or damaged that oxygen cannot move from the alveolus to the capillary. Diffusion block is seen with pulmonary fibrosis.

The $SaO_2$ of arterial blood depends on the effectiveness of oxygen transfer at the alveolar level but is also affected by the shunting of venous blood into the systemic arterial system through the heart or lungs. The addition of desaturated venous blood to oxygenated blood is called *venous admixture* and is the mechanism behind intrapulmonary shunt. The resultant saturation of the arterial blood is proportional to the amount and saturation of the combined blood volumes. It is the $SaO_2$ and oxygen content of the blood volumes that are being combined that influence the resultant saturation, not the $PaO_2$. Breathing 100% oxygen for a prolonged time can partially correct desaturation resulting from alveolar hypoventilation, diffusion block, or V/Q mismatching, but does not correct hypoxemia resulting from intrapulmonary shunt.

## ▶ PULMONARY VERSUS CARDIAC CYANOSIS

Distinguishing whether a sick newborn or child is cyanotic for pulmonary or cardiac reasons is challenging. Cyanotic heart disease may mimic respiratory disease and vice versa. Tachypnea, retractions, nasal flaring, and grunting point toward a pulmonary cause of cyanosis. Patients with anatomic cardiac lesions as the cause of cyanosis are generally somewhat distressed from a respiratory standpoint but to a somewhat lesser extent than found with purely respiratory disease. In cyanosis from PPHN, there may be a history of a difficult delivery, meconium-stained amniotic fluid, meconium aspiration, perinatal sepsis, asphyxia, and low Apgar scores. Because there is often a component of meconium aspiration pneumonia, these newborns demonstrate severe respiratory distress.

Pulse oximetry should be obtained immediately with any suggestion of cyanosis. A hyperoxia test (see following text) may help distinguish hypoxemia for respiratory reasons, such as pneumonia or neonatal respiratory distress syndrome, from hypoxemia caused by congenital heart disease or PPHN. Early in life, the $PaO_2$ may increase to greater than 100 mm Hg in infants with forms of cyanotic heart disease with high pulmonary blood flow such as total anomalous pulmonary venous return (TAPVR). If there is an inadequate rise in $PaO_2$ or oxygen saturation from a hyperoxia test, echocardiography should be performed immediately to ascertain the presence or absence of a congenital heart lesion. In general, echocardiography should be performed to assess for the possible presence of congenital cyanotic heart disease (CCHD) whenever hypoxemia is not responsive to supplemental oxygen or mechanical ventilatory support.

## ▶ CYANOSIS WITH PULMONARY DISEASE

Lower airway diseases, such as viral bronchiolitis, pneumonia, and status asthmaticus, can cause cyanosis from V/Q mismatching and small degrees of intrapulmonary shunt. Bronchiolitis, most often caused by respiratory syncitial virus (RSV), is a common disease process affecting infants in winter months. The airways become edematous and infiltrated with inflammatory cells, ultimately obstructing the lumens. In addition to signs and symptoms of respiratory distress such as tachypnea, retractions, grunting, and nasal flaring, RSV bronchiolitis is also associated with apnea that can induce deep cyanosis by hypoventilation.

Pertussis caused by *Bordetella pertussis* or *parapertussis* is often associated with cyanosis. In the paroxysmal phase, coughing paroxysms without an interceding breath can result in deep visible cyanosis. As the illness progresses over time, patients can turn blue after only a few coughs.

Upper airway obstruction presents with inspiratory symptoms often manifested as stridor, a harsh, sometimes high-pitched sound produced by vibration of upper airway structures upon inspiration. An infant with significant upper airway obstruction and stridor often demonstrates substernal retractions. Worrisome symptoms are change in voice, muffling or hoarseness, and difficulty in swallowing and handling secretions.

Croup, usually from infection with the parainfluenza virus, is the most common cause of stridor in children. Less common inciting agents include influenza, adenovirus, measles, and RSV. Croup usually occurs in children aged 6 months to 3 years. The pathophysiology involves endothelial damage, mucous production, loss of ciliary function, and edema of the subglottic region. Infants present with a history of a preceding upper respiratory infection, low-grade fever, characteristic barking cough, and inspiratory stridor. Airway radiographs may reveal subglottic narrowing.

Epiglottitis is a life-threatening bacterial infection of the epiglottis and supraglottic structures, usually caused by *Haemophilus influenzae.* Patients present with high fever, toxic appearance, and stridor. The incidence of epiglottitis has decreased significantly since the introduction of the *Haemophilus influenzae* vaccine.

Aspiration of foreign bodies is relatively common and can cause severe respiratory distress and cyanosis when an object is lodged in the trachea. Foreign body aspiration should be suspected in an afebrile infant with acute onset of coughing, choking, stridor, or wheezing. Many foreign bodies are not radiopaque, and physicians should thus have a high index of suspicion regardless of radiographic findings.

Laryngomalacia, choanal atresia or stenosis, subglottic stenosis, tracheomalacia, bacterial tracheitis, and obstructive sleep apnea are other causes of airway obstruction that may present with cyanosis.

## ▶ CYANOSIS WITH HEART DISEASE

Pediatric heart disease of several different types can result in cyanosis. CCHD results in cyanosis either from mixing of venous blood with arterial blood through intra- and extra-cardiac shunts or from insufficient pulmonary blood flow.

Heart disease that causes pulmonary venous congestion can result in cyanosis by leading to pulmonary edema, which forms when increased left atrial pressure is transmitted back to the pulmonary veins and further back to the pulmonary capillary bed. Increased pressure on the venous side of the pulmonary capillary bed results in transudation of fluid from the capillary to the interstitium and from there to the alveoli. The presence of edema fluid in the alveoli overwhelms the pulmonary lymphatics, deactivates pulmonary surfactant, and results in alveolar flooding and collapse. The resulting ventilation perfusion mismatching and intrapulmonary shunt can cause severe hypoxemia and even cyanosis. Diseases that can cause cyanosis by this mechanism include mitral stenosis and mitral regurgitation. With severe systolic and diastolic dysfunction of the left ventricle, such as may result from acute myocarditis, elevated left atrial pressure can lead to the formation of pulmonary edema as described above. In dilated cardiomyopathy, the left heart can dilate to the point that the mitral valve no longer effectively separates the left atrium from the left ventricle and, with each systole, there is retrograde flow of blood into the left atrium and pulmonary veins, leading to pulmonary edema. A similar effect occurs when the mitral valve leaflets are damaged by rheumatic heart disease.

A typically noncyanotic heart lesion such as a ventricular septal defect (VSD) can result in cyanosis with the development of Eisenmenger syndrome. With a VSD, blood flows from the left ventricle to the right ventricle because of the lower resistance of the pulmonary vascular system. There is no cyanosis. However, if the VSD is unrestrictive to flow and the lesion is not corrected over time, the extra volume of blood eventually induces hypertrophic changes in smooth muscles of the pulmonary arteries with a resultant increase in pulmonary vascular resistance. The pulmonary vascular resistance may become so high that the shunt reverses direction, with blood moving in a right-to-left direction through the VSD. This results in venous blood mixing with arterial blood in the left ventricle and the development of severe desaturation and cyanosis. Fortunately, with early repair of VSDs, Eisenmenger syndrome is seen very rarely. It may be seen, however, in parts of the world where access to repair of congenital heart lesions is not readily available.

### *Congenital Cyanotic Heart Disease*

Cyanosis in VSD and heart failure as described above is rare; but cyanotic heart disease always results in significant cyanosis. An infant with CCHD typically develops cyanosis in the first few hours of life. Initially, cyanosis may be noticeable with crying or feeding and generally without evidence of respiratory distress. In these lesions, a patent ductus arteriosus (PDA) serves either as a means to deliver blood from the aorta to the pulmonary artery so it can be oxygenated in the lungs (left-to-right shunt) or as a means of maintaining systemic blood flow (right-to-left shunt). In many cases, patients with cyanotic heart disease either deteriorate hemodynamically or become progressively more cyanotic as the PDA closes.

The lesions of CCHD can be placed into different groups. One group, consisting of tetralogy of Fallot (TOF), pulmonary atresia, tricuspid atresia, pulmonic stenosis, and Ebstein anomaly, creates cyanosis by obstructing pulmonary blood flow with resultant shunting of blood from the right to left side of the circulation. In dextro-transposition of the great arteries (d-TGA) and TAPVR, on the other hand, pulmonary blood flow may be normal or increased, but pulmonary venous return is anatomically separated from the systemic arterial circulation. In truncus arteriosus and double outlet right ventricle (DORV), there is mixing of arterial and venous blood with consequent cyanosis. Another group of lesions includes the left-sided obstructive lesions of hypoplastic left heart syndrome (HLHS), critical coarctation of the aorta and interrupted aortic arch that produce desaturation because of dependence on right-to-left shunting through a PDA to maintain systemic perfusion.

Simultaneous upper and lower extremity pulse oximetry measurements can be diagnostic. An $SaO_2$ that is higher in the right arm than in the umbilical artery or lower extremities indicates that venous blood has been added to the aorta at the level of the ductus arteriosus and is known as *differential cyanosis*. With d-TGA in the presence of pulmonary hypertension or coarctation of the aorta, the saturation in the right arm is less than in the lower extremities because oxygenated blood is added to desaturated blood at the level of the PDA; this is called *reverse differential cyanosis*.[11]

If the patient is not at a facility where echocardiography can be performed, immediate transport should be arranged to such a center. Stabilization should include initiation of an infusion of prostaglandin E1 (PGE1) at a dose of 0.05 mcg/kg/min if there is any suspicion of ductal dependent heart disease. PGE1 dilates the ductus arteriosus to provide adequate pulmonary or systemic blood flow. In that the benefits of prostaglandin are lifesaving and the drawbacks minimal, the threshold should be very low for initiating PGE1 therapy until ductal dependent heart disease is ruled out. The PGE1 infusion can be increased to a dose of 0.15 mcg/kg/min if no improvement in saturation and pulses is seen soon after initiation. It is appropriate to administer PGE1 to any infant in whom the diagnosis of CCHD is strongly suspected, even before a complete evaluation is performed. Potential side effects of PGE1 include apnea, jitteriness, seizures, and peripheral vasodilation with hypotension, as well as an increased risk of infection. Fluid administration may be necessary if vasodilation leads to hypotension, and respiratory support including intubation may be required if significant apnea occurs.[12]

### Abnormalities of the Right Ventricular Outflow Tract

Tetralogy of Fallot, the most common congenital heart lesion that can cause cyanosis, consists of VSD, pulmonic stenosis, right ventricular hypertrophy, and an overriding aorta. On examination, the systolic murmur of pulmonic stenosis might be appreciated. Chest radiographs reveal normal cardiac size, with a rounded, uplifted apex and concavity at the site of the pulmonary artery, a "boot-shaped" heart. There is diminished pulmonary vasculature. Electrocardiogram demonstrates right axis deviation and right ventricular hypertrophy.

With TOF, the degree of cyanosis depends on the severity of the right ventricular outflow tract obstruction. With more severe pulmonic stenosis, right ventricular pressure increases and blood is shunted across the septal defect from the right to the left ventricle, bypassing the lungs. In infants with mild obstruction, symptoms of heart failure from the large VSD are likely to predominate. Other infants may have severe cyanosis on closure of the ductus arteriosus. "Tet spells" may occur with vigorous crying or dehydration: affected infants initially become hyperpneic and restless as cyanosis increases; the murmur of pulmonic stenosis softens and then disappears as pulmonary blood flow decreases; and the spell may precipitate a syncopal episode. Treatment for an acute tet spell includes putting the patient in a knee-to-chest position to increase systemic vascular resistance and administering supplemental oxygen, sedation, and a beta blocker. Ultimately, only surgical repair can provide consistent pulmonary blood flow.

Pulmonary atresia with a VSD is a more severe form of TOF that presents with severe cyanosis shortly after birth. With atresia, the prominent murmur of pulmonic stenosis characteristic of TOF is absent. If there is sufficient pulmonary blood flow from collateral vessels from the descending aorta (identified by a continuous murmur heard over the back), the patient may not require treatment with PGE1.

Neonates with pulmonary atresia and an intact ventricular septum have severe cyanosis that progresses as the ductus arterious closes. Patency of the ductus arteriosus is necessary for pulmonary blood flow in this lesion.

### Abnormalities of the Tricuspid Valve

With tricuspid atresia, the only outlet for blood from the right atrium is a patent foramen ovale, through which blood travels from the right to the left atrium and then to the left ventricle. From the left ventricle, blood flows via an unrestrictive VSD to the right ventricle and from there to the pulmonary artery. Tricuspid atresia may be associated with normally related or transposed great arteries. Saturation, degree of cyanosis, and blood flow depends on the relationship of the great arteries, the size of the VSD, and the presence or absence of pulmonic stenosis. If pulmonary blood flow is unobstructed, patients may have tachypnea and heart failure with minimal to no cyanosis. Physical examination is significant for an increased left ventricular impulse as opposed to other cyanotic heart diseases with an increased right ventricular impulse. A murmur may or may not be present depending upon restriction of blood flow through the VSD (a holosystolic murmur at the left lower sternal border) and the semilunar valves (a systolic ejection murmur).

Ebstein anomaly of the tricuspid valve involves the downward displacement of the valve leaflets into the right ventricular cavity. The severity of the disease is dependent on the degree of displacement and the ability of the remaining portion of the right ventricle to generate sufficient force to pump blood into the pulmonary arteries. Newborns may have massive cardiomegaly on chest radiograph, marked cyanosis, a holosystolic murmur with a gallop rhythm, hydrops, and pulmonary artery hypoplasia. Infants with severe disease require PGE1 to maintain pulmonary blood flow until pulmonary vascular resistance has fallen and adequacy of the right ventricle and pulmonary valve can be assessed.

### Transposition of the Great Arteries

Transposition of the great arteries (TGA) is the most common cardiac lesion in neonates with cyanosis, with a male predominance. Neonates with TGA show severe cyanosis immediately after birth. There are 2 separate parallel circulations with oxygenated blood continuously circulating through the lungs and deoxygenated venous blood becoming increasingly deoxygenated as it flows through the systemic arterial circulation. Left untreated, affected neonates progress from cyanosis to tissue hypoxia, acidosis, and death. Unlike neonates with other cyanotic congenital heart lesions, these neonates have a normal volume of blood passing through the pulmonary bed. However, because their circulation is separated in parallel, neonates with TGA have very little effective pulmonary blood flow (deoxygenated blood from the systemic circulation reaching the pulmonary vascular bed) and little effective systemic blood flow (oxygenated blood that perfuses the systemic bed). The degree of mixing between the separate circulations depends on the number and size of the anatomic connections. Blood may shunt at the atrial, ventricular (if a VSD is present), or ductal level. The typical neonate with TGA and an intact ventricular septum becomes progressively more hypoxemic as the ductus arteriosus closes. Frequently, these neonates are given PGE1 until the atrial communication through the foramen ovale can be enlarged by balloon atrial septostomy performed in the cardiac catheterization laboratory or at the bedside. Clinically, the neonate with TGA is likely to appear cyanotic but otherwise healthy, with a weight appropriate for gestational age. Reverse differential cyanosis is rare but is indicative of TGA and a PDA with an associated aortic arch anomaly or pulmonary hypertension. In a neonate with TGA and an intact intraventricular septum, the chest radiograph may show a narrowed superior mediastinum with an egg-shaped cardiac silhouette (egg on a string), mild cardiomegaly, and increased pulmonary vascular markings. Surgical repair, typically by arterial switch operation, is often undertaken in the first week of life.

Truncus arteriosus is an uncommon lesion characterized by a single arterial trunk that originates from the heart and supplies the systemic, pulmonary, and coronary circulations. A large VSD is usually present, which allows total mixing of the 2 circulations. The degree of cyanosis depends on the amount of pulmonary blood flow, which is determined by the pulmonary vascular resistance and any concurrent pulmonic stenosis. Radiographs usually show cardiomegaly.

With TAPVR, pulmonary veins drain ectopically into the systemic venous circuit and ultimately into the right atrium, resulting in complete mixing of oxygenated and deoxygenated blood. The site of connection can be supracardiac, infracardiac, or cardiac. Maximal cyanosis occurs in neonates with an infradiaphragmatic connection, with pulmonary venous obstruction, and with a small atrial communication. Auscultation of the heart may not reveal any murmurs. Chest radiographs help by demonstrating pulmonary congestion in the absence of an enlarged cardiac silhouette.

### *Critical Left-Sided Obstructive Heart Lesions*

Newborns with critical obstructive cardiac lesions, such as critical coarctation of the aorta, interrupted aortic arch, and HLHS, often look pale and poorly perfused and may demonstrate abnormalities in regional oxygen saturation on pulse oximetry. Hypoperfusion from insufficient flow of blood into the systemic circulation results in hypotension and, with inadequate delivery of oxygen to the tissues, progressive metabolic acidosis. With ductal-dependent systemic circulation, as the ductus arteriosus starts to close, the affected patient clinically deteriorates. With HLHS, the diminished size and function of the mitral valve, left ventricle, aortic valve, and aortic arch result in a severely diminished systemic circulation that is dependent on a widely patent ductus arterious to supply blood to the body. In HLHS, not only are structures distal to the ductal insertion into the aorta dependent on the ductal flow, but, given the absence of forward blood flow through the aortic valve, the coronary arteries and the right arm are also dependent on the ductus via retrograde blood flow. Closure of the ductus with HLHS often results in rapid cardiac arrest and death.

In HLHS, the $SaO_2$ reflects mixing at the atrial level. Venous blood returning from the systemic veins mixes in the right atrium with oxygenated blood coming from the left atrium via an atrial septal defect. This mixed blood then travels through the right ventricle to the pulmonary artery and from there to the lungs and to the systemic circulation via the PDA. The measurement of $SaO_2$ becomes crucial in this circumstance of trying to balance 2 parallel circulations. In other words, blood in the pulmonary artery of patients with HLHS can flow either into the low-resistance pulmonary vasculature or into the high-resistance systemic vasculature. An ideal saturation in this situation is about 75%, representing an approximate balance of blood flow into the lungs and into the systemic vasculature. An acute rise in saturation could represent a preponderance of blood flow into the lungs to the detriment of systemic flow, resulting in acidosis and signs of systemic hypoperfusion despite the higher $SaO_2$.

## ▶ CYANOSIS WITH DYSHEMOGLOBINEMIAS

Dysfunctional Hgb that is unable to bind and deliver oxygen adequately is another cause of central cyanosis. Methemoglobinemia occurs when the iron in heme is in the 3+ oxidation state and cannot bind oxygen. Most often, methemoglobinemia results from the presence of an oxidizing substance that changes Hgb $Fe^{2+}$ to $Fe^{3+}$, combined with the deactivation of the usual process for reducing methemoglobin back to Hgb. The only accurate method of determining the concentration of methemoglobin is through co-oximetry.[13,14]

With carbon monoxide poisoning, significant tissue hypoxia can result from the increased affinity of Hgb for carbon monoxide compared to oxygen. However, cyanosis is not usually apparent. Direct determination of oxyhemoglobin and carboxyhemoglobin saturation by means of co-oximetry can reveal the true $SaO_2$. Standard pulse oximeters do not accurately measure $SaO_2$ in the presence of carbon monoxide, but special pulse oximeters are now available to determine carboxyhemoglobin saturation.[15]

Cyanide binds to the iron of cytochrome a3, not Hgb. Thus, cyanide poisoning does not directly cause cyanosis, but results in significant tissue hypoxia from the inhibition of oxidative phosphorylation. Even with Hgb 100% saturated, a person with cyanide poisoning is not able to use the oxygen that tissues draw from the blood. At the point when sufficient tissue hypoxia makes the muscles of respiration dysfunctional, cyanosis results from hypoventilation.[16]

## ▶ MISCELLANEOUS CAUSES OF CYANOSIS

Occasionally, children with significant gastroesophageal reflux will have paroxysmal acrocyanosis (especially perioral cyanosis) in association with brief episodes of limpness, stereotypical positioning or tonic clonic motions suggestive of a seizure, or apnea. This constellation of features is called Sandifer syndrome and often responds to treatment of the gastroesophageal reflux.[17]

Prolonged generalized seizures are often associated with impaired respiration and can result in cyanosis if respiration ceases for a prolonged period.

Neuromuscular disorders causing weakness of respiratory muscles, such as spinal muscular atrophy, botulism, congenital myopathies, or metabolic disorders, can result in hypoventilation followed by collapse of lung units that combine to result in hypoxemia that, if severe enough can, manifest as cyanosis.

In cyanotic breath-holding spells children present with a history of crying, typically followed by sudden breath-holding in forced expiration with apnea and cyanosis. These features may progress to limpness and loss of consciousness. Cyanosis can appear faster than anticipated with simple breath-holding, and the loss of tone is often striking. As the child resumes normal breathing, the cyanosis resolves. Cyanotic breath-holding spells most commonly occur around 1 year of age with a range of 6 months to 4 years. Up to 15% of cases may have an initial episode before the age of 6 months.

## ▶ CYANOSIS IN THE NEWBORN

Acrocyanosis of the hands and feet is common in the first 6 to 24 hours of life and is usually of little significance in an otherwise well newborn. Central cyanosis persisting beyond the first few minutes of life may indicate inadequate oxygen delivery and necessitates further evaluation. Newborns can have cyanosis over the lower half of the body in the presence of right-to-left shunting across a PDA. Newborns with persistent cyanosis or hypoxemia despite oxygen administration may have CCHD, primary lung disease, or pulmonary artery hypertension.

In utero, the fetus is markedly cyanotic because the placental circulation provides blood with an $SaO_2$ ranging from only 50% to 65% ($PaO_2$ 18–25 mm Hg). Even at this low saturation, oxygen delivery in the fetus is adequate for growth and development because of a high concentration of Hgb and the presence of fetal Hgb (Hgb F), which binds oxygen with a greater affinity than Hgb A. In utero, there is only minimal blood flow through the pulmonary artery into the lungs; instead, blood is shunted via the ductus arteriosus, the patent foramen ovale, and other anatomic channels from the right heart to the systemic circulation. At birth, with separation from the placenta and a rapid drop in pulmonary vascular resistance, blood flows from the right ventricle through the pulmonary artery and into the pulmonary capillary beds, where it is exposed to oxygen in the air. Within the first few breaths, the lungs become an extremely efficient gas exchange organ resulting in $SaO_2$ levels sufficient for the newborn to transition from cyanotic to centrally pink. In a healthy neonate, oxygen saturations continue to rise slowly over the initial few minutes of extrauterine life. The postductal oxygen saturations are usually lower than the preductal saturations for as long as 15 minutes, indicating persistence of elevated pulmonary vascular resistance with resultant mixing of venous blood in the aorta at the level of the ductus arteriosus. In the absence of a substantial pulmonary or cardiac defect, the arterial saturation continues to rise, and simultaneously, the channels that shunt blood from right to left in utero will close. By 24 hours of age, an Hgb oxygen saturation of less than 95% in the lower extremities is abnormal and warrants further investigation.[5]

In the period following birth, the persistence of Hgb F, with its higher affinity for oxygen, results in a leftward shift of the oxyhemoglobin dissociation curve so that cyanosis is observed only at lower oxygen tensions: 32 to 42 mm Hg, corresponding to saturations of 75% to 85%. Thus, in the presence of Hgb F, a greater degree of hypoxemia is required for cyanosis to be visible.

The best method for assessing cyanosis in a newborn is to look at the tongue. If central cyanosis persists for more than a few minutes after birth, a search for the cause should be undertaken. Comparing arterial blood saturation proximal to and distal to the entrance of the ductus ateriosus into the aorta is helpful in determining the origin of cyanosis in a newborn. In the presence of right-to-left shunting of blood through a PDA, blood in the aorta at the level of the ductal entry and more distally (left arm and lower extremities) is relatively desaturated from the admixture of venous blood entering the aorta via the PDA. In contrast, blood in the aorta proximal to the level of the PDA (right arm) will be more fully saturated because of a greater contribution of well-oxygenated blood that has returned to the left atrium and left ventricle via the pulmonary veins.

### Hyperoxia Test

In the presence of cyanosis, oxyhemoglobin desaturation, or low $PaO_2$, a hyperoxia test should be performed in a newborn to determine if the problem is with pulmonary oxygenation, from an anatomic shunting of blood through the PDA, or an intracardiac lesion.[8] In pulmonary causes of cyanosis or hypoxemia, there should be a significant increase in $SaO_2$ and $PaO_2$ with administration of 100% oxygen. A $PaO_2$ of less than 100 mm Hg in an enriched-oxygen environment is a strong indicator of CCHD or PPHN, and an echocardiogram should be obtained to evaluate for congenital heart disease. With a heart lesion in which some pulmonary blood flow is present, there can be a significant increase in $PaO_2$ or $SaO_2$ during a hyperoxia test. A $PaO_2$ greater than 250 mm Hg makes cyanotic heart disease unlikely, but a $PaO_2$ of 100 to 250 mm Hg does not completely rule out CCHD and warrants further investigation. When performing a hyperoxia test, simultaneous determinations of preductal and postductal $SaO_2$ or $PaO_2$ should be made to delineate the presence of a right-to-left ductal shunt or other shunting pattern. If desaturation is present, and especially if there is not a significant improvement in saturation with administration of 100% oxygen, the consultation of a neonatologist or pediatric cardiologist should be sought.

### Persistent Pulmonary Hypertension of the Newborn

In PPHN, high residual pulmonary vascular resistance reduces pulmonary artery blood flow to the lungs with concomitant persistence of shunting from the right to the left side of the circulation through the ductus arteriosus and foramen ovale. This is known as persistence of fetal circulation, and the oxygen content of blood in the left atrium is decreased as a result of mixing desaturated venous blood that has crossed the foramen ovale with whatever oxygenated blood has managed to traverse the pulmonary capillary bed. The blood leaving the left ventricle becomes further desaturated when mixed with blood entering the aorta through the ductus arteriosus, having bypassed gas exchange in the lungs. With blood distal to the ductal entrance to the aorta being more desaturated than the preductal blood, the oxyhemoglobin saturation measured by pulse oximetry or ABG in the right arm may be higher than in the left arm or legs; this is known as differential oxyhemoglobin saturation or differential cyanosis.

### Newborn Screening for Congenital Cyanotic Heart Disease

Current recommendations by the American Academy of Pediatrics state that newborns should be screened by pulse oximetry prior to discharge from the newborn nursery to ascertain the possible presence of CCHD that otherwise might be missed. Studies have shown that by 24 hours of life, an oxyhemoglobin saturation of less than 95% is not normal and supportive of a cyanotic or mixing cardiac lesion. A newborn should have oxyhemoglobin saturation measured in the right arm and in 1 leg at 24 hours of life, and if there is a gradient in saturation or if the saturation is 95% or lower, an echocardiogram should be obtained prior to discharge.[18–20]

## AAP POLICY STATEMENTS

Greer FR, Shannon M; American Academy of Pediatrics Committee on Nutrition, Committee on Environmental Health. Infant methemoglobinemia: the role of dietary nitrate in food and water. *Pediatrics.* 2005;116(3):784–786. Reaffirmed April 2009 (pediatrics.aappublications.org/content/116/3/784)

Kattwinkel JM, Perlman JM, Aziz K, et al. Neonatal resuscitation: 2010 American Heart Association guidelines for cardiopulmonary resuscitation and emergency cardiovascular care. *Pediatrics.* 2010;126(5):e1400–e1413 (pediatrics.aappublications.org/content/126/5/e1400)

Mahle WT, Newburger JW, Matherne GP, et al. Role of pulse oximetry in examining newborns for congenital heart disease: a scientific statement from the AHA and AAP. *Pediatrics.* 2009;124(2):823–836 (pediatrics.aappublications.org/content/124/2/823)

## REFERENCES


1. Stack AM. Etiology and evaluation of cyanosis in children. http://www.uptodate.com/contents/etiology-and-evaluation-of-cyanosis-in-children. Updated November 19, 2013. Accessed November 25, 2014
2. Lundsgaard C, Van Slyke DD. Cyanosis. *Medicine.* 1923;2:1
3. Goss GA, Hayes JA, Burdon JG. Deoxyhaemoglobin concentrations in the detection of central cyanosis. *Thorax.* 1988;43:212–213
4. Jubran A. Pulse oximetry. In: Tobin MJ, ed. *Principles and Practice of Intensive Care Monitoring.* New York, NY: McGraw-Hill; 1998:261–287
5. Mahle WT, Newburger JW, Matherne GP, et al. Role of pulse oximetry in examining newborns for congenital heart disease: a scientific statement from the AHA and AAP. *Pediatrics.* 2009;124(2):823–836
6. West JB. Normal physiology: exercise. In: *Pulmonary Physiology and Pathophysiology: An Integrated, Case-Based Approach.* Philadelphia, PA: Lippincott Williams & Wilkins; 2001:1–15
7. Lissauer T, Steer P. Size and physical examination of the newborn infant. In: Fanaroff AA, Fanaroff JM, eds. *Care of the High-Risk Neonate.* 6th ed. Philadelphia, PA: Elsevier; 2013:105–131
8. Sasidharan P. An approach to diagnosis and management of cyanosis and tachypnea in term infants. *Pediatr Clin North Am.* 2004;51:999–1021
9. Lumb AB. Hypoxia. In: *Nunn's Applied Respiratory Physiology.* 6th ed. Philadelphia, PA: Elsevier; 2005:334–341
10. West JB. Acute respiratory failure. In: *Pulmonary Physiology and Pathophysiology: An Integrated, Case-Based Approach.* Philadelphia, PA: Lippincott Williams & Wilkins; 2001:125–143
11. Phelps CM, Thrush PT, Cua CL. The heart. In: Fanaroff AA, Fanaroff JM, eds. *Care of the High-Risk Neonate.* 6th ed. Philadelphia, PA: Elsevier; 2013:368–409
12. Tabbut S, Helfaer MA, Nichols DG. Pharmacology of cardiovascular drugs. In: Nichols DG, Ungerleider RM, Spevak PJ, et al, eds. *Critical Heart Disease in Infants and Children.* 2nd ed. Philadelphia, PA: Mosby; 2006:173–203
13. Greer FR, Shannon M; American Academy of Pediatrics Committee on Nutrition, Committee on Environmental Health. Infant methemoglobinemia: the role of dietary nitrate in food and water. *Pediatrics.* 2005;116(3):784–786
14. Curry SC. Hematologic consequences of poisoning. In: Shannon MW, Borron SW, Burns MJ, eds. *Haddad and Winchester's Clinical Management of Poisoning and Drug Overdose.* 4th ed. Philadelphia, PA: Saunders; 2007:289–300
15. Lavonas EJ. Carbon monoxide poisoning. In: Shannon MW, Borron SW, Burns MJ, eds. *Haddad and Winchester's Clinical Management of Poisoning and Drug Overdose.* 4th ed. Philadelphia, PA: Saunders; 2007:1297–1307

16. Hall AH. Cyanide and related compounds—sodium azide. In: Shannon MW, Borron SW, Burns MJ, eds. *Haddad and Winchester's Clinical Management of Poisoning and Drug Overdose.* 4th ed. Philadelphia, PA: Saunders; 2007:1309–1316
17. Jung AD. Gastroesophageal reflux in infants and children. *Am Fam Physician.* 2001;64:1853–1860
18. Kemper AR, Mahle WT, Martin GR, et al. Strategies for implementing screening for critical congenital heart disease. *Pediatrics.* 2011;128:e1259–e1267
19. Peterson C, Ailes E, Riehle-Colarusso T, et al. Late detection of critical congenital heart disease among US infants: estimation of the potential impact of proposed universal screening using pulse oximetry. *JAMA Pediatr.* 2014;168:361–370
20. Mahle WT, Martin GR, Beekman RH, Morrow WR; American Academy of Pediatrics Section on Cardiology and Cardiac Surgery Executive Committee. Endorsement of Health and Human Services recommendation for pulse oximetry screening for critical congenital heart disease. *Pediatrics.* 2012;129:190–192

# Chapter 14

# Depression

*Lawrence S. Wissow, MD, MPH*

Symptoms of depression affect many children, including a large number whose symptoms do not rise to the level of a disorder. It is estimated that in the United States up to 3% of children younger than 13 years and up to 6% of adolescents experience depression at any given time. Estimates of lifetime prevalence of major depressive disorder (MDD) are significantly higher at up to 20%.[1]

Depression may remit on its own or after treatment but recur spontaneously at times of developmental transitions or with new stressors (both positive and negative). Depression is among the mental health problems associated with suicidal ideation, suicide attempts, and completed suicide. Other associated problems include negative effects on school performance, early pregnancy, and impairment of function in the work, social, and family environments.[2] Risk factors for the development of depression among children and adolescents include family history (heritability is approximately 40%), adverse childhood experiences, temperment/neuroticism, and the existence of a major nonmood disorder or a chronic or disabling medical condition.[3] Children who seem depressed may have relatives who have also experienced depression or other mental disorders. Finding such a history may reinforce the need to thoroughly evaluate concerns about the child, especialy if there is a family history of suicide. Knowing that there are other family members who have experienced the same problems can increase emphathy for the child's problems and may well provide role models for successful treatment.

There is some evidence that either initial onset or recurrence of depression may be preventable. Nurturing care during the critical first years of life, warm and confiding family relationships, learning active coping strategies for predictable stressors, promoting a sense of self-efficacy through learning to work through problems, and trying to maintain regular patterns of sleep and exercize may all be protective. If parents have mental health problems (especially depression), helping children understand and cope with changing parental mood and behavior may help prevent children themselves becoming depressed. If a child or youth has received treatment for depression, continuing treatment beyond the early stages of recovery is associated with a reduced risk of relapse or recurrence.

The guidance in this chapter applies to the care of children presenting with undifferentiated depression in pediatric clinical settings. It is based on the work of the World Health Organization, whose recommendations may be updated annually. The most up-to-date information can be found at www.who.int.

## ▶ FINDINGS SUGGESTING DEPRESSION

Though depression may come on without an apparent trigger, even among those who seem highly successful and privileged, it can often develop after 1 or more stresses or losses, or in conjunction with prolonged anxiety. Most children and adolescents will experience an event that induces sadness, such as breakup with a friend, the death of a loved one or pet, or other losses resulting from life changes such as a move, a family member's military deployment, or parents' separation. A sadness experience of greater intensity or duration than is typical for the child's peers is a cause for concern and may indicate depression. Symptoms of depression vary. A summary of the symptoms and clinical findings that suggest depression can be found in Box 14-1. For those familiar with the symptoms of depression in adults, it is important to remember that, among children, irritability may be a more prominent symptom than sadness. In some cases, withdrawal from usual activities or decreased interaction with friends and family may be the only obvious sign, possibly coupled with a change in appetite, sleep, or level of energy. Symptoms may be elicited from either parents or youth, but ideally from both. Children and youth may be better able to report on feelings that do not result in behavior change that is obvious to others; on the other hand, children and youth may not be aware of how their appearance or behavior has changed in ways that are apparent to others. Ideally, reports should be obtained from both youth and parents if there is a suspicion of depression.

## ▶ TOOLS TO ASSIST WITH IDENTIFICATION

Since many children do not spontaneously disclose their symptoms, standardized psychosocial screening instruments may be used to identify children with symptoms of depression. Several instruments have versions to collect information from the youth, parents, and teachers. Table 14-1 provides examples of general psychosocial screening results suggesting that a

**Box 14-1**

### *Symptoms and Clinical Findings Suggesting Depression*

#### INDICATIONS FROM HISTORY FROM YOUTH OR PARENT

- Low or sad mood present most days
- Loss of interest in school or other activities present most days
- Loss of pleasure in activities formerly enjoyed (When is last time he/you had fun?)
- Suicidal thoughts or acts
- Irritability (especially in adolescents)
- Academic difficulties
- Withdrawal from friends and family
- Physical symptoms such as headaches, abdominal pain, trouble sleeping, fatigue, or poor control of a chronic illness
- Hopelessness
- Poor concentration
- Poor or excessive sleep for developmental stage
- Weight loss (or failure to gain weight normally) or excessive weight gain
- Low self-esteem
- Loss of energy
- Agitation or slowing of movement or speech

#### RISK FACTORS FOR INCREASED SUSCEPTIBILITY

- Adverse childhood experiences (eg, mother experienced postpartum depression)
- Prior trauma or bereavement
- Family breakdown
- Shy personality
- Peer relationship problems
- Breakup of a relationship; setback or disappointment

**Table 14-1**
**General Psychosocial Screening/Results Suggesting Depression**

| SCREENING INSTRUMENT | SCORE SUGGESTING DEPRESSION |
|---|---|
| Pediatric Symptom Checklist (PSC)-35 | • Total score ≥24 for children 5 years and younger.<br>• ≥28 for those 6–16 years.<br>• ≥30 for those 17 years and older.<br>AND<br>• Further discussion of items related to depressive symptoms confirms a concern in that area. |
| PSC-17 | • Internalizing subscale is ≥5.<br>AND<br>• Further discussion of items related to depressive symptoms confirms a concern in that area. |
| Strengths & Difficulties Questionnaire (SDQ) | • Total symptom score of >19.<br>• Emotional symptom score of 7–10 (see instructions at www.sdqinfo.com).<br>• Impact scale (back of form) score of 1 (medium impairment) or ≥2 (high impairment).<br>AND<br>• Further discussion of items related to depression confirms a concern in that area. |

child may be depressed. Additional instruments such as the Patient Health Questionnaire for Adolescents (PHQ-A) or PHQ-A Depression Screen, Beck Depression Inventory-Primary Care (also known as Fast Screen), or the Modified Patient Health Questionnaire-9 (PHQ-9) can also be used to screen adolescents for depression or to help confirm findings of a general psychosocial screening.

It is important to differentiate the use of these tools as screening instruments at routine visits versus their use to refine concerns that have already been raised. When used as screening tools, they tend to have relatively low sensitivity and positive predictive value. That is, positive results need further discussion to understand the meaning of the result, and negative results may not be reassuring if the parent or youth are truly concerned. When used to follow up on existing concerns, results still need discussion with families, but are more likely be a fair indicator of the nature and severity of the child's problems. The use of a functional assessment tool such as the Strengths & Difficulties Questionnaire (SDQ) or Columbia Impairment Scale (CIS) will assist the clinician in determining whether the child's functioning is significantly impaired by the symptoms. Use of a tool to assess the impact of the child's problem on other members of the family may also be helpful; the Caregiver Strain Questionnaire (CGSQ) is one example.

## ▶ ASSESSMENT

Assessment begins by differentiating the child's symptoms from normal behavior. All children may be sad or irritable at times, but, for some children, these symptoms limit their adaptability to normal peer and family situations, interfere with learning, or precipitate suicidal thoughts. Of particular concern is major depressive disorder (MDD); *DSM-5* criteria for MDD are summarized in Box 14-2.

**Box 14-2**

## *Criteria for Major Depressive Episode* (DSM-5)

A. Five (or more) of the following symptoms have been present during the same 2-week period and represent a change from previous functioning; at least 1 of the symptoms is either depressed mood or loss of interest or pleasure. **Note:** Do not include symptoms that are clearly attributable to another medical condition.
   1. Depressed mood most of the day, nearly every day, as indicated by either subjective report (eg, feels sad, empty, hopeless) or observation made by others (eg, seems tearful). **Note:** In children and adolescents, can be irritable mood.
   2. Markedly diminished interest or pleasure in all, or almost all, activities most of the day, nearly every day (as indicated by either subjective account or observation).
   3. Significant weight loss when not dieting or weight gain (eg, a change of more than 5% of body weight in a month), or decrease or increase in appetite nearly every day. **Note:** In children, consider failure to make expected weight gain.
   4. Insomnia or hypersomnia nearly every day.
   5. Psychomotor agitation or retardation nearly every day (observable by others, not merely subjective feelings of restlessness or being slowed down).
   6. Fatigue or loss of energy nearly every day.
   7. Feelings of worthlessness or excessive or inappropriate guilt (which may be delusional) nearly every day (not merely self-reproach or guilt about being sick).
   8. Diminished ability to think or concentrate, or indecisiveness, nearly every day (either by subjective account or as observed by others).
   9. Recurrent thoughts of death (not just fear of dying), recurrent suicidal ideation without a specific plan, or a suicide attempt or a specific plan for committing suicide.

B. The symptoms cause clinically significant distress or impairment in social, occupational, or other important areas of functioning.

C. The episode is not attributable to the physiologic effects of a substance or to another medical condition. **Note:** Criteria A–C represent a major depressive episode. **Note:** Responses to a significant loss (eg, bereavement, financial ruin, losses from a natural disaster, a serious medical illness or disability) may include the feelings of intense sadness, rumination about the loss, insomnia, poor appetite and weight loss as noted in Criterion A, which may resemble a depressive episode. Although such symptoms may be understandable or considered appropriate to the loss, the presence of a major depressive episode in addition to the normal response to a significant loss should also be carefully considered. This decision inevitably requires the exercise of clinical judgment based on the individual's history and the cultural norms for the expression of distress in the context of loss.

D. The occurrence of the major depressive episode is not better explained by schizoaffective disorder, schizophrenia, schizophreniform disorder, delusional disorder, or other specified and unspecified schizophrenia spectrum and other psychotic disorders.

E. There has never been a manic episode or a hypomanic episode. **Note:** This exclusion does not apply if all of the manic-like or hypomanic-like episodes are substance-induced or are attributable to the psychological effects of another medical condition.

From American Psychiatric Association. *Diagnostic and Statistical Manual of Mental Disorders.* 5th ed. Washington, DC: American Psychiatric Publishing; 2013, with permission.

There are also some conditions that may mimic or co-occur with depression. Table 14-2 provides a summary of these conditions.

For a child with symptoms of depression, the psychosocial assessment process always includes determination of suicide risk, as described in Box 14-3.

**Table 14-2**
**Conditions That May Mimic or Co-occur With Depression**

| CONDITION | RATIONALE |
|---|---|
| Sleep deprivation | Sleep problems can cause irritability and labile mood; conversely, depression may contribute to difficulty sleeping. |
| Somatic complaints | Depressed children may present with a variety of somatic complaints (eg, gastrointestinal symptoms, headaches, chest pain). Conversely, acute or chronic medical conditions or pain syndromes may cause depression. |
| Learning problems or disabilities | If symptoms of depression are associated with problems of school performance, the child may be experiencing learning difficulties. See Chapter 49, Learning Difficulty, to explore this possibility. |
| Exposure to adverse childhood experiences (ACE) | Children who have experienced or witnessed trauma, violence, a natural disaster, separation from a parent, parental divorce or separation, parental substance use, neglect, or physical, emotional, or sexual abuse are at high risk of developing emotional difficulties such as adjustment disorder, post-traumatic stress disorder (PTSD), and depression. Denial of trauma symptoms does not mean trauma did not occur; questions about ACE should be repeated as a trusting relationship is established. See also Chapter 6, Anxiety. |
| Maltreatment | Children who have experienced neglect or physical, emotional, or sexual abuse are at high risk of developing emotional difficulties such as depression; this possibility should always be considered. |
| Anxiety | Depression often co-occurs with anxiety. See Chapter 6, Anxiety. |
| Bereavement | Most children will experience the death of a family member or friend sometime in their childhood. Other losses may also trigger grief responses—separation or divorce of parents, relocation, change of school, deployment of a parent in military service, breakup with a girlfriend or boyfriend, or remarriage of parent. Such losses are traumatic. They may result in feelings of sadness, despair, insecurity, or anxiety immediately following the loss and, in some instances, more persistent anxiety or mood symptoms or disorders. Furthermore, they may make the child more susceptible to impaired functioning at the time of subsequent losses. See also the discussion of PTSD in Chapter 6, Anxiety. |
| Physical illness and medication side effects | Medical issues that can mimic or provoke symptoms of depression include hypothyroidism, lupus, chronic fatigue syndrome, diabetes, and anemia. Children with any chronic medical condition are more likely to experience depression than their peers (and depression may contribute to poor management of the condition). Medications commonly used in adolescence can be associated with depression (eg, acne preparations, oral contraceptives, interferon, corticosteroids). |
| Substance use | Children with symptoms of depression may self-medicate with alcohol, nicotine, or other drugs. Conversely, children using substances may manifest depression and deteriorating school performance. See Chapter 75, Substance Use: Initial Approach in Primary Care. |
| Conduct or oppositional disorders | Oppositional children may manifest depressive symptoms. Children with conduct problems are at higher risk for suicide. See Chapter 16, Disruptive Behavior and Aggression. |
| Psychosis | Depression can be complicated by problems with thinking that go beyond the distortions or hopelessness of low mood. These problems include delusions (ie, strongly held and usually odd false beliefs about others, one's body, or one's self), paranoia (ie, strongly felt and unjustified concerns that others are following or intend harm), or hallucinations (ie, seeing or hearing things that others don't hear or see). Individuals often don't volunteer that they are having these sorts of thoughts; asking is important if the person's interactions seem unusual. (Do you ever feel your eyes or ears play tricks on you?) |

*Continued*

**Table 14-2**
**Conditions That May Mimic or Co-occur With Depression—cont'd**

| CONDITION | RATIONALE |
|---|---|
| Bipolar disorder | Adults and older adolescents with bipolar disorder may have markedly varying low mood (depression) or high mood (mania), cycling over weeks or months. Diagnosis of bipolar disorder in children remains controversial. It may be considered in children who cycle through low and high moods very rapidly and in children with explosive or destructive tantrums, dangerous or hypersexual behavior, aggression, irritability, bossiness with adults, driven creativity (sometimes depicting graphic violence), excessive talking, separation anxiety, chronic depression, sleep disturbance, delusions, hallucinations, psychosis, and talk of homicide or suicide. See also Chapter 45, Inattention and Impulsivity, Chapter 16, Disruptive Behavior and Aggression, and Chapter 6, Anxiety. |

**Box 14-3**

## *Determining Suicide Risk*

*Are there others in the family (present or past generations) who have had depression or bipolar disorder or who have attempted suicide?* Teens and parents may need opportunities to answer these questions confidentially because this is information that is not always shared among family members. Positive responses—especially a family history of suicide—increase concern. Other risk factors include substance use, a model among peers or famous individuals known to the youth, or a recent traumatic or shameful episode. A past attempt by the youth is the single strongest risk factor for future attempts and may warrant mental health referral for the current episode if the youth is not in ongoing care.

The severity of suicidal thoughts can be assessed with several questions (eg, Bright Futures, page 276) and tools (eg, SAD PERSONS; GLAD-PC). Examples include the following:

- *"Have you ever felt bad enough that you wished you were dead?"*
- *"Have you had any thoughts about wanting to kill yourself?"*
- *"Have you ever tried to hurt or kill yourself or come close to hurting or killing yourself?"*
- *"Do you have a plan?"*
- *"Do you have a way to carry out your plan?"*

One way of approaching suicidality is to think of your inquiry as a staged process. A significant minority of adolescents have transient suicidal thoughts or what psychiatrists call "passive death wishes"—thoughts that perhaps death would be a way out of problems or stresses but without thinking of a way to harm themselves. Absent the risk factors discussed above, these youth likely need exploration of stressors and assessment for depression or other mental health problems. A smaller group will have thought about ways of harming themselves but without a concrete plan or making any preparations. Again, absent past attempts, ongoing stressors, or substance use, these youth need support and further evaluation but are not at high risk of harming themselves. Youth with plans for harming themselves (no matter what the likelihood of success) or who have gathered or identified the means (ropes, medications, knives or other weapons) are at high risk of harming themselves. They require both a short-term plan for safety and an urgent mental health evaluation. For more information, see Chapter 68, Self-harm.

## ▶ PLAN OF CARE FOR YOUTH WITH DEPRESSION

Suicidal intent is an emergency requiring immediate treatment and close supervision of the youth at all times. The care of a youth experiencing depression can begin in the primary care setting from the time symptoms are recognized, even if the youth's symptoms do not rise to the level of a disorder and regardless of whether referral to a mental health specialist is ultimately part of the care plan.

### *Engage Youth and Family in Care*

Without engagement, most families will not seek or persist in care. The process may require multiple primary care visits.[4]

Reinforce strengths of the youth and family (eg, good relationships with at least 1 parent or important adult, prosocial peers, concerned or caring family, help-seeking, connection to positive organizations) as a method of engagement and identify any barriers to addressing the problem (eg, stigma, family conflict, resistance to treatment). Use "common factors" techniques[5] to build trust and optimism, reach agreement on incremental next steps, develop a plan of care, and collaboratively determine the role of the primary care physician. Regardless of other roles, the primary care physician can encourage a positive view of treatment on the part of the youth and family.

### *Provide Psychoeducation*

Depression is very common and not the result of lack of coping ability or personal strength. There is often a family history of the condition; talking about this may reduce stigma and increase empathy and a willingness to seek care, but may also be met with resistance. To assist family members in understanding the disorder, additional points to highlight include that the youth is not making the symptoms up, what looks like laziness or crossness can be symptoms of depression, and the hopelessness of depression is a symptom, not an accurate reflection of reality. However, this negative view of the world and of future possibilities can be hard to penetrate. In addition, the clinician can emphasize that treatment works, though it can take several weeks for improvement, and the affected individual is often the last person to recognize that it has taken place.

Families should be encouraged to address risk factors for maintenance of depression and for the risk of suicidal acts. Weapons should ideally be removed from the home or secured, and a careful survey should be made for potentially lethal medications or household chemicals including pesticides. Suicidal and depressive thoughts can be spread through social networks and, increasingly, through social media. Electronic communication has been found, paradoxically, to promote isolation at the same time as it seems to be increasing connectedness. Though not often easy, parents can be helped to both monitor and limit the use of e-mail, texts, and social media posts until the child has recovered.

The clinician may also, at this point, talk about how there is a variety of treatments for depression including various forms of psychosocial care, and, for teens, medications. It may be useful to ask about what the teen and family have thought of or heard about treatment;

in that way, the clinician can discover if they are anxious that the discussion is leading to a suggestion they would not be willing to accept.

### Encourage Healthy Habits

Encourage exercise, outdoor play, healthy diet, sleep, limiting screen time, 1-on-1 time with parents, praise for positive behavior, and acknowledgment of the youth's strengths. Caring for oneself can be presented honestly as therapeutic. One can "prescribe pleasure" by telling youth and families that caring for oneself, including engaging in activities that previously were pleasurable, is not weakness but rather an important part of self-care, just as athletes need to rest or stretch in addition to testing their limits in workouts.

### Reduce Stress

Consider the youth's social environment (eg, family social history, parental depression screening, results of any family assessment tools administered, reports from child care or school). Questions to raise might include the following:

- *Are there grief and loss issues in the youth or other family members?* Grief and loss are virtually universal childhood experiences. Children vary widely in their reactions to these events, depending on their developmental level, temperament, prior state of mental health, coping mechanisms, parental responses, and support system. Also helpful can be supportive counseling; explaining to children and adolescents what they might reasonably expect; inviting them to participate in the funeral or other ceremonies to the level they feel comfortable; active listening while allowing the child or adolescent to express his or her grief; providing guidance about the grief process; and identifying and addressing feelings of guilt. When a parent is also grieving, children and adolescents may need time alone with the clinician because they may be reluctant to increase parental sadness. Providing follow-up to see how the child and family are coping with a loss can help gauge how the family is doing and provide opportunities to assess for more serious reactions such as complicated bereavement, depression, or PTSD. Providing referral to community resources may also be helpful. The effects of profound losses, such as the death of a sibling or parent during childhood or removal from parents, last a lifetime. The clinician will need to view all future physical and mental health issues in the family through the prism of this loss. Overlooking such experiences and failing to follow up on the child and family's progress after a traumatic event are lost opportunities to connect with the child and family around important mental health issues.
- *Is the youth or family experiencing unusual stress?* The family can work to try to reduce stresses and increase support for the youth. This may involve reasonable and short-term changes in demands and responsibilities, including negotiating extensions for assignments or other ways of reducing stress at school; it can also include seeking help for others in the family who are distressed. If a parent is grieving a loss or manifesting symptoms of depression, it is particularly important that the parent address his or her own needs and find additional support for the youth and other family members.
- *Are there weapons or medications in the house?* Guns should be removed from the home; other weapons, medications (including over-the-counter preparations and acetaminophen), and alcohol should be removed from the home, destroyed, or secured. In farm communities, there may be toxic products (such as insecticides or fertilizers) that may need to be secured. Depressed individuals should be dissuaded from operating dangerous

machinery or engaging in other activities that require care and normal risk aversion to avoid injury.

### Offer Initial Intervention(s) to Address the Depression Symptoms

The strategies described in the following text are common elements of evidence-based psychosocial interventions for depression in children and adolescents. They are applicable to the care of children with mild or emerging depressive symptoms and to those with impairing symptoms that do not rise to the level of a disorder. They can also be used as initial management of children with a depressive disorder while readying them for or awaiting access to specialty care.

*Help the youth to develop cognitive and coping skills.* Find agreement with the youth and family on a description of the problem. Many negative thoughts can be empathetically challenged and looked at from another perspective. Helpful metaphors include, "Long journeys start with a single step" and "The glass is half full, not half empty." Relaxation techniques and visualization (eg, practicing relaxation cued by a pleasant memory, imagining being in a pleasant place) can be helpful for sleep and for anxiety-provoking situations. The clinician can also ask the youth what he or she does to feel better or relax and, if appropriate, prescribe more of that (*behavioral activation*). Encourage a focus on strengths rather than weaknesses and doing more of what the youth is good at. Distraction is also good therapy—if the youth is ruminating on a particular stressor, give permission to think about or engage with something else.

*Help the youth to develop problem-solving skills.* Determine what small achievable act would help the youth feel that he is on the way to overcoming his problems. Suggest that the youth list difficulties, prioritize them, and concentrate efforts on one issue at a time. Avoid downplaying social crises that are important to the young person even if, from an adult perspective, they seem trivial. Instead, offer to help the young person evaluate the options as he sees them, seeking, if there is an opening, permission to offer alternatives that may not have been raised.

*Rehearse behavior and social skills.* Reactions to particular situations or people often seem to trigger or maintain low mood. If these can be identified, assist the youth in developing and practicing means of avoidance or alternative responses. Practice doing things and thinking thoughts that improve mood.

*Create a safety and emergency plan.* Developed in partnership with the family, a treatment plan includes a listing of telephone numbers to call in the event of a sudden increase in distress. This listing should be specific to the child's community and circumstances (eg, the number for a suicide or depression hotline, on-call telephone number for the practice, or area mental health crisis response team contact information. The family should also be instructed to proactively remove lethal means and monitor for suicide risk factors such as increased agitation, stressors, loss of rational thinking, expressed wishes to die, previous attempts, and comorbid conduct disorder or aggressive outbursts.

### Provide Resources

Helpful handouts and Web sites are included in Tools for Practice: Engaging Patient and Family at the end of this chapter. Provide the family with contact numbers and resources in case of emergency.

### Monitor the Youth's Progress Toward Therapeutic Goals

Child care, preschool, or school reports can be helpful in monitoring progress. Screening instruments that gather information from multiple reporters (youth, parent, teacher), such as the SDQ and PSC, can be helpful in monitoring progress with symptoms and functioning.

It is important for the clinician to work with the family to understand that it is not uncommon for treatment to be successful for a period and then seem to lose effectiveness. This can happen when there are new stresses or demands, or when, after a period of success, there has been a letup on treatment. If troubleshooting existing treatment and ways of dealing with new stresses does not help get function back to baseline, new treatments, or new diagnoses, need to be considered. In particular, as school demands increase, learning issues may need to be considered even if they were not seen as contributing problems in the past.

### Involve Specialist(s)

Involve specialist(s) if the youth does not respond to initial interventions or if indicated by the following clinical circumstances:

- A preadolescent child manifests depression or suicidal ideation.
- An adolescent with depressive symptoms has made a prior suicide attempt, developed a plan (especially with means available), or known a friend or acquaintance who has committed suicide.
- An adolescent's functioning is significantly impaired.
- Symptoms are threatening the achievement of developmentally important goals (eg, attending school or spending time with friends.
- The adolescent has mental health comorbidities such as substance use or odd behavior suggestive of an emerging psychotic disorder.
- The adolescent also has symptoms of bipolar disorder—elevated (often more driven rather than positive) mood and energy associated with irritability and behavior that seems audacious for his or her age (grandiosity).
- Depressive symptoms were preceded by serious trauma.

For youth with a diagnosis of moderate to severe MDD, data indicate superior efficacy of a combination of cognitive behavior therapy (CBT) and a selective serotonin reuptake inhibitor (SSRI) compared with either CBT alone (which may not be sufficiently helpful for these more severe cases) or an SSRI alone.[6] Thus, youth with MDD would ideally receive treatment from a licensed therapist with training in CBT (see following text).

*When specialty care is needed, ensure that it is evidence-informed and assist the family in accessing it.* A variety of evidence-based and evidence-informed psychosocial interventions, and some pharmacologic interventions, are available for the treatment of depressive disorders in children and adolescents. Ideally, those referred for care in the mental health specialty system would have access to the safest and most effective treatments. Table 14-3 provides a summary of these interventions. Youth referred for mental health specialty care complete the referral process only 61% of the time, and a significantly smaller number persist in care.[7,8] Approaches to improving the referral process include making sure that the family is ready for this step in care, that they have some idea of what the specialty care will involve, and that they understand what the physician's ongoing role may be. If the specialty appointment is not likely to occur shortly, the physician can work with the child and family on a plan to manage the problem as well as possible in the meantime.

**Table 14-3**
**Psychosocial and Psychopharmacologic Treatments for Depression (as of November 2014)[a]**

| | PSYCHOSOCIAL TREATMENTS | |
|---|---|---|
| **CLUSTER AREA** | **LEVEL 1 (BEST SUPPORT)** | **LEVEL 2 (GOOD SUPPORT)** |
| Depressive or withdrawn behaviors[b] | • Cognitive behavior therapy (CBT)<br>• CBT and medication<br>• CBT with parents (includes parent and child, focusing on the child's concerns)<br>• Family therapy | • Client-centered therapy<br>• Cognitive behavioral psychoeducation<br>• Expressive writing/journaling/diary<br>• Interpersonal therapy<br>• Relaxation |
| Suicidality[b] | None | • Attachment therapy<br>• Counselors care<br>• Counselors care and support training<br>• Interpersonal therapy<br>• Multisystemic therapy<br>• Psychodynamic<br>• Social support |
| **US FOOD AND DRUG ADMINISTRATION–APPROVED PSYCHOPHARMACOLOGIC INTERVENTIONS[c]** | | |
| **DIAGNOSTIC AREA** | **PSYCHOPHARMACOLOGIC INTERVENTION** | |
| Major depressive disorder (MDD) | Selective serotonin reuptake inhibitor (SSRI) (fluoxetine and escitalopram are currently the only drugs approved by the FDA for treating MDD among youth). There are data that indicate superior efficacy of combination CBT and SSRI versus CBT or SSRI alone. | |

[a]For AAP policy, please visit pediatrics.aappublications.org/site/aappolicy.
[b]Excerpted from PracticeWise Evidence-Based Child and Adolescent Psychosocial Interventions. Reprinted with permission from PracticeWise. For updates and an explanation of PracticeWise determination of evidence level, please visit www.aap.org/mentalhealth.
[c]For up-to-date information about Food and Drug Administration (FDA)-approved interventions, go to www.fda.gov/ScienceResearch/SpecialTopics/PediatricTherapeuticsResearch/default.htm.

*Reach agreement on respective roles in the youth's care.* If the youth is referred to mental health specialty care for a depressive disorder, his or her primary care physician may be responsible for initiating medication or adjusting doses; monitoring response to treatment; monitoring adverse effects; engaging and encouraging the youth's and family's positive view of treatment; and coordinating care provided by parents, school, medical home, and specialists. In fact, the youth may improve just knowing that the clinician is involved and interested. Resources available to help clinicians in these roles are provided in Tools for Practice: Medical Decision Support.

Note that not all evidence-based interventions may be available in every community. If a particular intervention is not available, this becomes an opportunity to collaborate with others in the community to advocate on behalf of children. Increasingly, states offer both telepsychiatry services and consultation/referral support "warmlines" that help physicians provide initial treatment and locate resources. The availability of the latter form of help is tracked at www.nncpap.org.

### *ACKNOWLEDGMENT*

The author and editor wish to acknowledge the contributions of Linda Paul, MPH, manager of the AAP Mental Health Leadership Work Group.

### *TOOLS FOR PRACTICE*

#### Engaging Patient and Family

- *Childhood Depression: What Parents Can Do to Help* (fact sheet), American Academy of Pediatrics (www.healthychildren.org/English/health-issues/conditions/emotional-problems/Pages/Childhood-Depression-What-Parents-Can-Do-To-Help.aspx)
- *Help Stop Teenage Suicide* (fact sheet), American Academy of Pediatrics (www.healthychildren.org/English/health-issues/conditions/emotional-problems/Pages/Help-Stop-Teen-Suicide.aspx)
- *Teen Suicide, Mood Disorder, and Depression* (handout), American Academy of Pediatrics (patiented.solutions.aap.org)
- *Ten Things Parents Can Do to Prevent Suicide* (fact sheet), American Academy of Pediatrics (www.healthychildren.org/English/health-issues/conditions/emotional-problems/Pages/Ten-Things-Parents-Can-Do-to-Prevent-Suicide.aspx)

#### Medical Decision Support

- *Patient Health Questionnaire (PHQ) Screeners* (screen), Pfizer, Inc (www.phqscreeners.com)
- *Pediatric Symptom Checklist* (screen), Massachusetts General Hospital (www.massgeneral.org/psychiatry/services/psc_forms.aspx)
- *Strengths & Difficulties Questionnaire* (screen), Youth in Mind, Ltd (www.sdqinfo.com)
- *Adapted SAD PERSONS* (screen), American Academy of Pediatrics (pediatrics.aappublications.org/content/125/Supplement_3/S195.full.pdf)

### *REFERENCES*

1. Williams SB, O'Connor EA, Eder M, Whitlock EP. Screening for child and adolescent depression in primary care settings: a systematic evidence review for the US Preventive Services Task Force. *Pediatrics.* 2009;123:e716–e735
2. Fergusson DM, Woodward LJ. Mental health, educational, and social role outcomes of adolescents with depression. *Arch Gen Psychiatry.* 2002;59:225–231
3. American Psychiatric Association. *Diagnostic and Statistical Manual of Mental Disorders.* 5th ed. Washington, DC: American Psychiatric Publishing; 2013
4. Foy JM; American Academy of Pediatrics Task Force on Mental Health. Enhancing pediatric mental health care: algorithms for primary care. *Pediatrics.* 2010;125(Suppl 3):S109–S125
5. Kemper KJ, Wissow L, Foy JM, Shore SE. *Core Communication Skills for Primary Clinicians.* Wake Forest School of Medicine. nwahec.org/45737. Accessed January 9, 2015
6. Hodes M, Garralda E. NICE guidelines on depression in children and young people: not always following the evidence. *Psychiatric Bulletin.* 2007;31:361–362
7. Manfredi C, Lacey L, Warnecke R. Results of an intervention to improve compliance with referrals for evaluation of suspected malignancies at neighborhood public health centers. *Am J Public Health.* 1990;80:85–87
8. Friman PC, Finney JW, Rapoff MA, Christophersen ER. Improving pediatric appointment keeping with reminders and reduced response requirement. *J Appl Behav Anal.* 1985;18:315–321

# Chapter 15

# Diarrhea and Steatorrhea

*Martin H. Ulshen, MD*

Diarrhea, similar to vomiting, is a common symptom in young children, especially during infancy. Loosely defined, diarrhea is characterized by an increase in the frequency and water content of stools. Normal daily stool volume varies with the size of the child. Adults and older children have a normal daily stool weight up to 250 g (consisting of 60%–85% water); infants weighing fewer than 10 kg can have about 5 g/kg/day of stool. An intermediate range of 50 to 75 g/day is an appropriate approximation for the preschool-aged child. In infancy, the frequency and quality of normal stools depend very much on diet.

During the first weeks of life, breastfed infants commonly have up to 8 loose stools per day, which, at times, may contain mucus. These stools frequently follow feedings, as a result of the *gastrocolic reflex*, and do not constitute diarrhea. Infants receiving cow milk or soy formula usually have firmer and somewhat less frequent stools. After the first few weeks of life, normal breastfed infants tend to have less frequent stools, occasionally even less than once a week, although the stools remain soft. Commonly, the stool of the nursing infant becomes firm when solids or cow milk is introduced into the diet.

Steatorrhea signifies an excess of fat in the stool and is a symptom of malabsorption. However, disorders associated with malabsorption, such as gluten-sensitive enteropathy, do not always produce steatorrhea. Stools that contain an increased quantity of fat can be greasy, bulky, and foul smelling; however, with mild steatorrhea, the stool may appear normal. The stool can be evaluated quickly for fat content by using light microscopy with Sudan staining (known as qualitative analysis for stool fat). Fat excretion can be measured more precisely by quantitative chemical analysis of a 72-hour collection of stool. A record of the diet is kept during this period, and fat intake is calculated. The percentage of the ingested fat that is absorbed is called the *coefficient of absorption.*

$$\frac{\text{Fat Intake} - \text{Fat Output}}{\text{Fat Intake}} \times 100$$

Absorption of fat by infants varies with the type of fat that is fed and with the maturity of the infant. A healthy premature infant may absorb as little as 65% to 75% of dietary fat, but this amount improves to 90% in the term infant. Furthermore, neonates absorb vegetable fat much more efficiently than butterfat but human milk fat best of all. Children and adults typically absorb at least 95% of the fat in a normal diet.

## ▶ PATHOPHYSIOLOGIC FACTORS

Advances in the understanding of the pathophysiologic mechanism of diarrhea allow a more rational approach to diagnosis and treatment. Normally, the gastrointestinal tract processes a large volume of fluid (Figure 15-1 lists adult data). An infant can rapidly become fluid depleted from diarrhea when such large gastrointestinal fluid shifts take place each day. Under normal circumstances, about 90% of fluid absorption takes place in the small bowel. However, the colon has a reserve capacity for fluid absorption that must be overcome before diarrhea results. In adults, the colon can reabsorb as much as 2 L of ileal fluid daily without diarrhea occurring.

Movement of water across the gastrointestinal tract mucosa is passive, following osmotic gradients created by electrolytes and other osmotically active solutes such as glucose and amino acids. Nutrients are absorbed by active transport, facilitated transport, or passive diffusion; some solutes first require digestion to simpler compounds. The flux of electrolytes across the mucosa is bidirectional. The net result of absorption and secretion of these osmotically active solutes is net water retention or loss in the stool. In this sense, diarrhea can be considered the result of either malabsorption or net secretion of osmotically active substances.

Many nutrients, including glucose and most amino acids, are absorbed by active, carrier-mediated transport, which is coupled with sodium transport. The osmotic gradient created promotes the absorption of water. Movement of water, in turn, also carries small solutes such as sodium and chloride. This process is known as *solvent drag* and appears to be an important route for sodium absorption during normal digestion. These mechanisms of sodium movement associated with carrier-mediated nonelectrolyte transport are important to preserve

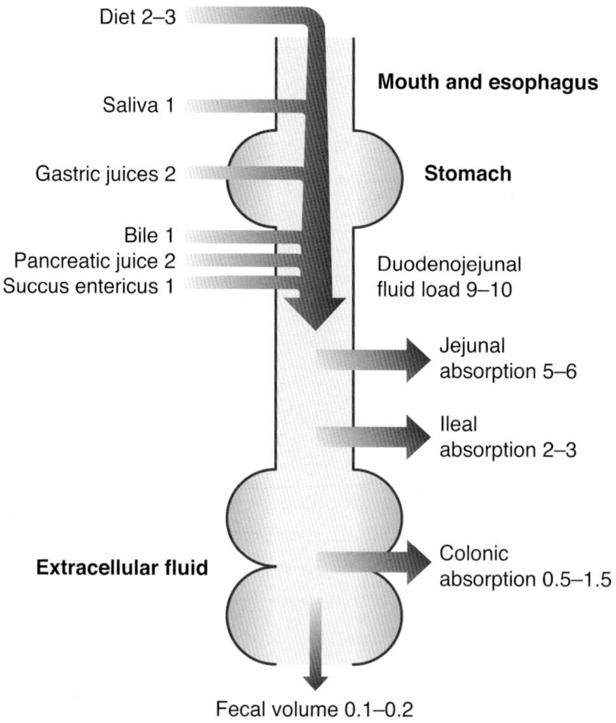


**Figure 15-1**
Ingestion, secretion, and absorption of water in the gastrointestinal tract of an adult. Numbers refer to liters of water.

normal fluid and electrolyte balance during some episodes of diarrhea (see discussion on oral rehydration).

Active absorption of chloride in exchange for bicarbonate takes place in the ileum and colon. Potassium moves passively along electrochemical gradients in the small intestine, but both active absorption and secretion of potassium occur in the colon. The permeability of the intestinal mucosa to passive fluid and electrolyte movement is high in the duodenum and proximal jejunum and decreases distally to the ileum and colon, which are poorly permeable. This feature allows the proximal intestinal contents to equilibrate rapidly with the isotonic extracellular fluid and facilitates the rapid absorption of water and small solutes by diffusion (ie, solvent drag). Conversely, the ileum and colon are poorly permeable and are able to absorb water and sodium against high electrochemical gradients.

The pathophysiologic mechanisms for diarrhea fall into 4 basic groups[1,2]: osmotic diarrhea, diarrhea resulting from secretion or altered absorption of electrolytes, exudative diarrhea, and diarrhea resulting from abnormal intestinal motility. Each mechanism has unique clinical characteristics and requires a different therapeutic approach. Therefore, for the physician considering an individual patient who has diarrhea, this framework provides a rational approach for both diagnosis and treatment. Frequently, more than one mechanism of diarrhea will be involved in an episode of diarrhea, but this variation will be apparent in the evaluation.

## Osmotic Diarrhea

The ingestion of a poorly absorbable, osmotically active substance and its presence in the bowel lumen create an osmotic gradient that encourages movement of water into the lumen and subsequently into the stool. Electrolyte losses increase because electrolytes will follow water into the lumen through solvent drag and will tend not to be reabsorbed because of unfavorable electrochemical gradients.

Two main groups of poorly absorbed solutes exist, the ingestion of which result in osmotic diarrhea. The first group includes normal dietary components that may be malabsorbed either transiently or permanently. For example, disaccharides are usually hydrolyzed to monosaccharides before they are absorbed. If a mucosal disaccharidase (eg, lactase) is deficient, then the disaccharide (in this case lactose) will be malabsorbed and will represent an osmotic load that will produce diarrhea. Similarly, monosaccharides may, at times, be poorly absorbed. Medium-chain triglycerides are also osmotically active and may lead occasionally to diarrhea when ingested in high concentration, such as when infants who have compromised mucosal function are given an elemental formula containing medium-chain triglycerides. Malabsorption of long-chain triglycerides (LCTs) does not lead to osmotic diarrhea because LCTs are large hydrophobic molecules and therefore have little osmotic activity. Malabsorption of LCTs, however, may lead to secretory diarrhea, as described later in this chapter. In addition, any osmotically active solute may produce diarrhea in healthy persons if given in quantities great enough to surpass the intestinal capacity for absorption. Thus some infants whose bowel function is normal will not tolerate the high osmolality of an elemental formula, especially if it is undiluted. Similarly, older children may develop functional gastrointestinal symptoms, including diarrhea, from ingesting large amounts of fructose in fruits and juices.[3] Patients who have decreased mucosal surface area may have decreased functional capacity and resultant osmotic diarrhea, a problem seen in infants after small bowel resection. Protein malabsorption does not appear to be associated with diarrhea, except in the rare instance of congenital trypsinogen or enterokinase deficiency. For example, Hartnup syndrome, with its malabsorption of primary amino acids, is not associated with diarrhea.

The second group of poorly absorbed solutes includes substances that are transported in limited amounts, even by healthy individuals. This group includes magnesium, phosphates, and sulfates. Because these ions invariably lead to diarrhea when given in large enough quantities, they are used as cathartics. The introduction of lactulose in the treatment of hepatic encephalopathy takes advantage of its being a nondigestible disaccharide that leads to acidification of colonic contents by bacterial fermentation of nonabsorbed sugar. Its side effect is diarrhea. In fact, lactulose has become a popular alternative for the treatment of constipation. Sorbitol, an artificial sweetener, causes osmotic diarrhea when ingested in large quantities.

The key characteristic of an osmotic diarrhea is its association with the ingestion of the offending solute. When a patient who has an osmotic diarrhea is given no oral or enteral feeding, the diarrhea will stop dramatically within 24 hours or less. If the agent is reintroduced, as in a lactose tolerance test, the diarrhea will reappear. The diarrhea is of a moderate volume compared with that in secretory diarrhea. The sodium and potassium ion concentrations in the stool fluid are useful in establishing a diagnosis. As ileal and colonic sodium absorption continue to function against a concentration gradient, stool sodium concentration will be lower than it is in the plasma. Normally, the electrolyte concentration in the stool is roughly twice its combined sodium and potassium concentration. When this number is much less than the total stool osmolality (usually about 290 mOsm/kg), osmotically active nonelectrolytes must be in the stool, and osmotic diarrhea is present.[4] An osmotic gap of more than 50 mOsm/kg indicates osmotic diarrhea. In some instances, the physician may be able to find the osmotic component in the stool, such as a reducing substance in lactose malabsorption.

### Diarrhea Secondary to Secretion or Altered Electrolyte Absorption (Secretory Diarrhea)

Under normal circumstances, opposing active and passive secretory and absorptive processes result in normal luminal electrolyte and water content. Secretory diarrhea occurs when a physiologic electrolyte secretory process is pathologically stimulated. Under such circumstances, a net increase in luminal electrolytes and, subsequently, a secondary increase in water occur. In addition, an associated decrease in absorptive processes may occur. The electrolytes that have been implicated are sodium, chloride, and perhaps bicarbonate. Diarrhea also may result from a decrease in active electrolyte absorption in the absence of any change in secretory function. Distinguishing increased electrolyte secretion from decreased absorption is clinically difficult; the results are similar.

The prototype for a secretory diarrhea is cholera. Cholera enterotoxin increases intestinal secretion of chloride and inhibits the absorption of sodium by stimulating surface epithelial adenylate cyclase, leading to an increase in cellular levels of cyclic 3'5'-adenosine monophosphate. The intestinal mucosa appears normal during cholera infection, without evidence of cell necrosis, inflammation, or local bacterial invasion; and other cell absorptive functions remain normal. The normal absorption of glucose provides a route for secondary sodium absorption; as a result, oral glucose- and electrolyte-containing solutions have gained wide use in the management of cholera. A growing number of infectious agents may be associated with secretory diarrhea. Toxigenic *Escherichia coli* produces at least 2 enterotoxins that activate adenylate cyclase or guanylate cyclase. Infantile diarrhea resulting from enterotoxigenic *E coli* is well known. Other bacteria that have been associated with stimulation of intestinal secretion are strains of *Shigella, Salmonella, Yersinia, Klebsiella, Clostridium perfringens, Staphylococcus aureus*, and *Pseudomonas* species. Experimental work with viral enteritis suggests that this diarrhea has a significant secretory component.[5] With rotavirus infection, secretion is the result of viral enterotoxin and only secondarily of damage to villous epithelial cells in the small intestine and repopulation of the villi with immature crypt cells.[6]

Noninfectious causes of secretory diarrhea exist as well. Malabsorbed bile acids and long-chain fats have been shown to stimulate a colonic secretory diarrhea.[7] Certain prostaglandins have been shown to activate adenylate cyclase and produce intestinal secretion in experimental models. Because prostaglandins are released during inflammation, researchers have hypothesized that diarrhea associated with certain inflammatory states may be caused by these hormones. This hypothesis is a particularly appealing way to explain the small bowel secretion that may take place with chronic inflammatory bowel disease. Prostaglandins have also been suggested as possible mediators for the activation of adenylate cyclase by *Salmonella* organisms in the absence of an enterotoxin. Secretory diarrhea may occur in association with increased levels of certain gastrointestinal hormones, most notably vasoactive intestinal polypeptide (VIP).

Isolated decrease of electrolyte absorption is much less frequent. The best-known example, although extremely rare, is congenital chloride-losing diarrhea. This autosomal recessive abnormality results from the apparent lack of normal, active chloride absorption by the distal small intestine. Great quantities of chloride are lost in the stool and lead to diarrhea from birth onward. A metabolic alkalosis results, in contrast to other causes of diarrhea.

The stool in secretory diarrheas tends to be watery and large in volume. Unlike osmotic diarrhea, secretory diarrhea persists despite discontinuing oral intake. The stool electrolyte concentration (ie, twice the sum of the sodium and potassium concentrations) is about equal to the stool water osmolality because no significant osmotic nonelectrolyte component is present.[4]

### Exudative Diarrhea

A break in the integrity of the mucosal surface of the intestine can result in water and electrolyte loss, driven by hydrostatic pressure in blood vessels and lymphatics. The exudate contains mucus, protein, and blood cells. Examples include infectious, allergic, or ulcerative colitis.

### Motility Diarrhea

The intestine has a cyclical, orderly pattern of motility. Increased, decreased, or disordered movement can lead to diarrhea. Rapid intestinal transit often occurs in association with osmotic and secretory diarrheas. Increased intraluminal volume has been implicated in stimulating increased peristaltic action. Increased motility may cause diarrhea by allowing less time for the contact of intraluminal contents with absorptive surfaces. When bowel function is compromised, as with short bowel syndrome, the time of contact with the limited functioning surface may be a crucial factor. In irritable bowel syndrome, disordered motility may also play a role.[8] Slowed transit and severely disordered motility lead to intraluminal stasis. In the normal bowel, steady, progressive movement of chyme is one of the mechanisms that prevents the development of bacterial overgrowth, whereas stasis encourages overgrowth. Certain bacteria deconjugate bile acids in the upper small bowel and produce fat malabsorption. In addition, bacterial proteases may damage the small bowel surface. Stasis may result from an anatomic obstruction, as well as from functional motor disorders. Disordered motility frequently is an associated factor in chronic inflammatory bowel disease. Stools associated with motility diarrhea, except those secondary to fatty acid malabsorption, tend to be small in volume. The response to feeding is variable, and the gastrocolic reflex may be heightened. Patients who have chronic inflammatory bowel disease may find that meals stimulate intestinal activity, resulting in postprandial abdominal cramps and bowel movements.

## ACUTE DIARRHEA

Acute diarrhea is common in children, is transient and usually self-limited, and is caused most often by infection. In the United States, children in the first few years of life average 1 or 2 episodes per year.[9] For most diarrheal infections, the incidence is greatest before 4 years of age. The role of the physician is to rule out causes that require specific treatment, to advise parents in supportive management, and to provide follow-up for possible complications. Box 15-1 lists some of the more frequent causes of acute diarrhea categorized by the usual presentation with or without gross blood in the stool. Transmission of diarrheal organisms is commonly by food, water, person-to-person spread, or exposure to animals at home, fairs, and petting zoos. Child care centers are likely sites for the spread of enteric pathogens. Pathogens that have been associated with epidemics include *Giardia lamblia*, rotavirus, *Norovirus*, *Shigella*, *Campylobacter*, *Cryptosporidium*, and *C difficile* organisms.[10–13]

**BOX 15-1**

### *Causes of Acute Diarrhea*

**USUALLY WITHOUT BLOOD IN STOOL**

- Viral enteritis rotavirus, orbivirus, noroviruses, other caliciviruses, enteric adenovirus, astrovirus, sapoviruses
- Enterotoxin *E coli*, *Klebsiella* organisms, cholera, *C perfringens*, *Staphylococcus* organisms, *Bacillus cereus*, and *Vibrio* species
- Parasitic *Giardia*, *Cryptosporidium*, *Cyclospora*, *Dientamoeba fragilis*, and *Blastocystis hominis* organisms
- Extraintestinal infection otitis media and urinary tract infection
- Antibiotic-induced and *C difficile* toxin (without pseudomembranous colitis)

**COMMONLY ASSOCIATED WITH BLOOD IN STOOL**

- Bacterial *Shigella*, *Salmonella*, and *Campylobacter* organisms, *Yersinia enterocolitica*, invasive *E coli*, gonococcus (venereal spread), enteroadherent *E coli*, enteroaggregative *E coli*, *Aeromonas hydrophilia*, and *Plesiomonas* shigelloides
- Cytomegalovirus (especially in immunocompromised individuals)
- Amebic dysentery, *Trichuris trichiura* (whipworm)
- Hemolytic uremic syndrome (enterohemorrhagic *E coli*—*E coli* O157:H7 and other Shiga toxin-producing *E coli*)
- Henoch-Schönlein purpura
- Pseudomembranous enterocolitis (*C difficile* toxin)
- Ulcerative or granulomatous colitis (acute presentation)
- Necrotizing enterocolitis (neonates)

### Neonatal Diarrhea

Neonates with acute diarrhea must be considered differently from older infants and children because of both lower tolerance to the associated fluid shifts and the greater likelihood of severe infection or of a congenital anomaly. In addition, signs of necrotizing enterocolitis, including gastric retention (frequently bilious), distention, and occult or bright red blood in the stool, should raise concern. Although this disease usually occurs in premature infants, it also has been reported in full-term infants. The presence of pneumatosis intestinalis, gas in the portal vein, or free intraperitoneal gas seen on abdominal radiographs supports this diagnosis. Epidemics of diarrhea associated with rotavirus, enteropathogenic *E coli*, salmonellae, and other organisms, including *Klebsiella* organisms, have been reported in nurseries. If the onset of diarrhea is associated with initial feedings, then the physician should consider congenital digestive defects, especially sugar intolerance. Hirschsprung disease may produce acute diarrhea and enterocolitis in the neonatal period and should be considered, especially in the infant who has not passed meconium in the first 24 hours. Bloody diarrhea that results from cow milk or soy protein intolerance may develop as early as the first few days of life. Resolution and exacerbation on removal and reintroduction of cow milk or soy formula, as well as an atopic family history, are clues to the diagnosis.

### Differential Diagnosis in the Older Infant and Child

Most episodes of acute diarrhea are transient and benign. On the initial visit, the physician must evaluate the course in terms of both possible causes and the status of hydration. The diarrhea is usually the result of viral enteritis, typically occurring with low-grade fever, vomiting, and frequent watery stools. Generally, the stools are without blood or white blood cells. Enterotoxin-producing organisms (eg, toxigenic *E coli*) are associated with watery stools and are without evidence of mucosal invasion (no high fever or blood in the stool). *G lamblia* produces watery diarrhea associated with intestinal gas and crampy abdominal pain. Diarrhea in association with extraintestinal infections, most notably otitis media and pyelonephritis, has been called *parenteral diarrhea*; its mechanism is obscure. An associated viral enteritis may occur in some cases of otitis media. Certain antibiotics, especially ampicillin, have been associated with transient diarrhea. Less common but of greater danger is antibiotic-associated pseudomembranous colitis,[10] which may occur acutely or as a more chronic illness of 1 or 2 months' duration.[14] *C difficile* toxin, the cause of most cases of pseudomembranous colitis, may also be associated with chronic childhood diarrhea in the absence of colitis.[15]

The presence of blood in the stool, especially with symptoms of colonic involvement (tenesmus, urgency, and crampy lower abdominal pain), should make the physician think of infection with *Campylobacter*, *Shigella*, or *Salmonella* organisms or with *C difficile* toxin-associated pseudomembranous colitis. The symptoms of dysentery may be less striking with *Salmonella*. When the *Shigella* is an enterotoxin-producing organism, watery diarrhea may actually precede the onset of dysentery.

Patients who have *Shigella* organisms tend to appear severely ill and may have meningismus or seizures. The stools tend to be foul smelling. Up to 40% of individuals who have Guillain-Barré syndrome have evidence of a *Campylobacter* infection occurring before the onset of neurologic symptoms.[16] *Yersinia* enterocolitis also may be associated with blood in the stool, but *Yersinia* appears to be incriminated less commonly as an etiologic agent in the United States. *E coli* can produce diarrhea by several pathogenic mechanisms; the enteroadherent, enteroinvasive, enterohemorrhagic, and enteroaggregative forms can all be associated with blood in the stool.[17] Hemolytic uremic syndrome is the result largely of enterohemorrhagic *E coli* (especially Shiga toxin–producing *E coli* O157:H7) and less commonly *Shigella* infections.

Amebiasis is unusual in the United States, but *Entamoeba histolytica* can produce a picture of acute colitis. Causes of bloody diarrhea that are not obviously infectious include intussusception and immune deficiencies. Chronic inflammatory bowel disease can produce an initial episode of acute dysentery, although the history may reveal previous episodes; arthralgia or growth failure may have preceded the diarrhea. A history of recent similar diarrheal illness in family members or friends suggests an infectious diarrhea.

Food-borne spread of organisms or toxins is an important cause of acute diarrheal illness.[18] Improperly prepared poultry and eggs are the major source for both campylobacteriosis and salmonellosis, and the major source for *E coli* O157:H7 infection is ground beef. Preventive measures include safe food-handling practices, pasteurization of in-shell eggs, and irradiation of ground meat and raw poultry. Explosive diarrhea after ingesting seafood is likely from infection with *Vibrio* species. Outbreaks of norovirus have occurred on cruises ships as well as college campuses.[19,20] The most common pathogens causing food-borne illness are listed in Box 15-2.

## Evaluation

At the initial evaluation (Box 15-3), the physician should establish the quantity of the diarrhea, the child's ability to maintain oral intake, and the presence of associated vomiting. On physical examination, the state of hydration should be estimated. The presence of tears and saliva is usually evidence of adequate hydration, but the most reliable reassurance comes from a normal heart rate and a brisk capillary refill. A simple guideline to hydration is that the absence of tears and the presence of a dry mouth suggest 5% dehydration; the addition of sunken eyes, sunken fontanelle, and poor skin turgor suggests 10% dehydration. Shock indicates at least 15% dehydration. In the presence of hypernatremia, the state of dehydration is typically more severe than suggested on physical examination inasmuch as extracellular fluid volume tends to be preserved at the expense of intracellular volume. A recorded weight is essential; it can be compared with previous weights and will also be available to reevaluate the state of hydration during the illness. Information about the frequency and quantity of urination is important. A history of good urine output is reassuring. Parents may underestimate or overestimate urine output (frequency and volume), especially when urine becomes mixed with liquid stool.

BOX 15-2

### *Top 5 Pathogens Causing Domestically Acquired Food-Borne Illnesses (CDC 2011 Estimates)*[a]

- *Norovirus*
- Salmonella, nontyphoidal
- *C perfringens*
- *Campylobacter* species
- *S aureus*

[a]The top five pathogens from among 31 pathogens known by the Centers for Disease Control and Prevention (CDC) to cause food-borne illness. However, unspecified agents account for 80% of the annual number of food-borne illnesses estimated by the CDC.[21,22]

BOX 15-3

## *Evaluation of Acute Diarrhea*

**HISTORY**

1. Length of illness
2. Characterization of stools: frequency, looseness (watery versus mushy), and presence of gross blood
3. Oral intake: diet, quantity of fluids and solids taken
4. Presence of vomiting
5. Associated symptoms: fever, rash, and arthralgia
6. Urine output: frequency and qualitative amount
7. Possible exposure to diarrheal illness

**PHYSICAL EXAMINATION**

1. Hydration status: weight (stable or loss), heart rate, capillary refill, mucosa (moist or dry), saliva and tears (present or absent), skin turgor (normal or poor), eyeballs and fontanelle (normal or sunken), and vital signs
2. Alertness
3. Infant: vigor of suck

**LABORATORY (PERFORMED AS INDICATED)**

1. Stool evaluation: test for viral etiology when available, culture, ova and parasites, smear for white blood cells, *C difficile* toxin assay, occult blood, and reducing substances
2. Complete blood count
3. If hydration status is in question: blood urea nitrogen (BUN) and serum electrolyte levels
4. Urinalysis
5. If child is lethargic or has had a seizure, culture for sepsis: measure the BUN and serum electrolyte and glucose levels and examine and culture the cerebrospinal fluid

A stool culture should be obtained if blood or leukocytes are noted in the stool and the child is severely ill. Examination of the stool for leukocytes is helpful in establishing the presence of colitis. In the presence of both infectious and noninfectious colitis, white blood cells (WBCs) are usually found in high numbers, frequently in sheets. Polymorphonuclear leukocytes usually account for at least 60% to 80% of the cells; the presence of only occasional cells is considered a negative finding. The absence of WBCs in grossly bloody diarrheal stool occurs with enterohemorrhagic *E coli* infection but should also direct attention to entities such as intussusception and Meckel diverticulum when these diagnoses seem clinically appropriate. Amebic colitis also may not be associated with WBCs in the stool, although the trophozoites and numerous red blood cells may be visible on a saline wet mount preparation of the stool. Invasive bacterial diarrhea frequently is associated with a peripheral blood leukocytosis.

### Treatment

The cornerstone of treatment in acute gastroenteritis is good fluid and electrolyte management (Box 15-4). Commercial oral hydration solutions provide more sodium and lower carbohydrate concentration than traditional clear liquids.[23] Human milk contains low concentrations of sodium (6–7 mEq/L); therefore, a supplemental rehydration solution should be used when diarrhea is persistent or severe.

BOX 15-4

## *Fluid and Electrolyte Management of Acute Diarrhea*

A. General rules for management of acute diarrhea
   1. Oral rehydration therapy with glucose-electrolyte solution (oral rehydration solution [ORS]) is the preferred treatment of fluid and electrolyte loss, except as noted below. These solutions generally contain 25 g/L glucose (or ≥30 g/L rice starch), 45–90 mEq/L sodium, 20–25 mEq/L potassium, and 30 mEq/L bicarbonate. The higher sodium concentration is appropriate for rehydration; the lower concentration is usually adequate for rehydration with mild diarrhea and is appropriate for maintenance.
   2. Moderate to high stool output should be replaced with ORS at 10 mL/kg/stool, if losses cannot be estimated. Losses from emesis should be replaced with ORS at 2 mL/kg/episode of emesis or replace estimated losses.
   3. The use of ORS is labor intensive. If a caregiver is not available to give small amounts of fluid frequently, then intravenous therapy may be necessary. If the child is not severely dehydrated, then oral rehydration may be completed at home with close follow-up. Otherwise, intravenous fluids should include replacement of deficit, ongoing losses, and maintenance fluids. Addition of intravenous potassium should wait until urine output is established.
   4. ORS therapy is effective for hypernatremic dehydration, as well as hyponatremic and isotonic dehydration.
   5. Age-appropriate feedings should be continued during acute diarrhea, except as noted below. Formula should be offered full strength. Diet may be better tolerated if fatty foods and foods high in simple sugars (eg, undiluted juices and soft drinks) are avoided.
   6. Breastfeeding should be continued when possible.
   7. Lactose-free diet is generally unnecessary. If stools worsen on reintroduction of lactose (human milk, cow milk, or lactose-containing formula), then lactose intolerance should be considered. If stools become acid and contain reducing substances, then lactose intolerance is likely.

B. No dehydration
   1. Continue age-appropriate feeding (see A.5, A.6).
   2. Use ORS only to replace excessive stool output (see A.2).

C. Mild-to-moderate dehydration (3%–9% of body weight)
   1. Correct dehydration with 50–100 mL/kg ORS over 3–4 hours, and replace continuing losses from stool and emesis with additional ORS (see A.2). See section E for special considerations for vomiting.
   2. Reevaluate hydration and replacement of losses at least every 1–2 hours. This process may require medical supervision (emergency department, hospital outpatient unit, or physician's office).
   3. Once dehydration is corrected, begin feeding (see A.5, A.6) and continue to correct losses as above.

D. Severe dehydration (at least 10%)
   1. Resuscitate with intravenous or intraosseous normal saline or lactated Ringer's solution 20 mL/kg of body weight over 1 hour. Monitor vital signs closely. Repeat until pulse and state of consciousness return to normal. Larger volumes and shorter periods of administration may be required. Delay giving intravenous potassium until urine output is established.
   2. Determine serum electrolyte levels.
   3. Lack of response to initial resuscitation suggests an underlying problem such as septic shock, toxic shock syndrome, myocarditis, myocardiopathy, or pericarditis. Persistently poor urine output may be a sign of hemolytic uremic syndrome.
   4. ORS may be initiated when the child's condition has stabilized and mental status is satisfactory. An intravenous line should be maintained until no

BOX 15-4

## *Fluid and Electrolyte Management of Acute Diarrhea—cont'd*

longer needed. See section E for special considerations for vomiting.

5. Feeding may be restarted when rehydration is complete (see A.1, A.2).

E. Special considerations
  1. Vomiting
     a. Vomiting occurs commonly during acute gastroenteritis.
     b. Children who are dehydrated and vomit usually tolerate ORS.
     c. Intractable, severe vomiting, unconsciousness, and ileus are contraindications to ORS treatment.
     d. ORS should be started at 5 mL every 1–2 minutes.
     e. Vomiting usually decreases as dehydration improves; larger amounts can be given at less frequent intervals.
     f. Nasogastric tube can be used for continuous ORS infusion for persistent vomiting or feeding refusal secondary to mouth ulcers (do not use in comatose child or one who has ileus or intestinal obstruction).
     g. Intravenous fluids should be used if ORS treatment is unsuccessful.
  2. Refusal to take ORS
     a. Children who are not dehydrated may not take ORS because of the salty taste. However, dehydrated children generally take it well.
     b. Giving ORS in small amounts at first allows the child to become accustomed to the taste.
     c. ORS can be frozen in ice-pop form.

Modified from American Academy of Pediatrics Provisional Committee on Quality Improvement, Subcommittee on Acute Gastroenteritis. Practice parameter: the management of acute gastroenteritis in young children. *Pediatrics.* 1996; 97:424–435; and King CK, Glass R, Bresee JS, et al. Managing acute gastroenteritis among children: oral rehydration, maintenance, and nutritional therapy. *MMWR.* 2003;52:1–16.

Electrolyte content in diarrheal stool varies widely, with the highest concentrations occurring in secretory diarrheas such as cholera. Fecal sodium levels may range from 40 to 100 mEq/L and may occasionally be as high as 150 mEq/L. In rotavirus diarrhea, fecal sodium concentration is typically 20 to 40 mEq/L.

Viruses cause at least 40% to 50% of acute diarrheal illnesses in childhood. Rotavirus is becoming less common with the widespread use of vaccine[24]; other viruses, in descending frequency, are noroviruses, astroviruses, and enteric adenoviruses. Viral enteritis has been shown to result in a transient, patchy, mucosal lesion of the small intestine, which may be associated with temporary lactose and fat malabsorption. Decreased mucosal lactase levels may be seen. In experimental viral diarrhea in piglets, intestinal glucose-stimulated absorption of sodium, and therefore water, is impaired.[5] Rotavirus produces an enterotoxin (known as NSP4), which is of much greater importance in the production of diarrhea than virus-induced mucosal damage.[5,6] Abnormal glucose absorption has also been observed in infants who have rotavirus enteritis. Nevertheless, secretion can be converted to net absorption in most children by providing oral glucose electrolyte solution because of the patchy nature of the lesion in viral gastroenteritis.

Oral rehydration solutions have been used safely and successfully to treat acute diarrhea with dehydration.[25,26] Infants who have diarrhea are usually able to drink large volumes of salty-tasting liquids ad libitum appropriate for the stool output. Episodes of diarrhea in previously healthy, well-nourished children are often mild; nevertheless, the use of oral rehydration solutions to replace diarrheal loss is encouraged in infants. Liquids can be offered ad libitum, although smaller volumes per feeding may be tolerated better when diarrhea is associated with vomiting. Guidelines for rehydration are described in Box 15-4. The most recent World Health Organization recommendation is for a lower-osmolarity (245 mOsm/L) solution for rehydration (containing 75 mEq/L sodium and 75 mmol/L glucose). The contents of commercially available rehydration solutions have evolved with advances in the understanding of optimal absorption during oral rehydration; thus, the physician should consult current manufacturer specifications before choosing a product. Continuing regular feedings with supplemental oral rehydration solution is generally tolerated and thought to lead to quicker recovery.[27] Vomiting is usually not a contraindication to oral rehydration.

Oral rehydration appears to be associated with shorter hospitalization and lower medical costs. Infants who have hypernatremic dehydration have fewer problems with seizures during oral rehydration compared with intravenous rehydration.[25] Oral rehydration therapy, however, requires the constant presence of a caretaker, although this individual need not have previous medical experience. The use of starches, amino acids, and probiotics in oral maintenance or rehydration solution to improve sodium and water absorption has been considered.

Indications for medications in the treatment of acute gastroenteritis in infants and children are limited. As already noted, the key mechanisms involved are intestinal secretion and transient malabsorption; physiologically, no apparent rationale exists for medications that slow gut motility (diphenoxylate, loperamide, and anticholinergics). In fact, pooling of fluid in the intestinal lumen after treatment may give a false impression that the diarrhea has improved. Slowing intestinal transit with drugs may allow greater mucosal contact with pathogens and thereby allow for local mucosal invasion. Bismuth subsalicylate, which may decrease the duration of diarrhea, has been shown to be a safe adjunct to oral rehydration but is not used routinely.[28] Antibiotics are useful in specific situations: *Shigella* dysentery, *Yersinia* or *Campylobacter* gastroenteritis, pseudomembranous colitis, *Salmonella* infections in infants younger than 6 months, and *Salmonella* infections in older patients who have enteric fever, typhoid fever, or complications of bacteremia.[29] *Campylobacter* gastroenteritis must be identified very early for antibiotics to shorten the illness. For the individual patient, the presence of an *E coli* serotype previously labeled enteropathogenic correlates poorly with the presence of diarrhea and is not alone an indication for antibiotic treatment.[17] *Lactobacillus* or other probiotics may be useful to prevent infectious diarrhea but are probably not effective as treatment.[30,31]

Most episodes of gastroenteritis are self-limited and of short duration. Symptoms of rotavirus enteritis typically last 4 to 10 days. However, prolonged secretion of rotavirus in stool (up to 8 weeks) has been demonstrated in association with severe gastroenteritis in immunocompetent children.[32] The current approach to treatment is to restart the previous full-strength formula and solids early after the onset of diarrhea. If diarrhea recurs on the introduction of lactose-containing formula, then the child may have transient lactose intolerance. In this situation, a lactose-free formula should be offered. (The sugar in this formula can be either sucrose or a glucose polymer.) Sugar malabsorption (see Malabsorption Syndromes) can be identified by the determination of reducing substance in the stool. (Sucrose must be hydrolyzed first with hydrochloric acid.) Transient lactose intolerance usually lasts only a week or less but can, at times, persist for months. If the degree of dehydration is 5% or greater, then use of oral rehydration solution should be instituted, if possible, in the manner presented in Box 15-4. For severe dehydration or shock, rapid intravenous administration of 10 to 20 mL/kg of isotonic fluid or colloid is required initially and may need to be repeated early. Hyponatremia and hypernatremia must be corrected slowly to prevent complications of the central nervous system. Oral solutions are better tolerated and result in fewer central nervous system complications than intravenous solutions in infants who have hypernatremia.[25] Potassium should not be added to intravenous fluids until adequate urine output is established. Urine specific gravity may be misleading inasmuch as kidney-concentrating ability may be poor as a result of reduced renal urea or whole-body potassium. Inability to acidify the urine during acute diarrhea occurs commonly in infants despite the presence of metabolic acidosis.[33] This finding is thought to be caused by sodium deficiency and the resulting inadequate delivery of sodium to the distal nephron.

## ▶ CHRONIC DIARRHEA

Although chronic diarrhea occurs in children of all ages, it is most frequent and often most challenging to diagnose in infants.[34] Both healthy and ill infants can develop diarrhea in response to a variety of stresses. The younger the infant is, the more likely he or she will be to enter the cycle of diarrhea and secondary malnutrition that leads to further diarrhea, malnutrition, and susceptibility to infection (known as protracted diarrhea of infancy). Many of the causes of chronic diarrhea may appear at any time during childhood. Certain diseases, however, occur more commonly in infancy; others are more likely to begin in later childhood. Dividing the causes of diarrhea between infancy and older childhood is arbitrary because the groups overlap, but this method is a helpful guide in initiating the evaluation of the child who has chronic diarrhea (Box 15-5).

### *Infants*

The physician confronted with an infant who is reported to have chronic diarrhea must decide first whether the stool pattern is abnormal. A nursing mother who has not been forewarned may become concerned about the appearance and frequency of her child's transitional stools. The infant's weight gain and healthy appearance, combined with an explanation about stools of breastfed infants, should dispel these concerns.

In the latter half of the first year and in the second year, the most common cause for persistent diarrhea is chronic nonspecific diarrhea (also called *toddler's diarrhea*).[3,35] Affected infants and toddlers have intermittent loose stools for no apparent reason. In many instances, the stools occur early in the day and typically not overnight. These children appear healthy and are thriving according to weight and length growth curves, unless inappropriate treatment with clear fluids has led to caloric deprivation. This condition represents a stool pattern rather than a pathologic state and requires minimal or no laboratory evaluation. Symptoms may begin initially after an apparent acute enteritis (postinfectious irritable bowel).

Treatment may include restricting the frequency of feedings, whether liquids or solids, in an effort to decrease stimulation of the gastrocolic reflex (in the toddler, 3 meals and a bedtime snack with nothing by mouth in between); restricting the volumes of fluids ingested when excessive; avoiding excessive intake of juices; and reassuring the parents of the benign nature of this entity. A high-fat diet may be helpful in some children, although

BOX 15-5

## *Causes of Chronic Diarrhea*

**COMMON CAUSES**

- Chronic enteric infection: *Salmonella* organisms; *Yersinia enterocolitica*; *Campylobacter, Giardia, Cryptosporidium*, and *Cyclospora* organisms; *C difficile* toxin; enteroadherent *E coli*; rotavirus (in immunodeficient patients); cytomegalovirus; adenovirus; and HIV
- Food allergy
- Chronic nonspecific diarrhea (toddler's diarrhea, irritable colon of childhood); postinfectious irritable bowel
- Disaccharide intolerance
- Chronic constipation with overflow diarrhea
- Cystic fibrosis
- Celiac disease (gluten-sensitive enteropathy)
- Inflammatory bowel disease: Crohn disease and ulcerative colitis
- Hirschsprung disease
- Immunodeficiency states
- Monosaccharide intolerance
- Eosinophilic (allergic) gastroenteritis
- Short bowel syndrome
- Urinary tract infection
- Postenteritis bile acid malabsorption
- Factitious causes

**LESS COMMON CAUSES**

- Autoimmune enteropathy
- Hormonal: adrenal insufficiency and hyperthyroidism
- Vasoactive intestinal polypeptide–secreting tumor
- Neural crest tumor and carcinoid
- Intestinal lymphangiectasia
- Acrodermatitis enteropathica
- Intestinal stricture or blind loop
- Pancreatic insufficiency with neutropenia
- Trypsinogen or enterokinase deficiency
- Congenital chloride-losing diarrhea
- Congenital sodium-secretory diarrhea
- Abetalipoproteinemia
- Microvillus inclusion disease
- Tufting disease
- Immunodysregulation, polyendocrinopathy, enteropathy, X-linked syndrome (IPEX)
- Intestinal pseudoobstruction
- Ileal bile salt receptor defect
- Congenital disorders of glycosylation

probably is of less importance.[35] Cholestyramine (2 g by mouth 1 to 3 times daily) is also effective at times; however, the duration of use should be restricted because of the potential for interference with fat-soluble vitamin absorption. In any event, this condition is self-limited and typically resolves by 3.5 years of age. The only danger is that well-intentioned parents may restrict oral intake to clear liquids repeatedly in an effort to treat the child; this action may result in poor weight gain. Bile acid malabsorption is an occasional sequela of gastroenteritis that can produce persistent, watery diarrhea. This condition also will respond to cholestyramine therapy.

## Protracted Diarrhea of Infancy

The syndrome of protracted diarrhea of infancy is poorly understood,[36] probably representing the final pathway for multiple causes, including gastrointestinal infections and, perhaps, food intolerances. This condition is defined somewhat arbitrarily as occurring in infants younger than 3 months and persisting for more than 2 weeks. Historically, this syndrome, previously called intractable diarrhea of infancy, has been associated with a high mortality from irreversible diarrhea and related malnutrition. However, the outcome has improved markedly with the advent of elemental diets and total parenteral nutrition. Now, intractable diarrhea is rare and related to more specific causes, such as microvillus inclusion disease.

Generally, malnutrition develops and, in concert with the protracted diarrhea, leads to alteration of gastrointestinal flora sometimes associated with bacterial overgrowth of the small intestine. Altered mucosal function of the small intestine and transient pancreatic insufficiency may occur with malnutrition and protracted diarrhea. Bile salts may be deconjugated as a result of bacterial overgrowth. In many instances, the initiating cause of protracted diarrhea is not found; it may likely be no longer present when the diarrhea has become chronic. The small bowel biopsy specimen may show patchy villous shortening with a decreased villus-to-crypt ratio and marked inflammation, as well as a damaged surface epithelium. However, the results of the small bowel biopsy also may be normal. Similarly, a rectal biopsy specimen may show evidence of inflammation, including crypt abscesses, or it may be normal. The presence or absence of these biopsy findings may not correlate with the severity of the clinical syndrome.[37] Affected infants are severely malnourished and have low serum protein and hemoglobin levels. In many instances, they have had repeated treatment with oral clear liquids and peripheral intravenous fluids, all of which provide inadequate nutrient intake.

When evaluating a young infant who has protracted diarrhea, the physician must rule out causes that require urgent treatment while correcting hydration and nutrition. Rehydration is similar to the treatment of acute diarrhea, although estimating the level of dehydration accurately is difficult in the presence of malnutrition, and initial oral therapy is less likely to be successful. Stool output should be measured. If the urine is collected in a urine bag, then diapers can be weighed before and after stools to give an accurate measure of stool output. Urine specific gravity and volume may be deceptive because of poor concentration by the kidneys in the presence of malnutrition and total-body hypokalemia. The infant should be weighed at least daily.

Infection should be ruled out as a cause of diarrhea early in the evaluation. Several stools should be collected for culture, for examination for parasites, and for *C difficile* toxin assay when indicated; blood and urine cultures should also be ordered. Consideration of Hirschsprung disease with enterocolitis is important because infants who have this disorder are prone to perforation of the colon unless a decompression colostomy is performed. In such infants, eliciting a history of early obstipation and of the absence of stools in the first 24 hours of life is usually possible. In Hirschsprung disease, a flat plate radiograph of the abdomen may show a dilated colon with absence of air in the rectum. Toxic megacolon may also be seen in infectious colitis or in chronic inflammatory bowel disease in infancy. Air-fluid levels throughout the bowel are common in infants who have gastroenteritis, and this sign is not helpful in defining a cause. A barium enema under low pressure in the unprepared patient may show the narrow distal segment of rectum; however, this finding may not be present in neonates, and evaluation for ganglion cells on rectal biopsy is often necessary. The transition zone of Hirschsprung disease may be more obvious on a delayed radiograph (24–48 hours after the barium enema).

For a child who has chronic diarrhea and has been fed recently, the presence of reducing substance or an acid stool pH (<5.3) suggests carbohydrate malabsorption.[4] The stool pH is not a good measure of the effect of diarrhea on total-body acid-base balance. If stool concentration of sodium and potassium minus chloride is greater than the plasma bicarbonate, then the infant is losing bicarbonate. WBCs or gross blood in the stool usually indicates colonic inflammation; occult blood in the stool suggests loss of blood across the mucosa anywhere in the gastrointestinal tract.

Nutritional rehabilitation should begin at once. The best choices are either enteral alimentation with an elemental or modular formula[38] or total parenteral nutrition (TPN), peripheral or central. In many instances, enteral nutrition is tolerated best by the continuous-drip method, and recovery may be more rapid when enteral alimentation is used.[39] Nevertheless, unsuccessful attempts at enteral feeding necessitate initiation of TPN therapy in some infants. Initial treatment with TPN and a gradually increasing, continuous enteral drip is a good approach to patients who do not tolerate elemental diet alone. Elemental formulas are composed of predigested components in fixed proportions; modular formulas allow the physician to vary the components. Stool output and weight gain may be measured to assess the infant's response.

During the treatment, further workup, including an upper gastrointestinal series with small bowel radiograph, barium enema, small bowel biopsy, proctoscopy, the measurement of sweat electrolytes, and other specific tests to rule out the entities noted later in this chapter, should be conducted as indicated. If disaccharidase levels are abnormal on small bowel biopsy, then disaccharides should be avoided.

## Malabsorption Syndromes

Infants and children who have malabsorption syndromes typically have diarrhea, steatorrhea, growth failure, or a combination of these conditions. Celiac disease and cystic fibrosis are the most common chronic disorders that cause malabsorption in children in the United States. Steatorrhea is much more striking with cystic fibrosis, resulting from pancreatic insufficiency and secondary maldigestion. Infants with cystic fibrosis who nurse or are fed soy formula, but not cow milk formula, may exhibit protein malabsorption in the first months of life.

Although cystic fibrosis is thought of primarily as a respiratory disease, some infants and children have malabsorption and little history of respiratory symptoms; these patients typically have voracious appetites. The diagnosis must be confirmed by sweat electrolyte studies or genetic testing. Other diseases much less common than cystic fibrosis may be associated with prominent steatorrhea in early infancy, including congenital pancreatic insufficiency with cyclic neutropenia (Shwachman-Diamond syndrome),[40] intestinal lymphangiectasia, and abetalipoproteinemia. Transient steatorrhea may follow an acute enteritis.[41] Measurement of stool pancreatic elastase level is a useful screening test for pancreatic insufficiency.

Celiac disease (gluten-sensitive enteropathy) is now appreciated to be a much more frequent disorder than previously recognized.[42,43] Presentation may occur at any age, and the manifestations may be subtle. In infancy, celiac disease becomes apparent within 1 to several months after the introduction of gluten-containing products (wheat, rye, barley) into the diet.[44] The classic symptoms in an infant with celiac disease are irritability, loose stools, poor appetite, and poor weight gain. Vomiting may occur as well. In older children, features such as growth retardation or iron deficiency anemia may be more striking than diarrhea.[43] In many patients, steatorrhea is not present, and results of absorptive studies such as the D-xylose tolerance test may be normal. Gluten-free dietary trials and antigliadin antibody studies may be misleading. The presence of endomysial antibody (EMA), tissue transglutaminase (tTG), or damidated gliadin peptide (DGP) antibody in the serum is a much more reliable predictor of celiac disease.[45] tTG has been identified as the antigen recognized by endomysial antibody. In individuals with total serum immunoglobulin A (IgA) deficiency, assay for tTG IgA, EMA, or DGP IgA is unreliable. A tTG or DGP IgG level can be measured. A diagnosis of celiac disease should be confirmed by small bowel biopsy. In the past, the diagnosis was often reconfirmed by a challenge with gluten and a repeat biopsy. Currently available antibody studies make this strategy unnecessary. Measuring endomysial IgA or tTG antibody may be useful in assessing the adequacy of a gluten-free diet or evaluating adherence to diet. *Giardia* infection can produce small bowel malabsorption that mimics celiac disease.

Carbohydrate (monosaccharide or disaccharide) intolerance may be primary or more commonly secondary to other gastrointestinal disorders.[46] The congenital form of lactase deficiency is much less common than congenital sucrase-isomaltase deficiency,[47] which typically appears after introduction of sucrose into the diet in solids. In carbohydrate intolerance, the extent of symptoms varies directly with the quantity of the offending sugar in the diet. Similarly, the age at presentation varies with the age at which the sugar is introduced into the diet. Infants who have congenital sucrase-isomaltase deficiency may have diarrhea when fed formula containing glucose polymers as well.[48] The diagnosis can be established by conducting standard sugar tolerance tests, measuring hydrogen excretion in the breath, or assaying the enzymes present in tissue obtained by a small bowel biopsy. Examination of the stool for reducing sugars is an imprecise screening test for stool carbohydrate content.[49] A stool pH less than 5.3 is suggestive of carbohydrate malabsorption, whereas a stool pH more than 5.6 is evidence against this diagnosis. Sorbitol,[50] a sugar substitute, as well as fructose,[51] may produce diarrhea when ingested in large amounts, and both are present in fruits. Oral enzyme supplements are available for both lactase and sucrase deficiency.

The congenital deficiency of trypsinogen, the zymogen precursor of the pancreatic protease trypsin, has been reported to be a very rare cause of congenital diarrhea. The absence of trypsin in the stool suggests the diagnosis (in the absence of cystic fibrosis and congenital pancreatic insufficiency), but evaluation of the pancreatic proteases in the duodenal aspirate is necessary to confirm this impression. Congenital deficiency of enterokinase, the intestinal enzyme that activates trypsinogen to trypsin, appears in a similar fashion to that of congenital trypsinogen deficiency but is reversed with very small amounts of pancreatic replacement.

A recently described congenital, autosomal recessive disorder of chronic malabsorption and diarrhea has been characterized by a lack of intestinal enteroendocrine cells. This disorder is associated with a mutation of a gene *(NEUROG3)* expressing a protein required for endocrine cell development in the pancreas and intestine. Individuals with this disorder have been identified to develop glucose intolerance as well.[52]

## Infection

Acute bacterial or viral enteritis may be an important initiator of protracted diarrhea in infancy.[53,54] If the initial infection is no longer present at the time of evaluation for chronic diarrhea, then this association will be difficult to prove. Infections at distant sites, especially urinary tract infections, have also been implicated as a cause of chronic diarrhea in infancy. A urinalysis and urine culture should be obtained routinely in the evaluation of children who have chronic diarrhea. *Salmonella* enteritis is commonly associated with a chronic asymptomatic carrier state, especially in infancy. *Salmonella* infection, however, may also be associated with persistent diarrhea in infants. *Y enterocolitica* enteritis has been associated with a chronic relapsing diarrhea, although not commonly in the United States; however, the microbiology laboratory must look specifically for this organism, or it will be missed. *Campylobacter* enteritis also may have a protracted course. Persistence of either rotavirus or enteric adenovirus excretion has been identified in immunocompromised individuals; rarely, rotavirus may be present in the stool of an immunocompetent child for a prolonged period after a severe gastroenteritis.[32] *Candida* has been described as a rare cause of persistent diarrhea in immunocompetent individuals.[55] However, the incidental finding of *Candida* is so common that the physician must be cautious before identifying it as the cause of diarrhea. A dramatic response to treatment for *Candida* would support this diagnosis.

## Parasites

The principal parasite that causes diarrhea in the United States is *G lamblia*, which may be associated with watery diarrhea and crampy abdominal pain and may occur in epidemic form. Stool testing for *Giardia* antigen is sensitive and has improved the ability to diagnose giardiasis. Evaluation of duodenal fluid aspirate or a small bowel biopsy is rarely necessary. Diarrhea from *Cryptosporidium* occurs in immunocompetent individuals and also can be recognized by stool antigen assay.[56,57] *Cyclospora* has been introduced into the United States on contaminated fruits. *B hominis* and *D fragilis* may cause persistent diarrhea. Amebic dysentery may be indistinguishable from the colitis of inflammatory bowel disease and must be considered along with bacterial colitis before a diagnosis of inflammatory bowel disease can be made.

## Hirschsprung Disease

Hirschsprung disease is a congenital abnormality involving the submucosal and myenteric plexuses of the colon (rarely involving the small intestine) and accounts for about 25% of intestinal obstructions in newborns. Affected neonates almost invariably fail to pass meconium early and have persistent obstipation and recurrent abdominal distention. These features may be overlooked, however, and the infants may subsequently have chronic diarrhea. The diarrhea is secondary to enterocolitis, which can be a surgical emergency that demands rapid diagnosis and treatment. A barium enema in the neonate may reveal false-negative findings. Anorectal manometric examination may be helpful, but an adequate rectal biopsy specimen showing absence of ganglion cells and presence of nerve fiber hypertrophy confirms the diagnosis. Calretinin staining is useful as well. Properly performed, suction biopsy of the rectum is highly reliable.[58]

## Food Allergy

Dietary protein hypersensitivity occurs in 6% to 8% of children during the first 5 years of life and most commonly is a hypersensitivity to cow milk protein. Food allergy is present in about 4% of the adult population. In 85% of children who have dietary protein intolerance, the symptoms resolve by 3 years of age.[59–61] This entity should be considered when an infant who has chronic diarrhea has any of the following manifestations:

- Occult or gross blood in the stool (colitis)
- Protein-losing enteropathy
- Peripheral eosinophilia
- Other extraintestinal manifestations of allergy such as eczema, hives, or asthma[62]

Continued or recurrent manifestations when the infant is fed a soy formula diet (free of cow milk) do not rule out the diagnosis, inasmuch as 30% to 50% of children who have cow milk protein intolerance will also be intolerant to soy protein. Typically, symptoms improve when the feeding is changed to a protein hydrolysate formula, although the response to specific protein hydrolysate formulas may not be equivalent. Occasionally, an amino acid formula will be necessary.[63]

Most food allergic reactions are IgE mediated and include immediate gastrointestinal hypersensitivity, with nausea, abdominal pain, and vomiting within 1 to 2 hours and diarrhea in 2 to 6 hours. Implicated food proteins include milk, egg, peanut, soy, cereal, and fish. Eosinophilic (allergic) gastroenteropathy is considered a mixed IgE-mediated and non–IgE-mediated disorder. It is characterized by infiltration of the stomach and intestine with eosinophils and often a peripheral eosinophilia. Symptoms include vomiting, abdominal pain, growth failure, and diarrhea (often with gross blood). Eosinophilic gastroenteropathy may respond to elimination diet, but corticosteroid treatment may be necessary. Non–IgE-mediated hypersensitivity food protein-induced enterocolitis syndrome (FPIES), which occurs most commonly in the first year of life but can occur at any age. Diet-induced proctitis causes gross blood in stool and often diarrhea in the first few days to months of life. Symptoms usually resolve within 72 hours with removal of the offending food allergen. Bloody diarrhea can develop in some infants while they are nursing; resolution may occur when cow milk is removed from the mother's diet or when a protein hydrolysate formula is substituted for nursing, suggesting an allergic basis.[64]

## Short Bowel Syndrome

Short bowel syndrome is associated with congenital anomaly of the small intestine or follows extensive resection of the small intestine, resulting in chronic malabsorption and diarrhea.[65] It begins most commonly in the newborn period in association with necrotizing enterocolitis or a congenital anomaly such as gastroschisis, intestinal atresia, or malrotation with secondary midgut volvulus. Recovery may be prolonged, requiring the use of TPN for the first several years of life.[66] The factors that appear to contribute to persistence of symptoms in neonates include the cause, decreased intestinal absorptive surface, altered intestinal motility, intraluminal bacterial overgrowth[67] (with secondary deconjugation of bile salts and hydroxylation of fatty acids), malabsorption of bile salts secondary to terminal ileal resection, and disaccharidase deficiency. Among neonates, infants with necrotizing enterocolitis or gastroschisis tend to have a more prolonged course than those with other causes of short bowel. In infants, symptoms of colitis may occur during the initiation of enteral feedings.[68] Later in life, volvulus, trauma, and Crohn disease are the most common causes of short bowel syndrome.

## Intestinal Lymphangiectasia

Intestinal lymphangiectasia is a syndrome of dilated intestinal lymphatic vessels and is associated with protein-losing enteropathy, steatorrhea, lymphocytopenia, and chronic diarrhea. As a result of the bowel protein loss, affected children may have hypogammaglobulinemia and hypoalbuminemia, usually with peripheral edema. Primary intestinal lymphangiectasia appears to be a developmental anomaly of unknown origin and is frequently associated with lymphatic abnormalities of the extremities. Secondary lymphangiectasia may result from chronic volvulus secondary to malrotation with malfixation of the bowel, constrictive pericarditis, tumor, lymphatic malformation, elevated right atrial pressure associated with the Fontan procedure for congenital heart disease, or any other factor that leads to obstruction of intestinal lymphatic flow. The diagnosis is suggested by a history of chronic diarrhea and poor growth and the presence of peripheral edema, hypoalbuminemia, hypogammaglobulinemia, and lymphocytopenia. The last 2 abnormalities may lead to a decreased immune defense and an increased risk for infections. A radiologic small bowel follow-through study may show generalized thickening of the intestinal folds. The diagnosis is confirmed by the presence of characteristically dilated lymphatics on a small bowel biopsy specimen. The treatment includes the dietary use of medium-chain triglycerides and avoidance of long-chain fat. Protection from and early treatment of infection also are important.

## Acrodermatitis Enteropathica

Acrodermatitis enteropathica is a rare autosomal recessive disease that typically appears when breastfed infants are weaned. The infant has chronic diarrhea, intermittent vomiting, and an intractable erythematous, raw, and crusty rash, which is most prominent in the perianal and perioral regions but may be seen on the extremities. Alopecia is characteristically present, and conjunctivitis and dystrophic changes of the nails may occur. Infants who have acrodermatitis enteropathica are usually irritable and unhappy. The disorder is associated with a zinc deficiency (perhaps secondary to malabsorption) and responds dramatically to zinc salts given orally.[69] A mutation of a gene that encodes a zinc-transporter protein has been identified in this condition. Nutritional zinc deficiency (eg, TPN without zinc supplementation or cystic fibrosis) may produce a syndrome similar to acrodermatitis enteropathica.

## Factitious Diarrhea

Factitious diarrhea is undoubtedly more common than pediatricians recognize. Screening a stool specimen for laxative abuse is reasonable when an infant has persistent diarrhea that does not seem to fit any known pattern. Surreptitious administration of laxative to an infant is a symptom of the caregiver's psychosocial dysfunction; problems in other areas often become apparent during the social history. Frequently, a parent is a medically knowledgeable person (eg, nurse, laboratory technician) and often seems to prefer staying in the hospital to being at home. These parents are usually helpful to the nursing staff, often to the degree of excessive involvement in the nursing care, and are commonly described by the nurses as caring and concerned parents. The pediatrician may note that the parent seems to encourage invasive diagnostic studies and treatment even beyond the medical plan and does not show an appropriate degree of hesitancy. A stool osmolality well below 290 mOsm/L can only occur by surreptitious dilution of stool with water. Another form of factitious diarrhea occurs among teenage girls who take laxatives surreptitiously to lose weight.

## Hormone-Related Diarrhea

Adrenal insufficiency caused by either adrenogenital syndrome or adrenal hemorrhage may be associated with significant diarrhea, as may congenital thyrotoxicosis. VIP-secreting tumors of the pancreas have been reported as a rare cause of diarrhea in adults and an even rarer cause in children.

Ganglioneuroma and ganglioneuroblastoma have been associated with chronic secretory diarrhea. The tumors are usually abdominal but have also been reported in the mediastinum. Although these tumors are catecholamine secreting, prostaglandins or VIP may be the mediator of the diarrhea. A workup of the infant who has persistent, undiagnosed, secretory diarrhea should include urinary catecholamine studies, prostaglandin and VIP levels, and computed tomography scans of chest and abdomen. Even when the results of these studies are negative, the physician must strongly consider further studies if severe secretory diarrhea persists. When a tumor is found and is completely excised, the diarrhea usually resolves abruptly.

## Immune Disorders

Immunodeficiency should be considered in any child who has chronic diarrhea. AIDS has become a major cause of immunodeficiency in childhood, and its first manifestation may be diarrhea. Several mechanisms of diarrhea have been described in infants and children who have AIDS.[70] In addition to the organisms the physician usually considers in individuals who have persistent diarrhea (especially *Giardia*), cytomegalovirus, *Mycobacterium avium-intracellulare, Cryptosporidium parvum, Isospora belli*, and *Enterocytozoon bieneusi* must also be considered. Astrovirus, calicivirus, and adenovirus have been associated with diarrhea in HIV-infected individuals and may be more important than rotavirus as agents of AIDS diarrhea.[71] HIV may be a primary pathogen in the bowel of these patients as well. Lactose intolerance occurs commonly in individuals who have AIDS, presumably occurring as a result of injury to small bowel mucosa. Pancreatic insufficiency with steatorrhea also has been noted in these patients.

The 2 major inborn disorders of immunity associated with diarrhea in early infancy are severe combined immunodeficiency and Wiskott-Aldrich syndrome. The most common primary disorder seen in later childhood is late-onset, variable hypogammaglobulinemia. Pure T-cell abnormalities (DiGeorge syndrome and other T-cell deficiencies) are also associated with diarrhea. Patients with selective IgA deficiency have an increased risk for celiac disease. Measurement of immunoglobulin levels should be a routine part of the workup of any patient who has chronic diarrhea. If the diagnosis remains unclear, then a T-cell evaluation should be conducted. Chronic parasitic, adenovirus, or rotavirus infection can be seen with immunodeficiencies. Diarrhea in association with granulomas of the intestinal tract has been noted in chronic granulomatous disease of childhood. These children may have perianal fistulas or gastric outlet obstruction; the disorder may initially be mistaken for Crohn disease.

The physician must consider the full range of enteric infections associated with immunosuppression in children who have received organ transplants. Diarrhea may also be the presentation of tacrolimus toxicity or of lymphoproliferative disease. In bone marrow transplant recipients, graft-versus-host disease is a common cause of diarrhea as well.

## Autoimmune Enteropathy

Autoimmune enteropathy is a poorly understood disorder, with chronic diarrhea beginning in the first year of life, and is often associated with failure to thrive.[72] Intestinal biopsies demonstrate villous atrophy and increased T-cell infiltrate in the lamina propria. Serum antienterocyte antibodies are identified in at least 50% of these patients. Extraintestinal autoimmune disorders (eg, diabetes mellitus, arthritis, thrombocytopenia, hemolytic anemia) are common and help make the diagnosis. Celiac disease, food allergy, and gastrointestinal infection must be ruled out. Treatment is immunosuppressive therapy, and a response confirms the diagnosis.[73]

## IPEX Syndrome

*I*mmune dysregulation, *p*olyendocrinopathy, *e*nteropathy, and *X*-linked inheritance (IPEX) syndrome exhibits a presentation similar to autoimmune enteropathy and similar biopsy findings.[72] This disorder is the result of a mutation in the *FOXP3* gene.

## Idiopathic Intestinal Pseudoobstruction

Idiopathic intestinal pseudoobstruction constitutes a group of rare disorders characterized by widespread gastrointestinal dysmotility. When this syndrome occurs in early infancy, vomiting and diarrhea are often major components. Diarrhea may alternate with constipation. In older children, the presentation is frequently more insidious; a long history of constipation may precede the onset of diarrhea. Persons who have this syndrome usually have intermittent or constant abdominal distention. The syndrome is characterized by the radiographic findings of bowel dilation with disordered motility; urinary bladder dysfunction is also often present. These disorders, which can be sporadic or transmitted in an autosomal dominant fashion, can result from a visceral myopathy or neuropathy or from a combination of both. Bacterial overgrowth is an important cause of diarrhea in this disorder.

## Microvillus Inclusion Disease

Microvillus inclusion disease (familial enteropathy) is a rare disorder that is present from birth and causes severe intractable secretory diarrhea with malabsorption.[72,74] It is the most common cause of intractable diarrhea in the neonatal period. Affected infants have small bowel villous atrophy in the absence of crypt hyperplasia. The villous surface epithelial cells lack a normal brush border, and on electron microscopic examination, the microvilli are absent or severely abnormal. The defective enterocytes and colonocytes contain intracytoplasmic inclusions, which, in turn, contain the components of the brush border. Microvillus inclusions are not found in every enterocyte. Fecal sodium and chloride concentrations are similar to those found in serum. Several families have been identified with more than 1 child with this disorder.

## Tufting Enteropathy

In contrast to microvillus inclusion disease, symptoms of tufting enteropathy are not present at birth. Affected infants develop chronic watery diarrhea in the first few months of life.[72] The name derives from a typical light microscopic *tufted* configuration of the small bowel mucosal epithelium.[75]

## Congenital Disorders of Electrolyte Absorption

Congenital chloride-losing diarrhea and congenital sodium-secretory diarrhea are very rare, autosomal recessive disorders associated with maternal polyhydramnios. The small bowel mucosa is histologically normal, and absorption of other nutrients is normal. Infants with congenital chloride-losing diarrhea have persistent diarrhea resulting from absence of the normal ileal mechanism for active absorption of chloride in exchange for bicarbonate. They have acidic stools and a chronic metabolic alkalosis instead of the metabolic acidosis usually seen in chronic diarrhea. Stool chloride concentration is high, usually exceeding the sum of concentrations of sodium and potassium. The stool chloride of children who have this disorder may be in the range of 100 to 150 mEq/L, although it may be 30 to 100 mEq/L in infants. (Adult stool chloride is normally <20 mEq/L.) Although no satisfactory treatment exists, support with oral fluids and potassium chloride is recommended. Congenital sodium diarrhea is also a rare cause of watery diarrhea from birth. However, these infants are acidotic, and stool chloride concentration is not excessive. The disorder is the result of defective mucosal $Na^+/H^+$ exchange in the small and large bowel.

## Congenital Disorders of Glycosylation

Congenital disorders of glycosylation exhibit in the first year of life, often with multisystem dysfunction.[76,77] In addition to hepatic, neurologic, cardiac, and optic manifestations, they can be associated with chronic diarrhea or severe protein-losing enteropathy, or both. Diagnosis is suggested if levels of serum glycoproteins such as haptoglobin and transferrin are low. Screening for this diagnosis has been performed with serum transferrin isoelectric focusing.

### *Infant of a Drug-Addicted Mother*

Diarrhea may be a prominent manifestation of neonatal drug abstinence syndrome, and this diagnosis should be entertained in newborns who have persistent diarrhea, especially when other symptoms of neonatal drug withdrawal are present.

### *Older Children*

A pediatrician will see fewer older children with chronic diarrhea than they will infants, but older children are more likely to have chronic diarrhea associated with significant underlying disease compared with toddler's diarrhea in young children. As in infancy, the association of poor growth, weight loss, or other systemic manifestations suggests a serious organic cause. Older children may deny symptoms, and the true effect of the disorder may not be immediately apparent. Clues may include subtle changes in personality, diminished sense of well-being, or loss of appetite. Children may hesitate to talk about their stooling pattern, and the degree of deviation from the norm may become apparent only after improvement occurs following initiation of appropriate therapy.

Causes of diarrhea differ somewhat after infancy, although many of the causes seen in infancy, even congenital anomalies, may exhibit first in childhood and therefore must still be considered. Factors that determine the age at diagnosis include variability of presentation of signs and symptoms, parental expectations of normality, and the index of suspicion of the physician who is consulted. However, certain diseases, including inflammatory bowel disease and chronic constipation with encopresis, are much more likely to be seen in childhood than in infancy. Symptoms of celiac disease may begin at any age, and the high occurrence rate of celiac disease is now recognized. Cystic fibrosis may be associated with only mild manifestations in infancy and may be overlooked until frequent, bulky, foul-smelling stools become intolerable at home. AIDS is seen in older children, as well as in infants.

## Irritable Bowel Syndrome

Irritable bowel syndrome (IBS) similar to that occurring in adults may be seen in children and adolescents.[8] Stools may alternate from diarrhea to constipation. In addition, the patient may have recurrent, crampy, abdominal pain. Late-onset lactose intolerance and fructose or sorbitol ingestion are important to rule out as causes of symptoms that may mimic IBS.[50,51] Symptoms of inflammatory bowel disease or celiac disease may also be mistaken at first for IBS. Standard treatment includes increased fiber in the diet and anticholinergics; the tricyclic antidepressants can be used for diarrhea-predominant IBS, under experienced supervision.

## Inflammatory Bowel Disease

The manifestations and presentation of Crohn disease and ulcerative colitis are so variable that these diseases should be considered whenever the physician sees an older child who has chronic diarrhea.[78] Systemic evidence of inflammation (fever, weight loss, and leukocytosis), abdominal pain, blood in the stool (gross or occult), perianal disease, anemia, or extraintestinal manifestations (arthralgia, arthritis, or erythema nodosum) are helpful in suggesting this diagnosis. Growth failure can occur with or precede other symptoms. An elevated sedimentation rate also is a clue; however, normal sedimentation rates may occur in as many as 50% of patients who have inflammatory bowel disease. Thrombocytosis and elevated C-reactive protein, both acute phase reactants, have been associated with inflammatory bowel disease as well and may be present in the absence of an elevated sedimentation rate. Suggestive signs and symptoms require evaluation, including a complete blood count, platelet count, erythrocyte sedimentation rate, serum protein levels, and possibly a stool assay for calprotectin. One would then consider imaging the small bowel by conventional contrast radiograms, computed tomography scan of the abdomen and pelvis, or MR enterography, as well as endoscopic examination of the upper gastrointestinal tract and colon with biopsy. Capsule endoscopy is useful when, despite negative radiographic and colonoscopic evaluation, a strong suggestion of small bowel Crohn disease is present. Serum antibody screening studies for IBD may be helpful in identifying the need for further evaluation for Crohn disease or ulcerative colitis, but may be misleading. Management of inflammatory bowel disease includes an array of medical, nutritional, and surgical measures.[78]

## Chronic Constipation

Chronic constipation with overflow incontinence may be mistaken for diarrhea. A thorough history and physical examination, including a rectal examination, should make the diagnosis apparent. A large amount of stool may be palpable in the abdomen, but a hard mass of stool is usually found in the rectal ampulla. This presentation is treated in the usual fashion of chronic constipation (as noted in Chapter 11, Constipation).

## When to Refer

- Persistent diarrhea when the workup for routine infectious causes is negative
- Steatorrhea
- Diarrhea or steatorrhea (or both), causing weight loss or failure to thrive
- Diarrhea associated with fevers, chronic anemia, or abdominal pain without an obvious explanation
- When inflammatory bowel disease is a consideration

## When to Admit

- Acute or chronic diarrhea with mild to moderate dehydration that cannot be managed successfully with outpatient rehydration solution
- Dehydration greater than 10% of body weight
- Diarrhea with intractable vomiting
- Severe electrolyte imbalance, including hypernatremic dehydration or serum potassium level less than 3 mEq/L
- Laboratory evidence suggesting hemolytic uremic syndrome
- Chronic diarrhea or steatorrhea (or both) with persistent signs of malnutrition that is unresolved with outpatient management
- Severe manifestations of inflammatory bowel disease, unresponsive to routine outpatient treatment

### *TOOLS FOR PRACTICE*

#### Engaging Patient and Family

- *Chronic Diarrhea* (fact sheet), Centers for Disease Control and Prevention (www.cdc.gov//healthywater/hygiene/disease/chronic_diarrhea.html)
- *Common Childhood Infections* (handout), American Academy of Pediatrics (patiented.solutions.aap.org)
- *Cryptosporidium Infection* (fact sheet), Centers for Disease Control and Prevention (www.cdc.gov/parasites/crypto/index.html)
- *Diarrhea* (fact sheet), American Academy of Pediatrics (www.healthychildren.org/English/health-issues/conditions/abdominal/Pages/Diarrhea.aspx)
- *Diarrhea and Dehydration* (handout), American Academy of Pediatrics (patiented.solutions.aap.org)
- *E coli (Escherichia coli)* (Web page), Centers for Disease Control and Prevention (www.cdc.gov/ecoli)
- *Entamoeba coli* (fact sheet), Centers for Disease Control and Prevention (www.cdc.gov/parasites/nonpathprotozoa/index.html)
- *Healthy Pets Healthy People—Salmonella from Pocket Pets* (fact sheet), Centers for Disease Control and Prevention (www.cdc.gov/healthypets/pets/pocket-pets/salmonella.html)
- *Healthy Pets Healthy People—Turtles Kept as Pets* (fact sheet), Centers for Disease Control and Prevention (www.cdc.gov/healthypets/pets/reptiles/turtles.html)
- *Healthy Swimming/Recreational Water* (Web page), Centers for Disease Control and Prevention (www.cdc.gov/healthywater/swimming)
- *Norovirus* (Web page), Centers for Disease Control and Prevention (www.cdc.gov/norovirus/about/index.html)
- *Parasites—Giardia (Web page)* Centers for Disease Control and Prevention (www.cdc.gov/parasites/giardia/index.html)
- *Rotavirus* (handout), American Academy of Pediatrics (patiented.solutions.aap.org)
- *Salmonella serotype Enteritidis* (fact sheet), Centers for Disease Control and Prevention (www.cdc.gov/nczved/divisions/dfbmd/diseases/salmonella_enteritidis)
- *Salmonella* (Web page), Centers for Disease Control and Prevention (www.cdc.gov/salmonella)
- *Shigellosis* (fact sheet), Centers for Disease Control and Prevention (www.cdc.gov/nczved/divisions/dfbmd/diseases/shigellosis)

### Medical Decision Support

- *Cryptosporidium* (Web page), Centers for Disease Control and Prevention (www.cdc.gov/dpdx/cryptosporidiosis/index.html)
- *Diarrheagenic Escherichia coli (non–Shiga toxin-producing E coli)* (fact sheet), Centers for Disease Control and Prevention (www.cdc.gov/ncidod/dbmd/diseaseinfo/diarrecoli_t.htm)
- *Giardiasis* (Web page), Centers for Disease Control and Prevention (www.cdc.gov/dpdx/giardiasis/index.html)
- *Managing Acute Gastroenteritis Among Children* (guideline), Centers for Disease Control and Prevention (www.cdc.gov/mmwr/PDF/RR/RR5216.pdf)
- *Norovirus* (Web page), Centers for Disease Control and Prevention (www.cdc.gov/norovirus/hcp/index.html)
- *Practice Guidelines for Management of Infectious Diarrhea* (guideline), Infectious Diseases Society of America (www.idsociety.org/Organ_System/#Diarrhea)
- *Rotavirus* (Web page), Centers for Disease Control and Prevention (www.cdc.gov/rotavirus/index/html)
- *Salmonella* (Web page), Centers for Disease Control and Prevention (www.cdc.gov/salmonella)
- *Shigellosis* (fact sheet), Centers for Disease Control and Prevention (www.cdc.gov/nczved/divisions/dfbmd/diseases/shigellosis)

## AAP POLICY STATEMENTS

American Academy of Pediatrics Committee on Nutrition. The use and misuse of fruit juice in pediatrics. *Pediatrics.* 2001;107(5):1210–1213. Reaffirmed August 2013 (pediatrics.aappublications.org/content/107/5/1210.full)

Centers for Disease Control and Prevention. Managing acute gastroenteritis among children: oral rehydration. *Pediatrics.* 2003;52(RR16):1–16. AAP Endorsed (www.cdc.gov/mmwr/pdf/rr/rr5216.pdf)

## REFERENCES

1. Phillips SF. Diarrhea: a current view of the pathophysiology. *Gastroenterology.* 1972;63:495–518
2. Field M. Intestinal ion transport and the pathophysiology of diarrhea. *J Clin Invest.* 2003;111:931–943
3. Lifshitz F, Ament ME, Kleinman RE, et al. Role of juice carbohydrate malabsorption in chronic nonspecific diarrhea in children. *J Pediatr.* 1992;120:825–829
4. Eherer AJ, Fordtran JS. Fecal osmotic gap and pH in experimental diarrhea of various causes. *Gastroenterology.* 1992;103:545–551
5. Kerzner B, Kelly MH, Gall DG, et al. Transmissible gastroenteritis: sodium transport and the intestinal epithelium during the course of viral enteritis. *Gastroenterology.* 1977;72:457–461
6. Morris AP, Estes MK. Microbes and microbial toxins: paradigms for microbial-mucosal interactions. VIII. Pathological consequences of rotavirus infection and its enterotoxin. *Am J Physiol Gastrointest Liver Physiol.* 2001;28:G303–G310
7. Oelkers P, Kirby LC, Heubi JE, et al. Primary bile acid malabsorption caused by mutations in the ileal sodium-dependent bile acid transporter gene (SLC10A2). *J Clin Invest.* 1997;99:1880–1887
8. Drossman DA, Camilleri M, Mayer EA, Whitehead WE. AGA technical review on irritable bowel syndrome. *Gastroenterology.* 2002;123:2108–2131
9. Glass RI, Lew JF, Gangarosa RE, LeBaron CW, Ho MS. Estimates of morbidity and mortality rates for diarrheal diseases in American children. *J Pediatr.* 1991;118:S27–S33
10. Alpert G, Bell LM, Kirkpatrick CE. Outbreak of cryptosporidiosis in a day-care center. *Pediatrics.* 1986;77:152–157
11. Bartlett AV, Reves RR, Pickering LK. Rotavirus in infant-toddler day care centers: epidemiology relevant to disease control strategies. *J Pediatr.* 1988;113:435–441

12. Bartlett AV, Moore M, Gary GW. Diarrheal illness among infants and toddlers in day care centers. I. Epidemiology and pathogens. *J Pediatr.* 1985;107:495–502
13. Hutson AM, Atmar RL, Estes MK. Norovirus disease: changing epidemiology and host susceptibility factors. *Trends Microbiol.* 2004;12:279–287
14. Schwarz RP, Ulshen MH. Pseudomembranous colitis presenting as mild, chronic diarrhea in childhood. *J Pediatr Gastroenterol Nutr.* 1983;2:570–573
15. Sutphen JL, Grand RJ, Flores A, Chang TW, Bartlett JG. Chronic diarrhea associated with Clostridium difficile in children. *Am J Dis Child.* 1983;137:275–278
16. Allos BM. Association between Campylobacter infection and Guillain-Barré syndrome. *J Infect Dis.* 1997;176(Suppl 2):S125–S128
17. Canadian Paediatric Society, Infectious Diseases Committee. Escherichia coli gastroenteritis: making sense of the new acronyms. *Can Med Assoc J.* 1987;136:241–244.
18. Centers for Disease Control and Prevention (CDC). Preliminary FoodNet data on the incidence of infection with pathogens transmitted commonly through food - 10 states, 2009. *MMWR Morb Mortal Wkly Rep.* 2010;59:418–422
19. Centers for Disease Control and Prevention (CDC). Norovirus outbreaks on three college campuses - California, Michigan, and Wisconsin, 2008. *MMWR Morb Mortal Wkly Rep.* 2009; 58:1095–1100
20. Vivancos R, Keenan A, Sopwith W, et al. Norovirus outbreak in a cruise ship sailing around the British Isles: Investigation and multi-agency management of an international outbreak. *J Infect.* 2010;60:478–485
21. Scallan E, Griffin PM, Angulo FJ, Tauxe RV, Hoekstra RM. Foodborne illness acquired in the United States-unspecified agents. *Emerg Infect Dis.* 2011;17:16–22
22. Scallan E, Hoekstra RM, Angulo FJ, et al. Foodborne illness acquired in the United States: major pathogens. *Emerg Infect Dis.* 2011;17:7–15
23. King CK, Glass R, Bresee JS, Duggan C; Centers for Disease Control and Prevention. Managing acute gastroenteritis among children: oral rehydration, maintenance, and nutritional therapy. *MMWR Recomm Rep.* 2003;52:1–16
24. Cortese MM, Tate JE, Simonsen L, Edelman L, Parashar UD. Reduction in gastroenteritis in United States children and correlation with early rotavirus vaccine uptake from national medical claims databases. *Pediatr Infect Dis J.* 2010;29:489–494
25. Santosham M, Duam RS, Dillman L, et al. Oral rehydration therapy of infantile diarrhea: a controlled study of well-nourished children hospitalized in the United States and Panama. *N Engl J Med.* 1982;306:1070–1076
26. Tamer AM, Friedman LB, Maxwell SRW, et al. Oral rehydration of infants in a large urban U.S. medical center. *J Pediatr.* 1985;107:11–19.
27. Duggan C, Nurko S. "Feeding the gut": the scientific basis for continued enteral nutrition during acute diarrhea. *J Pediatr.* 1997;131:801–808
28. Figueroa-Quintanilla D, Salazar-Lindo E, Sack RB, et al. A controlled trial of bismuth subsalicylate in infants with acute watery diarrheal disease. *N Engl J Med.* 1993;328:1653–1658
29. Wolfe DC, Giannella RA. Antibiotic therapy for bacterial enterocolitis: a comprehensive review. *Am J Gastroenterol.* 1993;88:1667–1683
30. DuPont HL. Prevention of diarrhea by the probiotic, Lactobacillus GG. *J Pediatr.* 1999;134:1–2
31. Costa-Ribeiro H, Ribeiro TC, Mattos AP, et al. Limitations of probiotic therapy in acute, severe dehydrating diarrhea. *J Pediatr Gastroenterol Nutr.* 2003;36:112–115
32. Richardson S, Grimwood K, Gorrell R, et al. Extended excretion of rotavirus after severe diarrhoea in young children. *Lancet.* 1998;351:1844–1848
33. Izraeli S, Rachmel A, Frishberg Y, et al. Transient renal acidification defect during acute infantile diarrhea: the role of urinary sodium. *J Pediatr.* 1990;117:711–716
34. Branski D, Lerner A, Lebenthal E. Chronic diarrhea and malabsorption. *Pediatr Clin North Am.* 1996;43:307–331

35. Cohen SA, Hendricks KM, Mathis RK, Laramee S, Walker WA. Chronic nonspecific diarrhea: dietary relationships. *Pediatrics.* 1979;64:402–407
36. Larcher VF, Shepherd R, Francis DE, Harries JT. Protracted diarrhoea in infancy. Analysis of 82 cases with particular reference to diagnosis and management. *Arch Dis Child.* 1977;52:597–605
37. Goldgar CM, Vanderhoof JA. Lack of correlation of small bowel biopsy and clinical course of patients with intractable diarrhea of infancy. *Gastroenterology.* 1986;90:527–531
38. Klish WJ, Potts E, Ferry GD, Nichols BL. Modular formula: an approach to management of infants with specific or complex food intolerances. *J Pediatr.* 1976;88:948–952
39. Orenstein SR. Enteral versus parenteral therapy for intractable diarrhea of infancy: a prospective, randomized trial. *J Pediatr.* 1986;109:277–286
40. Mack DR, Forstner GG, Wilschanski M, Freedman MH, Durie PR. Shwachman syndrome: exocrine pancreatic dysfunction and variable phenotypic expression. *Gastroenterology.* 1996;111:1593–1602
41. Jonas A, Avigad S, Diver-Haber A, Katznelson D. Disturbed fat absorption following infectious gastroenteritis in children. *J Pediatr.* 1979;95:366–372
42. Fasano A, Berti I, Gerarduzzi T, et al. Prevalence of celiac disease in at-risk and not-at-risk groups in the United States: a large multicenter study. *Arch Intern Med.* 2003;163:286–292
43. Tack GJ, Verbeek WH, Schreurs MW, Mulder CJ. The spectrum of celiac disease: epidemiology, clinical aspects and treatment. *Nat Rev Gastroenterol Hepatol.* 2010;7:204–213
44. Janatuinen EK, Pikkarainen PH, Kemppainen TA, et al. A comparison of diets with and without oats in adults with celiac disease. *N Engl J Med.* 1995;333:1033–1037
45. Hill ID, Dirks MH, Liptak GS, et al. Guideline for the diagnosis and treatment of celiac disease in children: recommendations of the North American Society for Pediatric Gastroenterology, Hepatology and Nutrition. *J Pediatr Gastroenterol Nutr.* 2005;40:1–19
46. Kahana DD, Ulshen MH, Martin MG. Carbohydrate absorption and malabsorption. In: Duggan C, Walker WA, Watkins J, eds. *Nutrition in Pedaitrics: Basic Science and Clinical Aspects.* Boston, MA: Little, Brown, and Co: 2008
47. Treem WR. Congenital sucrase-isomaltase deficiency. *J Pediatr Gastroenterol Nutr.* 1995;21:1–14
48. Newton T, Murphy MS, Booth IW. Glucose polymer as a cause of protracted diarrhea in infants with unsuspected congenital sucrase-isomaltase deficiency. *J Pediatr.* 1996;128:753–756
49. Ameen VZ, Powell GK, Jones LA. Quantitation of fecal carbohydrate excretion in patients with short bowel syndrome. *Gastroenterology.* 1987;92:493–500
50. Hyams JS. Sorbitol intolerance: an unappreciated cause of functional gastrointestinal complaints. *Gastroenterology.* 1983;84:30–33
51. Riby JE, Fujisawa T, Kretchmer N. Fructose absorption. *Am J Clin Nutr.* 1993;58:748S–753S
52. Wang J, Cortina G, Wu SV, et al. Mutant neurogenin-3 in congenital malabsorptive diarrhea. *N Engl J Med.* 2006;355:270–280
53. Mitchel DK, Van R, Morrow AL, et al. Outbreaks of astrovirus gastroenteritis in day care center. *J Pediatr.* 1993;123:725–732.
54. Yolken RH, Lawrence F, Leister F, Takiff HE, Strauss SE. Gastroenteritis associated with enteric type adenovirus in hospitalized infants. *J Pediatr.* 1982;101:21–26
55. Kane JG, Chretien JH, Garagusi VF. Diarrhoea caused by Candida. *Lancet.* 1976;1:335–336
56. Phillips AD, Thomas AG, Walker-Smith JA. Cryptosporidium, chronic diarrhoea and the proximal small intestinal mucosa. *Gut.* 1992;33:1057–1061
57. Wolfson JS, Richter JM, Waldron MA, et al. Cryptosporidiosis in immunocompetent patients. *N Engl J Med.* 1985;312:1278–1282
58. Andrassy RJ, Isaacs H, Weitzman JJ. Rectal suction biopsy for the diagnosis of Hirschsprung's disease. *Ann Surg.* 1981;193:419–424
59. Bock SA. Prospective appraisal of complaints of adverse reactions to foods in children during the first 3 years of life. *Pediatrics.* 1987;79:683–688
60. Scurlock AM, Lee LA, Burks AW. Food allergy in children. *Immunol Allergy Clin North Am.* 2005;25:369–388

61. Boyce JA, Assa'ad A, Burks AW, et al. Guidelines for the diagnosis and management of food allergy in the United States: summary of the NIAID-sponsored expert panel report. *J Allergy Clin Immunol.* 2010;126:1105–1118
62. Odze RD, Wershil BK, Leichtner AM, et al. Allergic colitis in infants. *J Pediatr.* 1995;126:163–170
63. Vanderhoof JA, Murray ND, Kaufman SS, et al. Intolerance to protein hydrolysate infant formulas: an underrecognized cause of gastrointestinal symptoms in infants. *J Pediatr.* 1997;131:741–744
64. Lake AM, Whitington PF, Hamilton SR. Dietary protein-induced colitis in breast-fed infants. *J Pediatr.* 1982;101:906–910
65. Goulet OJ, Revillon Y, Jan D, et al. Neonatal short bowel syndrome. *J Pediatr.* 1991;119:18–23
66. Goulet O, Ruemmele F, Lacaille F, Colomb V. Irreversible intestinal failure. *J Pediatr Gastroenterol Nutr.* 2004;38:250–269
67. Kaufman SS, Loseke CA, Lupo JV, et al. Influence of bacterial overgrowth and intestinal inflammation on duration of parenteral nutrition in children with short bowel syndrome. *J Pediatr.* 1997;131:356–361
68. Taylor SF, Sondheimer JM, Sokol RJ, Silverman A, Wilson HL. Noninfectious colitis associated with short gut syndrome in infants. *J Pediatr.* 1991;119:24–28
69. Neldner KH, Hambidge KM. Zinc therapy of acrodermatitis enteropathica. *N Engl J Med.* 1975;292:879–882
70. Winter H, Chang TI. Gastrointestinal and nutritional problems in children with immunodeficiency and AIDS. *Pediatr Clin North Am.* 1996;43:573–590
71. Grohmann GS, Glass RI, Pereira HG, et al. Enteric viruses and diarrhea in HIV-infected patients. Enteric Opportunistic Infections Working Group. *N Engl J Med.* 1993;329:14–20
72. Sherman PM, Mitchell DJ, Cutz E. Neonatal enteropathies: defining the causes of protracted diarrhea of infancy. *J Pediatr Gastroenterol Nutr.* 2004;38:16–26
73. Bousvaros A, Leichtner AM, Book L, et al. Treatment of pediatric autoimmune enteropathy with tacrolimus (FK506). *Gastroenterology.* 1996;111:237–243
74. Cutz E, Rhoads JM, Drumm B, et al. Microvillus inclusion disease: an inherited defect of brush-border assembly and differentiation. *N Engl J Med.* 1989;320:646–651
75. Patey N, Scoazec JY, Cuenod-Jabri, et al. Distribution of cell adhesion molecules in infants with intestinal epithelial dysplasia (tufting enteropathy). *Gastroenterology.* 1997;113:833–843
76. Jaeken J. Congenital disorders of glycosylation (CDG): update and new developments. *J Inherit Metab Dis.* 2004;27:423
77. Mention K, Michaud Left, Dobbelaere D, et al. Neonatal severe intractable diarrhea as the presenting manifestation of an unclassified congenital disorder of glycosylation (CDG-x). *Arch Dis Child Fetal Neonatal Educ.* 2001;85:F217–F219
78. Kim SC, Ferry GD. Inflammatory bowel diseases in pediatric and adolescent patients: clinical, therapeutic, and psychosocial considerations. *Gastroenterology.* 2004;126:1550–1560

# Chapter 16

# Disruptive Behavior and Aggression

*Lawrence S. Wissow, MD, MPH*

Disruptive and aggressive behaviors are common among children from toddlerhood through adolescence. They may be transient, influenced by temperament and environmental factors, or they may be persistent, rising to the level of oppositional-defiant disorder (ODD) or conduct disorder (CD) and causing significant impairment in the child's and family's functioning. ODD affects 1% to 16% of children, depending on the population studied; CD affects 1.5% to 3.4%. Male-to-female ratio varies with age and diagnosis from 3.2:1 to 5:1.[1] Some children progress from ODD to CD. They can be extremely challenging to manage and, if untreated, experience an increased risk of school failure, difficulty with legal authorities, substance abuse, and ultimately underemployment as adults. Those who go on to develop CD may be dangerous to themselves and others and, in some instances, require emergent treatment. All children manifesting disruptive or aggressive behaviors require intervention, education, support from parents and teachers, and careful monitoring.

There is accumulating evidence that some behavior problems can be prevented. Effective strategies include population-based interventions,[2] supporting parents' mood and reducing exposure to stresses, helping parents learn to both read and help modulate infant emotions, and helping parents learn ways to stimulate and have positive interactions with their infants and young children. As children get older, clinicians can offer anticipatory guidance about predictable parenting issues, written or online parenting materials, and referrals to parenting workshops. The Centers for Disease Control and Prevention (www.cdc.gov/ncbddd/childdevelopment/positiveparenting/index.html) offers colorful public-domain materials for children and youth of a wide range of ages and a new "Essentials" series of video modules for parents of children 2 to 4 years of age. The American Academy of Pediatrics (AAP) has published guidelines for effective discipline.[3]

The following guidance is based on the work of the World Health Organization (WHO), whose recommendations may be updated annually. The most up-to-date information can be found at www.who.int.

## ▶ FINDINGS SUGGESTING DISRUPTIVE BEHAVIOR OR AGGRESSION

Manifestations of disruptive behavior and aggression vary by age. In younger children, they include tantrums, defiance, fighting, and bullying. In older children and adolescents, they may include serious law breaking such as stealing, damage to property, or assault.

A summary of the symptoms and clinical findings that suggest disruptive behavior and aggression can be found in Box 16-1. These may be elicited from parents, teachers, others familiar with the child, or the children or youth themselves. Children, youth, and even parents may minimize problems, and parents and teachers may be unaware of conduct problems that happen when the child is out of their direct supervision. Thus, tactful but persistent discussion and comparing notes among observers may be required to get a full picture of the child's behavioral issues.

## ▶ TOOLS TO ASSIST WITH IDENTIFICATION

Because some children and parents do not spontaneously disclose their symptoms to their primary care clinician standardized psychosocial screening instruments may be used to identify children with symptoms of disruptive behavior or aggression. Several instruments have versions to collect information from youth, parents, and teachers. Table 16-1 provides examples of general psychosocial screening results suggesting that a child has disruptive behavior or aggression. Use of additional instruments, such as the Vanderbilt ADHD Rating Scale (developed for children 6–12 years of age) and the Modified Overt Aggression Scale

Box 16-1

### *Symptoms and Clinical Findings Suggesting Disruptive Behavior and Aggression*

#### INDICATIONS OF DISRUPTIVE BEHAVIOR AND AGGRESSION

- In younger children, marked tantrums, defiance, fighting, and bullying.
- In older children and adolescents, serious law breaking such as stealing, damage to property, or assault.
- Repetitive, persistent, excessive aggression or defiance; behaviors out of keeping with the child's development level, norms of peer group behavior, and cultural context indicating a disorder rather than a phase or transitional disruption.
- Aggression may be impulsive and associated with intense emotional states, or it may be predatory and premeditated. It is important to distinguish which pattern of aggression the child is showing.

#### BEHAVIORS CHARACTERISTIC OF OPPOSITIONAL-DEFIANT DISORDER (ODD)

- Symptoms may be confined only to school, home, or the community.
- Angry outbursts.
- Loss of temper.
- Refusal to obey commands and rules.
- Destructiveness.
- Hitting.
- Intentional annoyance of others, but without the presence of serious lawbreaking.

#### BEHAVIORS CHARACTERISTIC OF CONDUCT DISORDER

- Vandalism.
- Cruelty to people and animals (including sexual and physical violence).
- Bullying.
- Lying.
- Stealing.
- Truancy.
- Drug and alcohol misuse.
- Criminal acts.
- All the features of ODD.

**Table 16-1**
**General Psychosocial Screening/Results Suggesting Disruptive Behavior and Aggression**

| SCREENING INSTRUMENT | SCORE |
|---|---|
| Pediatric Symptom Checklist (PSC)-35 | • Total score ≥24 for children 5 years and younger.<br>• ≥28 for those 6–16 years.<br>• ≥30 for those 17 years and older.<br>AND<br>• Further discussion of items related to disruptive behavior and aggression confirms a concern in that area. |
| PSC-17 | • Externalizing subscale is ≥7.<br>AND<br>• Further discussion of items related to disruptive behavior and aggression confirms a concern in that area. |
| Strengths & Difficulties Questionnaire (SDQ) | • Total symptom score of >19.<br>• Conduct problem score of 5–10 (see instructions at www.sdqinfo.com).<br>• Impact scale (back of form) score of 1 (medium impairment) or ≥2 (high impairment).<br>AND<br>• Further discussion of items related to disruptive behavior and aggression confirms a concern in that area. |
| Ages & Stages Questionnaires: Social-Emotional (ASQ:SE) | • Cutoff score varies by age-specific questionnaire. |
| Early Childhood Screening Assessment | • Total score of ≥18.<br>AND<br>• Thorough emotional and behavioral history, family history, and close follow-up.<br>• Regardless of the total score, any items with a "+" circled should be explored further. These "+"s correlate with a child's emotional or behavioral problems, although, in some cases, parental reassurance is all that is necessary.<br>**Parent score**<br>• A score of 1 or 2 on questions 39 and 40 identify depression in adult primary care settings.<br>• Scores >0 on items 37 and 38 should be further investigated for maternal distress. |

(MOAS) (developed for adults, but sometimes used with adolescents), can help confirm findings of the initial screening; and the use of a functional assessment tool, such as the Strengths & Difficulties Questionnaire (SDQ) or Columbia Impairment Scale (CIS), will help the clinician determine whether the child is significantly impaired by the symptoms. For adolescents, consider assessing the extent of substance use. Use of a tool to assess the effect of the child's problem on other members of the family may also be helpful; the Caregiver Strain Questionnaire (CGSQ) is one example of such a tool. All of these instruments require consideration of their results in the context of other clinical information obtained in the process of discussing the results with the child/youth and family members.

## ▶ ASSESSMENT

Assessment begins by differentiating the child's symptoms from normal behavior. All children are defiant at times, and it is a normal part of adolescence to, at times, do or at least consider doing the opposite of what one is told. A problem or disorder may be present if the behaviors interfere with family life, school, or peer relationships, or put the child or others in danger. Children with disruptive behavior or aggression tend to exhibit repetitive and excessive aggression or defiance out of keeping with developmental and social norms. The behaviors persist, rather than appearing briefly as part of adaptation to a new situation or developmental period. Aggression may be impulsive and associated with intense emotional states, or may be predatory and premeditated. It is important to distinguish which pattern of aggression the child is showing.

Some conditions, such as depression (with prominent irritability), attention-deficit/hyperactivity (ADHD), or sleep deprivation, can mimic or co-occur with lesser degrees of disruptive behavior and aggression. Substance abuse may play a role in both minor and more severe forms of behavior problems. Having witnessed or experienced trauma, or currently living in a stressful or an anxiety-provoking situation may also provoke disruptive behavior. Table 16-2 summarizes these conditions.

In addition, perceptions of the child's symptoms may vary among caregivers or as a particular caregiver's circumstances change. A child whose behavior is perfectly acceptable in one setting may be seen as problematic in another where there are greater dangers or constraints, or where a caregiver may be experiencing other stressors. Recognizing the influence of context can be therapeutic by itself and can lead to development of a more holistic approach to intervention engaging the child, the primary caregiver, and others who support them.

## ▶ PLAN OF CARE FOR CHILDREN WITH DISRUPTIVE BEHAVIOR OR AGGRESSION

Suicidal or homicidal intent is an emergency requiring immediate treatment and close supervision of the youth at all times. Other emergencies may involve parents who feel that they can no longer tolerate the child's behavior, parents who have considered expelling the child from the home or feel that they could harm the child, or situations in which the child's behavior is related to past or ongoing trauma. Community social service agencies often have crisis services that may be of help in these situations and that can provide either respite care or emergency in-home intervention.

The care of a child exhibiting disruptive behavior or aggression can begin in the primary care setting from the time symptoms are recognized, even if the child's symptoms do not rise to the level of a disorder or if referral to a mental health specialist is ultimately part of the care plan.

### *Engage Child and Family in Care*

Without engagement, most families will not seek or persist in care. The process may require multiple primary care visits.[4]

Reinforce strengths of the child and family (eg, good relationships with at least 1 parent or important adult, prosocial peers, concerned or caring family, help-seeking, connection to positive organizations) as a method of engagement, and identify any

**Table 16-2**
**Conditions That May Mimic or Co-occur With Disruptive Behavior and Aggression**

| CONDITION | RATIONALE |
|---|---|
| ADHD | This is a common comorbidity. Association of ODD and ADHD confers a poorer prognosis and children tend to be more aggressive, have more behavior problems that are more persistent, suffer peer rejection at higher levels, and have more significant academic underachievement. See also Chapter 45, Inattention and Impulsivity. |
| Sleep deprivation | Sleep problems can cause irritability and contribute to outbursts of anger and poor impulse control. |
| Learning problems or disabilities | Unidentified learning difficulties can contribute to frustration and oppositionality. If disruptive or aggressive behavior is associated with problems of school performance, the child may have a learning disability. See Chapter 49, Learning Difficulty, to explore this possibility. |
| Developmental problems | Children with overall intellectual or social limitations may experience frustration and poor impulse control. |
| Exposure to adverse childhood experiences (ACE) | Children who have experienced or witnessed trauma, violence, a natural disaster, separation from a parent, parental divorce or separation, parental substance use, neglect, or physical, emotional, or sexual abuse are at high risk of developing emotional difficulties such as adjustment disorder or post-traumatic stress disorder (PTSD) and may manifest outbursts of disruptive or aggressive behavior; this possibility should always be borne in mind because PTSD requires specific trauma-focused interventions. The clinician should tactfully explore the possibility that harsh physical or emotional punishment is related to the child's behavior problem or that tensions might escalate to that point. Denial of trauma symptoms does not mean trauma did not occur; questions about ACE should be repeated as a trusting relationship is established. See Chapter 6, Anxiety. |
| Bereavement | Most children will experience the death of a family member or friend sometime in their childhood. Other losses may also trigger grief responses—separation or divorce of parents, relocation, change of school, deployment of a parent in military service, breakup with a girlfriend or boyfriend, or remarriage of parent. Such losses are traumatic. They may result in feelings of sadness, despair, insecurity, anger, or anxiety immediately following the loss and in some instances, more persistent anxiety or mood problems, including PTSD or depression. In some children, such losses trigger aggressive or disruptive behavior. See also Chapter 14, Depression. |
| Anxiety | Many children with disruptive or aggressive behaviors have anxiety. When faced with demands that make them anxious, they use oppositional behavior to manage their anxiety or avoid the expectations that triggered their anxiety. See Chapter 6, Anxiety. |
| Depression or bipolar disorder | Marked sleep disturbance, disturbed appetite, irritability, low mood, or tearfulness could indicate that a child is depressed. Symptoms of depression rapidly alternating with cycles of agitation may suggest bipolar mood disorder. Common symptoms of pediatric bipolar disorder include explosive or destructive tantrums, dangerous or hypersexual behavior, aggression, irritability, bossiness with adults, driven creativity (sometimes depicting graphic violence), excessive talking, separation anxiety, chronic depression, sleep disturbance, delusions, hallucinations, psychosis, and talk of homicide or suicide.[a] |

*Continued*

**Table 16-2**
**Conditions That May Mimic or Co-occur With Disruptive Behavior and Aggression—cont'd**

| CONDITION | RATIONALE |
|---|---|
| Substance use | All children exhibiting disruptive or aggressive behavior should be screened for substance use and abuse because drug effects or withdrawal from drugs may cause irritability and reduced self-control. |
| Autism spectrum disorders | Children with this developmental pattern also have problems with social relatedness (eg, poor eye contact, preference for solitary activities), language (often stilted), and range of interest (persistent and intense interest in a particular activity or subject). They often will have very rigid expectations for routine or parent promises and become anxious or angry if these expectations are not met. |

*ADHD,* attention-deficit/hyperactivity disorder; *ODD,* oppositional-defiant disorder.
[a]About pediatric bipolar disorder: a guide for families. Child & Adolescent Bipolar Foundation Web site. www.bpkids.org/site/PageServer?pagenamelrn_about. Accessed November 24, 2014

barriers to addressing the problem (eg, stigma, family conflict, resistance to treatment). Use "common factors" techniques[5] to build trust and optimism, reach agreement on incremental next steps, develop a plan of care, and collaboratively determine the role of the primary care physician.

Regardless of other roles, the primary care physician can encourage a positive view of treatment on the part of the youth and family. To do this, the physician will likely have to manage visits in which strong negative emotions are expressed. Parents and youth may accuse each other of instigating problems, or make derogatory remarks about each other. Either party may express hopelessness about improving the situation, and youth, in particular, may refuse to speak or otherwise collaborate in care. Techniques for making the best of these encounters include avoiding taking sides, acknowledging the legitimacy of feelings, acknowledging the frequency with which these problems occur, reminding that strong feelings often occur when people care about each other, and offering to have separate conversations with youth and parents so as to give both a chance to be fully heard.

### Provide Psychoeducation

Families can be assured that behavior problems are common and something for which the clinician is well-prepared to offer help. By the time families seek help, they are often discouraged and both angry and fearful of being criticized. Clinicians can help by emphasizing the great variation among children's temperament and personality, families' constantly evolving circumstances and stressors, and how these factors can combine to form challenges for any parent. Psychoeducation can often be tailored to a given situation by asking parents what they think are the causes of the child's behavior problems. Clinicians can acknowledge the validity of these beliefs and, to the extent necessary, begin to sketch out a range of other possible contributing factors that can be explored as treatment progresses. Usually, what parents are hoping to hear is a combination of reassurances that the behavior will improve over time and concrete plans that will work toward improvement in the short term.

### Encourage Healthy Habits

Encourage exercise, outdoor play, balanced and consistent diet, sleep (critically important to mental health), avoidance of exposure to frightening or violent media, limits on cell phone use and on TV and video games, positive and consistent (not punitive) experiences with parents, praise for good behavior, and reinforcement of strengths. This advice may extend to the parent; if the parent thinks that his ability to carry out normal activities is restricted by the child's behavior, it may be appropriate to see if there are ways the parent can feel more free to do routine or enjoyable activities.

### Reduce Stress

Consider the environment (eg, family social history, parental depression screening, results of any family assessment tools administered, reports from child care or school). Questions to raise might include the following:

- *Is stress on the parent(s) from causes other than the child leading to parental irritability or low mood, drinking, or greater demands for the child to behave? Are there ways for parents to get more support for themselves?* Explore parents' readiness to seek and accept help.
- *Do inconsistencies or differing beliefs about parenting among caregivers (eg, parents, grandparents) undermine attempts to create rules, limits, or consequences? Can caregivers agree on priority behavioral problems and how to address them?* Explore conflicts; seek agreement on common beliefs and achievable steps to help the child.
- *Are nonacademic issues such as the presence of bullying contribuitng to the behavior? Are there other social or behavioral challenges in school?* Collect information directly from the school to explore these issues.

If problems are mainly or exclusively at school, parents should request that the school assess the child for special educational needs and develop a plan to monitor behavior while at school. Primary care clinicians can often provide support in these situations by communicating to the school the degree to which the parents are actively engaged in finding help for their child's problems.

### Offer Initial Intervention(s)

The strategies described in the following text are common elements of evidence-based and evidence-informed psychosocial interventions for disruptive behavior and aggression. They are applicable to the care of children with mild or emerging problems with disruptive behavior and aggression and to the care of those with impairing symptoms that do not rise to the level of a disorder. They can also be used as initial primary care management of children with CD or ODD while readying them for referral or awaiting access to specialty care.

*Promote daily positive joint activities between parents and the child or teen.* The clinician can counsel parents to reinforce compliant, pro-social behavior using parental attention ("Catch 'em being good" [Ed Christopherson]). In addition, parents can encourage, praise, and reward specific, agreed-upon, and desired (target) behaviors. If appropriate, they can be monitored with a chart. Parents can negotiate rewards with the child. Change target behaviors every 2 to 6 weeks; change rewards more frequently. The choice of target behaviors and the time intervals for rewards should be developmentally appropriate. Parents can be encouraged to focus discipline on priority areas. Some minor unwanted behaviors can be ignored; often they will stop as the main focus of child-parent conflict improves. What is most important is that parents find a way to reduce the overall negative tone of interaction and find as many "successes" as possible about which to comment.

*Encourage parents to focus on prevention.* There are several ways for parents to do this. They can reduce positive reinforcement of disruptive behavior by not responding to negative bids for attention and by not engaging in discussion with the child when delivering a request or consequence. In contrast, when children seek attention in a prosocial way, parents should make every attempt to respond positively, even if the response is brief. When possible, parents can try to reorganize the child's day to avoid situations in which the child cannot control himself. Examples include asking a neighbor to look after the child while the parent goes shopping, ensuring that activities are available for long car journeys or other potentialy boring activities, and arranging activities in separate rooms for siblings who are prone to fight. In addition, parents can monitor the whereabouts of adolescents by telephoning the parents of friends whom they say they are visiting. All children appreciate age-appropriate advance notice of what will be expected of them and opportunities to make choices about how to meet those expectations.

Parents also can determine ways to limit contact with friends who have behavior problems and promote contact with friends who are a positive influence. If parents suspect the child's behavior may be caused or exacerbated by a learning problem, they can request that the school evaluate the child for learning problems.

*Encourage parents to be calm and consistent.* The clinician can suggest the following strategies to parents:

- Set clear house rules and give short, specific commands about the desired behavior, not prohibitions about undesired behavior (eg, "Please walk slowly," rather than "Don't run").
- Prioritize issues and target only a few key behaviors until things improve. Within these areas of behavior, make initial targets easily achievable.
- Provide consistent and calm consequences for misbehavior. Consequences should not be drastic or, in the case of young children, go on for so long that the child is likely to forget what he or she originally did wrong. "Time out" should be brief (the rule of thumb for preschoolers is 1 minute per year of age); consequences for older children can involve brief loss of privileges or parental attention. Ideally, these punishments are mirrored by inverse responses for good behavior, especially more parental attention.
- Find a way for children to make reparation for a negative behavior (eg, doing something nice for a sibling they have struck, cleaning up a mess they made while in a tantrum), followed by praise.
- When enforcing a rule, avoid getting into arguments or explanations, because this merely provides additional attention for the misbehavior; defer negotiations until periods of calm.
- If the behavior is taking place in public, quietly advise the child or youth that the problem has been noted but, if possible, defer a response until home or in a less public place.
- Consider parenting classes.
- See also the suggestions in Chapter 45, Inattention and Impulsivity, including Strategies for Working Constructively With a Child's School and Guidelines for Homework Battles.

*Create a safety and emergency plan.* When behavior problems are severe or involve threats of violence or running away, a care plan should be developed jointly with family, including a listing of telephone numbers to call for emergencies. This listing can include hotlines, the on-call telephone number for the practice, or area mental health crisis response team contact information, according to community protocol. The clinician should also instruct the family to proactively remove weapons from the home and monitor for situations that trigger outbursts.

### Provide Resources

Offer the child and parents educational resources to assist them with self-management. Helpful handouts, publications, and Web sites are included in Tools for Practice: Engaging Patient and Family. Provide the family with contact numbers and resources in case of an emergency.

### Monitor the Child's Progress Toward Therapeutic Goals

Child care, preschool, or school reports can be helpful in monitoring progress. Screening instruments that gather information from multiple reporters (youth, parent, teacher), such as the SDQ and PSC, can be helpful in monitoring progress with symptoms and functioning.

It is important for the clinician to help the family understand that it is not uncommon for treatment to be successful for a period and then seem to lose effectiveness. This can happen when there are new stresses or demands, or when, after a period of success, there has been a letup on treatment. If troubleshooting existing treatment and ways of dealing with new stresses does not help get function back to baseline, new treatments, or new diagnoses, need to be considered. In particular, as school demands increase, learning issues may need to be considered even if they were not seen as contributing problems in the past.

### Involve Specialist(s)

Consider involving specialist(s) if the child does not respond to initial interventions or if indicated by the following clinical circumstances:

- Child is younger than 5 years and problems go beyond what is expected developmentally.
- Family is not able to maintain a calm, consistent, or safe environment.
- Child's behaviors are injurious to other children or animals.
- Child has comorbid depression.
- Child is experiencing severe dysfunction in any domain.
- Child has comorbid anxiety. (The combination of shyness, anxiety, and behavior problems is thought to be particularly risky for future behavior problems of a more serious nature.)
- An adolescent has co-occurring problems with substance use.
- Problems at school are interfering with academic achievement or relationships.
- Child or adolescent is involved with legal authorities. (This situation requires coordination with probation officers and understanding the terms of probation; simply reminding the adolescent and family of the consequences of violating probation can help promote participation in treatment or changes to lifestyle.)

*When specialty care is needed, ensure that it is evidence-informed and assist the family in accessing it.* A variety of evidence-based and evidence-informed interventions are available for the treatment of emotional problems in young children and for CD and ODD in school-aged children and adolescents. Ideally, those referred for care in the mental health specialty system would have access to the safest and most effective treatments. Table 16-3 lists programs targeting young children and their families. Table 16-4 provides a summary of interventions for children and adolescents.

Approaches to improving the referral process include making sure that the family is ready for this step in care, that they have some idea of what the specialty care will involve, and that they understand what the clinician's ongoing role may be. If the specialty appointment is not likely to occur in the near future, the clinician can work with parents on a plan to manage the problem as well as possible in the meantime.

Note that not all evidence-based interventions may be available in every community. If a particular intervention is not available, this becomes an opportunity to collaborate with others in the community to advocate on behalf of children. Increasingly, states offer both telepsychiatry services and consultation/referral support "warmlines" that help physicians provide initial treatment and locate resources. The availability of the latter form of help is tracked at www.nncpap.org.

*Reach agreement on respective roles in the child's care.* If the child is referred to mental health specialty care, the primary care physician may be responsible for monitoring response to treatment through use of parent and teacher reports and communication with referral

**Table 16-3**
**Evidence-based Parenting Programs**

| CLUSTER AREA | PARENTING PROGRAM |
|---|---|
| For disruptive behavioral problems | • The Incredible Years (www.incredibleyears.com)<br>• Triple P Positive Parenting Program (www.triplep.net)<br>• Parent-Child Interaction Therapy (http://pcit.phhp.ufl.edu)<br>• "Helping the Noncompliant Child" parent training program (www.strengtheningfamilies.org/html/programs_1999/02_HNCC.html) |
| For high-risk pregnant women (First-time mother, refer before 28 weeks' gestation.) | • Nurse-Family Partnership (www.nursefamilypartnership.org) |
| For children in foster care | • Attachment and Biobehavioral Catch-up (www.infantcaregiverproject.com)<br>• Multidimensional Treatment Foster Care Program for Preschoolers (www.uoregon.edu/~snaplab/SNAP/Projects.html)<br>• Parent Child Interaction Therapy www.pcit.org |
| For parent-child relationship disturbances and high-risk parenting situations | • Circle of Security (www.circleofsecurity.net)<br>• Promoting First Relationships (www.pfrprogram.org)<br>• Parents as Teachers (www.parentsasteachers.org)<br>• Child Parent Psychotherapy www.childtrauma.ucsf.edu/resources/index.htm |
| For children exposed to trauma, including sexual abuse or domestic violence | • Child Parent Psychotherapy<br>• Trauma-focused cognitive behavioral therapy (http://tfcbt.musc.edu) |

**Table 16-4**
**Psychosocial and Psychopharmacologic Treatments for Disruptive Behavior and Aggression (as of November 2014)[a]**

| | PSYCHOSOCIAL TREATMENTS | |
|---|---|---|
| CLUSTER AREA | LEVEL 1 (BEST SUPPORT) | LEVEL 2 (GOOD SUPPORT) |
| Delinquency and disruptive behavior[b] | • Anger control<br>• Assertiveness training<br>• Cognitive behavior therapy (CBT)<br>• Contingency management<br>• Multisystemic therapy<br>• Parent management training<br>• Parent management training and problem solving<br>• Social skills | • CBT and teacher training<br>• Communication skills<br>• Functional family therapy<br>• Parent management training and CBT<br>• Parent management training and classroom management<br>• Problem solving<br>• Rational emotive therapy<br>• Relaxation<br>• Self-control training<br>• Therapeutic foster care<br>• Transactional analysis |
| US FOOD AND DRUG ADMINISTRATION–APPROVED PSYCHOPHARMACOLOGIC INTERVENTIONS[c] | | |
| DIAGNOSTIC AREA | PSYCHOPHARMACOLOGIC INTERVENTION | |
| Aggression | The US Food and Drug Administration (FDA) has no approved indications for aggression in children and adolescents apart from irritability-associated aggression in children with autism. In other populations, recent federally supported evidence-based reviews suggest efficacy for some psychotherapeutic agents. | |

[a]For AAP policy, please visit pediatrics.aappublications.org/site/aappolicy.
[b]Excerpted from PracticeWise Evidence-Based Child and Adolescent Psychosocial Interventions. Reprinted with permission from PracticeWise. For updates and an explanation of PracticeWise determination of evidence level, please visit www.aap.org/mentalhealth.
[c]For up-to-date information about Food and Drug Administration (FDA)-approved interventions, go to www.fda.gov/ScienceResearch/SpecialTopics/PediatricTherapeuticsResearch/default.htm.

sources or agencies involved in care; engaging and encouraging a positive view of treatment; coordinating care provided by parents, school, medical home, and specialists; and observing for comorbidities. Resources available to help clinicians in this role are provided at the end of this chapter in Tools for Practice: Medical Decision Support.

### ACKNOWLEDGMENT
The author and editor wish to acknowledge the contributions of Linda Paul, MPH, manager of the AAP Mental Health Leadership Work Group.

### TOOLS FOR PRACTICE

#### Engaging Patient and Family

- *Everybody Gets Mad: Helping Your Child Cope With Conflict* (Web page), American Academy of Pediatrics (www.healthychildren.org/English/healthy-living/emotional-wellness/Pages/Everybody-Gets-Mad-Helping-Your-Child-Cope-with-Conflict.aspx)
- *Parents' Roles in Teaching Respect* (handout), Bobbi Conner (www.brightfutures.org/mentalhealth/pdf/families/mc/parent_role.pdf)

- *Play Nicely* (video), Monroe Carell Jr Children's Hospital at Vanderbilt (www.playnicely.org)

### Medical Decision Support

- *Pediatric Symptom Checklist* (screen), Massachusetts General Hospital (www.massgeneral.org/psychiatry/services/psc_forms.aspx)
- *Strengths & Difficulties Questionnaires* (screen), Youth in Mind, Ltd (www.sdqinfo.com)
- *NICHQ Vanderbilt Assessment Scale* (scale), National Institute for Children's Health Quality (www.nichq.org/childrens-health/adhd/resources/vanderbilt-assessment-scales)
- *Modified Overt Aggression (MOAS) Scale* (scale) https://depts.washington.edu/dbpeds/Screening%20Tools/ScreeningTools.html
- *Practice Parameter for the Assessment and Treatment of Children and Adolescents With Oppositional Defiant Disorder* (article), *Journal of the American Academy of Child and Adolescent Psychiatry*, Vol 46, Issue 1, 2007 (www.aacap.org/App_Themes/AACAP/docs/practice_parameters/jaacap_adhd_2007.pdf)
- *Treatment of Maladaptive Aggression in Youth: CERT Guidelines I. Engagement, Assessment, and Management* (article), *Pediatrics*, Vol 129, Issue 6; 2012 (pediatrics.aappublications.org/content/129/6/e1562)
- *Treatment of Maladaptive Aggression in Youth: CERT Guidelines II. Treatments and Ongoing Management* (article), *Pediatrics*, Vol 129, Issue 6, 2012 (pediatrics.aappublications.org/content/129/6/e1577)

## REFERENCES

1. Loeber R, Burke JD, Lahey BB, Winters A, Zera M. Oppositional defiant and conduct disorder: a review of the past 10 years, part I. *J Am Acad Child Adolesc Psychiatry*. 2000;39:1468–1484
2. World Health Organization. *The World Report on Violence and Health*. Geneva, Switzerland: World Health Organization; 2002
3. American Academy of Pediatrics Committee on Psychosocial Aspects of Child and Family Health. Guidance for effective discipline. *Pediatrics*. 1998;101:723–728
4. Foy JM; American Academy of Pediatrics Task Force on Mental Health. Enhancing pediatric mental health care: algorithms for primary care. *Pediatrics*. 2010;125(Suppl 3):S109–S125
5. Kemper KJ, Wissow L, Foy JM, Shore SE. *Core Communication Skills for Primary Clinicians*. Wake Forest School of Medicine. nwahec.org/45737. Accessed January 9, 2015

# Chapter 17

# Dizziness and Vertigo

*Ruby F. Rivera, MD; Catherine R. Sellinger, MD*

*Dizziness* and *vertigo,* although often used interchangeably, refer to very different symptoms that have very different clinical implications. Distinguishing these symptoms in young children may be especially difficult because much of the distinction depends on the patient's account of the history.

## ▶ DIZZINESS

### Definition

Dizziness, a relatively common complaint in childhood and adolescence, is "an imprecise term commonly used by patients in an attempt to describe various peculiar subjective symptoms such as faintness, giddiness, light-headedness, or unsteadiness."[1] Patients who have simple dizziness do not describe the room spinning around them, and they do not have nystagmus.

### Causes of Dizziness

Dizziness is commonly seen as a symptom of presyncope in children and adolescents with fever, dehydration, orthostatic hypotension, and vasovagal syncope. It is also commonly associated with anemia, either from acute or chronic blood loss or from a congenital condition such as sickle cell disease.[2] Any heart disease or dysrhythmia that reduces cardiac output can cause dizziness; so too can hypertension. Hypoglycemia, which may be associated with altered mental status or seizures, can first manifest as dizziness.[3] Hyperthyroidism, hypothyroidism, and Addison disease can also cause dizziness. In female adolescents, pregnancy should be considered in the differential diagnosis of dizziness. Ocular disorders such as refractive errors, astigmatism, amblyopia, and strabismus can cause dizziness. Dizziness is often a symptom of anxiety and as part of panic attacks. Dizziness may also be caused by medications that affect the ear, such as aminoglycosides, phenytoin, loop diuretics, and nonsteroidal anti-inflammatory drugs. An algorithm to aid in narrowing the differential diagnosis of dizziness is shown in Figure 17-1.

When young children cannot describe dizziness or vertigo, observers tend to apply these terms to a child who is unsteady while standing. Disequilibrium in this age group may reflect acute cerebellar problems, such as postviral acute cerebellar ataxia and posterior fossa tumors. In adolescents, particularly girls, ataxia as part of multiple sclerosis may be described as dizziness. Another common cause of disequilibrium in young children is middle-ear disease. Several studies have shown deterioration in vestibular balance and motor function in children

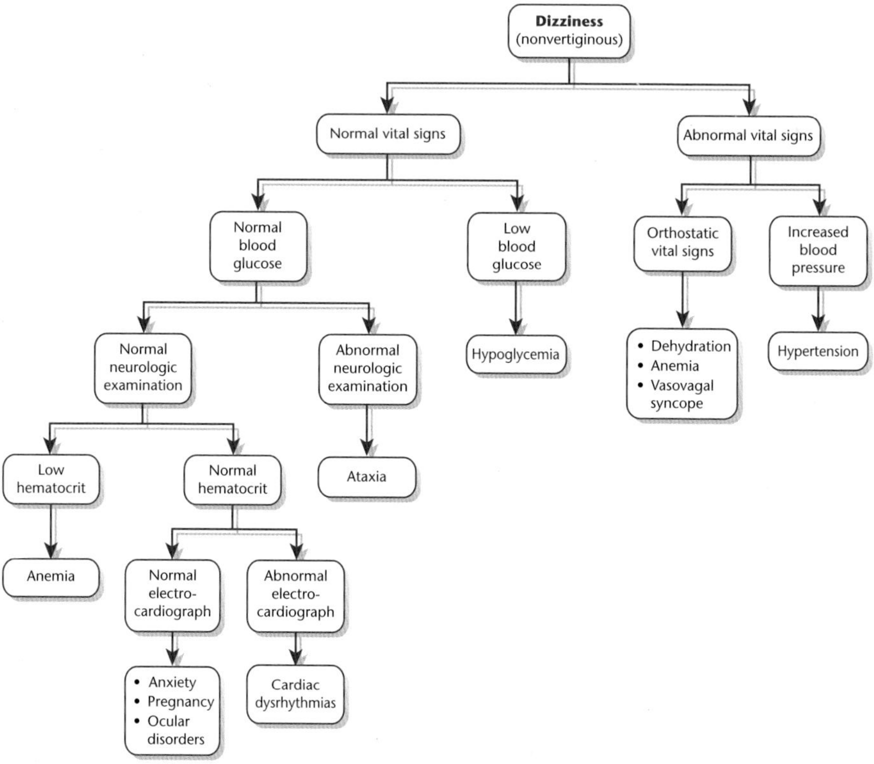


**Figure 17-1**
Algorithm for the differential diagnosis of dizziness.

with middle-ear effusion. If not self-limited, symptoms usually resolve after placement of tympanostomy tubes.

## ▶ VERTIGO

### *Definition*

Vertigo is "a sensation of spinning or whirling motion. Vertigo implies a definite sensation of rotation of the subject or of objects about the subject in any plane."[1] True vertigo almost always is accompanied by nystagmus, at least at the time of the episode.[5] Thus the primary care physician should ask observers about the presence of nystagmus and should ask them to watch for it in future episodes.

### *Causes of Vertigo*

The causes of vertigo can be differentiated based on 3 elements in the history: whether the vertigo is acute or chronic, whether episodes are recurrent, and whether it is accompanied by hearing loss. The causes of vertigo in children vary greatly from those in adults. Acute episodic vertigo is the most common type encountered by pediatricians and is usually not accompanied by hearing loss (Figure 17-2).

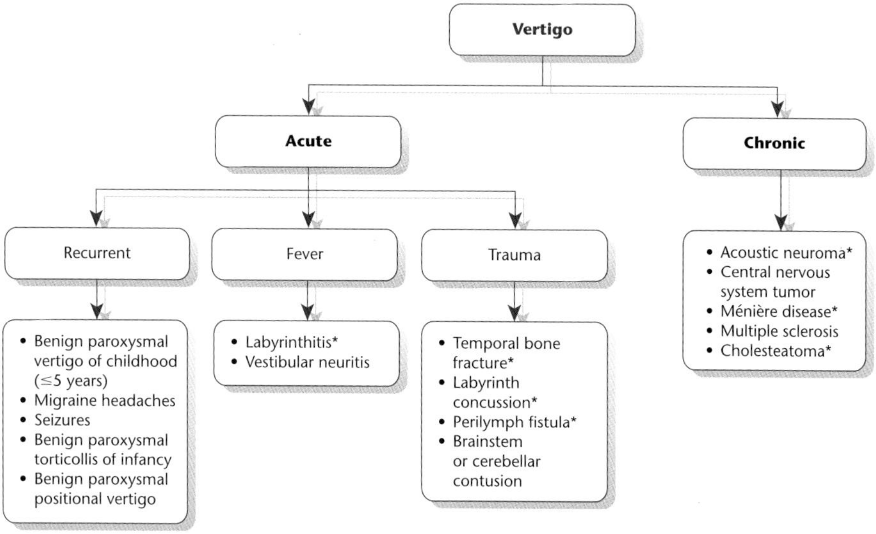


**Figure 17-2**
Algorithm for the differential diagnosis of vertigo. Asterisk denotes an associated hearing loss.

The most common causes of acute episodic vertigo are migraine headaches and related syndromes. Benign paroxysmal torticollis of infancy is thought to be a migraine variant that begins in infancy and generally resolves spontaneously by 2 to 3 years of age. It is characterized by episodes of recurrent head tilt, which may last for hours or days and is often associated with vomiting, agitation, pallor, and ataxia. Benign paroxysmal vertigo of childhood is also considered a migraine variant and is typically seen in children younger than 5 years. These children have the sudden onset of extreme unsteadiness and inability to stand, usually with nystagmus and sometimes with vomiting. The episodes last seconds to minutes. In many cases, the family has a history of migraine headaches, and many of these patients develop more typical migraine headaches in later life. Older children and adolescents may have episodic vertigo as a result of basilar artery migraines. Affected patients often have scintillating scotomas or visual obscuration, oral paresthesias, tinnitus, and occasionally drop attacks with or without loss of consciousness. These early symptoms are commonly but not always followed by a pounding headache. Other causes of acute recurrent vertigo include seizures, perilymph fistula, and benign paroxysmal positional vertigo. Seizures that are associated with vertigo are followed by an alteration or loss of consciousness. A perilymph fistula is an abnormal connection between the inner- and middle-ear spaces. Although some fistulas are congenital, most are acquired from trauma, such as direct penetrating trauma, head trauma, or barotrauma. Flying, diving, coughing, sneezing, or any type of excessive strain or exertion may tear the oval or round window, causing a sudden onset of vertigo associated with hearing loss. Benign paroxysmal positional vertigo (BPPV), although extremely common in adults, is rare in children. BPPV is believed to be caused by otoconia (debris or *ear rocks*) that have been deposited in a sensitive location in the semicircular canal. Acute episodes of severe vertigo are precipitated by a change of head position and are associated with nystagmus, nausea, and vomiting. The Epley and Semont maneuvers attempt to relocate the otoconia into a less-sensitive location. (A helpful Web site that illustrates these maneuvers is www.dizziness-and-balance.com/disorders/bppv/bppv.html). Vestibular neuritis exhibits similar symptoms to BPPV and, although uncommon in children, should be considered if vertigo is preceded by a viral infection. Neither BPPV nor vestibular neuritis is associated with hearing loss.

Vertigo with hearing loss in childhood is usually associated with severe otitis media leading to labyrinthitis. Affected patients are acutely uncomfortable, both from ear pain and from severe vertigo, usually with nausea, vomiting, and nystagmus. Less common causes of hearing loss with vertigo in children include head trauma or ear trauma. Ménière disease, consisting of vertigo, fluctuating hearing loss, pressure in the ear, and tinnitus, is rare in young children, usually occurring after 11 years of age.

Chronic persistent vertigo, especially if accompanied by neurologic signs, is usually indicative of central nervous system disease, including tumors, acoustic neuromas (seen in neurofibromatosis type II), and demyelinating and degenerative disorders.

## ▶ EVALUATION OF DIZZINESS AND VERTIGO

### *History*

Most episodes of dizziness and vertigo can be diagnosed on history and physical examination. Useful information, which may lead to a particular diagnosis, is listed in Table 17-1.

### *Physical Examination*

On physical examination, the physician should document orthostatic vital signs, look for evidence of anemia or dehydration, and pay particular attention to the head, neck, cardiac, and neurologic findings. The Dix-Hallpike maneuver (Nylan-Barany test) can help localize the source of nystagmus or vertigo. To provoke an episode, the child is moved rapidly from a sitting to supine position with the head 45 degrees below the edge of the table and turned 45 degrees to 1 side. The ear that is facing the floor when the nystagmus is elicited is the affected side. Nystagmus that resolves when the child fixates on an object is suggestive of a peripheral or vestibular disease, as opposed to persistent nystagmus, which is seen in central nervous system disorders.

The ears are examined for vesicles of herpes zoster (Ramsay-Hunt syndrome); a distorted tympanic membrane may be seen with otitis media, cholesteatoma, and perilymph fistula. Two useful maneuvers that may help in the diagnosis of perilymph fistula are applying pressure to the tragus to occlude the external auditory canal and pneumatic otoscopy; these may induce nystagmus or vertigo and transiently worsen a hearing loss.

### *Laboratory Testing and Imaging*

With a limited role in the evaluation of dizziness and vertigo, laboratory tests such as complete blood count, metabolic panel, thyroid function tests, electrocardiogram, electroencephalogram, and magnetic resonance imaging should be guided by the history and physical examination. In adolescent girls, a pregnancy test should also be considered. Formal audiometry and electronystagmography may be warranted for the evaluation of vertigo.

**Table 17-1**
**Differential Diagnoses of Dizziness and Vertigo**

| INFORMATION | POSSIBLE DIAGNOSES |
|---|---|
| **FAMILY HISTORY** | |
| Neurofibromatosis | Acoustic neuroma |
| Seizure disorder | Seizure |
| Migraines | Benign paroxysmal torticollis of infancy<br>Benign paroxysmal vertigo of childhood<br>Migraine |
| Unexplained syncope or sudden cardiac death | Dysrhythmias |
| Anxiety, panic disorders | Anxiety |
| **MEDICATION HISTORY** | |
| Aminoglycosides, loop diuretics, phenytoin, nonsteroidal anti-inflammatory drugs, chemotherapeutic agents, quinine | Ototoxicity<br>Intoxication |
| **MEDICAL HISTORY** | |
| Acute or chronic blood loss | Anemia |
| Palpitations or chest pain | Dysrhythmias<br>Anxiety, panic disorder |
| Recent life stressor | Anxiety |
| Last menstrual period | Pregnancy |
| Motion sickness | Benign paroxysmal vertigo of childhood<br>Migraine |
| Recent upper respiratory infection | Vestibular neuritis |
| Fever | Otitis media<br>Labyrinthitis |
| Ear trauma, barotrauma | Perilymph fistula |
| Headache | Migraine<br>CNS disease |
| Head trauma | Temporal bone fracture<br>Labyrinth or brainstem concussion<br>Cerebellar contusion<br>Perilymph fistula |
| Neurologic deficits | CNS tumor<br>Multiple sclerosis |
| Hearing loss | Cholesteatoma<br>Acoustic neuroma<br>Temporal bone fracture<br>Perilymph fistula<br>Labyrinth concussion<br>Labyrinthitis<br>Ramsay-Hunt syndrome (herpes zoster oticus)<br>Ménière disease |
| Triggered by change in head position | Benign paroxysmal positional vertigo<br>Perilymph fistula<br>Vestibular neuritis<br>Acute labyrinthitis |
| Loss of consciousness or altered mental status | Seizure<br>Dysrhythmia<br>Vasovagal syncope<br>CNS disease<br>Hypoglycemia |

*CNS,* central nervous system.

## ▶ MANAGEMENT OF DIZZINESS AND VERTIGO

For patients who have presyncopal or orthostatic dizziness, reassurance and instructions about adequate hydration, about care when arising suddenly, and about the necessity of putting the head lower than the heart when symptoms occur generally suffice for patient management. For patients in whom dizziness is part of a panic attack or a marker of significant stress, further history should be obtained, including any suicidal ideation, and referral for counseling considered.

Treatment for migrainous vertigo and its related syndromes should be symptomatic and targeted to the treatment of migraines (see Chapter 34, Headache).

Vestibular suppressants such as diazepam, meclizine (for children >12 years), and dimenhydrinate may be used to relieve the symptoms of vertigo and nausea. Antibiotics are required for treating labyrinthitis. Treatment for postinfectious vestibular neuritis is symptomatic and supportive, but evidence suggests that prednisone may be helpful.[6,7]

### When to Refer

- Acute ataxia
- A clear history of vertigo, especially with other neurologic signs, or after head trauma or barotrauma
- Suspected perilymph fistula or cholesteatoma
- Suspected seizure
- Complicated migraine

### When to Admit

- Bacterial or suppurative labyrinthitis
- Head trauma with temporal bone fracture
- Space-occupying lesions
- Potential life-threatening cardiac dysrhythmias
- Labile hypertension

### TOOLS FOR PRACTICE

#### Medical Decision Support

- *BPPV: Benign Paroxysmal Positional Vertigo* (Web page), Timothy C. Hain, MD (www.dizziness-and-balance.com/disorders/bppv/bppv.html)

### REFERENCES


1. *Stedman's Medical Dictionary*. 27th ed. Baltimore, MD: Lippincott Williams and Wilkins; 2000
2. Walker JS, Barnes SB. The difficult diagnosis. *Emerg Med Clin North Am*. 1998;16:846–875
3. Anoh-Tanon MJ, Bremond-Gignac D, Wiener-Vacher SR. Vertigo is an underestimated symptom of ocular disorders: dizzy children do not always need MRI. *Pediatr Neurol*. 2000;23:49–53
4. Casselbrant ML, Mandel EM. Balance disorders in children. *Neurol Clin*. 2005;23:807–829
5. Tusa RJ, Saada AA, Niparko JK. Dizziness in childhood. *J Child Neurol*. 1994;9:261–274
6. Goudakos JK, Markou KD, Franco-Vidal V, et al. Corticosteroids in the treatment of vestibular neuritis: a systematic review and meta-analysis. *Otol Neurotol*. 2010;31:183–189
7. Strupp M, Zingler VC, Arbusow V, et al. Methylprednisolone, valacyclovir, or the combination for vestibular neuritis. *N Engl J Med*. 2004;351:354–361

# Chapter 18

# Dysmenorrhea

*Linda M. Dinerman, MD, PC*

Dysmenorrhea, or painful menstruation, is a syndrome characterized by varying degrees of crampy, lower abdominal pain and other symptoms such as nausea, vomiting, urinary frequency, low back pain, diarrhea, fatigue, thigh pain, nervousness, dizziness, sweating, and headache. The pain typically begins just after menses and lasts for about 1 to 2 days, but it can also begin 1 to 2 days before the onset of menses and can last up to 4 days into menstruation.[1] Cramps may be more severe among teenagers who smoke. At least 40% to 60% of adolescent girls suffer some degree of discomfort during menstruation, with about 15% reporting severe symptoms and 14% reporting that they frequently miss school as a result of menstrual symptoms.[1] Most affected teenage girls have primary dysmenorrhea not associated with pelvic or other pathologic conditions; however, causes of secondary dysmenorrhea always should be considered when the patient is evaluated.

## ▶ PRIMARY DYSMENORRHEA

Increased amounts of prostaglandins $E_2$ and $F_{2\alpha}$ in the endometrium of women with dysmenorrhea[1] lead to smooth muscle contractions along with other symptoms such as vomiting and diarrhea. This biologic explanation correlates with the clinical observation that women who have anovulatory cycles usually do not have dysmenorrhea. Adolescent girls typically develop dysmenorrhea 1 to 2 years after menarche, correlating with the onset of ovulatory cycles.[2]

The incidence of dysmenorrhea increases with gynecologic age (as does the number of ovulatory cycles), with up to 31% of girls reporting dysmenorrhea in their first year of menses and 78% in their fifth year.[2] The increase in prostaglandin synthesis may be related to changes in serum progesterone levels not seen in anovulatory women. Additional confirmation comes from the dramatic response women experience with use of either prostaglandin synthetase inhibitors or oral contraceptives, which inhibit ovulation. Increased levels of prostaglandin activity are associated with increased uterine tone and high-amplitude myometrial contractions, both of which result in reduced uterine blood flow and pain.

The assessment of a teenager with dysmenorrhea should include the following:[1]

- Complete menstrual history
- Timing of cramps or pain
- Missed school or other activities
- Ability to participate in social events
- Presence of nausea, vomiting, diarrhea, dizziness, or other symptoms
- Medications used, including doses

- Factors that improve or worsen symptoms
- Family history of dysmenorrhea or endometriosis

In some cases, dysmenorrhea may be the presenting complaint when the true agenda is otherwise.[1] For example: Is the patient reluctant to attend school? Does the patient have a history of physical or sexual abuse? Does the patient have significant psychosocial problems? Is the teen secretly sexually active, and is this a way for her to obtain oral contraceptives for the purpose of contraception?

A careful history usually excludes most pathologic causes of dysmenorrhea. Physicians differ in their opinions regarding what examination is necessary to evaluate a patient with dysmenorrhea. In general, for a non–sexually active teenager who has mild to moderate menstrual cramps relieved by nonsteroidal anti-inflammatory drugs (NSAIDs), only an external genital examination to rule out hymenal abnormalities is indicated. Some physicians would also initiate oral contraceptive pills for a few cycles before performing a pelvic examination if the dysmenorrhea is unresponsive to NSAIDs. For any sexually active teenager or, in the opinion of some experts, for one who is having significant pain that is unresponsive to NSAIDs, a thorough pelvic examination is necessary. In sexually active teenagers, evaluation for sexually transmitted infections and pregnancy should be included. If a pelvic examination is not possible, then a rectoabdominal examination will provide some useful information about the presence of masses or adnexal tenderness. A pelvic ultrasound may be useful in defining uterine and vaginal abnormalities associated with obstruction but is not helpful in the detection of pelvic or abdominal adhesions or endometriosis.[1]

Although treatment of primary dysmenorrhea is likely to include drug therapy, the physician also should take the valuable opportunity to teach the patient about her body. Many teenagers do not understand the physiologic mechanisms of menstruation fully or may have inaccurate beliefs that have been passed on from mother to daughter.

Although teenagers who have very mild discomfort benefit from almost any analgesic, prostaglandin synthetase inhibitors in the form of NSAIDs are the treatment of choice for most young women with dysmenorrhea. Doses, both in terms of amount and timing, vary from patient to patient. Establishing not only prior use of specific medications but also doses is important, given that most patients use them in subtherapeutic amounts.[1] Some need medication only for part or all of the first day of menstruation; others require medication for up to 4 days or more.[1] Ibuprofen (200–800 mg every 6–8 hours) is highly effective for dysmenorrhea, as is naproxen sodium (550 mg immediately and then 275 mg every 6–8 hours). Mefenamic acid, an NSAID that blocks the effect of prostaglandin at the end-organ level and inhibits its production, can be used in a dose of 500 mg administered immediately, followed by 250 mg every 6 hours. Celecoxib, a cyclooxygenase inhibitor, in a dose of 200 mg every 12 hours, has been shown to be effective; however, intestinal bleeding and cardiovascular events have limited its use. In 1 study, 57% of adolescents used medications less often than the maximal daily frequency; thus, advising patients of the range of correct doses is important.[2] These medications are most effective if started at the first sign of menstrual bleeding; women who experience significant nausea with menses may benefit from starting treatment at the earliest symptom of menses, even before bleeding occurs. If the adolescent fails to respond to 1 type of NSAID (eg, ibuprofen), then another (eg, naproxen sodium) should be tried because variability is noted in response to different NSAIDs.[1] Between 70% and 80% of girls will respond to one NSAID or another. The patient should be reevaluated after 2 to 3 menstrual cycles to determine effectiveness of the treatment.

Some patients (perhaps as many as 20% to 30%) will not respond to these measures. In these young women, a trial of oral contraceptive pills (OCPs) used in the same way as for contraception usually provides relief. OCPs work by suppressing ovulation and decreasing endometrial prostaglandin production. Patients should be told that 2 to 3 cycles may elapse before contraceptives exert their maximal effect. If the patient is sexually active, then oral contraceptives are continued on a routine basis; for the non–sexually active teenager, therapy can be reassessed at 6- to 12-month intervals.

Low dose OCPs significantly decrease the symptoms of dysmenorrhea in adult women and adolescents.[3,4] After 3 cycles, adult patients using OCPs with 20 mcg of ethinyl estradiol and 150 mcg of desogestrel and adolescent patients using OCPs with 20 mcg of ethinyl estradiol and 100 mg of levonorgestrel experienced significant relief of dysmenorrhea compared with those using placebo.[3,4]

In a study of adolescent girls using the patch (Ortho Evra) for contraception, dysmenorrhea decreased in 39%, increased in 11%, and resulted in no change in 50%.[5] Depot-medroxyprogesterone acetate (Depo-Provera, DMPA) is also used to prevent ovulation and menstrual flow when OCPs are not tolerated or estrogen is contraindicated.[2] An extended oral contraceptive regimen in which OCPs are taken for up to 12 consecutive weeks followed by 1 hormone-free week is another treatment approach.[6] Continuous OCPs have also been well accepted and shown to be effective in eliminating menses, thereby reducing dysmenorrhea.[7] DMPA and extended oral contraceptive regimens decrease dysmenorrhea, and they decrease the frequency of menses.[8,9]

The efficacy of other treatments is still unproved. Some experts believe that heat, pelvic exercise, general exercise, biofeedback, relaxation therapy, massage, vitamin E, or various herbal remedies are effective; other authorities remain skeptical of these alternatives. Magnesium has been shown to be beneficial in some studies.[1] To the extent that smoking exacerbates dysmenorrhea, it provides yet another reason for physicians to urge their patients to stop smoking. The adolescent with dysmenorrhea should be encouraged to exercise, eat a well-balanced diet, decrease stress, and decrease caffeine consumption.[8]

Women who fail to respond to any of these measures should be referred to an adolescent medicine specialist or gynecologist for evaluation; they probably have secondary rather than primary dysmenorrhea.

## ▶ SECONDARY DYSMENORRHEA

Causes of secondary dysmenorrhea, such as pelvic inflammatory disease (PID), endometriosis, and conditions arising in a variety of other organ systems, can usually be excluded by a careful history and physical examination. Underlying pathologic conditions should be anticipated in a young woman whose pain begins after 20 years of age, who has a history of surgery related to the genitourinary or gastrointestinal tract, or who has pain that is dull and constant rather than crampy.

Endometriosis is the presence of functional endometrial glands and stroma outside the normal anatomic location in the uterus.[10] Patients who have endometriosis will have failed therapy with NSAIDs and oral contraceptives, and their pain may be acyclic rather than cyclic. Menstrual bleeding may be irregular, gastrointestinal symptoms may be present, and a family history of endometriosis can often be elicited. Endometriosis also may be associated with dyspareunia, tenesmus, and rectal pain. Some studies of teenagers with chronic pelvic pain show 25% to 38% of those undergoing laparoscopy have endometriosis. In yet other studies, 52% to 73% of teenagers with chronic pelvic pain have evidence of endometrial implants.[8,10] PID can cause dysmenorrhea acutely, and women often develop chronic pelvic pain as a consequence of PID. Even with assurances of confidentiality, some young women may still not admit to sexual activity. Hence, physicians must maintain a high index of probability if other historical and physical examination findings suggest PID. Teenagers who have a history of genital tract surgery, including abortion, may have outflow tract obstruction. A variety of müllerian anomalies with incomplete obstruction of the outflow tract also produce dysmenorrhea.[1] Depending on the type of obstruction, a pelvic mass may be palpable. Endometrial polyps or fibroids are rare in women younger than 20 years but should be anticipated if the menstrual bleeding is heavy, prolonged, or associated with the passage of clots. Whether these entities alone cause dysmenorrhea is unclear.

A pelvic examination that reveals cervical motion tenderness, or adnexal tenderness, or masses strongly suggests PID. If the cervical os is stenotic or the cervix or uterus feels atretic or abnormally shaped, then outflow obstruction is possible (eg, a uterus with a blind horn). Among adult women, physical findings such as small fixed nodules in the rectovaginal septum or cul de sac or fixation of the uterus indicated by the sensation of pain on stretching of the uterosacral ligaments suggest endometriosis. However, most adolescents generally have normal examinations; hence, endometriosis can be extremely difficult to detect on clinical grounds alone.[11] If a secondary cause of dysmenorrhea is thought to be present, then consultation with an adolescent medicine specialist or gynecologist is warranted. Ultrasound examination of the uterus will rule out uterine anomalies but cannot exclude endometriosis. Confirmation of endometriosis requires laparoscopy. Because the lesions of endometriosis in adolescents may differ from the typical lesions seen in adults, a gynecologist who is experienced in evaluating adolescents should perform this procedure. Endometriosis may be difficult to manage, and women who have this condition are at increased risk for infertility.

PID should be treated according to standard antibiotic regimens. Follow-up is critical because young women, once infected, are at risk for further episodes of PID as well as for chronic pelvic pain, ectopic pregnancy, and infertility.

## When to Refer

For dysmenorrhea, referral might be appropriate if

- Physician feels uncomfortable prescribing OCPs for the treatment of primary dysmenorrhea
- Patient fails to respond to NSAIDs and OCPs
- Clinical presentation or course suggests that the patient has secondary rather than primary dysmenorrhea
- Patient is sexually active and the physician feels uncomfortable performing a pelvic examination

## When to Admit

If the cause of the dysmenorrhea is determined to be PID, some physicians would recommend hospitalization of all adolescents for treatment. Others recommend hospitalization under certain but not all circumstances.

### *TOOLS FOR PRACTICE*

#### Engaging Patient and Family

- *Center for Young Women's Health* (Web site), (www.youngwomenshealth.org)
- *Menstrual Disorders* (Web page), American Academy of Pediatrics (www.healthychildren.org/English/health-issues/conditions/genitourinary-tract/Pages/Menstrual-Disorders.aspx)

### *REFERENCES*


1. Emans SJ, Laufer MR, Goldstein DP. *Pediatric and Adolescent Gynecology.* 5th ed. Philadelphia, PA: Lippincott Williams & Wilkins; 2005
2. Iglesias EA, Coupey SM. Menstrual cycle abnormalities: diagnosis and management. *Adolesc Med.* 1999;10:255–273
3. Callejo J, Díaz J, Ruiz A, García RM. Effect of a low-dose oral contraceptive containing 20 microg ethinylestradiol and 150 microg desogestrel on dysmenorrhea. *Contraception.* 2003;68:183–188
4. Davis AR, Westhoff C, O'Connell K, et al. Oral contraceptives for dysmenorrhea in adolescent girls. *Obstetr Gynecol.* 2005;106(1):97–104
5. Harel Z, Riggs S, Vaz R, et al. Adolescents' experience with the combined estrogen and progestin transdermal contraceptive method Ortho Evra. *J Pediatr Adolesc Gynecol.* 2005;18:85–90
6. Sulak PJ, Carl J, Gopalakrishnan I, Coffee A, Kuehl TJ. Outcomes of extended oral contraceptive regimens with a shortened hormone-free interval to manage breakthrough bleeding. *Contraception.* 2004;70:281–287
7. Archer DF, Jensen JT, Johnson JV, et al. Evaluation of a continuous regimen of levonorgestrel/ethinyl estradiol: phase 3 study results. *Contraception.* 2006;74:439–445
8. Greydanus DE, Patel DR, Pratt HD. *Essential Adolescent Medicine.* New York, NY: McGraw-Hill; 2006
9. Westoff C. Depot-Medroxyprogesterone acetate injection (Depo-provera): a highly effective contraceptive option with proven long-term safety. *Contraception.* 2003;68(2):75–87
10. Attaran M, Gidwani GP. Adolescent endometriosis. *Obstet Gynecol Clin North Am.* 2003;30:379–390
11. Schroeder B, Sanfilippo JS. Dysmenorrhea and pelvic pain in adolescents. *Pediatr Clin North Am.* 1999;46:555–571

# Chapter 19

# Dysphagia

*Mohammad F. El-Baba, MD*

Feeding and swallowing disorders are common complaints in children. Dysphagia is defined as difficulty swallowing, which derives from the Greek root, *dys,* meaning "difficulty," and *phagia,* meaning "to eat." It is not synonymous with the term *odynophagia,* which refers to painful swallowing.

## ▶ NORMAL DEVELOPMENT OF SWALLOWING

A sucking reflex, present as early as 18 weeks' gestation, is initially disorganized but becomes more organized and efficient for feeding by 34 to 36 weeks' gestation. For the term newborn the suck is mature and efficient for liquid feedings.[1,2] During early infancy, the infant develops a more rapid suck rate and higher suck pressure. Tongue movements are differentiated and become more coordinated, preparing the infant for pureed food by 5 to 6 months of age.[3] After this stage, sensory experience with food increases, and oral motor skills expand to handle more textured food. The gag reflex decreases to allow swallowing of an increasing amount of food with more texture. By age 2 years, chewing and tongue movements become more proficient.

## ▶ NORMAL PHASES OF SWALLOWING

Swallowing is divided into 3 phases: oral, pharyngeal, and esophageal.[4] These phases allow the food and liquid to move from mouth to stomach efficiently and safely. In the oral phase, the food is mixed with saliva and chewed if needed. A single bolus of food is collected between the roof of the mouth and tongue. The bolus is propelled to the posterior of the tongue and then to the pharynx. In infants and young children, the suckling swallow allows the liquid to fall from the mouth into the pharynx.

The pharyngeal phase is the actual reflexive swallow stimulated by the presence of food on the posterior tongue. During this phase the soft palate rises to keep the food from the nasal passage. The larynx moves up and forward, closing the glottis. The vocal cords come together, the epiglottis closes over the airway, and respirations cease. Food is propelled further by contraction of the pharyngeal muscles and relaxation of the upper esophageal sphincter.

During the esophageal phase, esophageal peristalsis moves the food down the esophagus into the stomach through the relaxed lower esophageal sphincter. The lower esophageal sphincter then returns to the closed tonic state to prevent regurgitation of gastric contents.

## ▶ CAUSES OF DYSPHAGIA

Any anatomic or functional disorder in the well-coordinated act of swallowing can result in dysphagia,[5] which can be for liquids, solids, or both. In general, mechanical or obstructive factors result in dysphagia for solids. Dysphagia for liquids is more pronounced in patients with neurologic disorders. The causes of dysphagia in children are widespread and include congenital, inflammatory, infectious, systemic, neoplastic, and traumatic reasons (Box 19-1).

Infants born before term or with a birth weight below the tenth percentile for gestational age are at increased risk for developing dysphagia and feeding difficulties. Improved survival

**Box 19-1**

### *Causes of Dysphagia in Children*

- Prematurity
- Congenital abnormalities
  - Congenital anomalies of the nasal and oral cavity
    - Cleft lip or palate
    - Choanal atresia or stenosis
    - Craniofacial anomalies (Crouzon syndrome, Apert syndrome, Möbius sequence, Pierre Robin sequence, Treacher Collins syndrome)
    - Congenital nasal masses (dermoids, encephaloceles)
  - Congenital anomalies of the larynx, trachea, and esophagus
    - Laryngomalacia
    - Laryngeal clefts
    - Laryngeal stenosis and webs
    - Vocal cord paralysis
    - Tracheoesophageal fistula
    - Esophageal atresia
    - Esophageal duplication
- Vascular rings
  - Double aortic arch
  - Right aortic arch with left ligamentum from a descending aorta
  - Innominate artery tracheal compression
- Infectious causes
  - Acute pharyngitis or tonsillitis
  - Peritonsillar and retropharyngeal abscesses
  - Epiglottitis
  - Esophagitis (cytomegalovirus, herpesvirus, *Candida albicans*)
- Inflammatory causes
  - Esophagitis secondary to gastroesophageal reflux disease
  - Eosinophilic esophagitis
- Neurologic or neuromuscular disorders
  - Hypoxic-ischemic encephalopathy
  - Head trauma
  - Cerebral palsy
  - Congenital malformations (Arnold-Chiari malformation, absent corpus callosum)
  - Degenerative diseases of white and gray matter
  - Brainstem tumors
  - Syringomyelia
  - Infantile spinal muscular atrophy (Werdnig-Hoffmann disease)
  - Diseases of neuromuscular junction
    - Myasthenia gravis
    - Guillain-Barré syndrome
    - Botulism
- Muscular
  - Congenital myopathies
  - Mitochondrial diseases
  - Glycogen storage diseases
  - Congenital muscular dystrophy and myotonic dystrophy
- Traumatic
  - External trauma
  - Intubation injury
- Neoplastic
  - Hemangioma
  - Lymphangioma
- Miscellaneous
  - Foreign-body aspiration
  - Caustic ingestion
  - Motor dysfunction of esophagus (achalasia)
  - Epidermolysis bullosa

of infants born prematurely has contributed to the increased incidence of dysphagia in children.[6]

Central nervous system impairment and developmental delay are common causes of dysphagia in infants and children. Almost all children with severe cerebral palsy are reported to suffer from some degree of dysphagia, and about 70% of children with severe traumatic brain injury present with dysphagia during the acute phase of care.[7] Children with gastroesophageal reflux disease often experience some feeding problems and food refusal.[8] Reflux can lead to nausea, vomiting, and esophagitis, all of which may cause feeding to be perceived as an aversive experience. Eosinophilic esophagitis has become a recognized entity that causes dysphagia in adults and children,[9] and it should be considered in the differential diagnosis of children with unexplained oral aversion, feeding difficulties, and poor weight gain.

Prolonged tube feeding in infancy or childhood can lead to long-term feeding difficulties. Several factors are implicated in such difficulties and include age at which oral feeding commences, underlying medical conditions, exposure to taste and textures during sensitive periods, aversive experiences, and different methods of delivering tube feeds.[10]

Infants and young children occasionally exhibit transient feeding difficulties such as selective eating, exceedingly slow eating, and tantrums. Some children without apparent risk factors show deviating feeding behaviors such as food refusal, aversion to feeding, low food intake, excessive gagging, and vomiting even before food is presented. Nonorganic feeding disorders are usually transient, but in 3% to 10% become persistent and carry the risk of inadequate growth. Early intervention and a multidisciplinary approach are crucial in the management of this group of children.[11]

## ▶ CLINICAL MANIFESTATION

Feeding disorders are commonly seen in early childhood. Minor feeding problems are reported in 25% to 35% of healthy young children, with major feeding disorders observed in 40% to 70% of infants born prematurely or children with chronic medical problems.[4,6] Affected infants or children commonly exhibit feeding difficulties, food refusal, failure to thrive, or sensation of food stuck in the throat or chest. These children may also have drooling, difficulty initiating swallowing, change in dietary habits, aversions to certain food textures, and unexplained weight loss.

Some children may experience change in voice, recurrent coughing, or noisy breathing during feeding. Oropharyngeal dysphagia should be considered in young children with recurrent aspiration or unexplained respiratory symptoms.[12] Respiratory symptoms that result from dysphagia vary and may be associated with coughing, chronic congestion, recurrent choking, acute life-threatening events, recurrent pneumonias, and chronic lung disease. The different symptoms of dysphagia in infants and children are summarized in Box 19-2.

## ▶ EVALUATION

### *History and Physical Examination*

A complete history and thorough physical examination of the child with dysphagia usually leads to the diagnosis and guides the selection of further diagnostic tests. Emphasis should be placed on birth history, neurodevelopmental history, and medical comorbidities. Detailed feeding history should include the type of current diet, texture, route of administration, meal

Box 19-2

## *Symptoms of Dysphagia in Infants and Children*

**ORAL PHASE**

- Failure to initiate or maintain sucking
- Prolonged feeding time
- Drooling

**ORAL HYPERSENSITIVITY**

- Exaggerated gag reflex
- Difficulty making the transition to textured foods
- Sensitivity to touch in and around mouth

**ORAL HYPOSENSITIVITY**

- Retaining food in the mouth
- Increased drooling

**PHARYNGEAL PHASE**

- Coughing
- Choking
- Noisy breathing during feeding
- Nasopharyngeal reflux

**ESOPHAGEAL PHASE**

- Spitting up or vomiting
- Irritability or arching during feeding
- Preference for liquid food
- Sensation of food stuck in the throat

duration, and specific food aversion or aversions. General examination should document any orofacial malformation. The combination of micrognathia and glossoptosis seen in Pierre Robin sequence may cause feeding difficulty in an infant. Cleft lip and palate, including submucous cleft, are important causes of dysphagia. Newborns with choanal stenosis may experience difficulty feeding because of the obligate nasal breathing in the first few months of life. Neurologic examination should include assessment of muscle tone and strength and evaluation of cranial nerve function.[1,13,14]

A clinical feeding evaluation should be performed by an experienced occupational therapist or speech pathologist. This clinical evaluation includes assessment of posture, positioning, oral structure and function, patient motivation, and interaction between the infant and feeder. A variety of foods, different positions, and adaptive utensils may be used during the examination. Specific symptoms observed during feeding can help identify the underlying disorder. Gagging, coughing, or emesis is usually present in infants with a structural or neurologic disorder. Repeated swallowing after feeding, fussiness, crying, or regurgitation are usually noted in infants with gastroesophageal reflux disease and require further investigation.

### Laboratory Evaluation

A complete blood count can be useful as a screening test for infectious or inflammatory conditions. Serum protein and albumen are useful for nutritional assessment. Chromosomal karyotyping, metabolic analysis, or specific DNA tests may be required for a specific diagnosis as directed by physical and neurologic examination. Electromyography, nerve conduction studies, and muscle biopsy may be needed in infants with suspected neuromuscular disorders.

### Imaging Studies

Chest radiography is indicated in patients with suspected pneumonia or chronic lung disease. Persistent pulmonary infiltrates on chest radiograph may be better elucidated by high-resolution chest computed tomography (HRCT). Computed tomography or magnetic resonance imaging of the brain may be especially helpful in patients with suspected central nervous system injury or structural abnormalities.

## *Diagnostic Studies*

### Upper Gastrointestinal Barium Study

Barium radiography plays a role in evaluating esophageal dysphagia. It is valuable in assessing anatomic or structural abnormalities, such as strictures, fistulas, masses, or intestinal rotational anomalies. Barium studies are usually more sensitive than endoscopy in the evaluation of patients suspected to have achalasia or vascular ring. In most cases, vascular rings appear as a persistent indentation of the esophagus.[15]

### Videofluorographic Swallowing Study

The videofluorographic swallowing study (VFSS), also known as the modified barium study, is considered the gold standard for assessment of the oral and pharyngeal stages of swallowing and allows the physician to determine the risk of aspiration.[15–17] Conducted jointly by a radiologist and a dysphagia-trained speech pathologist or occupational therapist, the VFSS provides evidence of all categories of oropharyngeal swallowing dysfunction, which include inability or excessive delay in initiation of pharyngeal swallowing, aspiration of food, nasopharyngeal regurgitation, and residue of food within the pharyngeal cavity after swallowing.

During this study the child will drink or eat foods mixed with barium while radiographic images are observed and recorded. Patients' difficulties with different food textures can be identified and compatible diets planned. The definitive finding of aspiration will permit the physician to make suggestions to avoid the offending consistency, usually thin liquids. Furthermore, the study allows for testing of the efficacy of compensatory dietary modifications, postures, and swallowing maneuvers so that the observed dysfunction can be corrected. Its disadvantages are those of exposure to ionizing radiation, hence a time limit on the study duration and a need for patient cooperation. Dose limiting techniques, such as pulsed fluoroscopy and tight coning, will be effective in eliminating unnecessary radiation.

### Fiberoptic Endoscopic Evaluation of Swallowing

In fiberoptic endoscopic evaluation of swallowing (FEES) a fiberoptic endoscope is introduced into the nose and advanced into the laryngopharyngeal area, permitting observation of the pharyngeal phase of swallowing. A swallowing assessment is performed with liquids and a variety of textures, if developmentally appropriate. Typically, dye is added to the food to provide better visualization and to determine residual pooling of food versus saliva. The feeding parameters evaluated in this study are laryngeal penetration and aspiration.[17] FEES, combined with laryngopharyngeal sensory testing, has shown that patients with a higher laryngopharyngeal sensory threshold are more likely to experience laryngeal penetration and aspiration during a feeding assessment.[18,19] The ability to initiate airway closure with stimulation demonstrates airway protection. FEES and sensory testing may be particularly valuable for the evaluation of swallowing safety in children who refuse to ingest adequate amounts of barium to perform VFSS.

### Esophagogastroduodenoscopy

Endoscopy is suggested for most patients with dysphagia of esophageal origin to establish or confirm a diagnosis, to seek evidence of esophagitis, and, when appropriate, to implement therapy.[20] It is particularly useful in evaluating patients suspected of having strictures, webs, mucosal inflammatory lesions, or specific infections. Endoscopic and histologic features are required for the diagnosis of eosinophilic esophagitis. A normal appearance of the esophagus during endoscopy does not exclude histopathological esophagitis; subtle mucosal changes such as erythema and pallor may be observed in the absence of esophagitis. During endoscopy, esophageal biopsy should be performed to detect microscopic esophagitis and to exclude causes of esophagitis other than gastroesophageal reflux.

### Esophageal Manometry

Esophageal manometry, the standard test for disorders of esophageal motility, is especially useful in establishing a diagnosis of achalasia and for detecting esophageal motor abnormalities associated with autoimmune diseases.

### Esophageal pH Probe Study

Esophageal pH monitoring, a valid and reliable measure of acid reflux, is useful to establish the presence of abnormal acid reflux, to determine whether a temporal association exists between acid reflux and frequently occurring symptoms, and to assess the adequacy of therapy in patients who do not respond to treatment with acid suppression. Most centers are currently replacing pH monitoring with combined multiple intraluminal impedance (MII) and pH monitoring. This test detects acid and nonacid reflux episodes. It is superior to pH monitoring alone for evaluation of the temporal relation between symptoms and GER.

### Scintigraphy

Scintigraphy is useful in the evaluation of gastric emptying and can also demonstrate episodes of aspiration detected during a 1-hour study or on images obtained up to 24 hours after the test feeding is administered. The role of scintigraphy in diagnosing gastroesophageal reflux disease in infants and children is unclear.

## ▶ MANAGEMENT

Management of children with dysphagia often involves a multidisciplinary approach, the aims of which are to identify and characterize dysphagia and identify the underlying cause whenever possible. Special emphasis should be placed on detection of treatable conditions, which include surgically or endoscopically treatable structural abnormalities, inflammatory conditions (eg, reflux esophagitis, eosinophilic esophagitis), specific infections, and underlying systemic conditions.

The goals of managing dysphagia are to reduce aspiration, improve the ability to eat and swallow, and optimize nutritional status. Feeding therapy for infants and children may include the strategies described below.[1,21]

#### *Normalization of Posture and Tone*

Head and trunk control are crucial to the development of oral motor skills. Children with neurologic abnormalities frequently have poor head control and poor trunk stability.

Occupational and physical therapy can be used to improve head control, neck and trunk tone, and posture as a basis for improved oral motor function.

### Adaptation of Food and Feeding Equipment

Food and feeding equipment may be adapted by changing the attributes of food and liquids, such as bolus volume, consistency, temperature, and taste. Adjustments in feeding schedule may be beneficial for children receiving continuous tube feeds with supplemental food orally. The feeds can be changed gradually to bolus feeds to stimulate the child's appetite. The rate of feeding should be paced to allow sufficient time to swallow before giving another bite. In addition, the bottle or utensils may be changed according to the child's needs.

### Oral Motor Therapy

Oral motor therapy is focused on improving the oral phase of feeding and may include stimulation with stroking, stretching, brushing, icing, tapping, and vibrating areas of the face and mouth.

### Nutritional Support

Management of dysphagia must focus on meeting the child's nutritional needs for adequate growth. When a patient is unable to achieve adequate nutrition and hydration by mouth, supplemental feedings through a nasogastric tube or a percutaneous endoscopic gastrostomy may be necessary. The presence of a feeding tube is not a contraindication for therapy. Many children with feeding disorders have neurologic or anatomic abnormalities that cannot be corrected, making oral feeding difficult or unsafe.

## ▶ MANAGEMENT OF ASSOCIATED DISORDERS

Associated disorders, such as gastroesophageal reflux disease, eosinophilic esophagitis, and chronic lung disease, may also need to be specifically managed. Application of synchronized neuromuscular electrical stimulation to cervical swallowing muscles (VitaStim therapy) has been shown to improve oral intake and help restore normal swallowing mechanism in adults,[22,23] but empirical data are lacking to support its use in children.

## When to Refer

A referral to a pediatric dysphagia center, if available, provides the most complete method to establish a diagnosis and render a management plan. Members of the team vary from center to center and usually include a gastroenterologist, otolaryngologist, pulmonologist, physical medicine and rehabilitation specialist, surgeon, occupational therapist, and pediatric dietitian. Referral is warranted

- When symptoms are persistent
- When the cause of dysphagia is unclear
- On evidence of aspiration

## When to Admit

- Severe feeding difficulties
- Malnutrition

- Failure to thrive
- Dehydration
- Aspiration

## REFERENCES


1. Dusick A. Investigation and management of dysphagia. *Semin Pediatr Neurol.* 2003;10:255–264
2. Bu'Lock F, Woolridge MW, Baum JD. Development of co-ordination of sucking, swallowing and breathing: ultrasound study of term and preterm infants. *Dev Med Child Neurol.* 1990;32:669–678
3. McGowan JS, Marsh RR, Fowler SM, Levy SE, Stallings VA. Developmental patterns of normal nutritive sucking in infants. *Dev Med Child Neurol.* 1991;33:891–897
4. Rudolph CD, Link DT. Feeding disorders in infants and children. *Pediatr Clin North Am.* 2002;49: 97–112, vi
5. Kosko JR, Moser JD, Erhart N, Tunkel DE. Differential diagnosis of dysphagia in children. *Otolaryngol Clin North Am.* 1998;31:435–451
6. Hawdon JM, Beauregard N, Slattery J, Kennedy G. Identification of neonates at risk of developing feeding problems in infancy. *Dev Med Child Neurol.* 2000;42:235–239
7. Morgan AT. Dysphagia in childhood traumatic brain injury: a reflection on the evidence and its implications for practice. *Dev Neurorehabil.* 2010;13:192–203
8. Mathisen B, Worrall L, Masel J, Wall C, Shepherd RW. Feeding problems in infants with gastro-oesophageal reflux disease: a controlled study. *J Paediatr Child Health.* 1999;35:163–169
9. Furuta GT, Straumann A. Review article: the pathogenesis and management of eosinophilic oesophagitis. *Aliment Pharmacol Ther.* 2006;24:173–182
10. Mason SJ, Harris G, Blissett J. Tube feeding in infancy: implications for the development of normal eating and drinking skills. *Dysphagia.* 2005;20:46–61
11. Romano C, Hartman C, Privitera C, Cardile S, Shamir R. Current topics in the diagnosis and management of the pediatric non organic feeding disorders (NOFEDs). *Clin Nutr.* 2014;pii:S0261–S5614
12. Lefton-Greif MA, Carroll JL, Loughlin GM. Long-term follow-up of oropharyngeal dysphagia in children without apparent risk factors. *Pediatr Pulmonol.* 2006;41:1040–1048
13. Garg BP. Dysphagia in children: an overview. *Semin Pediatr Neurol.* 2003;10:252–254
14. Kakodkar K, Schroeder JW. Pediatric dysphagia. *Pediatr Clin North Am.* 2013;60:969–977
15. Furlow B. Barium swallow. *Radiol Technol.* 2004;76:49–58; quiz 59–61
16. Palmer JB, Drennan JC, Baba M. Evaluation and treatment of swallowing impairments. *Am Fam Physician.* 2000;61:2453–2462
17. Cook IJ, Kahrilas PJ. AGA technical review on management of oropharyngeal dysphagia. *Gastroenterology.* 1999;116:455–478
18. Link DT, Willging JP, Miller CK, Cotton RT, Rudolph CD. Pediatric laryngopharyngeal sensory testing during flexible endoscopic evaluation of swallowing: feasible and correlative. *Ann Otol Rhinol Laryngol.* 2000;109:899–905
19. Willging JP, Thompson DM. Pediatric FEESST: fiberoptic endoscopic evaluation of swallowing with sensory testing. *Curr Gastroenterol Rep.* 2005;7:240–243
20. Spechler SJ. AGA technical review on treatment of patients with dysphagia caused by benign disorders of the distal esophagus. *Gastroenterology.* 1999;117:233–254
21. Arvedson JC. Management of pediatric dysphagia. *Otolaryngol Clin North Am.* 1998;31:453–476
22. Shaw GY, Sechtem PR, Searl J, et al. Transcutaneous neuromuscular electrical stimulation (VitalStim) curative therapy for severe dysphagia: myth or reality? *Ann Otol Rhinol Laryngol.* 2007;116:36–44
23. Miller CK, Willging JP. Advances in the evaluation and management of pediatric dysphagia. *Curr Opin Otolaryngol Head Neck Surg.* 2003;11:442–446

# Chapter 20

# Dyspnea

*Jay H. Mayefsky, MD, MPH*

Dyspnea is the uncomfortable feeling of not being able to satisfy *air hunger*. Patients may complain of not being able to catch their breath or of a suffocating feeling. As with any subjective complaint, the diagnosis of dyspnea and its cause in an infant or young child can be problematic. Therefore, to evaluate fully a child in respiratory distress, the pediatrician must be familiar with the pathophysiologic features, signs, and common causes of dyspnea. With the aid of the medical history, physical examination, and appropriate laboratory tests, the condition can be diagnosed and therapy initiated.

## ▶ PATHOPHYSIOLOGIC FEATURES

Dyspnea is seen most commonly with exercise because of the increased work of breathing necessary to keep up with the body's increased metabolic demands. The sensation is probably transmitted from stretch receptors in the chest wall muscles to the central nervous system (CNS). Chemoreceptors play a role, sensing changes in arterial pH, oxygen, and carbon dioxide concentrations, as well as chest wall proprioceptors, lung stretch receptors, and mechanoreceptors in the heart, skeletal muscles, and upper airway.[1] The transmission is processed in the CNS, causing the individual to experience the sensation of dyspnea. With exercise, the person who has dyspnea is aware of an increased ventilatory effort. Under these circumstances, the dyspnea is relieved after the exercise ceases and the pH and oxygen and carbon dioxide levels return to normal. Dyspnea also occurs when ventilation or gas exchange is compromised.

To satisfy their oxygen needs, children who have dyspnea must increase their minute ventilation ($\dot{V}E$), working harder to do so. In normal breathing, respiratory muscles work only during inspiration, and the diaphragm does most of the work. The work of inspiration is the sum of the work necessary to overcome the elastic forces of the lung, the tissue viscosity of the lung and chest wall, and airway resistance. When any of these factors is increased (eg, elastic force and tissue viscosity in restrictive pulmonary disease, resistance in obstructive airway disease), the work of inspiration must increase to maintain adequate $\dot{V}E$. The accessory muscles of inspiration (the sternocleidomastoid, anterior serratus, and external intercostal muscles) are recruited to accomplish this task. Contraction of these muscles causes forceful expansion of the thorax, resulting in an unusually large negative intrathoracic pressure. This negative pressure draws in the soft tissues of the chest wall and creates 1 of the classic signs of dyspnea, retractions, which may be seen in the suprasternal, infrasternal, intercostal, subcostal, and supraclavicular areas. An alternative way to maintain an adequate $\dot{V}E$ is to increase the rate of breathing; hence the second classic sign of dyspnea, tachypnea. Nasal flaring and grunting are other signs during respiration.

Little energy is expended during normal expiration. Relaxation of the diaphragm, elastic recoil of the lungs and chest wall, and compression of the lungs by the intra-abdominal organs force air from the lungs. In obstructive airway disease the force generated by these processes may not be great enough to effect adequate expiration. With tachypnea the elastic recoil may not be fast enough to allow adequate exhalation between breaths. In either instance the accessory muscles of expiration are used. The abdominal recti muscles contract and force the abdominal contents against the diaphragm to compress the lungs, and the internal intercostal muscles contract to pull the ribs downward and create a positive intrathoracic pressure to force the air from the lungs. The contractions of these muscles provide the most important expiratory sign of dyspnea.

Although dyspnea is a respiratory symptom, it may be caused by primary disorders in other body systems. Cardiac, hematologic, metabolic, circulatory, and psychogenic causes must be considered in the differential diagnosis of dyspnea. The child's age is also important, because the frequency of some disorders may vary with age.

## History

The history begins with a complete description of the dyspnea. The patient or parent should be asked whether the onset was sudden (eg, inhaled foreign body, lung collapse) or evolved over several hours (eg, asthma, diabetic ketoacidosis). The patient should also be asked about the duration of the illness, the frequency of attacks of dyspnea, and whether a trigger or event is apparent that is temporally related to the onset of dyspnea. An attempt should be made to quantify the severity of the dyspnea. This task may be accomplished by asking to what degree daily activities are restricted by shortness of breath. However, given that dyspnea is a subjective sensation, its perceived severity can be affected by the patient's anxiety level, previous experiences, perceived control over the symptom, perceived consequences of the symptom, and available coping resources.[2] The chronic use of medications such as inhaled corticosteroids and $\beta_2$-agonists has also been shown to have an effect on the patient's perception of dyspnea.[3,4] Therefore, whenever possible, objective measures as discussed here should be obtained.

An inquiry should be made as to whether the dyspnea is affected by the patient's position. With unilateral lung disease, dyspnea may get worse when the patient lies with the affected lung down. Dyspnea that worsens with recumbency is often caused by left-ventricular failure, obstructive airway disease, or muscle weakness. Dyspnea in the upright position relieved by lying down usually is caused by intracardiac, vascular, or parenchymal lung shunts.

The patient should also be asked about associated symptoms such as cough, wheezing, sputum production, and pleuritic pain. In addition, a history of other known illnesses, allergies, illnesses in the family, medication, and environmental exposure must be obtained.

## Clinical Evaluation

A thorough physical examination is always indicated, with special attention paid to the aforementioned systems. The most useful laboratory tests are the complete blood count and peripheral blood smear, arterial blood gas measurement, and radiographic studies of the airways and lungs. Measurement of arterial oxygen saturation by pulse oximetry is invaluable for its capacity to assess oxygenation status quickly and noninvasively. Pulmonary function tests are helpful but may not be immediately available for evaluation of an acutely ill patient.

# ▶ ETIOLOGY AND CLINICAL PRESENTATION

## Pulmonary Disease

Pulmonary disease that causes dyspnea can be classified as obstructive, restrictive, or vascular.

### Obstructive Pulmonary Disease

Obstructive disease is characterized by narrowing of airways that can be caused by intraluminal objects (mucus, foreign bodies, or tumor), intramural factors (smooth-muscle contraction, edema, or bronchomalacia), or extramural compression (tumor or lymph nodes). The narrowing increases both airway resistance and turbulent flow in the airways. If a fixed obstruction is present, then affected areas of the lungs will become atelectatic. With a ball valve–type obstruction (ie, air can get into the lungs but not out), air is trapped, and affected areas become hyperinflated. In either case, an imbalance occurs between pulmonary ventilation and perfusion, and oxygen exchange is adversely affected.[5] All of these processes force the patient to work harder to maintain adequate ventilation; dyspnea ensues.

During normal respiration, inspiration and expiration are of equal length. With a fixed degree of obstruction, both processes are equally prolonged. If the obstruction varies and is extrathoracic (ie, above the vocal cords), then inspiration is affected more because the negative intra-airway pressure during inspiration tends to collapse the extrathoracic airway. The characteristic sign of such an obstruction is inspiratory stridor (see Chapter 74, Stridor).

If the obstruction varies and affects the intrathoracic airways, then expiration is prolonged because the positive intrathoracic pressure tends to collapse these airways during expiration. If larger airways are involved, then rhonchi are present. Airflow across an obstruction in smaller airways generates wheezing.

A paradoxical pulse and cyanosis are sensitive, but nonspecific, signs of severe obstruction. Patients who have chronic obstructive disease may be barrel chested and have signs of chronic hypoxia such as clubbing. Children who have a systemic disease, such as cystic fibrosis, will also show the extrapulmonary manifestations of this disease. The common causes of obstructive airway disease in childhood are shown in Box 20-1. Obstruction in the nose or nasopharynx should not be overlooked, especially in infants who are obligatory nasal breathers.

Blood gas values may be normal with mild obstructive disease. As the disease progresses, hypoxemia is the first sign of abnormality. Hypocapnia, initially seen as a reflection of increased $\dot{V}E$, is replaced by hypercapnia as the maldistribution of ventilation and perfusion increases. The patient then tires, and respiratory failure occurs.

The chest radiograph may reveal whether the cause of the obstruction is inside or outside the airway. In many instances, hyperinflation with an increased anteroposterior chest diameter and flattened diaphragm are seen. Atelectasis may appear with a fixed obstruction. Fluoroscopic examination or inspiratory and expiratory radiographs may be useful in localizing a ball valve–type obstruction. However, an important point to remember is that many foreign bodies are radiolucent and will not be seen on radiographic examination. If a radiolucent foreign body is suspected, then laryngoscopy, bronchoscopy, or even esophagoscopy may be required.

### Restrictive Pulmonary Disease

The cardinal features of restrictive pulmonary disease are a reduction in lung volume and pulmonary compliance secondary to pathologic changes in the lung parenchyma or the

BOX 20-1

## *Causes of Obstructive Pulmonary Disease*

**NEWBORNS**

- Choanal atresia or stenosis
- Dermoid cyst
- Encephalocele
- Nasolacrimal duct cyst
- Hemangioma
- Vocal cord paralysis
- Pierre Robin sequence
- Ankyloglossia (tongue tie)
- Pertussis
- Tracheal stenosis (postintubation)

**INFANTS**

- Foreign body
- Vascular ring
- Tracheal web
- Bronchiolitis
- Asthma
- Cystic fibrosis
- Bronchomalacia
- Pyogenic thyroid
- Accessory thyroid

**CHILDREN AND ADOLESCENTS**

- Foreign body (airway or esophagus)
- Asthma
- Adenopathy
  - Lymphoma
  - Systemic lupus erythematosus
  - Tuberculosis
  - Sarcoidosis
- Croup
- Epiglottitis
- Retropharyngeal abscess
- Enlarged tonsils or adenoids
- Cystic fibrosis
- Anaphylaxis
- Laryngeal tumor
- Vocal cord tumor
- Tracheal tumors
- Mediastinal tumors
- Vocal cord polyp
- Laryngeal trauma
- Supraglottitis
- Diphtheria
- Bacterial tracheitis
- Ingestion of caustic substance
- Crack cocaine
- Trauma
- Environmental or occupational inhaled toxin exposure

pleura, deformities of the chest wall, or neuromuscular disease. Decreased volume necessitates an increase in respiratory rate to maintain a normal $\dot{V}E$. The work of breathing must be increased to overcome the reduced compliance. Because breathing rapidly with small tidal volumes is more energy efficient than breathing slowly and attempting to expand the chest against great restrictive forces, children who have restrictive diseases characteristically have rapid, shallow respirations.[6] The common pediatric causes of restrictive pulmonary disease are listed in Box 20-2.

Observation of the child often reveals skeletal and neuromuscular causes. Pleural and parenchymal diseases are detected best by palpation, percussion, and auscultation of the chest. Tactile fremitus can demonstrate pulmonary consolidation or pleural effusion. Careful percussion reveals effusions, consolidation, and abnormal diaphragmatic excursion. Auscultation can reveal rales characteristic of alveolar disease and changes in whispered pectoriloquy and egophony.

The complete blood count may be helpful in diagnosing an infectious cause. Arterial blood gases have a characteristic pattern of hypoxemia and hypocapnia. The chest radiograph is useful because it can demonstrate decreased lung volume, pleural thickening and effusions, increased interstitial markings, parenchymal consolidation, skeletal deformities, and abnormal movement of the diaphragm.

BOX 20-2

## *Causes of Restrictive Pulmonary Disease*

**NEWBORNS**

- Hyaline membrane disease
- Hypoplastic lungs
- Pulmonary agenesis
- Eventration of the diaphragm
- Meconium aspiration
- Pneumonia (group B streptococci or gram-negative organisms)
- Diaphragmatic paralysis
- Osteogenesis imperfecta
- Central nervous system depression
  - Hypoxia
  - Congenital
  - Maternal drugs
- Congenital myasthenia gravis
- Aspiration
- Pulmonary edema
  - Septicemia
  - Congenital heart disease

**INFANTS**

- Pneumonia
  - Bacterial
  - Viral
  - Aspiration
- Bronchopulmonary dysplasia
- Wilson-Mikity syndrome
- Hamman-Rich syndrome
- Pulmonary edema
- Infantile botulism
- Congenital lobar emphysema

**CHILDREN AND ADOLESCENTS**

- Skeletal
  - Kyphoscoliosis
  - Ankylosing spondylitis
  - Pectus excavatum
  - Crush chest injury
- Parenchymal
  - Pneumonia
  - Hypersensitivity pneumonitis
  - Systemic lupus erythematosus
  - Scleroderma
  - Fibrosis
  - Toxin inhalation
  - Granulomatous disease
  - Drugs (eg, antineoplastic agents, narcotics)
  - Carcinoma
  - Fat embolus
  - Pneumothorax
  - Pneumomediastinum
- Smoke inhalation
- Pulmonary infarction
- Pulmonary edema
  - Congestive heart failure
  - Sepsis
  - Intracranial disease
  - Croup
  - Epiglottitis
- Neuromuscular
  - Cord transection
  - Myasthenia gravis
  - Muscular dystrophy
  - Multiple sclerosis
  - Guillain-Barré syndrome
  - Pickwickian syndrome
  - Toxins
- Pleural effusion
  - Pneumonia
  - Malignancy
  - Cardiac disease
  - Hepatic disease
  - Renal disease
  - Rheumatologic disease
- Hypoproteinemia
- Renal failure
- Tumor
- Pulmonary infarction

## Vascular Pulmonary Disease

Vascular lung disease is characterized by a decrease in the size of the pulmonary vascular bed. In the neonate, this disease often results from persistent pulmonary hypertension of the newborn.[7] Microthrombi have also been reported in the lungs of infants who are in severe respiratory distress.[8] In older children, the most common cause of vascular pulmonary disease is intimal hyperplasia after persistent left-to-right shunting and resultant pulmonary hypertension. The size of the pulmonary vascular bed can also be reduced by obstruction caused by thromboembolic disease, obliteration (eg, vasculitis), or destruction, as in emphysema. The reduced blood flow through the lungs results in arterial hypoxemia and hypercapnia, which, in turn, lead to the symptoms and signs of dyspnea.

In addition to the common signs of dyspnea, the child who has vascular lung disease may have signs of pulmonary edema and pleural effusion. Systemic signs of right-sided heart failure caused by pulmonary hypertension or left-sided heart failure that was the cause of the pulmonary hypertension may be present. The cardiac findings observed with pulmonary hypertension are an accentuated $P_2$, paradoxical splitting of second heart sound, a third heart sound, a pulmonary ejection click, and a right-ventricular heave.

An electrocardiogram is helpful in the diagnosis of right-ventricular hypertrophy. A chest radiograph may reveal increased right ventricular size, enlargement of the pulmonary artery silhouette, decreased pulmonary blood flow in advanced disease, or increased flow early in the course of disease, with a left-to-right shunt.

### Exercise-Induced Dyspnea

As described earlier, dyspnea is a normal sensation felt during exercise, especially for children with a sedentary lifestyle and poor cardiovascular conditioning. However, if the dyspnea is severe, occurs after only minimal exertion, or is troublesome to the patient, then investigations into the cause of exercise-induced dyspnea (EID) are warranted.

Asthma is the most common cause of pathologic EID. However, when other signs and symptoms of asthma are absent, or when pretreatment with beta-agonistic medications does not prevent EID, then other causes must be considered. These causes include vocal cord dysfunction, exercise-induced laryngomalacia, exercise-induced hyperventilation, restrictive airway disease caused by skeletal abnormalities such as scoliosis and pectus deformities, and cardiac arrhythmias that occur only during exercise.[9,10]

### Cardiac Disease

Dyspnea occurs with cardiac disease when insufficient blood is pumped to the lungs as a result of congenital structural anomalies in the heart, pump failure (myocarditis or cardiomyopathy), restrictive pericarditis, arrhythmia, or, as already described, secondary pulmonary hypertension. Heart disease must be considered in all dyspneic newborns and older children who have a history of congenital heart disease. In the neonate, pulmonary disease can often be differentiated from cyanotic heart disease through a hyperoxia test. The nature of the cardiac defect can be delineated with the help of a thorough cardiac examination, an electrocardiogram, a chest radiograph, and an echocardiogram.

A trivial respiratory infection in a healthy child may cause severe respiratory insufficiency in a child who has cardiopulmonary disease. Indeed, the mortality of infants who have respiratory syncytial viral pneumonia and congenital heart disease has been shown to exceed significantly the mortality of children who have normal hearts.[11]

### Hematologic Disease

If the oxygen-carrying capacity of the blood is reduced sufficiently, then tissue hypoxia ensues. The resultant drop in arterial pH signals the CNS and stimulates the onset of dyspnea. Severe anemia, whether chronic or acute, congenital or acquired, can cause dyspnea. The oxygen-carrying capacity can also be lowered when the hemoglobin's ability to bind oxygen is reduced, seen most commonly with carbon monoxide poisoning but also with cyanide poisoning and methemoglobinemia. In any of these cases the child will not be cyanotic. The blue color of cyanosis is caused by at least a 5-g/dL reduction of oxygenated hemoglobin in the blood. Such a concentration of reduced hemoglobin is not found in anemia uncomplicated by other diseases or in the other conditions cited. Conversely, an infant with polycythemia whose blood is hyperviscous may have dyspnea from poor perfusion. Because such an infant has an increased hemoglobin concentration and more oxygen is removed from the hemoglobin as a result of decreased flow, the child may be cyanotic (having more than 5 g/dL unsaturated hemoglobin) and not hypoxic. An extreme elevation of leukocyte or platelet counts can also cause blood hyperviscosity and dyspnea.

Children with anemia, even though they may have tissue hypoxia and be dyspneic, are usually not hypoxemic; that is, the arterial oxygen tension measured by blood gas analysis is in the normal range.

### Metabolic Disease

Disorders that increase the body's rate of metabolism and therefore oxygen consumption can cause dyspnea. Examples are hyperthyroidism[12] and fever. Metabolic disorders associated with an increased production of hydrogen ion and carbon dioxide cause a dyspnea-like breathing pattern to help rid the body of the carbon dioxide. The classic example is Kussmaul breathing with diabetic ketoacidosis. Aspirin poisoning can be characterized similarly. In addition, children who have various muscle enzyme deficiencies, especially those affecting the mitochondria, may have dyspnea as a result of their increased acid production and decreased work tolerance.[13,14] In chronic renal failure the kidney's inability to remove acid from the blood adequately is the underlying cause of dyspnea. The history, physical examination, and appropriate laboratory tests should facilitate the proper diagnosis of these diseases.

If oxygen cannot reach the tissues, then the body responds with dyspnea, cardiovascular collapse, and shock.

### Obesity

Dyspnea, especially with exertion, is a common complaint of obese children because their metabolic requirement for a given amount of work is increased.[15,16] In addition, the diaphragm of an obese child must move against increased abdominal pressure, and the chest wall is heavier; thus, more energy must be expended to maintain $\dot{V}E$.

Asthma does not seem to play an important role as a cause of dyspnea in obese individuals. Although obesity is a risk factor for self-reported asthma, bronchodilator use, and dyspnea on exertion, obese individuals have a lower risk of objective airway obstruction as compared with persons who are not obese.[17]

Treatment of dyspnea in obesity should include dietary regulation and an exercise program graded to keep pace with the child's level of exercise tolerance.

### Pregnancy

Dyspnea is normal during pregnancy[18] and occurs during the first or second trimester. Seventy-six percent of women complain of dyspnea by the 31st week of gestation.

The sensation reflects a subjective awareness of the hyperventilation normally present during pregnancy.

The normal dyspnea of pregnancy can be differentiated easily from dyspnea arising from heart or lung disease. The woman who has dyspnea of pregnancy has no other symptoms of cardiac or pulmonary disease. Furthermore, dyspnea of pregnancy begins early and plateaus or improves as term approaches, while dyspnea resulting from heart disease begins during the second half of pregnancy and is worst during the seventh month. Finally, dyspnea of pregnancy is rarely severe, rarely occurs at rest, and does not interfere with the activities of daily life.

### Intravenous Drug Use

Several causes of dyspnea must be considered in patients with a history of intravenous drug use. Heroin can cause bronchospasm that responds to bronchodilator medications. In addition, heroin and other opioids may precipitate pulmonary edema.[19] Therapies consist of oxygen, diuretics, and naloxone.

Infections also may cause dyspnea in intravenous drug users. The most common infection is community-acquired pneumonia. However, opportunistic pulmonary infections, tuberculosis, and bacterial endocarditis with associated septic pulmonary emboli or heart failure must be considered.

Finally, talc granulomatosis, which can lead to chronic mild to moderate dyspnea, must be considered. It is caused by intravenous injection of dissolved opioid tablets, with deposition of foreign bodies in the pulmonary vasculature and granuloma formation.

### Psychogenic Cause

Stress or hysteria may cause dyspnea.[20] A complete history and thorough physical examination are keys to the diagnosis. Affected patients are tachypneic and complain of air hunger. When dyspnea is caused by pulmonary or cardiac conditions, the shortness of breath worsens with increasing activity and improves with rest. However, the dyspnea associated with hysteria does not improve with rest and may worsen. Affected patients also often complain of chest pain and sigh more frequently than normal. Contrary to previous belief, tetany is an uncommon accompaniment of hysterical dyspnea.

Findings on physical examination are usually normal. However, stress-induced paradoxical adduction of the vocal cords during inspiration has been reported.[21] Patients with this disorder may have either stridor or wheezing. In this instance the diagnosis of hysterical dyspnea is one of exclusion, and it can be made only after pathological lesions in the airways and lungs have been ruled out.

In most instances, the only laboratory abnormality found with hysteria-induced dyspnea is a diminished arterial carbon dioxide tension.

Treatment consists of calm reassurance and, occasionally, mild sedation. If the condition is chronic, then interventions to reduce stress and gain insight into the cause of the dyspnea, such as psychotherapy and hypnosis,[22] may be required. When paradoxical vocal cord motion is the cause, the patient should also be taught laryngeal relaxation techniques.

## ▶ MANAGEMENT

Severe acute dyspnea is a medical emergency. If not treated promptly, a child who has dyspnea may then progress rapidly to respiratory failure and death. First, the adequacy of the airway must be assessed. Foreign bodies must be removed and anatomic obstructions bypassed with endotracheal intubation or, in rare cases, tracheotomy. Bronchospasm, when present, should be treated with beta-agonistic drugs.

Subsequently, the efficacy of the child's ventilation must be evaluated. Normally, breathing uses 2% to 3% of the total body energy expenditure. When the work of breathing is increased during dyspnea, this amount may rise to 30% or more. Such a degree of energy expenditure cannot be continued indefinitely, and the child tires. Even after an obstruction is removed, the child may still be unable to effect adequate ventilation. In this instance, or in the case of neuromuscular disease, the child requires either noninvasive positive pressure ventilation or intubation and mechanical ventilation.

Once ventilation is established, the cardiovascular system's ability to deliver oxygen to the tissues must be appraised by evaluating the heart, peripheral circulation, intravascular volume status, and the blood's oxygen-carrying capacity. Therapy with vasopressors, fluids, blood transfusions, or diuretics should be initiated when indicated. Although not all children who have dyspnea require supplemental oxygen, every child should have oxygen administered until the cause of the dyspnea is known. Once the patient's condition has stabilized, the search for the underlying cause of the dyspnea should progress urgently, but calmly. At this point, a detailed history can be elicited, a full physical examination performed, and a chest radiograph and appropriate blood tests obtained. When the diagnosis is made, specific therapy can be initiated.

When dyspnea is caused by a chronic illness, no satisfactory therapy may be available to treat the underlying disease. However, simply relieving the dyspnea can significantly improve the child's functional ability and quality of life. Several modalities can be used to treat the symptom of dyspnea in a chronically ill child.[23] Sedatives and narcotics reduce $\dot{V}E$ and thereby diminish the intensity of the breathless feeling.[24,25] These medications are usually administered orally or by injection. However, they also may be effective when delivered by nebulization.[26] Beta-agonists may blunt the perception of dyspnea without affecting ventilation.[27] Theophylline may improve diaphragmatic contractility. Continuous supplemental oxygen reduces ventilatory drive. Noninvasive positive pressure ventilation is useful in assisting fatigued or dysfunctional respiratory muscles and in keeping small airways open. Children who have chronic obstructive pulmonary disease may be taught to breathe through pursed lips, reducing respiratory rate, increasing tidal volume, and diminishing the sensation of dyspnea. Hypnosis has proved useful in some patients, and others have reported a decrease in dyspnea when seated next to an open window or a blowing fan.[28]

Exercise and proper nutrition are helpful in maintaining or increasing inspiratory muscle mass and thereby reducing the perceived magnitude of dyspnea.[29] Finally, because dyspnea is a subjective complaint, the psychological contribution to its perceived severity is significant.[23] The child's emotional state, behavior, and personality must be monitored because psychosocial intervention may be indicated.

## When to Refer

- Chronic pulmonary disease
- Congenital or acquired heart disease
- Metabolic disease
- Conditions requiring endoscopy or surgical procedures

## When to Admit

- Respiratory failure
- Impending respiratory failure
- Hypoxia while breathing room air

### *REFERENCES*


1. Parshall MB, Schwartzstein RM, Adams L, et al. An official American Thoracic Society statement: update on the mechanisms, assessment, and management of dyspnea. *Am J Respir Crit Care Med.* 2012;185:435–452
2. Weinberger M, Abu-Hasan M. Perceptions and pathophysiology of dyspnea and exercise intolerance. *Pediatr Clin North Am.* 2009;56:33–48, ix
3. Ottanelli R, Rosi E, Romagnoli I, et al. Do inhaled corticosteroids affect perception of dyspnea during bronchoconstriction in asthma? *Chest.* 2001;120:770–777
4. Bijl-Hofland ID, Cloosterman SG, Folgering HT, et al. Inhaled corticosteroids, combined with long-acting beta(2)-agonists, improve the perception of bronchoconstriction in asthma. *Am J Respir Crit Care Med.* 2001;164:764–769
5. Cooper CB, Celli B. Venous admixture in COPD: pathophysiology and therapeutic approaches. *COPD.* 2008;5:376–381
6. Tsiligiannis T, Grivas T. Pulmonary function in children with idiopathic scoliosis. *Scoliosis.* 2012;7:7
7. Konduri GG, Kim UO. Advances in the diagnosis and management of persistent pulmonary hypertension of the newborn. *Pediatr Clin North Am.* 2009;56:579–600
8. Levin DL, Weinberg AG, Perkin RM. Pulmonary microthrombi syndrome in newborn infants with unresponsive persistent pulmonary hypertension. *J Pediatr.* 1983;102:299–303
9. Abu-Hasan M, Tannous B, Weinberger M. Exercise-induced dyspnea in children and adolescents: if not asthma then what? *Ann Allergy Asthma Immunol.* 2005;94:366–371
10. Seear M, Wensley D, West N. How accurate is the diagnosis of exercise induced asthma among Vancouver schoolchildren? *Arch Dis Child.* 2005;90:898–902
11. Thorburn K. Pre-existing disease is associated with a significantly higher risk of death in severe respiratory syncytial virus infection. *Arch Dis Child.* 2009;94:99–103
12. Leigh M, Holman G, Rohn R. Dyspnea as the presenting symptom of thyroid disease. *Clin Pediatr (Phila).* 1980;19:773–774
13. Robinson BH, De Meirleir L, Glerum M, Sherwood G, Becker L. Clinical presentation of mitochondrial respiratory chain defects in NADH-coenzyme Q reductase and cytochrome oxidase: clues to pathogenesis of Leigh disease. *J Pediatr.* 1987;110:216–222
14. Scholte HR, Busch HF, Luyt-Houwen IE, et al. Defects in oxidative phosphorylation. Biochemical investigations in skeletal muscle and expression of the lesion in other cells. *J Inherit Metab Dis.* 1987;10 (Suppl 1):81–97
15. Babb TG, Ranasinghe KG, Comeau LA, Semon TL, Schwartz B. Dyspnea on exertion in obese women: association with an increased oxygen cost of breathing. *Am J Respir Crit Care Med.* 2008;178:116–123
16. Sahebjami H. Dyspnea in obese healthy men. *Chest.* 1998;114:1373–1377
17. Sin DD, Jones RL, Man SF. Obesity is a risk factor for dyspnea but not for airflow obstruction. *Arch Intern Med.* 2002;62:1477–1481
18. Hegewald MJ, Crapo RO. Respiratory physiology in pregnancy. *Clin Chest Med.* 2011;32:1–13, vii
19. Sporer KA, Dorn E. Heroin-related noncardiogenic pulmonary edema: a case series. *Chest.* 2001;120:1628–1632
20. Tobin MJ. Dyspnea. Pathophysiologic basis, clinical presentation, and management. *Arch Intern Med.* 1990;150:1604–1613
21. Karaman E, Duman C, Alimoglu Y, Isildak H, Oz F. Paradoxical vocal cord motion—haloperidol usage in acute attack treatment. *J Craniofac Surg.* 2009;20:1602–1604

22. Anbar RD. Stressors associated with dyspnea in childhood: patients' insights and a case report. *Am J Clin Hypn.* 2004;47:93–101
23. Ullrich CK, Mayer OH. Assessment and management of fatigue and dyspnea in pediatric palliative care. *Pediatr Clin North Am.* 2007;54:735–756, xi
24. Williams SG, Wright DJ, Marshall P, et al. Safety and potential benefits of low dose diamorphine during exercise in patients with chronic heart failure. *Heart.* 2003;89:1085–1086
25. Cohen SP, Dawson TC. Nebulized morphine as a treatment for dyspnea in a child with cystic fibrosis. *Pediatrics.* 2002;110:e38
26. Brown SJ, Eichner SF, Jones JR. Nebulized morphine for relief of dyspnea due to chronic lung disease. *Ann Pharmacother.* 2005;39:1088–1092
27. O'Donnell DE, Sciurba F, Celli B, et al. Effect of fluticasone propionate/salmeterol on lung hyperinflation and exercise endurance in COPD. *Chest.* 2006;130:647–656
28. Galbraith S, Fagan P, Perkins P, Lynch A, Booth S. Does the use of a handheld fan improve chronic dyspnea? A randomized, controlled, crossover trial. *J Pain Symptom Manage.* 2010;39:831–838
29. Garcia-Aymerich J, Serra I, Gómez FP, et al. Physical activity and clinical and functional status in COPD. *Chest.* 2009;136:62–70

## ▶ PHYSICAL EXAMINATION

The presence of a fever (body temperature >101.3°F [38.5°C]) can indicate inflammation or an upper UTI such as pyelonephritis; cystitis and urethritis of any cause do not usually produce significant fever. Inspection of the skin may reveal vesicles with varicella or herpes simplex, or target lesions with Stevens-Johnson syndrome, which can be accompanied by conjunctival inflammation and oral lesions. Arthritis, particularly of the knee joint, in an adolescent should raise suspicion of Reiter syndrome.

In children of any age presenting with dysuria and a history of voiding dysfunction, particularly when accompanied by a history of chronic constipation, an occult spina bifida should be excluded by careful examination of the lower back looking for midline defects, such as a sacral cyst, a fistula, or a tuft of hair. The neurologic examination should include careful evaluation of the lower extremities for strength and reflexes, and, when suspicion is raised, the bulbocavernosal reflex should be evaluated as well.

Special attention should also be paid to the abdominal examination, which may reveal a flank or suprapubic mass, suggestive of urethral obstruction. Costovertebral tenderness suggests pyelonephritis, and suprapubic tenderness often accompanies cystitis.

On inspection of the genital area, the examiner should evaluate for discharge; if present, its character should be noted. In female patients, clear discharge may be a normal finding, whereas an odorless, cottage cheese–like appearance suggests an infection with *Candida* spp. A greenish discharge, suggestive of gonorrhea, should raise the possibility of pelvic inflammatory disease if accompanied by lower abdominal tenderness. Any discharge in male patients should be considered abnormal. Scratch marks around the mucosal area in females may suggest contact dermatitis or chemical irritation. Examination should include looking for labial adhesions and a urethral prolapse, which appears as a red circumferential protrusion of the mucosa from the urethral orifice. Attention should be paid to whether or not the male patient is circumcised; if not, note whether the foreskin is age-appropriately retractable. The location and the size of the meatus should be examined for hypospadias or stenosis.

## ▶ DIFFERENTIAL DIAGNOSIS

Dysuria can be caused by any inflammation, irritation, or obstruction of the bladder or urethra, but most often it is a symptom of a common disorder of childhood and adolescence, such as a UTI, urethritis, or a chemical or traumatic injury. Table 21-1 lists infectious and noninfectious causes of dysuria. Figures 21-1 and 21-2 depict a simplified algorithm allowing the physician to establish quickly whether the cause of dysuria is infectious/inflammatory or rather chemical/mechanical in male and female patients.

### *Common Conditions*

#### Urinary Tract Infection

UTIs are the most common cause of dysuria in children. The localization of the infection within the urinary tract may be challenging in young children because they tend to develop systemic symptoms such as fever, vomiting, and diarrhea even in the absence of pyelonephritis. Older children, who are likely to mount a fever with pyelonephritis rather than cystitis, can report suprapubic pain with cystitis or flank and costovertebral

**Table 21-1**
**Infectious and Noninfectious Causes of Dysuria**

| INFECTIOUS | NONINFECTIOUS |
|---|---|
| Pyelonephritis | Dysfunctional voiding |
| Cystitis | Chemical irritants |
| Urethritis | Trauma |
| Vulvovaginitis | Meatal stenosis |
| Balanitis and balanoposthitis | Labial adhesions |
| Pelvic inflammatory disease | Urethral strictures |
| | Urethral prolapse |
| | Hypercalciuria |

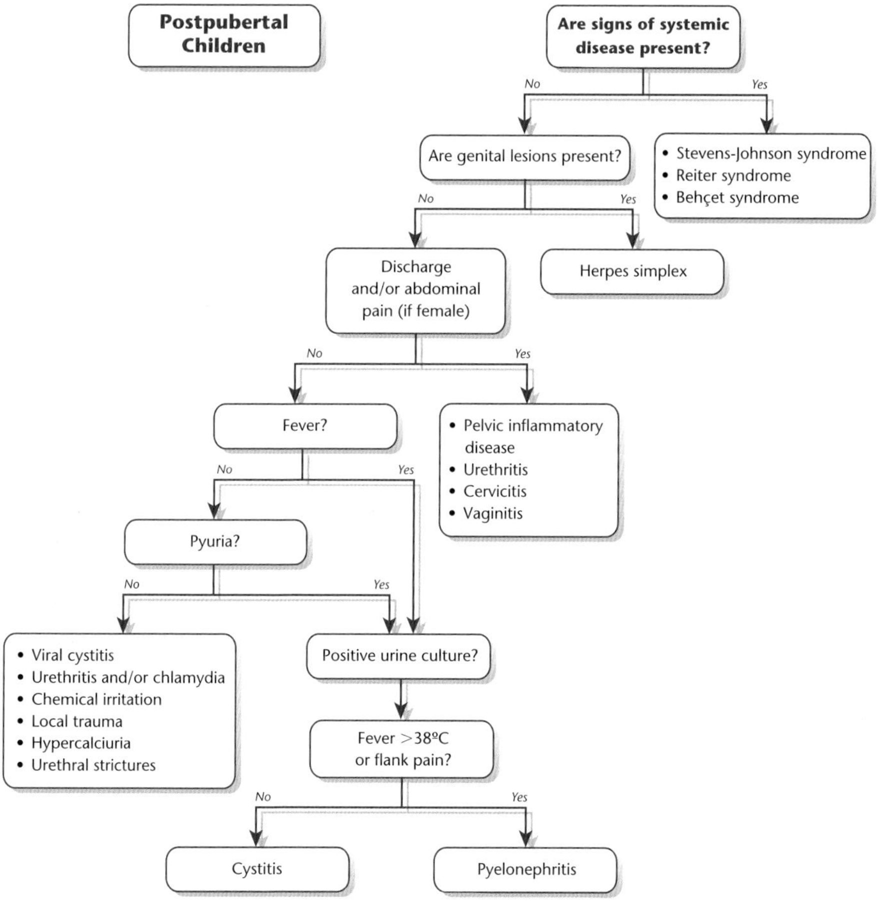


**Figure 21-1**
Algorithmic approach to dysuria in postpubertal males and females. *(Adapted with permission from Fleisher GR. Evaluation of dysuria in children. In: Bassow DS (ed);* UpToDate, *Waltham MA. Copyright © 2013 UpToDate, Inc. Available at: www.uptodate.com.)*

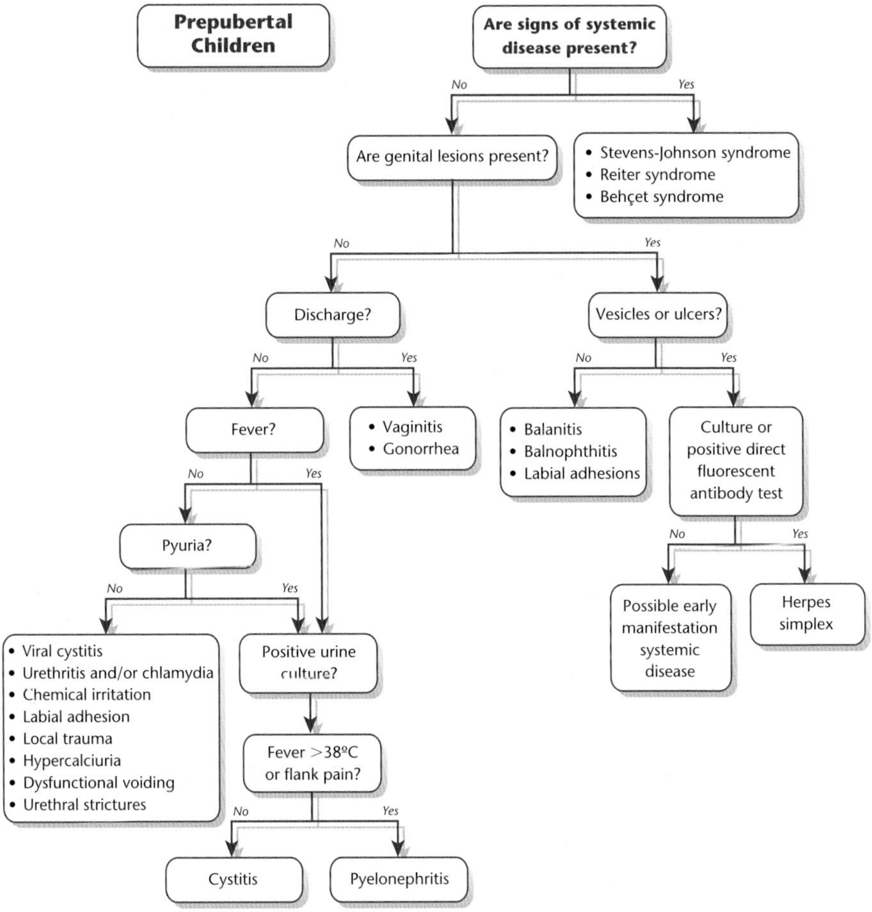


**Figure 21-2**
Algorithmic approach to dysuria in prepubertal males and females. *(Adapted with permission from Fleisher GR. Evaluation of dysuria in children. In: Bassow DS (ed);* UpToDate, *Waltham MA. Copyright © 2013 UpToDate, Inc. Available at: www.uptodate.com.)*

tenderness with pyelonephritis. All children younger than 2 years and boys of all ages should be evaluated for congenital anatomic abnormalities, such as vesicoureteral reflux, after the first UTI.[3]

## Urethritis

Urethritis can present with dysuria accompanied by discharge or blood spotting on the child's underwear. Causes of urethritis include infection, trauma, chemical irritation, and foreign body. Infectious causes in children are uncommon. Patients suspected of having infectious urethritis should have a urethral smear and urine culture included as part of their laboratory evaluation. Sexually transmitted infections are the major cause of urethritis in adults and adolescents. The finding of *Neisseria gonorrhea* or *Chlamydia trachomatis* in a child should prompt immediate investigation to rule out sexual abuse.[4]

## Irritants/Trauma

Irritants such as soap, bubble baths, and laundry detergents cause mild erythema at most. Localized trauma can result from foreign bodies, masturbation, voluntary sexual activity, or sexual abuse. Bicycle accidents and other traumas usually generate more extensive injuries than isolated genitourinary lesions.

## Meatal Stenosis

Meatal stenosis occurs relatively commonly in boys after circumcision. Typically, the urinary stream is deflected upward, and the boy has difficulty aiming. It may be accompanied by dysuria, increased frequency, and delayed bladder emptying. Consultation with a pediatric urologist is warranted.[5]

## Dysfunctional Voiding

Dysfunctional voiding can result from neuropathic or non-neuropathic voiding disorders. Neuropathic voiding is associated with conditions affecting the innervation of the muscles involved in coordinated micturition. Non-neuropathic voiding dysfunction encompasses all other causes of lack of coordination between the bladder, the bladder outlet, and the pelvic floor muscles. If the patient is also constipated, then the condition is referred to as *dysfunctional elimination syndrome,* which is an important cause of idiopathic urethritis in childhood; the history should focus on timing of completion of toilet training, episodes of bed wetting, and daytime incontinence.[1]

### *Uncommon Conditions*

## Labial Adhesions

Labial adhesions occur in prepubertal girls and are generally asymptomatic unless they cause secondary infections. The treatment is separation of the adhesion and topical estrogens to prevent readhesion.[6]

## Urethral Strictures

Urethral strictures in children can be congenital or acquired. Congenital strictures are rare. Acquired strictures occur after instrumentation, trauma, or processes accompanied by inflammation with production of an exudate and secondary sclerosis. The child presents with dysuria, infection, or a weak urinary stream. The diagnosis is made by voiding cystourethrogram or cystoscopy.[5]

## Urethral Prolapse

Urethral prolapse is the complete protrusion of the urethral mucosa beyond the meatus in girls. Although it is rare in the general population, there is an association with young age, black race or Hispanic ethnicity, and low socioeconomic status. The cause is unclear. Patients present with dysuria, gross hematuria, or blood spotting on the underwear. Treatment includes sitz baths, antibiotics, topical estrogens, or surgical repair. Left untreated, the prolapsed mucosa can become necrotic.[7]

## Pelvic Inflammatory Disease

Pelvic inflammatory disease primarily affects sexually active adolescent females, but should raise suspicion of sexual abuse in prepubertal girls. It presents with abdominal pain.[8]

## Vulvovaginitis

Vulvovaginitis, a rare cause of dysuria, more commonly presents with erythema of the vaginal mucosa and may be associated with discharge, which varies from clear to white to green, and may be odorless or foul smelling.

It occurs most often in sexually active adolescents, and sexually transmitted pathogens are the main cause. In prepubertal girls, the cause is often not apparent, but poor hygiene or allergies may play a role. Pathogens include local flora, such as group A streptococcus, or anaerobic bacteria, with concomitant decrease in the concentration of *Lactobacillus* spp. *Candida* spp. are commonly encountered in the setting of recent antibiotic treatment or diabetes mellitus. Herpes simplex infection can present with erythema alone; the absence of vesicles or ulcerative lesions does not rule it out. When erythema of the vaginal mucosa is observed, a Gram stain and culture, KOH, and a wet prep should be sent. Any vaginal discharge should be sent for pH testing. Screening for herpes simplex should be considered.[9]

## Balanitis and Balanoposthitis

Inflammation of the glans penis (balanitis) or both the glans and prepuce (balanoposthitis) occurs almost exclusively in young, uncircumcised boys with phimosis. Infection from entrapped smegma under the foreskin may result from trauma, allergies, or poor hygiene. Treatment consists of warm soaks as well as oral or local antibiotics. Topical steroids may alleviate the inflammation associated with balanitis from contact dermatitis.[10]

## Hypercalciuria and Urolithiasis

Urolithiasis rarely presents with dysuria, but rather is seen with flank pain and often with gross hematuria. Hypercalciuria, however, commonly manifests as dysuria caused by irritation of the uroepithelium by calcium-oxalate crystals. Patients typically have frequency, urgency, gross or microscopic hematuria, and dysuria. Examination of the urinary sediment may reveal crystals along with eumorphic red blood cells. The family history may be positive for urolithiasis.[11]

## When to Refer

- Voiding dysfunction
- Nephrolithiasis
- Girl younger than 2 years with a UTI for the first time
- Boy of any age with a UTI or meatal stenosis
- Genitourinary tract anomalies

## When to Admit

- Systemic inflammatory or infectious cause of dysuria
- Suspicion of sexual abuse

## TOOLS FOR PRACTICE

### Engaging Patient and Family

- *What Is a Pediatric Urologist?* (fact sheet), American Academy of Pediatrics (www.healthychildren.org/English/family-life/health-management/pediatric-specialists/Pages/What-is-a-Pediatric-Urologist.aspx)

## AAP POLICY STATEMENTS

American Academy of Pediatrics Subcommittee on Urinary Tract Infection, Steering Committee on Quality Improvement and Management. Urinary tract infection: clinical practice guideline for the diagnosis and management of the initial UTI in febrile infants and children 2 to 24 months. *Pediatrics*. 2011;128(3):595–610 (pediatrics.aappublications.org/content/128/3/595.full)

Finnell SME, Carroll AE, Downs SM; American Academy of Pediatrics Subcommittee on Urinary Tract Infection. Technical report: diagnosis and management of an initial UTI in febrile infants and young children. *Pediatrics*. 2011;128(3):e749–e770 (pediatrics.aappublications.org/content/128/3/e749.full)

## REFERENCES


1. Fleisher GR, Ludwig S. *Synopsis of Pediatric Emergency Medicine*. 4th ed. Philadelphia, PA: Lippincott Williams & Wilkins; 2002
2. Herz D, Weiser A, Collette T, et al. Dysfunctional elimination syndrome as an etiology of idiopathic urethritis in childhood. *J Urol*. 2005;173:2132–2137
3. Bensman A, Dunand O, Ulinski T. Urinary tract infections. In: *Textbook of Pediatric Nephrology*. 6th ed. Berlin, Germany: Springer Verlag; 2009:1299–1310
4. Best D, Ford CA, Miller WC. Prevalence of Chlamydia trachomatis and Neisseria gonorrhoeae infection in pediatric private practice. *Pediatrics*. 2001;108:E103
5. Farhat W, McLorie G. Urethral syndromes in children. *Pediatr Rev*. 2001;22(1):17–21
6. Baldwin DD, Landa HM. Common problems in pediatric gynecology. *Urol Clin North Am*. 1995;22:161–176
7. Desai SR, Cohen RC. Urethral prolapse in a premenarchal girl: case report and literature review. *Aust N Z J Surg*. 1997;67:660–662
8. Banikarim C, Chacko MR. Pelvic inflammatory disease in adolescents. *Semin Pediatr Infect Dis*. 2005;16:175–180
9. Arsenault PS, Gerbie AB. Vulvovaginitis in the preadolescent girl. *Pediatr Ann*. 1986;15(8):577–579, 583–585
10. Vohra S, Badlani G. Balanitis and balanoposthitis. *Urol Clin North Am*. 1992;19(1):143–147
11. Srivastava T, Schwaderer A. Diagnosis and management of hypercalciuria in children. *Curr Opin Pediatr*. 2009;21(2):214–219

# Chapter 22

# Edema

*Paul A. Levy, MD*

At birth, as much as 70% of the newborn's body weight is water. This decreases to approximately 60% of total body weight in older children. For adolescent and adult males, total body water is even lower, with only about 55% to 60% of their body weight being made up of water, and total body water is lowest in adolescent and adult females, who have only about 50% of their body weight contributed by water.[1] The body water is distributed into several compartments. Intracellular water represents two-thirds of the total volume. The remaining one-third is considered extracellular and is distributed between the vascular compartment (25%) and the interstitial spaces between the cells (75%). The distribution of water in these various body compartments is tightly controlled. Failure of this control can result in the accumulation of extra fluid in the interstitium, which is *edema.*

## ▶ PATHOPHYSIOLOGIC FEATURES

Water movement across a semipermeable membrane (osmosis) is governed by the number of particles (osmolarity) on either side of the membrane. Water moves to establish equilibrium between the 2 compartments. In blood vessels, such as capillaries, the osmolarity is generated, in part, by the electrolytes in plasma; however, because the concentrations of electrolytes in plasma and the interstitium are relatively equal, the osmotic force is largely determined by charged protein molecules, with albumin being the most predominant. The plasma proteins are referred to as *colloids,* and the osmotic force they generate is the *colloid osmotic pressure,* or *oncotic pressure.* Movement of fluid across a capillary wall is controlled by a combination of oncotic pressure, hydrostatic pressure, and the permeability of the capillary wall. The capillary oncotic pressure draws fluid into the capillary; the interstitial oncotic pressure draws capillary fluid out. The capillary hydrostatic pressure, which is related to blood pressure, is highest at the arteriole end of the capillary and drops off as blood moves toward the venule. The capillary hydrostatic force pushes fluid into the interstitium. Interestingly, systemic (arterial) hypertension does not result in edema because arteriolar sphincters protect the capillary bed from increased blood pressure.[2] The interstitial hydrostatic pressure is related to the pressure of the fluid in the interstitium, which depends on the lymphatic drainage, the amount of fluid present in the interstitium, and the compliance of the tissue. This force counteracts the capillary hydrostatic pressure and pushes fluid back into the capillaries. Finally, the permeability of the capillary wall contributes to the leakage of fluid into the interstitium.[2,3]

In normal circumstances, the interplay of these forces results in fluid exiting the capillaries at the arteriolar end and entering the capillaries at the venule end. Approximately 90%

of fluid that leaves the capillaries is reabsorbed before reaching the venule. The lymphatic system returns the remaining 10%, along with its associated proteins, to the circulation.

## ▶ CAUSES OF EDEMA

Fluid distribution between the intravascular compartment and the interstitial compartment results from the interplay of oncotic pressure, hydrostatic pressure, and capillary membrane permeability. Disruption of these forces can result in edema, but sodium concentration is usually the ultimate controller of this fluid movement[2,4–6] (Box 22-1).

### *Change in Capillary Membrane Permeability*

An increase in capillary membrane permeability is often the result of cytokines released from inflammation. Infections and burns tend to cause localized edema. An allergic reaction may cause more generalized edema. Hereditary angioedema can cause localized edema of the gastrointestinal tract and larynx. Trauma causes local edema.

### *Decreased Capillary Oncotic Pressure*

A decrease in the capillary oncotic pressure can be caused by decreased levels of protein, usually of albumin in the blood. Decreased synthesis of albumin occurs in cirrhosis or as a result of malnutrition or intestinal malabsorption. Protein loss by the kidneys in nephrotic

**Box 22-1**

***Causes of Edema (Systemic or Localized as Noted)***

**INCREASED CAPILLARY PERMEABILITY**

- Inflammation (localized or systemic edema)
- Burns (localized edema)
- Trauma (localized edema)
- Allergic reaction (localized or systemic edema)

**DECREASED CAPILLARY ONCOTIC PRESSURE**

- Protein loss (nephrotic syndrome, congenital lymphangectasia, inflammatory bowel disease)
- Decreased synthesis (cirrhosis, malabsorption, malnutrition)

**INCREASED CAPILLARY HYDROSTATIC PRESSURE**

- Systemic venous hypertension
  - Heart failure (myocarditis, cardiomyopathy, ischemic heart disease)
  - Constrictive pericarditis
  - Note: right-sided failure results in peripheral edema, left-sided failure results in pulmonary edema.
  - Cirrhosis/liver failure
  - High output failure [anemia (ABO and Rh incompatibility), arteriovenous fistulas, hyperthyroidism]
- Localized venous hypertension (localized edema)
  - Deep vein thrombosis, compression of venous return (localized edema)

**INCREASED PLASMA VOLUME**

- Heart failure
- Renal failure

**LYMPHATIC OBSTRUCTION AND INCREASED INTERSTITIAL ONCOTIC PRESSURE**

- Lymphedema, leakage of protein into the interstitium.

syndrome may also contribute to edema. Albumin levels below 2 mg/dL are usually associated with generalized edema.[2] The mechanism of edema formation with decreased oncotic pressure results in extravasation of fluid into the interstitium, but it also results in poor kidney perfusion, which activates renin-aldosterone secretion and results in increased sodium reabsorption and fluid retention. This fluid may then leak into the interstium because of the decreased oncotic pressure, compounding the edema.

### *Increased Capillary Hydrostatic Pressure*

#### Systemic Venous Hypertension

Systemic venous hypertension can be the result of heart failure (from cardiomyopathy, tricuspid valvular disease, or ischemic heart disease), constrictive pericarditis, or cirrhosis. In addition, high output failure (from anemia, hyperthyroidism, or arteriovenous fistulas) also leads to systemic venous hypertension. All of these conditions lead to increased capillary hydrostatic pressure and result in edema from increased extravasation of fluid into the interstitium. Left-ventricular heart failure results in pulmonary edema; right-ventricular heart failure results in venous congestion, hepatomegaly, and peripheral edema.

#### Localized Venous Hypertension

Localized edema may result from increased venous pressure with deep vein thrombosis or from compression of the inferior vena cava or iliac vein by a tumor. The increased venous pressure raises the capillary hydrostatic pressure.

#### Increased Plasma Volume

Glomerular nephritis increases plasma volume resulting from sodium retention. Renal failure can increase plasma volume from an inability to secrete sodium and water. Heart failure and liver disease (cirrhosis) result in decreased effective volume, which increases sodium reabsorption in the kidney by activation of the renin-angiotensin-aldosterone system. Sympathetic nervous stimulation can also result in increased sodium reabsorption in the kidney.

### *Increased Interstitial Hydrostatic Pressure*

Increased interstitial hydrostatic pressure, although rare, may result from lymphatic obstruction by a tumor or large lymph nodes, from damage to the lymphatic system by radiation or surgery, or from parasitic infections such as filariasis.

## ▶ EVALUATION

### *History*

A detailed history must be obtained to discover the cause of the edema. The time course of the edema—whether its onset is recent or chronic—is particularly important. If chronic, then the parents and child may report weight gain, tight clothing, or snug-fitting shoes, findings they may have attributed to the growth of the child. The history of a recent illness, such as pharyngitis, is important for the diagnosis of glomerulonephritis. In addition to the edema, other systemic complaints may be present, including shortness of breath, tachypnea, or cough, which may indicate the presence of heart failure and pulmonary edema. Ascites, a form of localized edema, is seen with liver failure or cirrhosis and with some congenital liver malformations. The child's nutritional status should be assessed, because malnutrition may result in hypoalbuminemia, which can, in turn, result in edema.

### Physical Examination

Edema may be generalized or localized. If localized, then it may be easily apparent when it affects an extremity (deep vein thrombosis, cellulitis, burn). If generalized, it may be more occult (pulmonary edema from left-ventricular heart failure, ascites from liver disease). Physical examination should begin with close observation of the vital signs. Tachypnea may indicate pulmonary edema. Increased blood pressure may be present in glomerulonephritis and renal failure. Fever and localized edema may be present with cellulitis.

Periorbital edema is generally found with nephrotic syndrome and glomerulonephritis. Crackles or rales may indicate the presence of pulmonary edema. A gallop may indicate heart failure. Abdominal distention, shifting dullness, or a fluid wave may be present with ascites. Generalized edema may include scrotal or labial edema. Findings related to generalized edema may depend on whether the patient has been lying down (sacral edema) or standing (feet and lower legs). Chronic edema may result in bedsores. A distinction may be made between pitting and nonpitting edema. Nonpitting edema is often the result of lymphedema, whereas pitting edema is the result of increased membrane permeability, increased hydrostatic pressure, or decreased oncotic pressure.[7]

### Laboratory Evaluation

Initial testing may include a urinalysis, complete blood count, electrolytes with blood urea nitrogen and creatinine, liver function tests with albumin, lipid studies and cholesterol, and thyroid function tests. The results of this initial evaluation may suggest further testing. Elevated blood urea nitrogen may suggest chronic renal injury. A renal ultrasound may be warranted to look for hydronephrosis because of congenital anomalies. With proteinuria, C3, C4 and antinuclear antibody (ANA) may be indicated. If heart failure is suspected, an electrocardiogram and chest radiograph can be obtained. Testing for fecal fat is appropriate if intestinal malabsorption is suspected, and $\alpha_1$-antitrypsin may be helpful for diagnosing protein-losing enteropathy. With angioedema, whether hereditary or acquired, levels of C1 esterase inhibitor are low.

## ▶ INTERPRETATION OF TESTS

### Hematologic Abnormalities

Severe anemia can result in edema, especially in a newborn. The anemia can be the result of hemolysis from ABO blood type or Rh incompatibility or from glucose-6-phosphate dehydrogenase deficiency. High-output cardiac failure leads to increased capillary hydrostatic pressure, resulting in edema.

### Renal Disease

The presence of proteinuria with low serum albumin is highly suggestive of nephrotic syndrome. If red cell casts and hematuria (especially cola-colored urine) are present, then glomerulonephritis may be the cause of the edema. C3 levels may be needed to help distinguish between the types of glomerulonephritis. Low C3 suggests poststreptococcal glomerular nephritis (PSGN) or membranoproliferative glomerular nephritis (MPGN). PSGN usually has improving C3 levels after several weeks. For nephrotic syndrome, low C3 with low C4 and a positive ANA suggest lupus nephritis. If uremia is present, a renal ultrasound may be indicated to look for dysplastic kidneys or hydronephrosis resulting from posterior urethral valves or other anatomic abnormalities. Children with undiagnosed reflux nephropathy may have severe hydronephrosis and renal failure.

### Liver Disease

Hypoalbuminemia without proteinuria suggests either a synthesis defect found with chronic liver disease or a protein-losing enteropathy. Prothrombin time, which is a good marker of the liver's ability to synthesize protein, should be assessed when hypoalbuminemia is present without proteinuria. Liver function tests may also provide helpful information. Analysis of stool $\alpha_1$-antitrypsin will help diagnose protein-losing enteropathy.

### Venous Thrombosis

If venous thrombosis is suspected, a Doppler ultrasound examination should be performed to assess the blood flow in the area that may be affected by the thrombosis. Clotting studies should then be conducted, especially if no predisposing factor, such as an indwelling catheter, is present.

### Enteropathy

The presence of increased fat in fecal matter strongly suggests intestinal malabsorption. Determining which intestinal disorder (cystic fibrosis, inflammatory bowel disease, milk protein allergy, enterokinase deficiency, celiac disease, or intestinal lymphangiectasia) may be the cause of the hypoalbuminemia requires further testing and consultation with a gastroenterologist.

## ▶ MANAGEMENT

Initial management involves determining whether the patient should be admitted to the hospital. Many causes of edema require admission. Patients with signs of respiratory distress that result from edema of the airway, heart failure with pulmonary edema, and tachypnea should be admitted. Renal causes, such as previously undiagnosed renal failure, acute glomerulonephritis, or nephrotic syndrome, may also require admission. Oliguria from renal failure or poor renal perfusion should result in emergent admission. Edema that results from cirrhosis may require admission if the cirrhosis had been unrecognized or if respiratory distress resulting from the ascites is present. Localized edema that results from venous thrombosis or lymphatic obstruction requires admission to assess and treat the underlying cause. Further management depends on the underlying cause of the edema.[2,7,8]

### Anemia

Severe anemia may need to be treated with transfusion. A hematologist should be consulted if the cause of the anemia is not readily apparent.

### Renal Disease

Most patients with renal disease benefit from a low-sodium diet. Fluid restriction may help, but it should be used cautiously on an individual-patient basis in consultation with a nephrologist. Diuretics may also be needed but should be used cautiously. If plasma volume is decreased, then fluid expansion with colloid followed by diuretics may be necessary.

### Liver Disease

A low-sodium diet is generally helpful if ascites is present. Diuretics, especially spironolactone, may also be beneficial. When possible, treating the underlying cause of the ascites is critical.

### Heart Disease

Treating heart failure may require inotropic medications such as digoxin or dobutamine. An angiotensin-converting enzyme inhibitor may help with afterload reduction. If congenital heart disease is causing the heart failure, then surgical repair of the underlying structural lesion is the ultimate treatment.

### Venous Thrombosis

When a venous thrombosis is present, anticoagulation therapy may be indicated. Consultation with a hematologist and possibly a vascular surgeon may be necessary. In the absence of an obvious predisposing factor, investigation for an underlying coagulopathy is appropriate.

### Enteropathy

Treatment depends on the cause of the enteropathy. A gastroenterologist should be consulted.

### Myxedema

Generally, myxedema is found with hypothyroidism and responds to treatment with thyroid hormone replacement.

## ▶ SUMMARY

Edema is the accumulation of fluid in the interstitial tissues resulting from disruption of the forces that control normal fluid movement out of and into capillaries and may be the result of many different disease states. The underlying cause is generally apparent, although sometimes subtle. Intervention may initially need to be supportive, but once a patient is stable, efforts to treat the underlying cause of the edema should be pursued, often with the help of a specialist.

## When to Refer

Many disorders that cause edema may require the assistance of a specialist. A referral to a specialist should be considered if evidence exists of

- Liver disease (ie, ascites)
- Renal disease (glomerulonephritis, nephrotic syndrome)
- Anemia
- Protein-losing enteropathy or increased fecal fat with malabsorption and secondary hypoalbuminemia
- Heart failure

## When to Admit

Many of the causes of edema are serious medical problems that often require admission. This approach may initially be for support. Once a diagnosis is established and the patient is stable, further treatment usually continues on an outpatient basis with the assistance of a specialist. Signs of any of the following may require admission:

- Respiratory distress
- Heart failure
- Tachypnea
- Renal failure
- Acute glomerulonephritis or nephrotic syndrome
- Oliguria from renal failure
- Edema caused by previously unrecognized cirrhosis
- Localized edema that results from venous thrombosis or lymphatic obstruction
- Anemia severe enough to require a transfusion

### *REFERENCES*


1. Ruth JL, Wassner SJ. Body composition: salt and water. *Pediatr Rev.* 2006;27:181–187; quiz 188
2. Cho S, Atwood JE. Peripheral edema. *Am J Med.* 2002;113:580–586
3. Starling EH. On the absorption of fluids from the connective tissue spaces. *J Physiol.* 1896;19:312–326
4. Cárdenas A, Arroyo V. Mechanisms of water and sodium retention in cirrhosis and the pathogenesis of ascites. *Best Prac Res Clin Endocrinol Metab.* 2003;17:607–622
5. Koomans HA. Pathophysiology of oedema in idiopathic nephrotic syndrome. *Nephrol Dial Transplant.* 2003;18(Suppl 6):vi30–vi32
6. Schrier RW. Water and sodium retention in edematous disorders: role of vasopressin and aldosterone. *Am J Med.* 2006;119:S47–S53
7. O'Brien JG, Chennubhotla SA, Chennubhotla RV. Treatment of edema. *Am Fam Physician.* 2005;71:2111–2117
8. Diskin CJ, Stokes TJ, Dansby LM, et al. Towards an understanding of oedema. *BMJ.* 1999;318: 1610–1613

# Chapter 23

# Epistaxis

*Miriam Schechter, MD; David M. Stevens, MD*

Epistaxis, from the Greek *epistazō*, to bleed at the nose (from *epi,* on, + *stazō*, to fall in drops) is defined as acute bleeding from the nostril, nasal cavity, or nasopharynx. A nosebleed is a relatively common and usually self-limited occurrence in childhood; however, when profuse or recurrent, it can be extremely distressing to children and parents and can at times be a sign of a more serious condition.

## ▶ EPIDEMIOLOGIC FACTORS

The incidence of epistaxis has a bimodal distribution with peaks in children younger than 10 years and in adults older than 50 years. It is more common in boys and men than it is in girls and women.[1] From 5% to 14% of Americans have a nosebleed each year, and approximately 10% of them seek care from a physician.[2] Although common in children, epistaxis is rare before the age of 2 years, peaks between the ages of 3 and 8 years, and is uncommon after puberty.[3,4] Nosebleeds also are more common in children living in dry climates and occur more often in winter months.[5] Approximately 30% of children from birth to age 5, 56% of children aged 6 to 10, and 64% of children aged 11 to 15 have had at least 1 nosebleed in their lifetime.[6] In a study of the epidemiology of epistaxis in US emergency departments from 1992 to 2001, approximately 1 in 200 emergency department visits were for epistaxis. Peaks were found in children younger than 10 years and in older adults between the ages of 70 and 79. A higher proportion of emergency department visits occurred during the winter months, and 83% of cases were from atraumatic causes.[7]

## ▶ DEFINITIONS AND ANATOMIC FEATURES

Nosebleeds are usually classified as anterior or posterior based on the location of the vessels that are the source of the bleed. The blood supply to the nose originates in both the internal and the external carotid arteries (Figure 23-1). The ophthalmic branch of the internal carotid gives off the anterior and posterior ethmoid arteries, which supply the superior nasal septum and the lateral nasal wall. The internal maxillary and facial arteries, which are branches of the external carotid, further divide to supply the nose. The internal maxillary artery splits into the sphenopalatine artery, the posterior nasal artery, and the greater palatine artery, and the facial artery gives off the superior labial artery. The branches of the sphenopalatine provide blood flow to the turbinates laterally and the anterior and posterior septum, the greater palatine supplies the anterior septum, and the superior labial artery supplies the anterior nose and anterior nasal septum.

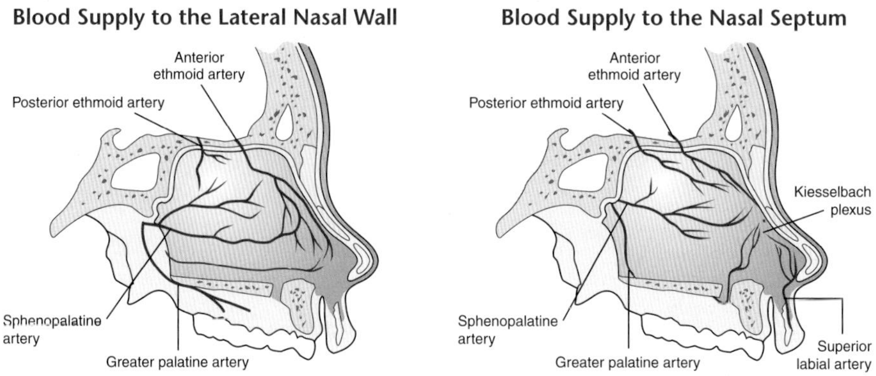


**Figure 23-1**
Blood supply to the nose (septum and lateral wall).

The anastomoses of vessels in the anterior 2 to 3 cm of the nasal septum, just 0.5 cm from the tip of the nose, also known as Little area, make up Kiesselbach plexus, the primary source of anterior nosebleeds. The delicate vessels that comprise Kiesselbach plexus include the septal branches of the anterior ethmoid, sphenopalatine, greater palatine, and superior labial arteries. These vessels are superficial because the nasal mucosa is closely adherent to the perichondrium and periosteum. Posterior bleeds usually originate in Woodruff plexus, a convergence of the sphenopalatine, posterior nasal, and ascending pharyngeal arteries, located over the posterior middle turbinate. Specifically, the sphenopalatine is the most frequent source of posterior epistaxis.

Anterior bleeds are by far the most common type, accounting for greater than 90% of epistaxis in children.[8] The rich vasculature under the thin mucosa in the area most exposed to trauma and dry air makes Kiesselbach plexus the most vulnerable to bleeding. During anterior epistaxis, almost all the blood exits anteriorly through the nares. However, with posterior epistaxis, most of the blood flows into the nasopharynx and mouth, making the degree of bleeding difficult to assess. Anterior bleeds are therefore much easier to visualize and easier to control than posterior bleeds, which are generally much more profuse and are more likely to lead to hemodynamic instability.

## ▶ DIFFERENTIAL DIAGNOSIS

The causes of epistaxis can be categorized into local and systemic causes (Box 23-1). More than 1 factor often plays a role in the bleeding.

Trauma from nose picking or nose rubbing accounts for most cases in children, particularly in association with inflammation from infection or allergy. Epistaxis from blunt external trauma is generally acute and self-limiting, but could result from child abuse in very young children.[3,9] Trauma from a foreign body is an occasional cause in toddlers, often resulting in unilateral bleeding accompanied by foul-smelling or bloody discharge.

Upper respiratory infection and allergic rhinitis are commonly associated with childhood epistaxis. The resultant rhinorrhea leads to digital manipulation or forceful sneezing and nose blowing, and the vascular congestion and mucosal irritation promote easy injury to

BOX 23-1

## Causes of Epistaxis in Children

**LOCAL**

- Trauma
  - Nose picking or rubbing
  - Blunt trauma or facial fractures
  - Foreign body
- Inflammation
  - Upper respiratory infection
  - Allergic rhinitis
- Dry air
- Neoplasms
  - Benign
    - Polyps
    - Hemangiomas
    - Juvenile nasopharyngeal angiofibroma
  - Malignant
    - Nasopharyngeal carcinoma
    - Rhabdomyosarcoma
- Nasal septal deviation
- Intranasal drugs
  - Steroids
  - Cocaine

**SYSTEMIC**

- Bleeding disorders
  - Thrombocytopenia
    - Immune thrombocytopenic purpura
    - Leukemia
  - Platelet dysfunction
    - Bernard-Soulier syndrome
    - Aspirin; nonsteroidal anti-inflammatory drugs
  - Coagulopathies
    - von Willebrand disease
    - Hemophilias
    - Liver disease
- Vascular abnormalities
  - Hereditary hemorrhagic telangiectasia (Rendu-Osler-Weber syndrome)

the blood vessels of the anterior septum. Positive allergy skin tests and recurrent epistaxis are associated in children.[10]

Exposure to low environmental humidity, especially in winter months, has clearly been associated with an increased frequency of nosebleeds.[5,7] A deviated nasal septum can contribute to recurrent epistaxis by causing a change in normal airflow, leading to mucosal drying and irritation.[11] Colonization with *Staphylococcus aureus* leading to chronic inflammation and neovascularization may contribute to recurrent episodes.[12]

Neoplasms (benign or malignant) are uncommon causes of epistaxis in children but should be considered in certain circumstances. Polyps in children are usually associated with cystic fibrosis. Juvenile nasopharyngeal angiofibroma is a benign vascular tumor originating in the lateral nasopharynx that occurs only in male adolescents because of its hormonal sensitivity. Although unilateral progressive obstruction or discharge are clues to this diagnosis, recurrent epistaxis is the most frequent presenting complaint in these patients.[13] Rhabdomyosarcoma of the nasal cavity or nasopharynx is a rare malignant cause of severe episodic epistaxis and may be associated with signs of eustachian tube dysfunction such as unilateral middle ear effusion. Nasal hemangioma is also a rare cause of epistaxis but should be considered in infants. Nasopharyngeal carcinoma is an extremely uncommon but serious disease in children[14]; epistaxis is the presenting complaint in approximately 50% of cases,[15] although it is nearly always accompanied by a neck mass or neck pain.[16]

Systemic causes of epistaxis should be considered whenever nosebleeds are recurrent or persistent in the absence of any obvious local cause. Hematologic disorders include platelet disorders and coagulation defects and may be either congenital or acquired.

Thrombocytopenia as a cause of epistaxis is almost always accompanied by petechiae or ecchymoses. The most common cause of isolated thrombocytopenia in otherwise healthy children is immune thrombocytopenic purpura, which presents as acute mucosal hemorrhage, often epistaxis, in approximately 30% of patients, although the bleeding is rarely severe.[17,18] By contrast, epistaxis rarely is the first symptom of leukemia, but this diagnosis should be considered in an ill-appearing child with epistaxis, especially with fever, pallor, lymphadenopathy, or hepatosplenomegaly. Thrombocytopenia can also be an adverse reaction to a variety of medications, including anticonvulsants such as carbamazepine and chemotherapeutic agents.

Platelet dysfunction from aspirin or nonsteroidal anti-inflammatory drugs can also predispose the individual to epistaxis. Bernard-Soulier syndrome, a disorder of platelet adhesion, is an occasional diagnosis in children evaluated for isolated epistaxis.[19,20] Primary coagulation defects may result in persistent and longstanding epistaxis; a positive family history is often present. Up to one-third of children with isolated recurrent epistaxis have a diagnosable coagulopathy.[20,21] Von Willebrand disease (vWD) is the most commonly identified inherited coagulopathy. In fact, 60% of patients with vWD suffer from recurrent epistaxis; other mucosal bleeding (eg, menorrhagia or postsurgical or postdental extraction) is also a common complaint in older children and adolescents. Much less common are the hemophilias, which in mild cases may cause isolated epistaxis (factors VII, VIII, IX or XI deficiency).[20]

Acquired coagulopathies are a rare cause of epistaxis in children, unlike adults, but include various liver diseases (eg, chronic active hepatitis) with consequent depletion of clotting factors. In addition, an acquired form of vWD has been described in children receiving valproic acid.[22]

Hereditary hemorrhagic telangiectasia (Rendu-Osler-Weber syndrome) is an autosomal-dominant disorder of blood vessel walls characterized by the progressive development of cutaneous and mucosal telangiectasias. More than 90% of affected patients have recurrent and progressively worsening epistaxis, presenting at a mean age of 12 years, although gastrointestinal bleeding and pulmonary arteriovenous malformations also occasionally occur in childhood.[23] Primary isolated hypertension has not been clearly associated with epistaxis in children, except in the context of renal failure. Finally, 1 recent study has shown a significant association between migraine headaches and recurrent epistaxis, suggesting a common pathogenesis.[24]

## ▶ EVALUATION

The evaluation of children with epistaxis should begin with a careful history and physical examination. The season and associated environmental conditions should be noted. The degree of chronicity may suggest an inherited systemic cause. Unilaterality may suggest a local anatomic cause. A history of nose picking or blunt trauma should be sought. One-half of children treated in an emergency room for intranasal foreign body admitted placing the object in the nose; therefore young children should be questioned.[25] A family history of bleeding symptoms or diagnosed disorder is useful in identifying children with a bleeding diathesis.[20]

Associated symptoms should be sought. Unilateral progressive obstruction suggests a mass. The presence and character of any associated rhinorrhea should be noted. Clear, watery rhinorrhea with associated sneezing suggests allergic rhinitis, and mucoid discharge with cough suggests upper respiratory infection. Unilateral foul smelling discharge in a young child may indicate a retained foreign body. A history of petechiae or easy bruising or other mucosal bleeding (eg, menorrhagia, postsurgical) may point to a bleeding disorder. Associated fever or pallor may suggest leukemia. A history of medication use, particularly of aspirin or nonsteroidal anti-inflammatory drugs, should be sought.

The physical examination should include a blood pressure and pulse if the history suggests significant acute or chronic blood loss. A careful examination of the nose should include an attempt to identify the source of any active bleeding (see Management later in this chapter) and to note any discharge, obstructing mass, or foreign body. The skin should be checked for petechiae or unusual location or number of ecchymoses. The neck should be examined for the presence of a mass. If the child is ill, a full examination, including a search for lymphadenopathy and hepatosplenomegaly, should be performed.

The need for and extent of laboratory testing should be guided by the history and physical examination. Frequent and prolonged episodes may warrant ruling out anemia caused by blood loss. Persistent or recurrent epistaxis in the absence of an obvious cause may warrant testing to search for an underlying pathologic condition. A complete blood cell count (CBC) is always indicated in the presence of petechiae or unusual ecchymoses to rule out thrombocytopenia. In an ill child with pallor, fever, lymphadenopathy, or hepatosplenomegaly, a CBC will help rule out leukemia.

The frequency, duration, amount, age at onset, and site of epistaxis have been used in an epistaxis scoring system (Table 23-1) to determine which patients should be evaluated for an underlying bleeding disorder.[26,27] Use of another pediatric bleeding questionnaire revealed that epistaxis of long duration, lacking seasonal correlation, and requiring medical intervention to stop was significantly associated with vWD. This is especially true if the child has bled excessively following circumcision, dental extraction, or with menses.[28] Age younger than 1 year or the need for cauterization have been suggested as reasons to perform an evaluation.[9,29] Prothrombin time and partial thromboplastin time are useful as initial screening tests. However, given that these results may be within the normal range in some patients with vWD, further evaluation with von Willebrand factor studies may be necessary. If this relatively common coagulopathy is being considered or a platelet dysfunction disorder is suspected, then referring the patient to a hematologist may be prudent.

Rarely, imaging studies are indicated, but plain films can rule out an associated fracture of the facial bones in the setting of blunt trauma. In children younger than 2 years, a child abuse evaluation for inflicted trauma may be warranted.[9] If a mass is thought to be present, then a computed tomography scan or referral to an otolaryngologist should be made.

## ▶ MANAGEMENT

Management of nosebleeds can be divided into 3 general phases. The initial first aid measures that often are performed at home should also be the first line of treatment on presentation to the physician. Next is the acute management of persistent bleeding, which may be initiated by a pediatrician in an office or emergency department but may have to be continued by an otolaryngologist if initial measures are unsuccessful. This phase may involve medical

**Table 23-1**
**Epistaxis Scoring System**

| COMPONENT | SCORE[a] |
|---|---|
| **Frequency** | |
| 5–15/yr | 0 |
| 16–25/yr | 1 |
| >25/yr | 2 |
| **Duration** | |
| <5 min | 0 |
| 5–10 min | 1 |
| >10 min | 2 |
| **Amount[b]** | |
| <15 mL | 0 |
| 15–30 mL | 1 |
| >30 mL | 2 |
| **Epistaxis history and age[c]** | |
| 33% | 0 |
| 33%–67% | 1 |
| >67% | 2 |
| **Site** | |
| Unilateral | 0 |
| Bilateral | 2 |

[a]Mild, 0–6; severe, 7–10.
[b]Estimation of average blood loss per episode, based on fractions or multiples of teaspoons, tablespoons, or cups.
[c]Proportion of the child's life that nosebleeds had been recurrent (>5/yr).
From Katsanis E, Luke K, Hsu E, et al. Prevelance and significance of mild bleeding disorders in children with recurrent epistaxis. *J Pediatr.* 1988;113:73–76. Copyright © 1988, Elsevier, with permission.

or surgical intervention, or both (Figure 23-2). Finally, long-term preventive treatment of recurrent epistaxis is necessary, including evaluation and treatment of underlying causes. Although most episodes of epistaxis in childhood are self-limited, they create parental concern and anxiety, and pediatricians must therefore be aware of the treatment options.

Many physicians and patients are unaware of the proper spot for applying direct pressure to the nose to stop a nosebleed.[30,31] Given that most bleeds originate anteriorly, in Little's area, the first step is to apply pressure to the alar nasi using the first and second fingers. Pressure should be held by pinching the nostrils without interruption for 5 to 10 minutes. The child should sit up with the head bent forward slightly, to minimize blood dripping posteriorly and being swallowed, which can cause nausea and hematemesis.[32] Some physicians suggest placement of ice packs to the forehead, bridge of the nose, nape of the neck, or upper lip to promote vasoconstriction, although only theory supports this practice.[33]

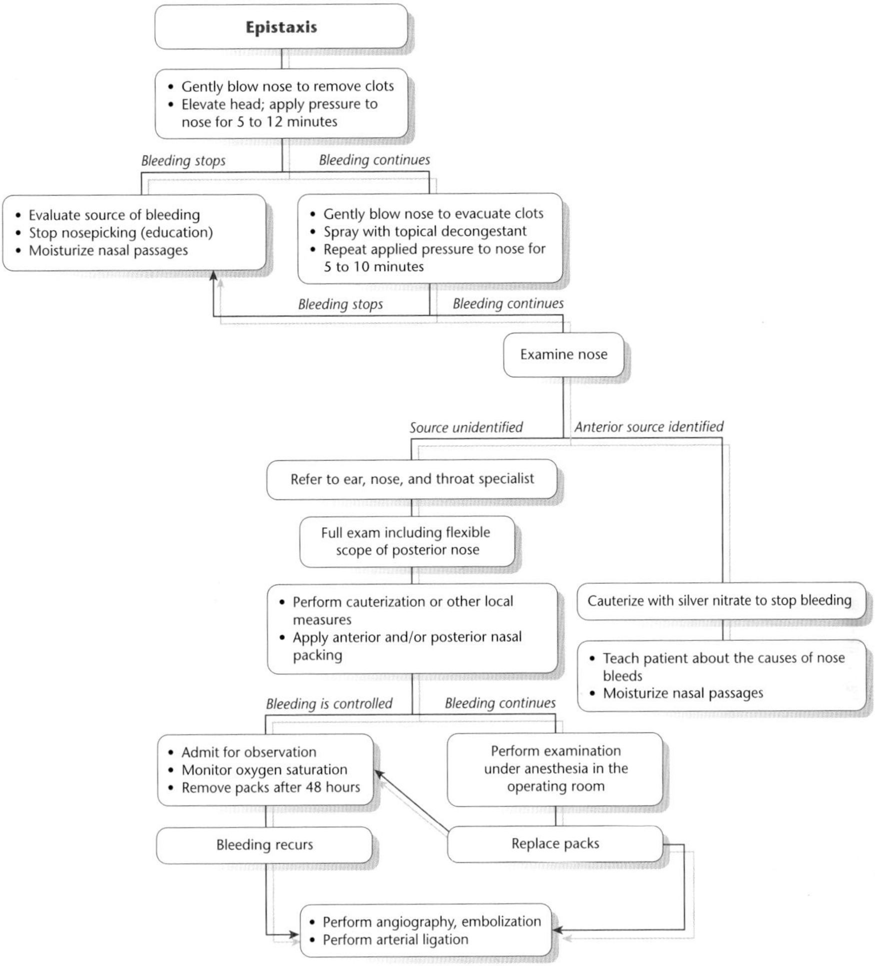


**Figure 23-2**
Treatment of epistaxis. *(From Rudolph AM, Rudolph CD, Hostetter MK, et al, eds.* Rudolph's Pediatrics. *21st ed. New York, NY: McGraw-Hill; 2003. Reprinted by permission of The McGraw-Hill Companies, Inc.)*

In the health care setting, initial treatment measures should occur simultaneously with assessment and history taking. Basic equipment should be readied (Box 23-2). Most anterior nosebleeds in children will stop after basic first aid. However, if bleeding persists, then additional measures are available. As in any acute situation, an initial CAB (Circulation, Airway, Breathing) assessment should be made. Evaluation for major hemorrhage includes evaluating for tachycardia, hypotension, and orthostasis. Although uncommon in children, airway compromise or hemodynamic instability (or both) requires emergency management.

A history should quickly be obtained (see discussion under Evaluation earlier in this chapter) and an attempt made to locate the source of bleeding. The bleeding has often stopped by the time medical attention is sought. The child should be asked to blow out all clots. If this is not possible, then blood in the nose can be suctioned out. To try to visualize the source of bleeding, 1 of the following 3 tools could be used: a flashlight, while applying

BOX 23-2

## *Equipment Used in the Initial Management of Anterior Epistaxis*

### EXAMINATION

- Flashlight *or*
- Otoscope with speculum *or*
- Headlight and nasal speculum
- Suction

### TOPICAL VASOCONSTRICTION

- Oxymetazoline 0.05% (Afrin) *or*
- Phenylephrine 0.25%, 0.5% (Neo-Synephrine) *or*
- Epinephrine 1:1,000 *or*
- Cocaine solution 3%–5%

### TOPICAL ANESTHESIA

- Lidocaine 4% *or*
- Cocaine solution 3%–5% *or*
- Ethyl chloride

### HEMOSTASIS

- Silver nitrate sticks
- Vaseline strip gauze
- Oxycellulose sponges (Surgicel) *or*
- Gelatin sponges (Gelfoam) *or*
- Nasal tampons/expandable nasal pack (Merocel, RhinoRocket)

### ADDITIONAL ITEMS

- Antibiotic ointment or cream (Naseptin; note: contains peanut oil)
- Cotton pledgets, gauze
- Gown, gloves, mask

gentle upward pressure to the nasal tip; an otoscope with speculum; or a headlight and nasal speculum. Because the anterior septum is the most common location of epistaxis in children, this area should be inspected first. Anterior bleeds on the septum, or lateral wall, should be evident by active bleeding, clots, crusts, ulcerations, or prominent blood vessels.[8] If an anterior source is not found and a posterior bleed is thought to exist, then an otolaryngologist should be consulted immediately because posterior bleeds are usually profuse and difficult to stop. Luckily, posterior bleeds are rare in children. If an anterior bleed has not ceased with application of pressure alone, then topical vasoconstrictors (Box 23-2) can be applied with a cotton pledget to shrink the nasal mucosa to improve visualization and possibly to slow down or even stop the bleeding. Use of topical thrombin may also help promote hemostasis.[32] Pressure, again by pinching, should be applied for another 5 to 10 minutes.

The next step to attempt to stop persistent hemorrhage is chemical cauterization, with silver nitrate on applicator sticks. First, local anesthesia should be administered (Box 23-2) with a cotton pledget for 5 minutes to reduce the discomfort of cauterization. After inserting and opening a nasal speculum, using adequate lighting, the silver nitrate is applied to the bleeding point and can be rolled over the site for 5 to 10 seconds. The procedure may have to be repeated 2 to 3 times to achieve hemostasis.[32] Silver nitrate does not work well in pools of blood; therefore, suction may be necessary to keep the area dry. A gray eschar will form at the cautery site. Excess silver nitrate should be removed with cotton or gauze to minimize dispersion by nasal secretions and resulting injury to intact mucosa.[34] Caution should be used to avoid cauterizing too large or too deep an area and to avoid cauterizing both sides of the septum because these measures can lead to septal perforation. After cauterization, the physician should prescribe antibiotic cream or ointment to apply to the area twice a day for 5 days to prevent crusting and infection.[11] Hydration with saline or ointment should continue until healing is complete, in approximately 1 to 3 weeks. Nasal trauma and forceful nose blowing should be avoided during this time. Otolaryngologists may use electrocautery as another hemostatic measure. This type of thermal cautery, however, cannot be performed with topical anesthesia alone.

If an anterior bleed persists despite direct pressure or nasal cautery, then anterior nasal packing may be required. This task can be accomplished with antibiotic impregnated petroleum jelly gauze, which is layered into the anterior nose and provides a tight pack. However, packing is uncomfortable and may require procedural sedation, requires subsequent removal (usually after 2 to 3 days), and can cause additional mucosal injury. Oxycellulose or gelatin sponges are absorbable and do not require later extraction. Although they do not apply a great deal of pressure to the bleeding site, these types of packing are usually adequate for most nosebleeds.[32] Commercially available nasal tampons made of a dehydrated polyvinyl polymer sponge can also be used. The tampons are inserted dry and then expand with blood or added saline partially to fill the nasal cavity. These products come in many sizes and can be cut to fit a child's nasal cavity. They must be removed, usually after 3 to 5 days, and have a tendency to adhere to the nasal lining.

All types of packing and sponges should be impregnated or coated with antibiotic ointment to prevent toxic shock syndrome, which is a reported complication of anterior and posterior nasal packing.[8,11] Although no clear evidence exists to prove that prophylactic antibiotics reduce the incidence of serious infection, studies have shown that they reduce gram-negative bacterial growth, and common practice is to prescribe them for any patient with nasal packing.[8,35] Antibiotics, such as amoxicillin-clavulanate, may also help prevent sinusitis that can result from stasis of nasal secretions when packing is in place.[32]

Identification of the source of a posterior bleed must be done by an otolaryngologist using a flexible fiberoptic nasopharyngoscope; sedation may be required for younger patients. In addition to locating a superior or posterior bleeding site, endoscopic visualization may also reveal causes such as foreign bodies, tumors, or sinusitis. In older, more cooperative patients, a rigid endoscope may be used. Cauterization of a posterior bleeding site can be performed under general anesthesia. Posterior packing can be done with gauze or even urinary catheter balloons. Other types of packing include premade nasal tampons or balloons.[8] All patients requiring posterior packing need sedation and must be admitted to the hospital and monitored in an intensive care unit for airway obstruction and respiratory compromise.[32] More invasive measures such as arterial embolization for refractory bleeds and arterial ligation for recurrent epistaxis are rarely indicated in children.[8]

Once the acute episode of epistaxis has resolved, attention can be focused on looking for predisposing factors or causes and respective preventive strategies or specific management. If a dry environment is present, then the use of normal saline nasal spray helps to humidify the nasal cavity. The spray should be used 4 to 5 times a day. A humidifier in the home may also be useful.[34] The increased moisture helps prevent the accumulation of crusts, which are often the impetus for nosepicking, and keeps scabs soft, allowing them to stay in place longer and thus promoting healing of underlying mucosal injury. Local trauma should be minimized by discouraging nosepicking, forceful rubbing, or blowing of the nose. Fingernails can be trimmed as well. Parents should be educated about the home management of an acute nosebleed; they should pinch the nasal tip for 5 to 10 minutes with the child sitting up, leaning slightly forward.[36]

If allergic rhinitis is a factor in epistaxis, then appropriate testing and medical management is indicated, including treatment with oral antihistamines or inhaled topical nasal steroids. For sinusitis, oral antibiotics are prescribed. If a bleeding disorder is thought to exist, then laboratory workup (see discussion under Evaluation earlier in this chapter) or referral to a hematologist is warranted. Otolaryngologists treat other uncommon lesions and conditions. For example, they will cauterize granulomas, monitor hemangiomas, and excise juvenile nasopharyngeal angiofibromas after hormonal therapy and embolization.[37] Patients with hereditary hemorrhagic telangiectasia (Rendu-Osler-Weber syndrome) are now treated with argon laser therapy along with septal dermoplasty.[38]

A common challenge for physicians is the management of recurrent nosebleeds. A recent Cochrane review of the literature on interventions for recurrent idiopathic epistaxis in children exposed the lack of evidence for current treatments of this problem.[39] The condition was defined as repeated nasal bleeding in patients younger than 16 years without identifiable cause. Consensus does not exist on the frequency or severity of the episodes of epistaxis that warrant medical intervention. However, common interventions for less severe cases include cautery with silver nitrate, application of antibiotic nasal creams, instillation of nasal saline spray, or coating the interior nose with ointments such as petroleum jelly. Less commonly advocated topical agents include oxymetazoline, desmopressin, antifibrinolytics, and, most recently, fibrin sealants. On review of the few studies that have been done, no single treatment (neomycin-chlorhexidine antiseptic cream, silver nitrate cautery, petroleum jelly) was found to be superior to another or to no treatment at all. No serious adverse effects were experienced, although silver nitrate cauterization caused pain in children despite topical anesthesia.[40–42] One small study suggested that cautery combined with antibiotic cream is more effective than cream alone.[43] Also, if cautery is used, 75% silver nitrate has been shown to be more effective in the short term (but not long term) and caused less pain for the children than 95%.[44] High-quality studies, with longer follow-up, are needed to ascertain which, if any, of these remedies for recurrent epistaxis in children are most optimal.

Nosebleeds occur commonly in children. Although quite upsetting and worrisome to parents, most epistaxis in childhood is anterior, is controlled by simple first aid measures, and results from benign causes. Epistaxis is therefore usually treated on an outpatient basis by general pediatricians. An understanding of all potential causes and acute and long-term management of nosebleeds will assist the pediatrician in appropriate treatment of this condition.

## When to Refer

Ear, Nose, and Throat

*Urgent Referral*

- Profuse, uncontrollable bleeding
- Inability to locate source of bleed
- Posterior bleeding
- Assistance with anterior packing
- Recurrence of bleed after initial emergency department measures

*Nonurgent Referral*

- Removal of anterior packing
- Recurrent epistaxis

- Evaluation for structural lesions (ie, granulomas, tumors, polyps)
- Treatment of specific lesions

Hematology

- Abnormal CBC or coagulation laboratory profile
- Severe, persistent, or recurrent bleeding
- Bleeding from more than 1 site, based on history or physical examination
- Bleeding that required blood transfusion or iron therapy
- Family history of coagulopathy

## When to Admit

- Hemodynamic instability on presentation
- Posterior nasal packing in place

## *TOOLS FOR PRACTICE*

### Engaging Patient and Family

- *Chronic Nosebleeds: What To Do* (fact sheet), American Academy of Pediatrics (www.healthychildren.org/English/health-issues/conditions/ear-nose-throat/Pages/Chronic-Nosebleeds-What-To-Do.aspx)

## *REFERENCES*


1. Kucik CJ, Clenney T. Management of epistaxis. *Am Fam Phys.* 2005;71:305–311
2. Quinn FB, Porter GT. Epistaxis. Grand rounds presentation. *UTMB Dept Otolaryngol.* April 2002
3. McIntosh N, Mok JY, Margerison A. Epidemiology of oronasal hemorrhage in the first 2 years of life: implications for child protection. *Pediatrics.* 2007;120:1074–1078
4. Guarisco JL, Graham HD III. Epistaxis in children: causes, diagnosis and treatment. *Ear, Nose, Throat J.* 1989;68:522–538
5. Nunez DA, McClymont LG, Evans RA. Epistaxis: a study of the relationship with weather. *Clinical Otolaryngol.* 1990;15:49–51
6. Petruson B. Epistaxis in childhood. *Rhinology.* 1979;17:83–90
7. Pallin DJ, Chng Y, McKay MP, et al. Epidemiology of epistaxis in US emergency departments, 1992 to 2001. *Ann of Emerg Med.* 2005;46:77–81
8. Manning S, Culbertson M Jr. Epistaxis. In: Bluestone C, Stool S, Kenna M, eds. *Pediatric Otolaryngology.* 4th ed. Philadelphia, PA: Saunders; 2003;925–931
9. Paranjothy S, Fone D, Mann M, et al. The incidence and aetiology of epistaxis in infants: a population-based study. *Arch Dis Child.* 2009;94:421–424
10. Murray AB, Milner RA. Allergic rhinitis and recurrent epistaxis in children. *Allergy Asthma Immunol.* 1995;74:30–33
11. Tan LKS, Calhoun KH. Epistaxis. *Med Clin North Am.* 1999;83:43–56
12. Whymark AD, Crampsey DP, Fraser L, et al. Childhood epistaxis and nasal colonization with Staphylococcus aureus. *Otolaryngol Head Neck Surg.* 2008;138:307–310
13. Malik MK, Kumar A, Bhatia BP. Juvenile nasopharyngeal angiofibroma. *Indian J Med Sci.* 1991;45:336–342
14. Komoroski EM. Nasopharyngeal carcinoma: early warning signs and symptoms. *Pediatr Emerg Care.* 1994;10:284–286
15. Bass IS, Haller JO, Berdon WE, et al. Nasopharyngeal carcinoma: clinical and radiographic findings in children. *Radiology.* 1985;156:651–654
16. Zubizarreta PA, D'Antonio G, Raslawski E, et al. Nasopharyngeal carcinoma in childhood and adolescence: a single-institution experience with combined therapy. *Cancer.* 2000;89:690–695
17. Buchanan GR. Thrombocytopenia during childhood: what the pediatrician needs to know. *Pediatr Rev.* 2005;28:401–409

18. Medeiros D, Buchanan GR. Major hemorrhage in children with idiopathic thrombocytopenic purpura: immediate response to therapy and long-term outcome. *J Pediatr.* 1998;133:334–339
19. Lubianca Neto JF, Brito LB, Santos EF. Epistaxis as a manifestation of Bernard-Soulier syndrome. *J Pediatr (Rio J).* 1997;73:111–114
20. Sandoval C, Dong S, Visintainer P, et al. Clinical and laboratory features of 178 children with recurrent epistaxis. *J Pediatr Hematol Oncol.* 2002;24:47–49
21. Kiley V, Stuart JJ, Johnson CA. Coagulation studies in children with isolated recurrent epistaxis. *J Pediatr.* 1982;100:579–581
22. Serdaroglu G, Tütüncüoglu S, Kavakli K, Tekgül H. Coagulation abnormalities and acquired von Willebrand's disease type 1 in children receiving valproic acid. *J Child Neurol.* 2002;17:41–43
23. Mei-Zahav M. [Osler-Weber-Rendu—a life-threatening disease in adults and children.] *Harefuah.* 2003;142:852–856, 876
24. Jarjour IT, Jarjour LK. Migraine and recurrent epistaxis in children. *Ped Neurol.* 2005;33:94–97
25. Ngo A, Ng KC, Sim TP. Otorhinolaryngeal foreign bodies in children presenting to the emergency department. *Singapore Med J.* 2005;46:172–178
26. Katsanis E, Luke KH, Hsu E, Li M, Lillicrap D. Prevalence and significance of mild bleeding disorders in children with recurrent epistaxis. *J Pediatr.* 1988;113:73–76
27. Callejo G, Velert Vila MM, Marco Algarro J. Recurrent epistaxis in children as an indicator of hemostatic disorders. *An Esp Pediatr.* 1998;49:475–480
28. Bowman M, Riddel J, Rand ML, et al. Evaluation of the diagnostic utility for von Willebrand disease of a pediatric bleeding questionnaire. *J Thromb Haemost.* 2009;7:1418–1421
29. Elden L, Reinders M, Witmer C. Predictors of bleeding disorders in children with epistaxis: value of preoperative tests and clinical screening. *Int J Pediatr Otorhinolaryngol.* 2012;76:767–771
30. Lavy JA, Koay CB. First aid treatment of epistaxis—are the patients well informed? *J Accid Emerg Med.* 1996;13:193–195
31. McGarry GW, Moulton C. The first aid management of epistaxis by accident and emergency department staff. *Arch Emerg Med.* 1993;10:298–300
32. Nadel F, Henretig F. Epistaxis. In: Fleisher G, Ludwig S eds. *Textbook of Pediatric Emergency Medicine.* 6th ed. Philadelphia, PA: Lippincott Williams & Wilkins; 2010:236–237, 1775–1777
33. Dost P, Polyzoidis T. [Benefit of the ice pack in the treatment of nosebleed.] *HNO.* 1992;40:25–27
34. Massick D, Tobin E. Epistaxis. In: Cummings C, Schuller DE, Thomas JR, et al, eds. *Otolaryngology/Head and Neck Surgery.* 4th ed. Philadelphia, PA: Elsevier Mosby; 2005
35. Derkay CS, Hirsch BE, Johnson JT, Wagner RL. Posterior nasal packing. Are intravenous antibiotics really necessary? *Arch Otolaryngol Head Neck Surg.* 1989;115:439–441
36. Shott SR. Epistaxis. In: Rudolph AM, Rudolph CD, Hostetter MK, et al, eds. *Rudolph's Pediatrics.* 21st ed. New York, NY: McGraw-Hill; 2002:1261–1262
37. Mulbury P. Recurrent epistaxis. *Ped Rev.* 1991;12:213–217
38. Lund VJ, Howard DJ. A treatment algorithm for the management of epistaxis in hereditary hemorrhagic telangiectasia. *Am J Rhinol.* 1999;13:319–322
39. Qureishi A, Burton MJ. Interventions for recurrent idiopathic epistaxis (nosebleeds) in children. *Cochrane Database Syst Rev.* 2012;9:CD004461
40. Kubba H, MacAndie C, Botma M, et al. A prospective, single-blind, randomized controlled trial of antiseptic cream for recurrent epistaxis in childhood. *Clin Otolaryngol Allied Sci.* 2001;26:465–468
41. Loughran S, Spinou E, Clement WA, et al. A prospective, single-blind, randomized controlled trial of petroleum jelly/Vaseline for recurrent paediatric epistaxis. *Clin Otolaryngol Allied Sci.* 2004;29:266–269
42. Ruddy J, Proops DW, Pearman K, et al. Management of epistaxis in children. *Int J Paediatr Otorhinolaryngol.* 1991;21:139–142
43. Calder N, Kang S, Fraser L, et al. A double-blind randomized controlled trial of management of recurrent nosebleeds in children. *Otolaryngol Head Neck Surg.* 2009;140:670–674
44. Glynn F, Amin M, Sheahan P, McShane D. Prospective double blind randomized clinical trial comparing 75% versus 95% silver nitrate cauterization in the management of idiopathic childhood epistaxis. *Int J Pediatr Otorhinolaryngol.* 2011;75:81–84

# Chapter 24

# Extremity Pain

*Michael G. Burke, MD, MBA; David C. Hanson, MD*

## DEFINITION OF TERMS

Extremity pain is a common complaint in primary care pediatric practice. Up to 16% of school-aged children report at least 1 episode of activity-limiting extremity pain annually.[1] Among surveyed 8- to 18-year-old Norwegian children, 38.9% of girls and 46.6% of boys reported lower extremity pain during the 3 months prior to survey, while 13.9% of girls and 18.4% of boys reported arm pain.[2] In a 9-year, 6-point, longitudinal survey, British researchers found that 56.6% of caregivers of 5- to 13-year-olds reported that their child often experienced extremity pain at the time of at least 1 survey.[3] Over the 9-year course of the study, caregivers reporting extremity pain in their child increased from 15.1% for 5-year-olds to 32.5% for 13-year-olds.[3] There is some evidence that extremity pain is more common in obese children than in controls.[4] Overall, approximately 6% of pediatric office visits are related to extremity pain.[5] Fortunately, most of these visits involve pain caused by minor trauma, overuse syndromes, and normal skeletal growth variants.[5] Occasionally, however, limb pain is the presenting complaint of a systemic illness, a neoplasm, an infectious process, a nutritional derangement, a specific orthopedic disorder, or a rheumatologic disease. The challenge for the physician is to determine when the pain is significant without exposing the child to excessive diagnostic studies and without delaying treatment or referral. For the most part, this determination is based on the history and physical examination alone.

## EVALUATION

### History

A thorough history from patients and parents often reveals the cause of extremity pain in children. Pain described as aching or cramping is likely to be muscular in origin. Bone pain is often described as deep and nerve pain as burning, tingling, or numbness. Referred pain is common in children; thus, although usually helpful, the location of pain may be deceiving. Migrating extremity pain is less likely to occur after trauma and is more typical of systemic illnesses such as leukemia, acute rheumatic fever, disseminated gonorrhea, and arthralgia or arthritis associated with inflammatory bowel disease. The mode of onset, variability, duration, and frequency of pain also help in determining its cause. Activities associated with worsening or relief of pain can also lead to a diagnosis. Similarly, color change associated with extremity pain may indicate inflammation (faint red), infection (intense red), or autonomic dysfunction (pallor, cyanosis, and erythema). Stiffness, especially with clinical evidence of arthritis not associated with trauma, should prompt concern about a rheumatologic process.

A history specific to trauma associated with extremity pain can be helpful. Trauma accompanied by an audible pop or snap is more likely the result of a dislocation, sprain, or fracture. Mild trauma that leads to a fracture might indicate some previous defect in the bone, as with a pathological fracture. If the physical findings of trauma are greater than would be expected from the history, then physical abuse must be considered.

The child's general health history completes the picture of extremity pain. For example, the differential diagnosis changes with age. Toxic synovitis of the hip is a common diagnosis in a child younger than 10 years; a slipped capital femoral epiphysis is more likely in an overweight adolescent.

As a screen for systemic disease, all systems should be reviewed briefly. Particular attention should be paid to a history of fever, recent weight loss, sweating, rashes, and gastrointestinal symptoms. A history of recent medications is important and might reveal a serum sickness–like illness. Even a short course of systemic steroids can cause aseptic necrosis of the hip or can result in demineralization of bone. Immunizations, particularly for rubella, may cause joint or extremity pain, and a history of exposure to viral illness might explain myalgia or arthralgia. Specifically, both parvovirus and hepatitis B can cause significant arthralgia.

The patient's family history may reveal a tendency toward autoimmune disease or recent exposure to infectious diseases. The family history is particularly helpful in identifying hemoglobinopathies. A family history of sickle cell anemia in a 6- to 24-month-old child whose hands and feet are painfully swollen may lead to the diagnosis of hand-foot syndrome and previously undiagnosed sickle cell disease. A sickle cell pain crisis must always be considered in a black child or a child of Mediterranean origin who has a painful extremity. Human leukocyte antigen B27 is associated with reactive arthritis (formerly called Reiter syndrome), psoriatic arthritis, inflammatory bowel disease, and ankylosing spondylitis, and has been described in association with enthesitis-related arthritis (inflammation of tendons, ligaments, or fascia at their attachments to bone).[6] Joint hypermobility syndrome and fibromyalgia also can be familial.

Extremity pain may be a symptom of a functional disorder and can serve as an entry to the physician's office. One large group of pediatric rheumatologists has estimated that 11% of their new patients suffer from psychosomatic musculoskeletal pain.[7] In cases of functional pain, the history may be either quite dramatic or highly understated. Pain in a nonanatomic distribution or that disturbs only unpleasant activities (waxing on school days and waning on weekends) should raise suspicion of a functional disorder. Eliciting a history of recent events at home, recent school performance, and other social history can be essential to determining the diagnosis.

### Physical Examination

A brief general physical examination is worthwhile even if the history points to extremity pain from minor local trauma. Abnormalities in blood pressure, heart rate, or growth pattern can reveal an endocrine cause. An elevated resting heart rate is associated with rheumatic fever. Pallor, fever, lymphadenopathy, or organomegaly may be clues to systemic disease. A rash may be particularly helpful. Dermatomyositis occurs with muscle pain and proximal weakness associated with a vasculitic rash on the extensor surfaces of knuckles, knees, and elbows (Gottron papules). Palpable purpura and extremity pain are associated with Henoch-Schönlein purpura. A photosensitive rash in a child who has limb pain might point to systemic lupus erythematosus, dermatomyositis, or parvovirus infection. Nail pitting is associated with psoriasis.

In a child with unexplained extremity pain, a thorough eye examination by an ophthalmologist may detect uveitis, sometimes associated with juvenile idiopathic arthritis. Photophobia, eye injection, or pain with accommodation associated with extremity pain warrants a consultation with a rheumatologist and ophthalmologist. A complete physical examination can reveal generalized joint laxity and hyperextensibility, differentiating benign hypermobility syndrome from a focal ligament injury. In benign hypermobility syndrome (Ehlers-Danlos syndrome type III), the joint laxity allows chronic hyperextension, which can cause pain, typically in weight-bearing joints. The pain often is worse in the evening. Dancing and gymnastics may exacerbate arthralgia, as can any other joint-impacting activity.

Claudication is a rare cause of extremity pain in children. However, in popliteal artery entrapment syndrome, vascular calf pain that radiates to the foot is associated with an anomalous popliteal artery or anomalous placement of the gastrocnemius muscle.[8] The pain begins with activity, sometimes more with walking than with running. This syndrome is suggested if normal pedal pulses are lost with simultaneous knee extension and foot plantar flexion.

Because referred pain is common in children, the physical examination should include areas proximal and distal to the site of the complaint. A slipped capital femoral epiphysis and Legg-Calvé-Perthes disease, both of which affect the hip, can produce knee or thigh pain, whereas an abscess of the psoas muscle may cause hip pain. Appendicitis and other intra-abdominal processes and diskitis can also cause pain that is referred to a lower extremity.

Examination of a painful extremity should include assessment of peripheral vascular status, muscle strength, soft-tissue swelling, and skeletal injury. Disruption of joint integrity may be shown by demonstration of abnormal range of motion of the joint with passive movement. Peripheral vascular status is assessed by palpating the pulses and determining the capillary refill time distal to the pain. Skin color and warmth, tenderness to palpation, and the extent of passive and active range of motion should all be assessed. Swelling, warmth, and erythema over a joint are signs of arthritis. Point tenderness over a bone raises suspicion of a fracture. Point tenderness in the absence of a clear history of trauma may indicate osteomyelitis. Comparing the opposite limb is helpful when assessing swelling, muscle wasting, or joint mobility. Observing the patient's gait or use of the painful limb when the patient is unaware of the observation helps in diagnosing a functional process. Isolated distal weakness is likely to be of neurologic origin, whereas proximal weakness is most likely from muscular disease. Finally, with chronic extremity pain, serial examinations of the patient over the course of weeks can be the key to diagnosis.

### Laboratory Examination

Laboratory studies are unnecessary for most extremity pain. However, if the history and physical examination do not lead to a definitive diagnosis, if they raise suspicion of a systemic or an infectious disease, or if the pain persists longer than anticipated, then screening laboratory tests are in order. A basic evaluation should include a complete blood cell count (CBC), a sedimentation rate, a C-reactive protein, and a sickle cell preparation or hemoglobin electrophoresis when indicated. Appropriate serologies should be considered if features of the physical examination are consistent with rheumatologic disease. An elevated sedimentation rate raises suspicion of an infectious or inflammatory disorder or, occasionally, of a neoplasm. A CBC may reveal anemia or may suggest an infectious disease. With leukemia, the white blood cell (WBC) count varies, but immature forms may be present in the differential WBC count or thrombocytopenia may be present. A creatine phosphokinase determination is occasionally indicated if muscular pain or weakness is suspected.

### *Imaging*

Radiologic studies are often unnecessary in evaluating limb pain. However, because of the plasticity of children's bones, traumatic injury that would ordinarily cause only a sprain in an adult is more likely to result in a greenstick or buckle fracture in a child. The presence of point tenderness or gross deformity in an extremity or pain on motion of the involved limb increases the likelihood of fracture. In an effort to minimize the use of radiographic studies after traumatic injury to the knee and ankle, The Ottawa Criteria have been developed for use in adults. These criteria have also now been validated for use in children older than 5 years[9,10] (Box 24-1). When no clear history of trauma is revealed, when symptoms persist, and when associated systemic complaints are present, radiographs can help identify bony tumors, pathological fractures, some metabolic defects, and a significant number of orthopedic conditions.

A bone scan is a useful diagnostic tool in evaluating limb pain and should be considered when a stress fracture, osteomyelitis, or malignancy is suspected. Bone scans are more sensitive than plain-film radiography for establishing these diagnoses. Increasingly, magnetic

**BOX 24-1**

## *Indication for Plain Radiograph Evaluation After Trauma Using the Ottawa Ankle and Knee Rules*

Radiograph of the knee is indicated after trauma if[a]

- Age older than 55 years
- Isolated tenderness of patella
- Tenderness at the head of the fibula
- Inability to flex the knee to 90 degrees
- Inability to bear weight both immediately and at medical evaluation

Radiograph of the ankle is indicated after trauma in cases of[b]

- Pain in the malleolar zone and (1) tenderness of the tip of the medial malleolus or bone tenderness of the distal 6 cm of posterior tibia, OR (2) tenderness of the tip of the lateral malleolus or bone tenderness of the distal 6 cm of the posterior fibula, OR (3) inability to bear weight immediately after injury and at the time of medical evaluation.

Radiograph of the foot is indicated after trauma in cases of

- Pain in the midfoot zone and (1) tenderness at the base of the fifth metatarsal, OR (2) tenderness at the navicular bone, OR (3) inability to bear weight immediately after injury and at the time of medical evaluation.

[a]Dowling S, Spooner CH, Liang Y, et al. Accuracy of Ottawa Ankle Rules to exclude fractures of the ankle and midfoot in children: a meta-analysis. *Acad Emerg Med.* 2009;16(4):277–287

[b]Vijayasankar D, Boyle AA, Atkinson P. Can the Ottawa knee rule be applied to children? A systematic review and meta-analysis of observational studies. *Emerg Med J.* 2009;26(3):250–253

resonance imaging (MRI) is being used as a replacement for bone scans in the diagnosis of osteomyelitis. The combined use of T1, T2, and short-tau inversion-recovery images effectively rules out osteomyelitis, with a negative predictive value approaching 100%.[11] MRI offers the additional advantage of excellent visualization of soft-tissue and joint disease. There may still be a role for bone scan in the evaluation for osteomyelitis when need for sedation is a concern and when the area of potential involvement cannot be adequately narrowed based on physical examination.

## Differential Diagnosis

The differential diagnosis of extremity pain is extremely broad (Box 24-2). However, most limb pain is benign, requires no intervention, and is self-limited. Characteristic patterns of pain and associated signs and symptoms signal the presence of certain diseases and conditions. A discussion of some of these disorders follows.

BOX 24-2

### *Extremity Pain in Childhood: Differential Diagnosis*

**IMMUNE-MEDIATED ORIGIN**

- Dermatomyositis
- Familial Mediterranean fever
- Guillain-Barré syndrome
- Henoch-Schönlein purpura
- Inflammatory bowel disease
- Juvenile idiopathic arthritis
- Kawasaki disease
- Mixed connective-tissue disease
- Polyarteritis nodosa
- Rheumatic fever
- Scleroderma
- Serum sickness
- Systemic lupus erythematosus

**CONGENITAL ORIGIN**

- Caffey disease
- Hemophilia
- Hypermobility syndrome (Ehlers-Danlos syndrome type III)
- Mucolipidosis
- Mucopolysaccharidosis
- Osteogenesis imperfecta
- Popliteal artery entrapment syndrome
- Sickle cell anemia, thalassemia

**ENDOCRINE ORIGIN**

- Hypercortisolism
- Hyperparathyroidism
- Hypothyroidism

**IDIOPATHIC ORIGIN**

- Fibromyalgia
- Growing pains
- Restless leg syndrome
- Sarcoidosis

**INFECTIOUS ORIGIN**

***Bacterial***

- Arthralgia or myalgia associated with streptococcal infection
- Diskitis, spinal epidural abscess
- Gonorrhea
- Osteomyelitis
- Pyogenic myositis
- Septic arthritis
- Enteric disease
- Meningococcal disease
- Syphilis: periostitis
- Tuberculosis

***Viral***

- Myalgia, arthralgia
- Myositis
- Toxic synovitis

***Other***

- Histoplasmosis
- Immunization reaction
- Trichinosis

*Continued*

BOX 24-2

## *Extremity Pain in Childhood: Differential Diagnosis—cont'd*

**METABOLIC ORIGIN**

- Carnitine palmityltransferase deficiency
- Fabry disease
- McArdle syndrome
- Phosphofructokinase deficiency

**NEOPLASTIC ORIGIN**

- Langerhans cell histiocytosis
- Leukemia
- Lymphoma
- Neuroblastoma
  - Chondrosarcoma
  - Ewing sarcoma
  - Osteoblastoma (benign)
  - Osteogenic sarcoma
  - Osteoid osteoma (benign)
- Tumors of soft tissue
  - Fibrosarcoma
  - Rhabdomyosarcoma
  - Synovial cell sarcoma
- Tumors of the spinal cord
- Tumors of bone

**NUTRITIONAL ORIGIN**

- Gout
- Hypercholesterolemia
- Hypervitaminosis A
- Osteoporosis
- Rickets (vitamin D deficiency)
- Scurvy (vitamin C deficiency)

**ORTHOPEDIC ORIGIN**

- Chondromalacia patellae
- Freiberg disease
- Inflexible flat feet, tarsal coalition
- Kohler disease
- Legg-Calvé-Perthes disease
- Osgood-Schlatter disease
- Osteochondritis dissecans
- Osteogenesis imperfecta
- Pathological fracture
- Sever disease
- Slipped capital femoral epiphysis

**PSYCHOSOCIAL ORIGIN**

- Behavior disorders
- Psychogenic pain
- Reflex neurovascular dystrophy
- School phobia

**TRAUMA OR OVERUSE**

- Compartment syndrome
- Fracture
- Myohematoma
- Myositis ossificans
- Nerve compression syndrome
  - Carpal tunnel syndrome
  - Cervical nerve root entrapment
- Other peripheral nerve root compression
- Physical abuse
- Shin splint
- Sprain
- Stress fracture
- Subluxed radial head
- Thoracic outlet syndrome

## Growing Pains

Growing pains are a time-honored pediatric disorder. They are intermittent, deep extremity pains that affect the lower more often than the upper extremities. The pain is nearly always bilateral, rarely involves the joints, and is almost universally worse at night, lasts fewer than 2 hours, and resolves completely in the morning. Despite their name, growing pains do not occur most frequently during periods of rapid growth. Instead, their onset is described at 3 to 5 or 8 to 12 years of age. For many children growing pains resolve in 12 to 24 months;

however, they may persist into adolescence. In a 5-year follow-up of 35 children with growing pains, half had resolution of the condition and nearly all had improvement.[12]

The cause of growing pains remains unclear. However, headache and abdominal pain, often associated with emotional illnesses, also have accompanied growing pains. In the 5-year follow-up study, only children with persistent growing pains had lower pain thresholds than controls.[12]

The diagnosis of growing pains is significant for its lack of associated physical signs. Thus, any abnormal finding on physical examination should provoke a search for another cause. Similarly, radiographs and the results of screening laboratory tests usually prove normal. Treatment involves heat, massage, and analgesics.

## Sprains

A sprain is a physical disruption of a ligament. In children, sprains occur less commonly than in adults because a child's open epiphyseal plate or plastic bony cortex tends to give way more easily than does a ligament. Therefore, Salter-Harris fractures and buckle fractures should be considered when the history indicates a sprain and when physical examination reveals tenderness on palpation or pain on stretching the ligament. Joint stability should also be assessed. Sprains can be graded according to the degree of associated ligament disruption. A mild, microscopic tear that results in no laxity of the involved joint is a grade I sprain. Grade II sprains involve macroscopic but incomplete ligament tears. Joint laxity is greater, but less than a 5-mm movement differential exists between the sprained and the contralateral joint. Grade III sprains result in more than 5 mm of increased mobility of the affected joint. The primary care physician can treat grade I sprains by icing and wrapping the involved joint to minimize swelling. Early range of motion exercises should be encouraged, with a gradual return to activity. The recurrence of pain indicates too rapid a return to a given level of activity. Grade II and grade III sprains should generally be referred to an orthopedist or sports medicine physician for immobilization and consideration of surgical repair of torn ligaments.

## Overuse Syndromes

Overuse injuries have become more common as organized sports for children have become popular nationwide and as the competitive level of some sports activities has increased. Localized, gradually increasing, and persistent extremity pain that worsens with weight bearing, exercise, and activity, but that diminishes with rest, can indicate a stress fracture. Stress fractures are rare in children younger than 12 years. They most commonly affect the second metatarsal, the proximal tibia, or the fibula. A radiograph may show normal findings, and although a bone scan or an MRI can help establish the diagnosis they are not routinely indicated because treatment consists mostly of rest and nonsteroidal anti-inflammatory agents. Casting or splinting is occasionally necessary.

*Little League elbow* is an overuse injury caused by the repetitive motion of pitching a baseball; this motion compresses the radial aspect of the elbow and stretches the ulnar aspect. The result is painful inflammation of the epicondyles. The range of joint motion also may be diminished. Fragments of bone splintered into the joint may cause the joint to catch or lock. Treatment consists of resting the arm by avoiding the repetitive movement. A change in pitching technique may reduce recurrences. To prevent this problem, some Little League systems limit both the number of innings a child may pitch in a game and the age at which certain pitches can be thrown.

Shin splints are also caused by overuse. The term originally referred to pain along the posteromedial aspect of the tibia as a result of irritation at the origin of the posterior tibial muscle. Shin splints now refer to any of a series of painful overuse syndromes of the lower portion of the leg, including irritation of the posterior or anterior tibial muscle, inflammation of the interosseous membrane located between the tibia and fibula, and both anterior and posterior compartment syndromes. All of these abnormalities can cause pain in the lower legs. The condition, which is exacerbated by running and jumping, occurs most commonly at the beginning of a training season. Although the pain occurs initially after activity, it may occur during or before activity as the syndrome progresses. On examination, tenderness may be felt over the posteromedial aspect of the tibia, over the proximal portion of the posterior tibia, or over the anterior tibia. Differential diagnosis includes Osgood-Schlatter disease with pain localized to the tibial tuberosity. Treatment of shin splints involves rest, application of ice, and anti-inflammatory agents. For runners, training on a softer surface or with better-quality running shoes may help.

### Subluxation of the Radial Head

Nursemaid's elbow is a common injury in toddlers. The injury usually follows sudden, forceful traction of the hand or forearm, which pulls the immature radial head briefly from the cuff formed by the annular ligament. Release of the force allows the radius to trap the ligament against the capitellum. A verbal patient usually localizes the pain to the elbow or, occasionally, to the wrist. More often, the child refuses to use the extremity and holds the arm with the elbow flexed, the forearm close to the chest, and the hand in pronation. The diagnosis is usually made by history alone. If the history is unclear, or if attempts to reduce the subluxation are unsuccessful, then radiographs may be obtained to rule out a fracture. Radiographic findings in subluxation of the radial head usually are negative. The physician can reduce the subluxation by using 1 hand to supinate the patient's forearm quickly while simultaneously exerting traction on the forearm and using the thumb of the other hand to create pressure over the patient's radial head. This maneuver is completed by placing the elbow through full extension and flexion while maintaining pressure over the radial head. Alternatively, the child's forearm can be fully pronated instead of supinated, and then either fully extended or flexed. With either maneuver, normal use of the extremity usually returns within 30 minutes. The rapid recovery is dramatic and rewarding to the parents and the physician. A prompt return to normal use of the affected arm may not occur if the subluxation has been present for some time because of swelling of the ligament. In such instances, the affected arm should be placed in a simple sling and positioned across the upper portion of the abdomen for 12 to 24 hours. Referral to an orthopedist is rarely required.

### Slipped Capital Femoral Epiphysis

A slipped capital femoral epiphysis is caused by a sudden or gradual dislocation of the head of the femur from its neck and shaft at the level of the upper epiphyseal plate. The characteristic pain occurs in the affected hip or the medial aspect of the ipsilateral knee. The displacement may be sudden, in which case the pain is usually severe and associated with the inability to bear weight. Gradual displacement is associated with slowly increasing, dull pain. This condition typically affects sedentary, obese adolescent boys. The physical examination may reveal diminished abduction and internal rotation of the hip. The diagnosis is made radiographically. Management involves surgical placement of a pin through the femoral head and the epiphysis to prevent further slippage. Avascular necrosis of the femoral head is a common complication, even with early recognition and treatment.

### Toxic Synovitis

Toxic synovitis, a self-limited inflammation of the hip joint, commonly occurs in children younger than age 10 years. The cause is unknown; however, because it often occurs within 2 weeks after an upper respiratory infection, a postviral inflammatory process is suspected. Typical presentation is that of a child who refuses to walk because of apparent pain in the hip. The hip is held in flexion, abduction, and external rotation. Findings may include a slight elevation in the WBC count and the sedimentation rate, a frustrating development for the physician, who hopes to rule out septic arthritis. A C-reactive protein of less than 1 mg/dL has been shown to have an 87% negative predictive value for septic arthritis.[13] This study may offer reassurance. However, persistent concern for septic arthritis may lead to consultation with an orthopedist. Treatment of toxic synovitis consists of bed rest, usually for fewer than 4 days. In rare instances, avascular necrosis of the femoral head may be a late complication.

### Osteochondroses

Osteochondroses include a group of disorders in which degeneration or aseptic necrosis of bone and overlying cartilage occurs at an ossification center and is followed by recalcification. The disorders vary in name and presentation according to their locations.

Legg-Calvé-Perthes disease, or osteochondrosis of the femoral head, results from compromise of the tenuous vascular supply to the area. The condition may be idiopathic or may result from a slipped capital femoral epiphysis, trauma, steroid use, sickle cell crisis, or congenital dislocation of the hip. Toxic synovitis also is associated with subsequent Legg-Calvé-Perthes disease, but not commonly. After compromise of the vascular supply, the bone underlying the articular surface of the head of the femur becomes necrotic. Collapse of the necrotic bone flattens the femoral head and causes a poor fit with the acetabulum, even after new bone is formed. The pain associated with Legg-Calvé-Perthes disease, which results from necrosis of the involved bone, is often referred to the medial aspect of the ipsilateral knee. A limp may be the presenting complaint. In many instances, an early diagnosis eludes the physician because radiographic findings may be normal or show only swelling of the joint's capsule. A bone scan may demonstrate diminished blood flow to the femoral head compared with the contralateral hip. Later, radiographs may show areas of bone resorption, irregular widening of the epiphysis, or dense new bone formation. The goal of therapy is to prevent flattening of the femoral head as it undergoes new bone formation by keeping the hip abducted so that the head of the femur is held well inside the rounded portion of the acetabulum. Either bracing or an osteotomy may accomplish this task; both require referral to an orthopedic surgeon.

Two similar processes can affect the knee joint. Osteochondritis dissecans involves degeneration of bone and cartilage at the articular surface of the knee, particularly at the lateral aspect of the medial condyle of the femur. Knee pain, crepitus, or a sensation of instability or locking caused by loose bone and cartilage fragments in the joint can result. Chondromalacia patellae occurs because of a painful softening or breakdown of the inner surface of the patella. The pain is localized to the knee and increases with activities that require prolonged knee bending and even with prolonged sitting. The pain is described as grinding and can sometimes be elicited by applying pressure over the patella. Moving the patella from side to side over the knee joint may cause crepitus and apprehension. Treatment is usually limited to pain relief and reassurance that, in time, the condition will resolve. Exercise to strengthen the medial quadriceps muscles and to stretch the hamstrings may promote better alignment of the patella with the knee and thereby diminish the pain. Rarely, in severe cases, the patella may have to be realigned surgically. Osteochondrosis of the growth plate of the calcaneus (Sever disease) can produce heel pain that worsens with activity. This usually mild process requires only rest, nonsteroidal anti-inflammatory agents, and padding of the heel to relieve the pain. Avascular necrosis and osteochondrosis of the tarsal navicular bone (Kohler disease) and of the head of the second metatarsal (Freiberg disease) can cause foot pain. Treatment usually requires only pain medication and rest.

Osgood-Schlatter disease is a painful degeneration of the tibial tubercle at the site of insertion of the quadriceps ligament. It is characterized by painful swelling of the anterior aspect of the tibial tubercle, usually occurring during adolescence. The degree of swelling may be alarming, and the area is tender to palpation. Pain is exacerbated by activity that involves increased use of the quadriceps muscles. The process is self-limited and resolves toward the end of adolescence when the epiphysis at the insertion site closes and the bone becomes stronger than the inserted ligament. Until it resolves, the condition is treated with rest, analgesics, and, occasionally, supportive patellar knee straps. In rare cases, casting or surgical attachment of the quadriceps ligament is required.

## Osteomyelitis

Osteomyelitis is a local infection of bone, usually involving 1 of the long bones. The highest incidence is in children 3 to 12 years of age. Although infection often occurs by hematogenous seeding, it can be caused by direct entry after local trauma. In both children and adults, the most commonly isolated organism is *Staphylococcus aureus.* Improved diagnostic testing has allowed identification of *Kingella kingae* as 1 of the primary pathogens of osteomyelitis (and septic arthritis) in children younger than 6 years.[14] Effective vaccination for *Haemophilus influenzae* type b has made this pathogen a rare cause of osteomyelitis in immunized children.[15] Other organisms, including *Salmonella* species and group A streptococci also infect the bone. Group B *Streptococcus* is more likely the cause of infection in newborns. Osteomyelitis caused by *Salmonella* tends to occur more often in children who have sickle cell anemia than in other children. In assessing trauma from a puncture wound to the foot, especially through a sneaker, *Pseudomonas aeruginosa* must be considered. In addition, tuberculous osteomyelitis still occurs and may become more common with the resurgence of tuberculosis.

Osteomyelitis can produce extremity pain alone or extremity pain with signs of a systemic infectious disease (fever, irritability, septic appearance). In the absence of systemic signs, distinguishing between osteomyelitis and a traumatic cause of the pain is often difficult. A period of 2 weeks or longer may be required for radiographic evidence of osteomyelitis to develop. A bone scan is usually, but not always, diagnostic. In rare cases, a reduction in perfusion caused by pressure from the exudative process may result in false-negative scans. MRI is now the preferred test for confirming this diagnosis. In addition, the WBC count and sedimentation rate are often elevated in osteomyelitis. The effectiveness of treatment can be monitored by repeating tests of the sedimentation rate or the C-reactive protein.

### *Neoplasms*

Although neoplasm is not commonly the cause of limb pain, the possibility of a tumor is a common concern for parents of children who have this complaint. Even if rare, benign and malignant bone tumors and systemic malignancies can cause limb pain.

Osteoid osteoma is a benign prostaglandin-secreting bone tumor that occurs most often in adolescents and usually involves a femur, tibia, or lumbar vertebral body. Pain, the presenting complaint, is initially dull and increases in intensity to deep and boring. The pain is more intense at night and with weight bearing. Radiographic findings of sclerotic bone around a lucent center are diagnostic of this condition; tomograms are sometimes required for confirmation. Surgical excision is curative.

Systemic neoplasms in which extremity pain occurs include leukemia and metastatic neuroblastoma. Childhood leukemia is an uncommon cause of extremity pain. However, up to one-third of children who have acute lymphocytic leukemia have bone pain at the time of diagnosis, and in one-fourth of children, joint or bone pain is a significant presenting complaint. Unrelenting, increasing pain that worsens at night or with rest and that is not relieved by analgesics, heat, or massage may indicate the presence of a metastatic bone tumor. Systemic signs (weight loss, pallor, lymphadenopathy, hepatosplenomegaly, or fever) may accompany the pain. In leukemia, examination of the extremity may reveal strikingly little to account for the degree of pain. Radiographic studies of the extremities may show lucent leukemic lines in the subepiphyseal area.

Primary malignant tumors of bone may cause severe unilateral pain, with swelling and tenderness at the tumor site. The possibility of this diagnosis supports the use of radiographic studies when unilateral limb pain is not explained adequately by a history of trauma and when pain from trauma does not resolve as expected. The peak incidence of both osteogenic sarcoma and the less common Ewing sarcoma occurs in late childhood and during adolescence. The radiograph of an osteogenic sarcoma may reveal a tumor in the metaphysis with the presence of both radiolucent and radiopaque areas. The characteristic sunburst results from extension of calcification into the overlying soft tissue. Although periosteal elevation may be present, it is not diagnostic of the disease.

## When to Refer

- Surgical procedure or subspecialist required for definitive treatment (eg, suspected anterior cruciate ligament tear, Ewing sarcoma, other associated conditions)
- Surgical procedure or subspecialist required for diagnostic evaluation (eg, suspected septic arthritis, juvenile idiopathic arthritis, systemic lupus erythematosus, other associated conditions)
- Extremity pain part of multisystemic signs and symptoms (eg, Fabry disease, Crohn disease, other associated conditions)

## TOOLS FOR PRACTICE

### Engaging Patient and Family

- *Growing Pains Are Normal Most of the Time* (fact sheet), American Academy of Pediatrics (www.healthychildren.org/English/health-issues/conditions/orthopedic/Pages/Growing-Pains-Are-Normal-Most-Of-The-Time.aspx)
- *Ankle Sprain Treatment* (fact sheet), American Academy of Pediatrics (www.healthychildren.org/English/health-issues/injuries-emergencies/sports-injuries/Pages/Ankle-Sprain-Treatment.aspx)
- *Nursemaid's Elbow* (fact sheet), American Academy of Pediatrics (www.healthychildren.org/English/health-issues/conditions/orthopedic/Pages/Nursemaids-Elbow.aspx)

## REFERENCES

1. Abu-Arafeh I, Russell G. Recurrent limb pain in schoolchildren. *Arch Dis Child.* 1996;74:336–339
2. Haraldstad K, Sørum R, Eide H, Natvig GK, Helseth S. Pain in children and adolescents: prevalence, impact on daily life, and parents' perception, a school survey. *Scand J Caring Sci.* 2011;25:27–36
3. Bishop JL, Northstone K, Emmett PM, Golding J. Parental accounts of the prevalence, causes and treatments of limb pain in children aged 5 to 13 years: a longitudinal cohort study. *Arch Dis Child.* 2012;97:52–53
4. Wilson AC, Samuelson B, Palermo TM. Obesity in children and adolescents with chronic pain: associations with pain and activity limitations. *Clin J Pain.* 2010;26:705–711
5. de Inocencio J. Musculoskeletal pain in primary pediatric care: analysis of 1000 consecutive general pediatric clinic visits. *Pediatrics.* 1998;102:E63
6. Olivieri I, Pasero G. Longstanding isolated juvenile onset HLA-B27 associated peripheral enthesitis. *J Rheumatol.* 1992;19:164–165
7. Sherry DD, McGuire T, Mellins E, et al. Psychosomatic musculoskeletal pain in childhood: clinical and psychological analyses of 100 children. *Pediatrics.* 1991;88:1093–1099
8. Cummings RJ, Webb HW, Lovell WW, Kay G. The popliteal artery entrapment syndrome in children. *J Pediatr Orthop.* 1992;12:539–541
9. Dowling S, Spooner CH, Liang Y, et al. Accuracy of Ottawa Ankle Rules to exclude fractures of the ankle and midfoot in children: a meta-analysis. *Acad Emerg Med.* 2009;16:277–287
10. Vijayasankar D, Boyle AA, Atkinson P. Can the Ottawa knee rule be applied to children? A systematic review and meta-analysis of observational studies. *Emerg Med J.* 2009;26:250–253
11. Tehranzadeh J, Wong E, Wang F, Sadighpour M. Imaging of osteomyelitis in the mature skeleton. *Radiol Clin North Am.* 2001;39:223–250
12. Uziel Y, Chapnick G, Jaber L, Nemet D, Hashkes PJ. Five-year outcome of children with "growing pains": correlations with pain threshold. *J Pediatr.* 2010;156:838–840
13. Levine MJ, McGuire KJ, McGowan KL, Flynn JM. Assessment of the test characteristics of C-reactive protein for septic arthritis in children. *J Pediatr Orthop.* 2003;23:373–377
14. Lundy DW, Kehl DK. Increasing prevalence of *Kingella kingae* in osteoarticular infections in young children. *J Pediatr Orthop.* 1998;18:262–267
15. Howard AW, Viskontas D, Sabbagh C. Reduction in osteomyelitis and septic arthritis related to *Haemophilus influenzae* type B vaccination. *J Pediatr Orthop.* 1999;19:705–709

# Chapter 25

# Facial Dysmorphism

*Robert W. Marion, MD; Joy Samanich, MD*

"It is my business to know things. Perhaps I have trained myself to see what others overlook."

Sherlock Holmes, "A Case of Identity"[1]

If someone were searching for a role model for the field of dysmorphology, the study of the recognition of patterns of congenital malformations and dysmorphic features that characterize particular syndromes, Sir Arthur Conan Doyle's famous detective, Sherlock Holmes, would be an excellent candidate. Like Holmes, the dysmorphologist, who is a subspecialist within the field of medical genetics, searches for clues when evaluating a patient: sometimes facts become available from a carefully obtained history; sometimes facial features that are in plain sight can lead to a diagnosis; and, similar to a detective solving a crime, the dysmorphologist attempts to assemble these bits of information into a single, unifying diagnosis. These clues may be obvious, or they may be so subtle that other physicians simply overlook them. Their diagnostic significance and the information they may provide about the developmental timing of a congenital anomaly, however, may prove invaluable.

## ▶ DEFINITIONS

Defined as clinically significant abnormalities in form or function, congenital *malformations* result from localized, *intrinsic* defects in morphogenesis that occur in embryonic or early fetal life. These defects, which include clefting of the lip or palate, congenital heart disease such as tetralogy of Fallot, and multicystic kidney disease, may result from an unknown cause, but increasingly can be traced to mutations in or deletions of single developmental genes. Malformations usually require surgical intervention.[2]

*Deformations* differ from malformations in that they arise from environmental forces acting on *normal tissue primordia*. For example, a fetus reared in a uterus in which a large fibroid is present may have limited space for the limbs to go through their normal range of motion; limitation of motion of the limbs leads to congenital contractures, a condition known as *arthrogryposis multiplex congenita*. Deformations occur later than malformations, usually after the first trimester of pregnancy is completed, and they often resolve with minimal therapy.[3]

A malformation such as a cleft lip or cleft palate or a deformation such as clubfoot deformity (Figure 25-1) may occur as an isolated feature or, in instances in which multiple malformations occur together, may be part of a *malformation sequence*, a *syndrome*, or an *association*.

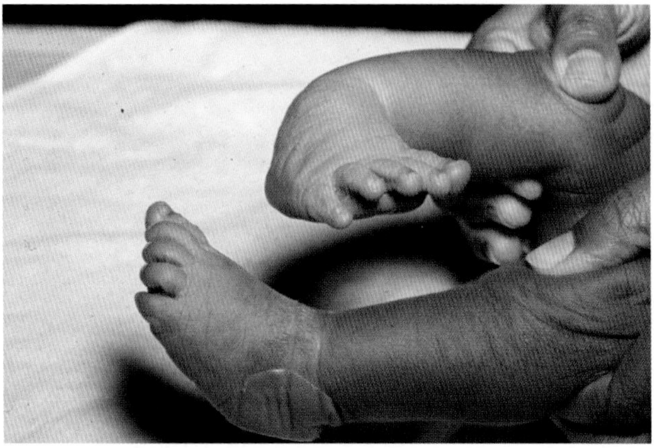

**Figure 25-1**
Club feet. (*From Hoyme HE. Assessing dysmorphology in primary care. In: Saul RA, ed.* Medical Genetics in Pediatric Practice. *Elk Grove Village, IL: American Academy of Pediatrics; 2013:135–174.*)

When a single malformation causes secondary effects on other structures later in development, a malformation sequence will result. For instance, in the Pierre Robin malformation sequence, the primary malformation, failure of the growth of the mandible during the first weeks of gestation, results in micrognathia (small jaw); because of the insufficient size of the jaw, the tongue, which is normal in size, is forced into an unusual position; the abnormally placed tongue blocks the fusion of the palatal shelves that normally come together in the midline, thus producing a *U*-shaped cleft of the palate; after delivery, the normal-sized tongue in the smaller-than-normal oral cavity leads to airway obstruction and obstructive apnea, a potentially life-threatening complication. Thus, 3 anomalies result from the single malformation.[2]

In clinical genetics, a syndrome is defined as a group of malformations that occur together and are caused by a clearly identifiable causative agent. This agent may be a single gene mutation; such is the case in Marfan syndrome in which a mutation in the *FBN1* gene on chromosome 15 leads to abnormally formed fibrillin, an important component of the myofibrillar array of connective tissue. The result is a characteristic set of abnormalities of the skeletal, cardiovascular, and ophthalmologic systems. Single gene mutations account for approximately 7.5% of all multiple malformation syndromes. A second cause of a syndrome can be a chromosomal abnormality, as in Down syndrome, in which an extra copy of chromosome 21 leads to craniofacial dysmorphic features, developmental disabilities, cardiac anomalies, and other abnormalities. Approximately 6% of infants with multiple malformation syndromes have a chromosomal abnormality. A third underlying cause of a syndrome can be a teratogenic agent—a drug, chemical, or environmental toxin that causes damage to the developing embryo or fetus. One example is valproic acid, an anticonvulsant that when given to a woman during the first trimester of pregnancy leads to spina bifida, a characteristic facial appearance, limb defects, and other anomalies in exposed embryos. Teratogens account for approximately 6% of cases of infants with multiple malformation syndromes.[4] Finally, a syndrome can result from unknown factors, as is the case with septo-optic dysplasia, which is characterized by midline brain abnormalities, optic nerve hypoplasia and pituitary endocrine dysfunction. Though a small number of patients (<1%) with septo-optic dysplasia have a mutation in the HESX1 gene, most individuals with this condition have no identifiable underlying cause.[5]

Associations differ from syndromes in that no single underlying cause has been identified to explain a recognizable pattern of anomalies that occur together more than would be expected by chance alone. One example is the VACTERL association (*v*ertebral anomalies, *a*nal atresia, *c*ardiac defects, *t*racheoesophageal fistula, *r*enal anomalies, and *l*imb anomalies). Because no single unifying cause that explains this condition has been identified, it is considered an association. When the cause of an association becomes known, the disorder is recategorized as a syndrome. This change recently happened with the CHARGE association (*c*oloboma, *h*eart disease, *a*tresia choanae, *r*etardation of growth or development, *g*enitourinary tract anomalies, and *e*ar anomalies) when, in 2004, this entity was found to be related to mutations in the *CHD7* gene on chromosome 8. Identification of mutations in this gene in patients with this condition allowed CHARGE association to become CHARGE syndrome.

Between 2% and 5% of newborns are found during the neonatal period to have 1 or more congenital malformations. This percentage increases at 1 year of age to between 7% and 8% because some malformations, such as congenital heart disease and renal anomalies, may remain clinically silent during the newborn period only to display later in life. In approximately one-half of children with congenital malformations, only a single malformation is identifiable; in the other half, multiple malformations are present.[6]

## ▶ APPROACH TO THE CHILD WITH DYSMORPHIC FEATURES

The birth of a child with dysmorphic features is a difficult and unsettling experience for the family, the physician, and the medical staff. In many instances, recognition of any problem in an infant will lead to a crisis for the family; the physician caring for the infant and the family may easily panic in such a situation. Therefore, establishing a standardized routine in a format that can routinely be followed when the physician is faced with such a situation is helpful for the evaluation of the child with dysmorphic features. This routine should include taking the history, including a 3-generational family history, and performing a careful physical examination. Following these steps, specific diagnostic laboratory tests can be ordered to confirm a diagnosis (Box 25-1).[6]

When approaching a child with dysmorphic features, physicians must be sensitive about the terminology used to describe the infant. The terms *funny-looking kid* and *funny-looking face* are derogatory, justifiably arouse parental indignation, and should be avoided at all times. In discussing dysmorphic features with parents or describing them in written or verbal communication with colleagues, the physician should describe the abnormal features as clearly and concisely as possible.[6]

### History

In taking the history, the following questions about the pregnancy should be asked:

1. *What was the birth weight?* A lower-than-expected birth weight can be associated with a chromosomal anomaly or exposure to a teratogen. Babies who are large for gestational age may be infants of diabetic mothers or have an overgrowth syndrome, such as

Box 25-1

## *Evaluation of the Individual Who Has Facial Dysmorphism*

- Review the pregnancy and medical history.
- Review the family history.
- Evaluate growth of the individual in height, weight, and head circumference.
- Evaluate the craniofacial region for dysmorphic features, and describe any such features that are found.
- Describe any other dysmorphic somatic features.
- Define the development of the individual.
- Develop a differential diagnosis and consider appropriate laboratory tests.
- Discuss the findings with the family and, if appropriate, offer genetic counseling.

Beckwith-Wiedemann syndrome. Infants who are accurate for gestational age may have a single gene mutation, a multifactorial condition, or, most likely, no genetic disease at all.

2. *Was the baby full term, premature, or postmature?* This information is especially important when evaluating an older child with developmental disabilities. Complications of extreme prematurity may be responsible for the patient's problems. Postmaturity is associated with some chromosome anomalies (such as trisomy 18) and anencephaly.
3. *Was the baby born by vaginal or cesarean delivery? If the latter, what was the indication?* These questions are helpful in evaluating the newborn with dysmorphic features and in older children with developmental disabilities. Cesarean delivery may be performed because of fetal distress, a risk factor for developmental disability caused by oxygen deprivation. Furthermore, babies born from breech presentation are approximately 4 times more likely than infants born from vertex presentation to have congenital malformations.
4. *How old were the parents at the time of the child's delivery?* Advanced maternal age is associated with an increased risk of nondisjunction leading to trisomies, such as Down syndrome (trisomy 21), whereas advanced paternal age may be associated with an increased risk of a new mutation leading to an autosomal dominant trait, such as achondroplasia.
5. *Did the pregnancy have complications? Does the mother have underlying medical problems? Does she take any medications? Did she smoke cigarettes, drink alcohol, or take any drugs?* Exposure of the embryo to teratogens—medications, or environmental agents known to cause birth defects—is a significant cause of congenital malformations.
6. *When did the mother feel quickening? Were fetal movements active?* Quickening, which normally occurs between 16 and 20 weeks' gestation, is delayed in hypotonic fetuses, who also have movements during fetal life that are not as vigorous as those of a fetus with normal muscle tone. Additionally, a mother's report of persistent hiccups in an infant found to have neonatal seizures suggests a prenatal onset of the condition.
7. *Was the amount of amniotic fluid normal?* An increased amount of amniotic fluid is associated with intestinal obstruction or a central nervous system anomaly that leads to poor swallowing, whereas a decreased amount of fluid may point to a renal or urinary tract abnormality that leads to failure to produce urine or a chronic amniotic fluid leak.

A 3-generation pedigree should be constructed, searching for similar and dissimilar abnormalities in first- and second-degree relatives; a history of pregnancy or neonatal losses should also be documented.[6]

### *Physical Examination*

In the process of evaluating the child with dysmorphic features, the physical examination is the most important element. Whenever possible, the patient should be examined using a standardized approach, described in the following sections.

## Growth

The height (length), weight, and head circumference should be carefully measured and plotted on appropriate growth curves. Growth that is appropriate for age may be consistent with the presence of a single gene disorder, a multifactorially inherited condition, or, most commonly, no genetic disease. Small size or growth restriction may be secondary to a chromosomal abnormality, a skeletal dysplasia such as achondroplasia, or exposure to toxic or teratogenic agents. Larger-than-expected size suggests an overgrowth syndrome (eg, Soto or Beckwith-Weidemann syndromes) or, if in the newborn period, of maternal diabetes.[6]

## Proportions

Do the limbs look appropriate for the head and trunk? If not, then are the limbs too short (implying the presence of a short-limbed bone dysplasia such as achondroplasia)? A trunk and head that are too small for the extremities may suggest a disorder affecting the vertebrae, such as spondyloepiphyseal dysplasia.[6]

## Craniofacial Features

Careful examination of the craniofacies is crucial for the diagnosis of many congenital malformation syndromes. Often, a careful observer can make a diagnosis simply by looking at the child's face.

In assessing the face, head shape and facial features should be systematically observed.

**HEAD SHAPE.** In the newborn period, molding may cause the head to be misshapen, the result of a late prenatal deformational process (see previous discussion). The examiner will need to allow a few days for the deformation to resolve before assessing the shape. The head should then be described using the following terms[6]:

- *Normocephaly* describes a normal head shape.
- *Dolichocephaly* or *scaphocephaly* describes a long, thin head.
- *Brachycephaly* describes a head that is narrow in the anteroposterior diameter and broad laterally.
- *Plagiocephaly* describes a head that is asymmetric or lopsided.

**FACIAL FEATURES.** A dysmorphic face may be appropriate in relation to the family's physiognomy, or it may indicate a particular syndrome. The child who has a large head who also has a parent with a large head does not prompt as much concern as the large-headed child whose parents have normal-size heads. Thus, the examiner must evaluate dysmorphic facial features in light of the child's genetic background. (Table 25-1 lists examples of genetic causes of facial malformation.)[7]

In evaluating the face, the examiner should first note the symmetry. Facial asymmetry may result from a deformation related to intrauterine or extrauterine positioning or a malformation of 1 side of the face, as is the case with *hemifacial microsomia* (also known as Goldenhar syndrome or *oculoauriculovertebral syndrome*).

**Table 25-1**
**Examples of Genetic Causes of Facial Malformation[a]**

| CAUSE | EXAMPLE | FACIAL DYSMORPHISM |
|---|---|---|
| Chromosomal | Down syndrome (trisomy 21) | Midface hypoplasia, upward obliquity of palpebral fissures, epicanthal folds, flat nasal bridge, anteversion of nares |
| Autosomal dominant | Treacher Collins syndrome | Dysplastic ears, maxillary hypoplasia |
| Autosomal recessive | Hurler syndrome | Corneal clouding, coarse facies |
| Teratogenic: intrauterine infection | Congenital rubella | Cataracts |
| Drug induced | Fetal alcohol syndrome | Smooth philtrum (Figure 25-2), small eyes |

[a]*Smith's Recognizable Patterns of Human Malformation* is the most valuable resource for this purpose; it also is helpful in determining if a particular condition is genetically based.

For purposes of evaluation, the face should be divided into 4 regions, each of which should be evaluated separately.

1. The *forehead* extends from the anterior hairline to the eyebrows.
2. The *midface* encompasses the region from the eyebrows to the upper lip and laterally from the outer canthus of each eye to the outer commissure of the lips.
3. The *malar region* extends on either side from the upper portion of the ear to the midface.
4. The *mandible* extends from lower ear to lower ear and including the lower lip.

By analyzing each of these 4 regions and determining which is typical and which is not, a clear description of the child's dysmorphic features can be made.[6]

The forehead may show overt prominence (as is the case with achondroplasia) or deficiency (often described as a *sloping* appearance, which occurs in children with primary microcephaly).

Hypoplasia of the midface is a common component of many syndromes, including Down syndrome and fetal alcohol syndrome. Evaluating the midface involves careful assessment, first by measurement and then through plotting those measurements on appropriate growth curves, of both the distance between the eyes (inner and outer canthal distances) and pupils (interpupil distance). Such assessment may confirm the impression of hypotelorism (eyes that are too close together), suggestive of a defect in midline brain formation (holoprosencephaly); or hypertelorism (eyes that are too far apart), suggestive of a syndrome such as *Opitz syndrome* (ocular hypertelorism, tracheal and esophageal anomalies, and hypospadias). The length of the palpebral fissure should be noted and plotted on the appropriate growth chart; palpebral fissures may be short in fetal alcohol syndrome or excessively long in Kabuki syndrome (short stature, intellectual disability, long palpebral fissures with eversion of lateral portion of lower lid).[3,4,8]

Other features of the eyes should be noted. The obliquity (slant) of the palpebral fissures may be upward (as in Down syndrome [Figure 25-3]) or downward (as in Treacher Collins syndrome [Figure 25-4] or Noonan syndrome [Figure 25-5]). The presence of epicanthal folds—flaps of skin covering the inner canthus of the eye, usually associated with flattening of the nasal bridge—may indicate Down syndrome or fetal alcohol syndrome.

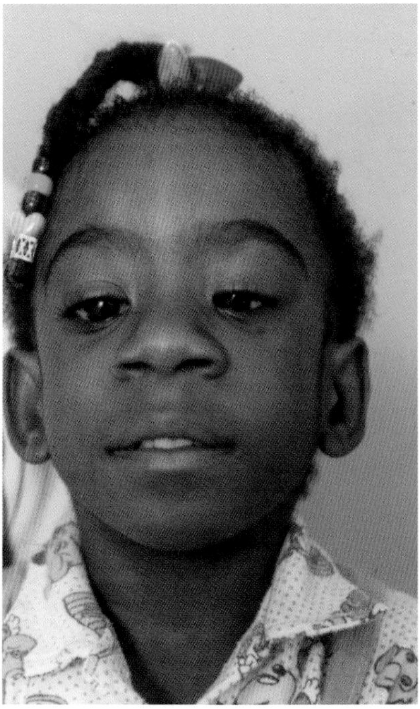

**Figure 25-2**
Smooth philtrum, characteristic of fetal alcohol syndrome. (*From Hoyme HE. Assessing dysmorphology in primary care. In: Saul RA, ed.* Medical Genetics in Pediatric Practice. *Elk Grove Village, IL: American Academy of Pediatrics; 2013:135–174. Courtesy of Greenwood Genetic Center, Greenwood, SC.*)

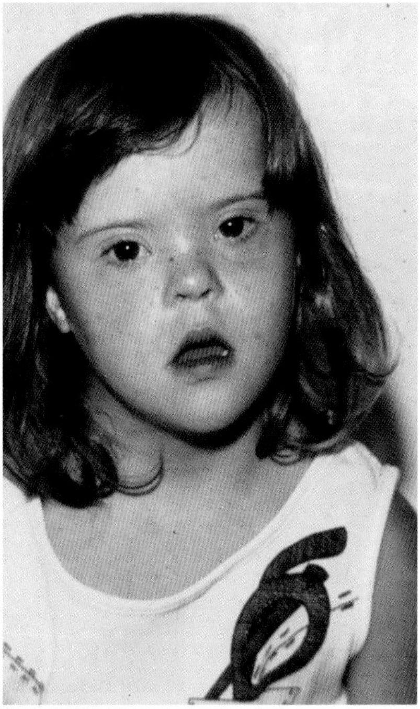

**Figure 25-3**
Upslanted palpebral fissures, characteristic of Down syndrome. (*From Hoyme HE. Assessing dysmorphology in primary care. In: Saul RA, ed.* Medical Genetics in Pediatric Practice. *Elk Grove Village, IL: American Academy of Pediatrics; 2013:135–174. Courtesy of Greenwood Genetic Center, Greenwood, SC.*)

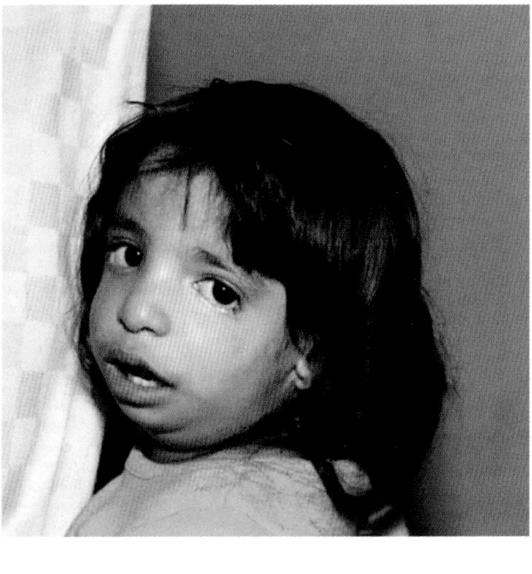

**Figure 25-4**
Treacher Collins syndrome. *(Courtesy of Marilyn Jones, MD)*

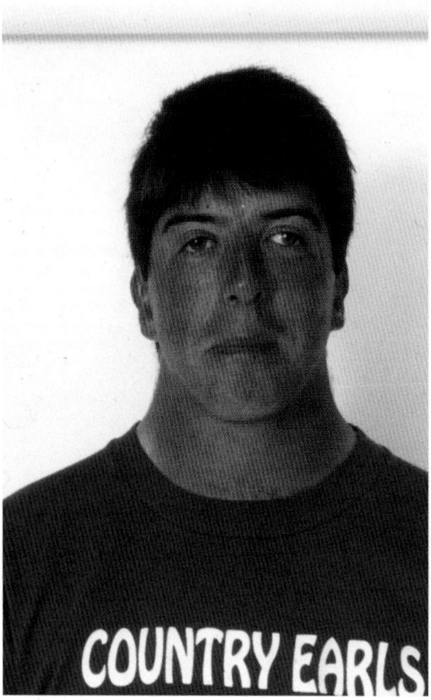


**Figure 25-5**
Downslanted palpebral fissures, characteristic of Noonan syndrome. (*From Hoyme HE. Assessing dysmorphology in primary care. In: Saul RA, ed.* Medical Genetics in Pediatric Practice. *Elk Grove Village, IL: American Academy of Pediatrics; 2013:135–174. Courtesy of Greenwood Genetic Center, Greenwood, SC.*)

Features of the nose—especially the nasal bridge, which can be flattened in Down syndrome or prominent as in velocardiofacial syndrome—should be noted. Are the nares oriented normally, or are they tipped back (a condition known as anteversion)? Is the body of the nose normal, or is it deficient?[6]

In evaluating the malar region, the ears should be checked for size (measured and plotted on growth charts that record length for age), shape (noting abnormal folding or flattening of the helices), position (ears are described as low set if the top of the ear is below a line drawn from the outer canthus to the occiput) and orientation (posterior rotation is present when the ear seems to be turned toward the rear of the head). Ears may be low set because they are small (or microtic) or because of a malformation of the mandibular region.

Finally, the examiner should evaluate the mandibular region, the area encompassing the lower portions of each ear and including the lower jaw. In most newborns, the chin is retruded (slightly set back behind the vertical line extending from the forehead to the philtrum). If the mandible itself is small, then it is described as micrognathic, whereas an unusually prominent mandible is described as prognathic. Significant micrognathia is seen in the Pierre Robin malformation sequence.[4]

## Remainder of the Body

Once facial dysmorphic features have been detected, the primary care physician must conduct a thorough examination looking for additional unusual findings. Again, findings may point to a specific diagnosis.

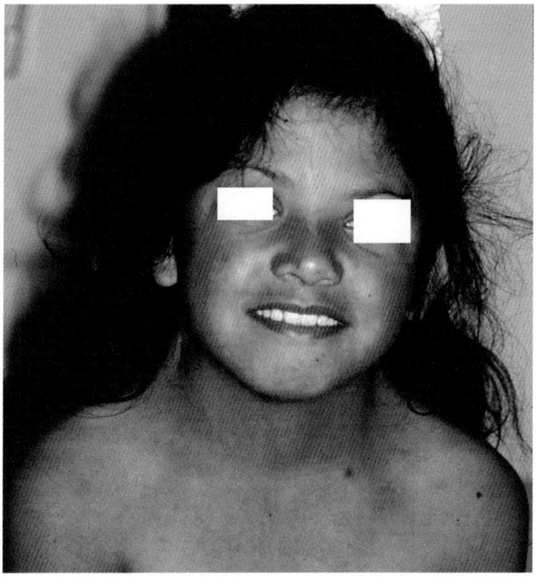

**Figure 25-6**
Webbed neck, characteristic of Turner syndrome. (*From Hoyme HE. Assessing dysmorphology in primary care. In: Saul RA, ed.* Medical Genetics in Pediatric Practice. *Elk Grove Village, IL: American Academy of Pediatrics; 2013:135–174. Courtesy of Lynne Bird, MD.*)

**NECK.** Examination of the neck may reveal webbing, a feature common in Turner (Figure 25-6) and Noonan syndromes, or shortening, as is occasionally seen in some skeletal dysplasias and in conditions in which anomalies of the cervical spine occur, such as Klippel-Feil syndrome. The position of the posterior hairline should also be evaluated, and the size of the thyroid gland should be assessed.[6]

**TRUNK.** The chest should be examined for shape (a shieldlike chest is found in Noonan and Turner syndromes) and symmetry (hypoplasia of the pectoralis major and minor muscles, leading to asymmetry, is a feature of the Poland malformation sequence). A pectus deformity of the chest (either pectus excavatum or pectus carinatum) is usually an isolated finding but is a cardinal feature of Marfan syndrome. Scoliosis, also usually an isolated feature, is often seen in individuals with Marfan syndrome, as well as in several other disorders.[6]

**EXTREMITIES.** Anomalies of the extremities are common in many congenital malformation syndromes. All joints should be examined for range of motion. The presence of single or multiple joint contractures suggests either intrinsic neuromuscular dysfunction, as in the case of some forms of muscular dystrophy, or external deforming forces that limited motion of the joint in utero. Radioulnar synostosis, an inability to pronate or supinate the elbow, occurs in fetal alcohol syndrome and in some X chromosome aneuploidy syndromes (such as *48, XXXX* and *48, XXXY syndromes*).[6]

Next, the hands should be examined. Polydactyly (the presence of extra digits) occurs in isolation as an autosomal dominant trait in up to 1% of all newborns, but can also be seen as part of a malformation syndrome such as trisomy 13. Oligodactyly (a deficiency in the number of digits) is seen in Fanconi syndrome (growth restriction, aplastic anemia, development of leukemia or lymphoma and associated heart, renal and limb defects, including radial aplasia and thumb malformation or aplasia), in which it is generally part of a more severe limb reduction defect, or secondary to intrauterine amputation that may occur with *amniotic band disruption sequence* (Figure 25-7). Syndactyly (a joining of 2 or more digits) is also common to several syndromes, including Smith-Lemli-Opitz syndrome.[6]

Dermatoglyphics, especially the palmar crease pattern, are also important to note. A transverse palmar crease (Figure 25-8), indicative of hypotonia during early fetal life,

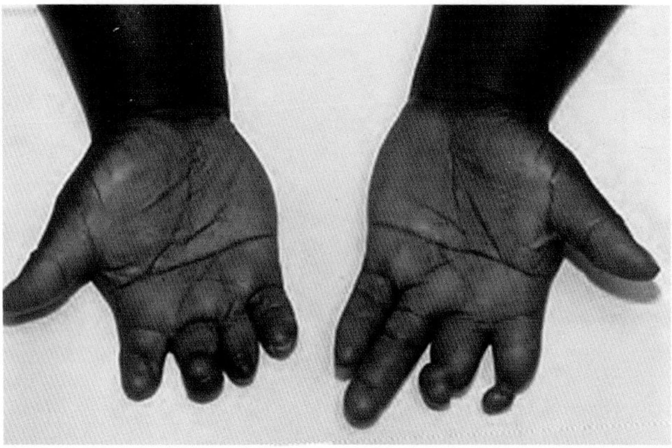

**Figure 25-7**
Amniotic bands. (*From Hoyme HE. Assessing dysmorphology in primary care. In: Saul RA, ed.* Medical Genetics in Pediatric Practice. *Elk Grove Village, IL: American Academy of Pediatrics; 2013:135–174.*)

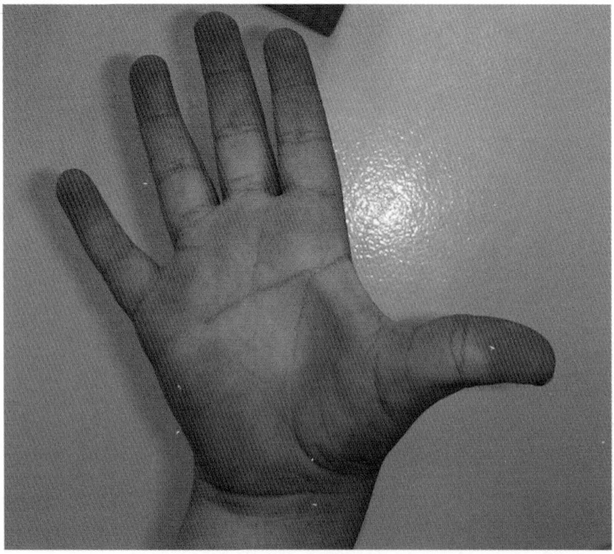

**Figure 25-8**
Single palmar crease. (*From Hoyme HE. Assessing dysmorphology in primary care. In: Saul RA, ed.* Medical Genetics in Pediatric Practice. *Elk Grove Village, IL: American Academy of Pediatrics; 2013:135–174. Courtesy of Lynne Bird, MD.*)

is seen in approximately 50% of children with Down syndrome (and 10% of individuals in the general population). A characteristic palmar crease pattern is also seen in fetal alcohol syndrome.[6]

**GENITALIA.** Genitalia should be examined for abnormalities in structure. In male infants, if the penis seems short, then it should be measured and plotted on an appropriate growth chart. Ambiguous genitalia can be associated with endocrinologic disorders such as congenital adrenal hyperplasia (female infants have masculinized external genitalia, but male genitalis may be unaffected), chromosomal disorders such as Turner syndrome mosaicism, or part of a multiple malformation disorder such as Smith-Lemli-Opitz syndrome. Although hypospadias, which occurs in 1 in 300 male newborns, is a common congenital malformation that often occurs as an isolated defect, if it is associated with other anomalies, then the possibility of a syndrome is strong.[6]

## Laboratory Evaluation

Following completion of the medical history, family history, and physical examination, the dysmorphologist takes the clues that have been gathered and attempts to solve the puzzle by assembling them into a diagnosis. The differential diagnosis is made up of conditions that feature some or all of the clues. Once this list has been assembled, a series of laboratory and imaging tests can be performed in an attempt to arrive at a definitive diagnosis. Typical tests used by the dysmorphologist are outlined here.

Chromosomal microarray analysis (CMA), should be routinely ordered for children with

- Multiple congenital anomalies
- The involvement of 1 major organ system and 2 or more dysmorphic features
- The presence of intellectual disability
- The presence of an autism spectrum disorder

Chromosome analysis (karyotype) will identify conditions caused by too much chromosomal material (ie, trisomies) or those with too little chromosomal material (ie, monosomies). However, karyotype will only identify large abnormalities. Chromosomal microarray uses DNA technology to identify smaller partial trisomies or monosomies than can be seen by karyotype, making it about 4 to 5 times more sensitive. This technique compares the amount of DNA from the patient to that of a control, looking for changes in the number of DNA copies. It is able to look for copy number changes throughout the genome. CMA will not identify balanced rearrangments such as translocations or inversions, so if this is suspected, karyotype should be ordered.

Fluorescent in situ hybridization (FISH) uses DNA technology to identify specific regions of the genome that are either missing or duplicated. FISH uses a DNA probe that is complementary to a specific region of the genome. After a fluorescent marker is attached to this probe, it is incubated with chromosomal DNA from the patient. If the sequence is present in the patient, then the probe will hybridize, its presence announced by the appearance of the bound fluorescent marker.

A FISH study is requested when a syndrome with a known chromosomal defect is suspected. Such disorders as velocardiofacial syndrome (deletion of *22q11.2*), Prader-Willi syndrome (deletion of *15q11.2*), Angelman syndrome (deletion of *15q11.2*), and Beckwith-Wiedemann syndrome (duplication of *11p15.2*) are included in this group. It may also be used to confirm findings of a CMA.

In a growing number of disorders, *direct DNA* analysis can be performed to identify specific mutations known to cause disease. Because the list of these disorders increases every day, using Web-based resources for the most recent information is necessary. An extremely helpful Web site is www.genetests.org. Frequently updated, Genetests provides information about the availability of testing for specific conditions and identifies laboratories performing the testing. Newer technologies, termed next-generation sequencing, are emerging that perform DNA analysis of multiple genes in a single test. These emerging techniques, including whole exome sequencing and whole genome sequencing, will allow for better diagnosis of disorders caused by multiple genes, and the identification of genes for disease in which the cause remains elusive.

Radiologic imaging plays an important role in the evaluation of children with dysmorphic features. Individuals found to have multiple external malformations should have a thorough evaluation to search for the presence of internal malformations. Testing might include ultrasound evaluations of the head and abdomen, the latter area to look for anomalies in the kidney, bladder, liver, and spleen. Skeletal radiographs should be taken if concern exists about a possible skeletal dysplasia. The presence of a heart murmur should trigger a cardiology consultation, and an electrocardiogram and echocardiogram may be indicated. Magnetic resonance imaging may be indicated in children with neurologic abnormalities or spinal defects. The presence of craniosynostosis indicates the need for a 3-dimensionally reconstructed computed tomographic *scan* of the head.

## ▶ DIAGNOSIS

Although the presence of characteristic findings may sometimes make the definitive diagnosis of a malformation syndrome simple, in most cases no specific diagnosis is immediately evident. Some constellations of findings are rare, and finding a match may prove difficult. In many cases, all laboratory tests are normal, and confirmation relies on subjective findings. Clinical geneticists have attempted to resolve this difficulty by developing scoring systems, cross-referenced tables of anomalies that help in developing a differential diagnosis, and even computerized diagnostic programs.

An accurate diagnosis is important for 3 reasons as follows:

1. It offers the family an explanation of why their child was born with congenital anomalies. This information may help allay feelings of guilt, given that parents often believe that they are responsible for their child's problem.
2. The natural history of many disorders is well described; as such, a diagnosis allows the physician to anticipate medical problems associated with a particular syndrome and to perform appropriate screening. A diagnosis may also provide reassurance that other medical problems are no more likely to occur than they might with other children who do not have the diagnosis.
3. It permits accurate recurrence risk for future progeny; only after a diagnosis is confirmed can genetic counseling and, eventually, preimplantation genetic diagnosis or prenatal diagnostic testing be performed.

Once a definitive diagnosis has been made, the dysmorphologist must meet with the family in person to explain the condition and the prognosis. Such meetings are often difficult, since this is the moment that the news is first delivered to the parents and the full effect of the child's condition is realized. A sufficient amount of time should be allotted for this meeting because families may have many questions, and each question should be answered in a thoughtful and considerate way. It is also often helpful to include social support professionals as participants in these meetings; genetic counselors, social workers and psychologists can help the family accept the news and begin moving on with the next phase of their lives.

The diagnosis also enables the physician to provide the family with educational materials about their child's condition. Additionally, many condition-specific support groups exist and the physician can provide the family with information about such groups in their area. These groups offer social and emotional assistance for the family of a child with a newly diagnosed genetic disorder. The Internet has become an important source for parents seeking information about their child's condition, but care should be exercised because information on the Internet is not always subject to editorial control, and some of the information may be inaccurate, or at times misleading or inappropriate. Physicians should try to screen Web sites before they suggest them to the family. Some recommendations of Web sites can be found in the Tools for Practice section at the end of this chapter.

## ▶ SUMMARY

The physician confronted with a patient who has dysmorphic facial features must decide whether the patient or family will benefit from a thorough evaluation or referral. The most important task initially is to determine whether the features are consistent with the individual's genetic background or whether they represent an abnormal phenotype. Through systematic gathering of information, the physician should attempt to establish an etiologic diagnosis and then convey the implications (including genetic counseling) to the appropriate family members.

### *TOOLS FOR PRACTICE*

#### Engaging Patient and Family

- *Congenital Abnormalities* (fact sheet), American Academy of Pediatrics (www.healthychildren.org/English/health-issues/conditions/developmental-disabilities/Pages/Congenital-Abnormalities.aspx)

#### Medical Decision Support

- *Genetests* (Web site), (www.genetests.org)
- *Genetic Alliance* (Web site), (www.geneticalliance.org/ws_display.asp?filter=home)
- *Management of Genetic Syndromes,* 3rd ed (book), John Wiley & Sons
- *March of Dimes* (Web site), (www.marchofdimes.com)
- *National Organization for Rare Diseases* (Web site), (www.rarediseases.org)
- *Online Mendelian Inheritance in Man* (Web site), National Center for Biotechnology Information (www.ncbi.nlm.nih.gov/entrez/query.fcgi?db=OMIM)
- *Smith's Recognizable Patterns of Human Malformations*, 6th ed (book), Elsevier

### *REFERENCES*


1. Aase JM. *Diagnostic Dysmorphology.* New York, NY: Plenum; 1990
2. Jones KL. *Smith's Recognizable Patterns of Human Malformation.* 6th ed. Philadelphia, PA: WB Saunders; 2005
3. Graham JM. *Smith's Recognizable Patterns of Human Deformation.* 3rd ed. Philadelphia, PA: WB Saunders; 2007

4. Hennakam RCM, Krantz ID, Allanson JE. *Gorlin's Syndromes of the Head and Neck.* 5th ed. New York, NY: Oxford University Press; 2010
5. Dattani MT, Martinez-Barbera JP, Thomas PQ, et al. Mutations in the homeobox gene HESX1/Hesx1 associated with septo-optic dysplasia in human and mouse. *Nat Genet.* 1998;19:125–133
6. Levy PA, Marion RW. Human genetics and dysmorphology. In: Marcdante KJ, Kliegman RM, Behrman RE, Jenson HB. *Nelson Essentials of Pediatrics.* 6th ed. Philadelphia, PA: Elsevier Saunders; 2011
7. Nuckolls GH, Shum L, Slavkin HC. Progress toward understanding craniofacial malformations. *Cleft Palate Craniofac J.* 1999;36:12–26
8. Winter RM. What's in a face. *Nat Genet.* 1996;12(2):130–136

# Chapter 26

# Failure to Thrive: Pediatric Undernutrition

*Andrew D. Racine, MD, PhD*

The unfortunate term *failure to thrive* has burdened generations of physicians and their patients as an unenlightening phrase that combines a heterogeneous group of infants and young children with nothing more in common than a growth pattern irreconcilable with a predetermined standard for age. Abnormalities ranging from congestive heart failure to psychosocial deprivation can eventually lead to the same place, called failure to thrive. To find a child in such a location, however, tells us little about the direction from which he or she strayed to come to our attention. Moreover, the term failure to thrive is as pejorative as it is devoid of content; thus, recent scholarship has favored phrases such as *pediatric undernutrition*, as used in the *Bright Futures in Practice* literature,[1] or *weight faltering,* as adopted by our British colleagues.[2]

Given the diversity of potential causes, evaluation and management of a child who fails to gain weight adequately represent a formidable challenge that requires of the physician:

- A determination to listen attentively and examine thoroughly, given that no adequate substitute has yet been found for a complete history and physical examination
- A broad familiarity with the many pathophysiologic sequences that can give rise to this condition
- An understanding of healthy infant behavior and development to identify aberrancies that may threaten weight gain at different ages
- A capacity to gather and synthesize information about the physical, psychological, emotional, familial, and social contexts of the patient's presentation
- A willingness to work with a team of other medical professionals to evaluate and manage the child
- The patience to persevere for as long as required to establish adequate weight gain

## ▶ DEFINITION

A diagnosis generally signals the culmination of a process of evaluation. By contrast, the diagnosis of failure to thrive merely serves to *initiate* the evaluation of a patient who has an abnormal pattern of weight gain. Deviation from normal weight gain has been defined conventionally by reference to age-adjusted nationally standardized norms of weight and rate of weight gain.[3] Infants or young children who either fall below a given weight-for-age or weight-for-height percentile, or whose rate of weight gain has declined across 2 major percentiles (ie, 90th, 75th, 50th, 25th, 10th, or 5th) invite close scrutiny. The Social Security Administration, for example, defines failure to thrive as a fall in weight to below the third percentile or to less than 75% of the median weight-for-height or weight-for-age percentile in children younger than 2 years.[4]

Static measurements of a child's weight-for-age or weight-for-height percentile that document a child's *size* should be distinguished from repeated measurements over time that record a child's *growth*. A deviation from the norm in size may or may not, depending on the clinical circumstances, indicate an abnormality of growth.

A clinical entity defined by reference to statistical norms merits some additional comment. First, although an occasional child may have obvious signs of severe malnutrition at the initial examination, a single observation of weight in a child is generally insufficient to make any diagnosis. The concern here, for the most part, is with children who exhibit abnormal patterns of weight gain over time.

Second, although the aim is to identify children whose weight or weight gain is abnormal, some children will fall into the extreme tails of the standard distributions, be it 10%, 5%, or 3%, of any cohort. The farther out on the curve we observe any individual child, however, the more likely the child is to be truly abnormal with respect to weight-for-age or weight-for-height percentile.

Third, the national reference charts for children's anthropometric measurements are constructed by using serial cross-sections of children, not longitudinal observations of cohorts as they grow. Therefore, the rate at which a child gains weight individually will differ from tracks across collections of different children at different ages that appear on these charts. Over time, children's weights generally regress toward the mean, with heavier infants gaining weight at slower rates than lighter infants. To account for this pattern, British researchers developed weight charts from a cohort of 3,418 full-term infants from Newcastle based on standard deviations of weight changes over time. These charts have wider percentile channels at upper weights and narrower channels at lower weights.[2]

Finally, statistical descriptions must not be allowed to obscure the salient feature common to most children who fail to gain weight adequately: they suffer from malnutrition and are therefore at risk for its attendant consequences. When acute malnutrition results in decreased weight-for-age percentile, the condition is referred to as *wasting*. If caloric deprivation is prolonged, it will eventually affect the child's linear growth, at which point the child is said to be *stunted*. Abnormalities in linear growth not accompanied by wasting (the child who has short stature alone) are not the subject of failure to thrive.

One common set of criteria defines failure to thrive in children younger than 2 years as[5]

- Weight consistently less than 80% of the median for age, or
- Weight on more than 1 occasion falling below the third percentile for age, or
- Weight that has fallen across 2 major percentiles on growth charts

Until 2006, the instruments most commonly used to track children's height, weight, and head circumference were growth charts published by the National Center for Health Statistics (NCHS) of the Centers for Disease Control and Prevention (CDC)[6] based on data collected on children in the United States between the years 1963 and 1994. These data reflected the actual growth of infants and children from a fairly homogeneous population with respect to its racial composition and also depicted the weights of a population most of whose members were formula fed.

In response to these and other shortcomings, in 2006 an expert panel with representatives from the CDC, the National Institutes of Health, and the American Academy of Pediatrics recommended adoption of the international growth charts for children 0 to 24 months of age released that year by the World Health Organization (WHO).[7] The data used to compile these charts were collected between 1997 and 2003 from six sites around the world. These charts are described as representing *standards,* meaning that they capture " . . . the growth of healthy children in optimal conditions," rather than the reference charts from the NCHS that they were designed to replace, which described " . . . how certain children grew in a particular place and time." The expert panel recommended continued use of the older NCHS charts for children 24 to 59 months, where discrepancies between the NCHS and WHO charts were felt to be negligible.

Common cutoff values used to identify children in need of more intense scrutiny differ between the NCHS charts and the WHO charts. The accepted value used with the NCHS charts is the 5th percentile, whereas the recommendation based on the WHO charts suggests concentrating on infants who fall below the 2.3rd percentile. Thus, although the older NCHS reference charts could have been anticipated to identify as many as 10% of children seen in outpatient settings[8] and 3% to 5% of hospital admissions, those fulfilling equivalent criteria using the WHO cutoffs are likely to be less numerous.[7,9] Children who exhibit weights from 61% to 75% of the median for age on the new charts are fewer still but require intensive outpatient monitoring. When a child's weight falls below 60% of the median for age on the new charts, the associated morbidity is severe and warrants inpatient hospitalization.[10] Children from lower socioeconomic backgrounds may be at heightened risk for malnutrition and consequent wasting.[11]

## ▶ HEALTHY WEIGHT GAIN IN INFANTS

Both the NCHS and the WHO growth charts have received widespread application as tools for plotting the growth patterns of healthy infants and children. The ease of their use makes them ideal screening instruments, but, as with all screening tools, their sensitivity and specificity are limited. They do not, for example, take into account parental size or the presence of preexisting chromosomal abnormalities, leading some researchers to argue for the use of standards that control for mean parental height or the presence of certain genetic conditions such as trisomy 21. The *Bright Futures* publication on nutrition provides references for growth charts based on specific disorders.[1]

Recent studies examined the rate at which infants gain weight[12] and how regression to the mean reflects the tendency of some heavier infants to gain weight more slowly and some lighter infants to gain weight more quickly over time.[2] The mean weight of a newborn is approximately 3.25 kg (±0.9 kg.). Many infants lose between 6% and 10% of this weight in the first week as they undergo the normal diuresis associated with adaptation to the extrauterine environment. Birth weight usually is regained by the age of 10 days. Because a newborn's weight at birth predominantly reflects the influence of maternal characteristics and the intrauterine environment, it is an imperfect reflection of genetic growth potential. By 4 to 8 weeks of age, however, much catch-up growth in babies born "light for dates" has already occurred; thus, an infant's weight at this time seems to be a more reliable predictor than birth weight or weight at 12 months.[13] In general, infants can be expected to gain a mean of 30 g (±15 g) a day during the first 3 months of life. Infants will usually triple their birth weight by 1 year of age, at which time the mean daily weight gain has declined to approximately 10 g (±3 g). Characteristics of maternal and child feeding behaviors may have important influence on the rate of weight gain in the first year of life among subpopulations of infants with feeding difficulties.[14]

## ▶ PATHOGENESIS

Infants and children grow in the presence of adequate amounts of 4 fundamental constituents: oxygen, substrate, hormones, and love. Deficiency of any one or a combination of these impedes normal weight gain. Oxygen deprivation at the tissue level from causes as diverse as congestive heart failure, chronic lung disease, or anemia will result in poor weight gain. Inadequate calories, protein, or micronutrients either from environmental deprivation, malabsorption, or inability to metabolize them at the tissue level also inhibit normal weight gain. Deficiencies in growth hormone, insulin-like growth factors, glucocorticoids, thyroid hormone, and other regulators of growth can result in failure to thrive. Finally, infants or children severely deprived of affection will often not grow despite what appears to be normal caloric intake.[15] Chronic disease from many causes will interrupt normal weight gain through the induction of anorexia, malabsorption, increased metabolic needs, and the elaboration of inflammatory mediators, including tumor necrosis factor. Children with chromosomal or other genetic abnormalities, although they may exhibit idiosyncratic growth patterns specific to their particular condition, will also attain their full growth potential only in the presence of these critical ingredients.

In the past, patients with inadequate weight gain were classified as a minority whose difficulty stemmed from a readily identifiable *organic* cause, and a majority whose problem was categorized as *nonorganic*.[5] Other researchers emphasized the overlapping nature of these distinctions and have suggested a third, or *mixed*, category of failure to thrive.[16] More recent approaches have tended to depart from the organic–nonorganic dichotomy in recognition of the somewhat arbitrary nature of this distinction.

A more useful categorization of infants and children who have inadequate weight gain acknowledges an imbalance between the energy needs of the organism that does not grow and the energy at its disposition. The largest share of energy consumed, about 55% to 60%, is devoted to maintaining a basal metabolic rate. An additional 5% to 10% of energy is lost in urine and stool, 5% is accounted for by specific dynamic action, 15% is used for normal physical activity above basal metabolic functions, and 15% is directed toward growth. To provide for all these functions, infants need approximately 100 to 110 kcal/kg/day.

An imbalance between energy needs and energy supplies can arise either from increases in the former or deficiencies in the latter. Box 26-1 lists conditions that increase the energy needs of the organism. Energy needs increase either with increases in the intensity of energy expenditure or decreases in the efficiency of energy use. Conditions that increase the intensity of energy expenditure include chronic heart disease, chronic lung disease, chronic anemia, chronic infection, certain endocrine abnormalities, malignancy, and intoxications. The efficiency of energy utilization can be compromised by chronic infection, chronic renal disease, hepatic insufficiency, inborn errors of metabolism, hormonal abnormalities, certain genetic syndromes, and deficiencies of various micronutrients, including iron, zinc, and carnitine.

BOX 26-1

## *Conditions That Increase Energy Needs*

**INCREASED INTENSITY OF ENERGY UTILIZATION**

- Chronic heart disease (congenital or acquired)
- Chronic lung disease (bronchopulmonary dysplasia, cystic fibrosis, pulmonary lymphangiectasis)
- Chronic anemia (hemoglobinopathies, enzyme deficiencies, membrane abnormalities)
- Chronic infection (urinary tract infections, respiratory infections, tuberculosis)
- Endocrine abnormalities (hyperthyroidism)
- Malignancy (neuroblastoma, ganglioneuroma)

**DRUGS OR TOXINS OR DECREASED EFFICIENCY OF ENERGY UTILIZATION**

- Chronic infection
- Chronic renal disease
- Hepatic insufficiency (cirrhosis)
- Metabolic disease (disorders of amino acid or carbohydrate metabolism, idiopathic hypercalcemia of infancy)
- Hormonal disturbances (hypopituitarism, hypoparathyroidism, chronic adrenocortical insufficiency, diabetes insipidus, hypothyroidism)
- Genetic conditions (Down syndrome, de Lange syndrome, cri du chat syndrome, Smith-Lemli-Opitz syndrome, familial dysautonomia)
- Micronutrient deficiencies (iron, zinc, carnitine)

Conditions leading to deficiency in energy supply are listed in Box 26-2. These conditions originate because calories are either withheld from or improperly presented to the child because they are refused, vomited, not ingested, or not absorbed.

In the category of caloric deprivation, nutritional deprivation in utero that may result in permanent growth restriction must be included. After delivery, a newborn may not receive sufficient calories because of parenting difficulties ranging from unfamiliarity with proper preparation of infant formula[17] or appropriate breastfeeding techniques, to psychosocial dysfunction, to maternal depression, and even to frank abuse or neglect.[18] Other conditions that fall into this category include economic deprivation, unsound parental beliefs regarding nutrition,[19] and subtle central nervous system abnormalities in the child causing him or her to be a difficult feeder.

Food refusal in children, beginning even in infancy,[20] can result from many causes, including pain (from reflux esophagitis), psychosocial adjustment disorders from emotional deprivation, anorexia from chronic infection or intoxication, and structural abnormalities resulting in dysphagia. Structural malformations of the nose or oropharynx, such as cleft palate, choanal atresia, or Treacher Collins syndrome, can lead to an inability to ingest nutrients properly, as can muscular weakness, cerebral palsy or other central nervous system abnormalities, and diseases that give rise to excessive dyspnea.

Vomiting caused by structural abnormalities of the gastrointestinal tract, increased intracranial pressure from any source, chronic acidosis, rumination, and gastroesophageal reflux may all impede growth through caloric deprivation.

The principal organ of nutrient absorption is the small bowel. Malabsorption can occur from gross structural abnormalities, inflammatory conditions, infectious agents, or disorders of organs that elaborate enzymes essential for digestion.

BOX 26-2

## *Conditions That Result in Deficient Energy Supply*

- Calories withheld
- In utero conditions
- Formula preparation mistakes
- Breastfeeding difficulties
- Parent–child psychosocial dysfunction
- Maternal depression
- Intentional abuse or neglect
- Poverty
- Unsound parental beliefs regarding nutrition
- Feeding difficulties
- Calories not properly ingested or digested
- Oral pain caused by dental disease
- Anorexia (reflux esophagitis, emotional deprivation, chronic infection, dysphagia)
- Structural abnormalities of the oropharynx or nasopharynx (cleft palate, choanal atresia, Treacher Collins syndrome, Pierre Robin syndrome, laryngeal web)
- Structural abnormalities of the gastrointestinal tract (stenosis or atresia of the esophagus or duodenum, tracheoesophageal fistula, vascular ring, strictures, achalasia, malrotation, antral web, pyloric stenosis)
- Neuromuscular disorders (cerebral palsy, hydrocephalus, myopathies)
- Conditions leading to excessive dyspnea (congestive heart failure, chronic lung disease)
- Vomiting and rumination
- Malabsorption
- Small bowel disease (celiac disease, inflammatory bowel disease, disaccharide malabsorption, intestinal lymphangiectasia, jejunal atresia, duplication cysts, chronic parasitic infections)
- Pancreatic disease (cystic fibrosis, Shwachman-Diamond syndrome, chronic pancreatitis)
- Liver disease (cirrhosis, intrahepatic cholestatic syndromes, biliary atresia)

In consideration of these potential causes for inadequate weight gain, 2 cardinal principles should be emphasized. First, most cases encountered in ambulatory practice will result from inadequate caloric intake, with most of these originating in a disturbance in the parent–child feeding behavior.[21,22] At one time, maternal mental health disorders were thought to account for the majority of these cases. The particular issue of maternal depression as a risk factor for failure to gain weight in infancy has received wide attention in the literature.[23] Although case-control studies have indicated a possible association between these 2 conditions,[24] more definitive population-based cohort studies have failed to confirm this finding.[25,26] Recent analysis dissected a more subtle web of causation.[27] The term *transactional model* allows for the complex interplay of social conditions,[28] family interactions,[29] and individual psychodynamics[30] in creating feeding abnormalities. The salient feature that distinguishes infants in this category who do not gain weight at the same rate as their peers is that they take in foods with less total energy.[31]

Second, a thorough history and physical examination is the surest route to diagnosis for the residual minority of cases not caused by caloric insufficiency. If the cause of the problem is not made clear by history and physical examination, then laboratory investigation is unlikely to reveal it.[9,32]

## ▶ EVALUATION

Prompt evaluation of infants and children who do not gain weight as expected is important. The history and physical examination should be directed toward certain areas (see later discussion), and in cases in which psychosocial features predominate, most laboratory tests may be unnecessary.

## ▶ HISTORY

### Initial Approach

Every evaluation of an infant or child who is not gaining weight must begin with a thorough history. Although the history and physical examination will usually be conducted in the office, a home visit affords the pediatrician an opportunity to observe the family interaction around feeding in the context in which it normally occurs. A history of the present illness should assemble all data available from previous anthropometric measurements of the patient, including weight, height, and head circumference. Premature infants should have their measurements corrected for gestational age until 18 months of age for head circumference, 24 months of age for weight, and 40 months of age for height.[33] The physician should begin by asking the principal caregivers how they think the baby is doing and what they believe is the problem. Knowledge of a parent's frame of mind may propel further evaluation toward or away from difficulty in parent–child interaction, including child neglect, as a potential explanation for a child's lack of weight gain.

### Feeding

A thorough feeding history is essential. Is the baby bottle fed or breastfed? How often does the child breastfeed, and for how long? Does the mother feel as though the child is sucking well, and does the baby appear sated after he or she feeds? If bottle fed, how in detail is the formula prepared and by whom? What is the baby's sleep pattern, and how many ounces will the baby take in a 24-hour period? Does the infant wet 6 to 8 diapers a day? Consider observing a feeding, which can be done while taking the history.

For older children, when were solids introduced? Does the parent find the child to be a *picky eater* or difficult to interest in food? Does the child drink excessive amounts of juice during the day, substituting for more calorie-rich nutrients? What are meal times like at home? Where does the child eat, and with whom? Are distractions, such as television or video games, present during meals? Is food being used for discipline or in battles over control? A 24-hour dietary recall of a typical day can often help quantify the caloric intake of the patient. If this information proves difficult to elicit, then the parents can be sent home with a nutritional diary to fill out prospectively and bring in at the next visit.

### Vomiting

The physician should inquire about any vomiting or spitting up, being sure to explore frequency, volume, and presence of blood or bile in the emesis. Gastric outlet obstructions (pyloric stenosis, antral web) often result in the generation of significant propulsive forces leading to projectile vomiting, whereas gastroesophageal reflux often results in less dramatic patterns of regurgitation. An obstruction distal to the ligament of Treitz will generally produce bilious vomiting, a symptom that must be taken with utmost seriousness in infancy because it may indicate the presence of a malrotation and midgut volvulus.

### Stools

The pattern and frequency of stooling must not be overlooked in the history of present illness. The child who has liquid stools may have a small-bowel pathologic condition, and bulky, foul-smelling stools may result from fat malabsorption. If mucus or blood is in the stools, an inflammatory condition may be present.

### Medical History

Additional information should be obtained as part of the medical history, beginning with the parents' attitudes regarding their decision to have a baby and what their experience with the pregnancy was like. Did the mother gain a reasonable amount of weight? Did she experience any illnesses during her pregnancy? Hypertension or preeclampsia will result in an infant who is small for gestational age; gestational diabetes may produce an infant with macrosomia who fails to gain weight because of postnatal cardiac complications.

The physician should ask about specific toxic exposures in utero, particularly to tobacco, marijuana, and alcohol. Tobacco may result in a small baby who rapidly catches up in weight with her peers, whereas marijuana and alcohol exert an influence on growth that may be sustained throughout childhood.[34] Recording the child's gestational age at birth, any unusual complications of the labor and delivery, and the presence of malformations or other obvious deformities will complete this portion of the history.

### Family History

A family history should document the growth patterns of siblings; record the occurrence of fetal loss or infant deaths; review the presence in the family of immune deficiencies, neurologic disorders, or metabolic derangements; and highlight any unexplained growth deficiencies in close relatives. These findings may provide clues to the cause of the growth abnormality in the child. The results of recent comprehensive longitudinal studies from England emphasize the extent to which mean parental height and parity overwhelm the influence of traditional markers of socioeconomic deprivation that includes parental education or occupational status on the weight gain of young infants.[25]

### Social History

The social history should focus on the availability of social supports for the parents, the existence of economic or legal circumstances that threaten the stability of the family, the nature of the relationship between the parents, and the presence of affective disorders, particularly depression, in either the mother or father. Is there substance abuse in the home, either of alcohol or drugs? Any recent disruptive events in the family's life should be explored to determine what effect they may have had on the parents' ability to care for the patient. Has there been any involvement of the family with child protective services? Finally, at this point, the physician may uncover unrealistic expectations that parents harbor regarding feeding patterns, dietary fads, or behavior in infancy, all of which provide clues to why feeding this infant developed into such a challenge.

## ▶ PHYSICAL EXAMINATION

Repeated anthropometric measurements over time constitute the most important component of the physical evaluation of children who are not gaining weight. On the initial examination, the physician should begin with observing the child's general relatedness to the parents and the examiner. Does the child appear listless, easily distractable, or irritable? Can he or she be engaged to make eye contact or to play with an age-appropriate toy? With the child completely undressed, a notation should be made of any evidence of wasting, of the presence and distribution of normal subcutaneous body fat, of muscle mass and tone, and of the presence of dysmorphic features. These observations will serve to set the stage for more detailed examination.

Particular attention should be paid to organ systems that may reflect evidence of malnutrition. The mucous membranes, hair, nails, and skin develop abnormalities in the presence of vitamin, protein, fat, and micronutrient deficiencies. The head, eyes, ears, nose, and throat may reveal conditions ranging from open fontanelles of hypothyroidism or craniotabes of nutritional rickets to the blurred disk margins of increased intracranial pressure in a child who has chronic emesis or a submucosal cleft of the hard palate in an infant who feeds poorly. Examination of the mouth may reveal extensive dental disease or a dental abscess that can be causing severe pain on oral intake.

The thyroid should be palpated gently and then auscultated for evidence of hyperthyroidism. Examination of the heart and lungs, with observation, palpation, and particularly auscultation, may reveal wheezing, rales, or heart murmurs suggestive of chronic conditions, which often result in substantial energy expenditures that outstrip the supply of nutrients available to the infant. Examination of the digits for clubbing in the older child should not be neglected. A thorough abdominal examination will identify organomegaly associated with tumor, infection, or storage disease. Intestinal distention can be associated with carbohydrate malabsorption from various causes. The neurologic examination may suggest explanations for an infant's inability to ingest adequate calories: disorders of mentation, cranial nerve abnormalities, generalized weakness, or spasticity should be carefully sought.

With infants who are not gaining weight, it can be very informative to observe a feeding. Does the parent make meaningful eye contact with the child and burp the baby appropriately? If there is any question about the adequacy of the baby's swallowing, an assessment by a speech therapist for the efficiency and safety of the swallow can be helpful.

## ▶ LABORATORY EVALUATION

In the absence of evidence from the history or physical examination indicating the need for specific laboratory testing, expectations of the yield of laboratory investigation should be modest. When charts of 185 patients who were hospitalized for failure to thrive at the Children's Hospital of Buffalo were reviewed, only 1.4% of the laboratory studies performed were found to be of diagnostic value.[32] A similar review of 122 infants who were hospitalized at the Boston Children's Hospital revealed that a mean of 40 laboratory tests were ordered, but only 0.8% revealed an abnormality that contributed to a diagnosis.[9]

If the cause of a child's failure to gain weight adequately remains uncertain after careful history and physical examination, then a limited number of screening studies might be considered, including a complete blood count, a blood pH, serum electrolytes, blood urea nitrogen and creatinine, a urinalysis and urine culture, and an examination of the stool for reducing substances, pH, occult blood, and ova and parasites.[35] More extensive testing for malabsorption, endocrine disorders, occult infection, malignancy, and cardiac, pulmonary, or renal abnormalities should be done only when historical or physical examination evidence of these diagnoses is present.

## ▶ THERAPY AND FOLLOW-UP

The therapeutic approach to children failing to gain weight adequately must be tailored to the individual needs of the family and the child. For infants and children in whom a specific diagnosis was identified, therapy should be directed toward the underlying disease or condition. A disturbance in the parent–child interaction will more often be recognized as the cause of the patient's inability to gain weight. Children exhibiting food avoidance behaviors may respond well to interventions that involve differential rewards aimed at extinguishing problematic interactions.[36] Regardless of the underlying cause, the family should be approached nonjudgmentally, and the severity of the child's condition should dictate the initial approach to therapy.

### *Mild to Moderate Undernutrition*

The pediatrician, with consultation from a nutritionist, can manage infants and children exhibiting mild degrees of malnutrition (greater than 80% of ideal body weight for age) as outpatients, with occasional consultation from subspecialist colleagues. Patients who have evidence of more severe caloric deprivation will require the involvement of a multidisciplinary team, including the pediatrician, nutritionist, mental health or behavioral therapist, and social worker.[37] Hospitalization may be necessary for a subset of these patients whose malnutrition is combined with or results from another significant medical condition. Home visitation using professionals[38] has been demonstrated to be a useful intervention in select circumstances. Others, however, have achieved less success in generating improved weight gain with this intervention despite its other notable benefits.[39,40] Child protective services must be alerted about any child thought to be the victim of neglect.

The goals of management must focus on nutritional rehabilitation, parental education, and behavioral intervention. Attempts to overfeed malnourished infants at the outset of therapy should be avoided because initially they may exhibit some degree of anorexia, and refeeding that is too vigorous may induce malabsorption and diarrhea. The refeeding regimen should be calculated to provide about 10% to 15% of calories from protein, 50% to 60% from carbohydrate, and 30% to 40% from fat.[41]

A typical 3-phase regimen[42] may begin with provision of 100% of daily age-adjusted energy and protein requirements based on the child's weight on day 1.

If this phase is well tolerated, in phase 2 intake is then increased to provide adequate nutrition to achieve catch-up growth. Multiplying the age-adjusted energy requirements (kcal/kg/day) by the ratio of the child's ideal body weight for height divided by the child's actual body weight at presentation will generate a reasonable estimate of the nutritional requirements for this stage. The same calculation can be made for protein requirements (Box 26-3). In most instances, the energy and protein requirements for these phases of infant refeeding can be accomplished with the use of a routine infant formula modified to increase its caloric density. Mixing 13 oz of concentrated formula with 10 oz of water rather than 13 oz of water will create a formula that is 24 cal/oz, as will mixing 3 scoops of powdered formula with 5 ounces of water. Alternatively, the use of carbohydrate in the form of glucose polymers or fat in the form of medium-chain triglycerides will add calories while avoiding the complications of overhydration. For older children, the repertoire of caloric supplements will include a wide variety of solid foods as well.

In the third, or consolidation, phase of nutritional rehabilitation, a varied diet is offered ad libitum as the child gradually approaches ideal body weight. Multivitamin and iron supplementation should be part of every refeeding regimen for undernourished children.

Initiation of nutritional rehabilitation is an ideal time to engage the parents in an educational program that focuses on family interactions, psychological vulnerabilities, and social needs.[43] Emphasis should be placed on appropriate nutritional information, and concrete

BOX 26-3

## *Sample Rehabilitation Schedule for Undernutrition*

Scenario: A 6-month-old boy with poor weight gain is referred for nutritional rehabilitation. He currently weighs 5.5 kg and is 67 cm in length. The 50th percentile weight for this length is 7.7 kg, putting the infant at 71% of the ideal body weight for height.

Normal adjustment catch-up requirements include the following:

| | REQUIREMENT | | FACTOR | | REQUIREMENT |
|---|---|---|---|---|---|
| Calorie supplementation | 100 kcal/kg/day | × | 7.7 / 5.5 | = | 140 kcal/kg/day |
| Protein supplementation | 2 g/kg/day | × | 7.7 / 5.5 | = | 2.8 g/kg/day |

Adding a multivitamin with iron to this child's regimen would be advisable.

suggestions should be offered about how to structure mealtime at home to minimize distractions in a relaxed social environment that encourages good eating habits. For families in need, access to community resources such as the Special Supplemental Nutrition Program for Women, Infants, and Children (WIC) and the Supplemental Nutrition Assistance Program (SNAP, formerly food stamps) must be facilitated. Pediatricians should be prepared to advocate vigorously for patients in need of supplemental nutrition or special infant formulas when families experience difficulties in obtaining these products.

### Severe Undernutrition

Children who are less than 60% of ideal body weight for height should be hospitalized, as should any less severely undernourished child who fails to respond to appropriate outpatient management with adequate weight gain. They should be cared for by a multidisciplinary team of nutritionists, social workers, pediatricians, and pediatric subspecialists, with attention to avoiding the refeeding syndrome with its attendant morbidity. The nutritional rehabilitation of these children will be more prolonged and may entail a period of tube feedings in addition to oral supplements. In cases in which the gastrointestinal tract is temporarily inaccessible, parenteral feedings with central venous access may be necessary. The laboratory evaluation of these patients will also need to be more intensive, with appropriate surveillance of potential electrolyte disturbances that can accompany initial refeeding if it is pursued too aggressively.[44]

### Follow-up

Once identified, poor weight gain in infancy should be followed up assiduously. Initial weekly visits for infants may be necessary to reassure the parents and physician that the therapy undertaken is having the desired effects. Studies of hospitalized children demonstrate that those younger than 6 months, when provided with adequate calories, begin to gain weight in a few days.[45] Older children may take longer than their younger counterparts before sustained weight gain is established. Ongoing developmental, behavioral, and social evaluations must be incorporated into any plan for follow-up. Abnormalities in these domains need to be monitored closely because they are frequently present in patients who gain weight poorly. Moreover, the lingering effects of calorie, protein, and micronutrient deprivation may show themselves in developmental and behavioral abnormalities,[46] particularly in families in which the mothers exhibit affective disorders.[47]

## ▶ PROGNOSIS

Outcomes for children who have abnormal weight gain patterns in infancy and childhood should be predicted cautiously in view of the variety of conditions that may give rise to this clinical picture and the lack of high quality data on which reasonable predictions might be sustained. A systematic review of 13 long-term longitudinal studies of children with failure to thrive lamented these methodologic challenges but concluded that the growth and neurocognitive outcomes in these children probably do not differ substantially from their unaffected peers.[48] A less sanguine view was taken by an extensive review of the literature conducted by the Agency for Healthcare Research and Quality, which concluded that children with failure to thrive in infancy are likely to suffer immunologic, behavioral, cognitive, and psychomotor developmental deficits that persist despite interventions.[4] Such disparate findings suggest that most children in the mild category will experience brisk nutritional rehabilitation and, with adequate follow-up, will do quite well. More severely affected children, depending on the cause of their condition, may require more prolonged or repetitive interventions and may be left with residual cognitive, behavioral, and educational consequences of their malnutrition. There is some evidence that intense interventions, including weekly home visitation programs, can, at least in controlled circumstances, attenuate the anthropometric deficiencies that might otherwise result from significant undernutrition in infancy.[49] In light of these findings, all children who exhibit faltering weight gain during infancy and childhood absolutely must receive early comprehensive evaluation and prompt treatment.

### When to Refer

- Diagnosis is made of a chronic disease pertaining to a subspecialty such as cardiology, pulmonary medicine, nephrology, gastroenterology, or endocrinology
- Psychosocial family dynamic indicates a need for psychiatric intervention for either or both parents
- Nutritional rehabilitation warrants the attention of a nutritionist
- Provider is concerned about intentional starvation or neglect, a referral to Child Protective Services must be made

### When to Admit

- Any child with a weight less than 60% of ideal body weight
- Any child who, despite appropriate outpatient management, continues to fail to gain weight at an acceptable rate
- Any child who presents with signs of marasmus or severe protein malnutrition (kwashiorkor)
- Any child for whom the provider believes a period of close, continuous monitoring would be helpful

## *TOOLS FOR PRACTICE*

### Engaging Patient and Family

- *Childhood Nutrition* (fact sheet), American Academy of Pediatrics (www.healthychildren.org/English/healthy-living/nutrition/Pages/Childhood-Nutrition.aspx)
- *Making Sure Your Child Is Eating Enough* (fact sheet), American Academy of Pediatrics (www.healthychildren.org/English/healthy-living/nutrition/Pages/Making-Sure-Your-Child-is-Eating-Enough.aspx)

### Medical Decision Support

- *Growth Charts–Girls* (chart), American Academy of Pediatrics (shop.aap.org)
- *Growth Charts–Boys* (chart), American Academy of Pediatrics (shop.aap.org)
- *Growth Charts–Interactive Tutorials* (Web site), Centers for Disease Control and Prevention (www.cdc.gov/growthcharts)

## *AAP POLICY STATEMENT*

Block RW, Krebs NF; American Academy of Pediatrics Committee on Child Abuse and Neglect and Committee on Nutrition. Failure to thrive as a manifestation of child neglect. *Pediatrics*. 2005;116:1234–1237. Reaffirmed May 2009 (pediatrics.aappublications.org/content/116/5/1234/full)

## *REFERENCES*


1. Holt K, Wooldridge N, Story M, Sofka D, eds. *Bright Futures: Nutrition.* 3rd ed. Elk Grove Village, IL: American Academy of Pediatrics; 2010
2. Wright CM, Avery A, Epstein M, et al. New chart to evaluate weight faltering. *Arch Dis Child.* 1998;78:40–43
3. Drotar D, et al. Early preventive intervention in failure to thrive: methods and early outcome. In: Drotar D, ed. *New Directions in Failure To Thrive: Implications for Research and Practice.* New York, NY: Plenum Press; 1985
4. Perrin E, Frank D, Cole C, et al. *Criteria for Determining Disability in Infants and Children: Failure to Thrive.* Evidence Report/Technology Assessment No. 72 (Prepared by Tufts-New England Medical center Evidence-based Practice Center under Contract No. 290-97-0019). AHRQ Publication No. 03-E026. Rockville, MD: Agency for Healthcare Research and Quality; March 2003.
5. Zenel JA Jr. Failure to thrive: a general pediatrician's perspective. *Pediatr Rev.* 1997;18:371–378
6. Centers for Disease Control and Prevention, National Center for Health Statistics. *CDC Growth Charts: United States.* Available at: www.cdc.gov/growthcharts. Accessed October 15, 2014
7. Grummer-Strawn LM, Reinold C, Krebs NF; Centers for Disease Control and Prevention. Use of World Health Organization and CDC growth charts for children aged 0-59 months in the United States. *MMWR Recomm Rep.* 2010;59:1–15
8. Mitchell WG, Gorrell RW, Greenberg RA. Failure-to-thrive: a study in a primary care setting. Epidemiology and follow-up. *Pediatrics.* 1980;65:971–977
9. Berwick DM, Levy JC, Kleinerman R. Failure to thrive: diagnostic yield of hospitalisation. *Arch Dis Child.* 1982;57:347–351
10. Gomez F, Ramos GR, Frenk S, et al. Mortality in second and third degree malnutrition. *J Trop Pediatr.* 1956;2:77–83
11. Massachusetts Department of Public Health. *The Massachusetts Growth and Nutrition Program—Summary Report FY 1996-FY 2002.* Boston, MA: Massachusetts Department of Public Health, Bureau of Family and Community Health; 2003. Available at: www.mass.gov. Accessed October 15, 2014
12. Guo SM, Roche AF, Fomon SJ, et al. Reference data on gains in weight and length during the first two years of life. *J Pediatr.* 1991;119:355–362

# Chapter 27

# Family Dysfunction

*Mary Iftner Dobbins, MD; Sandra Vicari, PhD, LCPC*

## ▶ INTRODUCTION

Theories of child development have long recognized that children in modern Western cultures require approximately 2 decades of life to achieve the self-sufficiency necessary for separation from their families. Because of this relatively prolonged dependency and because adverse childhood experiences negatively affect the developing brain and long-term health outcomes,[1–4] the functioning of the family is of utmost importance for optimal development and well-being of the child.

Complex sociocultural changes continue to redefine the family, with fewer "traditional" households that historically have consisted of 2 married biologic parents located near extended family members for support.[5,6] Single, divorced, remarried, same-gender, foster, and adoptive parents are commonplace. Children may also experience multiple, changing parental figures if grandparents assume their care or if biologic parents move on to new partners. Many children have half-, step-, or foster siblings. Particularly in times of economic hardship, families may move in together or experience frequent changes in composition.

In the case of separation or divorce, children often live between 2 different households. Children may also be separated from a caregiver for prolonged periods because of parental employment, illness, or incarceration. The mobility of Western society has resulted in the geographic isolation of many nuclear families from extended family support. Oftentimes, nonrelatives assume the roles of extended family members.

Many children have a family that changes dramatically over time. As a result, family may be defined less by composition and more by functional relationships. In fact, the American Academy of Family Physicians (AAFP) states, "The family is a group of individuals with a continuing legal, genetic and/or emotional relationship."[7] The AAFP additionally asserts, "Society relies on the family group to provide for the economic and protective needs of individuals, especially children and the elderly." When children are involved, the most important function of the family is to provide a safe and caring environment in which the child can grow and develop into a healthy adult.

## ▶ FAMILY CHARACTERISTICS

Families function in complex and multifaceted ways, with family members tending to assume various roles that interplay.[8] Changes in the functioning of an individual member affect the family unit, and changes in the family unit affect the individual members and their interactive roles. As a result, a variety of internal and external factors may influence the functioning of a family, and some families are more adaptable and resilient than others.

Healthy families have well-defined roles (ie, parent or child). Members freely ask for and provide attention, but boundaries are respected. Rules tend to be explicit and remain consistent, but with some flexibility to adapt to the individual. Communication is encouraged, and emotional expression is accepted. Security in relationships allows individuals to explore their own interests, and individuation is encouraged. As individual members grow and develop, the family as a unit adapts, also experiencing ongoing intrinsic growth and development over time, which is a sign of health.

All families experience misunderstandings, conflicts, and stressors at some time. Stressors may be internal (eg, illness, change in composition) or external (eg, financial insecurity, relocation). Healthy families cope with difficulties and maintain a sense of connectedness, which fosters a sense of security, self-worth, and competence in their children.

## ▶ PARENT CHARACTERISTICS

For the child, the most critical characteristic of a healthy family is an adult who functions as caregiver. In fact, the most important contributory factor regarding children's resilience is the presence in their lives of at least 1 consistent, caring adult.[9,10] This adult not only addresses safety and basic needs, but also shares an emotional connection with the child, conveying the sense that she has intrinsic value and is loved.

When 2 (or more) caregivers are involved, the relationship between them is exceptionally important. A supportive and flexible partnership fosters good parenting. Even those with very different backgrounds, knowledge, and attitudes can provide a consistent and united approach without undermining each other.

Specific parental practices do not have to be perfect. Although some are more intuitive than others, people with a variety of abilities, personal backgrounds, and personality types can be good parents. However, there are certain characteristics of maturity that are necessary for optimal caregiving—the ability to care for oneself, a sense of self-worth, the ability to emotionally connect with another person, a sense of responsibility, and a degree of selflessness.[8] Healthy parents do not desire a child to fix something in their own lives or relationships.

Parenting styles depend on many factors, including the parent's emotional health, experience in their own family of origin, and experience in the parental role, as well as the influence of or compromise with other adults assuming a co-parenting role, culture, and socioeconomic factors. Some traits are more enduring, but parenting styles may be dynamic because of these changeable influences.[11,12] The needs and temperament of a particular child may also result in variations in parenting. Conversely, children may vary in their response to parenting styles because of their developmental stage, temperament, and degree of resilience.

A parent who can maintain a healthy caregiver role helps the child develop a sense of self-worth and competence, learn to maintain appropriate interpersonal relationships, and plan for her independent future.

### *Effects of Parenting Styles*

Certain parenting styles are characteristic of healthy families. A caring yet authoritative parent will be attentive to the child and responsive to his needs, yet set consistent and developmentally appropriate expectations. Emphasis is placed on the parent-child relationship and communication, and discipline is provided in a constructive fashion that fosters the child's learning and self-control. Growing up in a context of guided yet growing autonomy, these children demonstrate more academic mastery, social and moral maturity, self-regulation, and sense of self-worth as they reach adulthood.[9]

Conversely, some parenting styles may have less favorable outcomes. Authoritarian parents satisfy their own need for control by granting little autonomy while also remaining less interpersonally involved with the child. Expectations for behavior give poor consideration to the needs or developmental abilities of the child, who learns over time that approval and affection may be conditional and unpredictable. Consequently, these children typically have poor self-esteem, are withdrawn and anxious, lack in resourcefulness, and are easily frustrated.[9] They reach adulthood with much less mastery, and often exhibit dependent or aggressive behaviors as adults. Not only are these children at high risk for maltreatment, but they are also at high risk for perpetuating the cycle of maltreatment when they have children of their own.[13–15]

Alternatively, parents may relinquish their authoritative parental role if they are distracted by their own needs or insecure in their parent-child relationship. The resultant permissiveness, whether arising through inattentiveness or overindulgence, grants the child developmentally inappropriate autonomy, adversely affecting their ability to delay gratification and work to meet their own needs. These children enter adulthood with less academic and interpersonal mastery, resulting in less self-control and more demanding and disruptive social behavior.[9]

Parents may also be relatively uninvolved, either from their own emotional detachment or from being overwhelmed by the stressors of their own lives. In the extreme form, this may present as true neglect, and the child may have developmental delays in a variety of areas, including interpersonal attachment. Growing up with little support or discipline, these children often reach adulthood with little emotional, academic, or interpersonal mastery, demonstrating poor self-esteem and antisocial behaviors.[9]

## ▶ FAMILY DYSFUNCTION

Difficult life circumstances may stress family functioning. If these circumstances are short-lived or less severe, healthier families adjust and persevere in their developmental tasks. When families become overwhelmed, composition is unstable, individual members are emotionally unhealthy, roles and boundaries are blurred, or communication is impaired, families may function in variations of chronically maladaptive patterns. When a parent figure fails to maintain a healthy parent role, the child's emotional health and development suffer, with potentially lifelong consequences.

Dysfunction can be subtle or severe. However, consequences of these problems affect almost all aspects of a child's life, including relationships, emotions, behavior, learning, the acquisition of coping skills, and psychological development.[1–4,16] Instead of developing a sense of self-worth and competence, the child incorporates self-doubt and insecurity. The child has difficulty developing trust and the balanced give-and-take of healthy relationships.[17,18] In severe cases, chronic disappointment and frustration lead to hopelessness and limited expectations for the future.[19]

## ▶ PATTERNS OF DYSFUNCTION

Parental dysfunction typically exists in certain core areas. The parent who lacks the desire or ability to emotionally connect with and appreciate the child causes the child to feel devalued and unlovable, undermining the development of healthy attachment. The insecure parent may be overcontrolling in an effort to demonstrate his or her authority, be permissive in an attempt to ensure the child's love, prioritize a partner over caring for the child, or use the child to meet her own needs. The parent who cannot consistently care for him/herself cannot consistently care for the child, resulting in the child's feeling insecure and frustrated. In severe cases, the roles may become reversed, with the child becoming parentified. These characteristics may manifest themselves in many circumstances, but are especially predictable in certain patterns.[8,9]

### Uninvolved Parent

The uninvolved or "inaccessible" parent may be preoccupied with his career, relationships, or community status. As our culture continues to change, even very committed parents may fall into routines that allow less time for their children. They may become caregivers for their own parents or seek new educational or employment opportunities. Families may easily become overscheduled, being "together" disproportionately in a social context rather than as a family unit. In addition, technology frequently replaces, rather than enhances, true interpersonal interaction and communication.

### Over-involved Parent

Conversely, parents may become over-involved for multiple reasons. Commonly, parents attempt to relive their own youth through their children's activities and status, and may allow little individuation or have unhealthy expectations. Additionally, societal factors have resulted in an extreme focus on achievement, and many children grow up in a culture of extreme competition. Even the possibility of failure may be perceived as an unbearable threat to self-worth, despite the fact that optimal development depends on the child's learning by trial and error. Less secure parents may become overprotective and try to lessen either the risks or the consequences for their children. As a result, the child tends to become less self-reliant, have unrealistically entitled expectations for life independent of the family, blame others rather than learn personal responsibility, paradoxically develop a decreased sense of competency, and consider self-worth to be conditional rather than intrinsic.[8,9]

### Divided Loyalties

When power struggles exist in the family, the child may be put in the middle of the conflict. This is especially true in cases of divorce, in which the parents or extended family members may harbor a great deal of unresolved hurt and animosity. The child, now especially vulnerable and insecure as the family restructures, may be considered a trophy, used as a conduit of information, or forced to choose sides. Children tend to blame themselves for the parents' divorce, and often learn to consider love and relationships as conditional. Frequently, they live with unresolved grief. If parents cannot model appropriate conflict resolution, children often become bullies or victims of bullying.[8,9]

### Blurred Roles or Boundaries

If a parent becomes vulnerable (ie, from illness, addiction, financial insecurity, loss of a relationship, or interpersonal violence), the child also becomes vulnerable. Not only has the child lost a degree of support, but the child often takes on a degree of worry about the parent. If stigma is associated with parental impairment (ie, addiction or mental illness), the child may receive little information or guidance to deal with their confusion, fear, and shame over the parent's circumstances. Many children are unable to develop close relationships because of feelings of loneliness and helplessness.[8,9,20,21]

Blurred parent-child roles or boundaries may occur in a variety of circumstances. When a parent is significantly impaired or when a child loses a parent through death or divorce, the child may become parentified, taking on tasks, concerns, and family roles more appropriately associated with an adult caregiver. This typically results in a tremendous amount of stress and can interfere with his or her developmental tasks.[8]

## ▶ PRESENTATIONS IN THE PRIMARY CARE SETTING

Physicians caring for children should be mindful of family functioning as it affects the well-being of the children both physically and emotionally. This is especially true in the setting of the medical home, where a physician with an ongoing relationship with the child and family coordinates continuity of care. The American Academy of Pediatrics (AAP) Task Force on Mental Health has recommended that children's health supervision visits routinely include psychosocial screening of the family, as well as the child.[22–25] However, any encounter provides an opportunity for assessment and intervention as indicated.

Family dysfunction may present in a wide variety of ways in the primary care setting. The appropriateness of physical care is typically more obvious, as the physician assesses safety, growth and development, general health, and medical care. The family who has trouble keeping appointments or completing treatment may be showing signs that the parent is overwhelmed or that there are other barriers to care.[26]

The child in a struggling family often develops signs of stress, which may manifest physically (eg, frequent somatic complaints) or emotionally (eg, mood or behavior changes). Changes in sleep, appetite, energy, motivation, self-care, school achievement, recreational pursuits, or social interactions are cause for some degree of further exploration. Often, parents are unaware of the child's internal distress until external behavior problems (eg, irritability, aggression, school failure, drug use, self-injury) arise.[27,28]

When family disturbance is severe, maltreatment may occur. Pediatricians and other physicians receive formal training in the detection of child abuse and neglect, and are uniformly considered to be mandated reporters for child welfare agencies. However, families (including the victim) often conceal abuse or neglect, necessitating a high index of suspicion. Chronic maltreatment, especially sexual abuse, may only be detected by specific investigation.[14,23]

The growing tendency of families to use emergency departments and urgent care centers in addition to (or instead of) a medical home setting (or even the practice of seeing more than 1 physician within a clinic) undermines continuity of care, and may also mask the degree of dysfunction. The use of multiple physicians should alert the physician to increase vigilance. Appropriate documentation is vital, and forms for release of information facilitate communication among treating physicians.[29]

## ▶ THE PHYSICIAN'S ROLE

Family dynamics are complicated, and patterns of interaction can become quite ingrained. However, support for families can have a profound, positive, and enduring effect for children and those in their lives. For the primary care physician, attention to family functioning is inextricably linked to practice,[5,6,30] providing many opportunities for supporting the development of healthy families as well as for addressing problems as they may arise.

Indeed, the physician-family relationship provides a unique opportunity for positive influence. Families are built on relationships, and the physician supports the family by first developing a therapeutic alliance with the child and caregiver. In this important position, the physician affirms intrinsic dignity and self-worth by modeling healthy, respectful interactions with each.

The preventive aspect of primary care integrates routine anticipatory guidance.[28] This helps parents understand their children, guides them through appropriate caregiving practices, and promotes healthy aspects of family development. Over time, the physician gains understanding of differences in personalities, expectations, and the culture of parenting within the family. This allows further customization of care, with recognition of strengths and anticipation of needed support.

In addition to office visits, most physicians provide supplemental educational material and refer families to parenting classes as available. Some physicians incorporate group checkups or classes of their own to facilitate discussion, involve extended family members, and engender parent-to-parent support.[31] When family problems are apparent, the physician may build on the above practices, remaining constructive and supportive.

The timing of well-child visits correlates with the transitional challenges of various developmental stages. Additional visits may be indicated for circumstances that challenge family members, such as the occurrence of night terrors or the experience of divorce. An up-to-date social history is invaluable.

The physician who is sensitive to parental development may prevent problems that arise from misinterpretation ("My baby cries because he doesn't like me"), unrealistic expectations ("He should be toilet-trained by now"), parental self-doubt ("I feel so guilty going back to work"), discipline ("He just needs a good spanking"), and cultural issues ("My father thinks we spoil her").

The need for anticipatory guidance remains dynamic, even as the child matures and seems to be more self-sufficient. Each child is unique, and may challenge a parent in ways a sibling did not. A new parental influence or attitude may be introduced (such as through a remarriage/new partner, more contact with a grandparent, or a new child care or classroom setting). Misinterpretation by a caregiver may become quite problematic (even to the point of maltreatment) if a child is labeled "oppositional," "bossy," "mean," "moody," or "lazy," especially if there is little consideration of the factors that may overwhelm the child and keep him from successfully adapting to the demands of his daily tasks. What seems to be "nothing" to an adult may mean much more to a child.

Many factors that influence parenting behavior may not be readily apparent, even to the parents themselves. A particular age or situation may present a special challenge to a parent who similarly struggled (ie, a mother who was assaulted, or a father who became overdependent on athletic competition for a sense of self-worth).

Typically, family roles are learned in the family of origin.[8,9] However, rapid cultural changes may result in much different family structures, needs, dynamics, and practices. Commonly, struggles within the family of origin resurface when the now grown child begins a family of her own. Even in the best of circumstances, there is some degree of differing opinion in regard to parental practices. Clearly, the physician who monitors family development and provides appropriate intervention provides a tremendous support to parental efficacy, child development and sense of self-worth, and overall family health.

For any clinical encounter, the interpersonal interaction is of great importance. However, it is even more so for a family that is struggling. The physician may be among the few consistent supports for the family. Although families typically place trust in the physician who cares for their child, this should not be taken for granted. In fact, there are many cultural stereotypes (ie, industry influence, overuse of medications) that may cause a family to be wary of their physician or treatment recommendations. One should always listen carefully to what the family is truly communicating and confirm shared understanding of the purpose of the visit.

Even if the child is the family member considered to need help, parents may be quite frustrated or ashamed of their perceived failure, and subsequently quite sensitive to any implied criticism. The physician should remain nonjudgmental, acknowledging the parents' care for their child and expressing the desire to problem-solve with them. The physician can both model respectful interactions and constructively guide interactions between family members during the office presentation.

Typically, several techniques are employed.[32–36] Emotional effect is acknowledged. ("That must have been quite upsetting.") Expectations are clarified. ("We won't use that type of language.") Communication is fostered. ("I feel that we pay attention to each other better if the cell phone is put away.") Positive actions are encouraged. ("I like the way that you followed through with the consequences.") Education is provided.

It is important to have the appropriate family members present and to ensure that each has a chance to be heard. Even if the physician disagrees with a statement or considers an emotion to be unwarranted, it is important to acknowledge an understanding of the perspective being communicated. Disagreement between any participants should be made transparent, with the goal of seeking a common point of agreement upon which to proceed. Problem-solving should be as concrete, achievable, and action-centered as possible. The "next steps" should be agreed upon and documented as specifically as possible ("We will turn off the computer an hour before bedtime.") It is important to acknowledge family strengths, efforts, and successes.

Physician-family interaction may range from a longer, prescheduled, and defined "family meeting" to a few minutes of conversation during a well-child or an acute-care visit.[37,38] If the allotted time does not seem to be sufficient to the task, this should be acknowledged, with agreement on the acute priority of the day. In this fashion, the physician can accommodate a variety of methods to work with families while still working within the schedule constraints of a clinical practice. By the end of a particular encounter, however, one should always try to understand the situation as clearly as is feasible, ensure safety, have an agreed-upon plan for the "next steps," and have scheduled follow-up.

Physicians vary a great deal in regard to personality, style of practice, experience, training, abilities, and motivation to work with families. This is especially true when working in challenging situations. Many already feel overtaxed by time constraints, documentation, and other work-related demands. Subsequently, it can be quite daunting to address additional levels of complexity when working with patients and their families. However, techniques can be customized across a variety of practice settings, presenting situations, and professional skill levels.

It is critical for the physician to understand, define, and communicate their own role. Caregivers by nature, physicians may have varied emotional responses to the patients and families in their care. Although families can be a source of joy, they may also engender sadness or other emotions that may not be as transparent. Professionals may feel frustrated with families who do not facilitate care or who challenge their skill level. They may feel anxious in sensitive or disagreeable situations, or feel dislike or anger towards certain patients or family members. They may be even more vulnerable to distress or countertransference in circumstances that resonate with their own life experiences. Often, the needs of the family seem insurmountable or can only be met with resources far outside of the physician's scope of practice. Subsequently, the effective physician needs a certain degree of self-reflection to provide insight into her own emotions and behaviors, and must acknowledge tendencies for minimization or avoidance, maintain appropriate boundaries, develop reasonable expectations for her work, and determine the need for additional resources and support.

As adult learners, physicians monitor their own "practice gaps" and seek information accordingly. A variety of resources is available to enhance the knowledge and skills that facilitate working with families.[10,14,15,22,23,37–49] In addition to the traditional written resources, organizational toolkits, workshops, and mentoring opportunities support the incorporation of knowledge and skills into clinical practice.

Physicians will be most effective if they also use educational and community resources for both children and the adults. There are many books, support groups, and Internet resources for common problems (eg, divorce, bereavement, alcoholism, violence). Families with significant and chronic dysfunction will typically benefit from the specific ongoing guidance of family therapy, and the physician should be aware of local mental health resources. When referral to additional physicians is warranted, personal attention to family engagement will greatly facilitate follow-through with the recommendation.[34,50]

The AAP Task Force on Mental Health has recommended that physicians develop "common factors" communication skills to elicit an accurate understanding, identify and address any barriers to the care and follow-up of identified problems, and build a therapeutic alliance with the child and family. Such skills have been shown to be readily acquired by experienced physicians and effective across a wide range of psychosocial problems presenting commonly in the primary care setting.[22,39,51]

## ▶ CONCLUSION

Family dynamics are complex and vulnerable to a variety of influences. Pediatric practice, however, provides a unique and powerful opportunity to guide not only the development of healthy children, but the development of healthy families as well. By understanding both adaptive and maladaptive patterns of behavior, the primary care physician can prevent problems, detect issues as they emerge, and intervene at early stages. By honing communication skills, using professional resources, and identifying community services, the physician can offer support, provide appropriate materials, and coordinate referrals for more specialized care. This results in profound benefits for children and their families, with the potential to affect generations to come.

## *TOOLS FOR PRACTICE*

### Engaging Patient and Family

- *Connected Kids (Violence Prevention)* (handouts), American Academy of Pediatrics (patiented.solutions.aap.org)

### Medical Decision Support

- *Addressing Mental Health Concerns in Primary Care: A Clinician's Toolkit* (toolkit), American Academy of Pediatrics (shop.aap.org)
- *Promoting Mental Health* (guideline), American Academy of Pediatrics (brightfutures.aap.org/3rd_Edition_Guidelines_and_Pocket_Guide.html)
- *The Resilience Project* (Web page), American Academy of Pediatrics (www.aap.org/en-us/advocacy-and-policy/aap-health-initiatives/Medical-Home-for-Children-and-Adolescents-Exposed-to-Violence/Pages/Medical-Home-for-Children-and-Adolescents-Exposed-to-Violence.aspx)

## *REFERENCES*


1. Garner AS, Shonkoff JP; Committee on Psychosocial Aspects of Child and Family Health, Committee on Early Childhood, Adoption, and Dependent Care, Section on Developmental and Behavioral Pediatrics. Early childhood adversity, toxic stress, and the role of the pediatrician: translating developmental science into lifelong health. *Pediatrics.* 2012;129:e224–e231
2. Felitti VJ. Adverse childhood experiences and adult health. *Acad Pediatr.* 2009;9:131–132
3. Anda RF, Felitti VJ, Bremner JD, et al. The enduring effects of abuse and related adverse experiences in childhood. A convergence of evidence from neurobiology and epidemiology. *Eur Arch Psychiatry Clin Neurosci.* 2006;256:174–186
4. Felitti VJ, Anda RF, Nordenberg D, et al. Relationship of childhood abuse and household dysfunction to many of the leading causes of death in adults. The Adverse Childhood Experiences (ACE) Study. *Am J Prev Med.* 1998;14:245–258
5. Schor EL; American Academy of Pediatrics Task Force on the Family. Family pediatrics: report of the Task Force on the Family. *Pediatrics.* 2003;111:1541–1571
6. American Academy of Pediatrics Committee on Early Childhood, Adoption, and Dependent Care. The pediatrician's role in family support and family support programs. *Pediatrics.* 2011;128:e1680–1684
7. Family medicine, definition of. American Academy of Family Physicians Web site. http://www.aafp.org/online/en/home/policy/policies/f/familydefinitionof.html. Published 1984. Accessed November 28, 2014
8. Nichols MP, Schwartz RC. *Family Therapy: Concepts and Methods.* 6th ed. Boston, MA: Pearson; 2004
9. Berk LE. *Child Development.* 7th ed. Boston, MA: Pearson Education, Inc; 2006
10. The Resilience Project: Tools for Communities, Families, Parents and Children. American Academy of Pediatrics Web site. www.aap.org/theresilienceproject. Accessed November 28, 2014
11. Belsky J. The determinants of parenting: a process model. *Child Dev.* 1984;55:83–96
12. Glascoe FP, Leew S. Parenting behaviors, perceptions, and psychosocial risk: impacts on young children's development. *Pediatrics.* 2010;125:313–319
13. Widom CS, Maxfield M. An update on the "cycle of violence." National Institute of Justice Research Brief. Washington, DC: National Institute of Justice; 2001:1–8
14. National Center for Injury Prevention and Control. Strategic direction for child maltreatment prevention: preventing child maltreatment through the promotion of safe, stable, and nurturing relationships between children and caregivers. Centers for Disease Control and Prevention Web site. http://www.cdc.gov/ViolencePrevention/pdf/CM_Strategic_Direction—Long-a.pdf. Accessed November 28, 2014
15. Merrick MT, ed. Interrupting child maltreatment across generations through safe, stable, nurturing relationships. *J Adolesc Health.* 2013;53(Suppl)

16. Shepherd S, Owen D, Fitch TJ, Marshall JL. Locus of control and academic achievement in high school students. *Psychol Rep*. 2006;98:318–322
17. Ainsworth MD. Patterns of infant-mother attachments: antecedents and effects on development. *Bull N Y Acad Med*. 1985;61:771–791
18. Bowlby J. Developmental psychiatry comes of age. *Am J Psychiatry*. 1988;145:1–10
19. Chapman DP, Whitfield CL, Felitti VJ, et al. Adverse childhood experiences and the risk of depressive disorders in adulthood. *J Affect Disord*. 2004;82:217–225
20. Wickrama KA, Conger RD, Lorenz FO, Jung T. Family antecedents and consequences of trajectories of depressive symptoms from adolescence to young adulthood: a life course investigation. *J Health Soc Behav*. 2008;49:468–483
21. Kahn RS, Brandt D, Whitaker RC. Combined effect of mothers' and fathers' mental health symptoms on children's behavioral and emotional well-being. *Arch Pediatr Adolesc Med*. 2004;158:721–729
22. Foy JM; American Academy of Pediatrics Task Force on Mental Health. Enhancing pediatric mental health care: report from the American Academy of Pediatrics Task Force on Mental Health. *Pediatrics*. 2010;125(Suppl 3):S69–S74
23. Preventing child maltreatment: a guide to taking action and generating evidence. World Health Organization Web site. http://www.who.int/violence_injury_prevention/publications/violence/child_maltreatment/en. Published 2006. Accessed November 28, 2014
24. Rush AJ, First MB, Blacker D. *Handbook of Psychiatric Measures*. Arlington, VA: American Psychiatric Publishing, Inc; 2008
25. Kemper KJ, Kelleher KJ. Family psychosocial screening instruments and techniques. *Ambul Child Health*. 1996;1:325–339
26. National Center for Medical Home Implementation Web site. http://www.medicalhomeinfo.org. Accessed November 28, 2014
27. Cluster guidance. In: *Addressing Mental Health Concerns in Primary Care: A Clinician's Toolkit*. Elk Grove Village, IL: American Academy of Pediatrics; 2010
28. Hagan JF, Shaw JS, Duncan PM. *Bright Futures: Guidelines for Health Supervision of Infants, Children, and Adolescents*. 3rd ed. Elk Grove Village, IL. American Academy of Pediatrics; 2008
29. Office of Civil Rights. A health care provider's guide to the HIPAA privacy rule. US Department of Health and Human Services Web site. http://www.hhs.gov/ocr/privacy/hipaa/understanding/coveredentities/provider_ffg.pdf. Accessed November 28, 2014
30. Rushton FE. *Family Support in Community Pediatrics*. Westport, CT: Praeger; 1998
31. Barlow J, Stewart-Brown S. Behavior problems and group-based parent education programs. *J Dev Behav Pediatr*. 2000;21:356–370
32. Providing culturally effective, family-centered care. In: *Addressing Mental Health Concerns in Primary Care: A Clinician's Toolkit*. Elk Grove Village, IL: American Academy of Pediatrics; 2010
33. Generic or common factors interventions: HELP. In: *Addressing Mental Health Concerns in Primary Care: A Clinician's Toolkit*. Elk Grove Village, IL: American Academy of Pediatrics; 2010
34. Engaging children and parents using patient activation techniques. In: *Addressing Mental Health Concerns in Primary Care: A Clinician's Toolkit*. Elk Grove Village, IL: American Academy of Pediatrics; 2010
35. Brief supportive interviewing technique. In: *Addressing Mental Health Concerns in Primary Care: A Clinician's Toolkit*. Elk Grove Village, IL: American Academy of Pediatrics; 2010
36. Motivational counseling. In: *Addressing Mental Health Concerns in Primary Care: A Clinician's Toolkit*. Elk Grove Village, IL: American Academy of Pediatrics; 2010
37. Coleman WL. *Family-Focused Pediatrics: Interviewing Techniques and Other Strategies to Help Families Resolve Their Interactive and Emotional Problems*. 2nd ed. Elk Grove Village, IL: American Academy of Pediatrics; 2011
38. Allmond BW Jr, Tanner JL, Gofman HF. *The Family Is the Patient: Using Family Interviews in Children's Medical Care*. 2nd ed. Baltimore, MD: Williams and Wilkins; 1999
39. American Academy of Pediatrics. *Addressing Mental Health Concerns in Primary Care: A Clinician's Toolkit*. Elk Grove Village, IL: American Academy of Pediatrics; 2010

40. Hagan JF, Shaw JS, Duncan PM. Promoting mental health. In: *Bright Futures: Guidelines for Health Supervision of Infants, Children, and Adolescents.* 3rd ed. Elk Grove Village, IL: American Academy of Pediatrics; 2008:77–107
41. Spivak H, Sege R, Flanigan E, Licenziato V. *Connected Kids: Safe, Strong, Secure Clinical Guide.* Elk Grove Village, IL: American Academy of Pediatrics; 2006
42. Langford J, Wolf KG. *Guidelines for Family Support Practice.* 2nd ed. Chicago, IL: Family Resource Coalition; 2001
43. Cheng MK. New approaches for creating the therapeutic alliance: solution-focused interviewing, motivational interviewing, and the medication interest model. *Psychiatr Clin North Am.* 2007;30:157–166
44. Gleason MM, Shah P, Boris N. Assessment and interviewing. In: Kliegman RM, Behrman RE, Jenson HB, Stanton B, eds. *Nelson Textbook of Pediatrics.* 18th ed. Philadelphia, PA: WB Saunders; 2008
45. Shah P. Interviewing and counseling children and families. In: Voigt RG, Macias MM, Meyers SM, eds. *Developmental and Behavioral Pediatrics.* Elk Grove Village, IL: American Academy of Pediatrics; 2011
46. Sommers-Flanagan J, Sommers-Flanagan R. Our favorite tips for interviewing couples and families. *Psychiatr Clin North Am.* 2007;30:275–281
47. Stuart MR, Lieberman JA. *The Fifteen-Minute Hour: Applied Psychotherapy for the Primary Care Physician.* Westport, CT: Praeger; 2008
48. Whitaker T, Fiore DJ. *Dealing With Difficult Parents and With Parents in Difficult Situations.* Larchmont, NY: Eye On Education; 2001
49. Ginsburg KR; American Academy of Pediatrics Committee on Communications, American Academy of Pediatrics Committee on Psychosocial Aspects of Child and Family Health. The importance of play in promoting healthy child development and maintaining strong parent-child bonds. *Pediatrics.* 2007;119:182–191
50. McKay M, et al. Integrating evidence-based engagement interventions into "real world" child mental health settings. *Brief Treatment and Crisis Intervention.* 2004;4(2):177–186
51. Wissow LS, Gadomski A, Roter D, et al. Improving child and parent mental health in primary care: a cluster-randomized trial of communication skills training. *Pediatrics.* 2008;121:266–275

# Chapter 28

# Fatigue and Weakness

*Philip O. Ozuah, MD, PhD; Marina Reznik, MD, MS*

## ▶ DEFINITIONS

Fatigue and weakness are ubiquitous complaints that may or may not be related to medical diagnoses but are used commonly in medical and colloquial language. Both terms are difficult to define. To add to the confusion, both patients and physicians often use the 2 concepts interchangeably. Moreover, adolescents and children often use other terms to describe their perceptions of somatic weakness and fatigue. Fatigue, in fact, is very different from true body weakness. Therefore, defining the 2 terms carefully is important, although the definitions must be modified for each age group.

*Fatigue* involves extreme and unusual tiredness, decreased physical performance, and an excessive need for rest. It often is accompanied by feelings of sleepiness, weariness, irritability, lassitude, boredom, and decreased efficiency. *Weakness,* in contrast, refers to diminished body or muscle strength, either the inability to generate force or maintain force (stamina), or both. True weakness can be identified only by demonstration of abnormal neurologic or muscular function based on history, physical examination, or laboratory techniques. Practically speaking, a history of weakness, on further questioning, will often suggest hypotonia in infants and will be expressed in older children as trouble running or keeping up in gym class, clumsiness, or lack of agility.

## ▶ ETIOLOGY

### Fatigue

Fatigue may be a normal result of any physical or mental work in which energy expenditure exceeds the restorative processes. The temporary fatigue that follows intense exercise involves several complex mechanisms, including increased central inhibition mediated by group III and IV muscle afferents along with a decrease in muscle spindle facilitation and suboptimal cortical output.[1,2] At the level of the muscle cell, fatigue results from a reduction in adenosine triphosphate caused by high utilization rates, as well as a depletion of glycogen.[3,4] Normal fatigue also follows activities such as cramming for examinations and occurs with food or sleep deprivation. In all of these instances, the degree of fatigue, even when prolonged, is usually appropriate for the amount of physical or mental exertion expended.

On the other hand, fatigue may be a pathologic state with an organic or psychological foundation. The lassitude associated with somatic illness, often with definable physical or laboratory abnormalities, is well known. Fatigue has also been shown to have a strong correlation with the psychiatric diagnoses of depression and anxiety disorder.[5-9] Any acute illness or trauma may be accompanied by fatigue, but only prolonged fatigue is usually noteworthy.

### Weakness

True weakness in a child should always be a cause of concern. Weakness is the result of a derangement of neuromuscular function at one of several levels, including the cerebral hemispheres, cerebellum, spinal cord, anterior horn cells, peripheral nerves, myoneuronal junction, or muscle.

## ▶ DIFFERENTIAL DIAGNOSIS

The differential diagnosis of prolonged fatigue is listed in Box 28-1. Box 28-2 lists some of the differential diagnoses for weakness in children.

### Fatigue in Infants

The term *fatigue* is rarely pertinent for infants. However, parents sometimes report that their infant tires easily during feedings or seems droopy. Infants who are in heart failure often appear to tire easily and sweat excessively with feedings. Infants who have other serious conditions, including severe anemia and hypothyroidism, may also be described by their parents as being listless.

BOX 28-1

### *Disorders Commonly Associated With Prolonged Fatigue in Different Age Groups*

**INFANCY**

- Cyanotic heart disease
- Congestive heart disease
- Severe anemia
- Hypothyroidism

**CHILDHOOD**

- Chronic upper respiratory tract infections
- Otitis media and sinusitis
- Tonsillitis
- Chronic asthma
- Chronic allergies
- Hepatitis
- Rheumatic fever
- Disseminated malignancy
- AIDS
- Immunologic disorders
- Chronic renal disease
- Obstructive sleep apnea

**ADOLESCENCE**

- *Mycoplasma* and other viral pneumonia
- Infectious mononucleosis
- Hepatitis
- Juvenile idiopathic arthritis
- Systemic lupus erythematosus
- Diabetes mellitus types 1 and 2
- Malignancy
- Inflammatory bowel disease
- Addison disease
- Drug abuse, including alcoholism
- Chronic pulmonary disease
- Juvenile primary fibromyalgia
- Obstructive sleep apnea
- Narcolepsy
- Depression
- Severe obesity

**BOX 28-2**

## *Differential Diagnosis of Weakness and Hypotonia*

- Down syndrome
- Spinal muscular atrophy
- Muscular dystrophies
- Congenital hypothyroidism
- Botulism
- Myasthenia gravis
- Guillain-Barré syndrome
- Juvenile dermatomyositis
- Polymyositis

## *Fatigue During Childhood*

Children complain only infrequently of feeling fatigued. Remarkably, even with chronic organic diseases, the child does not express fatigue itself verbally. Rather, concerned parents usually report that the child appears fatigued. Parents commonly make such statements as, "He has no energy," "She lies around all the time," "She seems bored and droopy," "He's sleeping a lot of the time," "She has no pep," "He drags around," or "I can't get her to do a thing." On questioning, younger children occasionally express a sense of lassitude and fatigue to their pediatrician. Much of the difficulty in the middle years of childhood (before adolescence), however, is children's inability to put into words what they feel. Fatigue, therefore, is usually exhibited in terms of a child's physical activity and performance in school, sports, and other organized activities. The younger the child, the more likely that the expressed or observed fatigue has a pathologic basis.

### Recurrent or Chronic Infection

The most common problem associated with fatigue in children is recurrent or chronic infection. Otitis media, sinusitis, and tonsillitis of a recurrent and smoldering nature are often overlooked for their systemic effects, among which fatigue may be prominent. Often mistakenly considered insignificant, upper respiratory tract allergies may cause impressive fatigue, irritability, and mild depression in children and adolescents.

### Endocrine Disorders

Of the common endocrine disorders, only hypothyroidism is likely to be associated with fatigue. Certainly, a child with hypothyroidism whose rate of growth has fallen off may exhibit increasing fatigue and lassitude, at first subtle, as the only symptoms. Thyrotoxicosis, in contrast, is uncommon in young children but occasionally produces isolated fatigue in adolescents.

### Diabetes Mellitus

Although any metabolic disorder can cause fatigue, only diabetes mellitus occurs with enough frequency to merit consideration. Fatigue almost always accompanies the initial or uncontrolled diabetic state.

### Inflammatory Diseases

Inflammatory diseases, especially juvenile idiopathic arthritis and other rheumatologic disorders, appear frequently in pediatric practice, and many children have significant fatigue, out of proportion to their musculoskeletal complaints. Lyme arthritis is a notable example.

## Pulmonary Disease

Cyanotic heart disease and chronic advanced pulmonary disease, as seen with cystic fibrosis, are commonly associated with marked fatigue; in these cases, however, the underlying disease is usually readily evident before the fatigue becomes severe. The pediatrician may occasionally see an older child for the first time who has severe fatigue caused by a previously undiagnosed hypoxic disorder.

## Anemia

Overall, the condition thought to be present most often as a cause of fatigue in both children and adults is anemia—usually, incorrectly so. Although fatigue is often ascribed to mild or moderate anemia, from whatever source, symptoms are usually not seen in children until the hemoglobin level falls to 6 or 7 g/dL; if red blood cell counts decrease gradually, then even lower hemoglobin levels may ensue without clinically evident symptoms. Irritability and attention problems may be present with mild to moderate iron deficiency anemia, but fatigue is usually not a common feature. Younger children especially seem to tolerate incredibly low hemoglobin levels with no symptoms at all.

## Malignancy

Malignancy, particularly leukemia or lymphoma, occasionally develops insidiously, with fatigue as the major symptom. Although always feared, these diseases are seen infrequently in pediatric office practice.

## Emotional Disorders

Many children who come to the pediatrician with unexplained chronic fatigue are found to have an emotionally related disorder. Before adolescence, the complaint usually centers on the parents' concern about a child's reduced activity level. A younger child will be noted to prefer sedentary activities—to "lie around the house a lot," appear tired, lack energy, and shrink from social contacts. These traits may have been longstanding, but a comment from grandparents or a teacher may arouse parental anxiety, precipitating the first visit to the pediatrician.

At this point, the family is often convinced that the child has a serious organic disease. Further evaluation, however, usually reveals that the child is performing very satisfactorily but not up to the family's excessive expectations. The child may be withdrawing because of failure to compete with an exceptional sibling or because of real or imagined failure in school. In other cases, a child may feel a lack of well-being because of parental discord. Similarly, lack of parental involvement with a child may lead to lassitude and boredom. Stress and anxiety in children often result in either hyperactivity or withdrawal, and the more common withdrawal reaction may express itself as chronic fatigue.

Most children experience transient periods of lassitude or fatigue, but such instances are brief and usually self-limited. At the opposite extreme is the child whose chronic fatigue is a sign of true psychiatric depression. In this case, as in the adolescent, the more protracted and severe the periods of withdrawal, the more likely that depression and fatigue are caused by a pathologic process.

### Fatigue in Adolescents

Complaints of chronic fatigue are encountered most often in adolescents. The normal swings in adolescent moods, from excessive exuberance to fatigue, are usually of more concern to parents and teachers than they are to the patient. In many instances, the adolescent may disagree vehemently with the parents' view and not share their concern. Adolescents, however, also initiate visits to their pediatrician because they feel fatigue. Parents may be unable or may refuse to recognize the adolescent's symptoms. Whereas a younger child who has a profound medical illness often does not experience fatigue, even minor illnesses often precipitate prolonged fatigue in adolescents.

## Viral Illnesses

*Mycoplasma pneumoniae* infection, often low grade and without fever, produces progressive fatigue. In addition, prolonged viral and parasitic illnesses (eg, infectious mononucleosis, hepatitis, cytomegalovirus infection, toxoplasmosis) commonly produce fatigue, especially in adolescents.

## Infectious Mononucleosis

The terms *chronic infectious mononucleosis* and *chronic fatigue syndrome* have become popular with both physicians and the media. This attention has led to misuse of these terms, as well as, undoubtedly, mild mass hysteria among young adults and adolescents who now are convinced they have one of these disorders. Most adults and many infants and children have been infected with the Epstein-Barr virus (EBV). The clinical manifestations in proved cases are extremely variable; some patients remain symptom free, whereas clinical, hematologic, and serologic findings support the diagnosis of infectious mononucleosis in others. The symptoms of infectious mononucleosis usually resolve in several weeks, but an occasional patient may have an atypical or a more prolonged course in which the initial clinical findings either persist or are intermittent over a period of months or, in rare cases, years. These unusual but documented cases of chronic infectious mononucleosis typically include complaints of chronic fatigue.[10] Another much smaller group of patients has been described as having a serious, sometimes lethal, illness associated with EBV infection. These patients usually do not exhibit the classic findings of infectious mononucleosis; their conditions are often proved to be either acquired or genetically determined immunologic abnormalities.

## Other Conditions

Always unpredictable and often insidious in its onset, inflammatory bowel disease may arouse concern initially with unexplained fatigue and a loss of sense of well-being. Although eventually accompanied by fever, abdominal symptoms, or abnormal stools, this disorder can continue for months, with fatigue as the only major symptom. The possibility of Addison disease should be considered in children or adolescents who have unexplained fatigue and associated weakness, anorexia, nausea, vomiting, or weight loss. Of more current importance in older children and adolescents are alcoholism and drug abuse—causes of chronic fatigue that are easily overlooked.

## Emotional Disorders

By far, adolescents are the patients who most commonly complain of fatigue. Pediatricians can expect to see a generous number of adolescents who characteristically appear each spring complaining of fatigue or lassitude and lack of energy and seem mildly depressed. This disorder usually appears during periods of greatest school-related stress, such as before examinations. Although the patient may have a fever, usually caused by infection (eg, infectious mononucleosis, influenza), the cause of fatigue is usually emotionally based.

In many instances, the adolescent collapses with fatigue after intense and exuberant activity involving schoolwork, extracurricular activity, sports, or social events. These individuals may also be short on sleep, have unhealthy eating habits, and complain of an additional variety of hypochondriacal symptoms. Burnout and fatigue are particularly common in overachieving high school and college students during late adolescence. The emotional reaction may actually be precipitated by a physical illness, particularly an infection. Most of these patients have normal findings on physical examinations and routine laboratory tests.

### *Chronic Fatigue Syndrome*

Since 1985, adolescents, adults, and, occasionally, children have been described as having a disorder referred to as *chronic fatigue syndrome* (CFS),[11,24] which most commonly involves persistent or relapsing severe fatigue, fever, headache, sore throat, tender lymphadenitis, nausea or vomiting, myalgia, arthralgia, and abdominal pain. Neurocognitive complaints, such as an inability to concentrate, sleep disturbances, episodic confusion and memory problems, depression, anxiety, and irritability, are also especially common in CFS.[5,17,18]

The neurocognitive complaints are the most difficult to evaluate in CFS because of the extreme difference in emotional perception from person to person. Furthermore, careful physical examinations by experienced physicians often fail to document any physical abnormalities, and extensive laboratory evaluations usually produce normal results. In addition, much of the difficulty surrounding both the diagnosis and the search for a cause of CFS is attributable to confusion about the use of the terms *chronic fatigue* and *chronic fatigue syndrome.* Consequently, in 1994, the Centers for Disease Control and Prevention (CDC) formulated strict criteria for the case definition of CFS.[26,27] Unfortunately, these criteria were based mainly on observations of adult populations and may not be completely pertinent to children and adolescents.

Nevertheless, the CDC criteria for CFS stipulate that the debilitating fatigue must last at least 6 months in addition to the presence of 4 or more symptoms (such as muscle pain, tender lymphadenopathy, headaches, arthralgia, pharyngitis, impaired memory or concentration, low-grade fever, postexertional malaise, and sleep disturbances). Although the CDC criteria exclude most past or current major psychiatric disorders, they allow some comorbid psychiatric symptoms, such as anxiety and nonmelancholic depression.[27] This allowance can be problematic because both anxiety and depression have an independent and well-established relationship with fatigue.[6,20]

Chronic fatigue syndrome quickly became a popular diagnosis. The syndrome was initially attributed to infection with the EBV, although few patients had documented physical findings or hematologic abnormalities consistent with the diagnosis of infectious mononucleosis. In addition, most patients had no serologic evidence of active EBV infection. Recently, however, a better understanding of the natural course of EBV antibody activity in healthy individuals months and years after an initial illness with infectious mononucleosis indicates that healthy patients who had mononucleosis years earlier could not be differentiated from fatigued patients who currently had the disease.

Until recently, the diagnosis of CFS in children and adolescents was based on adult criteria. However, children with the illness may exhibit a different symptomology than adults with CFS. In 2006, the International Association of Chronic Fatigue Syndrome published a Myalgic Encephalomyelitis/Chronic Fatigue Syndrome (ME/CFS) Pediatric Case Definition.[28] The main difference from the adult diagnostic criteria for CFS is a 3-month requirement for fatigue and other symptoms. Although few longitudinal data are available, the prognosis for pediatric patients with CFS is better than that for adults. Although symptoms may persist for months or several years, most children and adolescents with CFS have a good outcome, with approximately one-half reporting complete recovery.[14,29,30]

### Weakness

Infants with weakness are often brought to their pediatrician with a complaint of being floppy. A floppy infant is usually one who has hypotonia caused by a neuromuscular disorder. (See Chapter 44, Hypotonia.) In the newborn period, some of these patients may assume a *frog-leg* position. Chromosomal anomalies such as Down syndrome, congenital hypothyroidism, and the infantile form of spinal muscular atrophy (Werdnig-Hoffmann disease) are some of the more common causes of hypotonia in infancy. Infant botulism from ingesting *Clostridium botulinum* spores in honey can cause infants to appear floppy with a weak cry caused by muscle weakness, loss of head control, lethargy, inability to feed, and constipation.

Older children and adolescents who have weakness experience difficulty walking, running, and participating in athletic activities. Myasthenia gravis and Guillain-Barré syndrome (postinfectious polyneuropathy) are perhaps the 2 most common causes of weakness in this age group. A distinguishing clinical feature is that, in myasthenia gravis, deep tendon reflexes may be diminished but are rarely absent, whereas Guillain-Barré syndrome is remarkable for bilateral, symmetrically absent tendon stretch reflexes. Other causes of weakness in the older child include the muscular dystrophies, the juvenile form of spinal muscular atrophy, dermatomyositis, and polymyositis.

## ▶ EVALUATION

### Relevant History

Although the patient who is chronically fatigued may first appear to have an insignificant problem, great care must be taken to rule out underlying medical illness, to return the child to a state of well-being, and to relieve parental concerns. The pediatrician must remember that either the child or the parents are worried about the child's fatigue. Because family members may disagree about the significance of the symptoms, adequate time and concern are needed to evaluate the history. The symptoms of chronic fatigue cannot be dismissed casually over the telephone or with a quick office visit.

Because most patients who come to the physician complaining of fatigue have emotionally based problems, a careful history, with information from both child and parents (taken separately when appropriate), often helps narrow the differential diagnosis. An accurate assessment of sleep patterns, presence or absence of snoring, nocturnal awakenings, and daily exercise activities is essential. Discrepancies between the child's and the parents' observations soon become evident, and the diagnosis of emotionally related fatigue emerges in most cases based on the history alone. The information derived from a longstanding physician–patient relationship contributes enormously to reducing tensions during the evaluation. Although fatigue may be the only symptom, further questioning almost always uncovers other symptoms of somatic disease. Chronic fatigue, in the absence of other physical symptoms, is usually emotionally based. Other associated complaints are somnolence, depression, anxiety, boredom, decreased activity, and inappropriate affect. In many instances, emotional stress or some disruption in the patient's life is part of the history.

### *Physical Examination*

A physical examination, thoroughly performed, may be the only measure necessary and may reassure the anxious child or parent. The child's affect and appearance are most revealing. The impression that the child appears well invariably proves to be an accurate measure of the child's health. The condition of the adolescent, in contrast, may be more difficult to interpret. Although the physical examination may be benign, adolescents may be slovenly, uncommunicative, depressed, and unable to express their feelings; thus, at first, adolescents sometimes appear to be physically ill.

In all age groups, a search should be made for sites of chronic latent infection: adenopathy, enlargement or tenderness of the liver and spleen, and abdominal masses. Careful palpation for an enlarged or tender thyroid gland is essential. Mild scleral icterus and petechiae are easy to overlook. Similarly, a patient's pallor (a common finding, especially after long winters indoors) may evade even the most experienced physician. On the other hand, the characteristic facies of the chronically allergic child and signs such as clubbing and cyanosis are obvious. Examination of the oropharynx may reveal hyperpigmentation of gums and buccal mucosa, which may be present in Addison disease.

An assessment of the plotted height and weight should be an essential part of every routine health visit.[31] Failure of a child to progress along the expected growth parameters should draw the physician's attention to the possibility of an underlying systemic process affecting growth and causing unexplained fatigue. A normal linear growth velocity decreases the possibility of chronic cardiac, pulmonary, gastrointestinal, or renal disorders in children or adolescents who are excessively tired. An underlying endocrinopathy, such as hypothyroidism or Cushing syndrome, may cause fatigue in association with poor growth velocity and obesity. Poor weight gain over time may be a subtle manifestation of inflammatory bowel disease in adolescents with unexplained fatigue.

### *Laboratory Testing and Imaging*

A limited, well-selected group of laboratory tests should be performed on most patients who are chronically fatigued. These results will reassure the family, the patient, and the pediatrician and will usually erase any lingering doubt about the diagnosis.

## Other Diagnostic Tests

The laboratory evaluation should initially include a complete blood count with red blood cell indices, thyroid and liver function tests, a throat culture, and a stool examination for blood. The cold agglutinin test is often valuable as a simple initial screening test for a *Mycoplasma* species infection. Radiograms are rarely necessary and should be discouraged. Critical evaluation of data collected from the history, physical examination, and laboratory tests should enable the physician to detect quickly any organic causes of fatigue. Prolonged fever, however low grade, must always be viewed as significant and may suggest infection, inflammatory disease, or malignancy. Pallor points to the possibility of anemia or hypothyroidism. Hypertrophied tonsils or snoring and disturbed sleep might direct investigation toward a sleep study to evaluate airway competence during sleep and motor activity during sleep, and toward electroencephalogram tracings. In adolescence, a multiple sleep latency study may be considered in teens with fatigue and somnolence for early detection of narcolepsy.

## Viral Disease

Cervical adenopathy, even a single enlarged node in the absence of other findings, can be a clue to the diagnosis of infectious mononucleosis. In fact, in the autumn and early winter of each year, every physician begins to look for patients who have infectious mononucleosis. However, infectious mononucleosis is a protean illness, and the physical examination results are sometimes normal. Children and adolescents who have infectious mononucleosis may have no fever or signs of toxicity but may exhibit major fatigue. Furthermore, results of the heterophile antibody test for infectious mononucleosis may be negative in many young children and infants and in approximately 10% of older children and adolescents who have the disease. The reliability of EBV antibody testing has improved to the point at which the diagnosis of acute, active infectious mononucleosis can be confirmed. During the evaluation of chronic fatigue, EBV antibody titers can usually differentiate long-past infection from recent and active infection, thus eliminating EBV infection and infectious mononucleosis as causes for the fatigue and permitting a search for other likely neuropsychiatric causes. Toxoplasmosis and cytomegalovirus infections may mimic mononucleosis closely; these infections produce significant fatigue but with only minimal cervical adenopathy and fever. Positive results of a fluorescent antibody test for toxoplasmosis or cytomegalovirus with negative results of a heterophile antibody test will confirm the diagnosis. Similarly, fatigued children may have hepatitis and may be anicteric (or only slightly icteric), with little or no hepatic tenderness or enlargement. Other common viral infections, especially during convalescence, can cause a prolonged fatigue syndrome accompanied by depression.

## Chronic Fatigue Syndrome

The diagnosis of CFS should be restricted to patients who meet ME/CFS pediatric case definition criteria, including the new onset of persistent or relapsing fatigue lasting at least 3 months with no prior history of such fatigue and the exclusion of other clinical conditions that might produce similar symptoms. In addition, the children must have the concurrent occurrence of the classic ME/CFS symptoms, which must have persisted or recurred in the past 3 months of illness (symptoms may predate the reported onset of fatigue).[28,31–33]

## Autoimmune Disease

Children who have an autoimmune disease may have fatigue with little else at first. Mild articular or periarticular inflammation may be missed on examination. The emphasis must be on careful observation of subtle or minimal physical findings because children usually do not display fulminant findings initially. Children with inflammatory bowel disease, arthritis, or an arthritis-like illness, and some patients with a malignancy (monocytic leukemia, in particular), may have especially prolonged symptoms, including fatigue, without any physical findings whatsoever.

### Thyroid Disease

An enlarged, tender thyroid gland and fatigue may indicate thyroiditis with emerging hypothyroidism. However, the thyroid is often palpable and full in healthy adolescents. In any event, chronic fatigue from thyroid disease can usually be ruled out quickly with a thyroid-stimulating hormone and free thyroxine (free $T_4$) tests. Some patients who have hypothyroidism also demonstrate mild to moderate anemia, and those who have active thyroiditis may have an elevated sedimentation rate.

### Anemia

To be acceptable as an explanation for fatigue, the diagnosis of pure anemia requires marked reduction of hemoglobin. Red blood cell indices and a reticulocyte count will characterize the anemia and the probable cause. Anemia accompanied by thrombocytopenia, however, suggests leukemia or aplastic anemia. The white blood cell count may be normal in infectious mononucleosis or hepatitis, but lymphocytosis with atypical lymphocytes will most likely be present in the former. The heterophile antibody screening test (the *mono test*) is diagnostic in most such circumstances.

### Screening and Other Diagnostic Tests

The erythrocyte sedimentation rate is the most valuable screening test for inflammatory diseases of all varieties. A normal sedimentation rate is usually reassuring in ruling out autoimmune disease, inflammatory bowel disease, chronic smoldering infections, and disseminated malignancies. An elevated sedimentation rate requires further investigation. A routine urinalysis almost always reveals diabetes, and most patients who have chronic renal failure have abnormal urinalyses, as well as significant anemia. In these patients, the subsequent measurement of blood glucose in diabetes and of creatinine or blood urea nitrogen in renal disease can confirm these diagnoses. Hyperkalemia, hyponatremia, and hypoglycemia are useful diagnostic features of Addison disease, with the adrenocorticotropic hormone stimulation test being the most definitive diagnostic test.

### Weakness

The evaluation of a patient who has weakness may include chromosomal studies, muscle enzyme assays, nerve conduction studies, electromyography, edrophonium (Tensilon) challenge, muscle biopsy, and a lumbar puncture, depending on the suspected diagnosis. Consultation with a pediatric neurologist is often required.

## ▶ MANAGEMENT

After significant organic disease is ruled out in most patients, further management requires meaningful communication among the pediatrician, the patient, and the parents. In younger children, the variability in performance and behavior of healthy children must be put into perspective. Again, appropriate parental expectations must be emphasized. In addition, the child's and the family's daily schedule should be reviewed. A chaotic lifestyle that is frantic, with poorly structured activity and inadequate sleep patterns, is often revealed. Occasionally, true psychiatric depression is discovered, which calls for referral to a psychiatrist.

Older children and adolescents benefit from personal, warm attention. The value of a continuous relationship with a single physician becomes self-evident. An understanding, thorough session with the patient's pediatrician usually streamlines the evaluation and eliminates the need for excessive testing. Conversation after the physical examination should attempt to reassure children or adolescents about their basic health, reiterate the common and normal occurrence of fatigue, examine the daily routine and stresses on patients, and suggest modifications of patients' lifestyle and approaches to life's situations. This period is a time for respectful give and take. Attempting to establish the probable cause of the fatigue is the physician's responsibility before the patient is referred to a specialist. If emotional fatigue is thought to exist, then the adolescent, in particular, must be comfortable with the conclusion that organic diseases were ruled out. The patient then must be made aware of the emotional basis for the fatigue; if psychiatric referral is needed, then the reasons must be made clear. A knowledgeable pediatrician will be reassuring but firm in approaching the child or adolescent who needs referral. Fortunately, such a referral usually is not necessary.

## When to Refer

- Unexplained weight loss
- Hypotonia in infants
- Suspected major affective disorder
- Suspected malignancy

## When to Admit

- Severe depression or suicidal ideation
- Need for evaluation of neuromuscular disorders such as spinal muscular atrophy, Guillain-Barré syndrome, and myasthenia gravis

## *TOOLS FOR PRACTICE*

### Engaging Patient and Family

- *Building Resilience in Children and Teens,* 3rd ed (book), American Academy of Pediatrics (shop.aap.org)
- *Children, Teens, and Resiliency* (Web page), American Academy of Pediatrics (www.aap.org/stress)
- *Helping Children Handle Stress* (fact sheet), American Academy of Pediatrics (www.healthychildren.org/English/healthy-living/emotional-wellness/Pages/Helping-Children-Handle-Stress.aspx)
- *Helping Teens Handle Stress* (audio), American Academy of Pediatrics (www.healthychildren.org/English/healthy-living/emotional-wellness/Pages/Helping-Teens-Handle-Stress.aspx)
- *Kids and Stress* (audio), American Academy of Pediatrics (www.healthychildren.org/English/healthy-living/emotional-wellness/Pages/Kids-and-Stress.aspx)

- *Stress Management & Coping: Core to Resilience* (video), American Academy of Pediatrics (www.healthychildren.org/English/healthy-living/emotional-wellness/Pages/Stress-Management-Coping-Core-to-Resilience-Video.aspx)

## REFERENCES


1. Gandevia SC, Allen GM, McKenzie DK. Central fatigue. Critical issues, quantification and practical implications. *Adv Exp Med Biol.* 1995;384:281–294
2. Gandevia SC. Spinal and supraspinal factors in human muscle fatigue. *Physiol Rev.* 2001;81:1725–1789
3. Green HJ. Mechanisms of muscle fatigue in intense exercise. *J Sports Sci.* 1997;15:247–256
4. Baker JS, McCormick MC, Robergs RA. Interaction among skeletal muscle metabolic energy systems during intense exercise. *J Nutr Metab.* 2010;2010:905612
5. Smith MS, Martin-Herz SP, Womack WM, Marsigan JL. Comparative study of anxiety, depression, somatization, functional disability, and illness attribution in adolescents with chronic fatigue or migraine. *Pediatrics.* 2003;111:e376–e381
6. Epstein KR. The chronically fatigued patient. *Med Clin North Am.* 1995;79:315–327
7. Fuhrer R, Wessely S. The epidemiology of fatigue and depression: a French primary-care study. *Psychol Med.* 1995;25:895–905
8. Ridsdale L, Evans A, Jerrett W, et al. Patients with fatigue in general practice: a prospective study. *BMJ.* 1993;10:307(6896):103–106
9. Khalil AH, Rabie MA, Abd-El-Aziz MF, et al. Clinical characteristics of depression among adolescent females: a cross-sectional study. *Child Adolesc Psychiatry Ment Health.* 2010;4:26
10. Huang Y, Katz BZ, Mears C, Kielhofner GW, Taylor R. Postinfectious fatigue in adolescents and physical activity. *Arch Pediatr Adolesc Med.* 2010;164:803–809
11. Mears CJ, Taylor RR, Jordan KM, et al, and the Pediatric Practice Research Group. Sociodemographic and symptom correlates of fatigue in an adolescent primary care sample. *J Adolesc Health.* 2004;35(6):528e.21–528e.26
12. Jones JF, Nisenbaum R, Solomon L, Reyes M, Reeves WC. Chronic fatigue syndrome and other fatiguing illnesses in adolescents: a population-based study. *J Adolesc Health.* 2004;35:34–40
13. Farmer A, Fowler T, Scourfield J, Thapar A. Prevalence of chronic disabling fatigue in children and adolescents. *Br J Psychiatry.* 2004;184:477–481
14. Gill AC, Dosen A, Ziegler JB. Chronic fatigue syndrome in adolescents: a follow-up study. *Arch Pediatr Adolesc Med.* 2004;158:225–229
15. Patel MX, Smith DG, Chalder T, Wessely S. Chronic fatigue syndrome in children: a cross sectional survey. *Arch Dis Child.* 2003;88:894–898
16. Craig T, Kakumanu S. Chronic fatigue syndrome: evaluation and treatment. *Am Fam Physician.* 2002;65:1083–1090
17. Garralda E, Rangel L, Levin M, Roberts H, Ukoumunne O. Psychiatric adjustment in adolescents with a history of chronic fatigue syndrome. *J Am Acad Child Adolesc Psychiatry.* 1999;38:1515–1521
18. Richards J, Turk J, White S. Children and adolescents with chronic fatigue syndrome in non-specialist settings: beliefs, functional impairment and psychiatric disturbance. *Eur Child Adolesc Psychiatry.* 2005;14:310–318
19. Bou-Holaigah I, Rowe PC, Kan J, Calkins H. The relationship between neurally mediated hypotension and the chronic fatigue syndrome. *JAMA.* 1995;274:961–967
20. Carter BD, Edwards JF, Kronenberger WG, Michalczyk L, Marshall GS. Case control study of chronic fatigue in pediatric patients. *Pediatrics.* 1995;95:179–186
21. Dale JK, Straus SE. The chronic fatigue syndrome: considerations relevant to children and adolescents. *Adv Pediatr Infect Dis.* 1992;7:63–83
22. Sigler A. Chronic fatigue syndrome: fact or fiction. *Contemp Pediatr.* 1990;7:22–50
23. Smith MS, Mitchell J, Corey L, et al. Chronic fatigue in adolescents. *Pediatrics.* 1991;88:195–202

24. Wilson A, Hickie I, Lloyd A, Wakefield D. The treatment of chronic fatigue syndrome: science and speculation. *Am J Med.* 1994;96:544–550
25. Davies SM, Crawley EM. Chronic fatigue syndrome in children aged 11 years old and younger. *Arch Dis Child.* 2008;93:419–421
26. Fukuda K, Straus SE, Hickie I, et al. The chronic fatigue syndrome: a comprehensive approach to its definition and study. International Chronic Fatigue Syndrome Study Group. *Ann Intern Med.* 1994;121:953–959
27. US Department of Health and Human Services, Centers for Disease Control and Prevention. *Chronic Fatigue Syndrome: The Revised Case Definition (Abridged Version).* Available at www.cdc.gov/cfs/cfsdefinitionHCP.htm. Accessed July 17, 2006
28. Jason LA, Bell DS, Rowe K, et al. A pediatric case definition for ME/CFS. *J Chronic Fatigue Syndr.* 2006;13:1
29. Bell DS, Jordan K, Robinson M. Thirteen-year follow-up of children and adolescents with chronic fatigue syndrome. *Pediatrics.* 2001;107:994–998
30. van Geelen SM, Bakker RJ, Kuis W, van de Putte EM. Adolescent chronic fatigue syndrome: a follow-up study. *Arch Pediatr Adolesc Med.* 2010;164:810–814
31. Bright Futures Guidelines for Health Supervision. Available at www.brightfutures.org/bf2/pdf/index.html. Accessed October 15, 2014
32. Jason L, Porter N, Shelleby E, et al. Severe versus moderate criteria for the new pediatric case definition for ME/CFS. *Child Psychiatry Hum Dev.* 2009;40:609–620
33. Jason LA, Porter N, Shelleby E, et al. A case definition for chidren with myalgic encephalomyelitis/chronic fatigue syndrome. *Clin Med Pediatr.* 2008;1:53

# Chapter 29

# Fever

*Élise W. van der Jagt, MD, MPH*

For centuries, fever has been associated with illness. As many as 30% of all patients seen by primary care physicians and more than 5 million emergency department visits each year[1] have fever as their principal complaint, making it among the most common reasons children are taken to a physician. Add to this the numerous telephone calls about fever that physicians receive day and night, and it becomes evident that the proper evaluation and management of fever is a basic and necessary skill for everyone caring for children.

Even though physicians have long dealt with this common clinical sign, its mechanism, meaning, and management have remained sufficiently unclear and controversial that research on these matters continues. Although advances in neurochemistry and neurophysiology have improved the understanding of the pathophysiology of fever, clinical investigators continue to search for practical knowledge that will enhance the care of the febrile patient. Availability of such information can simplify the challenging role of the physician, who must evaluate a child quickly and effectively, arrive at a diagnosis, institute appropriate therapy, and both educate and support the parents and child during the entire process. The extent to which physicians accomplish these goals depends on their knowledge of the mechanisms of disease, the various clinical manifestations of disease, and their awareness of the social context in which the disease occurs.

## ▶ DEFINITION

The word *fever* is derived from the Latin *fovere,* meaning *to warm,* and commonly means an increase in body temperature. Although this general definition is acceptable in common parlance, fever is described more accurately as an adaptive response of thermoregulation. It must be differentiated from hyperthermia, an increased body temperature resulting from conditions that overwhelm the normal process of thermoregulation.

Normal rectal body temperature ranges between 97°F and 100°F (36.1°C and 37.8°C), although, on rare occasions, it may be as low as 95.5°F (35.3°C) or as high as 101°F (38.3°C). The *normal* temperature of 98.6°F (37°C) was derived from an 1868 study of more than 1 million axillary temperatures taken in adults.[2] This value may have no relevance for children, not only because adults were studied, but also because axillary and rectal temperatures correlate poorly. Young children seem to have higher body temperatures than adults, with temperatures slightly higher than 37.8°C occurring commonly in those younger than 2 years. The upper limits of the normal range for a rectal temperature are 100.4°F (38°C) for newborns younger than 1 month, 100.6°F (38.1°C) in 1-month-olds, and 100.8°F (38.2°C) in 2-month-olds. A total of 6.5% of well infants less than 3 months old have been reported to have rectal temperature of 100.4°F (38°C).[3] Nevertheless, because it is unknown which of these infants have these relatively high "normal" temperatures, it is safest to consider 100.4°F (38°C) as an abnormal temperature (fever) in this age group. Lowest body temperatures occur between 2 am and 6 am, and the highest ones occur between 5 pm and 7 pm, a diurnal variation that persists even during a febrile illness.

Because a range of normal body temperatures exists, it may be helpful in some instances to know a child's usual body temperature so that an abnormal increase can be recognized more easily. The extent to which body temperature is increased above normal may help determine the presence and significance of fever. This circumstance may be true especially in young infants, in whom even a mild fever may be associated with serious disease. Although the variability and range of normal temperatures in children have made it difficult to define fever precisely and consistently, a consensus panel of experts[4] has recommended that the lower limit of fever be defined as a rectal temperature of 100.4°F (38°C). This definition has become standard and is used both clinically and in research studies about fever.

## ▶ SIGNS AND SYMPTOMS ASSOCIATED WITH FEVER

The behavior of humans and animals is remarkably similar when fever is present.[5] When the set point in the hypothalamus is increased, patients attempt to adjust the environment to keep their bodies at this higher temperature. Young children usually seek close contact with a warm person (generally a parent), wish to be covered by a blanket, sit near a warm stove or register, and refuse cold liquids or foods. Although children may be quite comfortable at this higher body temperature, they interact less with others, have a decreased ability to concentrate, substitute quieter activities for energetic ones, and become less communicative except to indicate discomfort and distress. This adaptive withdrawal is often accompanied by loss of appetite and complaint of headache.

Such a combination of behavioral symptoms is a familiar indicator of illness to most parents and usually results first in placing the hand on the forehead, then measuring the temperature with a thermometer. Unfortunately, parents may not recognize the onset of fever in the younger child because the alterations in behavior are fewer and subtler. In a small infant, irritability and loss of appetite may be the sole evidence of fever and disease. If a parent is not familiar with these subtle cues, then recognition of serious illness may be significantly delayed.

In addition to the behavioral changes that may accompany fever, the general physical examination may reveal a pronounced hypermetabolic state. The child may have flushed cheeks, have an unusual sparkle in the eyes (likely from pupillary dilatation), and be either sleepy and lethargic or exceptionally alert and excited (particularly 5- to 10-year-olds). With rare exception, the pulse is increased by approximately 10 to 15 beats per 1°C of fever, and the respiratory rate is increased. (If the pulse rate is less than expected for the degree of fever, then typhoid fever, tularemia, mycoplasma infection, or factitious fever should be considered.) The skin may feel hot and dry ("burning up with fever"), although the distal extremities may be cold and pale (vasoconstricted), obscuring an extremely high core body temperature. Most children are not particularly uncomfortable, but some may shiver or sweat, mechanisms by which the body increases or decreases temperature. Sweating may be so severe that dehydration occurs, particularly if the intake of fluids has been poor. Thus, a dry mouth and lips may result not only from rapid mouth breathing, but also from dehydration. Finally, irritability of the central nervous system may increase, resulting in a febrile seizure.

The aforementioned signs and symptoms may be less obvious in a small infant. Shivering does not occur in the first few months of life, and diaphoresis is seen less often than in the older child. Because irritability and pallor may be the only suggestions of illness, a careful measurement of the temperature should be taken if the parent mentions these signs.

## ▶ PRESENTATION

A febrile child may come to the attention of a primary care physician in several ways. Probably the most dramatic and frightening manifestation of fever in a child is the sudden occurrence of a seizure. A generalized tonic or tonic-clonic seizure, usually lasting less than 15 minutes and occurring within 24 hours of the onset of fever, may begin without warning. Most parents are not aware that a fever is present and often feel guilty for not having noted it. The primary care physician may be called immediately after the seizure has occurred or after the child has been transported to the emergency room. There the child is likely to be postictal and have a rectal temperature of 102°F to 104°F (39°C−40°C). A thorough assessment of the patient is indicated because a seizure may be the first sign of meningitis or encephalitis.

Although some experts have suggested that every patient who has a first febrile seizure should routinely undergo a lumbar puncture (LP), the American Academy of Pediatrics (AAP) recommends an approach that takes the age and immunization status of the child into consideration.[6] The younger the child is, the more difficult it is to diagnose meningitis clinically (eg, meningismus, Kernig sign, Brudzinski sign), and strong consideration should be given to performing an LP. In infants younger than 6 months, an LP should be strongly considered because clinical signs of meningitis may be absent. In children between 6 and 12 months of age, when clinical manifestations of meningitis still may be subtle, an LP should be considered if the infant has not received the recommended immunizations for *Haemophilus influenzae* and *Streptococcus pneumoniae* or immunization status is unknown. Infants xho have received the 3 *H influenzae* and *S pneumoniae* immunizations are unlikely to develop meningitis from these organisms. In children older than 12 months, an LP is not routinely warranted except in the presence of signs and symptoms suggestive of meningitis or other intracranial infection. Because antibiotic treatment can mask meningitis, an LP should also be considered in a child with a fever and a seizure who has received antibiotics. Reexamination of the child after the convulsive episode may also help determine whether an examination of the cerebrospinal fluid is needed.

More commonly, a patient with fever is first examined when the fever has been present for longer than 24 hours and is associated either with nonspecific symptoms or with symptoms referable to a particular organ system. Inasmuch as many evaluations of febrile children take place over the telephone (the first contact with the physician), the physician must be able to take an accurate and pertinent history. Of particular significance are the age of the patient (the younger the child is, the more thorough the evaluation will need to be), any associated signs and symptoms, exposure to illness in the family or community, history of recent immunizations, and a history of any recurrent infections (eg, urinary tract infections [UTIs], streptococcal infections, otitis media). The time of year also should be considered, because certain viral illnesses are more prevalent at particular times of the year. For example, respiratory syncytial virus (RSV) and influenza virus infections are more common during the winter, parainfluenza virus infections (the most common cause of croup) are more common during the spring and especially in the fall, and enterovirus infections occur primarily during the summer. In addition, questions should be asked about the duration and height of the fever. A low-grade fever that has been present for many days usually does not need to be evaluated as urgently as a temperature of 106°F (41°C) that has been present for a few hours. The former is more likely to indicate a chronic or benign illness; the latter is more likely to be a potentially rapidly progressive infectious disease. Unfortunately, the height of the fever is often not very reliable in distinguishing viral from bacterial illness or even serious from nonserious disease. Young infants especially may not have much of a fever or even be hypothermic during a serious infection.

A visit or telephone call for minimal fever and little evidence of disease should prompt a thorough assessment of the psychosocial factors that may be contributing to parental concern. Is the main concern about something else—a hidden agenda? Is the caregiver anxious about the fever because of lack of knowledge about its significance? Has the caregiver had a previous traumatic experience with disease, resulting in excessive anxiety? Might the patient be a vulnerable child? Is this family dysfunctional, in which minor illness either cannot be dealt with or is used as a means to meet other needs? Answers to these questions and others may clarify the situation.

## ▶ DIFFERENTIAL DIAGNOSIS

Because many conditions may cause fever, an extensive discussion about each condition is beyond the scope of this chapter. However, classifying conditions associated with fever into broad categories is useful (see Box 29-1). In addition to specific etiologies, dehydration, excessive muscle activity, autonomic dysfunction, and heat exposure all may cause hyperthermia.

Although any disease in these categories may cause fever at any age, some diseases are more likely to occur at some ages than at others. Autoimmune disease and inflammatory bowel disease, for example, are unusual in infants but become progressively more common with increasing age. Similarly, febrile immunization reactions are much more common during the first year of life when most immunizations are administered.

Infections affecting the respiratory and gastrointestinal tracts account for most fevers in all age groups. Most of these infections have a viral origin (eg, enteroviruses, influenza virus, parainfluenza virus, RSV, adenovirus, rhinovirus, rotavirus) and are generally self-limited. Knowledge of the seasonality of these viruses promotes correct and efficient diagnoses. In addition, knowledge of the typical physical findings in these infections and their course may help distinguish them from bacterial diseases. For example, high fever, irritability, posterior cervical adenopathy, and painful vesicles on the gums and tongue are characteristic of herpes gingivostomatitis. Failure to examine the tongue and gums may result in an unnecessary workup in search of a possible bacterial infection. On the other hand, assuming that a high

**Box 29-1**

### *Differential Diagnosis of Fever*

- Infection
- Autoimmune disease
- Neoplastic disease
- Metabolic disease (eg, hyperthyroidism)
- Chronic inflammatory disease
- Hematologic disease (eg, sickle cell disease, transfusion reaction)
- Drug fever and immunization reaction
- Poisoning (eg, aspirin, atropine)
- Central nervous system abnormalities
- Factitious fever

fever in a 2-month-old infant is from roseola (exanthem subitum) would be erroneous because this infection (human herpesvirus type 6) usually does not occur at such an early age.

## ▶ EVALUATION

Failure to evaluate the fever further might result in missing a serious bacterial infection. Although viral infections may cause significant morbidity and mortality, the more aggressive course and serious outcomes of bacterial infections make early diagnosis especially important, particularly because effective antibiotic treatment is usually available. Bacterial infections may be especially devastating in younger children who are relatively immunocompromised because of their immature immune systems. An infection that remains localized in the older child may disseminate rapidly in the infant and toddler, particularly to the blood (bacteremia), the lungs (pneumonia), the meninges (meningitis), the bones (osteomyelitis), and the joints (arthritis). Because these infections may be seriously debilitating or even fatal if not recognized, the physician must be able to differentiate bacterial infections from the more benign viral infections.

At greatest risk are those children who present with fever or hypothermia and have severe sepsis or septic shock, because the mortality, although better than in adults, is still as high as 8% to 12%.[7] These children typically have a constellation of symptoms and signs collectively called systemic inflammatory response syndrome (SIRS), along with evidence of organ dysfunction. The Worldwide Pediatric Surviving Sepsis Campaign[8] has standardized (by consensus of experts) the definitions of SIRS, sepsis, severe sepsis and septic shock as outlined in Table 29-1, Table 29-2, and Table 29-3.

**Table 29-1**
**Systemic Inflammatory Response Syndrome Criteria**

| SIGN | AGE | VALUE |
|---|---|---|
| Temperature | All ages | <36°C or >38.5°C |
| Heart rate (bpm) | 0 days–1 mo<br>1 mo–1 yr<br>2–5 yr<br>6–12 yr<br>13–18 yr | <100 or >180<br><90 or >180<br>>140<br>>130<br>>110 |
| Respiratory rate (rpm) | 0 days–1 wk<br>1 wk–1 mo<br>1 mo–1 yr<br>2–5 yr<br>6–12 yr<br>13–18 yr | >50<br>>40<br>>34<br>>22<br>>18<br>>14 |
| White blood cell count ($\times 10^3$/mm) | 0 days–1 wk<br>1 wk–1 mo<br>1 mo–1 yr<br>2–5 yr<br>6–12 yr<br>13–18 yr<br>all ages | >34<br>>19.5 or <5<br>>17.5 or <5<br>>15.5 or <6<br>>13.5 or <4.5<br>>11 or <4.5<br>>10% bands (immature WBC) |

*WBC,* white blood cell.

From Goldstein B, Giroir B, Randolph A; International Consensus Conference on Pediatric Sepsis. International pediatric sepsis consensus conference: definitions for sepsis and organ dysfunction in pediatrics. *Pediatr Crit Care Med.* 2005;6(1):2–8, with permission from Wolters Kluwer Health.

**Table 29-2**
**Sepsis-Related Definitions**

| | |
|---|---|
| Systemic inflammatory response syndrome (SIRS) | The presence of at least 2 of the following SIRS criteria, 1 of which must be an abnormal white blood cell (WBC) count or abnormal temperature: (1) temperature abnormality; (2) tachycardia/bradycardia; (3) increased respiratory rate; (4) abnormal WBC count. |
| Sepsis | SIRS + evidence or suspicion of infection. |
| Severe sepsis | Sepsis + (cardiovascular dysfunction OR acute respiratory distress syndrome OR 2 other organ dysfunctions [see Table 29-3]). |
| Septic shock | Severe sepsis + cardiovascular dysfunction as defined in the organ dysfunction. |
| Refractory shock | *Fluid Refractory*: Cardiovascular dysfunction persists in spite of >60 mL/kg of fluid over 1 hr. *Catecholamine Refractory*: Cardiovascular dysfunction persists in spite of >10 mcg/kg/min of dopamine and/or need for epinephrine/norepinephrine. |

**Table 29-3**
**Severe Sepsis—Organ Dysfunctions**

| | |
|---|---|
| Cardiovascular | Despite >40 mL/kg fluid in an hour, there is systolic hypotension OR need for vasoactive drugs to keep BP within normal limits OR 2 of the following: capillary refill >5 sec; unexplained metabolic acidosis (base deficit >5 meq/dL); oliguria (<0.5 mL/kg/hr urine); lactate >2× upper limit of normal; >3 degrees between peripheral and core temperature. |
| Respiratory | Any of the following: $Pao_2/Fio_2$ <300 in absence of cyanotic heart disease or preexisting lung disease; >50% $Fio_2$ to maintain $O_2$ sat >92%; $Pco_2$ >65 or >20 mm Hg over baseline; need for nonelective mechanical or noninvasive ventilation. |
| Neurologic | Glasgow Coma Scale ≤11 or an acute change in Glasgow Coma Scale with decrease of ≥3 from baseline. |
| Hematologic | Platelets <80,000 or >50% decrease from previous 3-day baseline OR INR >2. |
| Hepatic | Total bilirubin ≥4 mg/dL OR ALT >2× upper limit of normal. |
| Renal | Serum creatinine ≥2× upper limit of normal or 2× baseline. |

*ALT,* alanine aminotransferase; *BP*, blood pressure; *$FiO_2$*, inspired fraction of oxygen; *Hg*, mercury; *INR*, international normalization ratio; *$PaO_2$*, partial pressure of oxygen in arterial blood; *$PcO_2$*, partial pressure of carbon dioxide.

Early recognition and aggressive, goal-directed therapy can decrease mortality significantly. This means that careful clinical and laboratory assessment is necessary to identify patients, give antibiotics within an hour, and provide early and rapid fluid administration (eg, 20 mL/kg boluses of crystalloid given over 5–10 minutes), along with early use of inotropic agents as appropriate to normalize the patient's physiology. Both the International Surviving Sepsis Guidelines for pediatric patients and the American Heart Association's Pediatric Advanced Life Support Sepsis algorithm provide guidance to the management of these patients.[8]

The younger the child is, the more difficult it is to recognize bacterial infection. Complaints cannot be verbalized, and physical signs and symptoms are more subtle and easily missed unless a high index of suspicion is maintained. Serious bacterial disease is especially difficult to diagnose in children with no obvious focus of infection. For this reason, many attempts have been made during the last 30 years to identify children in whom fever is a sign of a serious bacterial infection,[9] particularly pneumococcal disease and infections caused by *Haemophilus influenzae* type b (Hib). Children between birth and 36 months of age have been of special interest because fever is most common in this age group, and they may be difficult to assess, particularly during the first 3 to 6 months of life. Efforts to improve the ability to diagnose a serious bacterial infection have focused on 3 areas: data from the history and physical examination,[10,11] laboratory data,[12] and response to antipyretics.[13] Of the 3 areas, the response to antipyretics has been shown most clearly to be unhelpful in distinguishing between patients who have a serious bacterial infection and those who have a more benign viral infection.[13] Children who have a serious infection respond to antipyretics no differently from those whose illness is less significant. In fact, some children who have viral illnesses do not defervesce either.

Many studies have attempted to delineate the precise combination of clinical or laboratory variables that might identify the febrile child at risk for serious disease. Defined clinical observational scales (eg, Yale Observation Scale, Young Infant Observation Scale, Severity Index) are not sufficiently discriminatory and predictive to be used alone.[14,15] Laboratory studies continue to be necessary as well.

During the early 1990s, specific practice guidelines were published to facilitate the initial management of febrile infants and children without an obvious source of infection.[16] Although these guidelines remain controversial,[17–21] as many as one-third of primary care physicians found them to be helpful and changed the way they evaluated young children with fever.[22] Nevertheless, each patient continues to require individual assessment, with application of the recommendations as appropriate to the individual context of the patient. Considerations of the inconvenience, discomfort, and cost of laboratory testing and the increasing resistance to antibiotics in the community must be weighed carefully against the risk of missing a serious bacterial infection, with its subsequent morbidity and mortality. Therefore, physicians must make the best decisions possible in an environment of incomplete certainty about the presence of serious disease. Parents need to be part of these discussions, and adequate follow-up of all patients is crucial, no matter what is decided in the initial visit.

Although the early practice guidelines were helpful during the 1990s, they were formulated before the introduction in 2001 of the heptavalent pneumococcal vaccine for infants. This vaccine provides protection against pneumococcal serotypes 4, 6B, 9V, 14, 18C, 19F, and 23F, and is administered at 2, 4, and 6 months and between 12 and 15 months of age. With the introduction of the vaccine, a decline of 60% to 80% in pneumococcal disease occurred in children younger than 24 months.[23] In 2010, a more comprehensive pneumococcal vaccine was introduced, covering 13 serotypes including serotype 19A, with similar recommendations for administrating it 4 times in the first 15 months.[24] Because occult pneumococcal bacteremia and other pneumococcal infections made up most of the serious bacterial infections in young children with high fever (>102°F [>39°C]), the use of this vaccine greatly lowered the incidence of serious bacterial infections in children at greatest risk—those between 2 to 3 months and 3 years of age. A similar effect occurred when the Hib vaccine was introduced in the 1980s, nearly eliminating Hib meningitis, epiglottitis, and bacteremia. Given the marked decrease in pneumococcal and Hib serious bacterial infections, the likelihood of a serious bacterial infection when high fever (>102°F [>39°C]) is present in infants and toddlers is now even smaller, and a fairly limited assessment may be more suitable at this time.[25] In addition, with an increased ability to diagnose specific viral illnesses (RSV, influenza, enterovirus) by rapid diagnostic testing with polymerase chain reaction (PCR) methodology, and the increased use of inflammatory markers more typically associated with bacterial infections (procalcitonin, C-reactive protein), the likelihood of missing a seriouis bacterial infection is even lower. Thus, even the revised, updated practice guidelines of 2000[26] are no longer as useful as they once were (figures 29-1 and 29-2).

Fever during the first 4 days of life has been associated with a high incidence of bacterial disease.[27] A temperature above 98.6°F (37°C) occurs in 1% of all newborns; of these children, 10% have a bacterial infection, usually caused by group B streptococcal or gram-negative enteric pathogens. A full workup is indicated in these children, including a complete blood count and differential count, a urine analysis, and cultures of the blood, urine, and cerebrospinal fluid (CSF); antibiotics (usually intravenous ampicillin and gentamicin, or ampicillin and cefotaxime) should be administered until the results of cultures are known.

Similarly, neonates up to 28 days of age with fever have a significant risk of a bacterial infection (approximately 12% in some studies[17,28]). Pneumococcal infection is uncommon; *Escherichia coli* (*E coli),* group B *Streptococcus,* and other enteric pathogens are more usual; *E coli* is by far the most common and Listeria monocytogenes has become very uncommon.[29] Urinary tract infection (UTI) and occult bacteremias are the most common types of infection; however, with group B *Streptococcus* infection, the risk of accompanying meningitis is as high as 39%.[30] Low-risk criteria, such as the Rochester criteria, may not be consistently reliable to differentiate young patients with serious bacterial infection from those who have more benign disease. Although some studies have demonstrated only a 0.2% incidence of bacteremia or meningitis in neonates satisfying the low-risk criteria,[31,32] others have found that up to 6% of neonates who satisfy low-risk criteria have a serious bacterial infection.[33,34] Of note, neonates with RSV infection do not have a lower incidence of serious bacterial infection when they have fever but these are typically UTIs and not meningitis or bacteremia.[35] Concomitant UTIs are especially common, occurring in 5% to 7% of patients.[36] In addition to bacterial infection, herpes simplex virus (HSV1/HSV2) infection, especially meningoencephalitis, should be considered in any neonate who has risk factors for HSV infection (maternal primary HSV infection, prolonged rupture of membranes, fetal scalp electrode use) or clinical evidence (temperature elevation/depression or instability, seizures, lethargy, skin/oral/ocular vesicles, CSF pleocytosis, or hemorrhage).[37] Acyclovir is the treatment of choice while awaiting an HSV PCR test on spinal fluid/blood/surface cultures to confirm the diagnosis.

Fever of 100.4°F (38°C) or higher in infants between 28 and 60 days of age is associated with a 5% to 10% incidence of serious bacterial infection.[17,33,38] Unfortunately, neither height of fever nor apparent degree of toxicity has been a reliable predictor by itself of bacteremia or serious bacterial infection.[39,40] Instead of using a single predictor, a combination of clinical and laboratory criteria seems to be more useful in identifying infants who are at low risk for having a bacterial infection. The most well known of these combinations are the Rochester criteria[41] (Table 29-4). The infants must satisfy all of the following conditions: previously healthy (as defined in Table 29-4), no clinical signs of toxicity (in some studies[33] defined by an infant observation score of ≤10), no focal bacterial infection found at physical examination, a white blood cell (WBC) count between 5,000 and 15,000 cells/mm$^3$ with 1,500 bands or fewer, a normal urinalysis (≤5 WBCs per high-power field [HPF] with few or no bacteria

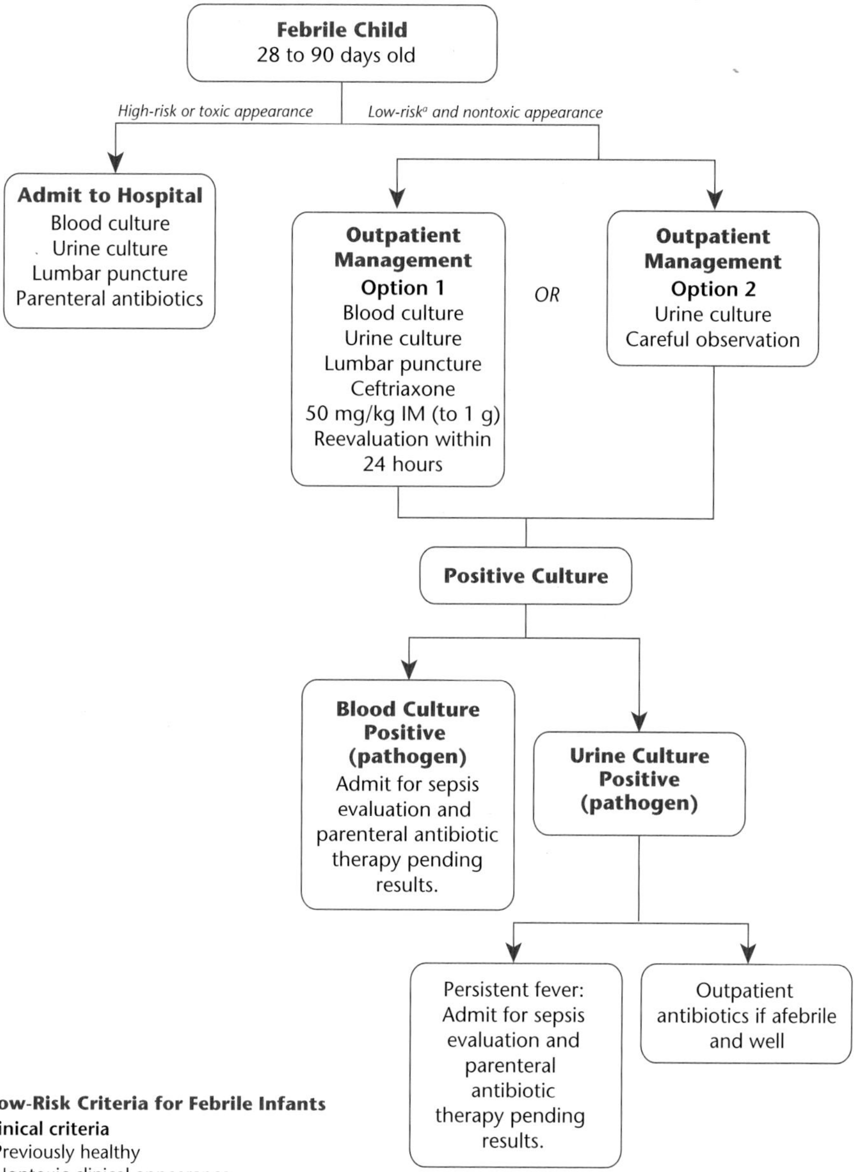


**[a]Low-Risk Criteria for Febrile Infants**

**Clinical criteria**
- Previously healthy
- Nontoxic clinical appearance
- No focal bacterial infection on examination (except otitis media)

**Laboratory criteria**
- White blood cell (WBC) count 5,000 to 15,000/mm$^3$, <1,500 bands/mm$^3$
- Normal urinalysis (<5 WBCs/high-power field [HPF]) or Gram-stained smear
- When diarrhea is present: <5 WBCs/HPF in stool

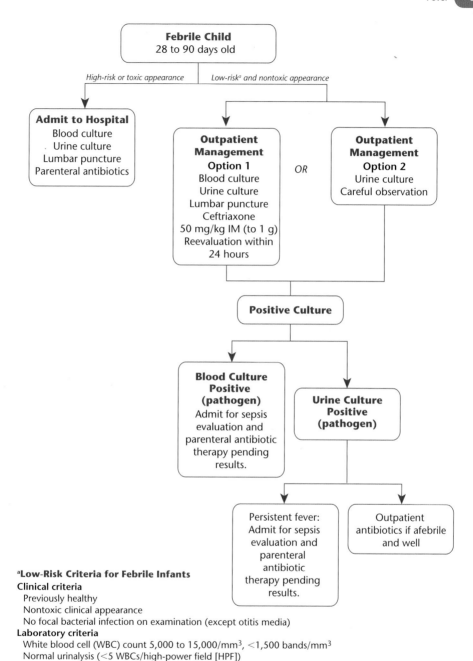

**Figure 29-1**
Algorithm for the management of a previously healthy infant 28 to 90 days of age with fever without source at least 100.4°F (38°C). *(From Baraff LJ. Management of fever without source in infants and children.* Ann Emerg Med. *2000;36:602–614. Copyright © 2000, Elsevier, with permission.)*

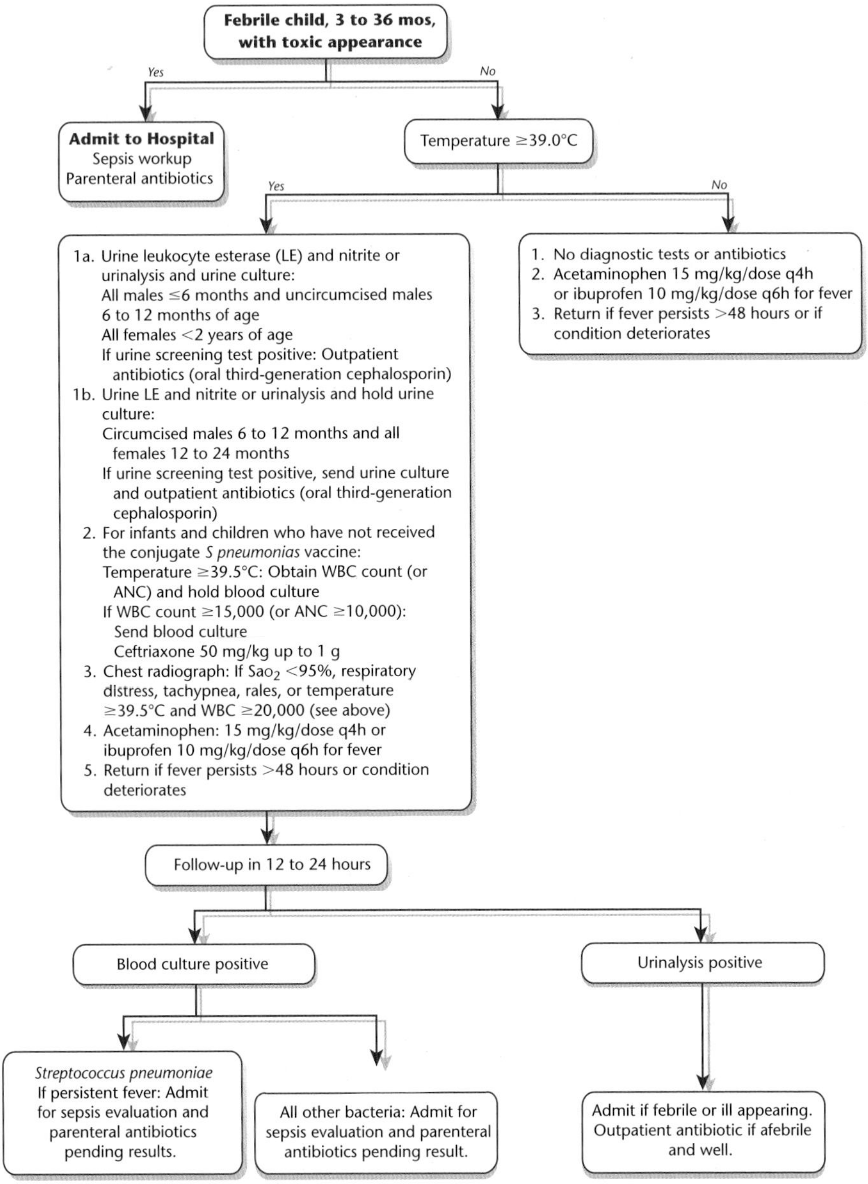


**Figure 29-2**
Algorithm for the management of a previously healthy child 91 days to 36 months of age with fever without source. *(From Baraff LJ. Management of fever without source in infants and children.* Ann Emerg Med. *2000;36:602–614. Copyright © 2000, Elsevier, with permission.)*

found in centrifuged urine and a Gram-stained smear of stool demonstrating fewer than 5 WBCs/HPF if diarrhea is present. If cerebrospinal fluid is obtained, then the cell count should be 8 WBCs/HPF or fewer.[41] One- to 2-month-old infants who satisfy these criteria have only a 1.1% probability of having a serious bacterial infection, and a 0.5% probability of having meningitis.[42]

**Table 29-4**
**Rochester Criteria**

| | |
|---|---|
| 1 | Infant seems generally well. |
| 2 | Infant has been previously healthy.<br>Born at term (≥37 weeks' gestation).<br>Did not receive perinatal antimicrobial therapy.<br>Was not treated for unexplained hyperbilirubinemia.<br>Had not received and was not receiving antimicrobial agents.<br>Had not been previously hospitalized.<br>Was not hospitalized longer than mother. |
| 3 | No evidence of skin, soft tissue, bone, joint, or ear infection. |
| 4 | Laboratory values:<br>Peripheral blood white blood cell (WBC) count 5.0 to 15.0 $\times$ $10^{11}$ cells/L (5,000 to 15,000/mm$^3$).<br>Absolute band form count ≤1.5 $\times$ $10^{11}$ cells/L (≤1,500/mm$^3$).<br>≤10 WBC per high-power field (×40) on microscopic examination of a spun urine sediment.<br>≤5 WBC per high-power field (×40) on microscopic examination of a stool smear (only for infants with diarrhea). |

From Jaskiewicz JA, McCarthy CA, Richardson AC, et al; Febrile Infant Collaborative Study Groups. Febrile infants at low risk for serious bacterial infection—an appraisal of the Rochester criteria and implications for management. *Pediatrics.* 1994;94:390–396.

Because of the difficulty in determining solely by the degree of fever whether an infant younger than 3 months is at a low or high risk for bacterial disease (septicemia has occurred even in infants who have low-grade fevers[43]), evaluation should be prompt and thorough whenever a fever of at least 100.4°F (38°C) exists, paying particular attention to obtaining the data necessary for classifying the child as low or high risk. Such a comprehensive evaluation should generally include a complete physical examination, total and differential WBC count, urinalysis[44] and urine culture, a Gram-stained smear of stool if diarrhea is present, blood culture, and possibly examination and culture of cerebrospinal fluid. A urine culture is especially important because UTIs are the most common bacterial infections in this age group, even in the absence of pyuria.[31,45,46]

If the infant seems nontoxic and meets the low-risk criteria, then examination and culture of the cerebrospinal fluid and blood might reasonably be avoided as long as good observation and follow-up can be made within 24 hours and antibiotics are not administered. If antibiotics are to be administered, then a full workup, including blood and cerebrospinal fluid cultures, should always be performed.

After obtaining a thorough history, including queries about illness of a similar nature in other family members and queries about whether the child has been immunized with the Hib and pneumococcal vaccines, the physician should assess the child for toxicity. If the child seems toxic (eg, lethargic or irritable, noninteractive, poor perfusion), then hospitalization should be considered along with further diagnostic tests to assess for serious bacterial infection. If the child does not seem toxic, a WBC count should be considered; if this count is greater than 15,000/mm,$^3$ then a blood culture should be considered. In the pre–pneumococcal vaccine era, children with WBC counts >15,000/mm$^3$ were 5 times as likely to experience bacteremia as those who had WBC counts <15,000.[19] In addition, an absolute neutrophil count of at least 10,000/mm$^3$ correlated with an increased (8.2%) risk of pneumococcal bacteremia. Practically, obtaining the WBC and blood culture at the same time is easiest, with the blood sent for culture only if the WBC count warrants doing so. Procalcitonin and C-reactive protein blood levels might have better sensitivity and specificity than the WBC count in predicting serious bacterial infection, but findings from various studies still vary widely with respect to the best cutoff levels to use.[47,48]

Given the lower incidence of pneumococcal disease now, avoiding blood tests altogether might be more cost-effective[49] and reasonable as long as the child has received at least 3 doses of the Hib and pneumococcal vaccines, does not seem toxic, has no obvious focus of infection, and has reliable physicians with excellent follow-up capabilities.

Approximately 5% to 8% of children in the 3- to 36-month-old age group who have an undifferentiated febrile illness have a UTI.[50] Two groups of patients in this age group are especially at risk. Female infants with temperatures greater than 39°C (102.2°F) have a UTI incidence of 16% to 17%.[44,50] Uncircumcised boys in the first 12 months of life have an 8- to 9-fold higher rate of UTI than circumcised boys.[51] Because of the high rate of UTIs in this age group, a urine culture is suggested for febrile boys younger than 6 months of age. A urinalysis alone is generally not adequate as a screening tool to determine which child should have a urine culture; 20% of children who have a UTI have a normal urinalysis, including a negative test for urinary nitrites or leukocyte esterase. However, a more recent study suggests that the urine dipstick may be an adequate screen for ruling out a UTI, with a negative predictive value of over 98%.[52] A chest radiograph is generally necessary only if clinical symptoms or signs suggest pneumonia (eg, cough, tachypnea, dyspnea, rales, decreased breath sounds, dullness to percussion).[10] However, at least 1 study has suggested that up to 20% of children with fever of at least 102.2°F (39°C) and a WBC count of more than 20,000/mm$^3$ have pneumonia by chest radiograph, even in the absence of respiratory symptoms and signs.[53]

If one considers all of the above, it is obvious that one must attempt to predict the risk of a serious bacterial infection in different age groups and circumstances. The advent of immunizations directed to serious bacterial pathogens with a subsequent decline in serious illness caused by these agents, and the possibilities of diagnosing viral infection very early, even in the emergency room, make it imperative that a balanced approach be taken in diagnostic testing, hospitalization, and treatment. One way of doing this has been outlined by Ishimine[54] and is shown in Figure 29-3.

A further consideration in the approach to a febrile infant or child in the first 3 years of life is the increased availability of rapid diagnostic viral testing. Rapid tests are now available for influenza A and B, RSV, and enterovirus. Although sensitivity and specificity vary with individual tests, a positive test may be helpful in decreasing the number of other tests that need to be performed to rule out a bacterial infection.[55,56] Including neonates younger than 28 days, the rate of serious bacterial infections in febrile patients is lower if they are infected with influenza[57] and RSV.[58] When this rate of infection is coupled with a generally lower incidence of serious pneumococcal and *H influenzae* infections because of the advent of vaccines given at a young age, a reasonable strategy might be to use positive viral tests as a way to reduce blood and urine tests in vaccinated children older than 2 to 3 months who do not seem toxic.

Children older than 3 years are more likely to have signs and symptoms consistent with a recognizable illness. If they have nonspecific symptoms, an urgent consultation with a physician is probably unnecessary; however, regardless of age, all febrile children with localized signs and symptoms, such as swollen joints, meningismus, labored respirations, chest

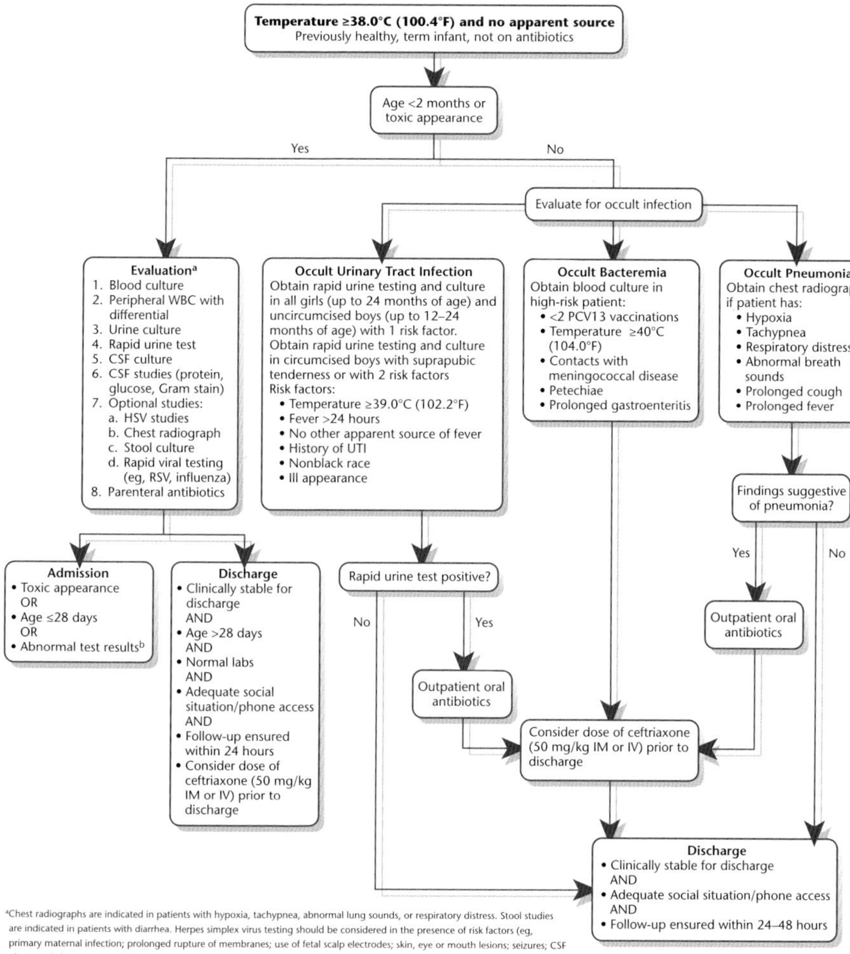


[a]Chest radiographs are indicated in patients with hypoxia, tachypnea, abnormal lung sounds, or respiratory distress. Stool studies are indicated in patients with diarrhea. Herpes simplex virus testing should be considered in the presence of risk factors (eg, primary maternal infection; prolonged rupture of membranes; use of fetal scalp electrodes; skin, eye or mouth lesions; seizures; CSF pleocytosis; hemorrhagic CSF). HSV testing is best accomplished by polymerase chain reaction or viral culture. Neonates should receive both ampicillin (50 mg/kg IV; 100 mg/kg IV if concern for meningitis) and ceftriaxone (50 mg/kg IV; 100 mg/kg IV if concern for meningitis). Older children should receive ceftriaxone (50 mg/kg IV if concern for meningitis).

[b]**Abnormal labs**

- Peripheral WBC count: <5,000/mm³ or >15,000/mm³ or band-to-neutrophil ratio >0.2
- Urine testing: ≥10 WBC/HPF, bacteria on Gram stain, or positive leukocyte esterase or nitrate
- CSF: ≥8 WBC/mm³ or bacteria on Gram stain
- Stool specimen: ≥5 WBC/HPF
- Chest radiograph: infiltrate on chest radiograph

**Figure 29-3**

Fever without apparent source in children 0 to 24 months old. (*From Ishimine P. Risk stratification and management of the febrile young child.* Emerg Med Clin N Am. *2013;31:601–626. Copyright © 2013, Elsevier, with permission.*)

pain, dysuria, petechiae, alteration of consciousness, and severe abdominal pain, should be examined immediately. Moreover, any child with fever or hypothermia who satisfies the criteria for SIRS should be immediately evaluated.

Although many febrile children do not have signs and symptoms pointing to an obvious cause, a complete physical examination may reveal important clues to the origin of the fever. Because most infections involve the respiratory tract, this area must be examined carefully. In all instances, the tympanic membranes should be examined for otitis media, the pharynx for pharyngitis, the nose for the discharge of sinusitis or a viral upper respiratory tract infection, and the lungs for evidence of pneumonia or bronchiolitis. Conjunctivitis may be a clue to adenovirus, influenza or RSV infection, conjunctivitis-otitis syndrome, or Kawasaki disease.

The skin is no less important and may demonstrate typical viral exanthems, such as those associated with rubella, roseola, or chickenpox, or it may show the erythema marginatum of rheumatic fever or the rose spots of typhoid fever.

Generalized lymphadenopathy often occurs with viral illnesses, such as infectious mononucleosis, hepatitis, or cytomegalovirus infection, but it also may be a clue to the diagnosis of leukemia or lymphoma. Localized enlargement of lymph nodes should prompt a search for a skin infection or for a tumor. Isolated cervical lymphadenopathy may be associated with tuberculosis infection or cat scratch disease (*Bartonella* infection).

The musculoskeletal system must be examined with care. Localized bone tenderness may suggest osteomyelitis, and a restricted range of motion in a warm joint may suggest arthritis. Although the latter finding may occur in many different diseases, a meticulous examination of the heart is always indicated to detect the carditis of rheumatic fever or infective endocarditis. The spine should be palpated for any evidence of diskitis, and any costovertebral angle tenderness should prompt an examination of the urine for evidence of a UTI.

Although uncommon, factitious fever is a final consideration and a well-described entity. Children as young as 8 years have been known to increase the thermometer reading artificially by rubbing the mercury thermometer bulb on the sheets or by exposing it to warm liquids. Clues at physical examination include a pulse that is not correlated with the increase in temperature, inability to document fever when it is measured rectally, and an absence of sweating during defervescence. Investigation of psychosocial disturbances within the family is usually necessary.

## ▶ SUMMARY

Although fever may be associated with serious illness, treatment of the fever itself is much less crucial than the evaluation and treatment of the illness causing the fever. Health care professionals are responsible for educating parents about the proper management of their febrile children, emphasizing their role in the observation for signs and symptoms that are more likely to be associated with serious disease. Fever as a harbinger of severe sepsis is especially important and both physicians and parents need to be educated on how to differentiate patients who are septic from those who have a more benign illness. Fever is but a single sign that should be evaluated in the total context of the care of the patient.

### *TOOLS FOR PRACTICE*

#### Engaging Patient and Family

- *Fever and Your Child* (handout), American Academy of Pediatrics (patiented.solutions.aap.org)
- *How to Take a Child's Temperature* (fact sheet), American Academy of Pediatrics (www.healthychildren.org/English/health-issues/conditions/fever/Pages/How-to-Take-a-Childs-Temperature.aspx)
- *Medications Used to Treat Fever* (fact sheet), American Academy of Pediatrics (www.healthychildren.org/English/health-issues/conditions/fever/Pages/Medications-Used-to-Treat-Fever.aspx)

## AAP POLICY STATEMENTS

American Academy of Pediatrics Subcommittee on Urinary Tract Infection, Steering Committee on Quality Improvement and Management. Urinary tract infection: clinical practice guideline for the diagnosis and management of the initial UTI in febrile infants and children 2 to 24 months. *Pediatrics*. 2011;128(3):595–610 (pediatrics.aappublications.org/content/128/3/595)

American Academy of Pediatrics Subcommittee on Febrile Seizures. Clinical practice guideline: febrile seizures: guideline for the neurodiagnostic evaluation of the child with a simple febrile seizure. *Pediatrics*. 2011;127(2):389–394 (pediatrics.aappublications.org/content/127/2/389)

## REFERENCES

1. McCaig LF, Burt CW. National Hospital Ambulatory Medical Care Survey: 2002 emergency department summary. *Adv Data*. 2004;(340):1–34
2. Wunderlich C. *Das Verhalten der Eigenwarme in Krankenheiten*. Leipzig, Germany: Otto Wigard; 1868
3. Herzog LW, Coyne LJ. What is fever? Normal temperature in infants less than 3 months old. *Clin Pediatr (Phila)*. 1993;32(3):142–146
4. Callanan D. Detecting fever in young infants: reliability of perceived, pacifier, and temporal artery temperatures in infants younger than 3 months of age. *Pediatr Emerg Care*. 2003;19:240–243
5. Donaldson JF. Therapy of acute fever: a comparative approach. *Hosp Pract (Off Ed)*. 1981;16(9):125–129, 133, 136–138U
6. American Academy of Pediatrics Subcommittee on Febrile Seizures. Clinical practice guideline—febrile seizures: guideline for the neurodiagnostic evaluation of the child with a simple febrile seizure. *Pediatrics*. 2011;127:389–394
7. Goldstein B, Giroir B, Randolph A; International Consensus Conference on Pediatric Sepsis. International pediatric sepsis consensus conference: definitions for sepsis and organ dysfunction in pediatrics. *Pediatr Crit Care Med*. 2005;6:2–8
8. Dellinger RP, Levy MM, Rhodes A, et al. Surviving sepsis campaign: international guidelines for management of severe sepsis and septic shock: 2012. *Crit Care Med*. 2013;41:580–637
9. Teele DW, Marshall R, Klein JO. Unsuspected bacteremia in young children: a common and important problem. *Pediatr Clin North Am*. 1979;26:773–784
10. Heulitt MJ, Ablow RC, Santos CC, O'Shea TM, Hilfer CL. Febrile infants less than 3 months old: value of chest radiography. *Radiology*. 1988;167:135–137
11. McCarthy PL, Sharpe MR, Spiesel SZ, et al. Observation scales to identify serious illness in febrile children. *Pediatrics*. 1982;70:802–809
12. McCarthy PL. Controversies in pediatrics: what tests are indicated for the child under two with fever. *Pediatr Rev*. 1979;1:51–56
13. Baker RC, Tiller T, Bausher JC, et al. Severity of disease correlated with fever reduction in febrile infants. *Pediatrics*. 1989;83:1016–1019
14. Bonadio WA. The history and physical assessment of the febrile infant. *Pediatr Clin North Am*. 1998;45(1):65–77
15. Kupperman N, Fleisher GR, Jaffe DM. Predictors of occult pneumococcal bacteremia in young febrile children. *Ann Emerg Med*. 1998;31(6):679–687
16. Baraff LJ, Schriger DL, Bass JW, et al. Commentary on practice guidelines. *Pediatrics*. 1997;100:128–134
17. Baker MD, Bell LM. Unpredictability of serious bacterial illness in febrile infants from birth to 1 month of age. *Arch Pediatr Adolesc Med*. 1999;153:508–511
18. Bauchner H, Pelton SI. Management of the young febrile child: a continuing controversy. *Pediatrics*. 1997;100:137–138
19. Finkelstein JA, Christiansen CL, Platt R. Fever in pediatric primary care: occurrence, management, and outcomes. *Pediatrics*. 2000;105:260–266
20. Kramer MS, Shapiro ED. Management of the young febrile child: a commentary on recent practice guidelines. *Pediatrics*. 1997;100:128–134

# Chapter 30

# Fever of Unknown Origin

*Élise W. van der Jagt, MD, MPH*

Fever without a discernible cause poses several difficulties for the physician. Since fever suggests disease, the inability to identify its cause can create anxiety for the family and the physician, undermine the physician's credibility, and affect patient rapport. The longer the fever persists, the more concerned parents are and the higher their level of anxiety. A fever of only a few days' duration, not associated with any localizing signs or symptoms, usually does not even come to a physician's attention unless the child also appears ill. Fever that continues beyond 5 to 7 days, or that occurs repeatedly, almost always will prompt a medical consultation. This discussion focuses on these prolonged fevers including their evaluation and management.

## ▶ DEFINITION

In 1961, Petersdorf[1] proposed the classic definition for a fever of unknown origin (FUO): fever that is higher than 38.3°C (101°F) on several occasions, that is present for more than 3 weeks, and that has a cause that is still unexplained after 1 week of evaluation in the hospital. Since then, researchers have suggested that these criteria are inappropriate for immunocompromised patients and that the third criterion—evaluation—be changed either to reflect the increased emphasis on ambulatory assessment (unexplained fever after 3 days of in-hospital evaluation or 3 ambulatory visits) or to make the evaluation more quantitative by requiring specific tests that should have been performed before applying the label of FUO.[2,3] The latter definition is more acceptable to most primary care physicians, who usually don't wish to delay evaluation for 3 weeks or require a week of hospitalization. In children, an FUO has been defined as a daily rectal temperature greater than 38.3°C (101°F), lasting for at least 2 weeks, the cause of which has not been determined by simple diagnostic tests, including a complete history and thorough physical examination.[4] Some experts suggest that 1 of the 2 weeks of fever should be documented in the hospital.

Careful and precise documentation of fever is necessary before using the label of FUO. A thorough awareness of the range of normal core body temperature for age, with its diurnal variation, may help to exclude patients who are actually not febrile but, instead, have a high normal body temperature. The physician should teach the parents how to take a rectal temperature and define a day of fever as a 24-hour period in which a temperature greater than 38.3°C (101°F) occurs at least once. All medications taken, the activities in which the child has participated, and the environmental temperature during this time should be recorded because each of these may affect body temperature.

Although much importance has been attached to fever patterns in the past (ie, remittent, intermittent, sustained), detailing them may not be useful because they are rarely diagnostic of a specific disease.[5] Nevertheless, some inflammatory diseases do have recognizable fever patterns (eg, double quotidian fever of systemic idiopathic juvenile arthritis). In addition, it should be carefully determined if even 1 or 2 days of normal temperature have been interspersed between days of fever: children with this pattern may have a series of rapidly sequenced brief febrile illnesses, which are masquerading as a single febrile illness. Careful documentation of fever should also help exclude the so-called *pseudo-FUO* or factitious fever.[6] Children who have a pseudo-FUO not only do not have a true fever if their body temperature is measured accurately and consistently (sometimes this needs to be done under hospital supervision), but also exhibit a specific and recognizable constellation of findings that is often diagnostic (Box 30-1). In addition to the inability to corroborate fever, and in the setting of a completely normal physical examination, the parents may relate a previous serious illness and their concerns about its possible recurrence or lasting effect on the child (vulnerable child syndrome). Their child may have missed an excessive amount of school, given the general degree of illness described; school absence is often prompted by the presence of fatigue, abdominal pain, and headache in the morning—symptoms that are conspicuously absent during the rest of the day. Others have noted a similar pattern of findings and called it *deconditioning syndrome,* which occurs after an acute, easily definable febrile illness and usually occurs in children who are older than 12 years. The syndrome includes significant fatigue, sedentary habits, absence of depression, and a normal neurologic and musculoskeletal exam. Treatment is directed towards establishing required physical activity in a graduated way while acknowledging that fatigue is present.[7]

Another category of FUO is periodic fever. Instead of a single episode of prolonged fever, affected children have shorter episodes of fever that recur in a regular (periodic) fashion, accompanied by a predictable constellation of symptoms. Patients with this pattern of fever are said to have *periodic fever syndrome.*[7] Many of these periodic fevers are now known to be

**BOX 30-1**

## *Characteristics of the Child Who Has Pseudo-Fever of Unknown Origin*

- Absence of documented, persistent fever
- Lack of objective, abnormal physical findings
- History of significant or near-fatal illness
- Parental fear of malignant or crippling disease
- Frequent environmental exposure to illness
- Absence of persistent weight loss
- Normal erythrocyte sedimentation rate and platelet count
- Many missed school days because of subjective morning complaints
- Discordance of fever and pulse rate
- Medical or paramedical family background
- One or more of mild self-limited diseases, behavioral problems, parents who have misconceptions concerning health and disease, or families under stress

From Kleiman MB. The complaint of persistent fever. *Pediatr Clin North Am.* 1982;29(1):201–208. Copyright © 1982, Elsevier, with permission.

genetically based and can be diagnosed by sophisticated genetic testing. Unfortunately, the most common periodic fever (periodic fever, aphthous stomatitis, pharyngitis, and cervical adenopathy [PFAPA]) is not known to be genetic.

## ▶ DIFFERENTIAL DIAGNOSIS

Box 30-2 lists the common causes of FUO in children. The causes are subdivided into 5 main categories: (1) infectious diseases—bacterial/viral/fungal/parasitic, (2) autoimmune diseases, (3) malignancies, (4) periodic fever syndromes, and (5) miscellaneous. This list suggests that most FUOs eventually are found to be caused by common pediatric illnesses that are either self-limited or treatable.

An infectious illness is the most common cause for an FUO in children, comprising between 40% and 60% of the reported cases[4,8–11]; the second most common cause is autoimmune disease, comprising between 7% and 20% of the cases. Children younger than 6 years are most likely to have an FUO from an infection; autoimmune diseases become more common after 6 years, although infection remains the most frequent cause of FUO overall (Table 30-1).[9,11]

Although most infections that present themselves as an FUO are atypical or incomplete manifestations of common infectious diseases, less common infections should also be considered. Epstein-Barr virus is the most common infectious cause of FUO,[8,12] followed by osteomyelitis and bartonellosis. The advent of serologic testing (indirect immunofluorescent antibodies) for Epstein-Barr virus and *Bartonella* infections has made these diagnoses easier to make. Although bartonellosis (caused by *Bartonella henselae*) usually presents as classic cat-scratch disease, it may also manifest as atypical cat-scratch disease, producing prolonged fever and hepatosplenic abscesses,[13] lymphadenopathy, or central nervous system disease.[14] Thus, when exposure to kittens and cats can be documented, serologic testing for *Bartonella* should be obtained; if positive, an abdominal ultrasound should be considered. Tick-borne diseases should also be considered, especially in areas of the United States where ticks are plentiful. These diseases include Lyme disease, tularemia, tick-borne relapsing fever and ehrlichiosis.[15] Osteomyelitis, particularly of the axial skeleton (intervertebral disk space and vertebral body) and the pelvis, should also be a consideration, especially in young children who are more difficult to examine.

Another interesting syndrome likely initiated by a variety of viruses, and first described in 1972 in adults, is Kikuchi-Fujimoto disease or histiocytic necrotizing lymphadenitis, which is most common in the Far East. Kim[16] recently described a series of 40 children, noting that 90% of them had fever (>37.5°C) lasting for a mean of 18 days with tender unilateral cervical lymphadenitis (<3 cm, often multiple). Leukopenia was present in 45%, elevated LDH (>500 U/L) in 88%, and ANA was weakly positive in 30% of patients in whom it was measured. All patients completely recovered.

The appearance during the 1980s and the subsequent increased incidence of HIV infection and acquired immunodeficiency syndrome (AIDS) should encourage primary care physicians to look for characteristic physical signs and symptoms, as well as known risk factors, including parental intravenous drug abuse, parental sexual contact with individuals who may be HIV positive, an HIV-positive mother, and hemophilia requiring transfusion of blood products. Fortunately, in the United States, hemophilia poses less of a risk, since screening for HIV is very sensitive and more synthetic factors are also being used. In addition,

BOX 30-2

## *Causes of Fever of Unknown Origin in Children*

### INFECTIOUS DISEASES

#### *Bacterial*

- Bacterial endocarditis
- Bartonellosis
- Brucellosis
- Chlamydia
  - Lymphogranuloma venereum
  - Psittacosis
- Dental infections
- Ehrlichiosis
- Leptospirosis
- Liver abscess
- Lyme disease (*Borrelia burgdorferi*)
- Mastoiditis (chronic)
- Osteomyelitis
- Mycoplasma infections
- Pelvic abscess
- Perinephric abscess
- Pyelonephritis
- Salmonellosis
- Sinusitis
- Subdiaphragmatic abscess
- Tuberculosis
- Tularemia

#### *Viral*

- Cytomegalovirus
- Epstein-Barr virus (infectious mononucleosis)
- Hepatitis viruses
- Human immunodeficiency virus
- Rickettsial diseases
  - Q fever
  - Rocky Mountain spotted fever

#### *Fungal*

- Blastomycosis (nonpulmonary)
- Histoplasmosis (disseminated)

#### *Parasitic*

- Malaria
- Toxoplasmosis
- Visceral larva migrans
- Visceral leishmaniasis

### AUTOIMMUNE DISEASES

- Polyarteritis nodosa
- Sarcoidosis
- Systemic idiopathic juvenile arthritis
- Systemic lupus erythematosus

### MALIGNANCIES

- Hodgkin disease
- Leukemia
- Lymphoma
- Neuroblastoma
- Pheochromocytoma

### PERIODIC FEVER SYNDROMES

- Cyclic neutropenia
- Familial Mediterranean fever
- Hyperimmunoglobulinemia D and periodic fever syndrome (HIDS)
- Periodic fever, aphthous stomatitis, pharyngitis, and cervical adenopathy (PFAPA)
- Tumor necrosis factor receptor–associated periodic syndrome (TRAPS)
- Other periodic fever syndromes

### MISCELLANEOUS CAUSES

- Colitis, granulomatous
- Colitis, ulcerative
- Diabetes insipidus—central
- Diabetes insipidus—nephrogenic
- Drug fever
- Ectodermal dysplasia
- Familial dysautonomia
- Hemophagocytic lymphohistiocytosis
- Infantile cortical hyperostosis
- Kawasaki disease
- Kikuchi-Fujimoto disease
- Münchausen by proxy
- Pancreatitis
- Pseudo-fever (factitious fever)
- Serum sickness
- Thyrotoxicosis

Modified from Feigin RD, Cherry JD. *Textbook of Pediatric Infectious Diseases.* 5th ed. Philadelphia, PA: WB Saunders; 2004. 

**Table 30-1**
**Diagnoses of Prolonged Fever in Children**

| DIAGNOSIS | AGE <6 YEARS | AGE ≥6 YEARS | TOTAL |
|---|---|---|---|
| ***Infection*** | | | |
| Viral | 14 (27%) | 7 (15%) | 21 |
| Nonviral | 20 (38%) | 11 (23%) | 31 |
| ***Other*** | | | |
| Collagen | 4 (8%) | 16 (33%) | 20 |
| Malignancy | 4 (8%) | 2 (4%) | 6 |
| Miscellaneous | 7 (13%) | 3 (6%) | 10 |
| No diagnosis | 3 (6%) | 9 (19%) | 12 |
| Total | 52 | 48 | 100 |

From Pizzo PA, Lovejoy FH, Smith DH. Prolonged fever in children: review of 100 cases. *Pediatrics.* 1975;55(4):468–473.

infant screening for HIV is also occurring now. Fever is not usually the sole manifestation of HIV infection. However, HIV infection should be strongly considered and the appropriate laboratory tests performed if the fever has been present for more than 2 months and is associated with 1 or more of the following:

- Failure to thrive or a weight loss of more than 10% from baseline
- Hepatomegaly
- Splenomegaly
- Generalized lymphadenopathy (lymph nodes measuring at least 0.5 cm in 2 or more sites, with bilateral site involvement counting as 1 site)
- Parotitis
- Persistent or recurrent diarrhea[17]

Of the autoimmune diseases, systemic-onset juvenile idiopathic arthritis (formerly known as systemic juvenile rheumatoid arthritis) is the most common. Fever is almost always associated with this illness, and it frequently precedes the joint manifestations by weeks or months. The typical double quotidian fever (2 fever spikes in 24 hours with a normal temperature in between) is a helpful clue to this diagnosis. Other common autoimmune diseases that should be considered are lupus erythematosus and chronic regional enteritis. These latter conditions are more common in children older than 6 years.

Malignancy, the diagnosis that provokes the most anxiety, is present in only a small percentage of patients in most studies (1.5%–6%).[4,8,9,12] This is in significant contrast to adults with FUO, of whom between 7% and 16% have a neoplastic process.[3,18] The most common malignancy in children is leukemia, although solid tumors such as lymphoma, neuroblastoma, hypernephroma, pheochromocytoma[19] and hepatoma have been reported to present as FUO. The exact reason for fever in these diseases is unclear but seems to be related to various endogenous pyrogens such as interleukin-1, interleukin-6 and other cytokines produced by the neoplastic cells. A large variety of miscellaneous diseases may cause prolonged fevers (see Box 30-2). However, a clear diagnosis is never obtained in 25% to 67% of patients who have persistent fever.[8,12,20] These fevers are the genuine FUOs. Most of these patients seem to do well, and the fever eventually disappears after months or even years.[21]

Some patients have fevers that do not satisfy the classic definition of FUO. Instead, they have recurrent fevers that are associated with a well-defined constellation of symptoms each time. The most common of these periodic fever syndromes is PFAPA.[7] This nonhereditary autoinflammatory syndrome has its onset before the age of 3 years, is associated with a sudden fever to 39°C to 40°C (102°F–104°F) lasting 3 to 5 days. Also present are anorexia, mild oral ulcerations with pharyngitis, cervical lymphadenopathy, an increased white blood cell count, and an increased erythrocyte sedimentation rate (ESR). This constellation of symptoms returns every 3 to 6 weeks. A single dose of corticosteroids may quickly resolve the symptoms of individual episodes.[22] In the longest follow-up study available,[23] the average time until resolution of symptoms was 6.3 years, but some patients still had symptoms 18 years later. Removal of adenoids/tonsils has been associated with resolution but it is not always effective.

Other periodic fever syndromes include cyclic neutropenia, familial Mediterranean fever, hyperimmunoglobulinemia D and periodic fever syndrome (HIDS, or mevalonate kinase deficiency), and tumor necrosis factor receptor–associated periodic syndrome (TRAPS). These syndromes are found in various populations around the world and are associated with known gene mutations.[7,24] The primary care physician should therefore know the patient's race, ethnicity, and country of origin because these factors may provide clues to a specific periodic fever syndrome.

## ▶ EVALUATION

### History

Whether the child has a true FUO or a pseudo-FUO cannot be determined without a precise history and thorough physical examination, with the physician paying close attention to behavioral, social, familial, and environmental factors. Information regarding travel, patient residence if outside the United States, animal exposure, frequency of exposure to other persons who have common febrile illnesses, previous illness, hospitalizations, medications, family history of disease, race and ethnicity, and the precise course of the exhibiting symptoms must be obtained methodically and efficiently. Meticulous documentation of dates is especially important. To this end, having the family record on a calendar both the daily time and height of the fever, along with associated symptoms, is usually helpful.

For children older than 11 to 12 years, a separate interview should be conducted alone with the child to obtain the child's perspective on the illness and to elicit information that may be difficult to express in the presence of parents. School, peer relationships, family functioning, and sexual identity and activity should be explored.

### Physical Examination

A full physical examination must be performed. Rectal temperature, respiratory rate, heart rate, and blood pressure measurements should be obtained. Any discrepancy between heart rate and temperature may imply factitious fever. A thorough examination of the respiratory tract is indicated. Inspection of the tongue and gums for aphthous ulcers, pharynx for hyperemia and exudate, the tympanic membranes for chronic otitis media, and the nose for a purulent nasal discharge, and auscultation of the chest for localized wheezing are all important.

In the older child, an examination of the teeth to exclude dental caries and periodontal disease should be included. A new cardiac murmur may be a clue to rheumatic fever or infective endocarditis. A careful abdominal exam may demonstrate an enlarged and/or tender liver, splenomegaly, generalized tenderness, or a mass. Lymphadenopathy, especially if generalized, may suggest a viral infection, such as infectious mononucleosis, cytomegalovirus infection, toxoplasmosis, or HIV infection, but could also suggest leukemia. If lymphadenopathy is limited to the cervical areas, the physician should consider periodic fever syndrome, Kawasaki disease, Kikuchi-Fujimoto disease, and cat-scratch disease. Joints must be examined meticulously for swelling, restricted range of motion, and tenderness. Skin rashes may suggest a viral disease, a tick-borne disease, infectious mononucleosis, or an autoimmune disease such as juvenile idiopathic arthritis. The absence of sweating and the presence of a smooth tongue are consistent with familial dysautonomia, a rare genetic disorder of thermoregulation. Finally, a rectal examination in the older child and a stool guaiac test are imperative; finding pararectal lymphadenopathy may suggest a pelvic infection, and a positive stool guaiac test may be consistent with inflammatory bowel disease.

### Laboratory Evaluation

If the history and physical examination disclose no specific findings and growth is normal, then only simple diagnostic tests are indicated. Routine blood counts and urinalyses have not been shown to be particularly useful, although no one advocates their elimination from the workup. A purified protein derivative tuberculin skin test or interferon-gamma release assay (IGRA) should be done to detect tuberculosis. Negative blood, urine, and throat cultures exclude infections of these areas. One should be careful to recognize that if there is a group A strep positive throat culture without symptoms or physical findings of pharyngitis, one should assume that the throat is colonized with group A strep and this is not the etiology of the fever.

Probably the most useful laboratory tests are the ESR, C-reactive protein (CRP), albumin-globulin ratio, LDH, and uric acid. If the ESR is more than 30, the CRP is elevated, or the albumin-globulin ratio is inverted, then a higher probability of serious disease exists, particularly an autoimmune vascular disease or a malignancy. Significantly elevated LDH and uric acid suggest tissue breakdown often associated with lymphoproliferative disease or other malignancy. A significantly elevated ferritin is usually present in hemophagocytic lymphohistiocytosis (HLH) and juvenile arthritis with macrophage activation syndrome, but affected children are usually very ill and clearly require hospitalization. Further evaluation should be vigorously pursued.

The remainder of the evaluation should be individualized based on historical and clinical findings. Because infectious causes are the most common, pursuing specific serologic tests for such diseases as hepatitis A and B, Epstein-Barr virus infection (infectious mononucleosis), bartonellosis, toxoplasmosis, and cytomegalovirus infection are reasonable. A radioactive gallium (or other isotope) scan may be useful in detecting occult abscesses and infections, although this scan has been found to be less helpful in children than in adults.[25] Total body computed tomographic scans may help find tumors; however, if the abdomen is of primary concern, an abdominal ultrasound may detect significant abnormalities and would avoid the significant radiation associated with computed tomography.[20] Radiologic studies of the sinuses, the gastrointestinal tract, and the chest all may be appropriate in certain individuals but should not be routine. A bone marrow examination may occasionally help in the diagnosis of tuberculosis, leukemia, metastatic cancer, or fungal infections, but should be considered only in children who have either a clinical or laboratory finding suggestive of malignancy or who are immunocompromised.[26] More recently, with the advent of sophisticated imaging technology, a $^{18}$F-FDG PET or PET/CT scan has been found especially helpful in diagnosing sytemic-onset idiopathic juvenile arthritis, obviating further workup.[27] The PET scans demonstrate areas where there is high glucose consumption, typically areas of tumor or inflammation. Further evaluation of the benefit of these types of scans is necessary.

If the ESR, CRP, albumin-globulin ratio, LDH, and uric acid are normal and no signs and symptoms are present that are specific to a particular disease, little can be gained from any of the tests previously mentioned. Observation and periodic evaluation are the only measures that are required while the physician remains alert for the occurrence of new symptoms or signs that might lead the investigation in a specific direction. Fortunately, most FUOs for which a cause cannot be found resolve over time.

Since it is likely that the parents and patient will be anxious about an undiagnosable problem, the primary care physician must be ready to provide all family members with a clear explanation of the evaluative process, any normal results, and reassurance. Referrals to pediatric infectious disease specialists, rheumatologists, specialized diagnosticians, or any combination of these professionals may occasionally be necessary for additional assistance in determining a diagnosis. However, over-referral may accentuate the anxiety of the family.

## ▶ SUMMARY

The evaluation of the child who has FUO must be individualized and depends on a careful assessment of the history, the physical examination, and the social context of the child. An initial and often repeated meticulous examination of all these factors is the physician's responsibility and is the first stage of managing the patient. Whether hospitalization is part of this approach ultimately depends on the amount of parental anxiety, the necessity to document fever, and the need for diagnostic tests that cannot be done on an outpatient basis. A minimal number of diagnostic tests is usually sufficient to rule out serious disease that requires aggressive intervention and/or treatment by specifc subspecialists.

Frequent assessment of children with persistent FUO is necessary so that subtle clues for diagnoses are not missed, diagnostic testing is timed carefully, and the family continues to maintain confidence in the physician. In the absence of any alarming symptoms, physical findings, or results of diagnostic tests, it is important to emphasize to families and the patient (where appropriate) that even though the fever may last for weeks or months, children with FUOs generally do well.

### When to Admit

Consider admission for the following patients:

- Patients in whom the accuracy of reported temperature is unclear or questionable; temperatures must be taken by hospital staff or under their direct supervision.
- Patients who need multiple tests, many of which require procedural sedation. Coordinating these tests together over a period of 24 to 48 hours may be more efficient than performing them individually as an outpatient.

## TOOLS FOR PRACTICE

### Engaging Patient and Family

- *Fever* (handout), American Academy of Pediatrics (patiented.solutions.aap.org)
- *Fever* (Web page), American Academy of Pediatrics (www.healthychildren.org/English/health-issues/conditions/fever/Pages/default.aspx)
- *Fever and Your Child* (handout), American Academy of Pediatrics (patiented.solutions.aap.org)

### Medical Decision Support

- *Red Book: 2012 Report of the Committee on Infectious Diseases,* 29th ed (book), American Academy of Pediatrics (shop.aap.org)

## REFERENCES

1. Petersdorf RG, Beeson PB. Fever of unexplained origin: report on 100 cases. *Medicine (Baltimore).* 1961;40:1–30
2. Durack DT, Street AC. Fever of unknown origin—re-examined and redefined. *Curr Clin Top Infect Dis.* 1991;11:35–51
3. Vanderscheuren S, Knockaert D, Adriaenssens T, et al. From prolonged febrile illness to fever of unknown origin—the challenge continues. *Arch Intern Med.* 2003;163(9):1033–1041
4. Feigin RD, Shearer WT. Fever of unknown origin in children. *Curr Probl Pediatr.* 1976;6:1
5. Musher DM, Fainstein V, Young EJ, Pruett TL. Fever patterns. Their lack of clinical significance. *Arch Intern Med.* 1979;139:1225–1228
6. Kleiman MB. The complaint of persistent fever. Recognition and management of pseudo fever of unknown origin. *Pediatr Clin North Am.* 1982;29:201–208
7. Long SS. Distinguishing among prolonged, recurrent, and periodic fever syndromes: approach of a pediatric infectious diseases subspecialist. *Pediatr Clin North Am.* 2005;52:811–835, vii
8. Jacobs RF, Schutze GE. Bartonella henselae as a cause of prolonged fever and fever of unknown origin in children. *Clin Infect Dis.* 1998;26:80–84
9. Pizzo PA, Lovejoy FH, Smith DH. Prolonged fever in children: review of 100 cases. *Pediatrics.* 1975;55:468–473
10. Lohr JA, Hendley JO. Prolonged fever of unknown origin: a record of experiences with 54 childhood patients. *Clin Pediatr.* 1977;16(9):768–773
11. Cogulu O, Koturoglu G, Kurugol Z, et al. Evaluation of 80 children with prolonged fever. *Pediatr Int.* 2003;45:564–569
12. Pasic S, Minic A, Djuric P, et al. Fever of unknown origin in 185 paediatric patients: a single-centre experience. *Acta Paediatr.* 2006;95:463–466
13. Ventura A, Massei F, Not T, et al. Systemic *Bartonella henselae* infection with hepatosplenic involvement. *J Pediatr Gastroent Nutr.* 1999;29(1):52–56
14. Tsujino K, Tsukahara M, Tsuneoka H, et al. Clinical implication of prolonged fever in children with cat scratch disease. *J Infect Chemother.* 2004;10:227–233
15. Antoon JW, Bradford KK. Fever of unknown origin in a child. *Clin Pediatr (Phila).* 2013;52:99–102
16. Kim TY, Ha KS, Kim Y, et al. Characteristics of Kikuchi-Fujimoto disease in children compared with adults. *Eur J Pediatr.* 2014;173(1):111–116
17. Centers for Disease Control (CDC). Classification system for human immunodeficiency virus (HIV) infection in children under 13 years of age. *MMWR Morb Mortal Wkly Rep.* 1987;36:225–230, 235–236
18. Bleeker-Rovers CP, Vos FJ, de Kleijn EM, et al. A prospective multicenter study on fever of unknown origin. *Medicine (Baltimore).* 2007;86(1):26–38
19. Yarman S, Soyluk O, Altunoglu E, Tanakol R. Interleukin-6-producing pheochromocytoma presenting with fever of unknown origin. *Clinics (Sao Paulo).* 2011;66:1843–1845

20. Steele RW, Jones SM, Lowe BA, Glasier CM. Usefulness of scanning procedures for diagnosis of fever of unknown origin in children. *J Pediatr.* 1991;119:526–530
21. Miller LE, Sisson BA, Tucker LB, et al. Prolonged fevers of unknown origin in children: patterns of presentation and outcome. *J Pediatr.* 1996;129(3):419–423
22. Marshall GS, Edwards KM, Butler J, Lawton AR. Syndrome of periodic fever, pharyngitis, and aphthous stomatitis. *J Pediatr.* 1987;110:43–46
23. Wurster VM, Carlucci JG, Feder HM, Edwards KM. Long-term follow-up of children with periodic fever, aphthous stomatitis, pharyngitis, and cervical adenitis syndrome. *J Pediatr.* 2011;159:958–964
24. Hofer M, Mahlaoui N, Prieur AM. A child with a systemic febrile illness—differential diagnosis and management. *Best Pract Res Clin Rheumatol.* 2006;20:627–640
25. Buonomo C, Treves ST. Gallium scanning in children with fever of unknown origin. *Pediatr Radiol.* 1993;23:307–310
26. Hayani A, Mahoney DH, Fernbach DJ. Role of bone marrow examination in the child with prolonged fever. *J Pediatr.* 1990;116:919–920
27. Jasper N, Däbritz J, Frosch M, et al. Diagnostic value of [(18)F]-FDG PET/CT in children with fever of unknown origin or unexplained signs of inflammation. *Eur J Nucl Med Mol Imaging.* 2010; 37:136–145

# Chapter 31

# Foot and Leg Problems

*Benjamin Weintraub, MD*

## INTRODUCTION

Parents frequently come to the physician with concerns about their children's feet and legs, such as "my son is pigeon-toed," or "my daughter is knock-kneed." In most cases, these findings are purely normal developmental stages seen in the growth of the lower extremities. For example, it is entirely normal for a toddler just starting to walk to be "bowlegged" or "pigeon-toed," or for a 3-year-old to have "knock-knees." However, it may be pathologic for a 10-year-old to have significant genu valgus (knock-knees) or a 5-year-old to have severe genu varum (bowed legs). The physician, then, needs to understand the normal changes seen during growth and development to judge properly when a finding is pathologic and requires further evaluation, treatment, and referral to a specialist.

## NATURAL GROWTH OF LOWER EXTREMETIES

During the course of gestation, the lower extremities of the fetus undergo vast changes. Lower limb buds develop at 4 weeks' gestation. During week 6, the lower limbs begin to flex toward the parasagittal plane, and then proceed to rotate medially so that the knee points cranially and the great toe is brought to the midline. By term, 80% of babies are in the classic fetal position with knees and hips flexed, hips externally rotated, and ankles plantar-flexed and internally rotated. This tightly packaged position conveniently helps drive the femoral head into the acetabulum, thereby aiding in the development of the hip socket. It also leads to a number of transient conditions that self-resolve over time but until then may cause significant parental anxiety: pigeon toeing and bow legs, or more precisely, internal tibial torsion, metatarsus adductus, and medial femoral anteversion.

Of the remaining 20% not in the usual fetal position, most are in a position with hips and knees flexed, ankles dorsiflexed, and legs and feet externally rotated, which can lead to external tibial torsion, calcaneovalgus feet, and out-toeing.

After birth, the first of these "packaging defects" to self-correct is metatarsus adductus. This medial deviation of the forefoot usually either self-resolves or can be corrected by 1 year of age with simple stretching. Tibial bowing is next to resolve by about age 2 to 4 years. Bowing is usually followed by the appearance of an increasingly knock-kneed or genu valgus stance from 3 to 5 years of age. By the end of the first decade of life, tibial torsion goes from a mean of 5 degrees medial torsion to 10 degrees lateral torsion, and femoral anteversion decreases from about 40 degrees at birth to about 10 degrees. The result is a lateral rotation of the lower extremity during growth and a gradual decline

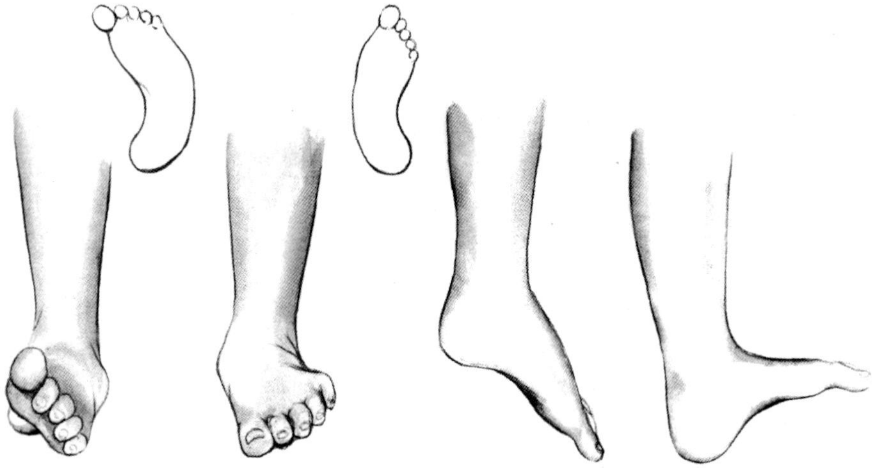

**Figure 31-1**
Positional deformities of the foot and ankle. **A,** Varus. **B,** Valgus. **C,** Equinus. **D,** Talipes calcaneus.

in the degree of genu valgus until the normal adult stance of minimal genu valgum is reached at maturity (Figure 31-1).

Most functional deformities of the legs and feet are self-correcting in time through this normal developmental progression of the lower extremities. In the past, many of these rotational and positional deformities were treated with stretching, bracing, and even casting. However, studies of these functional deformities comparing treated versus untreated paired-control groups have demonstrated the relative ineffectiveness of treatment for these conditions. Therefore, most physicians choose watchful waiting for these conditions because children naturally grow out of them. A more detailed discussion of these conditions follows.[1-3]

## ▶ ORTHOPEDIC TERMINOLOGY

Orthopedists use a standard terminology to describe positional and structural variations of the lower extremities. In general, the joint that is primarily involved in the condition constitutes the first word; the subsequent word or words relate to the positioning of the extremity relative to the midline of the body. For example, coxa vara is a condition of the hip (coxa) that results in a deviation of the leg toward the midline (varus position). The orthopedic terms in Box 31-1 have special reference to abnormalities of the feet and legs.

## ▶ ROTATIONAL DEFORMITIES

### *In-toeing and Out-toeing*

Rotational deformities of the lower extremities are the most common cause of in-toeing and out-toeing. With in-toeing (pigeon toe), the foot turns inward more than expected during walking or running relative to the line of progression; with out-toeing, the foot turns outward more than expected. Parents, seeing either in-toeing or out-toeing, often become concerned that some intervention is needed. In most cases, these deformities are physiologic, related to normal growth and development, and the appropriate intervention is reassurance.

BOX 31-1

## *Glossary of Terms That Refer to Foot and Leg Abnormalities*

- *Abduction:* deviation away from the midline of the body
- *Adduction:* deviation toward the midline of the body
- *Cavus:* medial longitudinal arch of the foot elevated
- *Equinus:* foot plantar-flexed, placing the toes below the level of the heel
- *Pes:* the foot
- *Planus:* medial longitudinal arch of the foot flattened
- *Talipes:* congenital deformity describing a foot that is twisted out of shape or position
- *Talipes calcaneus:* a deformity of the foot in which the foot is dorsiflexed
- *Torsion:* excessive or abnormal twisting along the long axis
  - *Internal torsion:* excessive or abnormal inward twisting
  - *External torsion:* excessive or abnormal outward twisting
- *Varus:* medial or inward deviation of the distal segment of an extremity relative to the proximal (previous) segment
- *Valgus:* lateral or outward deviation of the distal segment of an extremity relative to the proximal (previous) segment
- *Version:* physiologic or normal twisting along the long axis
  - *Inversion:* physiologic or normal twist inward
  - *Eversion:* physiologic or normal twist outward
  - *Anteversion:* physiologic or normal twist forward
  - *Retroversion:* physiologic or normal twist backward

In-toeing and out-toeing may be seen at all ages and are caused by a variety of conditions affecting the feet, ankles, legs, knees, and hips. In general, with in-toeing, if the child's patellae are rotated inward (kissing knees) while walking, then the underlying problem will be found above the knee—most commonly femoral anteversion. If the patellae face straight forward, then the underlying problem is likely below the knee—most commonly medial tibial torsion or metatarsus adductus.[4] Less common causes of in-toeing include talipes equinovarus, metatarsus varus, and spasticity of the internal rotator muscles of the hip, as seen in cerebral palsy.

Excessive out-toeing, less common than in-toeing, may be seen with excessive external tibial torsion and femoral retroversion, or with posterior maldirection of the acetabulum, rigid flat feet, and flaccid paralysis of the internal rotator muscles of the hip. Most adults have a mild degree of physiologic out-toeing when standing and walking.

Parents can be reassured that most cases of in-toeing and out-toeing will resolve spontaneously as the lower extremities finish growing. Although in-toeing or out-toeing may reflect a variety of underlying orthopedic diseases, no evidence has been found to suggest that uncorrected in-toeing or out-toeing of normal developmental origin leads to any functional disabilities.[5]

An orthopedic or neurologic evaluation should be made for any child with severe in-toeing or out-toeing, or for an unsteady gait (especially while running) that causes stumbling. A referral may also be advised if a child's condition does not follow the expected physiologic progression with growth.[6,7]

## Metatarsus Adductus and Deformities of the Forefoot

### Clinical Conditions

Deformities of the forefoot are among the earliest causes of in-toeing noted by parents. The most common and generally benign cause is *metatarsus adductus* (Figure 31-2), a condition in which the only finding is a flexible adduction of the metatarsals at the tarsometatarsal joints. The incidence of metatarsus adductus is generally reported to be approximately 1 in 1,000 live births, but in some studies it is reported to be as high as 1 in 100. There is a slightly higher incidence in the left foot than the right, and 50% to 60% of cases occur bilaterally.[8]

The differential diagnosis of metatarsus adductus includes the uncommon conditions talipes varus, metatarsus varus, and clubfoot. *Talipes varus* (Figure 31-3) is a condition in which the entire foot is inverted and the forefoot is adducted. In *metatarsus varus* (Figure 31-4), the forefoot is inverted and adducted while the hindfoot and heel are in the normal position. Talipes varus and metatarsus varus have been considered lesser degrees of clubfoot and are fixed deformities of the foot that require early treatment.[2]

## Evaluation

### Relevant History

Although its exact cause has not been established, metatarsus adductus is widely considered a packaging defect. There may be a history of oligohydramnios, uterine fibroids, multiple

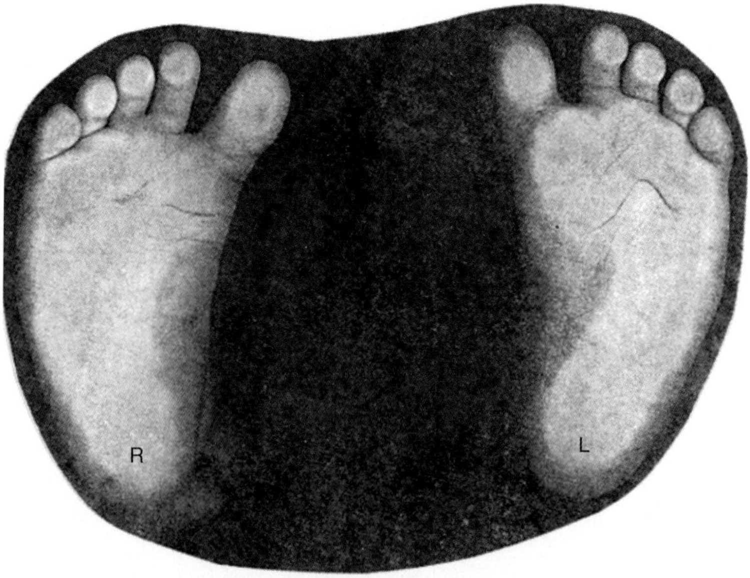


**Figure 31-2**
Photocopy of the feet of a 9-month-old infant with bilateral metatarsus adductus. *(From Greene WB. Metatarsus adductus and skewfoot.* Instr Course Lect. *1994;43:161–177. Reproduced with permission from American Academy of Orthopaedic Surgeons.)*

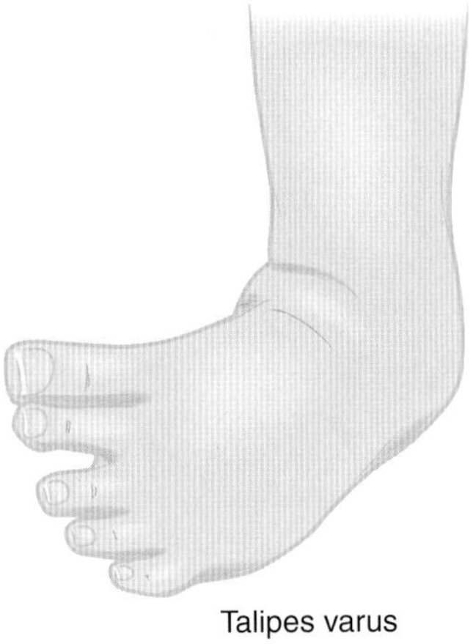


**Figure 31-3**
Talipes varus. The entire foot is twisted inward on its longitudinal axis, and the forefoot is adducted.

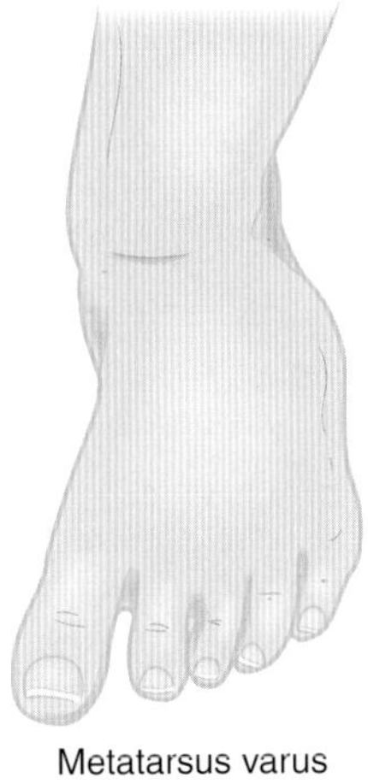


**Figure 31-4**
Bilateral metatarsus varus. The forefoot is inverted and adducted, and the lateral border of the foot is convex. The hindfoot is in a neutral position.

gestation, or other cause of a crowded intrauterine environment; but such a history is not necessary for making the diagnosis. Metatarsus adductus was previously thought to be associated with developmental hip dysplasia. However, more recent studies do not support the association, and an ultrasound of the hips is no longer required as part of the workup of metatarsus adductus.[3]

## Physical Examination

Metatarsus adductus is graded by both the degree of adduction and the flexibility of the deformity. The severity of adduction is graded by the heel bisector method. Normally, a line bisecting the heel and sole longitudinally lines up approximately with the second toe. In mild metatarsus adductus, the heel bisector line falls through the third toe, whereas in severe metatarsus adductus, the line falls between the fourth and fifth toes. The heel bisector line can be assessed directly on the child's foot, or the child may be stood up on a photocopy machine to take a photograph of the soles of the feet. A bisector line can then be drawn on the photocopy. An advantage of this method is that it allows for easy tracking of the condition over time.

Next, flexibility of the forefoot should be assessed by holding the heel and abducting the forefoot. With a flexible foot, the second toe can be easily brought in line with or even past the heel bisector line. If the foot is not flexible, then the defect is more consistent with metatarsus varus or talipes varus, and referral should be made to an orthopedist.[8,9]

### Imaging

Radiographic examination is necessary only when there is limited flexibility of the forefoot to evaluate for talipes varus and metatarsus varus.

## *Management*

Metatarsus adductus is a functional deformity and requires minimal if any treatment because most cases correct spontaneously during the first year of life. Parents may be instructed to perform simple stretching exercises of the child's foot. The parent holds the heel in place and puts gentle pressure on the medial side of the foot with the other hand, stretching the midfoot and bringing the foot into normal or even slightly overcorrected position. This stretch can be held for several seconds and repeated 5 to 10 times with each diaper change. About 85% to 90% of cases will resolve by 8 to 12 months of age with this simple management. If some improvement is not seen by 6 months of age, referral to a specialist should be made. Most of these refractory cases can be treated successfully with serial casting. Whether through spontaneous resolution or with treatment, nearly all cases of metatarsus adductus resolve without any long-term complications.[2,3]

Talipes varus and metatarsus varus are fixed deformities of the foot that require early referral and treatment. Treatment consists of serial casting, long-leg splints that abduct the forefoot, or both. Abduction stretching exercises and outflare shoes may be used as an adjunct to cast treatment but should not be relied on as the only therapy. The sooner therapy is initiated, the better the outcome.

## *Tibial Torsion*

### Natural History and Presentation

*Tibial torsion* is the rotation of the tibia on its longitudinal axis. Most infants are born with internal tibial torsion resulting from normal growth and the classic fetal position in utero. This turning inward results in mild in-toeing at birth for many infants. The average tibial torsion in infancy is −5 degrees (5 degrees of internal tibial torsion). An increased degree of internal tibial torsion is a common cause of in-toeing in toddlers up to age 3 or 4 years. As the child grows, the tibia externally rotates until a mild degree of external tibial torsion is reached in later childhood. Adults have an average external tibial torsion of +15 to +25 degrees, which accounts for the standard mild out-toeing position seen in adulthood. There is no evidence that patients with unresolved internal tibial torsion experience any increased incidence of knee pain, arthritis, or other conditions later in life. External tibial torsion in early childhood is much less common. It may be idiopathic, or it can be seen with calcaneovalgus foot deformities, as compensation for persistent severe femoral anteversion, or associated with tight iliotibial bands. As the tibia normally undergoes external rotation during growth, external tibial torsion may actually worsen over time rather than improve.

Pathologic degrees of internal and external tibial torsion are rare and may occur with other significant deformities of the hips or lower extremities, or as a result of improperly applied casts or braces.[6,8,10]

## Evaluation

### Physical Examination

The easiest way to assess tibial rotation is to measure the thigh–foot angle, which is the axis of the foot relative to the axis of the thigh (see Figures 31-5 and 31-6). The infant or child should be placed prone on the abdomen with the knees together and bent to 90 degrees and the ankles in neutral position. The acute angle made between the axis of the femur and the heel bisector is the thigh–foot angle. An internal or negative angle indicates internal rotation; an external or positive angle indicates external rotation. The normal thigh–foot angle at birth ranges widely from −35 degrees to +40 degrees, with a mean of −5 degrees. Thigh–foot angles of +10 degrees and +15 to +25 degrees are the average seen in older children and adults, respectively.[2,9,10]

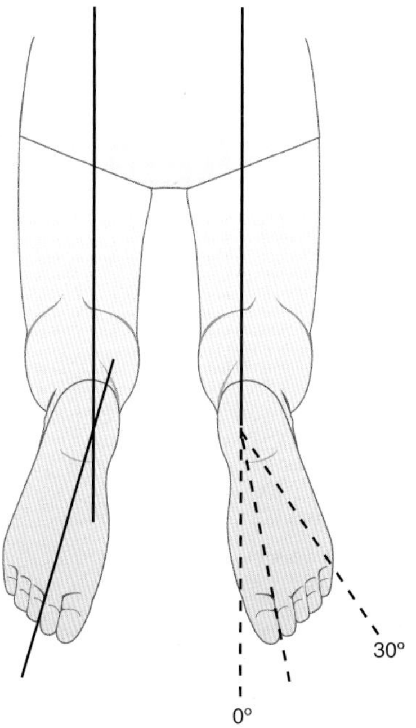


**Figure 31-5**
Thigh-foot angle: normal range. *(From Alexander IJ.* The Foot: Examination and Diagnosis. *New York, NY: Churchill Livingstone; 1990. Copyright © 1990, Elsevier, with permission.)*

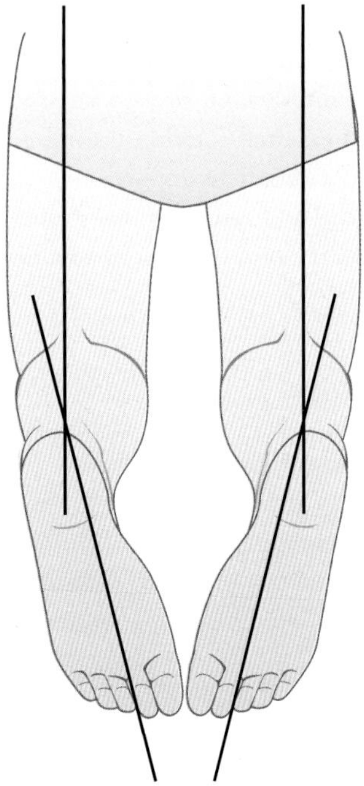

**Figure 31-6**
Bilateral internal tibial torsion. *(From Alexander IJ.* The Foot: Examination and Diagnosis. *New York, NY: Churchill Livingstone; 1990. Copyright © 1990, Elsevier, with permission.)*

## Imaging

Although studies have shown computed tomography scanning to be an excellent method for measuring the exact degree of tibial torsion, imaging is not required in most cases: physical examination is generally sufficient.

### *Management*

In the past, various forms of bracing, such as Denis Browne splints, were used to treat internal tibial torsion. However, because it is now understood that this condition resolves on its own over time, treatment of primary internal tibial torsion is no longer recommended. Even toddlers who may occasionally trip over their toes as a result of increased internal tibial torsion generally do not need treatment and outgrow the condition by age 6 years. The mainstay of treatment is parental reassurance and education about the natural growth and development of the legs. In very rare cases, when severe residual internal tibial torsion is affecting function, derotational osteotomies may be required. Surgery should be delayed until at least 8 to 10 years of age to ensure that the issue does not self-correct. Surgery may also be required for the rare case of significant external tibial torsion that interferes with function.[10]

### *Femoral Anteversion*

*Femoral anteversion* is the increased internal rotation or twisting of the femoral neck anteriorly relative to the femoral condyles; *femoral retroversion* is the extreme twisting of the femoral neck posteriorly relative to the femoral condyles. Femoral anteversion is greatest at birth (about 40 degrees) and gradually declines to adult values of 10 to 15 degrees by age 8 years. Femoral anteversion is the most common cause of in-toeing seen in preschool-aged children. Conversely, femoral retroversion is an uncommon condition that results in an out-toeing gait. New onset of femoral retroversion may occur in older children in the setting of slipped capital femoral epiphysis (SCFE).[8]

## Natural History and Presentation

In utero and postnatal positioning of the legs and hips produces stresses that are thought to bring about these rotational deformities of the femoral neck. The true incidence of excessive anteversion and retroversion is not known. However, femoral anteversion is much more common and occurs twice as frequently in girls as in boys.

### *Evaluation*

## Physical Examination

Parents of a child with femoral anteversion may express concerns about kissing knees, in-toeing, or a clumsy gait, or they may note that the child will not or cannot sit in the modified lotus position but rather prefers to "W" sit.

The best manner in which to assess for femoral anteversion or retroversion is to place the child in the prone position with the knees flexed to 90 degrees. To measure hip rotation, the lower leg is used as a pointer, and the legs are rotated through the axis of the hip joint (Figures 31-7 and 31-8). Normally the examiner should be able to move the hip through approximately 50 degrees of internal and 40 degrees of external rotation. With excessive femoral anteversion, there will be increased internal rotation of the hip of at least 60 to 65 and sometimes as much as 80 to 90 degrees, along with a decrease in external rotation to less than 20 degrees. With excessive femoral retroversion, there will be increased external rotation and decreased internal rotation. Until 1 or 2 years of age, the clinical measurement of hip rotation using this method is limited by the physiologic tightness of the hip joint capsule.[5]

## Imaging

Imaging is only required with severe femoral anteversion. New-onset, severe, or worsening femoral retroversion, however, can be associated with SCFE or other hip disorders, and radiographs should be obtained.

### *Management*

Most femoral torsion deformities correct themselves by 7 years of age. Children with pronounced femoral anteversion often are noted to sit in a "W" position with the child's bottom firmly planted between the feet. It is unclear if this sitting position contributes to the development of femoral anteversion, or if children with preexisting femoral anteversion find this position to be more comfortable. Parents who feel the need to intervene can encourage their child to sit in a modified lotus or Indian-style position, while discouraging sitting in the "W" position. They should be informed that these interventions are more anecdotal than evidence based. The use of splints is contraindicated, and corrective shoes are of no value.

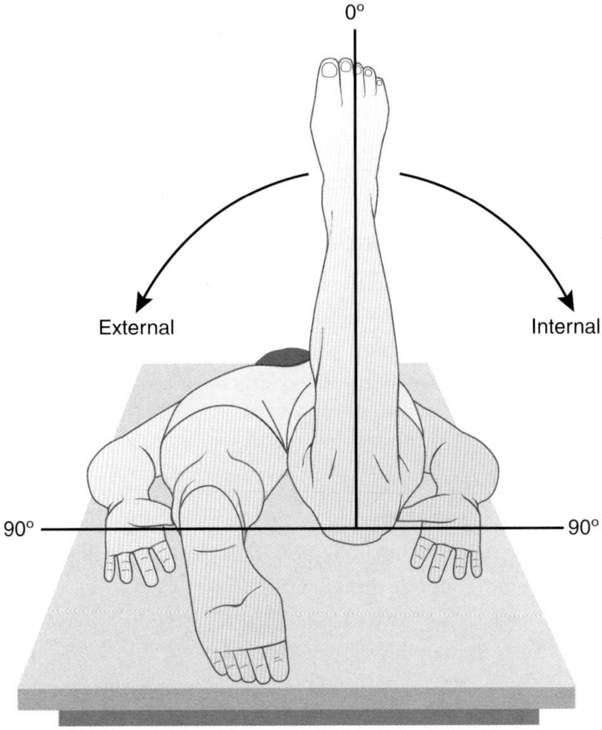


**Figure 31-7**
Starting position for measuring hip rotation with the hip extended while the child is in the prone position. *(Reprinted with permission from* Joint Motion Method of Measuring and Recording. *Rosemont, IL: American Academy of Orthopedic Surgeons; 1965.)*

An orthopedist should be consulted if the femoral anteversion does not follow the typical pattern of improvement with growth, if it is associated with difficulty walking or running, or if significant asymmetry of the anteversion exists between the 2 legs. Orthopedic treatment may consist of the use of a bivalve lower trunk and leg cast during sleeping hours or, in rare cases, a derotation osteotomy of the middle or lower femoral shaft. It remains unclear whether untreated excessive femoral anteversion contributes to early degenerative changes and osteoarthritis of the hip. Stronger evidence indicates that persistent excessive femoral retroversion may be associated with degenerative changes, and therefore referral to an orthopedist may be warranted. With femoral retroversion, immediate referral should be made if radiographs reveal SCFE.[7,10]

## ▶ PATHOLOGIC BOWED LEGS AND KNOCK-KNEES

Genu varum (bowed legs) is an angular deformity at the knee with the tibia adducted (varus) in relation to the femur. Genu valgum (knock-knees) is characterized by alignment of the knee with the tibia abducted (valgus) in relation to the femur. These conditions are generally part of the normal growth and development of the lower extremities. Bowed legs, normal at birth, start to correct once children begin to walk and are usually fully resolved by 2 to

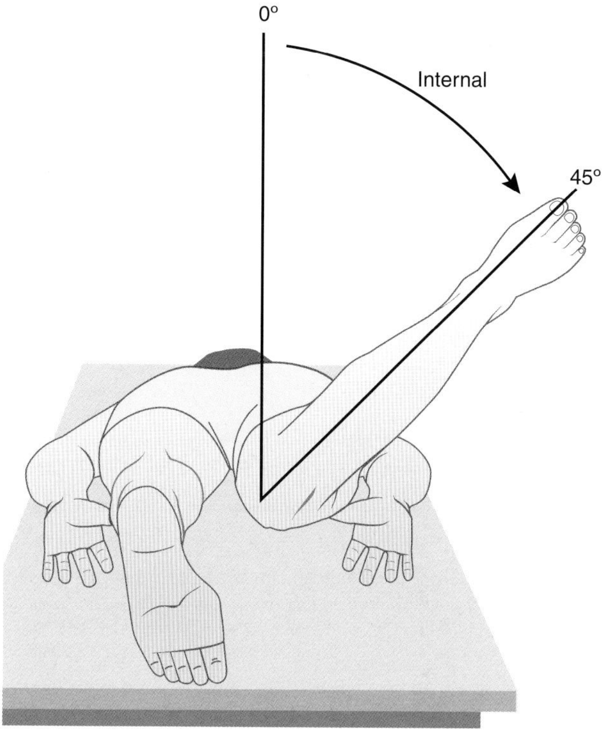


**Figure 31-8**
Internal rotation. *(Reprinted with permission from* Joint Motion Method of Measuring and Recording. *Rosemont, IL: American Academy of Orthopedic Surgeons; 1965.)*

3 years of age. Children then become increasingly knock-kneed by age 3 to 4 years, with ultimate resolution over the next several years.[2]

## *Differential Diagnosis*

Although bowed legs and knock-knees are normal at various stages of growth and development, extremes of either of these conditions, unilateral presentation, or their persistence beyond the normal time of resolution may indicate an underlying pathology. Extreme degrees of physiologic bowing of the legs may occur in the young child, and although even this usually resolves over time without treatment, a basic evaluation should be performed to ensure there is no underlying pathology (Figure 31-9).

Genu varum (bowed legs), when extreme, unilateral, or persistent, may result from a variety of conditions, including rickets, chondroplasia, osteogenesis imperfecta, osteochondritis, neuromuscular disorders, or Blount disease. In addition, trauma, infection, or tumor involving the medial proximal epiphysis of the tibia can result in genu varum.

Genu valgum (knock-knees) is often associated with pronation and is more frequently seen in the overweight child. Causes of severe bilateral genu valgum include rickets, renal osteodystrophy, and skeletal dysplasia. Unilateral genu valgum may be a result of trauma, infection, or tumors involving the lateral proximal epiphysis of the tibia (Figure 31-10).[9]

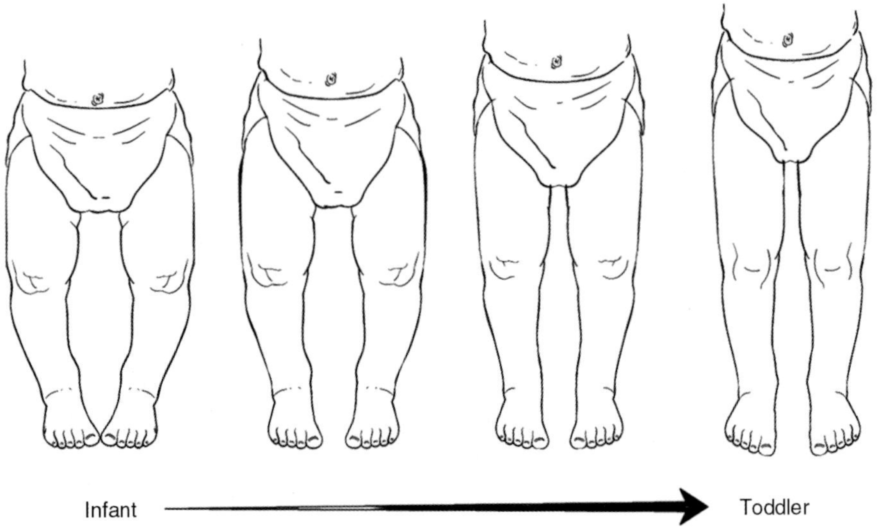


**Figure 31-9**
Normal progression from bowlegs of infancy through slow evolution to a physiologic valgus angle of about 12° at 3 years of age. *(From Gómez JE. Growth and maturation. In: Harris SA, Anderson SJ, eds.* Care of the Young Athlete. *2nd ed. Elk Grove Village, IL: American Academy of Pediatrics; 2010:18)*

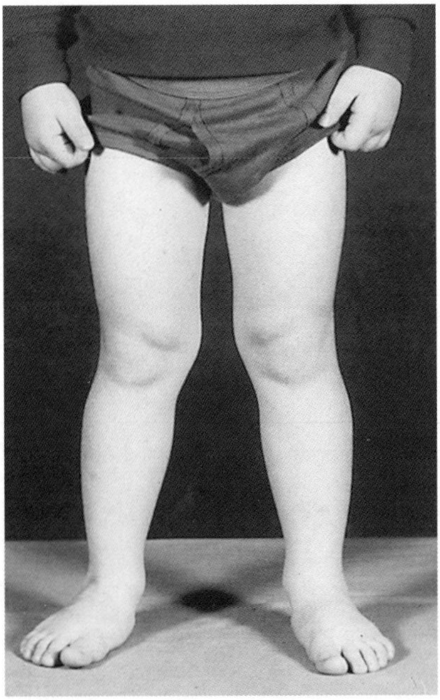

**Figure 31-10**
Clinical photograph of boy referred for evaluation of "knock-knees." The patient was considered to be within normal limits. *(From Greene WB. Genu varum and genu valgum in children.* Instr Course Lect. *1994;43:151–159. Reproduced with permission from American Academy of Orthopaedic Surgeons.)*

### Evaluation

#### Pertinent History

When evaluating severe or abnormal genu varum or valgus, a family history of metabolic, renal, or skeletal diseases should be elicited, along with any history of prior trauma, endocrine, metabolic, or bone abnormalities.

#### Physical Examination

The best way to track the progression of genu varum is to lay the patient down supine, place the ankles together, and measure the distance between the knees. This distance can be followed over time and can be used as a simple way to demonstrate to a parent that the issue is self-resolving. Similarly, the degree of genu valgum can be tracked by measuring the distance between the medial malleoli when the child is standing with the knees together.

#### Imaging

With extreme or unilateral genu valgum or genu varum, radiographic examination should be obtained to exclude rickets, chondroplasia, osteogenesis imperfecta, osteochondritis, Blount disease, injury to the proximal epiphysis of the tibia, or other pathologic process. Additional targeted laboratory evaluation for underlying metabolic conditions may also be indicated.

### Management

Simple observation and reassurance are all that are required for physiologic genu varum and genu valgum because these conditions spontaneously correct 99% of the time. When identified, underlying causes of extreme varus or valgum deformities must be effectively treated to improve angulation. Treatment of severe bowing or knocking of the knees caused by underlying disease is determined by the nature of the condition and may include wedge osteotomy, epiphyseal stapling, or nutritional, hormonal therapy. Treatment of mild cases of Blount disease may be attempted with bracing; more severe cases often require surgery.[3]

## ▶ CLUBFOOT

### General

*Clubfoot* or *talipes equinovarus* is a pathologic condition in which the foot and ankle are rigidly inverted, adducted, and plantar-flexed, resulting in a clubbing appearance (Figure 31-11). Clubfoot can easily be distinguished from benign packaging deformities of the foot that frequently occur in newborns; whereas functional deformities can be placed into normal physiologic position and usually even overcorrected, clubfoot is a rigid deformity that cannot be placed into normal alignment.

The differential diagnosis of clubfoot includes severe metatarsus adductus, talipes varus and metatarsus varus, and *calcaneovalgus* foot, which is characterized by eversion of the heel and forefoot, abduction of the forefoot, and dorsiflexion of the entire foot (Figure 31-12). Calcaneovalgus foot generally resolves in time with stretching exercises.

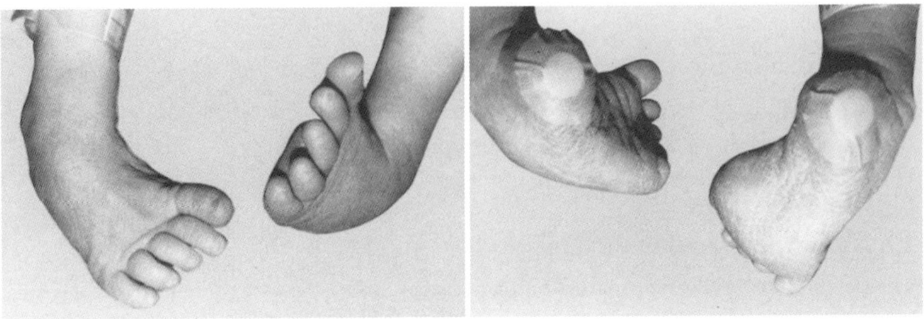

**Figure 31-11**
Bilateral congenital clubfoot seen in a newborn. *(From Sarwark JF, ed.* Essentials of Musculoskeletal Care. *4th ed. Rosemont, IL: American Academy of Orthopaedic Surgeons; 2010. Reproduced with permission.)*

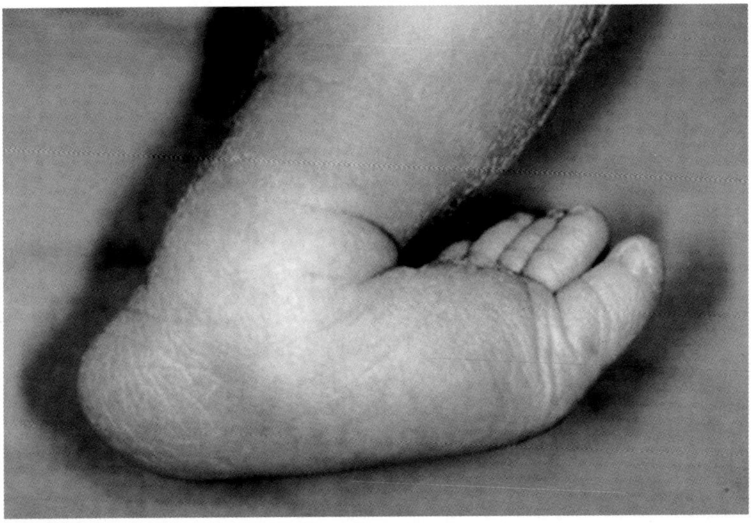

**Figure 31-12**
Clinical photograph of a calcaneovalgus foot in a neonate. *(From Sarwark JF, ed.* Essentials of Musculoskeletal Care. *4th ed. Rosemont, IL: American Academy of Orthopaedic Surgeons; 2010. Reproduced with permission.)*

## Evaluation

### Relevant History

The cause of congenital clubfoot is unknown. Although it can be associated with conditions such as spina bifida, trisomy 18, or congenital constriction band syndrome, clubfoot occurs as an isolated deformity in otherwise normal newborns in 80% of cases. Inheritance of idiopathic clubfoot seems to be multifactorial, and a specific genetic cause has not yet been identified. The incidence of clubfoot is approximately 1 in every 1,000 live births. It occurs bilaterally in 50% of cases and affects boys twice as frequently as girls. There is a 3% to 4% risk for recurrence in a family if a prior sibling had clubfoot. When a parent and sibling are affected, future children have upward of a 25% risk. Clubfoot can also develop later in life as a result of neuromuscular conditions such as arthrogryposis and meningomyelocele, and even as a neurologic complication of Wilson disease.[9]

### Physical Examination

Four main components combine to form the defective foot and ankle of a clubfoot: significant and uncorrectable plantar flexion of the ankle; heel and hindfoot adduction; high arch (cavus) at the midfoot; and severe adduction of the forefoot. All combined, the result is a rigidly plantar-flexed, medially rotated, and twisted foot and ankle that cannot be passively manipulated into a normal foot position.

When clubfoot is present, an evaluation for associated neurologic, muscular, or other skeletal anomalies should be performed.[3,9]

### Imaging

Although radiographic examination is not generally required for diagnosis, it is useful to delineate the pathologic findings and guide management.

### *Management*

For pediatricians, treatment of clubfoot entails early and immediate referral to a pediatric orthopedist for either serial casting or surgery. Some institutions report extremely high success rates with serial casting beginning in the first weeks of life and continuing through several months of age. Rates of recurrence vary after correction by manipulation alone. Recurrence after casting is most common within the first 2 to 3 years but may still happen as late as 5 to 7 years of age. Surgical correction (tenotomy, muscle transplantation, and arthrodesis) may be required in severe cases, when conservative management fails, or as a result of recurrence when the child is older. Recurrence is much less likely after surgical correction, although functional outcomes are not necessarily improved compared with more conservative measures. Even with successful treatment, the affected foot is generally smaller and less mobile than a normal foot. Early initiation of therapy increases the success rate of manipulative or conservative management and therefore decreases the need for surgical intervention.[3]

## ▶ FLATFOOT

*Pes planus*, or flatfoot, is a very common condition in childhood characterized by the loss or absence of the medial longitudinal arch when weight bearing. It is associated with a pronated gait and stance, eversion of the calcaneus and valgus position of the heel, and prominence of the medial talar head. The condition is best divided into 2 main categories: flexible flatfoot and rigid flatfoot. There is significant disagreement about the clinical importance of flexible flatfoot, if any, and its treatment. Rigid flatfoot is more likely to be clinically significant and to require treatment, although disagreement exists about this condition as well.

### *Flexible Flatfoot*

Infants are born with flat feet. The normal medial longitudinal arch does not begin forming until about 3 years of age and continues to develop for several years. The prevalence of flexible flatfoot in one study was shown to decrease on average from 54% at 3 years to 24% by 6 years of age. Boys seem twice as likely as girls to have flatfoot at 6 years of age. Overweight and obesity also increase the risk for flexible flatfoot.[11] By adulthood, the prevalence of flatfoot is closer to 10% to 20%.

Prevailing opinion in the past was that flatfoot was a cause of foot, leg, and back pain, and that it interfered with physical activity. This, however, is now not so clear. Some studies suggest that people with flatfoot walk more slowly and have decreased physical performance, whereas other studies, one involving military recruits and one involving teenagers, showed neither disadvantages in performance nor increased injury rates with flatfoot. In short, there remains a lack of general consensus on the clinical significance of this condition.[12,14]

### Physical Examination

The diagnosis of flexible flatfoot is made clinically; imaging is not required. The patient's foot should be examined while he or she is standing. If flatfoot is present, the examiner will notice a collapse of the medial longitudinal arch and ankle pronation with valgus heel position (Figure 31-13). When viewed from behind, the Achilles tendon is noted to bend medially before arcing back laterally toward the everted calcaneus. To be certain that the condition is flexible, the examiner should have the patient stand on tiptoe: in flexible flatfoot, the medial longitudinal arch of the foot will return; with rigid flatfoot, the sole remains flat.

### Treatment

Treatment of flexible flatfoot remains controversial. If flatfoot is not causing any problems, no treatment is needed beyond parental reassurance. In cases in which the condition seems to be contributing to pain and discomfort or impairing function, flatfoot can be managed conservatively with arch support inserts. If the condition is associated with tight Achilles tendons, stretching may be a beneficial part of treatment.[15]

## Rigid Flatfoot

Unlike flexible flatfoot, rigid flatfoot is more likely to represent a pathologic condition. It can result from tarsal coalition (fusion of 1 or more of the tarsal bones) or vertical talus. Two types of tarsal coalitions have been identified: *calcaneonavicular coalition,* which involves the calcaneus and the navicular bones; and *talocalcaneal coalition,* in which the calcaneus is coalesced to the talus. Congenital rigid flatfoot occurs in approximately 1% of the

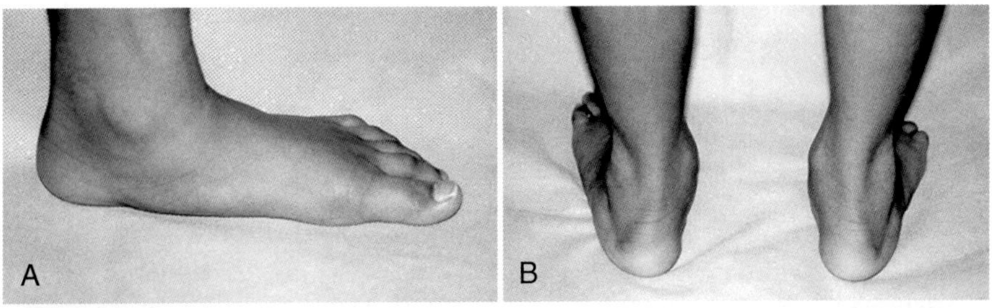


**Figure 31-13**
Medial (A) and posterior (B) views of flatfoot. *(From Sarwark JF, ed.* Essentials of Musculoskeletal Care. *4th ed. Rosemont, IL: American Academy of Orthopaedic Surgeons; 2010. Reproduced with permission.)*

population and frequently is bilateral. Rigid flatfoot may also be acquired from trauma, infection, an arthritic process, or neuromuscular disease. In these cases, the condition may be progressive, and any underlying condition should be treated as part of the management of the rigid flatfoot.[9,16]

### Physical Examination

Examination of a rigid flatfoot reveals a foot with a stiff, flattened arch in both weight-bearing and non–weight-bearing positions. There is no return of a normal arch when standing on tiptoe. This condition is generally associated with a significant degree of ankle pronation. Vertical talus and accessory tarsonavicular can usually be detected in the newborn by the presence of a bony prominence on the medial and plantar aspects of the foot, with limitation of plantar flexion and inversion of the forefoot.

Tarsal coalitions are not usually detected until late childhood or adolescence, when the initially fibrous or cartilaginous bar connecting the hindfoot bones becomes ossified, producing pain with walking and an inability to invert the foot. The foot is held in a pronated position with eversion of the forefoot. The peroneal tendons stand out prominently when attempts are made to invert the foot. Calcaneonavicular coalition tends to develop between 9 and 13 years of age, whereas talocalcaneal coalition develops later, typically at 13 to 16 years of age.[16]

### Imaging

Radiographs may be useful in identifying the exact cause of rigid flatfoot in a patient.

### Treatment

Treatment in most cases of rigid flatfoot is with orthopedic shoes. Surgical correction is required only for accessory tarsonavicular or tarsal coalition if symptoms cannot be relieved through conservative means (only about 10% of cases) and is usually performed in adulthood. Vertical talus usually requires surgical correction early in infancy.[16]

## ▶ PES CAVUS

Pes cavus (cavus foot deformity) is an equinus deformity of the forefoot relative to the hindfoot, producing a very high medial longitudinal arch (Figure 31-14). It is referred to as clawfoot when associated with flexion deformities of the toes. The primary pathologic condition is neuromuscular rather than bony, with weakness or paralysis of the intrinsic muscles of the foot and its dorsiflexors leading to the deformity over time. Pes cavus is not seen at birth. Depending on the underlying neuromuscular disease, it usually does not develop until late childhood or adulthood. Pes cavus may be seen in muscular dystrophy, peripheral neuropathies, and diseases of the spinal cord, brainstem, and cerebral cortex. Cerebral palsy, meningomyelocele, poliomyelitis, Charcot-Marie-Tooth disease, and Friedreich ataxia are some neurologic conditions that may produce pes cavus as a late manifestation.[17]

### *Evaluation*

### Pertinent History

Because pes cavus is not seen at birth but rather develops over time, parents may say they have begun finding it difficult to fit shoes on their child's feet, or they may note that the

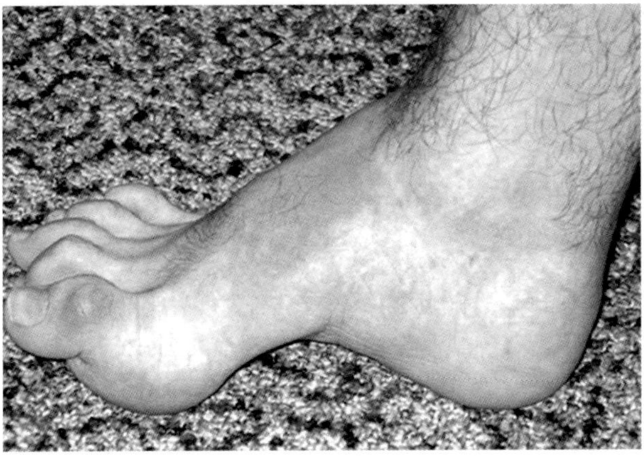

**Figure 31-14**
Clinical photograph demonstrating pes cavus. *(From Sarwark JF, ed.* Essentials of Musculoskeletal Care. *4th ed. Rosemont, IL: American Academy of Orthopaedic Surgeons; 2010. Reproduced with permission.)*

foot is different in appearance. A review of symptoms may reveal problems with bowel or bladder control consistent with spinal cord pathology.[9] There may be a family history of pes cavus because many of the conditions producing this deformity are inherited.[17]

### Physical Examination

A high-arched foot is the main finding in this condition. Pes cavus takes 1 of 2 forms: cavovarus, in which the calcaneus is inverted with tightness of the heel cord; or calcaneo-cavus, in which a high arch with normal heel alignment is present, usually from weakness of the calf muscles resulting in increased ankle dorsiflexion and increased plantar flexion of the forefoot.

### Imaging

Radiographic examination may be necessary if surgical management is being considered.

### *Management*

Early treatment includes exercises designed to strengthen the affected muscles and application of metatarsal pads to the innersoles of the shoes or metatarsal bars to the outer soles. Surgical correction of the fixed deformities may be required if contractures develop.

## ▶ TOE DEFORMITIES

### *Hallux Valgus*

Hallux valgus is a common problem in which the great toe is deviated laterally and the first metatarsal bone is deviated medially, causing a prominence to form on the medial aspect of the first metatarsophalangeal (MTP) joint (Figure 31-15). The condition is more common in females than males, and most cases are asymptomatic and do not require treatment other than counseling to wear shoes with adequate toe room and to avoid high heels. Persistent irritation of the overlying bursa from rubbing against a shoe can lead to inflammation and

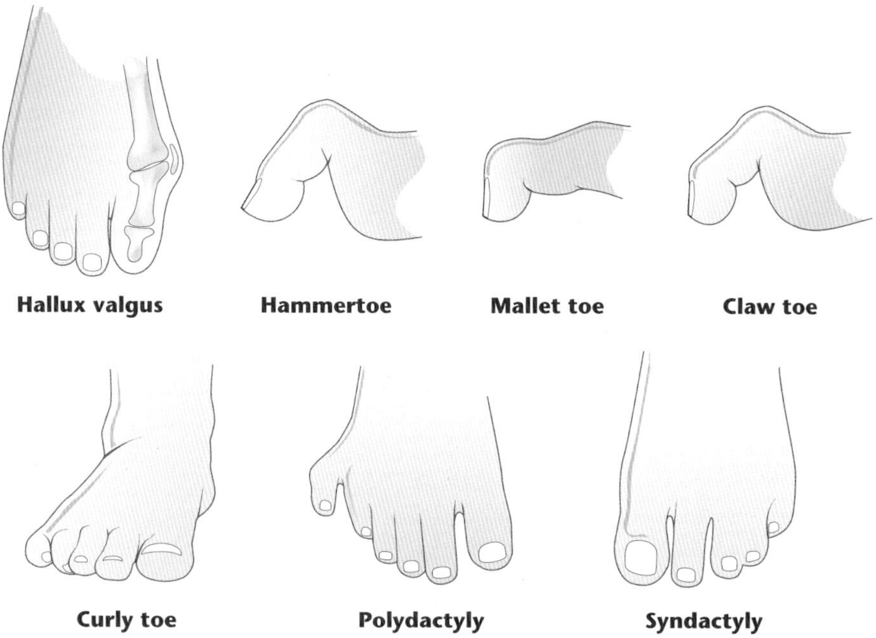


**Figure 31-15**
Common toe anomalies.

a painful bunion. Frequently, some degree of ankle pronation and flat foot is associated with hallux valgus, in which case a shoe insert may help prevent progression. In severe cases, surgical correction may be necessary.

### Hammertoe

Hammertoe describes a contracture of the proximal interphalangeal joint (PIP) in the second, third, fourth, or fifth toe (Figure 31-15). In an infant, hammertoe is usually hereditary; in an older child, it usually results from ill-fitting shoes. Most cases of hammertoe are mild, cause no pain, and can be left alone. Parents should make sure that the child has roomy shoes that allow the toes to stretch. More severe cases can cause pain, corns (an area of thickened skin overlying an area of pressure on the toes), inflammation, and worsening contractures. In severe cases, surgical correction may be needed.

### Mallet Toe

Mallet toe occurs less frequently than hammertoe. It is a chronic flexion deformity of the distal interphalangeal joint (DIP) (Figure 31-15) that causes pressure on the tip of the toe resulting in callouses or nail deformities. It usually occurs at the second digit but may affect the third to fifth toes as well. Generally caused by improperly fitting shoes, it may also be idiopathic or congenital, result from trauma, or rarely result from a neuromuscular problem. Most cases of mallet toe are mild, flexible, and need no treatment. When a corn develops over the deformity, shaving and padding will help. In the more severe cases, surgical correction can be performed.

### *Claw Toe*

Claw toe involves all joints of the toe—fixed hyperextension of the MTP joints and flexion contractures at both the PIP and DIP joints (Figure 31-15). Claw toe is a rare condition but usually occurs in conjunction with a cavus foot, is present in neuromuscular diseases such as Charcot-Marie-Tooth disease, and can occur in inflammatory conditions such as rheumatoid arthritis.

### *Curly Toe*

In a child with a curly toe, the fourth or fifth toe is usually flexed downward and twisted underneath the adjacent toe (Figure 31-15). Curly toe is quite common in infancy and childhood. If curly toe does not cause symptoms, no treatment is needed. When the condition is severe and causes irritation with shoe wear, surgical transfer of the toe flexor can correct the problem.

### *Polydactyly*

Polydactyly, the presence of an extra digit (Figure 31-15), may exist as an isolated finding or as part of a more extensive syndrome of congenital anomalies (5% of cases) such as trisomy 13, trisomy 21, or Ellis–van Creveld syndrome. There is a family history of polydactyly of the toes in 30% of cases, and 50% of case occur bilaterally. In 80% of cases, the extra digit occurs postaxially. If the extra toe is not causing problems with walking and shoe wear, no treatment is needed. However, the extra toe usually does cause difficulty and is cosmetically unacceptable for most families. In these cases, surgical excision of fully formed digits is generally performed after 9 to 12 months of age, whereas vestigial digits can be removed by suture ligation at birth.

### *Syndactyly*

Syndactyly, the presence of webbed digits (toes) (Figure 31-15), may exist as an isolated finding or, in rare cases, as part of a more extensive syndrome of congenital anomalies. A family history of the same anomaly is often found. Syndactyly is quite common and rarely causes problems. The interconnection between 2 or more toes can vary from thin skin that partially connects the digits to a bony attachment (synostosis) between parts of the phalanges. Unlike with fingers where surgical separation is needed to obtain finer hand functions, syndactyly in the toes does not necessitate treatment.

### *Bunionette (Tailor Bunion)*

Whereas a bunion forms on the great toe in association with hallux valgus, the less common bunionette occurs at the fifth MTP joint. When a bunionette develops, the bursa over the lateral aspect of the fifth MTP joint becomes prominent, inflamed, and painful. When padding does not help relieve the discomfort of a bunionette, surgical correction is needed.

## ▶ TOE-WALKING

Walking on the toes or the ball of the foot is a variation of normal gait often seen between 10 and 18 months of age as toddlers begin to walk. This variation usually progresses to a toe–heel gait and eventually to the normal heel–toe gait pattern several months later.[11] By parental report, as many as 25% of children continue to exhibit some degree of toe-walking later in development.

## Differential Diagnosis

Bilateral toe-walking beyond 2 years of age may be idiopathic or habitual toe-walking, but the differential diagnosis includes spastic diplegia, tethered cord, and diastematomyelia, muscular dystrophy, and other neuromuscular diseases. Unilateral toe-walking may be caused by spastic hemiplegia, a congenitally short Achilles tendon, a shortened limb, a dislocated hip, or significant tibial bowing on the affected side. Children with idiopathic toe-walking are able to place their feet flat on the ground and even have normal dorsiflexion. However, they prefer to use a toe-walking gait. In rare, extreme cases, this can lead to Achilles contractures and an equinus deformity.[19]

## Evaluation

### Pertinent History

A full history should be obtained, including birth history, developmental history and milestones, and history of stooling and bladder control to help find cases with underlying pathology. Children with idiopathic or habitual toe-walking exhibit otherwise normal development, whereas those with a spastic diplegia usually exhibit delays in attaining gross motor skills and walking.

### Physical Examination

A thorough examination is required to rule out underlying conditions. The legs should be examined for evidence of any leg-length discrepancies, joint abnormalities, or limitation in range of motion. A neuromuscular examination should be performed to evaluate for spasticity or abnormal bulk, tone, or sensation that could indicate cerebral palsy, muscular dystrophy, tethered cord, or other neuromuscular disorders. In males, look for hypertrophy of the calf muscles and Gower sign as part of the examination for Duchenne muscular dystrophy. Children with simple idiopathic or habitual toe-walking will have normal neurologic and musculoskeletal examinations.[10]

### Imaging

Radiographic examination is not indicated in most cases of toe-walking. Neuroimaging or other testing may be necessary if the toe-walking is acquired (develops after a period of normal gait) or underlying pathology is suggested by history or examination.

## Management

The only treatment generally required for idiopathic toe-walking is parental reassurance. However, in the child with idiopathic toe-walking beyond 2 to 3 years of age, stretching exercises or a dorsiflexion-assist ankle–foot orthosis may be of benefit. Older children who have developed mild Achilles tendon contractures from toe-walking may require serial casting. If any underlying pathologic cause of toe-walking is found, then treatment for the specific disorder should be initiated. Additional stretching and bracing, the use of ankle–foot orthoses, or casting may also be required for these children.[18–20]

## ▶ SHOES

The foot grows to conform to the shape of the shoe. Improperly fitted or manufactured shoes may be the primary cause of acquired foot deformities and problems. Shoes that do not fit properly can deform an otherwise normal foot, resulting in hammertoes, hallux valgus, bunionettes, corns, and, ultimately, the need for surgery.

### *Functions of Shoes*

Parents often ask the physician when their child should begin wearing shoes and what kind of shoe should be worn. The shoe has 2 functions, the most important of which is protecting the feet from trauma and extreme temperatures. The second function of the shoe is to provide style. Older children will often sacrifice comfort for style despite parental or medical advice to the contrary.

Support to the foot and ankle is not a function of the shoe except when a pathologic condition is present. Athletes in all sports that place the feet and ankles under severe strain wear low shoes that have soft uppers. Ski boots are worn not to support the foot and ankle but to make them one with the ski, to ensure response to movements originating in the knee and lower leg. Babies and toddlers usually wear ankle-high shoes, not to provide support to the foot and ankle but to make removing the shoes more difficult for the child.

Style is the only reason for a baby to wear shoes at all until the child begins walking outdoors or is taken out in cold weather. Some babies may gain a certain degree of stability from hard-sole shoes when beginning to stand, but this circumstance has not been shown to enhance learning to walk. In fact, shoes that are rigid prevent foot motion and may diminish the development of the intrinsic musculature of the feet. Properly fitting shoes that have flexible, smooth soles and soft uppers should be recommended. They need not be expensive. Toddlers can go barefoot in a protected environment such as indoors. Sneakers are perfectly adequate for summer wear and for winter indoor wear for older children, but toddlers may stumble in sneakers, which can stick to the floor during the stance and step-off phases of the toe–heel gait that typifies this age group.[21]

### *Fitting Shoes*

Determining the proper fitting of shoes involves no great science. Given that the foot widens while standing and through the day, these measurements should be made later in the day with the child standing. Both feet should be measured so that the shoes can be fitted to the larger foot. The counter should hug the heel snugly; the length should allow a fingerbreadth (½ inch) between the tip of the great toe and the top of the toe box. The foot should fit snugly into the widest part of the shoe; the width should not crowd the ball of the foot and should allow the toes to extend without wrinkling the upper. While still in the store, parents should have the child walk in the shoes to ensure comfort. The shoes should not be expected to stretch to fit. If shoes do not fit, they should not be purchased. Shoes in good condition can be handed down to a younger sibling.

The frequency with which shoes should be changed depends on the rate of growth of the feet, the quality of the shoes, and the degree of their use. Parents are usually able to tell when shoes become too small (or rather, feet become too large) without professional advice. The toes will be felt to press against the toe box, and getting the shoes on or having the child keep them on will be increasingly difficult.

## When to Refer

In-toeing and out-toeing
- Severe in-toeing
- Unsteady gait (especially while running) that causes stumbling
- Condition that does not follow the expected physiologic progression with growth

Metatarsus adductus and metatarsus varus
- Forefoot with limited flexibility
- Condition that appears to be progressing or is not improving with growth

Tibial torsion
- Extreme rotation (especially when associated with difficulty walking or running)
- Significant asymmetry
- Sudden proximal tibial deviation
- Condition that does not follow the typical pattern of improvement with growth

Femoral anteversion
- Extreme rotation (especially when associated with difficulty walking or running)
- Significant asymmetry of the femoral anteversion
- Condition that does not follow the typical pattern of improvement with growth
- New-onset femoral retroversion

Bowed legs and knock-knees
- Severe, asymmetrical, or unilateral genu varum or genu valgus
- Condition that does not follow the expected physiologic progression with growth

Clubfoot
- Immediate referral to an orthopedist on diagnosis of clubfoot

Flatfoot
- Presence of a rigid flatfoot
- Symptoms not relieved through conservative management

Pes cavus
- Referral for evaluation by a neurologist, physiatrist, or orthopedist, individually or in collaboration

Toe anomalies
- Referral to a podiatrist or orthopedist if the anomaly leads to pain, uncomfortable shoe wear, or ambulation, and if these symptoms do not respond to conservative management

Toe-walking
- Persists beyond 3 to 4 years of age
- Abnormal neuromuscular examination
- Leg-length discrepancy of >1 cm or other significant physical abnormality on examination

### *TOOLS FOR PRACTICE*

#### Engaging Patient and Family

- *Flat Feet and Fallen Arches* (fact sheet), American Academy of Pediatrics (www.healthychildren.org/English/health-issues/conditions/orthopedic/Pages/Flat-Feet-Fallen-Arches.aspx)
- *Shoes: Finding the Right Fit* (fact sheet), American Academy of Orthopaedic Surgeons (orthoinfo.aaos.org/topic.cfm?topic=A00143&return_link=0)

### Medical Decision Support

- *Essentials of Musculoskeletal Care,* 4th ed (book), American Academy of Orthopaedic Surgeons and American Academy of Pediatrics (shop.aap.org)
- *Wheeless' Textbook of Orthopaedics* (book), Duke Orthopaedics (www.wheelessonline.com)
- *Children* (Web page), American Academy of Orthopaedic Surgeons (orthoinfo.aaos.org/menus/children.cfm)
- *National Library of Medicine and the National Institutes of Health: Medline Plus* (Web site), (medlineplus.gov)
- *Orthoseek* (Web site), (www.orthoseek.com)
- *Pediatric Orthopaedic Society of North America* (Web site), (www.posna.org)

## REFERENCES

1. Craig CL, Goldberg MJ. Foot and leg problems. *Pediatr Rev.* 1993;14:395–400
2. Sass P, Hassan G. Lower extremity abnormalities in children. *Am Fam Physician.* 2003;68:461–468
3. Scherl SA. Common lower extremity problems in children. *Pediatr Rev.* 2004;25:52–62
4. Kling TF, Hensinger RN. Angular and torsional deformities of the lower limbs in children. *Clin Orthop Relat Res.* 1983;(176):136–147
5. Staheli LT, Corbett M, Wyss C, King H. Lower-extremity rotational problems in children. Normal values to guide management. *J Bone Joint Surg Am.* 1985;67:39–47
6. Dietz FR. Most torsional variations of tibia, femur resolve spontaneously. *AAP News.* 2000;16(1):35
7. Heinrich SD, Sharps CH. Lower extremity torsional deformities in children: a prospective comparison of two treatment modalities. *Orthopedics.* 1991;14:655–659
8. Smith BG. Lower extremity disorders in children and adolescents. *Pediatr Rev.* 2009;30:287–293
9. American Academy of Orthopaedic Surgeons, American Academy of Pediatrics. *Essentials of Musculoskeletal Care.* Sarwark J, ed. 4th ed. Rosemont, IL: American Academy of Orthopaedic Surgeons, American Academy of Pediatrics; 2010
10. Schwend RM, Geiger J. Outpatient pediatric orthopedics: common and important conditions. *Pediatr Clin North Am.* 1998;45(4):943–971
11. Pfeiffer M, Kotz R, Ledl T, Hauser G, Sluga M. Prevalence of flat foot in preschool-aged children. *Pediatrics.* 2006;118:634–639
12. Cowan DN, Jones BH, Robinson JR. Foot morphologic characteristics and risk of exercise-related injury. *Arch Fam Med.* 1993;2:773–777
13. Lin CJ, Lai KA, Kuan TS, Chou YL. Correlating factors and clinical significance of flexible flatfoot in preschool children. *J Pediatr Orthop.* 2001;21:378–382
14. Tudor A, Ruzic L, Sestan B, Sirola L, Prpic T. Flat-footedness is not a disadvantage for athletic performance in children aged 11 to 15 years. *Pediatrics.* 2009;123:e386–e392
15. Harris EJ. The natural history and pathophysiology of flexible flatfoot. *Clin Podiatr Med Surg.* 2010;27:1–23
16. Harris EJ, Vanore JV, Thomas JL, et al. Diagnosis and treatment of pediatric flatfoot. *J Foot Ankle Surg.* 2004;43:341–373
17. Duke Orthopaedics. Pes cavus: Charcot-Marie tooth. *Wheeless' Textbook of Orthopedics.* Available at: www.wheelessonline.com/ortho/pes_cavus_charcot_marie_tooth. Accessed October 16, 2014
18. Sala DA, Shulman LH, Kennedy RF, Grant AD, Chu ML. Idiopathic toe-walking: a review. *Dev Med Child Neurol.* 1999;41:846–848
19. Tidwell M. The child with the tip-toe gait. *Int Pediatr.* 1999;14(4):235–238
20. Hirsch G, Wagner B. The natural history of idiopathic toe-walking: a long-term follow-up of fourteen conservatively treated children. *Acta Paediatr.* 2004;93:196–199
21. Bleck EE. The shoeing of children: sham or science? *Dev Med Child Neurol.* 1971;13:188–195

# Chapter 32

# Gastrointestinal Hemorrhage

*Jeffrey R. Avner, MD*

Most causes of gastrointestinal (GI) bleeding in children, unlike in adults, are relatively benign and involve small amounts of blood loss. Although rare, some GI lesions may cause severe bleeding and lead to life-threatening conditions. In addition, GI bleeding may be a symptom of systemic illness or serious underlying chronic disease.

Evaluation of GI bleeding must be systematic. The age of the child, the history, the physical examination, and associated symptoms help focus the workup and allow the physician to identify the source of the bleeding in most cases. Endoscopy and new radiologic techniques are particularly useful for diagnosis and management of many conditions.

Bleeding can occur at any point along the length of the GI tract, from the mouth to the anus. Multiple folds, coils, and villous borders of the GI mucosa provide a large surface area for secretion of enzymes and absorption of water and nutrients. A large vascular supply to the GI tract accounts for an appreciable fraction of the cardiac output, especially after meals. Bleeding may be arterial, venous, or both. Although most bleeds are slow and involve oozing from the mucosal surface, massive bleeding can result from lesions involving high-pressure arteries or a large, engorged venous plexus.

Acute GI bleeding may occur with or without symptoms and can originate in either the upper or the lower GI tract. Chronic bleeding is usually slow and intermittent and may be identified only by occult blood in the stool. The slow nature of these bleeds allows the body ample time to compensate and preserve cardiac output. Signs of chronic bleeding include compensatory tachycardia, iron deficiency anemia, fatigue, pallor, or change in stool color.

## ▶ DEFINITION OF TERMS

It is helpful to divide GI bleeding as originating from either the *upper* GI tract (proximal to the ligament of Treitz) or the *lower* GI tract (distal to the ligament of Treitz). In addition, a variety of terms describe specific characteristics of GI bleeding that may also give clues to the nature, location, and duration of the bleeding. Hematemesis is bloody vomitus, which usually represents bleeding proximal to the ligament of Treitz. Blood that is altered by gastric acid becomes dark and coffee ground–like in appearance. Bleeding that has little or no contact with gastric acid will be bright red. GI bleeding that occurs proximal to the ileocecal valve and is passed rectally will usually appear as melena: black, tarry, sticky stools that result from the denaturing of hemoglobin by intestinal bacteria and enzymes. Hematochezia (red, bloody stool passed rectally) usually results from distal GI bleeding. Blood is usually mixed with the stool or passed just before or just after defecation. Occasionally, rapid bleeding from an upper GI source combined with the cathartic action of blood can speed transit time and cause hematochezia. Specific types of hematochezia include maroon-colored stools, seen with significant bleeding usually from the distal small bowel, and currant-jelly stools, indicative of intestinal vascular congestion and hyperemia.

## ▶ DIFFERENTIAL DIAGNOSIS

### *Identification of True Bleeding*

Red color appearing in the stool is often assumed to be blood. However, many other substances cause change in stool color. Foods that contain a high concentration of red pigments, such as tomatoes, cranberries, beets, and red fruit juices and gelatin (Jell-O), can cause red stools. Similarly, red-colored medications such as acetaminophen and amoxicillin can be passed in the stools, especially if diarrhea is present. Spinach, licorice, iron, and bismuth (Pepto-Bismol) often lead to dark, black stools, which can be confused with true melena. In infants, *Serratia marcescens* can cause *red diaper syndrome* as a result of the formation of red pigment in soiled diapers stored for longer than 1 day.

Several biochemical tests are available to detect blood in the stool. The most common test, the stool guaiac, uses the peroxidase activity of hemoglobin to catalyze a color change on a test card or paper strip. This highly sensitive test is able to identify even trace amounts of blood. Foods that have peroxidase activity may cause false-positive results if eaten within 3 days of testing: red meat, liver, processed meats, and raw fruits and vegetables, especially melon, turnip, radishes, and horseradish. High vitamin C intake interferes with the peroxidase reaction and can cause false-negative results. Similarly, outdated guaiac cards and prolonged storage may affect the accuracy of the test. Stool guaiac cards are not accurate for testing emesis for the presence of blood because gastric acid can affect the reaction that causes the color change. Therefore, heme testing of emesis should be done with guaiac cards that use a buffered stabilized hydrogen peroxide solution (eg, Gastroccult).

### *Nongastrointestinal Source of Bleeding*

Although blood is present in the GI tract, the bleeding may originate from a peripheral source. The most common example of this phenomenon occurs in the newborn period. The infant may swallow maternal blood either during delivery or when breastfeeding if the mother has bleeding nipples. The Apt-Downey test is helpful in differentiating maternal blood from infant blood. One part of the bloody stool (or gastric aspirate) is mixed with 5 parts of water to lyse the red blood cells. After the mixture is centrifuged, 1 mL of 0.2 normal sodium hydroxide is added to the supernatant hemoglobin solution. After 2 minutes, fetal hemoglobin, which resists the alkaline reduction, remains pink, whereas maternal hemoglobin turns yellow-brown. Melena contains denatured hemoglobin and therefore cannot be used for the Apt-Downey test.

Swallowed blood by a child is usually the result of nosebleeds or bleeding mouth lesions. These nasopharyngeal bleeds can mimic hematemesis or melena. Although rare in children, pulmonary hemorrhage may exhibit acutely as hematemesis or more chronically as melena and anemia. Vaginal bleeding in a newborn with estrogen withdrawal may be mistaken for rectal bleeding. In the menstruating teenager, vaginal blood may affect the accuracy of stool guaiac testing. The possibility of blood being added to the stool by a caregiver suggests Münchausen syndrome by proxy.

## Age at Presentation

### Newborn

GI bleeding in newborns usually appears as rectal bleeding or blood suctioned from the stomach during routine postnatal care. In many instances, no lesion is readily discernible, and the bleeding resolves spontaneously and permanently. Common causes of GI bleeding in the first 24 hours of life include maternal blood swallowed during delivery and local trauma after nasogastric suctioning. Hemorrhagic disease of the newborn as a result of inherited deficits of coagulation factors or delay in administration of postnatal vitamin K occasionally produces GI bleeding, although it is more common for these disorders to show as diffuse bleeding from venipuncture sites.

Premature infants and newborns who have low Apgar scores are at increased risk for having gastric ulcerations and erosions that can bleed. These lesions are rarely primary, usually resulting from asphyxia associated with a difficult delivery, a cardiac lesion, or sepsis. The diagnosis is made by radiograph or upper GI endoscopy. Newborns who have persistent or severe gastroesophageal reflux can develop esophagitis. Although esophageal bleeding is upper GI bleeding, hematemesis is rare. Rather, the slow bleeding is occult and exhibits more commonly with signs of anemia or guaiac-positive stools. Because a barium swallow has poor sensitivity, pH probe manometry and esophagoscopy are better tests for identifying gastroesophageal reflux. Treatment usually involves histamine-2 ($H_2$) receptor blockers.

Newborns with necrotizing enterocolitis (NEC) usually have a sudden onset of bilious vomiting, abdominal distention, lethargy, and lower GI bleeding. These symptoms usually occur after the first feeding but may be delayed for a few weeks. NEC is most common in premature infants but can occasionally occur in stressed full-term infants. Up to 5% of neonates in intensive care units develop NEC, and the overall mortality rate may be as high as 30%.[1] Complications of NEC include sepsis and shock. The diagnosis is confirmed by the presence of pneumatosis intestinalis on abdominal radiograph, but this finding is variable. These neonates remain hospitalized for bowel rest and intravenous antibiotics, and they occasionally need surgical intervention.

Intrinsic structural lesions of the GI tract are also a serious cause of lower GI bleeding in the newborn. Intestinal duplication, a tubular structure lined with normal GI mucosa adjacent to the true intestine, can be present anywhere along the GI tract. Duplications can cause lower GI bleeding, either acute or chronic, along with abdominal distention and vomiting. The diagnosis is confirmed by radiograph, computed tomography (CT) scan, or ultrasound. Unrepaired duplications may lead to obstruction, volvulus, or perforation. A volvulus or malrotation of the GI tract should be suspected in any infant who has abdominal pain, bilious vomiting, and melena. However, because these symptoms and signs are often unreliable, the diagnosis should be considered in any newborn who vomits and has guaiac-positive stools. An abdominal radiograph may show loops of small bowel overriding the liver shadow, with paucity of air in the GI tract distal to the volvulus. An upper GI series, barium enema, or both are sometimes needed to confirm the diagnosis. Midgut volvulus may also be diagnosed on CT scan or ultrasound by noting duodenal dilation, fixed midline bowel, and the wrapping of the bowel and the superior mesenteric vein around the superior mesenteric artery (whirlpool sign). Immediate surgical repair is necessary. Vascular malformations can occur anywhere along the GI tract and produce slow or diffuse lower

GI bleeding. The bleeding is usually painless, and the color of the blood in the stool will vary depending on the level of the lesion. Vascular malformations may be associated with cutaneous hemangiomas or cardiac defects.

Milk or soy protein allergy can begin as early as the first week of life and exhibit as severe diarrhea, gross blood in the stool, abdominal distention, and vomiting. Older infants may have occult lower GI bleeding and mucus in the stool. The diagnosis is made by clinical response to withdrawal and rechallenge with the offending protein. Infectious enteritis, although rare in the newborn, may appear later in the first month of life. In very young infants, bacterial gastroenteritis, especially that caused by *Salmonella* spp, can cause bloody diarrhea with or without fever; 8% to 13% of infants may have associated bacteremia.[2] Bright-red blood streaks on the surface of the stool suggest an anal fissure. Often associated with hard stools, anal fissures are the most common cause of rectal bleeding. Visual inspection of the anus usually confirms the diagnosis. Medications, such as indomethacin and dexamethasone, can cause mucosal erosion and GI bleeding.

## Infants and Young Children

Upper GI bleeding in a young child is usually caused by mucosal lesions in the esophagus and the stomach. Infectious esophagitis is usually viral, but fungi can be the cause of disease in immunocompromised children. As infants become more mobile and dexterous, they are at higher risk for foreign body and toxic ingestions. Coins and small toys, when lodged in the esophagus, can cause drooling, vomiting, and chest pain. Persistent or unrecognized esophageal foreign bodies lead to edema and erosion of the esophagus and may cause hematemesis. Caustic ingestion severe enough to burn the esophageal mucosa can also result in painful swallowing, drooling, oral burns, and hematemesis. Children who have forceful or prolonged vomiting may develop a rent at the gastroesophageal junction known as a Mallory-Weiss tear. The emesis becomes streaked with bright-red blood and may develop into coffee-ground emesis if the tear persists. Although the bleeding is minor and usually resolves spontaneously, an $H_2$-blocker may be needed to prevent continued irritation by stomach acid.

Gastroesophageal varices can occur at any age but usually occur in children younger than 8 years. Variceal bleeding can range from slow, persistent oozing to acute massive hematemesis. Physical examination usually reveals signs of portal hypertension, such as enlarged liver or spleen, or both. Most cases result from the cavernous transformation of the extrahepatic portion of the portal vein, which has been associated with umbilical vessel catheterization, omphalitis, or neonatal conditions associated with hypoxia, prolonged jaundice, or sepsis. Intrahepatic causes of cirrhosis, leading to portal hypertension that may first show during childhood, include Wilson disease (>6 years of age), $a_1$-antitrypsin deficiency, biliary cirrhosis, and metabolic, infectious, or anatomic forms of chronic liver disease. These chronic liver diseases also may be associated with coagulopathy and thrombocytopenia from the hypersplenism that usually accompanies them. If the cause of the portal hypertension is extrahepatic, then the bleeding may be tolerated remarkably well, in contrast to that in patients who have cirrhotic liver disease, in whom rapid hepatic decompensation may occur. Fortunately, most variceal bleeding stops spontaneously, but the incidence of rebleeding is high. Endoscopy confirms the diagnosis.

Juvenile polyps are the most common cause of lower GI bleeding, reaching a peak incidence in children aged 3 to 7 years. Typically, polyps are located in the colon and are simple, solitary, benign hamartomatous lesions that may irritate the GI tract and cause intermittent, painless, bright-red rectal bleeding. Many of these polyps will autoamputate if left alone and are passed with the stool. Because most polyps are located within 25 cm of the anus, they can often be identified by digital examination, air-contrast barium enema, or sigmoidoscopy and can be removed with snare electrocautery.

Adenomatous polyps may produce rectal bleeding as early as infancy, but they are managed differently from juvenile polyps. Juvenile polyps are benign inflammatory lesions that do not cause later complications. Adenomatous polyps, conversely, are premalignant tumors, which may transform into a malignancy over an average period of 10 years.[3] Familial polyposis and Gardner syndrome are associated with adenomatous polyps. Juvenile polyposis coli (JPC) is suggested by the presence of 5 to 10 juvenile polyps; 10 or more polyps is considered diagnostic. JPC, which occurs in about 10% of patients who have colonic polyps, is associated with anemia, right-colon polyps, and adenomas.[3]

Meckel diverticulum, a remnant of the omphalomesenteric duct found within 2 feet of the ileocecal valve, is present in up to 2% of the population. The acid secreted by ectopic gastric mucosa, which is usually present in diverticula that bleed, causes peptic ulceration of the ileal mucosa. Meckel diverticulum typically occurs in children younger than 3 years and causes painless, maroon- or red-colored lower GI bleeding. Typically, the bleeding is severe enough to cause the hemoglobin level to fall to about 8 g/dL. Diagnosis is made by technetium-99 scan, which identifies the ectopic gastric mucosa. This test is fairly sensitive but only during active bleeding; thus, a repeat scan is sometimes necessary when the suspicion is high. Treatment requires surgical excision.

Intussusception, the telescoping of an intestinal segment, is seen typically in children 6 to 24 months of age. The occurrence is often idiopathic and usually involves invagination of the distal ileum through the ileocecal valve into the colon. Older children who have intussusception and those who have multiple recurrences may have pathologic lesions that serve as lead points (Meckel diverticulum, polyp, and tumor). The classic presentation begins with intermittent, severe, crampy abdominal pain, with vomiting following shortly thereafter. As the intussusception progresses, lethargy or paradoxical irritability develops. Guaiac-positive stools are seen as the bowel becomes ischemic and may progress to the passage of red bloody mucus, classically referred to as *currant-jelly stools*. The use of screening ultrasound has decreased unnecessary enemas for clinically suspected intussusception.[4] Diagnosis can be confirmed on ultrasound by identification of the layering of intestinal mucosa as a *bull's-eye* or *coiled-spring* lesion. Confirmation of diagnosis, followed by hydrostatic reduction with barium or air enema, is successful in about 70% to 80% of cases, even in those with symptoms for more than 24 hours.[5] Complications include intestinal perforation, peritonitis, and significant bleeding.

Lymphonodular hyperplasia on the mucosa of the terminal ileum or colon may cause painless, blood-streaked stools. Lymphonodular hyperplasia is usually seen in children younger than 6 years and may be associated with food allergy.[6] Diagnosis is made by endoscopic examination and histologic confirmation.

Symptoms associated with infectious enterocolitis range from mild diarrhea to fever, abdominal cramping, and watery or mucoid stools (or both forms) with or without blood. *Salmonella, Shigella, Yersinia,* and *Campylobacter* spp are the most common bacterial causes of bloody diarrhea. Pseudomembranous colitis, caused by *Clostridium difficile,* also causes fever, diarrhea, abdominal cramping, and bloody stools. In many instances, a history of recent hospitalization and antimicrobial therapy exists, but the onset of symptoms can be delayed for weeks. A variety of parasites, such as *Entamoeba histolytica* and *Trichuris trichiura*, can cause bloody diarrhea.

Systemic disease, in particular vasculitis, may be accompanied by bloody stools. The constellation of arthritis, hematuria, purpura, intestinal cramping, and bloody stools suggests Henoch-Schönlein purpura (HSP). Children with HSP are at increased risk for intussusception, or they may have severe GI bleeding. Hemolytic uremic syndrome (HUS) often has a prodrome of hemorrhagic colitis caused by Shiga toxin–producing *Escherichia coli* with a serotype O157:H7. The classic triad of HUS includes thrombocytopenia, hemolytic anemia, and renal disease. Milk protein allergy, anal fissures, and congenital anatomic anomalies of the GI tract can also occur in this age group.

### Older Children and Adolescents

Peptic ulcer disease can occur at any age but is more common in older children and adolescents. Symptoms usually begin with epigastric or periumbilical pain accompanied by nausea. GI bleeding is evident in about 50% of children either as hematemesis or as melena. *Helicobacter pylori,* bacteria found in the gastric mucous layer or adherent to the epithelial lining of the stomach, has been causally associated with ulcers. *H pylori* infection is diagnosed by culture of biopsy specimens from the stomach and duodenum. Serologic tests, which measure specific *H pylori* immunoglobulin G antibodies, are often unreliable and, therefore, should be reserved for children with endoscopically diagnosed, or radiographically definitive, duodenal or gastric ulcers. Treatment, when indicated, consists of a 7- to 14-day course of any of a variety of antibiotic regimens together with a proton pump inhibitor.

Hemangiomas and other vascular lesions, such as hereditary hemorrhagic telangiectasia (Rendu-Osler-Weber syndrome), must be considered in the evaluation for painless rectal bleeding. Its most common form is the larger cavernous hemangioma, either polypoid or diffuse, extending several centimeters through the submucosa of the small or large intestine. The large bowel, specifically the rectum, is the area usually involved in the diffuse type. Cutaneous vascular malformations are often present but may require scrupulous searching to detect. Selective arteriography or digital subtraction angiography may aid in demonstrating the abnormal vessels if they are not visible on direct inspection.

Inflammatory bowel disease may appear in the adolescent age group as episodes of bloody diarrhea, cramping, and tenesmus. The course may be atypical in children, making the diagnosis difficult. Growth failure, weight loss, or anemia with evidence of recurrent bouts of GI bleeding should alert the physician to the diagnosis, which colonoscopy and biopsy usually confirm.

## ▶ EVALUATION OF PATIENTS WHO HAVE GASTROINTESTINAL BLEEDING

When evaluating a patient who has GI blood loss, the physician should keep 2 goals in mind. First, the severity of the blood loss must be assessed quickly to expedite appropriate resuscitative measures. Second, the physician must consider the most likely causes so that problems requiring immediate surgery can be separated from those requiring medical evaluation and management. The workup is based on the patient's age and history, the clinical appearance, and the physician's familiarity with the patient. A list of lesions commonly associated with GI bleeding is provided in Box 32-1.

## Relevant History

A detailed history may help the physician determine the location and duration of the bleeding. Particular attention should be paid to the color of the stool and emesis and whether a change has occurred in the preceding days or weeks. Massive amounts of red blood from the mouth or rectum are readily apparent to the parent and the patient. However, the importance of maroon or tarry stools as a sign of GI bleeding may not be appreciated unless the physician asks.

Antecedent symptoms are also a key to identifying many diseases. Vomiting that progresses from bile stained to bloody is seen with intestinal obstruction (volvulus, intussusception, NEC)

BOX 32-1

### *Causes of Gastrointestinal Bleeding*

**NEWBORNS**

***Upper GI Bleeding***

- Hemorrhagic disease of the newborn
- Gastritis
- Stress ulcer
- Esophagitis

***Lower GI Bleeding***

- Necrotizing enterocolitis
- Duplication
- Volvulus, malrotation
- Vascular malformations
- Milk allergy
- Infectious enteritis
- Anal fissure

**INFANTS AND YOUNG CHILDREN**

***Upper GI Bleeding***

- Nasopharyngeal bleeding
- Esophagitis
- Acid reflux
- Viral, fungal, caustic sources
- Esophageal foreign body
- Mallory-Weiss tear
- Gastroesophageal varices
- Gastritis

***Lower GI Bleeding***

- Juvenile polyps
- Meckel diverticulum
- Intussusception
- Infectious enterocolitis
- Pseudomembranous colitis
- Vasculitis (HSP, HUS)
- Milk allergy
- Lymphonodular hyperplasia
- Anal fissure or trauma (abuse)
- Duplication
- Vascular malformation

**OLDER CHILDREN AND ADOLESCENTS**

***Upper GI Bleeding***

- Nasopharyngeal bleeding
- Esophagitis
- Mallory-Weiss tear
- Gastroesophageal varices
- Gastritis
- Aspirin, NSAIDs
- *Helicobacter pylori*
- Peptic ulcer disease

***Lower GI Bleeding***

- Polyps
- Infectious enterocolitis
- Inflammatory bowel disease
- Vasculitis
- Vascular malformation
- Meckel diverticulum
- Hemorrhoids
- Anal fissure

*GI,* gastrointestinal; *HSP,* Henoch-Schönlein purpura; *HUS,* hemolytic uremic syndrome; *NSAIDs,* nonsteroidal anti-inflammatory drugs.

or with Mallory-Weiss tears. Bloody diarrhea may accompany infectious enteritis, food allergy, and inflammatory bowel disease, or it may precede HUS. Painless lower GI bleeding, if substantial, is seen with Meckel diverticulum or GI vascular anomalies, whereas a smaller amount of painless bleeding suggests polyps or lymphonodular hyperplasia. Fever is common in infectious or inflammatory disorders. Arthritis and rash are seen with HSP. Abdominal pain, fever, and weight loss suggest inflammatory bowel disease. Lower rectal disorders, such as hemorrhoids or anal fissures, produce blood-streaked stools and painful defecation. Young children who have upper GI bleeding should be questioned about foreign body or caustic ingestion. Medication use, especially of aspirin, nonsteroidal anti-inflammatory drugs, steroids, and tetracycline, is a frequent cause of gastritis. A family history of polyps, bleeding disorders, or GI diseases is important. Neonatal history should focus on risk factors for NEC or varices, including umbilical vein catheters, liver disease, and birth asphyxia. Sexual activity or abuse involving anal penetration should alert the physician to anal and rectal trauma.

### Physical Examination

The physical examination should be complete and systematic because clues to the diagnosis may be present in any organ system. The general appearance and vital signs can be helpful in determining the duration of bleeding. Slow, chronic bleeding allows time for physiologic changes such as tachycardia, orthostasis, and decreased pulse pressure. Children may initially appear comfortable but tired and have some degree of pallor. Patients who have acute, rapid bleeds may be in various stages of shock depending on the amount of blood loss. The nose and mouth should be examined for bleeding lesions or burns. The abdominal examination should evaluate for tenderness, bowel sounds, masses, and hepatosplenomegaly. The physician must also look for signs of chronic liver disease, such as the presence of telangiectasias, jaundice, hepatosplenomegaly, and a prominent abdominal venous pattern. With lower GI bleeding, a thorough rectal examination should be performed, with special attention paid to the perianal region, observing for skin tags, abscesses, fissures, bleeding points, or much less commonly, hemorrhoids; the character of the stool; and the presence of occult blood by guaiac testing. Palpation for polyps and pelvic masses must be part of the rectal examination. Eczema may be associated with food allergy. Finally, skin lesions such as purpura and petechiae suggest a bleeding disorder, HSP, or HUS.

### Laboratory Testing

In the setting of GI bleeding, laboratory testing should focus on determining the amount and duration of the bleeding, assessing for coagulopathy, and evaluating for other laboratory abnormalities that may be associated with the underlying disease process. Hemoglobin determination can help assess the level of blood loss, with the caveat that acute bleeding may not lower the hemoglobin level until some intravascular equilibration takes place. An elevated white blood cell count may occur in infectious colitis. Coagulation studies should be obtained, including prothrombin and partial prothrombin times, as well as the platelet count. The prothrombin time may be elevated as a sign of a bleeding disorder or as a result of abnormalities in liver synthetic function. Liver function tests are useful in evaluating suspected liver disease. Serum chemistries can be used to assess renal function, although an elevation in the blood urea nitrogen may result from increased intestinal absorption of blood with longstanding upper GI bleeding. Any patient with significant bleeding or a low hemoglobin level should have blood sent immediately for blood type and screen in the event of the need for blood transfusion. If bloody diarrhea is present, a stool specimen should be sent for culture and, if appropriate, ova and parasites.

### Imaging

Most children with GI bleeding require some type of imaging study to locate the source of the bleeding or confirm a suspected diagnosis. The type of study will depend on the age of the child, clinical presentation, and possible diagnosis. Plain radiographic films are generally nonspecific and usually require additional imaging to confirm a diagnosis. Two-view (flat and upright) abdominal radiographs may show signs of intestinal obstruction such as air-fluid levels and dilated bowel loops. Some specific radiographic findings include pneumatosis intestinalis in NEC and intestinal obstruction with absence of gas in the right colon in intussusception. Barium studies can be used to identify intestinal foreign bodies, polyps, lymphonodular hyperplasia, and inflammatory bowel disease, although, in many cases, endoscopy remains the procedure of choice for diagnosis. Color Doppler ultrasound is becoming increasingly useful as a diagnostic aid in both intussusception and malrotation, but its usefulness depends on the skill of the operator. CT scans are occasionally helpful in defining related anatomic features if the child is hemodynamically stable and either cooperative or sedated. Nuclear medicine imaging studies (Meckel scan, radioactively labeled colloid or red blood cells) or direct angiography can often identify the source of an acute, ongoing bleed.

Wireless capsule endoscopy (WCE) is a relatively new technical innovation used for evaluation of the small intestine, primarily in adult patients but now with increasing frequency in pediatrics. As in adults, a common use of WCE in children is for evaluation of obscure gastrointestinal bleeding. In one recent study, more than 50% of children had the source of obscure bleeding identified with WCE, including ulcerative jejunitis, polyps, angiodysplasia, blue rubber bleb nevus syndrome, and Meckel diverticulum.[7] Some of the limitations of WCE use in pediatrics include the size of the standard capsule that needs to be swallowed and the risk for capsule retention in strictured areas of the small bowel (more common in Crohn disease). However, several studies show that WCE is a practical and safe technique, even in children as young as 2 years.[7,8]

## ▶ MANAGEMENT

For a child who has acute massive GI bleeding, the approach must be the same as that in any other emergency. The physician must approach the patient with an efficient, rational plan in mind that will allow obtaining the pertinent historical information, performing a brief but adequate examination, stabilizing the patient clinically, arriving at a working diagnosis, and instituting appropriate therapy or consultations. Massive upper GI bleeding may lead to vomiting, aspiration, and airway obstruction that requires stabilization of the airway with endotracheal intubation. Administration of oxygen is always indicated. Evaluation of peripheral perfusion, quality of pulses, and capillary refill time assesses the adequacy of circulation. In children, the initial response to hypovolemic shock is tachycardia. In acute bleeds, adequate blood pressure may be maintained with blood loss of up to 30% without replacement.

Tachycardia and capillary refill time are essential criteria in determining the nature of the resuscitation required. Skin turgor and the color of the mucous membranes also should be noted. If signs of shock are present (eg, orthostasis or frank hypotension, tachycardia, poorly perfused extremities, pale mucous membranes, altered mental status), then at least 1 (preferably 2) large-bore intravenous catheters should be placed. Initial laboratory studies include complete blood count, hematocrit, reticulocyte count, coagulation times, electrolytes, blood urea nitrogen, creatinine, liver function tests, and blood typing and cross-matching. If percutaneous venous access is not obtained within a few minutes, then an intraosseous line should be placed, and 20 mL/kg of normal saline should be given rapidly to reexpand the vascular volume. This fluid bolus may need to be repeated several times. Additional fluid should be given as needed to allow equilibration of these solutions with the extravascular space. With more than 30% to 40% acute blood loss, packed red blood cells should be given as soon as possible.

An appropriately sized nasogastric (NG) tube, preferably of the vented sump type, helps determine the source of bleeding and helps estimate the volume of ongoing blood loss. The tube should be left in place and attached either to low-pressure continuous suction, if vented, or to intermittent suction, if nonvented. The only instance in which NG tube placement may aggravate bleeding is in a patient who has varices. Nonetheless, even in this case, an NG tube may be required to quantitate blood loss adequately.

Controlling the bleeding and determining the specific diagnosis are the next steps in management. If the NG aspirate contains blood, or if the patient has hematemesis, then saline irrigation may be instituted in an attempt to decrease mucosal blood flow and thereby stop profuse bleeding. Although the efficacy of lavage in decreasing and controlling gastric bleeding has not been demonstrated conclusively, it allows easier assessment of the rate of bleeding and helps in removing clotted blood. At the same time, prolonged lavage (>10 minutes) may not allow fibrin clots to form at the bleeding site. Saline at room temperature should be used because irrigation with water can lead to hyponatremia, and iced or cold fluid may cause hypothermia. The saline is instilled through an NG tube and is withdrawn after 3 to 5 minutes. Aspirate returns that do not clear in 10 minutes suggest continued GI bleeding and should prompt additional evaluation.

If the bleeding ceases, then gastroduodenoscopy should be performed to demonstrate the bleeding source and to determine the type of lesion present. Upper GI fiberoptic endoscopy can establish the diagnosis in 75% to 90% of patients. If the bleeding is massive and cannot be controlled with saline lavage, then adequate visualization is not likely to be achieved with the fiberoptic endoscope. If the bleeding is not immediately life-threatening, then arteriography, which can demonstrate bleeding that occurs at a rate of 1.0 mL/min or more, should be considered. More sensitive than arteriography, and less invasive, a sulfur-colloid isotopic study can demonstrate active bleeding at rates as low as 0.1 mL/min.[9] This method demonstrates active bleeding by using a tracer with a very short half-life. In small infants, a large uptake of the isotope by the liver may mask the right upper quadrant. An additional isotopic method of determining the bleeding site consists of injecting the patient with technetium-99 pertechnetate–labeled red blood cells. These labeled cells may remain in the circulation for more than a day and allow repeated imaging to locate the site of intermittent bleeding.

If the lesion is one of mucosal erosion or inflammation, then antacid therapy with or without the concomitant use of an $H_2$-blocker may be instituted. For bleeding ulcers, intravenous therapy with a proton pump inhibitor reduces the risk for ulcer rebleeding but does not appear to influence the overall mortality rate.[10] If the bleeding source is variceal, then the cause of the lesions must be determined, with appropriate treatment of the underlying disease. In particular, liver or portal venous disease should be sought. Clotting factors and platelets should be replaced as indicated.

Variceal bleeding requires special mention because of the many settings in which varices may be seen. The treatment of variceal bleeding in children has evolved over the past 2 decades. Use of balloon tamponade with a Sengstaken-Blakemore tube (an NG tube with additional lumina for a gastric balloon and an esophageal balloon in which the gastric balloon is inflated and traction is applied so that the balloon abuts the gastroesophageal junction and tamponades the variceal bleeding) was effective in controlling most cases of bleeding but had a high incidence of complications. This treatment has been replaced, in most cases, with the use of vasoactive drugs and endoscopy. Previously, the major medical therapy included the use of intravenous vasopressin as a mesenteric vasoconstrictor to reduce portal blood flow and thus decrease variceal pressure. Octreotide, a synthetic peptide similar in properties to somatostatin, decreases splanchnic blood flow, which thereby decreases portal pressure, has less effect on systemic blood flow and is associated with fewer side effects than vasopressin. Pediatric studies (with no control groups) have shown octreotide to be 50% to 63% effective in controlling acute variceal bleeding.[11,12] Initially, a 1-mcg/kg (maximum of 50-mcg) bolus is infused, preferably through a central or intraosseous line, followed by an infusion of 1 mcg/kg/hr, which may be increased by 1 mcg/kg/hr up to 4 mcg/kg/hr.[13]

Endoscopy is the preferred intervention for variceal bleeding because it can provide both diagnosis and therapy. The most commonly used techniques are endoscopic injection sclerotherapy (EIS), which uses an injection of a sclerosing solution into the varices, and endoscopic variceal band ligation (EVL), in which elastic bands are placed around the varices in the distal esophagus. Endoscopy has been found to be 80% to 100% effective in controlling variceal bleeding.[11,12,14,15] In a randomized controlled trial in 49 children, EVL achieved variceal eradication faster than EIS, with a lower rebleeding rate and fewer complications.[12] Endoclips are a newer technique used in severe GI bleeding; metal devices, applied to the GI mucosa through a flexible endoscope, are used to compress the tissue around a bleeding vessel.[13] In all cases, endoscopy should be performed by an experienced gastroenterologist, with the availability of general anesthesia and endotracheal intubation, if necessary, especially when performed in small children.

Studies in adults and experience in pediatrics, although limited to date, suggest that octreotide should be used as the initial treatment for bleeding varices, followed by endoscopic therapy, either EVL or EIS.[14,16] If the bleeding continues despite vasoactive and endoscopic therapies, then balloon tamponade can be attempted.

Evaluation for lower GI bleeding differs in several aspects from that for upper GI bleeding. The abdomen, perineum, and rectum are thoroughly examined. Stool must be analyzed for the presence of blood and, when appropriate, for enteric pathogens and for ova and parasites. If diarrhea is present, then the stool should be examined microscopically for polymorphonuclear leukocytes and mucus, both of which are evidence of bacterial infection. Digital rectal examination should follow in an attempt to discover the presence of anal fissures, rectal polyps, or hemorrhoids. Sigmoidoscopy may be necessary for children who have persistent rectal bleeding to identify polyps or mucosal lesions. The presence of blood originating from above the reach of the sigmoidoscope indicates the need to proceed with other diagnostic studies.

Several different imaging studies are used to evaluate persistent lower GI bleeding. An upright and supine view of the abdomen will reveal signs of obstruction or calcifications. For severe, life-threatening bleeds, angiography can be both diagnostic and therapeutic, depending on the ability to embolize the bleeding vessels. Because angiography has limited sensitivity in detecting slow or past bleeding, it is best performed when bleeding is active.

Children with persistent, active bleeding who are clinically stable should have a radionuclide scan, which identifies accumulation of an isotope at the bleeding site. With a sulfur-colloid isotopic scan, the isotope is extracted rapidly so that background radioactivity is low. Although high-contrast resolution can be found around the bleeding site, it is effective only for identifying rapid bleeding. An isotope-labeled red blood cell infusion has a lower contrast ratio but is better at detecting slower or intermittent bleeds than a sulfur-colloid isotopic scan. A Meckel scan uses technetium-99 pertechnetate, which is secreted by ectopic gastric mucosa, to identify the diverticulum. If the rate of bleeding does not permit the time necessary to perform these studies, then vasopressin or octreotide may be administered parenterally in an attempt to control the bleeding and to stabilize the patient. Air-contrast barium studies or endoscopy can identify sources of more chronic, low-grade bleeding. However, a barium enema or an upper GI series with small bowel follow-through should be the last study performed because they each make the further use of arteriography, isotope scans, and endoscopy impossible for several days thereafter. In cases in which the intestine is compromised vascularly, or when the rate of bleeding is excessive and uncontrollable by more conservative methods, prompt surgical intervention is required. Fortunately, however, conservative measures control most acute episodes of GI bleeding relatively easily; patients who eventually require surgical intervention can usually undergo elective surgery at a later time.

## When to Refer

- Upper GI bleed
- Lower GI bleed that is of moderate amount, persistent, or intermittent

## When to Admit

- Any nontrivial upper GI bleeding, such as that associated with active bleeding, moderate amount of blood, anemia, and abdominal pain
- Significant lower GI bleeding
- Hemodynamic instability
- Anemia (hematocrit)
- Severe abdominal pain
- Associated systemic symptoms (eg, HUS, inflammatory bowel disease)
- Altered mental status or lethargy
- Suggestion of surgical etiology (eg, Meckel diverticulum, intussusception, volvulus)

## REFERENCES


1. Caplan MS, Jilling T. New concepts in necrotizing enterocolitis. *Curr Opin Pediatr.* 2001;13:111–115
2. Lin PY, Huang YC, Chang LY, Chiu CH, Lin TY. C-reactive protein in childhood non-typhi Salmonella gastroenteritis with and without bacteremia. *Pediatr Infect Dis J.* 2000;19:754–755
3. Hoffenberg EJ, Sauaia A, Maltzman T, et al. Symptomatic colonic polyps in childhood: not so benign. *J Pediatr Gastroenterol Nutr.* 1999;150:175
4. Henrikson S, Blane CE, Koujok K, et al. The effect of screening sonography on the positive rate of enemas for intussusception. *Pediatr Radiol.* 2003;33:190–193
5. van den Ende ED, Allema JH, Hazebroek FW, Breslau PJ. Success with hydrostatic reduction of intussusception in relation to duration of symptoms. *Arch Dis Child.* 2005;90:1071–1072
6. Kokkonen J, Karttunen TJ. Lymphonodular hyperplasia on the mucosa of the lower gastrointestinal tract in children: an indication of enhanced immune response? *J Pediatr Gastroenterol Nutr.* 2002; 34:42–46
7. Fritscher-Ravens A, Scherbakov P, Bufler P, et al. The feasibility of wireless capsule endoscopy in detecting small intestinal pathology in children under the age of 8 years: a multicentre European study. *Gut.* 2009;58:1467–1472
8. Shamir R, Eliakim R. Capsule endoscopy in pediatric patients. *World J Gastroenterol.* 2008;14:4152–4155
9. Lefkovitz Z, Cappell MS, Lookstein R, Mitty HA, Gerard PS. Radiologic diagnosis and treatment of gastrointestinal hemorrhage and ischemia. *Med Clin North Am.* 2002;86:1357–1399
10. Leontiadis GI, Sharma VK, Howden CW. Systematic review and meta-analysis of proton pump inhibitor therapy in peptic ulcer bleeding. *BMJ.* 2005;330:568
11. Heikenen JB, Pohl JF, Werlin SL, Bucuvalas JC. Octreotide in pediatric patients. *J Pediatr Gastroenterol Nutr.* 2002;35:600–609
12. Zgar S, Javid G, Khan B, et al. Endoscopic ligation compared with sclerotherapy for bleeding esophageal varices in children with extrahepatic portal venous obstruction. *Hepatology.* 2002;36:666–672
13. Boyle JT. Gastrointestinal bleeding in infants and children. *Pediatr Rev.* 2008;29:39–52
14. Molleston JP. Variceal bleeding in children. *J Pediatr Gastroenterol Nutr.* 2003;37:538–545
15. McKiernan PJ, Beath SV, Davison SM. A prospective study of endoscopic esophageal variceal ligation using a multiband ligator. *J Pediatr Gastroenterol Nutr.* 2002;34:207–211
16. Bañares R, Albillos A, Rincón D, et al. Endoscopic treatment versus endoscopic plus pharmacologic treatment for acute variceal bleeding: a meta-analysis. *Hepatology.* 2002;35:609–615

# Chapter 33

# Gender Expression and Identity Issues

*Robert J. Bidwell, MD*

Throughout history and across many cultures, children and adolescents have, through their gender expression and gender identity, transcended cultural expectations about the meaning of being a girl or a boy.[1–4] In some times and places, as these children and youths grew into adulthood, they became respected and even revered members of their societies. In others, including the current culture in many parts of the United States, they have been seen as legitimate targets of discrimination and persecution. Issues related to gender expression and gender identity are highly controversial, and the understanding of them is evolving based on increased research and societal changes. In 2013, the American Academy of Pediatrics (AAP) issued a policy statement and accompanying technical report on office-based care of lesbian, gay, bisexual, transgender and questioning (LGBTQ) youth.[5,6] These give physicians the basic understanding and skills to work in a respectful and relevant manner with children and youths facing issues related to sexual orientation and gender identity. A similar position paper has been issued by the Society for Adolescent Health and Medicine.[7] While sexual orientation (whom one is attracted to) is distinct from gender identity (one's inner sense of being female, male, or another gender), in practice these 2 concepts are often interrelated, as the following section will explain.

## ▶ DEFINITIONS

Gender is a complex concept that is still not well understood. Researchers and theorists have attempted to study and explain various aspects of gender to improve their understanding of this important part of being human. *Gender role* represents a set of behaviors, attitudes, and interests that a society or culture believes are typically female or male. A child internalizes these cultural gender role expectations by the age of 3 to 5 years. *Gender expression* refers to how an individual signifies gender in terms of dress, speech, interests, and other outward signs. When a child displays behaviors, attitudes, or interests outside the cultural norm for the child's biologic (genetic or anatomic) sex, it is referred to as *gender nonconforming* or *gender variant* expression. More recent terms include *gender creative* and *gender expansive* expression. For example, boys with gender nonconforming behavior may prefer playing house to playing football, enjoy dressing up in their mothers' clothes or trying on their makeup, prefer long hair, and be more stereotypically feminine in their mannerisms and speech, as determined by a particular culture. Girls with gender nonconforming behavior may avoid wearing clothes that are culturally more associated with girls, enjoy more physically aggressive play with boys, prefer short hair, and have more stereotypically masculine mannerisms.

In contrast, *gender identity* refers to a person's deepest inner sense of being female or male (or even something other than female or male) and is often established early in childhood. For most individuals, gender identity is congruent with biologic or birth-assigned sex. For some, it is not. Although their bodies seem to tell them and the world around them that they are female or male, their inner identity is either of the opposite gender or a sense of gender separate from female or male. These individuals are referred to as *transgender*.

Gender identity is distinct from *sexual orientation*, which refers to an individual's affectional, romantic, or sexual attraction to others of the same sex (homosexual), opposite sex (heterosexual), or both sexes (bisexual).

*Transgender* also is used sometimes as a broader umbrella term encompassing those who do not conform to cultural norms of being female or male. This group includes individuals whose gender identity is incongruent with their biologic gender and who may seek to change their bodies to make them more consistent with their inner sense of gender. These individuals are sometimes referred to as *transsexual*, but more commonly are referred to as transgender in the narrower sense of the term as described above. Transgender in its broader sense recently has been referred to as the *trans* spectrum*. In addition to those who experience an incongruence between their bodies and their inner gender identity, the trans* spectrum also includes those who cross culturally defined gender boundaries, including crossdressers (transvestites), drag kings and queens, and persons who perceive themselves to be of both genders (bigender), all genders (pangender) or no gender (agender). It also includes those who may refer to themselves as *genderfluid* or *genderqueer*, or who are routinely gender nonconforming in terms of their attitudes, interests, and behaviors. The term *transgender* is not used in referring to prepubertal children with gender dysphoria or gender nonconforming behavior.

In this chapter, *transgender* is used in its narrower sense, referring to gender identity. Transgender individuals often refer to themselves as *trans*, *trans**, *TG*, or *T*. Many transgender people, but not all, experience significant *gender dysphoria*, a persistent discomfort with the gender assigned to them at birth and the societal gender role expectations that accompany it. These dysphoric feelings often begin in early childhood and increase with the appearance of unwanted physical changes at puberty. Many transgender individuals gradually let go of the need to conform to societal expectations attached to their birth-assigned gender and increasingly present themselves to the world in a manner consistent with their gender identity. This process is known as *transition*. The transition process may be facilitated medically by pubertal suppression, cross-gender hormonal treatment, and/or gender-affirmation surgery (also referred to as sex-reassignment surgery or SRS). However, it not only is a physical process but also takes place on psychological, social, and spiritual levels. The terms *male-to-female* (MTF) and *female-to-male* (FTM) transgender are used to describe the direction of transition from biologic gender to actual gender identity. An FTM transgender person is often referred to as a *trans-man* and an MTF person as a *trans-woman*.

Most gender nonconforming children and youths do not experience gender dysphoria nor do they have gender identities that differ from their birth-assigned sex. The prevalence of gender nonconfomity in children and youth is uncertain, although studies have shown that gender nonconforming behavior is common.[8–10] Persistent gender nonconforming behavior or expressed wishes to be another gender are less common.[11–13] In a 2011 population-based survey of middle school students in San Francisco, when given a choice of identifying themselves as male, female, or transgender, 1.3 percent chose the latter response. The World Professional Association for Transgender Health (WPATH) estimates that the prevalence of MTF transgender identity is 1 in 11,900 to 1 in 45,000 individuals and of FTM transgender identity is 1 in 30,400 to 1 in 200,000.[14] Some believe that these estimates are low because they are based on individuals seeking hormonal and surgical transition services: some transgender individuals do not have access to or do not want sex-reassignment services and so are not represented in the data.

One of the most controversial issues related to gender expression and gender identity during childhood and adolescence is whether gender nonconformity and transgenderism are causes for concern.[15–19] Do they represent a pathologic abnormality, or are they simply part of the continuum of normal human expression and identity? Similar debates occurred around homosexuality until it was officially removed from the American Psychiatric Association's list of mental disorders in 1973. Although controversial, until 2013 transgenderism (in the narrower sense) and transsexualism were represented in the fourth edition of the *Diagnostic and Statistical Manual of Mental Disorders* (*DSM-IV*) under the diagnostic category of *gender identity disorder* (GID).[20] Based on the work of the *DSM-5* Workgroup on Sexual and Gender Identity Disorders, the APA fifth edition (*DSM-5*) introduced several important changes in terminology and diagnostic criteria related to gender identity, with separate criteria for children and for adolescents and adults.[21] The diagnostic category of GID was replaced by the less stigmatizing designation *gender dysphoria*. The controversy surrounding these diagnoses is well documented.[22,23] The diagnostic criteria for both childhood and adolescent/adult gender dysphoria require a marked difference between an individual's experienced or expressed gender and the gender assigned at birth. For a diagnosis of gender dysphoria to be made, this gender incongruence must have persisted for at least 6 months and resulted in significant distress or impairment in social, school, occupational, or other important areas of functioning.

At a basic level, the move from GID to gender dysphoria emphasizes that no longer is cross-gender *identity* considered disordered. Instead, it is the distress related to having a cross-gender identity, which is often caused in significant measure by growing up and living in a nonaccepting, often aggressively hostile societal environment. Much of the controversy arising from the creation of both GID and gender dysphoria as DSM diagnostic categories is the observation that any gender-nonconforming child or adolescent raised in a society that enforces a binary view of gender will predictably experience some degree of discomfort or distress related to gender expression and identity. Given the overt discrimination and violence that have occurred against transgender individuals in the United States, distress or impairment in social and other areas of functioning is not surprising. Evidence suggests that transgender individuals growing up in more accepting societies experience less discomfort and distress related to their gender identity and gender expression.[24]

Several developmental trajectories have been described for children with GID, which presumably are relevant for those now diagnosed with gender dysphoria. The diagnostic rubric of gender dysphoria is too recent to be reflected in a substantial body of literature. The studies on which these proposed trajectories are based are small and inconclusive. Taken as a whole, however, they suggest that many children diagnosed with GID (and more recently gender dysphoria) eventually self-identify as gay or bisexual as adolescents or adults and no longer experience gender dysphoria. A smaller percentage later self-identify as heterosexual and also experience no gender dysphoria. A small but significant percentage continue to experience discomfort with their biologic sex and self-identify as transgender.[25]

## ▶ ETIOLOGY

Considerable controversy exists around possible causes for the development of persistent gender nonconforming expression, cross-gender identity, and gender dysphoria, which are related yet distinct phenomena. Theories proposed have suggested psychosocial, biologic, and genetic factors, or varying combinations thereof. However, research data are very limited, often narrowly focused, and sometimes contradictory. Therefore, to date there are no scientifically supported explanations for how gender nonconforming expression, gender identity, or gender dysphoria arise. Nevertheless, among all theories offered, those suggesting a biologic or genetic basis for cross-gender expression and identity are gathering the most robust scientific interest and support. Recent reviews have documented what little is known and how much still needs to be learned about the origins of gender identity and expression and the developmental trajectories experienced by gender nonconforming and gender dysphoric children and youths.[26]

Psychosocial theories seeking to explain gender nonconforming expression and gender dysphoria often focus on familial, and particularly parental, psychopathology, and aberrant parenting practices that may interact with biologic factors and predispose a child to gender dysphoria.[18,27] Zucker, for example, posits that some children may experience subtle biologically or genetically related prenatal events affecting areas of the brain that lead to gender nonconforming behavior or personality traits.[27] This may in turn interact with parenting styles or psychopathology that encourages persistent gender nonconforming behaviors and possibly the development of gender dysphoria. Much of the controversy around such theories, in addition to a lack of robust scientific evidence to support them, is that many feel they are similar to earlier theories related to the origins of homosexuality, later discredited, that saw aberrant parenting and familial psychopathology as probable etiologies. This is especially relevant because research demonstrates that most gender dysphoric children and many gender nonconforming children later to come to recognize a lesbian, gay, or bisexual orientation in adolescence or adulthood. Psychosocial theories are no longer generally accepted as primary causal explanations for variances in gender expression and identity, while their role in informing the treatment approach to gender dysphoria remains highly controversial.[19,28,29] Some have suggested that a more likely route to gender dysphoria for some children is growing up in a home and community that pathologizes their gender expression and identity,[29] although this theory, like all others, lacks robust research support at this time.

Most recent scientific attention has focused on possible biologic, genetic, and neurologic explanations for gender nonconforming expression, cross-gender identity, and gender dysphoria. No clear unequivocal biologic markers for these have been identified, but early limited findings are intriguing and invite further research. One area of inquiry has examined the possible influence of prenatal maternal androgens on those areas of the developing fetal brain associated with sexual dimorphism.[30] There is some evidence that prenatal androgen exposure may predispose an individual to male gender identity, but not always; among 46,

XY intersex children exposed to increased androgens prenatally but raised as girls, only 40% to 50% developed male gender identity. Also, MTF transgender individuals with presumed normal male prenatal levels of androgen exposure override this influence and develop a female gender identity. Recent studies examining 46, XX individuals exposed to higher levels of prenatal androgens demonstrated marked masculine gender expression but no evidence of male gender identity or gender dysphoria. In this area of inquiry, data suggest that for some gender nonconforming and transgender individuals, prenatal exposure to androgens may be influential, but it seems not to be applicable to the broader transgender community.

Recent research provides incomplete but increasing evidence for a genetic component to gender nonconformity and cross-gender identity. Hare and colleagues have identified an association between longer androgen receptor (AR) gene polymorphism and MTF transsexualism, perhaps caused by inhibition of the ability of testosterone to masculinize the fetal brain.[31] A similar gene anomaly has been associated with FTM transsexualism.[32] Familial and twin studies have documented increased occurrence of gender nonconforming expression and cross-gender identity within families and between twins, providing further evidence of a possible genetic component to the development of cross-gender identity and expression.[33]

Another focus of biomedical inquiry has been comparison studies of transgender and nontransgender individuals looking at sex-related anatomic dimorphism in terms of brain structure and functioning.[34–36] Differences have been reported, but most of these studies have not been replicated and therefore the significance of their findings is uncertain. However, documenting brain differences between transgender and nontransgender individuals would suggest a possible neurologic component to the development of cross-gender identity, at least for some individuals.

Given the complexity of gender as a concept, and the diverse ways in which it is experienced and expressed within a population, continuing research may find that the origins of gender expression and identity are multifactorial, with genetics, biology, and environment each playing a role in varying combinations and degrees of influence. Since gender nonconfomity and cross-gender identity do not appear in the *DSM-5*, and therefore may be considered part of the normal spectrum of human experience, perhaps the most valuable research will be that which examines the factors contributing to gender dysphoria among children and adolescents. With this increased understanding, physicians and other providers will be better able to prevent the onset of dysphoria or to ameliorate its effects in the child where it already exisits.

## ▶ ADVERSE EFFECTS

Due in large part to the experience of societal stigma and ostracism, gender nonconforming and transgender youths may be at high risk on many fronts, as outlined in the paragraphs that follow. Nevertheless, there are reasons for immense optimism because these young people are coming of age on the cusp of enormous and positive societal change. This change is marked by an increased understanding and celebration of the diversity of gender expression and identity and an awareness of how this diversity can enrich families, schools, workplaces, and the broader community. In many parts of the United States, primary care physicians (PCPs) have begun to recognize the amazing creativity and resilience of these youths as they navigate changing societal currents. They have met parents who love their children unconditionally and who confidently and passionately work to make the world a safer, more accepting place for them. They have joined with educators, social workers, mental health professionals, and others to create empowering transgender youth programs, including youth leadership workshops, mentorship programs, music/poetry/art events, speakers' panels, and many others. Such programs help develop important life skills but just as importantly validate the rightful place of gender nonconforming and transgender youth among other happy, healthy, and hopeful young people. These exciting changes have not yet arrived in many parts of the United States, but they are on the horizon. The risks described below are still very real for many children and youths. But is important to recognize that they are an aberration, a result of living in the presence of stigma and ostracism. They are not part of the natural history of being gender nonconforming or transgender.

In those communities where the societal change described above has not yet arrived, transgender youths often experience a profound isolation that intensifies their feelings of confusion and distress. They and most people in their lives, including parents, teachers, counselors, clergy, and physicians, often know little about gender identity or what it means to be transgender. In many instances, gender identity is confused with sexual orientation, a much different concept. Many PCPs and counselors were trained at a time when gender nonconforming behaviors and transgender identity were seen as aberrant or pathologic, and some continue to conduct their practices accordingly. Many transgender youths have few adult role models or mentors for support or validation, and many know no other transgender youth. When transgender youths have little access to accurate information, supportive counselors, or physicians, and when they have no opportunity for healthy interactions with transgender peers and adults, the negative messages that surround them in their daily lives go unchallenged. Although this continues to be true in many communities across the United States, over the past decade there have been major advances in increasing the understanding of families, health and social service providers, educators, and others about the importance of recognizing, validating, and empowering gender nonconforming and transgender youths.[15,37] PCPs have often been at the forefront of the movement to increase public awareness, developing creative programs for youths and their families, and providing needed advocacy on their behalf. With the growing love and support of families and communities, many gender nonconforming and transgender youths no longer struggle under the burden of stigma and ostracism.

For those many children and youths who grow up in families and communities still untouched by this societal change, the most harmful reality they face is society's disapproval of who they are and how they present themselves to the world. Social stigma, and the violence and discrimination it engenders, permeate their daily lives. It makes completing the expected developmental tasks of childhood and adolescence related to identity and self-esteem enormously difficult. Many of these children and youths are viewed by their families with shame and disgust. They are often forced to change their behaviors and renounce their declared inner sense of gender. Many of them are taken to therapists for the express purpose of changing their gender expression or identity. Many transgender adolescents and adults recall being ridiculed, ostracized, or beaten for being true to who they were, including within their own families. Many gender nonconforming and transgender youths drop out of school and run away or are thrown out of their homes; some seek survival on the streets; many contemplate or attempt suicide.[38] As a result, many end up in the child welfare or juvenile justice systems.[39–41] The harassment and abuse against gender nonconforming and transgender young people often continue in these settings, perpetrated both by other youths and by staff members. Fortunately, state judiciaries across the country as well as organizations such as the Child Welfare League of America and the Equity Project, with the active involvement of pediatricians and other advocates, have developed training, model policies, and other tools to meet the needs of transgender youths in out-of-home care and address the societal antecedents that bring them into these systems.

Schools often are especially dangerous places for gender nonconforming children and transgender youths.[42–44] Many of them experience daily verbal, physical, and sexual harassment on the playground and in the classroom. In many instances, this harassment is not addressed by teachers, counselors, or other school staff, or it is dealt with by blaming the victim. Sometimes, disapproving teachers and other school staff members engage in harassing behaviors themselves. Many schools have no specific policies prohibiting harassment or bullying based on gender identity or expression, even though these, along with sexual orientation, are among the most common targets of harassment on school campuses. An increasing number of school systems, however, are adopting rigorous anti-bullying programs and antiharassment policies that specifically include harassment based on gender identity and expression. Many have included transgender issues in regular teacher trainings and have worked with national organizations such as the Gay, Lesbian and Straight Education Network (GLSEN) to ensure that school campuses are safe places for transgender students. Many school systems have encouraged the establishment of gay-straight alliances in schools to support LGBT students and their friends. Many schools also routinely invite PCPs to join in the development of individualized education programs (IEPs) and participate in other discussions related to addressing the needs of individual gender nonconforming and transgender students.

Societal stigma also may be reflected in the daily discrimination experienced by some children and youths. Children may be admonished for playing with toys or displaying interests that are considered inappropriate for their presumed gender. They are told by what names they will be called and by what pronouns they will be referred to, in spite of their protests that these names and pronouns do not reflect who they really are. Their genitalia rather than their inner identity as female or male are referenced in assigning them to bathrooms, lockers, physical education classes, athletic teams, graduation ceremonies, and other school activities in which gender is still considered relevant. School dress codes often limit transgender students' ability to wear clothes that are consistent with their gender identity. Many PCPs have begun to work with individual schools on behalf of their gender nonconforming and transgender patients, advocating policies and accommodations that ensure safety, respect, and validation for their patients in the school setting.

As transgender youths grow older, they begin to experience broader societal forms of discrimination. Their driver's licenses and other forms of identification, as well as their school, employment, and health records, usually reflect their biologic sex rather than their gender identity. Because fear, embarrassment, and potential humiliation accompany the presentation of these documents to others, many transgender adolescents may avoid applying for school or a job or accessing health care. Transgender individuals have been denied access to educational opportunities, community programs, social services, and health care simply because of their gender identity. Fortunately, each year more states and municipalities enact laws and ordinances that prohibit discrimination based on gender identity and expression in the areas of housing, employment, public accommodations, and health care, providing transgender individuals, including adolescents, legal recourse when faced with discrimination. In addition, LGBT communities have made great strides in recognizing that LGBT social and health services should be as welcoming and accessible to transgender individuals as they are to members of the lesbian, gay and bisexual communities.

The risks described above are not inherent in being a gender nonconforming child or transgender youth. They are the common experience of any young person who is stigmatized, fearful, and alone. The genuine distress experienced by some children diagnosed with GID (and presumably gender dysphoria) and some transgender youths over the perceived dissonance between their biologic sex and gender identity should not be dismissed or minimized. Nevertheless, evidence from other cultures and the experience of many counselors and physicians suggest that when provided love, support, and validation, these young people thrive and can expect to grow into happy, healthy, and productive adults. Perhaps the most important role that PCPs can play in the lives of gender nonconforming children and transgender youths is to go beyond the confines of their offices and engage with schools, social service agencies, faith communities, and others to ensure that these young people grow up in safe and nurturing environments.

## ▶ EVALUATION

The AAP, the American Academy of Child and Adolescent Psychiatry, and the Society for Adolescent Health and Medicine have each issued official guidelines related to providing supportive care to children and adolescents facing issues of gender identity and gender expression.[5,7,37] In addition, several resources are available to PCPs on providing culturally sensitive and relevant care to gender nonconforming children and transgender adolescents and adults.[45,46]

PCPs should not presume the sexual orientation or gender identity of any patient. Children with gender nonconforming behaviors, many of whom will later identify as LGB, have often learned or have been pressured to change their behaviors, particularly in public settings such as schools and health clinics. Many transgender youths will also hide their true gender identity. Even when asked in a sensitive and nonjudgmental manner about their inner feelings of being female, male, or another gender, they often will deny these feelings because they are fearful of PCP disapproval, uncertain about confidentiality, or still confused about the meaning of their emerging feelings. Perhaps one of the greatest barriers to appropriate health care for gender nonconforming and gender dysphoric children and transgender youth is physicians' assumption that they have no patients in their practices who are dealing with issues of gender identity and expression. Another mistaken assumption is that significant gender nonconforming behavior in childhood accurately predicts sexual orientation. Although some children with persistent gender nonconforming behaviors will later identify as LGB, many will not. Few PCPs may consider that some may also later identify as transgender. Many transgender youths are thought by their PCPs, and sometimes by themselves, to be LGB. However, the distinction between sexual orientation and gender identity is important for the provision of care because the different issues related to each require different responses from a PCP. In addition, transgender identity does not predict sexual orientation. Transgender youths may be gay, lesbian, heterosexual, or bisexual. For example, an MTF-transgender adolescent who is attracted to boys may be considered a heterosexual trans-woman, if she so considers herself. Some, however, may describe themselves as "gay," either because it feels like the appropriate term to them or because it is easier for others to understand.

The goal of PCPs is not to identify every child with gender nonconforming behaviors or transgender identity; instead, it is to create a safe and accepting clinical setting where children, adolescents, and their families know they can discuss any topic of concern, including gender identity and expression, without discomfort or disapproval on the part of the physician. Some patients and parents do not know that PCPs may have expertise in discussing issues of sexual and gender development. Specific messages can be provided through clinic posters and brochures informing patients that these issues are appropriate topics of discussion. The most important signal that these topics are a natural part of pediatric practice is in the PCP's own history taking and anticipatory guidance, in which issues of child and adolescent sexuality and gender should be routinely discussed.

After patients have identified themselves as transgender, the PCP should create an accepting and supportive clinical environment by using pronouns consistent with their patients' gender identity and asking by what name they would like to be called by clinic staff. Although medical records must retain the patient's legal name, the notice "Also Known As [preferred name]" can be added to the front of the chart, and all clinic staff members should use this name in personal encounters with the patient. Patients should use either a unisex restroom or a restroom consistent with their gender identity while in the clinic. As with all adolescents, transgender patients should be seen alone for at least part of each visit and their confidentiality should be respected. An adolescent patient's gender identity should not be revealed to parents without the patient's permission. Patients should also be asked how they would like their gender identity recorded in the chart, if at all, because medical records containing confidential information are sometimes accessible to parents.

PCPs should reflect on their own feelings about gender nonconforming behaviors and gender identity issues. As products of their own society, many physicians may initially approach these issues with discomfort or disapproval. However, such an approach to gender nonconforming children or transgender youths will diminish the PCP's ability to care for these patients. Most transgender patients have had profoundly negative experiences with the health care system.[46,47] In the past, these patients have been labeled as disordered and were often treated accordingly. Transgender patients report how staff in clinical settings often display fear or open disapproval of them or joke about them, even within hearing of the patient. At times, these patients have been refused medical care. PCPs who receive little training about transgender health issues often do not understand the transgender adolescent's unique life experiences and needs. Most PCPs are unfamiliar with community resources that might help their transgender patients. Most health insurance companies refuse to pay for transition treatments, including hormone therapy, surgery, and the laboratory studies needed to monitor treatment. Fortunately, this refusal of payment for necessary, even lifesaving, care is slowly beginning to change.

PCPs are in a position of power relative to their transgender patients. As gatekeepers, PCPs decide who does or does not receive transition treatments. Many, often through disapproval or lack of knowledge, have barred transgender patients from passing through that gate, preventing them from receiving necessary transition treatment and care. PCPs must understand the history of tension between the transgender and medical communities. PCPs can improve this strained relationship by listening carefully and respectfully to their patients' life stories and expressions of need and by providing care that addresses these needs in a compassionate, comprehensive, and timely manner.

### *History*

Gender and sexuality are important parts of a child's life. At each well-child visit, beginning in early childhood, the PCP should ask parents how they think their child is developing compared with other children. Parents and child should be asked how the child is getting along with siblings and peers. Does their child seem happy? Is the child teased or harassed by other children, and over what issues? All parents should be asked if they have any concerns over their child's sexual development or gender expression. Many parents who have such concerns are hesitant to bring them up on their own but are often relieved when the PCP does so. If a child with gender nonconforming behavior is happy and safe from teasing and parents have no concerns about these behaviors, no reason exists for the PCP to question further. However, as a child grows older and has more social contacts beyond the family, issues will likely arise related to being gender nonconforming or transgender in a society that is often nonaccepting. PCPs should remain attuned to this likelihood and reopen the door to discussion of these issues in future visits.

If parents express concerns about their child's gender expression or gender identity, then the PCP should ask what they have noticed or heard from the child and what their concerns or fears might be. Parents' concerns are often related to their own embarrassment because of their child's behavior; they may also fear for their child's safety in a nonaccepting world. Many of them fear that their child's behavior or verbal expressions of wanting to be the opposite gender signal an eventual lesbian or gay sexual orientation or transgender identity. PCPs may gently question gender nonconforming children if they feel safe from teasing at home and school and about their feelings of being more like a girl, a boy, or another gender inside. Care must be taken to avoid conveying the message that anything is wrong with the child because of the child's gender nonconformity. In addition to the well-child visit, any visit suggesting an unhappy child or a child in distress should lead the PCP to consider discussing issues of gender nonconforming expression and gender identity with the parents and child.

Transgender adolescents may come to the PCP's office either because of parental concerns or through school or child welfare agency referral. Transgender youths may also seek care themselves, often to discuss issues of safety and acceptance at home or school or concerns about sexually transmitted infections (STIs), or to request hormone treatment. However, many transgender patients see their PCPs not through referrals or acute care visits but rather in the context of routine well-teen evaluations. Many transgender patients hide any evidence of their inner gender identity; others are presumed, perhaps even by themselves, to be lesbian or gay. PCPs should initiate discussion of sexuality and gender with all adolescents at each well-teen visit. Although many PCPs routinely discuss sexual activity and safer sex practices, fewer discuss sexual orientation, and almost none of them address gender identity. However, as noted earlier, most transgender adolescents face significant confusion and distress related to their gender identity and major risks from growing up in an often nonaccepting world. PCPs must be willing to open the door to discussion of gender in order to reduce the turmoil and dangers that these youths face.

The PCP can begin to approach the issue of gender identity in the broader context of obtaining a HEADSSS (home, education, activities, drugs, sexuality, suicide, and safety) interview.[48] This approach will provide a sense of how things are going in various aspects of an adolescent's life, recognizing that many transgender youths face serious issues in each of these areas. Throughout this conversation, it is essential that the PCP use non-heterosexist, gender-neutral language, reflecting that no assumptions are being made about a youth's sexual orientation or gender identity, or that of family members or friends. To address gender identity within a broader sexual history, the PCP might say, "Sexuality and sexual feelings can be confusing sometimes. During puberty, bodies change in lots of different ways. Sexual feelings are changing as well. Some of my patients are not sure if they are attracted to guys or girls or maybe both; and some of my patients even wonder if they're more like a girl or a boy inside. All of this is completely normal but can be really confusing. So I'm wondering what it's been like for you." After asking about attractions (sexual orientation), the PCP can simply ask, "And how about inside? Do you feel more like a girl or a boy or maybe something else?" For the patient who is not dealing with gender identity issues, these questions may seem odd. This can be addressed by a simple statement such as, "These are questions I ask all my patients, and for some, they're really important." For transgender youths, the questions may be life saving. Even if they decide not to acknowledge their gender identity concerns at the current visit, they have learned that someone is available with whom they can talk when the time is right. If youths do acknowledge cross-gender feelings, the PCP can ask whether they have defined themselves in terms of gender. Some may refer to themselves as transgender while others may self-define as pansexual, pangender, bigender, genderfluid, genderqueer, or another designation. Some may refer to themselves as gay or lesbian. It is appropriate to ask each teen what their particular self-designation means to them. This demonstrates respect on the part of the PCP and can foster a sense of empowerment in the youth.

If adolescents acknowledge a transgender, pangender, or other-gendered identity, the PCP should thank them for their trust in sharing this important and personal part of who they are. As a demonstration of understanding and respect, the PCP should then ask about preferred name and pronouns and use these through the remainder of the interview and subsequent visits. Patients should be reassured that the discussion of gender identity will remain confidential unless they give permission to share it with others or unless a risk of danger to someone exists. It is essential to ask, at an appropriate time in the interview, "Do you have any periods of feeling very sad? How long do they last? Have you ever had feelings of wanting to hurt yourself or kill yourself? Have you ever actually tried to do this?" If the PCP is not comfortable with the depth of interviewing suggested in the following paragraphs, she or he has a responsibility to refer the adolescent to someone else who can have this conversation.

The subsequent history may then focus on the adolescent's path to recognizing their transgender identity. When were they first aware of feeling more like a girl, a boy, or another gender? What was this experience like? How comfortable are they with their transgender identity now? What do they know about gender identity and what it means to be transgender? What are their hopes and dreams for the future? Do they see their futures as enhanced or limited by being transgender? The history may focus on the adolescent in the context of the world around them. Have they told others (family, peers, teachers, or counselors) about their inner feelings of gender? Have these people responded in a supportive or negative way? Have they been bullied, harrassed, scolded, ridiculed, or teased because of their gender identity? With whom do they spend time, and what kinds of things do they do together? Have they met other transgender adolescents or adults? Have they been in relationships, and have these relationships been healthy ones? Have they been sexually active, and do they use safer-sex practices? How have they met their sexual and romantic partners? Have they ever been pregnant, impregnated anyone, or had an STI? How many different sexual partners have they had, and what have been their genders? Have they ever been touched sexually or forced to have sex without their permission?

Understanding that transgender youths often are subjected to harassment and rejection at home and school, the PCP should ask about their treatment in these settings and whether they have ever run away from home or dropped out of school. Have they needed to sell their bodies, deal drugs, or engage in other illegal activities to survive on the streets? Have they been involved with the child welfare or juvenile justice systems, and how have they been treated within them? Have they ever used drugs or contemplated suicide? How do they believe their physical health has been, and do they have any health needs they believe are not being addressed? What do they know about gender transitions and is that something they have thought about? Have they actually begun the transition process? Have they begun to cross-dress? Have they begun puberty blockers or cross-gender hormone therapy, and, if so, where have they obtained their treatment? Have they injected silicone? Have they thought about gender affirmation surgery (sex-reassignment surgery) or other transition-related procedures in the future?

Other questions to consider include, "What have you found on the internet or in various forms of media about transgender people?"; "Do you know any transgender or LGB people?"; and "Who do you have as supports?" Because eating disorders are common among sexual minorities and especially among transgender populations where malnutrition can suppress pubertal progression, it is also important to ask, "Do you restrict your diet, binge and then purge, or use laxatives or make yourself vomit?"

Not all of these questions need to be addressed at the first visit. Follow-up visits should be made to address these issues on an ongoing basis. The PCP should be aware that the history, beyond providing specific information about the experience and needs of a transgender adolescent, is an opportunity for the PCP to interact with the patient in a comfortable, respectful, and caring manner that validates who the adolescent is as a human being. Many transgender adolescents have never experienced such acceptance before, and providing it is among the most fundamentally important things a PCP can do.

### Physical Examination

The physical examination of children with gender nonconforming behaviors or who express the desire to be other than their anatomic gender is the same as that for other children. A complete examination, including the genitals, should be a routine part of every well-child visit. On occasion, the PCP may observe a child wearing clothes or exhibiting behaviors or interests that are more typical of another gender. These behaviors or interests may or may not relate to the child's gender identity.

Similarly, the content of the physical examination of transgender adolescents does not differ significantly from that of other adolescents. It should be guided by a comprehensive and accurate health history, including sexual and other risk behaviors. The PCP should remember that transgender youths may be heterosexually, homosexually, or bisexually active or not sexually active at all. Many transgender youths hide all public expressions of their gender identity. Some may have already begun the transition process and come to clinic displaying dress, hairstyles, makeup, and mannerisms usually associated with another gender but consistent with their gender identity. Occasionally, transgender patients may wear non–gender-defining street clothes but underwear appropriate for their gender identity. If patients have begun pubertal suppression, they will generally remain at Tanner Stage 2 or 3 and depending on the duration of suppression may eventually show delay in pubertal development relative to their peers. If patients have already begun transition hormone treatment, they may show evidence of breast development (MTF), appearance of facial hair (FTM), and other expected changes of estrogen and testosterone treatment.

PCPs should understand and respect the significant discomfort that many transgender youths have related to their pubertal changes, such as development of facial hair, deepening of the voice, breast development, and menstrual periods, which feel alien to their gender identity. Some MTF-transgender adolescents may tuck their genitals, placing their penis and testes between their legs so they are less visible. Some FTM-transgender youths may wear chest binders or baggy tops to make their breasts less visible. Some may also wear a "packer," which is padding or a phallic-shaped object worn in the front of the underwear or pants to give the appearance of having a penis.

In preparing for the examination, the PCP should discuss the rationale for suggesting the parts of the examination that might be particularly uncomfortable for a transgender adolescent, especially the breast and genital examinations. PCPs should explain that their intention is to make the examination as comfortable as possible for the patient and to elicit the patient's guidance in how best to accomplish this task. The patient should be informed that they have a right to refuse any part of the examination. The PCP should ask transgender patients what words they would like used in referring to various body parts—for example, *genitals* instead of *penis* or *vagina*. An FTM-transgender patient may prefer the term *chest* rather than *breast*. MTF-transgender patients should be treated the same as other female patients, and FTM-transgender patients like other male patients in conducting the examination. Conducting all comprehensive physical examinations of MTF- and FTM-transgender patients with the patient in a gown and draped appropriately to minimize exposure is best. At the same time, acknowledging that the patient's anatomic features may suggest gender-specific evaluation such as breast, testicular, or pelvic examinations is appropriate. For example, suggesting a pelvic examination for an FTM adolescent with unexplained vaginal discharge or bleeding might be appropriate. Most transgender patients will agree to the suggested examination if the medical rationale is presented in a factual and respectful manner, inviting the patient's questions and input on how to make the examination as comfortable as possible. All aspects of the physical examination should be for the purpose of medical necessity, not to satisfy physician curiosity about possible genital or breast changes related to hormonal or surgical transition therapy. As for all adolescents, a chaperone should be present during a breast, genital or anorectal examination. The gender of the chaperone should be based on patient preference.

## Laboratory Evaluation

The child with gender nonconforming behaviors who has an unremarkable history and normal physical examination requires no special laboratory evaluation. Laboratory evaluation of transgender adolescents should be based on an accurate and comprehensive history, including sexual and other risk behaviors, and physical examination, not on gender identity. Several clinical guidelines provide information on the appropriate laboratory evaluation and monitoring of those patients who elect to begin hormonal transition therapy.[49,50]

## ▶ MANAGEMENT

The goal of care in working with gender nonconforming children and transgender youths is to promote optimal physical, developmental, emotional, and social well-being. The challenge faced by PCPs is to achieve this goal within a context of nonacceptance and stigmatization by many people in society. In this sense, gender nonconforming children and transgender youths have life experiences and needs that are similar to those of LGB youths.

Another challenge faced by PCPs is how to advise and support families of gender nonconforming and gender dysphoric children and youths when there is a considerable lack of professional consensus on appropriate treatment approaches and goals in these age groups. Because there has been insufficient research in these and related areas, treatment approaches and goals rely in large part on "expert opinion" rather than scientific data. This has allowed a number of different treatment approaches to be proposed, particularly for preadolescent children, that are sometimes based on differing philosophical foundations but very little science. This lack of evidence-based best practice standards can present a dilemma for PCPs and families in trying to decide which of the varying approaches best meets the needs of a particular child. Fortunately, a 2012 issue of the *Journal of Homosexuality* was dedicated to assisting PCPs and parents by offering a comprehensive review of what is known and what has yet to be learned about gender nonconformity and gender dysphoria in childhood, as well as various treatment approaches and their specified goals.[26] It also provided detailed descriptions of a number of well-established clinical programs and identified areas of consensus and disagreement among them.[51–53] Ethical implications of the various approaches also were discussed.[28] Since most PCPs work in communities without specialized child and adolescent gender clinics, it is imperative that PCPs become familiar with these issues, understand where they themselves stand philosophically on the continuum of treatment approaches, and be willing to reach out to experts at nationally recognized child and adolescent gender centers for consultation as the need arises.[54]

Although relatively little is known about gender nonconformity, cross-gender identity, and gender dysphoria in childhood, the area that is best understood is the likely developmental trajectories of children with gender dysphoria. It also serves as an excellent example of how robust, reproducible research data can result in a greater degree of consensus around certain aspects of treatment approach. We now know, for example, that the dysphoria of most younger children with gender dysphoria does not persist into adolescence.[18] These children are referred to as *desisters*, and their dysphoria usually disappears in later childhood at about age 7 to 9 years. Research has shown that most desisters will go on to self-identify as lesbian or gay during adolescence, and a small percentage will identify as heterosexual. Children with gender dysphoria that persists into adolescence are referred to as *persisters*, and most eventually identify in adolescence and adulthood as transgender. At this point, there is no way to accurately predict which children will end up desisting or persisting in their gender dysphoria. Another unknown is whether treatment aimed at promoting a child's desistance is effective, or more importantly, ethical. This is among the more disputed aspects related to the treatment of gender nonconforming expression, cross-gender identity, and gender dysphoria in preadolescent childhood. While there is some controversy related to the treatment of transgender adolescents in terms of timing and length of various transition treatments, most clinical experts support medical transition treatments in adolescence and adulthood, such as pubertal suppression, hormone therapy, and eventual gender affirmation surgery. This is because research has shown that most transgender adolescents have a gender identity that will perisit into adulthood. Furthermore, there is a robust body of evidence that demonstrates that transition treatments are safe and lead to significant improvements in physical and emotional well-being.[55–58] There is no similar body of research definitively supporting a single treatment approach over another in addressing gender dysphoria and gender nonconformity in preadolescent children, thus leading to the confusing and sometimes contradictory choices facing PCPs and the parents and children they are trying their best to support.

Despite controversy, several shared themes can be found across most treatment programs for preadolescent gender dysphoric and gender nonconforming children.[28] Since research findings related to persistence and desistence among children are well-accepted, with an understanding that most gender dysphoric children will be desisters and no longer gender dysphoric as they move into adolescence, it is generally agreed that the appropriate approach is to provide support and counseling to parents and children, but not to provide medical transition treatment in childhood. There is also a widely held view that social transition in terms of living full-time as a child of another gender or use of name and pronouns consistent with inner gender identity should probably be deferred until adolescence. Since so many preadolescent gender dysphoric children eventually desist, many feel that encouraging them to transition socially and then later "de-transition" might cause unnecessary trauma to the child, although there are no research data to support this. Another area of general agreement is that, ideally, support and counseling should be provided to gender dysphoric children and their families by a multidisciplinary team consisting of the PCP, a psychiatrist or other mental health professional, and a social worker. These professionals can be valuable additions to the treatment plan in exploring a child's or youth's sense of gender identity, social and academic functioning, family relationships, cultural expectations, and self-esteem. They can help assess and support parents through the process of acceptance and, it is hoped, eventual celebration of their child. They also can address parental fears, concerns, and misconceptions, which likely will change in nature as a child grows older and moves into adolescence. Most treatment programs emphasize that their goal is not to prevent homosexuality or cross-gender identity. Instead, the stated goal for most is to prevent or ameliorate gender dysphoria, recognizing that not all children with cross-gender identity are gender dysphoric.

Despite these common themes among most programs, there are also significant and often controversial differences regarding what "support and counseling" actually mean among varying programs. These often reflect underlying philosophical differences and varying understandings of gender nonconformity and gender identity, their etiologies, and the degree to which they are felt to reflect possible underlying pathology or simply another way of "being" in the world. At one end of the spectrum are programs that are prepared to focus on perceived psychopathology in a child, a parent, or family dynamics that either cause gender nonconforming expression or cross-gender identity and dysphoria or allow them to persist.[51] Treatment often involves trying to help a child "work through" his or her cross-gender identity with the goal of decreasing gender dysphoria, even if it means engaging in efforts to decrease a child's desire to be another gender. Parents are asked to put limits on their child's cross-gender behaviors and to create more opportunities for their child to have interactions with temperamentally compatible same-sex peers, feeling that these kinds of interactions help solidify a child's appropriate sense of gender consistent with natal sex, and perhaps counteract pathologic influences contributing to the creation or persistence of cross-gender identity. At the other end of the spectrum are those professionals who believe the appropriate approach is to validate and celebrate the unique gender identity of each child,[59] respecting the child's right to express their gender as they wish, while keeping them safe in an often nonaccepting and hostile world. Most programs working with gender nonconforming and gender dysphoric children fall somewhere in the middle of the spectrum.[52,53,60] They tend not to focus on looking for sources of psychopathology as factors contributing to a child's gender identity or gender dysphoria. Most feel that a good measure of the dysphoria experienced by children and youths comes from the negative responses of family, peers, and community to their cross-gender identity and expression. Therefore, a significant part of providing support to a child is to determine how safe and supportive that child's environment is and to work with extended families, schools, places of worship, and other settings to ensure that a child is safe and validated in all areas of his or her life. Parents are provided information about gender dysphoria and its possible developmental trajectories, as well as the understanding, skills, and resources to support their child effectively, no matter what their gender identity or sexual orientation might eventually be. Most physicians take a "watchful waiting" approach toward the child, allowing the child to express their gender, although sometimes suggesting certain limits (for example, being allowed to cross-dress at home but not when they go to school). As a child approaches adolescence they are especially watchful for evidence that a child's gender dysphoria, if present, may persist or desist. If it looks like it may persist then discussions with parents and child about possible future choices related to transition take place (for example, the initiation of pubertal suppression early in puberty). If it seems that the child's gender dysphoria may desist, then there are other discussions to be had, including considering the possibility that a child may later recognize a lesbian or gay identity, and providing family and child supportive resources in preparation for this possibility.

When faced with such a diverse and often contentious array of opinion and practice, what is a PCP to do when a family arrives in their clinic expressing concerns about their young child's gender nonconforming behaviors, expressed cross-gender identity, or gender dysphoria? First, it is important to be familiar with the areas of consensus and controversy outlined above. Secondly, it is important to keep in mind the replacement of the GID diagnosis with gender dysphoria in the *DSM-5*. This means that gender nonconforming expression and cross-gender identity per se are now considered part of the normal spectrum of human diversity. Discomfort and distress over gender should be the focus of concern, and the goal of treatment is to prevent or ameliorate that distress, whether its origins are within a person's psyche, in their environment, or perhaps both. It is important to remember that the goal of treatment is not to prevent homosexuality, and most physicians would agree that it is also not to change a child's expressed gender identity. PCPs should be aware of and willing to access local and national resources that can support them in the provision of informed care to these children and youths and their families. If possible, it is very helpful to bring together a multidisciplinary team as described above, to support both the patient and the patient's family over time, from childhood through adolescence and possibly into adulthood.

It is important to be open with parents about the varying approaches to working with gender nonconforming and gender dysphoric children, and about their underlying assumptions and goals. It is also important for PCPs to let parents know where they are on the spectrum of professional opinion about the appropriate treatment approach to these children and their families. PCPs or other team members should open the opportunity for a discussion of parental concerns, fears, and degree of comfort related to their child's gender identity and expression. They should also be asked what their hopes and expectations around treatment might be. Parents should be informed clearly that the goals of treatment are to prevent or diminish a child's distress around gender, but not to change their gender identity or sexual orientation. Often parents fear that their child might someday be lesbian or gay, and may or may not have thought about the possibility of their child being transgender. The PCP should gently remind parents that any child might be gay, lesbian, bisexual or transgender, and let them know of the medical profession's position that all these possibilities are considered normal developmental outcomes, while recognizing that not all segments of society yet agree. The PCP should also share, in lay terms, what is known about the developmental trajectories of children experiencing gender dysphoria—that in adolescence many do come to realize their lesbian or gay identities, while a much smaller number are transgender. Over time, as a child gets older, this issue should be revisited, offering parents an opportunity to share their thoughts or concerns and allowing the PCP to correct misconceptions and connect parents, childen, and youths to supportive resources.

Above all, PCPs should remind parents of the importance of expressing their unconditional love for their child and refraining from comments or actions that demonstrate disapproval of their child's gender expression or identity. The Family Acceptance Project at San Francisco University has conducted research demonstrating the important role that parents play keeping their lesbian, gay, bisexual, and transgender children healthy and safe through the provision of acceptance and love.[61] The PCP should share this understanding with all families, and provide them the skills and resources to accept and support their children no matter what their gender identity or sexual orientation might be.

The following sections continue the discussion by focusing on how PCPs can recognize and address the needs of transgender adolescents.

## *Physical Well-being*

Gender nonconforming children and transgender youths face the same health issues as other young people. The health care they receive should be based on a comprehensive history, physical examination, and evaluative studies, not on their gender expression or identity. Nevertheless, the PCP should recognize that these children and youths often grow up in hostile environments that may have a negative effect on their physical well-being. Among these negative effects are the physical sequelae of substance use, poor nutrition caused by homelessness or disordered eating, unprotected sexual behaviors, self-harm, injuries from physical and sexual victimization, and hormonal or surgical transition treatments accessed outside of health care settings.

## Developmental, Social, and Emotional Well-being

In most ways, children with gender nonconforming expression and transgender youths are exactly the same as their peers. They have the same needs for protection, nurturance, and love and the same hopes and dreams for the future. They grow up in the same families and communities and attend the same schools and places of worship. Similar to other children, they face the fundamental task of achieving a sense of identity that integrates all aspects of who they are, including their sexual orientation and gender identity. This integration of sexual and gender identity, accompanied by a growing sense of comfort with that identity, is essential for the optimal health and well-being of each child and adolescent.

However, the experience of growing up as a child with gender nonconforming expression or as a transgender youth is different in several important ways.[15,62,63] Unlike their peers, these young people face an often lonely and sometimes frightening journey of self-discovery, attempting to understand 2 of the most fundamental aspects of who they are as human beings—their gender identity and their sexual orientation. Some of these children will recognize, often at a young age, that their inner sense of being female, male, or another gender differs from the gender that was assigned to them at birth. Some children and adolescents accommodate themselves to this growing awareness. Most, however, experience significant confusion and distress, wondering what their feelings mean and uncertain of who they are. Growing up in a society that believes that a person is either male or female and that gender expression and identity must strictly reflect biologic sex undoubtedly intensifies their sense that something inside them has gone wrong. Many of these individuals become filled with an overwhelming mix of confusion, shame, anger, self-hatred, and despair. It is important to remember that most gender-dysphoric children eventually self-identify as lesbian, gay, or bisexual and no longer experience gender dysphoria as adolescents. Being lesbian, gay, or bisexual in an often-disapproving society may bring its own distinct set of developmental challenges.

The PCP's role as educator and counselor is as important as that of medical physician in caring for gender nonconforming children, transgender youths, and their families. The PCP should avoid assumptions based on stereotypes and listen carefully to understand each patient's unique experience and needs. In general, the counseling of nonconforming and transgender youths will address 6 areas: (1) self-acceptance and validation of gender expression and identity, (2) safety, (3) connectedness to supportive others, (4) self-disclosure or *coming out,* (5) healthy relationships and sexual decision making, and (6) optimism for the future. Addressing each of these areas is essential in ensuring their healthy development. These should be addressed over time and not all at an initial presentation or single visit.

### Self-acceptance and Validation

The PCP can play an important role in countering the effects of disapproval and the pathologizing of gender nonconforming expression and identity. For the gender nonconforming child, the PCP should state that although being different in this society can be painful, the child's gender nonconforming behavior can be healthy for that child. For transgender youths, the PCP should acknowledge the controversy around the use of gender dysphoria as a diagnostic category. PCPs should present being transgender as part of the tapestry of normal human identity and clarify that the primary issue of concern is distress that can often come from having a transgender identity in a society that is unaccepting. This validating reassurance of healthiness and normalcy is perhaps the most powerful statement a PCP can make to gender nonconforming children and transgender youths and their families.

A growing number of older gender nonconforming children and transgender adolescents know a significant amount about gender, gender identity, and gender expression. Many have done extensive research on the Internet, accessing YouTube videos and Web sites that are easily searchable, or connecting with other gender nonconforming and transgender youth on social media. Others, however, continue to be very isolated and know little or nothing about the nature and meaning of their emerging sense of identity. Therefore, the PCP should conduct an initial inquiry into what the youth knows and has seen or read, and focus on correcting misconceptions, providing validation, and supporting empowerment. Gender nonconforming children can be reassured that many ways exist of being a boy or a girl and that their way is one of these many ways. They can also be told that some children feel more like a girl inside and some more like a boy, or perhaps another gender, and that however they feel in terms of gender identity is all right. Transgender youths should be provided information on sexual orientation, gender identity, and what it means to be transgender. Some of these adolescents may go through a period of confusion, not knowing whether they are gay, lesbian, bisexual, straight, transgender, or a combination of these. The PCP should inform the adolescent that such uncertainty is normal and that over time they will have a clearer understanding of who they are. The PCP may also provide brochures to adolescents facing issues of gender identity or refer them to supportive Web sites.[64]

Ethnic and other minority youths who are transgender may have an especially difficult time. The PCP should discuss these issues with their patients openly and connect them to appropriate supportive resources within their communities and online.

## Safety

Because gender nonconforming children and transgender youths endure higher rates of physical and sexual assault, harassment, discrimination, and social rejection, PCPs should ask gender nonconforming children and transgender youths about their safety in their home, school, place of worship, and broader community. If harassment or other harmful treatment is acknowledged, then the PCP should work with the youth and family to identify and implement appropriate strategies to end the violence. Many of these children and youths feel shame and are afraid to advocate for their own safety. They may think they deserve the harm inflicted on them, or they may simply accept that this is the way the world is. The PCP should tell children and adolescents that they do not deserve such treatment and that they should expect and demand safety and respect from everyone in their lives and in all settings. Because gender nonconforming children and transgender youths have so few advocates, the PCP should offer to join with them in approaching every venue in which they experience violence, including the home and school, to work out a plan to end violence immediately and completely. Parents, PCPs, teachers, and others should also work together to ensure that schools and other community organizations create and implement policies and practices that ensure respectful treatment and appropriate accommodations for these children. The state of Massachusetts, for example, has developed a detailed policy statement about the responsibilities of schools to accept and support gender nonconforming and transgender students, which can serve as a model for other states. (See Tools for Practice at the end of this chapter.) Many states also have specifically designated offices, often within state departments of education, to combat bullying and harassment, including that specifically based on gender identity and expression. If necessary, the PCP should call on the state child welfare services office or advocacy organizations such as the American Civil Liberties Union to join in the effort to keep these young people safe.

## Isolation

Because gender nonconforming children and transgender youths experience profound isolation and loneliness, their physical and emotional health may be compromised. PCPs should address the issue of isolation by giving accurate information about gender expression and gender identity. They should provide supportive and reassuring counseling, or they should refer the child or adolescent to colleagues who have the time, comfort, and expertise to provide them accepting and supportive care and counseling. PCPs should connect these children and youths to local community resources such as support groups and other youth programs. Children, youths, and families who do not have access to local programs should be informed about national organizations and Web sites created specifically for gender nonconforming children, transgender youths, and their families (see Tools for Practice). PCPs can also point out positive gender nonconfoming and transgender role models in the community or nationally. In certain circumstances, it is appropriate for transgender PCPs to present themselves as role models to transgender youths and their families.

## Self-disclosure and Coming Out

Transgender adolescents often reach a point in their development at which they feel a strong urge to disclose their gender identity to others. Transgender youths often have a history of gender nonconforming expression as children. Therefore others may have already assumed or sensed that they may be transgender or lesbian or gay. Some transgender youths, however, successfully conceal their gender identity, either by adapting their gender expression to fit societal expectations consistent with their biologic sex or by labeling themselves or allowing others to perceive them as gay or lesbian. The process of disclosure to family and friends is often emotional and traumatic. Transgender youths who disclose their gender identity (come out) risk condemnation and rejection by family and peers. Therefore, coming out should be considered carefully, weighing the risks and benefits. It is sometimes suggested that if an adolescent expects a negative response from parents, then the adolescent should wait to disclose until legally and financially independent. However, many adolescents think that continuing to live a lie is intolerable and harmful to their self-esteem, and they come out earlier. A PCP should never reveal an adolescent's gender identity to parents without permission unless imminent risk of harm exists. A PCP can play an important role in the process of disclosure by helping adolescents decide whether they are ready to come out to family or friends and helping them choose an appropriate time, place, and approach for disclosure. PCPs who feel they do not have the skills to provide such counseling effectively should refer to or collaborate with a therapist who can guide the teen and support the family through the coming out process.

## Relationships and Sexual Decision Making

Most transgender youths have difficulty in meeting other transgender adolescents to establish friendships and share mutual support. PCPs should help connect transgender youths to local LGBT teen support groups and LGBT-supportive programs in the community, if they exist. This task can be accomplished ethically without parental notification. PCPs can suggest national telephone hotlines or Web sites where transgender youths can receive accurate information and supportive counseling and can communicate with other transgender youths (see Tools for Practice). If these options are not available, then the PCP can serve as a supportive and reassuring lifeline until the adolescent is old enough to become independent and possibly move away to attend school or work in a community more accepting of transgender people.

Transgender adolescents may be heterosexual, homosexual, or bisexual in their attractions and behaviors. Given the prevailing societal disapproval of transgender individuals, however, many transgender youths are afraid to reveal their gender identity to those with whom they might be interested in establishing a relationship. Therefore, some transgender youths find that their only options for exploring emotional and physical intimacy are through anonymous sexual encounters on the streets, in parks, or through Internet hookups. In addition to being potentially dangerous, these encounters are often accompanied by feelings of shame and degradation, which are harmful to an adolescent's sense of identity and self-worth. That many transgender youths are eager to engage in the typical courting practices of adolescence, which normally take place in safer and more affirming circumstances, is evidenced in the great popularity of LGBT youth proms and other social gatherings in a growing number of communities across the United States.

Transgender youths who are in relationships face many of the same questions as their nontransgender peers: "Am I in love?" "What do I want from a relationship?" "Do I really want to be in this relationship?" "How do I know if this is a good relationship?" "How do I get out of this relationship?" In addition, transgender youths face the exceedingly difficult questions of how and when to tell their potential boyfriend or girlfriend about their gender identity. A transgender-supportive PCP or therapist can help adolescents reflect on and find answers to these questions.

As with other adolescents, many transgender youths know little about sexuality and how to make healthy sexual choices. Abstinence is always the appropriate option for adolescents who do not feel ready for a sexual relationship. Transgender adolescents should understand that when they are ready for a sexual relationship, they can expect to lead healthy and fulfilling sexual lives. All adolescents who have decided they are ready for a sexual relationship should be advised to limit their number of sexual partners and avoid mixing sex and alcohol or drugs so as to reduce their risk for infection, trauma, and sexual assault. Transgender youths, like other adolescents and depending on the sexual behaviors they engage in, are at risk for unplanned pregnancy and should be counseled on contraception. Not only could pregnancy lead to medical risks but it often can be extremely psychologically traumatizing to a gender nonconforming or transgender youth. Safer sex practices related to oral, vaginal, and anal sex should be reviewed in detail. Transgender youths should also be aware that *no* always means *no* in negotiating sex, and any forced or coerced sexual experience represents sexual assault.

## Optimism for the Future

PCPs should not only focus on the risks that transgender youths face, but also identify specific strengths that have allowed them to survive and sometimes thrive in the face of an often hostile environment. They should also challenge the belief of many transgender adolescents that their futures will be significantly limited by their gender identity. Although some communities are more accepting of transgender people than others, many transgender adults lead happy, healthy, and productive lives. Although growing up transgender is often challenging, the future should be seen as hopeful and exciting.

## ▶ TRANSITION CARE

Transition represents the emotional, psychological, social, physical, and legal processes transgender persons experience to assume a body and gender role consistent with their gender identity. The transition process often begins in childhood and continues through adolescence into adulthood. Pubertal suppression, hormone therapy, and surgery are often the final medical steps in this process. PCPs play an essential role in facilitating the patient's transition from female to male, male to female, or perhaps to another gender. They often have known their gender nonconforming and gender dysphoric patients since early childhood. As puberty approaches and it seems that gender dysphoria may persist into adolescence, they are in an advantageous position to provide patient and parents with detailed and accurate information about the nature and timing of transition, its limitations and benefits, and the choices that lie ahead. It is also important to share with families that, just as there is significant controversy around the understanding and management of gender dysphoria and gender variance in childhood, there is also controversy around certain aspects of the provision of medical transition care from early puberty through adolescence. This understanding is essential in order for patients and parents to give informed consent to treatment. At the same time, it is imperative for the PCP to be clear about where she or he stands within the spectrum of opinion on the medical management of transition, including pubertal suppression, hormonal treatment, and gender-affirmation surgery.

The PCP has an important role in helping patients and families identify possible natural transition points for initiating hormone therapy, such as when a patient is changing schools (for example, from middle school to high school) or a family is planning to move to a new home and neighborhood. Whether or not such transition points are identified, it is important that the PCP work with school personnel before transition begins, educating them about what it means to be transgender and the social and psychological benefits of transition. The potential risk of harassment by other students or by school staff should also be addressed. In order to ensure both respectful treatment and safety in the school setting, the PCP should advocate for the development of an IEP or other formal assurance that the transgender student's preferred name and pronouns will be used in all school settings, both inside and outside the classroom and whether the student is present or not, and that appropriate restrooms and changing rooms are identified and accessible.

In addition to facilitating and monitoring social and psychological aspects of transition, PCPs are playing an increasingly central role in the initiation and management of physical transition, including both pubertal suppression and hormonal therapy. Many PCPs still feel they do not have the training, experience, or time to do so effectively. Therefore, they refer their patients with significant gender nonconformity or gender dysphoria to gender specialists and other colleagues whom they feel have greater expertise in assessing gender issues and providing transgender care. At the same time, they retain their role as PCP and provider of a medical home. Many larger communities have endocrinologists and adolescent medicine, family practice, and internal medicine physicians, as well as mental health physicians, who are experienced in providing medical care and counseling to gender dysphoric youths considering transition. Such physicians often can be located through local LGBT community centers or national organizations such as the Gay and Lesbian Medical Association. Many PCPs, however, practice in smaller communities with few or no physicians with such expertise. These physicians should reach out to regional or other gender experts, through telemedicine and other means, to request their guidance in the evaluation and management of children and youths experiencing significant gender nonconformity or gender dysphoria. Thus, through necessity, many PCPs have become experts on transgender care. They recognize that for most gender dysphoric youths entering puberty, the provision of transition-related treatments such as pubertal suppression and hormonal therapy (outlined below) is not elective but instead represents a standard of care, with the early institution of treatment predicting optimal improvement in both physical and psychological well-being.[55,57,58]

Guidelines are available to help PCPs and other physicians facilitate the transition process. WPATH in 2011 published the seventh edition of *Standards of Care for Transsexual, Transgender, and Gender Non-conforming People*, which is considered to be among the most authoritative guides to providing medical and mental health transition counseling, treatment, and support.[14] The Endocrine Society also has developed detailed clinical practice guidelines on hormonal transition treatment for transgender adolescents and adults.[56] In addition, several health centers experienced in providing comprehensive transgender health care have developed their own clinical guidelines.[49,50] These latter guidelines often approach transgender care based on an informed-consent model, which is premised on a belief in the ability of patients (and if a minor, their parents as well) to determine their own transition path if provided complete and unbiased information about transition choices and their benefits and limitations. This model differs markedly from the traditional approach to transition care, including those represented in earlier versions of the WPATH standards of care, which presented a very prescriptive and linear path to transition. Under these earlier standards, transition was presided over by medical and mental health gatekeepers who could decide who was eligible for transition treatments, as well as the nature, sequence, and timing of those treatments. The latest edition of the WPATH standards of care differs significantly from previous versions. It is much more patient centered and allows for a flexible approach in which recommendations related to transition care may be modified on a case-by-case basis in order to address a patient's specific needs and circumstances. The ultimate goal of the current WPATH standards of care is to reduce gender dysphoria and maximize physical and psychological well-being. It explicitly emphasizes that efforts to change an individual's gender identity or expression are considered unethical.

Regarding physical interventions for adolescents considering transition, WPATH suggests an approach consisting of 3 stages: (1) fully reversible interventions, using gonadotropin-releasing hormone (GnRH) analogs in early puberty to suppress estrogen and testosterone production, thereby delaying the progression of puberty; (2) partially reversible interventions, consisting of hormone therapy to masculinize or feminize the body; and (3) irreversible interventions such as gender-affirmation surgery, generally occuring in adulthood. WPATH advocates a staged approach in order to allow the adolescent and parents time to adjust to one stage before moving on to the next. The involvement of a multidisciplinary team to support the adolescent and family through the significant changes of physical, psychological, and social transition is highly recommended, with the understanding that the role of each team member is to facilitate the process of timely transition and not to stand as a gatekeeper obstructing the path to receiving appropriate care, as has occurred in the past.

Despite WPATH's staged model of transition care, it is important to recognize that the path of transition is not the same for everyone. Some individuals are satisfied to live their lives consistent with their gender identity in a social sense but have no urge to initiate hormone therapy or undergo surgery. Others seek hormone treatment but feel that surgical alteration of their bodies is unnecessary. Still others may choose partial surgical gender reassignment; for example, many FTM transgender individuals choose mastectomy but not genital reconstruction. In addition, the transition process is not necessarily a linear one. Some individuals move back and forth between feelings of being more feminine or masculine and may present themselves differently to the world at different times in terms of gender role and expression. This fluidity of identity should be expected and supported by the PCP.

### Pubertal Suppression

Pubertal suppression has become the standard of care for children entering puberty with persistent gender dysphoria, and it is advocated by both WPATH and the Endocrine Society. Puberty is suppressed through the administration of GnRH analogs, very similar to the treatment of precocious puberty in younger children. Pubertal suppression as treatment for gender dysphoria represents an off-label use of this medication. GnRH analogs suppress the secretion of lutenizing hormone (LH) from the pituitary, resulting in suppressed levels of testosterone and estrogen, thereby postponing the development of secondary sexual characteristics. One proposed benefit of pubertal suppression is that it allows an adolescent additional time to better understand his or her gender identity and with increasing maturity be able to make more informed decisions about whether to proceed with gender transition or not. A second benefit is that pubertal suppression can prevent or postpone the emotional trauma that can accompany the development of secondary sexual characteristics reflecting natal sex for most transgender youths, resulting in decreased gender dysphoria. A third benefit is that pubertal suppression prevents the development of secondary sexual characteristics that often makes later physical transition much more difficult. Hormonal therapy is much more effective in bringing about desired physical changes if the undesired pubertal changes reflecting natal sex have not taken place. Suppression of unwanted pubertal changes may also decrease the need for more invasive interventions later, such as breast surgery, electrolysis, and tracheal shaving.

For a child experiencing persistent or emerging gender dysphoria, pubertal suppression should be initiated when the first signs of puberty appear (which may occur as early as age 9).[56] Suppression should continue until the adolescent is able to confidently specify his or her gender identity. If an adolescent decides that his or her gender identity is consistent with natal sex, pubertal suppression is ended and puberty allowed to proceed. The hormonal influences of suppression are completely reversible with no compromise to subsequent pubertal development. If an adolescent confirms a transgender identity, pubertal suppression is ended and cross-gender hormonal treatment is begun.

During pubertal suppression, the involvement of a supportive pediatric endocrinologist is recommended. Research on the use of GnRH analogs suggests the possibility of decreased bone mineral density in some patients during suppression treatment. However, current research suggests that children who have been on suppressive therapy catch up on bone growth once they progress through puberty or are started on cross-gender hormone therapy.[56] Suppression therapy may also lead to irregular menses in biologic females, particularly if started later in pubertal development. An endocrinologist can help address these issues and can monitor attainment of gender-appropriate height, making appropriate adjustments to treatment as necessary. The few potential risks of suppression treatment must be weighed against the growing body of research documenting the positive outcomes on physical and psychological well-being resulting from the use of pubertal suppression in the management of gender dysphoric youth in early puberty and adolescence.[58]

Gender dysphoric youths whose natal sex is male should be informed, along with their parents, that pubertal suppression could result in insufficient penile tissue if later penile-inversion vaginoplasty is desired. However, skin grafts and colonic tissue may be used instead. PCPs should also have detailed discussions with patients and their parents about the effects of both pubertal suppression and cross-gender hormone therapy on future fertility. Youths who receive only pubertal suppression treatment should progress to full fertility once pubertal suppression is discontinued and pubertal development resumes. Those who move from pubertal suppression directly to cross-gender hormone treatment likely will experience some degree of impaired fertility. Some patients may chose to have a hormone-free interval between pubertal suppression and the initiation of cross-hormone therapy in order to permit collection of sperm and oocytes for cryopreservation. Others have interrupted cross-gender hormone therapy later in life for the same purpose. The important thing is that this essential conversation take place, and that patients and their families are made aware of fertility experts that they may turn to for further consultation. Finally, families should be informed that pubertal suppression treatment is expensive and may not be covered by some insurance plans, although this likely will change as such treatment increasingly is recognized as a standard of care.

The primary controversy related to pubertal suppression therapy relates to when it should be started. Gender specialists agree that for children who have long-standing or emerging intense gender dysphoria at the onset of puberty, pubertal suppression should be initiated early. While some guidelines suggest beginning therapy at Tanner Stage 2 or 3, many advocate beginning treatment with the first physical or hormonal evidence of puberty, early in Tanner Stage 2.[56]

### *Hormone Therapy*

The offering of hormonal therapy, like pubertal suppression, represents a standard of care for adolescents experiencing gender dysphoria. A number of protocols are available that address the evaluation and hormonal treatment of transgender adolescents.[14,49,50,56] There is uniform agreement across protocols on the appropriateness of hormonal treatment for transgender adolescents, supported by research showing the significant benefits of hormonal transition in terms of both physical and psychological well-being.[55,58] Certain aspects of these protocols, however, continue to be quite controversial. The most significant among these reflects a debate among physicians about the appropriate age for initiating hormonal therapy. Historically, the age of 16 was most often cited, accompanied by a belief that a 16-year-old would be better able than a younger adolescent to make informed, mature decisions around treatment that could lead to irreversible physical changes. In fact, age 16 was initially recommended solely because the age of majority in the Netherlands, where most early treatment protocols were developed, was 16, and represented the age at which adolescents in that country could consent to their own care. The latest edition of WPATH's standards of care as well as the recommendations of others working in the field of transgender health allow for flexibility in determining the age of hormonal treatment initiation, advising that such decisions should be made on a case-by-case basis, with age 16 set only as a guideline and with allowances made for earlier initiation.[14,57,65] In fact, many families and children seek care much earlier than age 16, and many centers initiate hormone therapy much earlier than 16 and sometimes as young as age 12. These centers see no reason to delay treatment unnecessarily, because the trauma of experiencing puberty reflecting natal sex or being told to wait for years in a suspended peripubertal state as peers continue to develop, is significant, and may even be life threatening. PCPs should discuss these issues openly with families and youths, considering the question, "For this particular child, what is the rationale for suppressing puberty for 3 to 5 years? Does this child in fact display uncertainty regarding his or her gender identity that dictates waiting this long to end suppressive treatment or initiate hormonal therapy?"

While many centers operate under a belief that mental health support is an essential component of transition, it should not delay or become a barrier to accessing appropriate and timely treatment. WPATH's standards of care state directly that "refusing timely medical interventions for adolescents might prolong gender dysphoria and contribute to an appearance that could provoke abuse and stigmatization. As the level of gender-related abuse is strongly associated with the degree of psychiatric distress during adolescence... withholding puberty suppression and subsequent feminizing and masculinizing hormone therapy is not a neutral option for adolescents."[14]

## Male-to-Female Hormone Treatment

Estrogen is the mainstay of MTF-transgender hormone therapy. For adolescents, most physicians prescribe estrogen sublingually or transdermally, to avoid first-pass metabolism. Protocols also cite oral and injectable forms as options. For transgender individuals, many of the "side effects" of estrogen therapy are in fact desirable effects. Expected changes include breast development, softening of skin, increase in subcutaneous fat and its redistribution to the thighs and buttocks, diminished body hair, fewer erections, and testicular atrophy. Patients may also experience decreased libido, weight gain, and emotional changes. Some of these changes may be irreversible, continuing even after possible discontinuation of treatment. Fertility will be impaired while on estrogen therapy and possibly even if estrogen treatment is discontinued. This should be discussed openly with patients and their parents, as should the option of cryopreservation of sperm if desired. Estrogen treatment is generally safe in adolescents.[66] Although PCPs should be aware of the precautions generally noted for estrogen therapy,[49] including the possibility of blood clots in high-risk populations such as smokers, medical contraindications to estrogen treatment in adolescents are rare. Antiandrogens, such as spironolactone, finasteride, and GnRH analogs, are routinely added to the regimen to suppress the action of endogenous testosterone, augment breast development, and soften facial and body hair. Gonadectomy serves a similar purpose although generally is not considered until age 18 or older as part of gender affirmation surgery.

## Female-to-Male Hormone Treatment

The FTM transition is facilitated through the use of testosterone administered through injection, patch, or topical gel. Testosterone treatment is generally safe in adolescents. Among the potentially desirable "side effects" of testosterone treatment for these patients are increased facial and body hair, clitoral enlargement, vagina atrophy, cessation of menses, male pattern baldness, deepening of voice, decreased fat mass, increased muscle mass and strength, a more masculine body shape, increased weight, more prominent veins, coarser skin, and mild breast atrophy. Patients may also notice increased acne, mood changes, and increased libido. Some of these changes may be irreversible. Fertility will likely be impaired during testosterone treatment, although it may return if treatment is interrupted. PCPs should discuss this openly with patients and their families, and should also discuss options for cryopreservation of oocytes before treatment is begun.

### *Other Treatments*

Some transgender individuals will seek other treatments to facilitate physical and psychosocial transition to their appropriate gender. Often these treatments will occur after the adolescent years, partly because these procedures are expensive and not yet covered by many insurance plans. Because many of these treatments involve irreversible changes, most protocols recommend deferring them until at least age 18, especially those that represent gender affirmation surgery. MTF-transgender individuals may seek reconstructive surgery, including penectomy, orchiectomy, vaginoplasty, clitoroplasty, vulvoplasty, breast and gluteal augmentation, tracheal shaving, and facial reconstruction. Electrolysis or other hair-removal procedures may be sought. Silicone injections also may be sought to obtain a more feminine body contour. FTM-transgender individuals may seek chest reconstruction surgery, hysterectomy, oophorectomy, phalloplasty, and other genital reconstruction. Both MTF and FTM individuals may seek voice therapy and professional guidance in how to present themselves as male, female or another gender through body language, facial expression, gait, posture, and mannerisms. Although these surgical, cosmetic, and other procedures often take place after adolescence, discussing these options and their benefits and limitations and making appropriate referrals should be part of the PCP's anticipatory guidance of transgender youths.

## ▶ PARENTS

Parents who come to recognize their child's gender nonconforming behavior or transgender identity may experience a variety of emotions: confusion, fear, sadness, concern, embarrassment, guilt, anger, or disgust, but also acceptance and celebration. These feelings should be discussed openly and with compassion. Many parents fear for their child's safety and happiness. Many of them fear that their child may eventually self-identify as lesbian or gay. In many instances these concerns and fears are not raised on visits to the PCP or are referred to only indirectly ("My son is a sensitive child," or "My daughter is definitely a tomboy"). The PCP should be sensitive to any cues of parental worry about gender nonconformity and ask parents simply, "Do you have any concerns about your child's behaviors?" or even better, "Have you had any concerns that your son's [daughter's] behaviors or interests are more feminine [masculine] than other children's his [her] age?" Most concerned parents, although perhaps embarrassed, are relieved to have such a discussion. The PCP's primary role in working with parents is to help them understand and celebrate their gender nonconforming child and support them in their efforts to keep their child happy, healthy, and safe.

Parents should be referred to Web sites, books, brochures, and media resources geared to parents of gender nonconforming children.[67]

Parents should be assured that with love, validation, and support their children should grow up to be happy, healthy, and productive adults, no matter what their gender expression, gender identity, or sexual orientation might be. The National Children's Medical Center has developed guidelines to help parents in their provision of support for their children.

Box 33-1 lists ways parents can support their child, and Box 33-2 lists pitfalls parents should try to avoid.

**BOX 33-1**

### *Children's National Medical Center Outreach Program Guidelines for Parents of Gender-variant and Transgender Youth*

- Love your child for who your child is. Love, acceptance, understanding, and support are especially important when peers and society are often intolerant of difference.
- Question traditional assumptions about gender roles and sexual orientation. Do not allow societal expectations to come between you and your child.
- Create a safe space for your child, allowing your child always to be who the child is, especially in the child's own home.
- Seek out socially accepted activities (sports, arts, hobbies) that respect your child's interests while helping your child fit in socially.
- Validate your child and your child's interests, supporting the idea that more than one way exists to be a girl or boy. Speak openly and calmly about gender variance with your child. Talk about these subjects in positive terms, and listen as your child expresses feelings of being different.
- Seek out supportive resources (books, videos, Web sites, support groups) for parents, families, and children.
- Talk about gender variance with other significant people in your child's life, including siblings, extended family members, babysitters, and family friends.
- Prepare your child to deal with bullying. Let your child know that he/she does not deserve to be hurt. Be aware of behaviors that suggest bullying may be occurring, such as school refusal, crying excessively, or complaining of aches and pains.
- Be your child's advocate. Expect and insist on acceptance, respect, and safety wherever your child is. Parents may need to educate school staff and others about the special experience and needs of gender-variant children.

Adapted from Children's National Medical Center. *If you are concerned about your child's gender behaviors: a guide for parents.* (http://childrensnational.org)

**BOX 33-2**

### *Children's National Medical Center Pitfalls to Avoid as Parents of Gender-variant and Transgender Youth*

- Avoid finding fault. No blame exists. Your child's gender variance came from within, not from you as parents. Blame will get in the way of enjoying your child.
- Do not pressure your child to change, because this will cause much pain and harm.
- Do not blame the victim. Do not accept bullying as *just the way things are.* No one has the right to torment or criticize others because they are different.

Adapted from Children's National Medical Center. *If you are concerned about your child's gender behaviors: a guide for parents.* (http://childrensnational.org)

## ▶ ADVOCACY

Because of their expertise and position of respect, PCPs are in an advantageous position to advocate on behalf of children with gender nonconforming behaviors, transgender youths, and their families. PCPs should encourage parents, siblings, and extended family to accept and love these young people unconditionally. The PCP should also be willing to meet with school personnel, child and youth welfare program staff, and others to share information about gender nonconformity and transgenderism. Because schools are a major part of a child's or adolescent's life, and because they are often the site where significant harassment and bullying of gender nonconforming and transgender youths take place, it is especially important that PCPs provide advocacy at all levels of local educational systems. This includes advocacy for the adoption of antiharassment policies specifically addressing harassment based on gender identity and expression as well as sexual orientation. It also includes advocating for mandated training of teacher and social service providers and policies that ensure that transgender youths are safe and treated respectfully, such as through the use of preferred names and pronouns, designation of appropriate bathrooms and changing rooms, and allowing a student to participate in graduation ceremonies and other activities based on gender identity rather than natal sex.

For PCPs seeking to advocate for societal change, encouraging the development and implementation of policies, procedures, and programs that recognize and respect the individuality of these children and youths and address their special needs for validation and safety is esssential. The PCP may also provide testimony at official meetings and hearings on proposals to add gender identity and expression to laws and school policies prohibiting discrimination, bullying, and harassment. The PCP may also advocate for the inclusion of meaningful medical school, residency training, and continuing medical education curricula on the life experience and health needs of children with gender nonconforming behaviors and transgender individuals and how to meet these needs in a respectful and effective manner. Finally, the PCP should encourage professional organizations to develop policy statements and clinical guidelines to support them in their work with these young people and their families.

### When to Refer

Refer to a child behavioral, adolescent, or gender specialist whenever a child or adolescent

- Shows significant gender nonconforming behaviors, particularly if they are concerning to parents or have resulted in rejection or mistreatment by family members, peers, or others. Ideally, referral will be made before possible dysphoria arises.
- Shows signs or symptoms of gender dysphoria, including expression of dissatisfaction or distress related to their birth-assigned gender or insistence that they are of another gender.
- Refer to a child and adolescent psychiatrist or other mental health professional whenever a child or adolescent.
- Experiences persistent or recurrent depressed or anxious mood that interferes with function.
- Has acute or recurrent suicidal ideation or self-injury.
- Evidences isolation from peers or family members.
- Engages in substance use or other high-risk behaviors.

It should be noted that referrals for therapy to change an adolescent's gender identity or expression are considered unethical.[14]

## TOOLS FOR PRACTICE

### Community Advocacy and Coordination

- *FORGE* (Web page), FORGE (forge-forward.org)
- *Guidance for Massachusetts Public Schools: Creating a Safe and Supportive School Environment* (article), Massachusetts Department of Elementary and Secondary Education (www.doe.mass.edu/ssce/genderidentity.pdf)
- *TransYouth Family Allies* (Web page), (www.imatyfa.org)

### Engaging Patient and Family

- *Camp Aranu'tiq* (Web site), Harbor Camps, Inc. (www.camparanutiq.org)
- *Family Acceptance Project* (Web site), Marian Wright Edelman Institute, San Francisco State University (familyproject.sfsu.edu)
- *Get Support* (Web page), Parents, Families, and Friends of Lesbians and Gays (PFLAG) (community.pflag.org/staff/transgender)
- *I Think I Might Be Transgender, Now What Do I Do?* (booklet), Youth Resource (www.advocatesforyouth.org/component/content/article/731-i-think-i-might-be-transgender-now-what-do-i-do)
- *If You Are Concerned About Your Child's Gender Behaviors: A Guide for Parents* (booklet), Children's National Medical Center: Outreach Program for Children with Gender-Variant Behaviors and Their Families (childrensnational.org/~/media/cnhs-site/files/departments/gender-and-sexuality-development-program/gvparentbrochure.ashx?la=en)
- *Legal Resources* (Web page), Trans Youth Equality Foundation (www.transyouthequality.org/legal-resources)
- *Resources: Parenting and Family* (Web page), Gender Spectrum (www.genderspectrum.org/resources/parenting-and-family-2/#more-432)
- *Resources: Teens* (Web page), Gender Spectrum (www.genderspectrum.org/resources/teens-2/#more-428)
- *The Transgender Child: A Handbook for Families and Professionals* (book), Cleis Press
- *The Trevor Project* (Web site), (www.thetrevorproject.org)
- *Transparenthood* (blog), (www.transparenthood.net)
- *Youth and Education* (Web page), Trans Youth Equality Foundation (www.transyouthequality.org/youth-and-education)

### Medical Decision Support

- *Guidelines for Care of Lesbian, Gay, Bisexual, and Transgender Patients (guideline),* Gay and Lesbian Medical Association (glma.org/_data/n_0001/resources/live/GLMA%20guidelines%202006%20FINAL.pdf)
- *Patient Health Questionnaire (PHQ) Screeners* (screen), Pfizer Inc. (www.phqscreeners.com)
- *Pediatric Symptom Checklist* (screen), Massachusetts General Hospital (www.massgeneral.org/psychiatry/services/psc_forms.aspx)
- *Standards of Care for the Health of Transsexual, Transgender, and Gender Nonconforming People* (article), International Journal of Transgenderism, Vol 13, 2011 (www.wpath.org/uploaded_fi les/140/fi les/IJT%20SOC,%20V7.pdf)

- *Strengths & Difficulties Questionnaires* (screen), Youth in Mind, Ltd. (www.sdqinfo.com)
- *Transgender Persons* (Web page), Centers for Disease Control and Prevention (www.cdc.gov/lgbthealth/transgender.htm)

## AAP POLICY STATEMENTS

American Academy of Pediatrics Committee on Adolescence. Sexual orientation and adolescents. *Pediatrics.* 2004;113(6):1827–1832 (pediatrics.aappublications.org/content/113/6/1827.full.html)

American Academy of Pediatrics Committee on Adolescence. Office-based care for lesbian, gay, bisexual, transgender, and questioning youth. *Pediatrics.* 2013;132(1):198–203 (pediatrics.aappublications.org/content/132/1/198.full.html)

## REFERENCES


1. Peletz MG. Transgenderism and gender pluralism in Southeast Asia since early modern times. *Curr Anthropol.* 2006;47:309–340
2. Lang S. Lesbians, men-women, and two-spirits: homosexuality and gender in Native American cultures. In: Blackwood E, Wieringa S, eds. *Female Desires: Same-Sex Relations and Transgender Practices Across Cultures.* New York, NY: Columbia University Press; 1999
3. Matzner A. *'O Au No Kea: Voices from Hawai'i's Mahu and Transgender Communities.* Philadelphia, PA: Xlibris; 2001
4. Green R. Mythological, historical, and cross-cultural aspects of transsexualism. In: Denny D, ed. *Current Concepts in Transgender Identity.* London, United Kingdom: Routledge Press; 1998
5. American Academy of Pediatrics Committee on Adolescence. Office-based care for lesbian, gay, bisexual, transgender, and questioning youth. *Pediatrics.* 2013;132:198–203
6. Levine DA; Committee on Adolescence. Office-based care for lesbian, gay, bisexual, transgender, and questioning youth. *Pediatrics.* 2013;132:e297–e313
7. Society for Adolescent Health and Medicine. Recommendations for promoting the health and well-being of lesbian, gay, bisexual, and transgender adolescents: a position paper of the Society for Adolescent Health and Medicine. *J Adolesc Health.* 2013;52(4):506–510
8. Achenbach TM. *Manual for Child Behavior Check List/4-18 and 1991 Profile.* Burlington, VT: University of Vermont Department of Psychiatry; 1991
9. Sandberg DE, Meyer-Bahlburg HF, Ehrhardt AA, Yager TJ. The prevalence of gender-atypical behavior in elementary school children. *J Am Acad Child Adolesc Psychiatry.* 1993;32:306–314
10. Steensma TD, van der Ende J, Verhulst FC, Cohen-Kettenis PT. Gender variance in childhood and sexual orientation in adulthood: a prospective study. *J Sex Med.* 2013;10(11):2723–2733
11. Achenbach TM, Edlebrock C. *Manual for the Youth Self-Report and Profile.* Burlington, VT: University of Vermont Department of Psychiatry; 1987
12. Meyer WJ 3rd. Gender identity disorder: an emerging problem for pediatricians. *Pediatrics.* 2012;129(3):571–573
13. van Beijsterveldt CE, Hudziak JJ, Boonsma DI. Genetic and environmental influences on cross-gender behavior and relation to behavioral problems: a study of Dutch twins at 7 and 10 years. *Arch Sex Behav.* 2006;35:647–658
14. World Professional Association for Transgender Health. Standards of care for the health of transsexual, transgender, and gender nonconforming people. *Int J Transgend.* 2011;13:165–232
15. Mallon GP, DeCrescenzo T. Transgender children and youth: a child welfare practice perspective. *Child Welfare.* 2006;85:215–241
16. Richardson J. Response: finding the disorder in gender identity disorder. *Harvard Rev Psychiatry.* 1999;7:43–50
17. Zucker KJ, Spitzer RL. Was the gender identity disorder of childhood diagnosis introduced into DSM-III as a backdoor maneuver to replace homosexuality? A historical note. *J Sex Marital Ther.* 2005;31:31–42

18. Zucker KJ. Gender identity development and issues. *Child Adolesc Psychiatr Clin North Am.* 2004;13:551–568
19. Pleak R. Ethical issues in diagnosing and treating gender-dysphoric children and adolescents. In: Rottnek M, ed. *Sissies and Tomboys: Gender Nonconformity and Homosexual Childhood.* New York, NY: New York University Press; 1999
20. American Psychiatric Association. *Diagnostic and Statistical Manual of Mental Disorders (DSM-IV).* 4th ed. Washington, DC: American Psychiatric Association; 2000
21. American Psychiatric Association. *Diagnostic and Statistical Manual of Mental Disorders.* 5th ed. Arlington, VA: American Psychiatric Publishing; 2013
22. Drescher J. Controversies in gender diagnoses. *LGBT Health.* 2013;1:1
23. Zucker KJ, Cohen-Kettenis PT, Drescher J, et al. Memo outlining evidence for change for gender identity disorder in the DSM-5. *Arch Sex Behav.* 2013;42:901–914
24. Vasey PL, Bartlett NH. What can the Samoan "fa`afine" teach us about the Western concept of gender identity disorder in children. *Perspect Bio Med.* 2007;50:481–490
25. Green R. *The "Sissy Boy Syndome" and the Development of Homosexuality.* New Haven, CT: Yale University Press; 1987
26. Drescher J, Byne W. Gender dysphoric/gender variant (GD/GV) children and adolescents: summarizing what we know and what we have yet to learn. *J Homosex.* 2012;59:501–510
27. Zucker KJ. Gender identity disorders. In: Lewis M, ed. *Child and Adolescent Psychiatry: A Comprehensive Textbook.* Philadelphia, PA: Lippincott Williams & Wilkins; 2002
28. Stein E. Commentary on the treatment of gender variant and gender dysphoric children and adolescents: common themes and ethical reflections. *J Homosex.* 2012;59:480–500
29. Menvielle EJ. Gender identity disorder. *J Am Acad Child Adolesc Psychiatry.* 1998;37:243–245
30. Gooren L. The biology of human psychosexual differentiation. *Horm Behav.* 2006;50:589–601
31. Hare L, Bernard P, Sánchez FJ, et al. Androgen receptor repeat length polymorphism associated with male-to-female transsexualism. *Biol Psychiatry.* 2009;65:93–96
32. Bentz EK, Hefler LA, Kaufmann U, et al. A polymorphism of the CYP17 gene related to sex steroid metabolism is associated with female-to-male but not male-to-female transsexualism. *Fertil Steril.* 2008;90:56–59
33. Coolidge FL, Thede LL, Young SE. The heritability of gender identity disorder in a child and adolescent twin sample. *Behav Genet.* 2002;32:251–257
34. Zhou J-N, Hofman MA, Gooren LJG, Swaab DF. A sex difference in the human brain and its relation to transsexuality. *Nature.* 1995;378:68–70
35. Kruijver FP, Zhou JN, Pool CW, et al. Male-to-female transsexuals have female neuron numbers in a limbic nucleus. *J Clin Endocrinol Metab.* 2000;85:2034–2041
36. Berglund H, Lindström P, Dhejne-Helmy C, Savic I. Male-to-female transsexuals show sex-atypical hypothalamus activation when smelling odorous steroids. *Cereb Cortex.* 2008;18:1900–1908
37. Adelson SL; American Academy of Child and Adolescent Psychiatry (AACAP) Committee on Quality Issues (CQI). Practice parameter on gay, lesbian, or bisexual sexual orientation, gender nonconformity, and gender discordance in children and adolescents. *J Am Acad Child Adolesc Psychiatry.* 2012;51: 957–974
38. Grossman AH, D'Augelli AR. Transgender youth and life-threatening behaviors. *Suicide Life Threat Behav.* 2007;37:527–537
39. Wilber S, Ryan C, Marksamer J. *CWLA Best Practices Guidelines for Serving LGBT Youth in Out-of-Home Care.* Washington, DC: CWLA Press; 2006
40. Ray N. *Lesbian, Gay, Bisexual, and Transgender Youth: An Epidemic of Homelessness.* New York, NY: National Gay and Lesbian Task Force Policy Institute and National Coalition for the Homeless; 2006. www.thetaskforce.org/static_html/downloads/HomelessYouth.pdf. Accessed January 30, 2015
41. Majd K, Marksamer J, Reyes C. *Hidden Injustice: Lesbian, Gay, Bisexual, and Transgender Youth in Juvenile Courts.* Washington, DC: Legal Services for Children, National Juvenile Defender Center, National Center for Lesbian Rights; 2009

42. Toomey RB, Ryan C, Diaz RM, et al. Gender-nonconforming lesbian, gay, bisexual, and transgender youth: school victimization and young adult psychosocial adjustment. *Developmental Psychology.* 2010;46(6):1580–1589
43. Ryan C, Rivers I. Lesbian, gay, bisexual and transgender youth: victimization and its correlates in the USA and UK. *Cult Health Sex.* 2003;5:103–119
44. Greytak EA, Kosciw JG, Diaz EM. *Harsh Realities: The Experience of Transgender Youth in Our Nation's Schools. Gay, Lesbian and Straight Education Network.* New York, NY: GLSEN; 2009. www.glsen.org/sites/default/files/Harsh%20Realities.pdf. Accessed January 30, 2015
45. Gay and Lesbian Medical Association. *Guidelines for the Care of Lesbian, Gay, Bisexual, and Transgender Patients.* 2006. glma.org/_data/n_0001/resources/live/GLMA%20guidelines%202006%20FINAL.pdf. Accessed January 30, 2015
46. Kaiser Permanente National Diversity Council, Kaiser Permanente National Diversity Department. *A Provider's Handbook on Culturally Competent Care: Lesbian, Gay, Bisexual, and Transgendered Population.* 2nd ed. Oakland, CA: Kaiser Permanente; 2004
47. Dean L, Meyer IH, Robinson K, et al. Lesbian, gay, bisexual, and transgender health: findings and concerns. *J Gay Lesbian Med Assoc.* 2000;4:101–151
48. Goldenring JM, Rosen DS. Getting into adolescents' heads: an essential update. *Contemp Pediatr.* 2004;21:64–90
49. Tom Waddell Health Center Protocols for Hormonal Reassignment of Gender. 2013. https://www.sfdph.org/dph/comupg/oservices/medSvs/hlthCtrs/TransGendprotocols122006.pdf. Accessed February 5, 2015
50. Center of Excellence for Transgender Health, University of California, San Francisco. Primary Care Protocol for Transgender Patient Care. transhealth.ucsf.edu/tcoe?page=protocol-00-00. Accessed December 19, 2014
51. Zucker KJ, Wood H, Singh D, Bradley SJ. A developmental, biopsychosocial model for the treatment of children with gender identity disorder. *J Homosex.* 2012;59:369–397
52. Menvielle E. A comprehensive program for children with gender variant behaviors and gender identity disorders. *J Homosex.* 2012;59:357–368
53. de Vries AL, Cohen-Kettenis PT. Clinical management of gender dysphoria in children and adolescents: the Dutch approach. *J Homosex.* 2012;59:301–320
54. Hsieh S, Leininger J. Resource list: clinical care programs for gender-nonconforming children and adolescents. *Pediatr Ann.* 2014;43:238–244
55. Gorin-Lazard A, Baumstarck K, Boyer L, et al. Hormonal therapy is associated with better self-esteem, mood, and quality of life in transsexuals. *J Nerv Ment Dis.* 2013;201:996–1000
56. Hembree WC, Cohen-Kettenis P, Delemarre-van de Waal HA, et al. Endocrine treatment of transsexual persons: an Endocrine Society clinical practice guideline. *J Clin Endocrinol Metab.* 2009;94:3132–3154
57. Spack NP, Edwards-Leeper L, Feldman HA, et al. Children and adolescents with gender identity disorder referred to a pediatric medical center. *Pediatrics.* 2012;129:418–425
58. de Vries AL, McGuire JK, Steensma TD, et al. Young adult psychological outcome after puberty suppression and gender reassignment. *Pediatrics.* 2014;134:696–704
59. Ehrensaft D. From gender identity disorder to gender identity creativity: true gender self child therapy. *J Homosex.* 2012;59:337–356
60. Edwards-Leeper L, Spack NP. Psychological evaluation and medical treatment of transgender youth in an interdisciplinary "Gender Management Service" (GeMS) in a major pediatric center. *J Homosex.* 2012;59:321–336
61. Ryan C, Huebner D, Diaz RM, Sanchez J. Family rejection as a predictor of negative health outcomes in white and Latino lesbian, gay, and bisexual young adults. *Pediatrics.* 2009;123:346–352
62. DeCrescenzo T, Mallon GP. *Serving Transgender Youth: The Role of Child Welfare Systems.* Arlington, VA: Child Welfare League of America; 2002
63. Woronoff R, Estrada R, Sommer S. *Out of the Margins: A Report on Regional Listening Forums Highlighting the Experience of Lesbian, Gay, Bisexual, Transgender, and Questioning Youth in Care.* Washington, DC: Child Welfare League of America Inc, and New York, NY: Lambda Legal Defense and Education Fund Inc; 2006

64. Advocates for Youth. *I Think I Might Be Transgender, Now What Do I Do?* Washington, DC: Advocates for Youth; 2004. www.advocatesforyouth.org. Accessed December 19, 2014
65. Olson J, Forbes C, Belzer M. Management of the transgender adolescent. *Arch Pediatr Adolesc Med.* 2011;165(2):171–176
66. van Kesteren PJM, Asscheman H, Megens JAJ, et al. Mortality and morbidity in transsexual subjects treated with cross-sex hormones. *Clin Endocrinol.* 1997;47:337–342

# Chapter 34

# Headache

*Jack Gladstein, MD*

For a pediatrician, a chief complaint of headache can be daunting. Although the outcome is most often benign, the worry of both the parent and the clinician centers on the fear of missing a tumor or other serious condition. Given the constraints of time in a busy office, an efficient but caring approach will allay the anxiety of both the family and the physician.

## ▶ CLINICAL APPROACH

### *Part 1: Establish the Right Pattern*

All headaches in the pediatric age group fall into 4 patterns as described by Rothner[1] (see Figure 34-1). The most common pattern is called *acute and recurrent*, characterized by periods of normalcy between attacks. Severe attacks accompanied by autonomic symptoms (nausea/vomiting, photophobia and/or phonophobia) ensure the diagnosis of migraine. Milder attacks are called *tension type* headaches. The migraine patient may also have milder tension type headaches, and because these headaches still respond to triptans the distinction in a migraine patient is basically irrelevant. Children who *never* get autonomic symptoms but have this pattern have pure tension type headache, and do not respond to triptan medications. In children, location of the headache is less important diagnostically than in adults. Ninety percent of migraine in the pediatric age group is bilateral. Pain can be under the eyes or even in the neck area. If the pattern is still acute and recurrent, and there are autonomic symptoms, the diagnosis is migraine. Most children and teens have migraine without aura. Children who have migraine with aura often describe wavy lines at the periphery of their vision.[2]

In the context of headache, a *simple acute headache* is less of a diagnostic dilemma. It can be caused by meningitis, encephalitis, systemic viral or bacterial infection. Subarachnoid hemorrhage features a severe headache that gets to full force instantly. Patients describe feelings of being shot or punched in the head. There can sometimes be accompanying fever or neck stiffness. The speed of headache onset is what is important here.

The pattern of *chronic progressive headache*, where symptoms get worse and worse over weeks, should alert the physician that a tumor or other serious pathology looms. Pain is often worse in the morning and gets a little better as the day goes on. Systemic or neurologic signs and symptoms further add to the worry. Posterior fossa tumors are often accompanied by wobbly gait. Frontal tumors may present with unilateral weakness. Tumors of the pituitary area manifest with changes in visual acuity or problems with growth; adolescent girls may have secondary amenorrhea.

*Chronic nonprogressive headache* either evolves from a previous headache pattern or presents without previous headache history. In *transformed* or *chronic migraine* there is a history

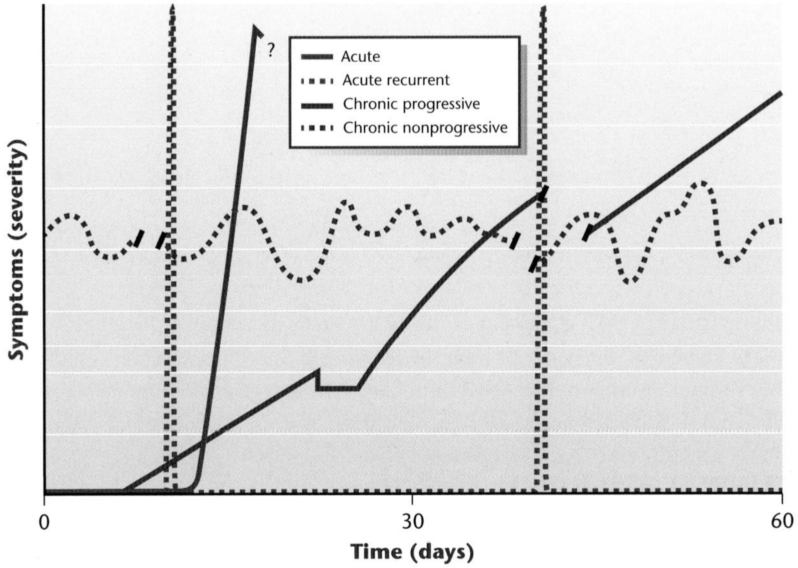


**Figure 34-1**
All headaches fit in this diagram. The severity of the headache is on the Y axis, and time measured in days is on the X axis. *(From Rothner AD. The evaluation of headaches in children and adolescents.* Semin Pediatr Neurol. *1995;2(2):109–119, with permission from Elsevier.)*

of prior acute intermittent headache accompanied by autonomic symptoms. Over time, the pain has become almost daily, with intermittent spikes in headache resembling bad migraine. In *chronic tension type headache* (CTTH), there is a history of episodic tension type headaches. With no history of migraine attacks, triptans have no role in this condition. In *new daily persistent headaches* (NDPH), the daily headache comes out of nowhere, often after a viral syndrome or mild head trauma. Whereas TM or CTTH responds well to a multidisciplinary approach, NDPH is more of a troublesome problem, often puzzling even the most experienced headache specialist. Patients with the chronic nonprogressive pattern of headache require imaging because there is no return to normalcy between attacks.

## Part 2: Establish Disability With 2 Questions

Since an acute headache is not, from the point of view of headache, a diagnostic dilemma, and chronic progressive headaches warrant timely evaluation for serious intracranial pathology, the issue most commonly facing the physician is how to proceed artfully and efficiently to manage most patients who come to attention with headaches. For both intermittent migraine and chronic daily headache the first priority is to assess how disabled the child is, using as meaures *absenteeism* and *presenteeism*. Absenteeism refers to the number of days missed from school, work or after-school activities. Presenteeism refers to days when, although present, the child cannot learn or fully participate because of headaches. Worsening of school grades can result either from the child being absent or, if present, having performance adversely affected by headache. The more disabled the child is, the heftier the required intervention.

Having properly categorized the headache from the initial history, decided whether or not serious underlying pathology is a consideration, and assessed how disabling the headaches are for the child's normal functioning, the physician can next fill in details, including family history of headache, medications tried, comorbidities, "stuff" going on at home, triggers, level of stress, and sleep and eating patterns. This information will set the table for the assessment to be shared with the family at the end of the visit, when it is important to reinforce healthy habits for headache prevention. At this point, if worry level has dropped, it is a good time to say something like, "nothing so far makes me worried about a brain tumor."

### *Part 3: Physical Examination*

With the physical examination, the physician should look particularly for arrest of growth, puberty, or menstruation. Examination of the skin should be thorough, looking for lesions suggestive of a neurocutaneous disorder such as neurofibromatosis. The neurologic examination should include looking for abnormalities of the optic discs, impaired extraocular movements, visual field defects, evidence of ataxia on gait and rapid nose-to-finger movement, and asymmetric reflexes. When the history has already established a pattern of headaches that does not raise concern about serious underlying illness, the physical examination offers the opportunity for the physician to reinforce how reassuring are the benign findings: "With something serious, like a brain tumor, we would expect this part of the examination to be abnormal." If all is normal, a summary statement is appropriate to reassure that nothing in the history or physical examination raises concern about a tumor or anything else serious.

### *Part 4: Imaging*

Children and adolescents with a history consistent with migraine, who have a normal neurologic examination, do not need magnetic resonance imaging (MRI). Patients with either systemic symptoms (arrested growth, puberty, or menstruation), abnormal neurologic features on history or physical examination, abrupt onset of severe headache, or a change in pattern to a more chronic headache, should have an MRI.

### *Part 5: Management*

The following sections will discuss the principles for treatment of migraine and chronic daily headache (see Figure 34-2).

## Migraine Principles

**PRINCIPLE 1: PATIENTS WITH MIGRAINE HAVE A MORE SENSITIVE BRAIN.** Children with migraine are more sensitive to internal and external triggers than children without headaches.[3] Therefore, migraine sufferers must not miss meals, must sleep at regular intervals, must exercise regularly, and must learn to manage their stress. When alerted, children are adept at figuring out what causes their headaches, often making it possible to modify or eliminate their identified triggers. Some strategies may include having a snack at school, cutting out some extracurricular activities, or assessing for an undiagnosed learning disability.[4]

**PRINCIPLE 2: TREAT ATTACKS AT FIRST TWINGE.** With bee sting allergy, one does not wait until anaphylaxis sets in before seeking treatment. Similarly with migraine, medications work best the earlier they are given. Once a migraine is full blown, medication that previously was effective often will not work.

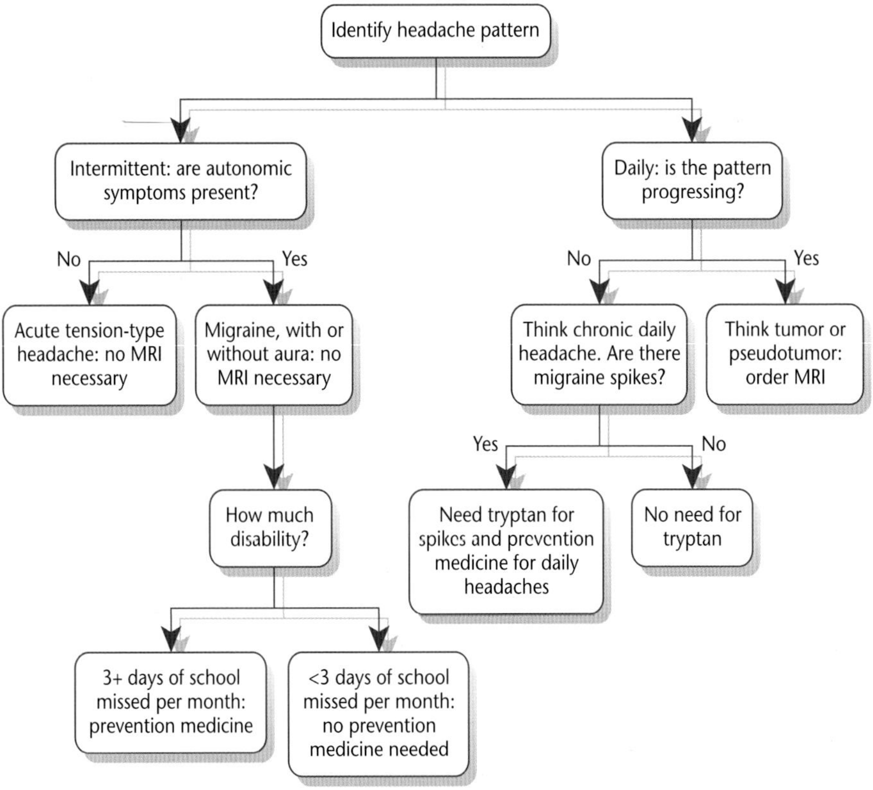


**Figure 34-2**
Algorithm for pediatric headache.

**PRINCIPLE 3: TREAT ATTACKS WITH HIGH DOSES OF ORAL MEDICATION.** A migraine starts a few hours before the patient notices. In particular, the stomach has delayed emptying. Therefore by the time headache is apparent, acute medication should be given in sufficient dose to ensure that a reasonable amount passes through the gastroparetic stomach.[5] For most patients attacks are episodic, so there is no harm if high doses of the medication are used to treat a migraine attack.

**PRINCIPLE 4: DON'T WAIT UNTIL YOU ARE SURE IT IS A MIGRAINE.** Children with migraines who have a tension type headache still respond to triptans; so treating at the first twinge, even if that results in a few headaches being overtreated, offers more benefit than risk. The alternative, waiting too long and compromising the effectiveness of treatment, is far worse.

**PRINCIPLE 5: INVOLVE TEACHER AND NURSE.** Children are in school for a large portion of their lives. If a migraine strikes during the school day, the "alarm bell" should go off for that child, and the teacher and nurse should know to respond with treatment immediately.

**PRINCIPLE 6: TRIPTANS ARE OK.** Once principles 1 to 5 have been addressed, the child with migraines should go home with a plan to include healthy lifestyle changes, urgings to treat early, an explanatory letter to the school with authorization to treat, and a prescription for medication. Only a few triptans (sumatriptan nasal spray and eletriptan tabs) have thus far received FDA approval for use in children. Although studies have demonstrated excellent efficacy, they have not been able to prove benefit over placebo (see Table 34-1 and Table 34-2). Triptans are safe, with no negative outcomes in any of the studies,[6] and are available in low doses for preschool and school-aged children, and for adolescents.

**PRINCIPLE 7: WHO NEEDS PROPHYLAXIS?** A follow-up visit should be scheduled within 2 to 6 weeks to evaluate whether or not progress has been made. At the follow up, if absenteeism and presenteeism have not diminished to an acceptable level despite the initial interventions described above, the child should receive either a nonpharmacologic or pharmacologic long-term treatment plan. Since they require substantial practice and a large time commitment, nonpharmacologic treatments work well only for patients invested in their recovery. Relaxation techniques, biofeedback, cognitive behavior therapy, and acupuncture can all be effective. The appropriate strategy is to try to treat comorbidities while avoiding medications that will make other conditions worse. Obese patients should use topiramate and avoid valproate, amitriptyline, and cyproheptadine. A patient with an eating disorder should avoid topiramate. A child with a sleep disorder may benefit from amitriptyline, while for patients with seizures either topiramate, gabapentin, or valproate may be appropriate. With hypertension, either propranolol or verpapmil might be effective. Propranolol should not be prescribed for a child with depression. Whichever medication is selected, begin slowly and gradually increase the dose until either therapeutic effect is reached or side effects ensue

**Table 34-1**
**Short-acting Triptans**

| TRIPTAN | TABLET (mg) | MELT (mg) | NASAL (mg) | SUBCUTANEOUS (mg) |
|---|---|---|---|---|
| Almotriptan | 6.25; 12.5 | — | — | — |
| Eletriptan | 20; 40 | — | — | — |
| Rizatriptan | 5; 10 | 5; 10 | — | — |
| Sumatriptan | 25; 50; 100 | — | 5; 20 | 4; 6 |
| Zolmitriptan | 2.5; 5 | 2.5; 5 | 5 | — |

**Table 34-2**
**Longer Acting and Combination Triptans**

| TRIPTAN | TABLET (mg) | MELT (mg) | NASAL (mg) | SUBCUTANEOUS (mg) |
|---|---|---|---|---|
| Frovatriptan | 2.5 | — | — | — |
| Naratriptan | 1; 2.5 | — | — | — |
| Sumatriptan/Naproxen | 85/500 | — | — | — |

Frovatriptan and naratriptan have longer half-lives than other triptans and may be used for menstrual migraine prophylaxis, or for migraine recurrence.

Box 34-1

## *Dose Ranges of Preventive Medications*

- Amitriptyline 10–75 mg qhs
- Cyproheptadine 2–18 mg qd
- Divalproex sodium 125–500 mg tid
- Gabapentin 300–1,200 mg tid
- Propranolol 40–120 mg tid
- Topiramate 25–200 mg bid
- Verapamil 80–240 mg tid

*bid,* twice daily; *qd,* every day; *qhs,* every night at bedtime; *tid,* 3 times per day.

(see Box 34-1). In the absence of side effects, the medication should be given time to become effective before deciding to change.

**PRINCIPLE 8: WHEN TO REFER.** A primary care physician should be able to prescribe medication, and recommend lifestyle changes and a prevention modality. If improvement is not reported, then referral to a headache specialist is indicated.

## Chronic Daily Headache Principles

**PRINCIPLE 1: RULE OUT INTRACRANIAL PATHOLOGY.** Unlike migraine, which does not require neuroimaging, chronic daily headache does. Because migraine is so common, with an estimated yearly prevalence of 10% to 25% (at least among adults),[7] many people diagnosed with brain tumors will have also had migraines. The change in the pattern of the headaches to daily chronic is what necessitates the MRI. Computed tomography scanning is not adequate because it does not delineate the posterior fossa well enough.

**PRINCIPLE 2: IDENTIFY PATTERN: TRANSFORMED MIGRAINE VS CHRONIC TENSION TYPE HEADACHE VS NEW DAILY PERSISTENT HEADACHE.** Transformed or chronic migraine will still have migraine spikes with autonomic symptoms, and these will respond to triptans. Sufferers of CTTH do not have migraine, and will not respond to triptans. Patients with NDPH may or may not have migraine spikes: if present, use triptans; if not, then no.

**PRINCIPLE 3: REMOVE ACUTE MEDICATIONS OVERUSED ON A DAILY BASIS.** Overuse of analgesics can itself lead to headaches. Stopping an overused medication can be done "cold turkey" or gradually over a month or so. If an analgesic is removed acutely, the physician should provide comfort measures, knowing that the headache will get worse for a few days. Such comfort measures might include intranasal dihydroergotamine, or a long-acting drug like frovatriptan or naratriptan. Families should be told to begin the transition over a weekend, preferably a long one, to avoid unnecessary absence from school. If the medication is tapered gently over a month, the patient and family must be warned there will be spikes in headache activity during the withdrawal.

**PRINCIPLE 4: START OR REINFORCE HEALTHY HEADACHE HABITS.**

**PRINCIPLE 5: STAY IN SCHOOL.** Try to avoid health related home schooling, which will only make it harder to reintegrate once the child is better. School attendance forces the child to get up early and have a daily routine. Sleep patterns are easier to regulate, and tendencies towards isolation and depression are lowered.

**PRINCIPLE 6: START A NONPHARMACOLOGIC AND/OR PHARMACOLOGIC INTERVENTION.** Someone with daily headache needs an intensive approach, as described in migraine Principle 7.

**PRINCIPLE 7: WATCH OUT FOR UNDETECTED DEPRESSION OR ANXIETY.** Consider referral for counseling as part of the comprehensive approach to the child with chronic headache.

**PRINCIPLE 8: WHEN TO REFER.** Ideally, all children and adolescents with chronic daily headache should be seen by a specialist. Many communities do not have an expert in pediatric headache, or even a pediatric neurologist with an interest in chronic headache. In such a setting, the principles listed above can guide the initiation of treatment, with a timely follow up in a month or so to confirm that progress has been made. If not, then referral is necessary. The primary care physician should also be familiar with local community mental health resources, as well as acupuncturists, physical therapists, and therapists with expertise in biofeedback and relaxation training.

## ▶ PROGNOSIS

Short-term studies show great improvement for both episodic and chronic headache with appropriate treatment. However there are no long-term studies tracking either childhood migraine or chronic daily headache cohorts over a long period of time. The goal of the pediatrician should be to prevent chronic headaches by treating migraine early and effectively.

## ▶ SUMMARY

This approach allows the physician to diagnose, assess, and treat headache effectively while addressing the concerns of the child and family. Identifying benign patterns of headache reassures the family and the physician, whereas identifying a worrisome pattern directs the child with a potentially serious condition to a diagnostic MRI. Promoting healthy headache activities, identifying comorbidities, and assessing the degree of disability will guide the prescription of acute or chronic medications and nonpharmacologic interventions. The pediatrician can properly manage most patients with headache, but referral to a specialist is indicated when improvement is not seen after these measures have been implemented.

### *TOOLS FOR PRACTICE*

#### Engaging Patient and Family

- *Headaches* (Web page), American Academy of Pediatrics (www.healthychildren.org/English/health-issues/conditions/head-neck-nervous-system/Pages/Headaches.aspx)

#### Medical Decision Support

- http://pediatrics.aappublications.org/content/132/5/e1173.abstract
- http://pediatrics.aappublications.org/content/132/1/e9.abstract
- http://pediatrics.aappublications.org/content/132/1/e1.abstract

### *ADDITIONAL RESOURCES*


1. *Pediatric headaches in Clinical Practice* Hershey AD, Powers SW, Winner P, Kabbouche MA. Eds. Wiley Blackwell, Hoboken NJ, 2009
2. *Headache in Children and Adolescent* Winner P, Rothner AD. Eds. BC Decker, Ontario, Canada, 2001

3. AmericanHeadacheSociety.org
4. ACHE.org
5. Gladstein J, Rothner AD. Pediatric headache: Introduction. *Semin Pediatr Neurol.* 2010;17(2):87
6. Gladstein J, Rothner AD. Chronic daily headache in children and adolescents. *Semin Pediatr Neurol.* 2010;17(2):88–92
7. Pakalnis A, Gladstein J. Headaches and hormones. *Semin Pediatr Neurol.* 2010;17(2):100–104

## REFERENCES


1. Rothner AD. The evaluation of headaches in children and adolescents. *Semin Pediatr Neurol.* 1995;2:109–118
2. Gladstein J, Holden EW, Peralta L, Raven M. Diagnoses and symptom patterns in children presenting to a pediatric headache clinic. *Headache.* 1993;33:497–500
3. Welch KM, D'Andrea G, Tepley N, Barkley G, Ramadan NM. The concept of migraine as a state of central neuronal hyperexcitability. *Neurol Clin.* 1990;8:817–828
4. Martin VT, Behbehani MM. Toward a rational understanding of migraine trigger factors. *Med Clin North Am.* 2001;85:911–941
5. Aurora SK, Kori SH, Barrodale P, McDonald SA, Haseley D. Gastric stasis in migraine: more than just a paroxysmal abnormality during a migraine attack. *Headache.* 2006;46:57–63
6. Lewis DW, Winner P, Wasiewski W. The placebo responder rate in children and adolescents. *Headache.* 2005;45:232–239
7. Stewart WF, Linet MS, Celentano DD, Van Natta M, Ziegler D. Age and sex-specific incidence rates of migraine with and without aura. *Am J Epidemiol.* 1991;134:1111–1120

# Chapter 35

# Hearing Loss

*Anne Marie Tharpe, PhD; Douglas P. Sladen, PhD; Ann Rothpletz, PhD*

Pediatricians are usually the first health care practitioners approached by parents when they have concerns about their child's hearing, and in the course of a typical practice a pediatrician will encounter approximately a dozen children with severe-to-profound hearing loss.[1] Although when the hearing loss is severe parents become concerned about their child's hearing rather early (at approximately 6 months of age), milder degrees of hearing loss typically do not generate concern until the child reaches school age. As such, it is imperative that pediatricians recognize the signs, symptoms, and risk factors for hearing loss in children and become aware of appropriate referral paths. It is also important to note that despite the widespread implementation of newborn hearing screening, such programs are designed to identify moderate and greater degrees of hearing loss, not mild degrees of loss. Therefore, even a child who passed a hearing screening in the newborn period might still have hearing loss that was missed by or acquired after the screening. This chapter addresses permanent hearing loss in children, not transient losses that often accompany otitis media.

## ▶ DEMOGRAPHICS

Rubella and meningitis were once leading causes of severe-to-profound hearing loss in children; but the advent of vaccines for these disorders has virtually eliminated hearing loss caused by congenital rubella and dramatically reduced hearing loss resulting from meningitis. Genetic mutations are now the most common cause of congenital hearing loss, accounting for 50% to 60% of all cases. Consequently, severe-to-profound hearing losses are not as common as they once were, and milder degrees of hearing loss are more prevalent.[2]

Although the prevalence of severe bilateral hearing loss in newborns is estimated to be 1 per 1,000, estimates for mild or minimal losses approach 1 per 20 in school-aged children.[2] In the neonatal intensive care unit (NICU), estimates of hearing loss range from 20 to 40 per 1,000.[1] Minimal hearing loss is defined as thresholds greater than 25 dB HL at 2 or more frequencies above 2,000 Hz, pure tone average between 15 and 25 dB HL bilaterally, or unilateral hearing loss of any degree.[2] This increase in reported prevalence from the newborn period to school age is the result, in part, of not including minimal and mild losses as targets of newborn hearing screening, as well as the addition of losses that progress or are acquired later in childhood (eg, meningitis).

Figure 35-1 is the audiogram of a child with normal hearing sensitivity in both ears such that all the speech sounds fall within the range of audibility. Two of the more typical patterns of minimal-to-mild hearing loss are demonstrated in Figure 35-2 and Figure 35-3.

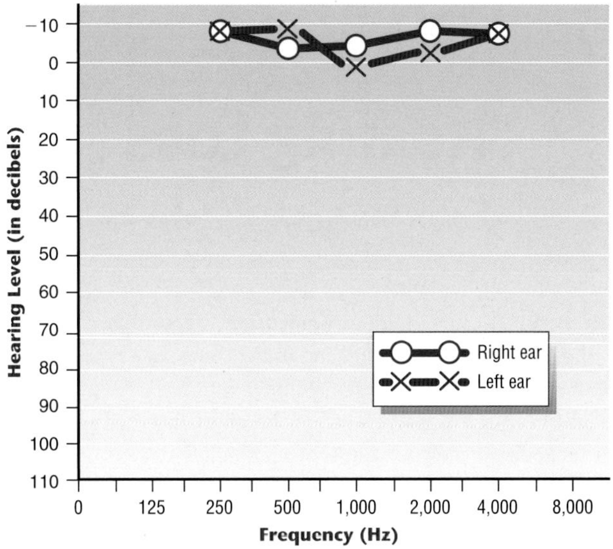


**Figure 35-1**
An audiogram reflecting normal hearing sensitivity in both ears.

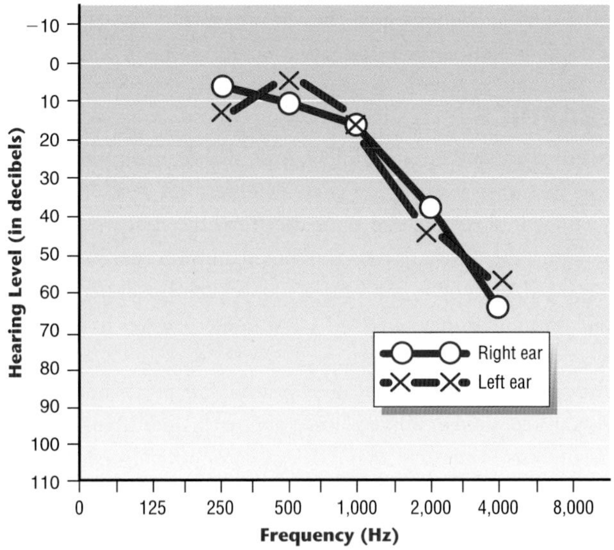


**Figure 35-2**
An audiogram reflecting a high-frequency hearing loss bilaterally.

Figure 35-2 is the audiogram of a child with normal hearing sensitivity for all frequencies through 1,000 Hz but a high-frequency hearing loss, a pattern typical with ototoxic drug use or perinatal anoxia. Although this child would be expected to develop speech and language in a timely manner, distortions or omissions of the high-frequency consonant sounds of speech are expected. Parents may report that the child has difficulty hearing in the presence

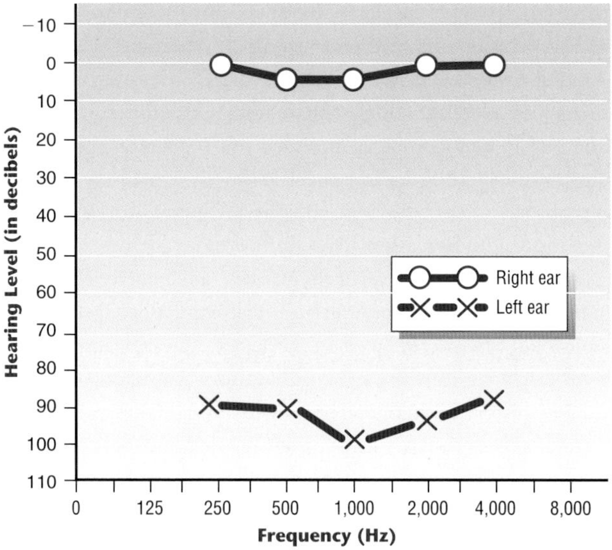


**Figure 35-3**
An audiogram reflecting a profound hearing loss of the left ear.

of background noise but seems to have little difficulty in quiet settings. The hearing loss depicted in Figure 35-3 is a profound unilateral loss of the left ear that is not typically identified until a child enters school unless the child receives a hearing screening in the newborn period. A child with unilateral hearing loss may reach age-appropriate speech and language milestones but experience difficulty hearing in the presence of background noise. In addition, children with unilateral hearing loss typically demonstrate difficulty localizing sound sources.

Although these patterns of hearing loss are termed *mild* or *minimal,* building evidence suggests that their effect is far from benign. School-aged children who have minimal and mild losses have been found to experience greater academic, communicative, social, and emotional difficulty than normally hearing children. In fact, approximately 35% of children with minimal hearing losses fail at least 1 grade in school compared to an overall failure rate of approximately 3%.[2,3]

## ▶ ASSOCIATED SIGNS AND SYMPTOMS

The Joint Committee on Infant Hearing (JCIH) has published a list of risk factors that provides an excellent starting place when attempting to identify hearing loss in children.[4] However, approximately 35% to 50% of children with hearing loss will not have any known risk factors,[5,6] making a complete history and keen observation accompanied by hearing screening essential if hearing loss is to be identified early. Although most congenital hearing loss is hereditary, a negative family history is common: 80% of inherited hearing loss results from autosomal-recessive transmission, 18% from autosomal-dominant transmission, and approximately 2% from X-linked recessive transmission. Furthermore, even children with dominantly inherited hearing loss may have families who demonstrate incomplete penetrance. Evidence of the gene expression can be highly variable. In addition, most children with inherited hearing loss are nonsyndromic, providing no additional clues and potentially limiting the pediatrician's level of suspicion. However, 20% of children with congenital sensory hearing loss have an associated syndrome (eg, Alport syndrome, Waardenburg syndrome) or progressive loss (eg, Usher syndrome). Children with Down syndrome are at high risk for conductive hearing loss, as well as a higher-than-average risk for sensory loss.

Infants in the NICU may also be at increased risk for neural conduction or auditory brainstem dysfunction, including auditory neuropathy/dyssynchrony, a disorder characterized by a unique constellation of behavioral and physiologic auditory test results.[7,8] Children with auditory neuropathy/dyssynchrony have normal outer cochlear hair cell function, but dyssynchronous signal firing at the level of the VIIIth cranial nerve. They exhibit a range of sensitivity from normal hearing to profound hearing loss and poor speech perception ability (often worse than would be expected based on the degree of hearing loss). Infants who receive intensive neonatal care are at increased risk for auditory neuropathy/dyssynchrony, as are children with a family history of childhood hearing loss and infants with hyperbilirubinemia. However, some children with auditory neuropathy/dyssynchrony have no history of these risk factors. Currently, neither the prevalence of auditory neuropathy/dyssynchrony in newborns nor the natural history of the disorder is clearly understood, and treatment options are not well defined. Many children with auditory neuropathy/dyssynchrony do not benefit from the use of hearing aids but do benefit from cochlear implantation. Audiologic and medical monitoring of infants at risk for auditory neuropathy/dyssynchrony is recommended.

The significant speech and language delays associated with severe to profound childhood hearing loss are typically obvious to parents and physicians; but because identification of milder degrees of hearing loss may prove more elusive, children who exhibit behavioral, social, or academic difficulties should be screened for hearing loss in addition to those with speech and language delays or disorders. Some of the concerns expressed commonly by parents of children with milder forms of hearing loss are included in Table 35-1.

## ▶ IDENTIFICATION APPROACHES

The 2007 position statement of the JCIH recommended that identification of and intervention for congenital hearing loss in children should follow a 1-3-6 rule. That is, all infants should have access to hearing screening no later than 1 month of age, confirmation of hearing loss by 3 months of age, and early intervention services no later than 6 months of age.[4] The recommendations of the JCIH are widely accepted, although significant concerns remain with follow-up. A significant percentage of infants who fail the screening do not return for follow-up testing. According to the Centers for Disease Control and Prevention, only 70% of infants with hearing loss receive appropriate diagnostic testing by 3 months of age and only 56% receive intervention prior to 6 months of age.[9] The pediatrician plays an important role in the identification of childhood hearing loss for several reasons. First, many infants lost to follow up can be recaptured when they are seen in pediatricians' offices for well- or sick-baby visits. Second, even if infants have passed a hearing screening at birth, many children with hearing loss acquire their deficits after the newborn period. Finally, the JCIH recommends that universal newborn hearing screening programs target permanent, bilateral, or unilateral hearing loss averaging 40 dB or greater, a target level that will necessarily miss some minimal and mild hearing loss. The obvious implication is that, even for children who have passed their newborn hearing screenings, pediatricians should be vigilant in monitoring hearing status and, with any suspicion of

**Table 35-1**
**Explanations for Parental Concerns Regarding Their Child's Hearing Acuity**

| PARENTAL COMMENTS | EXPLANATIONS |
|---|---|
| "He can hear me when he wants to hear me. Sometimes he just ignores me." | Children who have mild hearing losses may have little or no difficulty listening in quiet settings. However, if background noise is present they may have more difficulty. |
| "When I call her, she has to look around for me. She never seems to know where I am in the house." | Children who have unilateral hearing loss often have difficulty localizing a sound source. |
| "When we are in crowds, I have to call his name several times before he responds." | Children who have high-frequency or other mild hearing losses often have difficulty hearing in the presence of background noise. |
| "My child is exhausted when she comes home from school." | Children who have minimal or mild hearing loss may be fatigued by the effort exerted to listen throughout the day. |
| "His speech is very difficult to understand. I don't think it's his hearing, because he always responds when I call him." | Children who have high-frequency hearing loss may have poor speech production because they are unable to hear high-frequency speech sounds (consonants) even though they can hear low- and mid-frequency sounds clearly. |
| "My child is doing poorly in school, but I know she understands the material because we go over her homework at night." | Children who have minimal hearing loss may have difficulty hearing in school settings because of the background noise. When working at home in a 1-on-1 situation, they may demonstrate no hearing difficulties because the acoustic conditions are good. |

hearing loss by parents or others, should arrange for hearing assessments by audiologists experienced in working with children.

When an infant or child fails a hearing, speech, or language screening measure in the pediatrician's office, referral for a full audiologic evaluation is recommended. Unfortunately, at least 1 study suggested that more than half of children who failed hearing screenings in primary care practices did not receive rescreenings or referrals for further testing.[10] Audiologists with pediatric experience can define the degree of hearing loss and distinguish among conductive, sensory, and neural types of loss in children of all chronologic ages and developmental levels. Evaluation of hearing in infants and young children consists of a combination of physiologic and behavioral measures. For infants younger than approximately 6 months, testing is typically limited to physiologic measures because their behavioral responses are not yet reliable enough for defining the extent of hearing loss.

## ▶ MANAGEMENT

The early identification of hearing loss in children is of little value if timely intervention does not follow. Many children have conductive and sensorineural hearing losses that are not amenable to medical treatment. For these children, several options remain, the most familiar being traditional hearing aids, which are devices designed to pick up sounds in the child's environment and convert them to electrical signals that are amplified, filtered, and converted back to acoustic signals by a receiver. For children in noisy settings (eg, child care centers, classrooms), frequency-modulated (FM) systems can be used alone or in combination with hearing aids. These systems use a microphone worn by the teacher to amplify only the teacher's voice while minimizing the interfering background noise. The signal is transmitted to the child via an FM signal, which is received by a hearing aid or loudspeaker.

Most children who have hearing loss benefit from some form of amplification. However, in cases of severe-to-profound hearing loss, conventional amplification might not be enough. An alternative to traditional hearing aids for these children is the cochlear implant, a surgically implanted device with electrodes that are coiled into the cochlea to stimulate the auditory nerve with electrical current. Although cochlear implants do not restore normal hearing and children vary markedly in the benefits they derive from the implant, most experience at least an awareness of sound, and some reach a high level of speech recognition, enabling the development of normal speech and language skills.[11] Children are eligible for cochlear implants at age 1 year, although some exceptions for earlier implantation can be made. Children who receive their cochlear implants at an early age (ie, prior to 3 years of age) tend to benefit more from the implant than children who receive their implants at older ages. All children who have cochlear implants are considered at risk for pneumococcal meningitis. Pediatricians should ensure these children are up to date on the pneumococcal vaccine recommendations. All vaccines should be administered at least 2 weeks or more prior to cochlear implant surgery.[9]

As the gatekeepers for children's health care, pediatricians are responsible for recognizing the signs and symptoms of hearing loss in their young patients. Only through the vigilance of pediatricians and other health care practitioners will the age of identification of hearing loss in children be lowered, thus avoiding delays in intervention.

For infants with permanent hearing loss, communication with the state's coordinator for early hearing detection and intervention should ensure that the child and family are enrolled in appropriate early intervention services as soon as possible following identification of hearing loss. Such services can include speech-language and communication intervention, behavioral therapy, and family counseling or support. The pediatrician should also ensure that the child has received a thorough medical evaluation to determine the cause of the hearing loss, including a genetics consultation. Furthermore, because of the high incidence of vision problems in children with hearing loss, a referral for ophthalmologic evaluation may be warranted. Children with permanent hearing loss are especially vulnerable to the effects of otitis media with effusion because additional hearing loss secondary to the effusion can negatively affect the audibility of speech through hearing aids. Accordingly, pediatricians must closely monitor and manage children who have persistent otitis media with effusion. Finally, approximately 30% to 40% of children with hearing loss have additional disabilities. Therefore periodic developmental screening and surveillance, as recommended by the JCIH,[4] is an integral part of the management of these children.

## When to Refer

The 2007 position statement of the JCIH lists risk indicators for delayed-onset hearing loss. In addition to any babies who do not pass their newborn hearing screenings, children whose medical history includes 1 or more of the following indicators should be referred for audiologic testing:

- Caregiver concerns regarding hearing, speech, language, or developmental delay
- Family history of permanent childhood hearing loss

- Neonatal intensive care of more than 5 days or any of the following regardless of length of stay: ECMO, assisted ventilation, exposure to ototoxic medications (gentimycin and tobramycin) or loop diuretics (furosemide), hyperbilirubinemia that requires exchange transfusion
- In utero infections, such as CMV, herpes, rubella, syphilis, and toxoplasmosis
- Craniofacial anomalies, including those that involve the pinna, ear canal, ear tags, ear pits, and temporal bone anomalies
- Physical findings such as white forelock that are associated with a syndrome known to include a sensorineural or permanent conductive hearing loss
- Syndromes associated with hearing loss or progressive or late-onset hearing loss such as neurofibromatosis, osteopetrosis, and Usher syndrome; other frequently identified syndromes include Waardenburg, Alport, Pendred, and Jervell and Lange-Nielson
- Neurodegenerative disorders such as Hunter syndrome, or sensory motor neuropathies such as Friedreich ataxia and Charcot-Marie-Tooth syndrome
- Culture-positive postnatal infections associated with sensorineural hearing loss, including confirmed bacterial and viral meningitis
- Head trauma, especially basal skull/temporal bone fractures that require hospitalization
- Chemotherapy

## *TOOLS FOR PRACTICE*

### Engaging Patient and Family

- *Your Baby Needs Another Hearing Test* (handout), Maternal Child Health Bureau, Health Resources and Services Administration and American Academy of Pediatrics (www.medicalhomeinfo.org/downloads/pdfs/Anotherhearingtest.pdf)

### Medical Decision Support

- *Hearing Loss in Children* (Web page), Centers for Disease Control and Prevention (www.cdc.gov/ncbddd/hearingloss/index.html)
- *Hearing Loss in Children: Information About Early Hearing Detection and Intervention (EHDI) State Programs* (Web page), Centers for Disease Control and Prevention (www.cdc.gov/ncbddd/hearingloss/ehdi-programs.html)
- *NIDCD Fact Sheet: When a Newborn Doesn't Pass the Hearing Screening* (fact sheet), National Institute on Deafness and Other Communication Disorders (www.medicalhomeinfo.org/downloads/pdfs/NIDCDFactSheetHowMedicalandOtherProfessionals.pdf)

## *AAP POLICY STATEMENT*

American Academy of Pediatrics Joint Committee on Infant Hearing. Year 2007 position statement: principles and guidelines for early hearing detection and intervention programs. *Pediatrics.* 2007;120(4):898–921 (pediatrics.aappublications.org/content/120/4/898.full)

## *REFERENCES*

1. US Department of Health and Human Services, Public Health Service. *Healthy People 2000, National Health Promotion and Disease Prevention Objectives for the Nation.* (DHHS [PHS] Publication No. 91-50212). Washington, DC: US Government Printing Office; 1990
2. Bess FH, Dodd-Murphy J, Parker RA. Children with minimal sensorineural hearing loss: prevalence, educational performance, and functional status. *Ear Hear.* 1998;19:339–354
3. Bess FH, Tharpe AM. Unilateral hearing impairment in children. *Pediatrics.* 1984;74:206–216

4. American Academy of Pediatrics Joint Committee on Infant Hearing. Year 2007 position statement: principles and guidelines for early hearing detection and intervention programs. *Pediatrics*. 2007;120:898–921
5. Davis A, Wood S, Healy R, Webb H, Rowe S. Risk factors for hearing disorders: epidemiologic evidence of change over time in the UK. *J Am Acad Audiol*. 1995;6:365–370
6. Stein LK. Factors influencing the efficacy of universal newborn hearing screening. *Pediatr Clin North Am*. 1999;46:95–105
7. Sininger YS, Hood LJ, Starr A, et al. Hearing loss due to auditory neuropathy. *Audiology Today*. 1995;7:10–13
8. Starr A, Picton TW, Sininger Y, Hood LJ, Berlin CI. Auditory neuropathy. *Brain*. 1996;119(Pt 3): 741–753
9. Centers for Disease Control and Prevention. Vaccines and immunizations. Cochlear implants and meningitis vaccination. Q&A for healthcare professionals. www.cdc.gov/vaccines/vpd-vac/mening/cochlear/dis-cochlear-faq-hcp.htm. Updated April 8, 2014. Accessed December 11, 2014
10. Holloran DR, Wall TC, Evans HH, et al. Hearing screening at well-child visits. *Arch Pediatr Adolesc Med*. 2005;159:949–955
11. Geers AE, Nicholas JG. Enduring advantages of early cochlear implantation for spoken language development. *J Speech Lang Hear Res*. 2013;56:643–655

# Chapter 36

# Heart Murmurs

*Christine Tracy, MD; Christine A. Walsh, MD*

A heart murmur is a common finding during the physical examination of children. However, few children with heart murmurs have structural cardiac disease. The challenge for the pediatrician lies in distinguishing innocent murmurs from those that indicate a cardiac abnormality.

## ▶ CARDIAC CYCLE AND ASSOCIATED HEART SOUNDS

The pediatrician needs to understand the events of the cardiac cycle and its associated heart sounds when determining the significance of a heart murmur. Heart sounds are directly related to the hemodynamic events of systole and diastole (Figure 36-1).

The first heart sound ($S_1$) is related to the closure of the mitral and tricuspid valves at the end of diastole, when the ventricles are completely filled. The ventricles then undergo a period of isovolumic contraction, followed by opening of the aortic and pulmonary valves. Rapid systolic ejection ensues, followed by a phase of reduced ejection later in systole.

The second heart sound ($S_2$) is created by the closure of the aortic and pulmonary valves at the end of systole. The first component of $S_2$ is created by the closure of the aortic valve ($A_2$), and the second component of $S_2$ is created by the closure of the pulmonary valve ($P_2$). During inspiration, $P_2$ occurs after $A_2$, generating an audibly split $S_2$ ($A_2$-$P_2$). During exhalation, the closures of the aortic and pulmonary valves are nearly coincident, creating a single $S_2$. Abnormal splitting of $S_2$ can be a clue to structural heart disease, but splitting of $S_2$ can be difficult to appreciate in infants or children with accelerated heart rates.

Wide splitting of $S_2$ is associated with prolonged ejection from the right ventricle, as occurs with conditions such as an atrial septal defect (ASD), in which $S_2$ is widely split and fixed. A narrowly split $S_2$ is associated with pulmonary hypertension, in which closure of the pulmonary valve is early, or aortic stenosis, when closure of the aortic valve is delayed. Failure of $S_2$ to split at all can be the result of simultaneous closure of the aortic and pulmonary valves during all phases of the respiratory cycle, found with conditions that result in high pulmonary artery pressure. A single $S_2$ can also be associated with certain congenital cardiac anomalies, such as truncus arteriosus and tetralogy of Fallot, or with a single ventricle after the bidirectional Glenn shunt or the Fontan operation.

Third and fourth heart sounds may also be appreciated during physical examination. The third heart sound ($S_3$) is heard early in diastole, during the initial phase of passive rapid ventricular filling. It is a low-frequency sound that can be best heard at the left lower sternal border or at the apex. An apical $S_3$ can frequently be heard in healthy children, particularly in competitive athletes. Usually pathologic, the fourth heart sound ($S_4$) is also a low-frequency sound but is heard late in diastole, just before $S_1$. It results from rapid filling of the ventricle caused by atrial contraction. An $S_4$ gallop is associated with decreased ventricular compliance (as is seen in cardiomyopathy) and congestive heart failure. Auscultation of an $S_4$ gallop warrants an evaluation by a pediatric cardiologist.

Clicks may also be audible during the cardiac cycle. Ejection clicks are heard in systole; the timing of the click in the cardiac cycle helps elucidate the cause. An early systolic click, heard just after $S_1$, is associated with semilunar valve stenosis (aortic stenosis or pulmonary stenosis) or dilation of the great arteries (the aorta or pulmonary artery). Aortic valve clicks, best heard at the apex or right upper sternal border, do not vary in intensity with respiration. Pulmomary valve clicks increase in intensity with exhalation, and they are best heard along the left sternal border. A midsystolic apical click is heard with mitral valve prolapse and may be accompanied by a late systolic murmur.

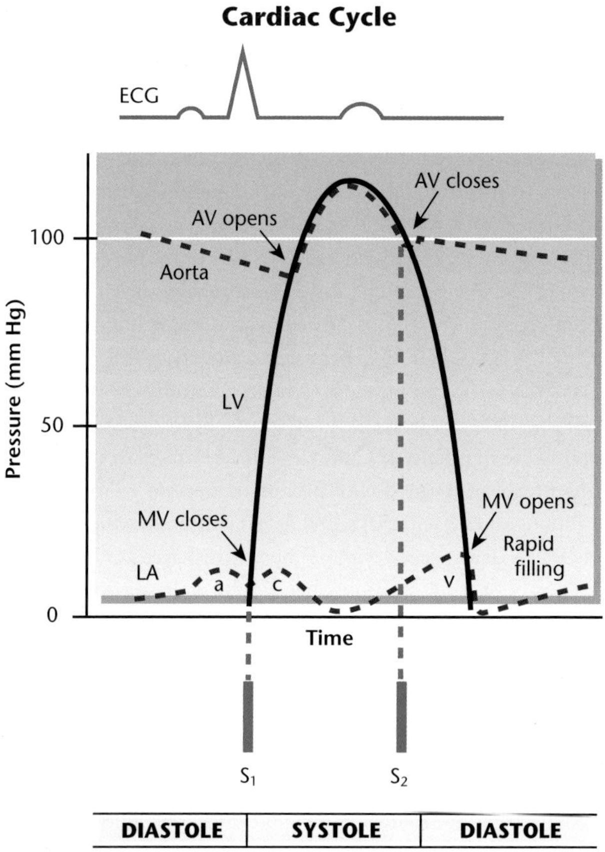


**Figure 36-1**
Pressure time relationships of the left-sided heart chambers are illustrated during the normal cardiac cycle. *AV,* aortic valve; *ECG,* electrocardiogram; *LA,* left atrium; *LV,* left ventricle; mm *Hg,* millimeters of mercury; *MV,* mitral valve; $S_1$, first heart sound; $S_2$, second heart sound. (*From Lilly LS.* Pathophysiology of Heart Disease. *3rd ed. Philadelphia, PA: Lippincott Williams & Wilkins; 2003. Used by permission.*)

## ▶ CARDIAC ANATOMY

In evaluating a child with a heart murmur, the physician must understand the anatomy of the heart and its position in the chest. The location of the heart murmur on the chest wall can serve as an important tool in deciding whether the murmur is innocent or pathologic. Figure 36-2 demonstrates the location of the valves of the heart in relation to their position on the chest wall.

## ▶ PATIENT EVALUATION

### *History*

A complete and accurate history is one of the most important aspects of evaluating a cardiac murmur in children because the clinical context in which the murmur occurs provides clues to the cause of a heart murmur. The history should include the patient's chief complaints and medical history, including the birth history and family history (Box 36-1).

### *Physical Examination*

Evaluation of a cardiac murmur involves much more than auscultation of the heart. A complete physical examination in the child or adolescent with a heart murmur is needed to put the murmur in perspective. Pertinent aspects of the physical examination in a patient with a heart murmur are outlined in Table 36-1.

## ▶ CARDIAC EVALUATION

A detailed cardiac examination includes thorough inspection, palpation, and auscultation.

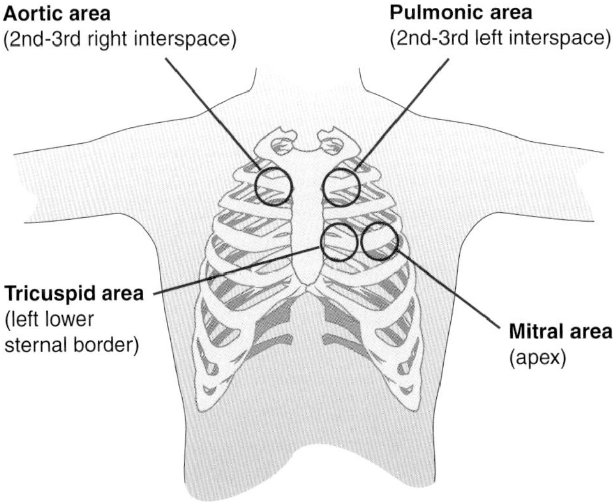


**Figure 36-2**
Areas of cardiac auscultation are governed by the location of the heart valves in relation to their position on the chest wall. (*From Lilly LS.* Pathophysiology of Heart Disease. *3rd ed. Philadelphia, PA: Lippincott Williams & Wilkins; 2003. Used by permission.*)

BOX 36-1

## *Raised Index of Suspicion for Cardiac Disease*

**PATIENT HISTORY**

- Poor weight gain or difficulty feeding
- Frequent respiratory difficulties or respiratory distress
- Cyanosis
- Exercise intolerance
- Chest pain with exercise
- Unexplained syncope (especially syncope resulting in injury)
- Concurrent syndromic disorder or genetic disease
- Concurrent metabolic disorder or storage disease
- Sickle cell anemia or blood dyscrasias resulting in anemia
- History of cardiotoxic chemotherapy
- Concurrent human immunodeficiency virus disease
- Hypertension

**BIRTH HISTORY**

- Maternal diabetes
- Maternal TORCH (*t*oxoplasmosis, *o*ther agents, *r*ubella, *c*ytomegalovirus, *h*erpes simplex) infections during pregnancy
- Multiple gestation pregnancy
- In vitro fertilization pregnancy
- Maternal drug use (either legal or illicit), known teratogens
- Abnormal amniocentesis
- Abnormal fetal ultrasound
- Maternal history of congenital heart disease

**FAMILY HISTORY**

- Congenital heart disease
- Sudden cardiac death or unexplained death in young people
- Hypertrophic cardiomyopathy
- Infantile Marfan syndrome

### *Inspection*

Inspection begins with a general assessment of appearance, nutritional status, genetic abnormalities, color, and comfort. The chest wall should then be inspected for abnormalities, including deformities such as a pectus excavatum, asymmetry, and surgical scars.

### *Palpation*

Palpation should include more than the chest, beginning with the extremities to assess perfusion, pulses, capillary refill, and temperature. The precordium is then palpated to identify the point of maximal impulse (PMI) and to detect thrills. Under normal conditions, the PMI represents the activity of the left ventricle and is palpated in the left fourth or fifth intercostal space in the midclavicular line. Activity of the right ventricle is appreciated in the fourth to fifth intercostal space along the left lower sternal border. Abnormal intensity or location of the PMI or of the right ventricle's activity is suggestive of a cardiac anomaly. Thrills can be palpated in the suprasternal notch (suggesting aortic valve disease or coarctation of the aorta), along the left upper sternal border (suggesting pulmonary valve disease), along the right upper sternal border (suggesting aortic valve disease), or along the left lower sternal border (in association with ventricular septal defects [VSDs]). A thrill is an abnormal finding and warrants referral to a pediatric cardiologist.

### *Auscultation*

A systematic approach to auscultation of the heart ensures that each major anatomic area of the heart is heard in systole and diastole. The major areas of auscultation on the precordium

**Table 36-1**
**Physical Examination to Evaluate a Heart Murmur**

| SITE | FINDING |
|---|---|
| Vital signs | Temperature, heart rate, respiratory rate, height, weight<br>Blood pressures in the right arm, left arm, leg<br>Pulse oximetry on room air (right hand and either foot if infant) |
| General | Cyanosis, pallor, dysmorphic features, overall distress<br>Breathing pattern: retractions, grunting, nasal flaring |
| Head and neck | Jugular venous distention<br>Thyromegaly, thyroid nodules |
| Chest | Chest wall deformity, asymmetry, surgical scars<br>Lung aeration<br>Rales, rhonchi, wheezes, stridor |
| Cardiac | Inspection<br>Palpation<br>Auscultation |
| Abdominal | Liver span<br>Tenderness<br>Distention, ascites |
| Extremities | Perfusion: capillary refill, temperature, quality of pulses<br>Clubbing, cyanosis, edema<br>Arachnodactyly, joint laxity (Marfan syndrome)<br>Increased arm span, upper-to-lower body ratio (Marfan syndrome) |

are the apex, the left lower sternal border, the left mid or upper sternal border, and the right upper sternal border. These areas correspond to each atrioventricular and semilunar valve, as well as the outflow tracts of the right and left ventricles (see Figure 36-2). The physician should also auscultate the left and right infraclavicular areas, the axillae, and the back. Auscultation for systolic or continuous blood flow noises (bruits) should be performed over the liver and fontanelle. A bruit suggests an arteriovenous malformation. The patient should be examined in the supine, sitting, and left lateral decubitus positions. Other postural maneuvers, such as squatting or standing, or performing a Valsalva maneuver, may be useful during auscultation. Auscultation includes an assessment of $S_1$ and $S_2$, including the nature of the splitting of $S_2$. Noting any $S_3$ and $S_4$, murmurs, clicks, and rubs completes the auscultation.

## ▶ EVALUATION OF HEART MURMUR

A heart murmur is usually the result of turbulent blood flow. Random fluctuations in velocity and pressure during blood flow result in vibration of the surrounding tissue, which is auscultated as a murmur. A complete description of a heart murmur includes its intensity, timing, location, radiation, and quality.

### *Intensity*

Murmur intensity is graded on a scale of I to VI for murmurs in systole (Table 36-2). Some cardiologists use a scale of I to IV for murmurs in diastole (Table 36-3). The intensity of a

**Table 36-2**
**Intensity of Systolic Murmurs**

| GRADE | DESCRIPTION |
|---|---|
| I | Barely audible |
| II | Soft, but easily audible |
| III | Moderately loud without a thrill |
| IV | Moderately loud with a thrill |
| V | Loud with a thrill, heard with stethoscope partly on the chest |
| VI | Loud with a thrill, heard with stethoscope off the chest |

**Table 36-3**
**Intensity of Diastolic Murmurs**

| GRADE | DESCRIPTION |
|---|---|
| I | Barely audible |
| II | Soft, but immediately heard |
| III | Easily heard |
| IV | Very loud |

murmur does not necessarily reflect the severity of the abnormality. For example, a small VSD may have a very loud murmur, but critical aortic stenosis may have a very soft murmur if cardiac output is low.

### *Timing*

Timing refers to the point in the cardiac cycle at which the murmur is heard. Murmurs are described as being systolic, diastolic, or continuous.

Systolic murmurs occur between atrioventricular valve closure ($S_1$) and semilunar valve closure ($S_2$). Systolic murmurs are further divided into ejection (crescendo–decrescendo) murmurs, holosystolic (pansystolic) murmurs, and late systolic murmurs (Figure 36-3).

Ejection murmurs, which may be innocent or pathologic, begin shortly after $S_1$, peak in intensity, and then end at or before $S_2$. All innocent systolic ejection murmurs are grade I to III. Pathologic ejection murmurs can be of any intensity. They may result from obstructed blood flow across a semilunar valve (aortic or pulmonary stenosis), in which case an ejection click may usher in the murmur. Other pathologic ejection murmurs without associated clicks arise from excessive volume crossing a normal semilunar valve (ASD). Holosystolic murmurs start with $S_1$ and continue to $S_2$ at the same level of intensity, sometimes obscuring $S_2$. These murmurs result from movement of blood from a higher-pressure chamber to a lower-pressure chamber, such as with a VSD or mitral regurgitation. Late systolic murmurs are associated with mitral valve prolapse and resultant mitral regurgitation; they are classically preceded by a mid- or late-systolic click.

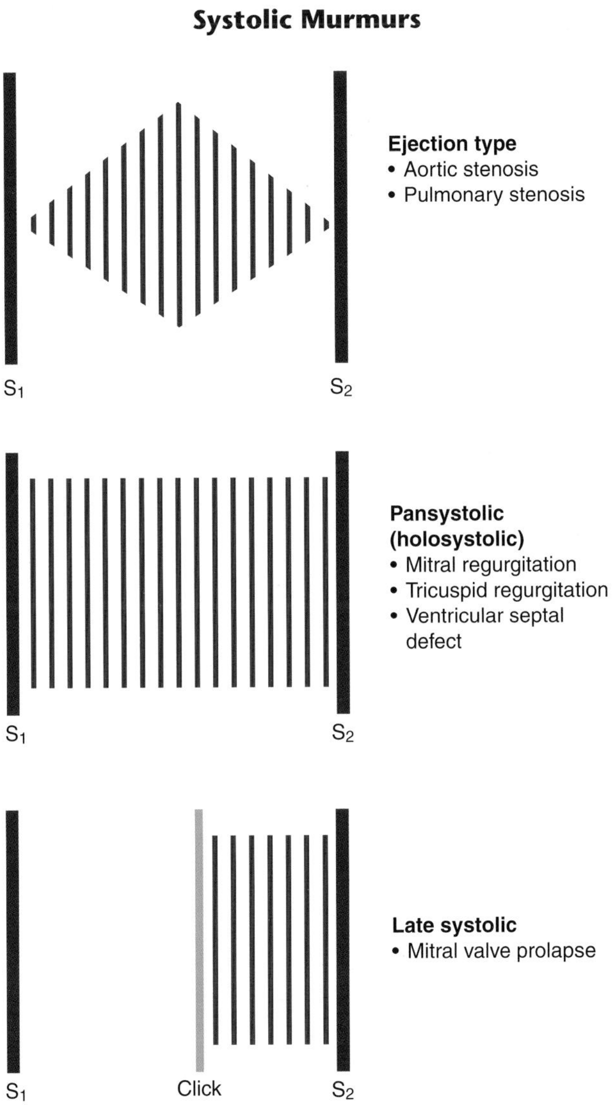


**Figure 36-3**
Classification of systolic murmurs. $S_1$, first heart sound; $S_2$, second heart sound. (*From Lilly LS.* Pathophysiology of Heart Disease. *3rd ed. Philadelphia, PA: Lippincott Williams & Wilkins; 2003. Used by permission.*)

Diastolic murmurs occur between semilunar valve closure ($S_2$) and atrioventricular valve closure ($S_1$); they are further divided into early-, mid-, and late-diastolic murmurs (Figure 36-4). Diastolic murmurs are all pathologic and require referral to a pediatric cardiologist. Early-diastolic murmurs begin immediately after $S_2$ and are decrescendo in nature; they become less audible as the ventricle fills. Aortic insufficiency and pulmonary insufficiency are heard in early diastole. Mid-diastolic murmurs occur during rapid ventricular filling. Murmurs of mild mitral and tricuspid stenosis are heard in mid diastole. Late-diastolic

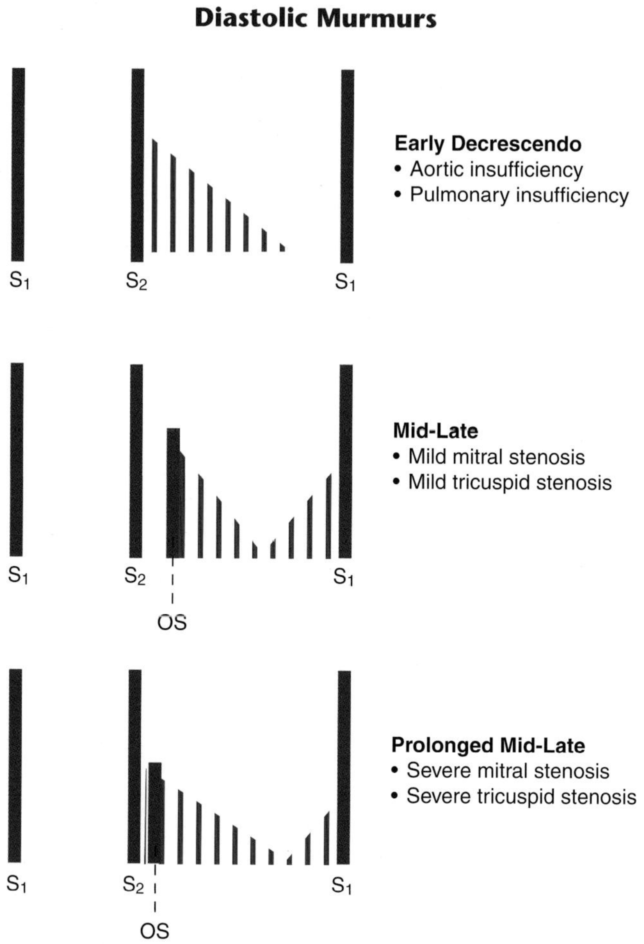


**Figure 36-4**
Classification of diastolic murmurs. *OS*, opening snap; *$S_1$*, first heart sound; *$S_2$*, second heart sound. (*From Lilly LS.* Pathophysiology of Heart Disease. *3rd ed. Philadelphia, PA: Lippincott Williams & Wilkins; 2003. Used by permission.*)

(presystolic) murmurs occur near the end of diastole, during atrial contraction. Severe mitral stenosis or tricuspid stenosis murmurs increase in late diastole.

Continuous murmurs extend across portions of systole and diastole. They are almost always vascular in origin and are caused by aortopulmonary (eg, patent ductus arteriosus) or arteriovenous (eg, arteriovenous malformation) connections, turbulent flow in collateral arteries (eg, coarctation of the aorta), turbulent flow in veins (eg, venous hum), or a surgical shunt. With the exception of the innocent venous hum (Table 36-4), continuous murmurs are pathologic. They tend to wax and wane in intensity through the cardiac cycle, often diminishing in late diastole (Figure 36-5). A somewhat different auscultatory phenomenon from the continuous murmur, the to-and-fro murmur describes an ejection murmur heard in systole, coupled to a decrescendo murmur early in diastole. Combined aortic stenosis and

**Table 36-4**
**Common Innocent Murmurs**

| MURMUR | INTENSITY | TIMING | LOCATION | QUALITY |
|---|---|---|---|---|
| Still | I–III/VI | Early–mid systolic | LM–LLSB or apex | Vibratory, musical |
| Pulmonary | I–III/VI | Early–mid systolic | LUSB | Low pitched, ejection |
| Venous hum | I–III/VI | Continuous | Right (rarely left) infra- or supra-clavicular | Low pitched, disappears with head turn, supine position, jugular compression |

*LM–LLSB,* left mid to left lower sternal border; *LUSB,* left upper sternal border.

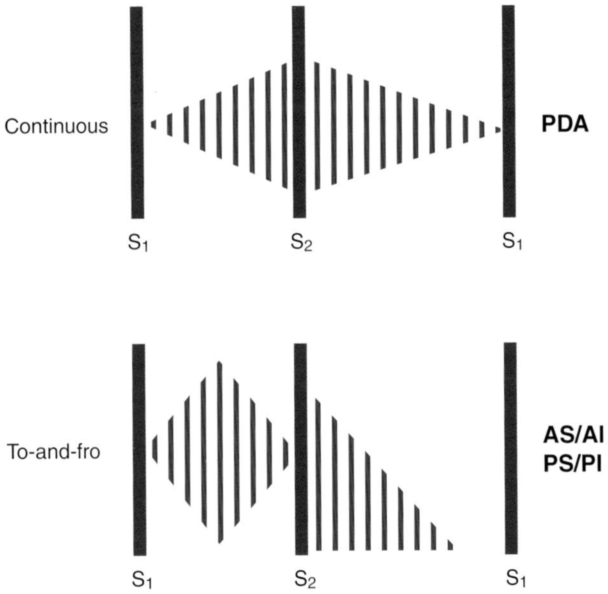


**Figure 36-5**
Continuous murmur versus to-and-fro murmur. *AS/AI,* aortic stenosis and aortic insufficiency; *PDA,* patent ductus arteriosus; *PS/PI,* pulmonary stenosis and pulmonary insufficiency; $S_1$, first heart sound; $S_2$, second heart sound. (*From Lilly LS.* Pathophysiology of Heart Disease. *3rd ed. Philadelphia, PA: Lippincott Williams & Wilkins; 2003. Used by permission.*)

aortic insufficiency or combined pulmonary stenosis and pulmonary insufficiency produces to-and-fro murmurs.

### *Location and Radiation*

Location refers to the area where the murmur is heard the best. Radiation means the murmur is also audible with unexpected intensity at some distance from its location. As seen in Figure 36-2, location helps narrow the differential diagnosis of the murmur. Radiation of the murmur can also be very helpful diagnostically. For example, murmurs that radiate to the neck tend to be of aortic or left ventricular outflow tract origin, whereas a murmur heard best at the left upper sternal border with radiation to the axillae and back is more likely to be pulmonary in origin.

### *Quality and Behavior With Maneuvers*

Quality refers to the pitch and nature of a murmur. Pitch is generally described as either high or low. High-pitched murmurs occur when the pressure differential involved is large. For example, aortic insufficiency is a high-pitched murmur. Low-pitched murmurs occur when a lower pressure differential is involved. Pulmonary insufficiency is a low-pitched murmur. Systolic murmurs are described as harsh, blowing, musical, or vibratory. Diastolic murmurs are described as blowing, rumbling, crescendo, or decrescendo.

Postural maneuvers are useful in distinguishing among different types of murmurs. Innocent murmurs tend to become louder when the patient moves from an upright to a supine position. Placing the patient in the left lateral decubitus position increases the murmur of mitral stenosis. A Valsalva maneuver, by decreasing venous return, makes the murmur of aortic stenosis softer, but it makes the murmur of hypertrophic obstructive cardiomyopathy louder. Valsalva maneuver also decreases the murmurs associated with a VSD and mitral regurgitation and can nearly eliminate innocent Still murmurs (Table 36-4). Squatting increases venous return and makes the murmur of hypertrophic obstructive cardiomyopathy softer. Standing up after squatting can accentuate the murmur or click of mitral valve prolapse by moving the murmur and click closer to $S_1$. Recumbent positioning and/or turning the head can eliminate the innocent continuous murmur of a venous hum.

## ▶ CONCLUSION

Pediatricians commonly evaluate childhood murmurs. Most murmurs in children and adolescents are innocent. They do not reflect cardiac disease, and they do not require referral to a pediatric cardiologist, prophylaxis against endocarditis, or exercise restriction. Innocent murmurs are generally short systolic murmurs and are less than grade IV. They are often low pitched, vibratory, or musical; are best heard in the supine position; and often diminish when the patient is upright or during a Valsalva maneuver. Most innocent murmurs can be recognized with confidence based on the clinical history and careful physical examination. Further evaluation is required for any murmur for which suspicion persists that it may be pathologic.

### When to Refer

- Patient, maternal, or family history raising index of suspicion for heart disease
- All diastolic murmurs
- Continuous murmurs, except venous hum
- All systolic murmurs grade IV or higher
- All systolic murmurs not clearly fitting the pattern of innocent murmur
- Ausculatation of an S4 gallop
- A thrill is an abnormal finding and warrants referral to a cardiologist
- Cyanosis, clubbing
- Higher blood pressure in one or both arms than a leg
- Congestive heart failure—rales, respiratory distress, hepatomegaly, edema
- Abnormal electrocardiogram
- Symptoms that suggest reactive airway disease that do not improve with appropriate medical therapy

## *TOOLS FOR PRACTICE*

### Engaging Patient and Family

- *Heart Murmurs* (fact sheet), American Academy of Pediatrics (www.healthychildren.org/English/health-issues/conditions/heart/Pages/Heart-Murmur.aspx)

### Medical Decision Support

- *American Heart Association* (Web site), (www.americanheart.org)

## *SUGGESTED READINGS*

Allen HD, Gutgesell HP, Clark EB, et al. *Moss and Adams' Heart Disease in Infants, Children, and Adolescents.* 6th ed. Philadelphia, PA: Lippincott Williams & Wilkins; 2001

Berne RM, Levy MN. *Physiology.* 4th ed. St Louis, MO: Mosby; 1998

Park MK. *The Pediatric Cardiology Handbook.* 3rd ed. Philadelphia, PA: Mosby; 2003

Chapter 37

# Hematuria

*Kimberly J. Reidy, MD; Marcela Del Rio, MD*

Hematuria may manifest as a dramatic change in the color of a child's urine, with the appearance of blood on a diaper or underwear, or as a finding on a urinalysis. Red or brown (cola-colored) urine with red blood cells (RBCs) seen on microscopy is typical of macroscopic (or gross) hematuria. In general, urologic causes of gross hematuria often present with red or pink urine, while glomerular hematuria presents with brown-, tea-, or cola-colored urine. In a retrospective study of children presenting to a pediatric emergency department, gross hematuria had an incidence of 1.3 per 1,000 visits.[1] Microscopic hematuria (defined as >5 RBCs per high power field seen on microscopy of centrifuged urine) is more common. On routine screening urinalysis, studies suggest up to 32 per 1,000 girls and 14 per 1,000 boys will have microscopic hematuria. The American Academy of Pediatrics (AAP) currently does not recommend routine screening urinalyses in asymptomatic children.[2]

The most likely causes of macroscopic and microscopic hematuria differ (Figure 37-1 and Box 37-1). Macroscopic hematuria may originate from any component of the genitourinary tract, and the differential diagnosis, in addition to infection, includes glomerular, interstitial, and tubular diseases and bleeding from trauma, stones, or coagulopathy. Many of the causes of macroscopic hematuria, such as infection, nephrolithiasis, and glomerulonephritis, may also present with microscopic hematuria. Overall, the most common causes of asymptomatic isolated microscopic hematuria are thin basement membrane disease, idiopathic hypercalciuria, immunoglobulin A (IgA) nephropathy, and sickle cell disease or trait.[3]

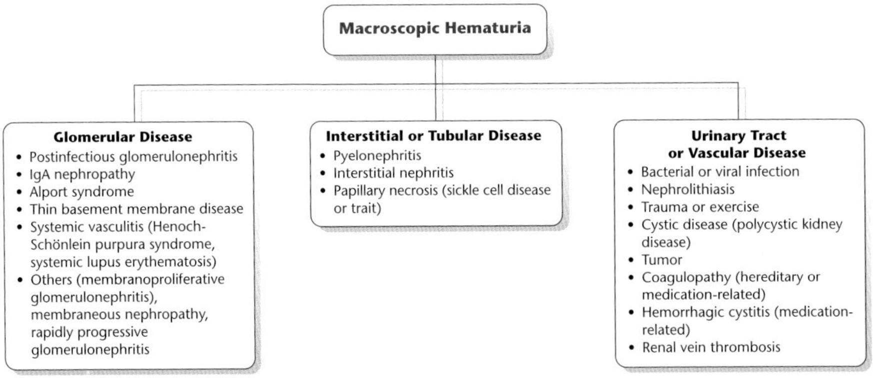


**Figure 37-1**
Differential diagnosis of macroscopic hematuria in children.

## ▶ MACROSCOPIC HEMATURIA

The first and most important step in evaluating macroscopic hematuria is obtaining a detailed description of the urine (Figure 37-2). Renal or glomerular causes of hematuria result in tea- or cola-colored urine, as opposed to hematuria of lower-tract origin, which causes red or pink urine. In addition to color, highly turbid urine may indicate the presence of cells

**Box 37-1**

### *Causes of Microscopic Hematuria*

- Transient
- Thin basement membrane disease
- Idiopathic hypercalciuria
- Immunoglobulin A (IgA) nephropathy or Alport syndrome
- Sickle cell anemia or trait
- Trauma or exercise
- Postinfectious glomerulonephritis
- Nephrolithiasis
- Other glomerular disease or glomerulonephritis
    - Focal and segmental glomerulosclerosis
    - Henoch-Schönlein purpura syndrome
    - Systemic lupus erythematosis
    - Membranoproliferative glomerulonephritis
    - Membranous glomerulonephritis
- Congenital abnormality
    - Ureteropelvic junction obstruction
    - Cystic disease
- Pyelonephritis or infection
- Vascular malformation
- Drugs or toxins

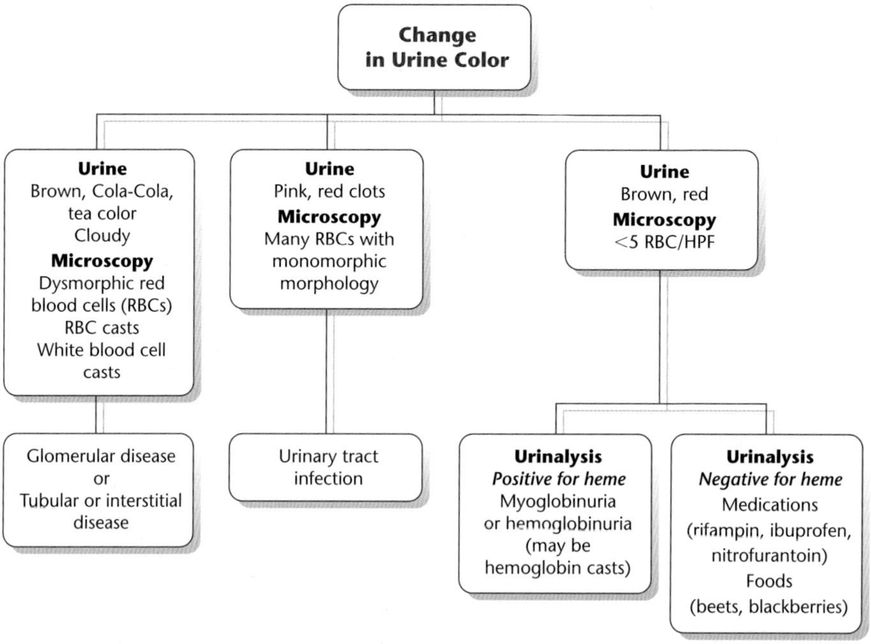


**Figure 37-2**
Evaluation for macroscopic hematuria begins with the examination of the urine.

and suggests glomerular disease or infection. Blood clots suggest urinary tract bleeding. The timing of the bleeding may be helpful (eg, if it occurs only with the onset of micturation, then the source of the bleeding is likely to be in the lower urinary tract.

Associated signs and symptoms from a detailed history and physical examination will dictate laboratory and radiologic evaluation. Important historical elements include associated urinary symptoms, such as dysuria, frequency, urgency, or enuresis. A decrease in urine output should prompt particular concern and rapid evaluation and treatment. A review of systems should include associated symptoms of abdominal pain or colic, upper respiratory infection symptoms, swelling of extremities, or blurry vision or headaches suggestive of hypertension. The history should be explored for prior episodes of hematuria, preceding infections (either documented group A streptococcal throat infection or a history of sore throat or skin infection), history of trauma, or other illnesses, such as the presence of sickle cell trait or disease. Systemic illnesses may be suggested by a history of fever, malaise, weight loss, alopecia, rash, or joint pains, which may be seen in rheumatologic disease. The age of the patient is an important factor to consider—certain causes of hematuria, such as renal vein thrombosis and tumors, are more common in infants. Important points on the family history include other family members with hematuria, kidney or rheumatologic disease, and any history of deafness, which may occur with Alport syndrome.

A thorough physical examination should include measurement of blood pressure, abdominal or costovertebral angle tenderness, a search for evidence of local trauma to the genitourinary tract, inspection and palpation for periorbital, genital, or extremity edema, and examination of the skin for rashes. Hematuria in association with edema and hypertension suggests glomerulonephritis.

Laboratory evaluation begins with a urinalysis with microscopic examination of a fresh-spun urine sample to confirm the presence of red blood cells. Dysmorphic red blood cells and red blood cell casts are pathognomonic of hematuria of glomerular origin (see Figure 37-3).[4] If the urine dipstick is positive for blood and fewer than 5 red bloods cells are found on microscopy, then the diagnosis is hemoglobinuria or myoglobinuria

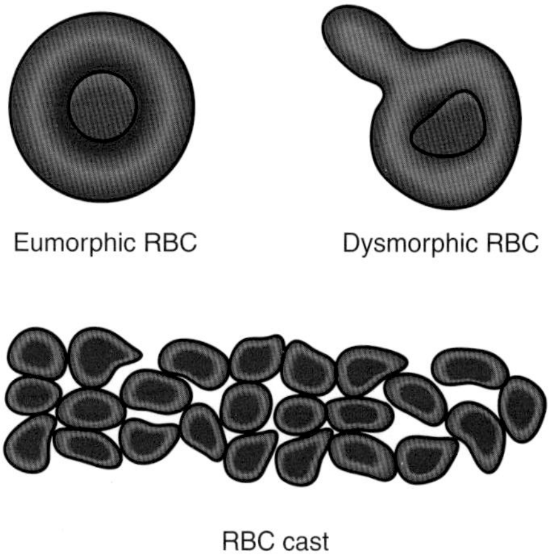


**Figure 37-3**
Urinary findings in hematuria

rather than hematuria. Several drugs, including rifampin, ibuprofen, and nitrofurantoin, as well as foods such as beets and blackberries, can discolor urine to give it the appearance of hematuria, but urinalysis will be negative for blood. The presence of calcium, uric acid, or cystine crystals in the urine is suggestive of nephrolithiasis. Identification of white blood cell casts on microscopy or leukocyte esterase or nitrate positivity on urine dipstick point to infectious causes of hematuria.

Further evaluation is determined by the most likely cause of the blood in the urine. For example, a workup for suspected glomerular hematuria might include evaluation of serum electrolytes, blood urea nitrogen, creatinine, calcium, and phosphorus to assess renal function and liver function tests if there is a nephrotic component. Antinuclear antibody test, complement studies (C3, C4, and total complement), streptozyme (deoxyribonuclease B) and streptolysin O antibody titers may help determine the etiology of a glomerulonephritis. Throat culture or rapid testing for group A β-hemolytic streptococci is indicated with a history of sore throat. A urine culture should be performed on all patients with urinary symptoms or on infants, because infection is a common cause of hematuria. Proteinuria on urinalysis should be further evaluated with a first-morning void for protein-to-creatinine ratio. In patients with suspected nonglomerular macroscopic hematuria, a renal-bladder sonogram is indicated to evaluate for cystic disease, congenital obstruction, tumors (including Wilms tumor), nephrolithiasis, or parenchymal renal disease. A renal doppler study is needed to evaluate for suspected vascular thrombosis, renal infarcts, or renal artery stenosis.

Evaluation of glomerular hematuria may be continued as an outpatient or inpatient. Indications for admission include decreased urine output, hypertension, azotemia, or renal insufficiency. Renal biopsy is absolutely indicated in cases of hematuria with nephrotic syndrome, recurrent hematuria, azotemia, or renal insufficiency. Renal biopsy may be considered if a family history of hematuria exists or if the history or laboratory evaluation is suggestive of rheumatologic disease, such as systemic lupus erythematosus.

Management of glomerular disease will depend on the cause of the glomerulonephritis. The most common glomerulonephritis is postinfectious, an entity characterized by a prodromal infection (often a streptococcal skin or throat infection but also viral infections, such as varicella, cytomegalovirus, Epstein-Barr virus, hepatitis B and C, and parasitic infections such as toxoplasmosis) between 1 and 6 weeks before the onset of hematuria. Other causes of acute postinfectious glomerulonephritis include ventriculoperitoneal shunt infections (shunt nephritis) and acute or subacute endocarditis. Low complement (C3) and elevated streptolysin O antibodies are characteristic of post-streptococcal glomerulonephritis. Post-streptococcal glomerulonephritis is typically self-limited with a good prognosis for long-term renal function. Admission may be required for renal insufficiency, oliguria, or acute hypertension (the latter requiring aggressive management with fluid and salt restriction and antihypertensive medications).

Other types of glomerulonephritis often require management by a nephrologist. The most common chronic glomerulonephritis worldwide is IgA nephropathy, although it is more often diagnosed in adults than children. IgA nephropathy characteristically results in persistent microhematuria with intermittent episodes of gross hematuria associated with upper respiratory infections. Long-term outcome is variable, with 20% to 40% of children progressing to end-stage kidney disease. Proteinuria and hypertension are poor prognostic indicators. Henoch-Schönlein purpura (HSP), a common systemic vasculitis in children, is often associated with crampy abdominal pain, arthralgia, and palpable purpura, and can produce glomerulonephritis with hematuria.[5]

Management of nonglomerular hematuria depends on the cause. Further imaging with computed tomography may be indicated. Patients with sickle-cell disease and macroscopic hematuria from papillary necrosis may require admission for intravenous hydration. Trauma, tumors, cystic disease, congenital obstruction, hemorrhagic cystitis, and lower urinary tract bleeding often require urologic evaluation, which may include direct visualization by cystoscopy. Children with nephrolithiasis benefit from both nephrologic and urologic evaluation.

## ▶ MICROSCOPIC HEMATURIA

The evaluation of microscopic hematuria involves a thorough history and physical examination. A family history of deafness or kidney disease and the presence of hypertension, proteinuria, or edema should prompt referral to a pediatric nephrologist for further evaluation. In the absence of any other signs and symptoms, microhematuria is often benign and, in many cases, resolves spontaneously (transient hematuria). Therefore, in an asymptomatic, normotensive child with isolated microhematuria, repeating a urinalysis on 1 or more occasions is often prudent before further evaluation. School-aged children may be observed in excess of 2 years before more extensive testing is undertaken. Figure 37-4 shows a proposed algorithm for the evaluation of microscopic hematuria.[6,7] Significant proteinuria or the occurrence of gross hematuria should prompt referral to a pediatric nephrologist.

Hereditary nephritis includes a spectrum of familial hematuria that ranges from benign thin basement membrane nephropathy (TBMN) to progressive Alport syndrome. TBMN is a common cause of persistent microhematuria.[8] TBMN is characterized by painless microscopic hematuria with minimal proteinuria and normal renal function. Renal biopsy reveals uniform thinning of the glomerular basement membrane. TBMN is also called thin basement membrane disease, hereditary hematuria, benign familial hematuria, and benign hereditary nephritis. Because it is transmitted in an autosomal-dominant fashion, a family history of microscopic hematuria without symptomatic renal disease, or an asymptomatic parent testing positive for hematuria, suggests the diagnosis of TBMN. The overall prevalence is estimated at 1% to 10% of the population. It is more common in females than in

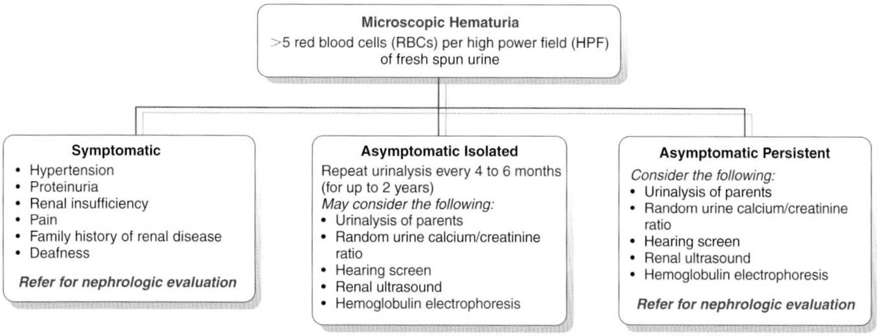


**Figure 37-4**
Evaluation of microscopic hematuria.

males and has been diagnosed in children as young as 1 year of age. Between 5% and 22% of affected individuals will have an episode of gross hematuria associated with an infection or exercise. No evidence has been found to support treatment of TBMN, which is typically nonprogressive. However, affected children should be monitored for with a yearly urinalysis and blood pressure check throughout their lives, because they are at higher risk of hypertension, proteinuria, and renal insufficiency in later adulthood.

Another common cause of microscopic hematuria is hypercalciuria, defined as a urine calcium-to-creatinine ratio of greater than 0.21 or more than 4 mg/kg/day of excreted calcium on a 24-hour urine collection. Children with hematuria and underlying hypercalciuria are at risk for nephrolithiasis, with the risk seeming to be greater in older children, in children with gross rather than microscopic hematuria, and when there is a family history of stone formation.[9]

Significant proteinuria or the occurrence of gross hematuria should prompt referral to a pediatric nephrologist.

## BLOOD ON A DIAPER OR UNDERWEAR

Blood on a diaper or underwear most commonly occurs with trauma to or manipulation of the genital area. Localized irritation of the meatus in boys is the most frequent cause and responds to treatment with petroleum jelly and reassurance to the parent without further evaluation. Sexual abuse is on the differential diagnosis. Nonurethral sources of bleeding, such as perineal or vaginal bleeding, should be considered. Again, a urinalysis is useful to confirm that hematuria is the source of the discoloration. "Red diaper syndrome" can result from infection with *Serratia marcescens* (deposits of reddish pigment), or uric acid crystals (reddish/brown or pink crystals) that can be found in the normal or dehydrated newborn.

## CONCLUSION

Key points for the primary care physician include the following:

- Gross hematuria is a common sign of glomerular and urologic disease.
- Hematuria of glomerular origin presents with tea- or cola-colored urine.
- Hematuria arising from the urinary tract is usually red-pink, with or without clots.
- Red blood cell casts are the hallmark of hematuria of glomerular origin.
- Proteinuria is a more important prognostic finding than gross hematuria.
- Every child with gross hematuria should have a renal ultrasound to rule out nephrolithiasis, tumor, or urologic abnormalities, such as cystic disease and obstructive uropathy.
- Gross hematuria rarely is a cause of anemia.
- Most children with isolated microscopic hematuria do not have a serious or treatable cause for the hematuria and do not require an extensive workup.
- Hematuria of glomerular origin is typically painless.

### When to Refer

- Macroscopic hematuria
- Hematuria associated with pain
- Persistent microscopic hematuria, especially with associated proteinuria, hypertension, hearing loss, or family history of renal disease or deafness

## When to Admit

When hematuria (with or without proteinuria) is associated with the following:

- Severe abdominal or flank pain
- Congestive heart failure or fluid overload indicative of oliguria or anuria
- Hypertension
- Renal insufficiency
- Anasarca (generalized edema)

### TOOLS FOR PRACTICE

#### Engaging Patient and Family

- *Blood in Urine (Hematuria)* (fact sheet), American Academy of Pediatrics (www.healthychildren.org/English/health-issues/conditions/genitourinary-tract/Pages/Blood-in-Urine-Hematuria.aspx)
- *Proteinuria* (fact sheet), American Academy of Pediatrics (www.healthychildren.org/English/health-issues/conditions/genitourinary-tract/Pages/Proteinuria.aspx)

### AAP POLICY STATEMENTS

Finnell SME, Carroll AE, Downs SM; American Academy of Pediatrics Subcommittee on Urinary Tract Infection. Diagnosis and management of an initial UTI in febrile infants and young children. *Pediatrics.* 2011;128(3):e749–e770 (pediatrics.aappublications.org/content/128/3/e749)

Downs SM. Technical report: urinary tract infections in febrile infants and young children. *Pediatrics.* 1999;103:e54 (pediatrics.aappublications.org/content/103/4/e54)

### REFERENCES

1. Ingelfinger JR, Davis AE, Grupe WE. Frequency and etiology of gross hematuria in a general pediatric setting. *Pediatrics.* 1977;59:557–561
2. Simon GR, Baker C, Barden GA 3rd, et al; American Academy of Pediatrics Committee on Practice and Ambulatory Medicine, Bright Futures Periodicity Schedule Workgroup. 2014 recommendations for pediatric preventive health care. *Pediatrics.* 2014;133(3):568–570
3. Meyers KE. Evaluation of hematuria in children. *Urologic Clin North Am.* 2004;31(3):559–573
4. Crompton CH, Ward PB, Hewitt IK. The use of urinary red cell morphology to determine the source of hematuria in children. *Clin Nephrol.* 1993;39:44–49
5. Lau KK, Wyatt RJ. Glomerulonephritis. *Adolesc Med Clin.* 2005;16(1):67–85
6. Feld LG, Meyers KE, Kaplan BS, Stapleton FB. Limited evaluation of microscopic hematuria in pediatrics. *Pediatrics.* 1998;102:E42
7. Wood EG. Asymptomatic hematuria in childhood: a practical approach to evaluation. *Indian J Pediatr.* 1999;66:207–214
8. Tryggvason K, Patrakka J. Thin basement membrane nephropathy. *J Am Soc Nephrol.* 2006;17:813–822
9. Garcia CD, Miller LA, Stapleton FB. Natural history of hematuria associated with hypercalciuria in children. *Am J Dis Child.* 1991;145:1204–1207

# Chapter 38

# Hemoptysis

*Scott A. Schroeder, MD*

*Hemoptysis,* the spitting or coughing of blood that originates within the thorax, can vary from flecks of blood in the sputum to massive, life-threatening bleeding that can lead to respiratory distress or death. Unlike in adults, for whom more than 100 different causes of hemoptysis have been described, hemoptysis is a rare occurrence in children; it is most commonly associated with previously diagnosed congenital heart disease or cystic fibrosis (CF), although other causes include infectious respiratory illnesses and, rarely, neoplasms.[1] Acute hemoptysis, respiratory failure, and cyanosis may be the result of exposure to mold growing in water-damaged homes or to environmental tobacco smoke. Affected children need to be hospitalized and placed on mechanical ventilation.[2,3]

Four important considerations should be kept in mind when evaluating children who have hemoptysis. First, it is necessary to determine whether the bleeding requires an emergency resuscitative effort. Second, what seems to be hemoptysis may actually be bleeding from the upper airway or gastrointestinal tract; thus, the source of the bleeding should be established. Third, children without chronic diseases who develop hemoptysis with associated symptoms of a lower respiratory tract infection usually have mild, self-limited bleeding that requires no specific treatment other than management of the underlying acute illness. Fourth, the management of hemoptysis that arises from a localized site differs from that which causes a diffuse alveolar hemorrhage, because the latter may be the presenting sign of an underlying immunologic or rheumatologic disorder.

## ▶ PATHOGENESIS

Hemoptysis can result from the disruption of either arm of the dual pulmonary vascular system or from damage to the alveolar endothelial junction. The low-pressure, high-capacitance pulmonary arterial system accepts the entire cardiac output from the right ventricle and carries blood to be oxygenated at the pulmonary capillaries before returning the oxygenated blood to the left atrium through the pulmonary veins. Although the pulmonary arteries travel alongside the bronchial tree, they interact with the airways only at the level of the terminal bronchioles. The second arm of the blood supply within the lungs is the high-pressure bronchial system. The bronchial arteries originate from the aorta or, less commonly, the intercostal arteries, and they receive only 1% to 2% of the cardiac output. The bronchial arteries enter the lungs at the hilum, and as they branch with the bronchi they anastomose and penetrate the bronchial mucosa, forming an extensive submucosal plexus. The high-flow, low-pressure pulmonary capillary bed allows the exchange of gases between the alveoli and the capillaries to occur with little risk for hemorrhage in the normal state.

Localized hemoptysis, in most cases, is the result of bleeding from the high-pressure bronchial circulation in inflamed airways. The pulmonary circulation is rarely to blame for hemoptysis except in necrotic infarcts and from pulmonary arterial aneurysms in tubercular cavities. Both of these conditions are extremely rare in children. Inflammation within the lungs, pulmonary vascular obstruction, and neoplasia can all cause an increase in the bronchial circulation. In chronic inflammatory conditions, such as bronchiectasis, the cardiac output to the bronchial circulation can triple, and bronchopulmonary anastomoses are increased, thereby increasing the potential for erosion of vessels in the presence of superimposed infection. The pathogenesis of disease states with diffuse pulmonary hemorrhage—for example, necrotizing granulomatous vasculitis—is not entirely understood, but the bleeding into the alveoli seems to result from neutrophil-mediated injury to pulmonary capillaries with interstitial and air-space fibrosis from the chronic hemorrhage.

## ▶ ETIOLOGY

### *Hemoptysis in Children Without a Preexisting Medical Condition*

In children who do not have a preexisting medical condition, the most common causes of hemoptysis are acute infections of the tracheobronchial tree, acute infectious pneumonias, and the aspiration of a foreign body. A child with a pneumococcal pneumonia who is old enough to expectorate is classically febrile, seems ill, and has a cough that is productive of rusty sputum. Certain other bacterial and viral lower respiratory tract infections can cause hemoptysis; in these cases, the hemoptysis usually occurs early in the course of the illness, is self-limited, and consists of only blood-tinged sputum. Globally, tuberculosis, echinococcus, and paragonimiasis are probably the most common causes of hemoptysis in children (Table 38-1).

After acute infectious processes, the most common cause of hemoptysis in a previously healthy child is the aspiration of a foreign body. In many children who aspirate foreign bodies, the initial choking episode is not observed or not remembered. A bout of paroxysmal coughing may occur after the initial event, but as the cough receptors in the bronchi or trachea adapt, the coughing will stop. Over time, and depending on the location and composition of the foreign object, subsequent inflammation will occur, which may result in airway obstruction, with wheezing or recurrent pneumonitis. If neovascularization of granulation tissue in the airways occurs, or if bronchiectasis develops, then hemoptysis can occur weeks to months after the initial event. Only 40% of children with a foreign-body aspiration will exhibit the classic triad of wheezing, cough, and decreased breath sounds distal to the site of obstruction.[4] The chest radiograph will be normal in 25% of children with bronchial foreign bodies and in more than 50% of children with tracheal foreign bodies.[5]

Because only 10% of aspirated foreign bodies are radiopaque, a normal chest radiograph does not preclude aspiration. Inspiratory and expiratory films, decubitus films, and fluoroscopy may be necessary to confirm the diagnosis. If the evidence for aspiration is definitive, then referral for rigid bronchoscopy to a pediatric surgeon or otolaryngologist experienced in retrieving foreign bodies is indicated. If the diagnosis is uncertain, then referral to a pediatric pulmonologist or other physician skilled in the use of the fiberoptic bronchoscopy is appropriate to determine whether a foreign body is present.

**Table 38-1**
**Common, Less Common, and Uncommon Causes of Hemoptysis**

| POPULATION | CAUSE | DIAGNOSTIC CLUES |
|---|---|---|
| Common causes in children who have no preexisting medical problems | Pneumonia | Usually rusty-colored sputum early in the course of the illness |
| | Foreign-body aspiration | Needs a high index of suspicion; may have a normal chest radiograph; localized wheezing that does not respond to medical therapy |
| Less common causes in children who have no preexisting medical problems | Pulmonary tuberculosis | Usually with systemic manifestations, such as anorexia and weight loss; may have negative purified protein derivative test |
| | Autoimmune disorders | Diffuse pulmonary hemorrhage, often with weight loss or other systems involved, including the kidneys and joints |
| | Congenital malformations | Symptoms depend on the nature of the lesion; may be associated with massive hemoptysis or respiratory distress in newborns |
| Rare causes in children who have no preexisting medical problems | Primary pulmonary neoplasms | Primary pulmonary cancers reported in fewer than 500 children; usually present with cough and recurrent pneumonitis |
| | Pulmonary embolism | Associated with pleuritic pain, cough, and dyspnea; oral contraceptive use; recent abortion; trauma to lower extremities |
| | Parasitic lung infections | Travel to endemic areas or sheep-raising areas; peripheral eosinophilia |
| | Arteriovenous malformations | Recurrent epistaxis, a positive family history for hereditary hemorrhagic telangiectasia (Rendu-Osler-Weber syndrome), or cutaneous telangiectasia |
| | Idiopathic pulmonary hemosiderosis | Cough, wheezing, iron-deficiency anemia, and diffuse pulmonary hemorrhage on chest radiograph |
| | Catamenial hemoptysis | Hemoptysis occurs with onset of menses |
| | Factitious hemoptysis | Form of Münchausen syndrome |
| Common causes in children who have a preexisting medical problem | Bronchiectasis | Blood-tinged sputum, clubbing, signs of increasing airway inflammation |
| | Congenital heart lesions | Seen with Eisenmenger complex and pulmonary venous congestion |
| Less common causes in children who have a preexisting medical problem | Sickle cell anemia | Hemoptysis associated with acute chest syndrome or pulmonary infarction |
| | Aspergillosis | Seen in association with CF or asthma; peripheral eosinophilia and fungi seen on Gram stain of sputum |

*CF*, cystic fibrosis.

## Diffuse Pulmonary Hemorrhage

Children with acute hemoptysis, cough, wheezing, or crackles, diffuse patchy infiltrates on chest radiograph, and bronchoscopic evidence of blood in all lobes or hemosiderin-laden macrophages should be assumed to have diffuse pulmonary hemorrhage or hemosiderosis. The 4 categories of diffuse hemorrhage syndromes that occur in children are those associated with antiglomerular basement membrane antibodies in serum or tissue (eg, Goodpasture syndrome), those associated with an autoimmune-mediated disease (eg, systemic lupus erythematosus), those without any immunologic abnormalities but associated with antibodies to cow's milk, and idiopathic pulmonary hemosiderosis (IPH). All of these conditions are exceedingly rare.

*Goodpasture syndrome,* which occurs most commonly in men in their second and third decades, is characterized by diffuse pulmonary hemorrhage, antiglomerular basement membrane antibodies in serum or tissue, and glomerulonephritis. The autoimmune diseases, which are more common in girls and women, rarely produce hemoptysis alone; more commonly, systemic manifestations occur, including fever, weight loss, malaise, anorexia, amenorrhea, rashes, or hypertension, as well as hemoptysis. Treatment for the pulmonary hemorrhage in these disorders should be directed at the underlying disease process.

In *Heiner syndrome,* or pulmonary hemosiderosis associated with cow milk allergy, infants and children exhibit failure to thrive, vomiting, gastrointestinal bleeding, and upper respiratory tract congestion, in addition to hemoptysis.[6] Although the mechanism whereby the milk causes the multisystem damage is unclear, elimination of milk from the diet results in a dramatic improvement in the children.

In IPH, no evidence for an immune-mediated mechanism is found. Most children with IPH are diagnosed before the age of 7 years or after the age of 16 years. They usually have respiratory distress, bilateral alveolar infiltrates, and iron-deficiency anemia. The treatment of the acute exacerbations of IPH includes the use of high-dose oral or intravenous corticosteroids, as well as supportive care for the acute bleeding into the lungs. Controversy exists regarding the need for chronic immunosuppressive therapy, but most physicians caring for children with IPH use azathioprine, chloroquine, or cyclophosphamide to help maintain normal lung function and prevent further episodes of hemoptysis.

## Primary Pulmonary Neoplasms

Unlike in adults, primary pulmonary neoplasms are extremely rare in children, especially immunocompetent children. Fewer than 5% of tumors reported in the literature were associated with hemoptysis. The most common presentations of primary pulmonary neoplasms in children are fever, cough, and pleural pain.[7]

### *Hemoptysis in Children With a Preexisting Medical Condition*

The most common chronic disease associated with hemoptysis is CF. Hemoptysis in CF, which usually begins in the second or third decade of life, can range from the production of blood-tinged sputum with excessive coughing to massive bleeding. Mild hemoptysis can be treated with conservative medical therapy, which includes bed rest, intravenous or oral antibiotics, withholding of chest physiotherapy, and administration of vitamin K. Massive hemoptysis has an annual incidence of 1% among patients with CF and carries a high mortality rate. Massive or recurrent hemoptysis in CF and other diseases is now treated with bronchial artery embolization. Despite a moderately high rate of recurrent bleeding, embolization can relieve symptoms for a significant period. A team composed of a pulmonologist, thoracic surgeon, and interventional radiologist should evaluate these patients before bronchial artery embolization.

Although the number of children with bronchiectasis has declined because of the decline of tuberculosis and the use of effective vaccines against measles and pertussis, children with immunodeficiencies, recurrent aspiration, and ciliary dyskinesias may develop bronchiectasis and have episodes of hemoptysis. In most cases, a history of a chronic, productive cough with purulent sputum and changes on the lung examination precede the hemoptysis. The diagnosis is made by high-resolution chest tomography, and management is similar to that of CF.

Hemoptysis is a well-recognized complication of congenital heart disease but is becoming an uncommon problem because of advances in corrective cardiac surgery. Hemoptysis in primary or secondary pulmonary hypertension occurs as a result of thromboembolic events. In right ventricular outflow obstruction with increased bronchial arterial circulation, hemorrhage from enlarged and tortuous bronchial arteries can produce hemoptysis. Pulmonary vascular obstructive disease can lead to hemoptysis because of pulmonary hypertension, as well as to thrombosis. These vascular changes take years to develop and are usually first observed in adolescents.

## ▶ EVALUATION

As with any potential emergency, the first question to be answered about hemoptysis is, "Is it life threatening?" Because the expectoration of blood understandably arouses anxiety and fear, and because the blood can be mixed with saliva or phlegm and swallowed or aspirated, accurately determining the amount of blood is often difficult for children and their parents. In adults, the quantity of expectorated blood does not correlate with the seriousness of the underlying disease. In children, the gravity of the hemoptysis is determined more by the child's clinical status and ability to keep the airway clear than by the amount of blood expectorated. The greatest danger to a child with hemoptysis is not exsanguination but rather asphyxiation from aspirated blood. The management of the child with life-threatening hemoptysis is beyond the scope of this chapter. However, if the child has evidence of cardiorespiratory distress, hypotension, orthostatic changes, poor perfusion, pallor, tachypnea, tachycardia, mental status changes, arterial hypoxemia, or hypercarbia, then the stabilization and evaluation of the child should occur simultaneously in a pediatric intensive care unit.

Before summoning the bronchoscopist, echocardiographer, and interventional radiologist and scheduling pulmonary arteriography and radionuclide scanning, the primary care physician must ascertain whether the source of bleeding is indeed within the thorax. Thorough inspection of the oropharynx and nasal passages may identify an upper airway source of bleeding. Infants and young children with hemoptysis may not cough up blood but instead swallow the blood and vomit it later. Therefore, in infants, distinguishing hematemesis from hemoptysis is difficult. Examination of the blood-stained secretions may help differentiate the bleeding site so that it can be established whether the bleeding is from the respiratory tract or not. Table 38-2 describes how to differentiate hemoptysis from bleeding from other sources.

### *History*

As is the case for any sign or symptom with many possible causes, a detailed history of both pulmonary and nonpulmonary symptoms will often allow a tentative diagnosis to be made. The presumptive diagnosis can then be proved or disproved by the findings of

**Table 38-2**
**Differentiation of Hemoptysis From Hematemesis and Upper Airway Hemorrhage[a]**

| CHARACTERISTIC | HEMOPTYSIS | HEMATEMESIS AND UPPER AIRWAY HEMORRHAGE |
|---|---|---|
| pH | Alkaline | Acidic |
| Color | Bright red | Dark red or brown |
| Consistency | Clotted, liquid, or frothy | Coffee ground |
| Symptoms | Cough | Nausea and vomiting |
| Gram stain | Macrophages | Food particles and epithelial cells |

[a]Younger children and infants may swallow blood that originates from the lungs, which may seem to have a nonpulmonary source of bleeding.

specific laboratory tests and procedures. For a child or adolescent without any preexisting medical condition who displays a first episode of hemoptysis, the most common causes are acute infections of the tracheobronchial tree, pneumonias, and foreign-body aspirations.[8–10] Hemoptysis can be the presenting symptom for an autoimmune disorder or other immunologic abnormality, although this circumstance is rare. Travel to or from developing countries and areas that raise sheep may necessitate evaluation for mycobacterial, mycotic, or parasitic lung infections. Recurrent pneumonitis, sinus infections, and chronic sputum production may be indicative of bronchiectasis from CF, foreign-body aspiration, ciliary dyskinesias, or other chronic lung diseases. Other aspects of the history that will help focus the evaluation include recent trauma, easy bruising, changes in urine color, weight loss, arthralgias, previous heart disease or surgery, medication use, substance abuse, family history of bleeding disorders, surgical procedures, pica, fever, pleuritic chest pain, menstrual irregularities, and asthma not responsive to appropriate medical therapy. In adolescents with unusual or perplexing symptoms and normal findings at evaluation, factitious hemoptysis and Münchausen syndrome should also be considered. Factitious hemoptysis has been reported in children who underwent numerous invasive procedures, and, ultimately, the determination was made that these children were biting their oral mucosa to simulate hemoptysis.[9,11,12]

## Physical Examination

Physical examination begins with a determination of the vital signs to decide the rapidity at which the examination should be conducted. A thorough inspection of the nasal passages and oropharynx is conducted to rule out a nonpulmonary cause of the hemoptysis. As the examination proceeds caudally, certain findings on inspection and auscultation may suggest a specific diagnosis. Cutaneous telangiectases with a murmur or bruit over the lung fields suggest hereditary hemorrhagic telangiectasia (Rendu-Osler-Weber syndrome). Clubbing with or without adventitial breath sounds suggests bronchiectasis. A saddle nose and stridor suggestive of subglottic stenosis are often seen in patients with necrotizing granulomatous vasculitis. A pleuritic rub, acute pleuritic chest pain, and a history of oral contraceptive use or recent abortion suggest a pulmonary embolic event or other pleural-based lesion. Localized homophonous wheezing over a major airway or decreased breath sounds, with or without a cough, suggest an intraluminal obstruction such as an aspirated foreign body. Evidence of trauma to the thorax may be subtle and not always obvious. Thirty percent of children who experience major trauma to other organ systems will be found to have thoracic trauma as well.[13] Examination of the heart may provide evidence of pulmonary hypertension or a new murmur. Lymphadenopathy and hepatosplenomegaly should raise the possibility of a lymphoproliferative disease with an associated bleeding diathesis.

### Laboratory Evaluation

Numerous laboratory tests may be helpful, but they should be focused depending on the history and physical examination. If the patient has a compromised airway, then arterial blood gas measurement may help in the decision of how quickly the intensive care unit needs to be called. Urinalysis or specific serologic markers will help determine if the child has an immunologic disease that involves the basement membranes of both the kidneys and the lungs. A complete blood count with an eosinophil count may help differentiate a bacterial from a parasitic pneumonia. Although clotting studies are routinely ordered, they will invariably be normal because bleeding disorders do not generally cause spontaneous hemoptysis. Although skin tests for mycobacteria should always be performed, other skin tests, or serologic testing for fungi or other infectious agents, should be guided by clinical acumen. If sputum is produced or bronchoscopy is performed, then these pulmonary fluids should be cultured for bacteria, fungi, ova, parasites, and mycobacteria and stained for the presence of hemosiderin-laden macrophages. If warranted, early-morning gastric aspirates can be cultured and stained for microorganisms and macrophages.

### Imaging Studies

The history and physical examination should allow a tentative diagnosis and help decide what imaging studies or procedures need to be undertaken to make a definitive diagnosis. If the child is stable, then a chest radiograph should be obtained. Any abnormality on a chest film should be considered as a potential source for the hemoptysis, but a normal radiograph does not exclude the thorax as the source of bleeding. In approximately one-third of children with hemoptysis, the initial chest radiographic examination will reveal nothing abnormal.[14] Findings on the chest film that help focus the evaluation include hilar adenopathy, an air-fluid level in an abscess, a mass, a cavitary lesion, mediastinal widening, or alveolar infiltrates. Alveolar infiltrates in a child with hemoptysis are a common finding with autoimmune diseases that involve the lungs. Thickening of the bronchial walls with ring shadows and tramlines suggests bronchiectasis. If a foreign body is suspected to be the cause, then inspiratory and expiratory films or left and right lateral decubitus films may help localize the foreign body. If the foreign body is present and causes obstruction of an airway, then the side of the thorax that does not deflate normally on expiration or when dependent is the side with the foreign body. If the foreign body is embedded within the mucosa of the airway, or if only partial obstruction is present, then the standard chest radiograph may be normal.

The next imaging studies depend on the presumptive diagnosis because not every child with hemoptysis needs special radiographic studies. If the chest radiograph is normal or does not add any information to that obtained from the history and physical examination, then computed tomography (CT) or high-resolution computed tomography (HRCT) may be contributive. CT is effective for detecting parenchymal disease, and HRCT has replaced bronchography for diagnosing bronchiectasis. CT can identify airway abnormalities, elucidate abnormalities seen on chest radiographs, define mediastinal structures, and help categorize congenital pulmonary malformations and pulmonary vasculitis syndromes. CT may also serve as a road map for subsequent bronchoscopy.

Magnetic resonance imaging (MRI) is useful in looking for congenital vascular malformations and for the differentiation of structures within the mediastinum and hilum. Perhaps in the future MRI will supplant CT in the evaluation of hemoptysis, but for now the advantages of MRI do not outweigh its disadvantages, especially if excessive respiratory motion is present or the child's condition is unstable.

### *Bronchoscopy*

The timing and need for bronchoscopy, either rigid or flexible, depend on the stability of the child's condition and the suspected cause of the hemoptysis. Not every child with hemoptysis needs to undergo bronchoscopy; research indicates that hemoptysis is rarely the primary indication for bronchoscopy.[9] If a child has rapid and complete resolution of hemoptysis after medical therapy, then bronchoscopy need not be performed. Indications for bronchoscopy include a diagnosis that is in question, massive hemoptysis, or an incomplete response to therapy.

No studies have compared the use of fiberoptic versus rigid bronchoscopy for evaluating hemoptysis in either adults or children. Both instruments can be used to administer therapeutic agents to the airways, sample bronchial fluids, and take biopsy samples. With the rigid bronchoscope, bronchoscopists have complete airway control: they can suction through a larger channel, sample suspicious lesions, and insert packing material to tamponade the bleeding. The rigid bronchoscope is the preferred instrument for removing foreign bodies from the airway. On the other hand, fiberoptic bronchoscopy does not require the use of general anesthesia; the scope is usually passed transnasally (so that the upper airways can also be examined), and it can be easily maneuvered into the upper lobes and more distal airways. If a child with hemoptysis needs bronchoscopy, then fiberoptic bronchoscopy may be used for the initial evaluation. If an anatomic lesion or foreign body is discovered, then rigid bronchoscopy will be needed.

## ▶ HEMOPTYSIS IN THE NEWBORN PERIOD

Neonates who have a variety of congenital defects can develop localized hemoptysis and diffuse pulmonary hemorrhage in the newborn period. Arteriovenous malformations, extralobar sequestration, or hereditary hemorrhagic telangiectasia (Rendu-Osler-Weber syndrome) can exhibit in the nursery as respiratory distress or mild to massive hemoptysis. All of these vascular malformations cause bleeding as a result of the abnormal connections between the bronchial and pulmonary circulations. The diagnosis of these lesions is made by CT scan with contrast, and children with these defects need to be hospitalized in a center that has a pediatric surgeon and an interventional radiologist.

Diffuse pulmonary hemorrhage is not an uncommon occurrence in infants of very low birth weight. The more premature the infant, the higher is the likelihood of hemorrhage. The pathogenesis of the diffuse bleeding is thought to be from effects of barotrauma on an immature pulmonary capillary endothelium. The risk for pulmonary hemorrhage increases slightly with the administration of exogenous surfactant therapy. Many nonpulmonary conditions have also been associated with diffuse hemorrhage in premature newborns, including central nervous system insults and coagulation and metabolic defects.[14]

## When to Admit

- Evidence of hemodynamic instability
- Mental status changes
- High suspicion of tuberculosis
- Known heart disease
- Chronic lung disease (eg, CF, ciliary dyskinesias, immunodeficiencies)
- High suspicion of pulmonary neoplasm
- Sickle cell anemia, vaso-occlusive crisis, or acute chest syndrome
- Inability to protect airway
- Risk for pulmonary embolism
- Lung abscess
- Children younger than 1 year
- Foreign-body aspiration
- Pulmonary hypertension

### REFERENCES


1. Coss-Bu JA, Sachdeva RC, Bricker JT, Harrison GM, Jefferson LS. Hemoptysis: a 10-year retrospective study. *Pediatrics.* 1997;100:E7
2. Etzel RA, Montaña E, Sorenson WG, et al. Acute pulmonary hemorrhage in infants associated with exposure to Stachybotrys atra and other fungi. *Arch Pediatr Adolesc Med.* 1998;152:757–762
3. Brown CM, Redd SC, Damon SA; Centers for Disease Control and Prevention. Acute idiopathic pulmonary hemorrhage among infants. Recommendations from the Working Group for Investigation and Surveillance. *MMWR Recomm Rep.* 2004;53:1–12
4. Dore ND, Landau LI, Hallam L, Le Souef PN. Haemoptysis in healthy children due to unsuspected foreign body. *J Paediatr Child Health.* 1997;33:448–450
5. Pyman C. Inhaled foreign bodies in childhood. A review of 230 cases. *Med J Aust.* 1971;1:62–68
6. Heiner DC, Sears JW, Kniker WT. Multiple precipitins to cow's milk in chronic respiratory disease. A syndrome including poor growth, gastrointestinal symptoms, evidence of allergy, iron deficiency anemia, and pulmonary hemosiderosis. *Am J Dis Child.* 1962;103:634–654
7. Hancock BJ, Di Lorenzo M, Youssef S, et al. Childhood primary pulmonary neoplasms. *J Pediatr Surg.* 1993;28:1133–1136
8. Fabian MC, Smitheringale A. Hemoptysis in children: the hospital for sick children experience. *J Otolaryngol.* 1996;25:44–45
9. Godfrey S. Pulmonary hemorrhage/hemoptysis in children. *Pediatr Pulmonol.* 2004;37:476–484
10. Tom LW, Weisman RA, Handler SD. Hemoptysis in children. *Ann Otol Rhinol Laryngol.* 1980;89:419–424
11. Batra PS, Holinger LD. Etiology and management of pediatric hemoptysis. *Arch Otolaryngol Head Neck Surg.* 2001;127:377–382
12. Sood M, Clarke J, Murphy M. Covert biting of the buccal mucosa masquerading as haemoptysis in children. *Acta Pediatr.* 1999;88:1038–1040
13. Sinclair MC, Moore TC. Major surgery for abdominal and thoracic trauma in childhood and adolescence. *J Pediatr Surg.* 1974;9:155–162
14. Pianosi P, al-sadoon H. Hemoptysis in children. *Pediatr Rev.* 1996;17:344–348

# Chapter 39

# Hepatomegaly

*Philip O. Ozuah, MD, PhD; Marina Reznik, MD, MS*

## ▶ DEFINITIONS AND CLINICAL MANIFESTATIONS

Hepatomegaly is an enlargement of the liver resulting from an increase in the number or size of cells and structures within the liver. Although hepatomegaly usually manifests clinically as a palpable liver, not all palpable livers result from hepatomegaly. In healthy children, the liver edge may be palpable up to 2 cm below the right costal margin at the midclavicular line. Clinical estimation of the liver span has a much stronger correlation with hepatomegaly than does reporting the liver projection below the costal margin as a single indicator of liver size.[1] The liver span is the distance between the upper and lower margins of the liver at the right midclavicular line. The upper margin should be determined by percussion and the lower edge by either percussion or palpation. Liver span has a curvilinear relation to age, height, weight, and body surface area.[2–4] Studies have demonstrated no consistent sex differences in liver size.[5–8] A normal liver span ranges from 5.9 cm (±0.8 cm) in the first week of life to 6.5 to 8 cm by 15 years of age.[1–3] The upper edge of liver dullness is usually at the level of the fifth rib in the right midclavicular line. Radiographic assessment of liver size can be a helpful adjunct to the clinical examination. Ultrasonography, computed tomography (CT), magnetic resonance imaging (MRI), and sulfur colloid scintigraphy have all been demonstrated to measure liver size reliably.[5–13]

## ▶ DIFFERENTIAL DIAGNOSIS

The differential diagnoses of a palpable liver and hepatomegaly are presented in Box 39-1.

### *Palpable Liver Without Hepatomegaly*

Several intrathoracic conditions may push the right hemidiaphragm down and thereby result in a palpable liver. For example, asthma, bronchiolitis, and pneumonitis may produce a palpable liver through hyperinflation of the lungs. Tension pneumothorax usually has other accompanying clinical features, including dyspnea, tachycardia, tracheal deviation, and hypotension. Congenital diaphragmatic hernias often manifest in the neonatal period with a scaphoid abdomen and the presence of bowel sounds in the chest. Other thoracic space–occupying lesions also can displace the diaphragm.

Abdominal sepsis with a subdiaphragmatic abscess may push the liver caudally. Riedel lobe is an occasional tonguelike process extending downward from the right lobe of the liver lateral to the gallbladder. A palpable liver without hepatomegaly also may be a normal variant.

BOX 39-1

## *Differential Diagnosis of a Palpable Liver Without Hepatomegaly and With Hepatomegaly*

**PALPABLE LIVER WITHOUT HEPATOMEGALY**

- Downward displacement of right hemidiaphragm
  - Hyperinflated lung (eg, asthma, bronchiolitis, pneumonitis)
  - Tension pneumothorax
  - Congenital diaphragmatic hernia
  - Thoracic tumors
- Subdiaphragmatic lesions (eg, abscess)
- Normal variant
- Aberrant lobe of liver (Riedel lobe)

**PALPABLE LIVER WITH HEPATOMEGALY**

- Inflammatory disorders
  - Viral hepatitis
  - Bacterial hepatitis (eg, abscess, sepsis)
  - Toxic hepatitis (eg, drugs)
  - Neonatal hepatitis
  - Autoimmune hepatitis (eg, systemic lupus erythematosus, sarcoidosis)
- Infiltrative disorders
  - Primary tumors
    - Hepatoblastoma
    - Hepatocellular carcinoma
    - Hemangioma
    - Focal nodular hyperplasia
  - Metastatic tumors
    - Lymphoma
    - Leukemia
    - Neuroblastoma
    - Wilms tumor
    - Histiocytosis
- Storage disorders
  - Fat accumulation
    - Obesity
    - Malnutrition
    - Reye syndrome
    - Cystic fibrosis
    - Diabetes mellitus
    - Lipid infusion
    - Metabolic liver disease
    - Lipidoses (eg, Niemann-Pick, Gaucher, Wolman diseases)
  - Glycogen excess
    - Glycogen storage diseases
    - Infant of mother who has diabetes
    - Beckwith-Wiedemann syndrome
    - Total parenteral nutrition
  - Copper accumulation
    - Indian childhood cirrhosis
    - Wilson disease
  - Miscellaneous
    - $\alpha_1$-Antitrypsin deficiency
    - Hypervitaminosis A
- Vascular congestion
  - Suprahepatic
    - Congestive heart failure
    - Cardiac tamponade
    - Constrictive pericarditis
  - Intrahepatic
    - Hepatic vein thrombosis (Budd-Chiari syndrome)
    - Hepatic vein web
    - Vascular malformations
      - Cavernous hemangioma
      - Capillary hemangioma
      - Hemangioendothelioma
- Biliary obstruction
  - Congenital biliary atresia
  - Congenital hepatic fibrosis
  - Caroli disease

### *Palpable Liver With Hepatomegaly*

#### Inflammatory Disorders

Inflammatory liver disorders frequently manifest clinically with jaundice and a liver that is firm and tender to palpation. Viral hepatitis (including hepatitis A, B, C, D, and E) may be fulminant or insidious in onset. Hepatitis A may be anicteric in 50% of infected children younger than 4 years and in more than 80% of children younger than 2 years.[14]

Bacterial sepsis may result in hepatomegaly as part of a generalized process or a localized liver abscess.[15,16] Toxic hepatitis may result from exposure to a variety of therapeutic and other chemical agents. Idiopathic neonatal hepatitis occurs with direct hyperbilirubinemia and may be difficult to distinguish clinically from congenital biliary atresia without a liver biopsy.[17] Idiopathic neonatal hepatitis is characterized by marked infiltration with inflammatory cells in contrast to bile duct proliferation found in biliary atresia. Giant cell transformation is found in both conditions. In rare instances, autoimmune diseases such as systemic lupus erythematosus and sarcoidosis may involve the liver, leading to a hepatitis with hepatomegaly.

## Infiltrative Disorders

Primary or metastatic neoplasia may infiltrate the liver and is often associated with other clinical findings. Malignant hepatic tumors manifest clinically with a hard, palpable liver. Benign tumors include large hemangiomas, which occasionally lead to a platelet consumption coagulopathy (Kasabach-Merritt syndrome) as a result of excessive trapping and destruction of platelets within the vascular bed. Clinically, a bruit may be heard over the liver in patients who have hemangiomas and arteriovenous shunts.

## Storage Disorders

Several genetic enzyme defects result in excessive accumulation of metabolites in the liver. These conditions produce a smooth, distended liver. Many of these syndromes are also associated with other clinical features besides hepatomegaly. Fat and glycogen accumulation are well-known causes of hepatomegaly.[18,19] Less frequently, copper accumulation results in Indian childhood cirrhosis or Wilson disease.[20–27] Indian childhood cirrhosis, caused by genetic and environmental factors, produces jaundice and hepatomegaly predominantly in middle-income, rural Hindu children, but it also has been described in other parts of the world.[24,25] Its onset is at approximately 1 to 3 years of age, usually with rapid evolution to cirrhosis and hepatic failure if left untreated. This disorder was previously thought to be uniformly fatal, but chelation therapy has shown promising results. Wilson disease, an autosomal recessive inherited disorder of copper metabolism, occurs with hepatomegaly in young children but does not generally manifest clinically until after 5 years of age. Children older than 10 years often have neuropsychiatric symptoms; they may also have hemolytic anemia.[28] $\alpha_1$-Antitrypsin deficiency may occur with hepatomegaly, icterus, and acholic stools in the first week of life. Signs of chronic liver disease and portal hypertension are seen in older children. Excessive ingestion and accumulation of vitamin A can also result in hepatomegaly.

## Vascular Congestion

Congestive heart failure, cardiac tamponade, and constrictive pericarditis all lead to impaired cardiac filling and pressure backup into the inferior vena cava and portal vein, all of which produce a smooth, distended, and tender liver. Other signs of cardiac decompensation, including dyspnea, cough, chest pain, and tachycardia, are usually present.

Budd-Chiari syndrome may be caused by a thrombus, mass, or web occluding the inferior vena cava or the hepatic veins and tributaries, resulting in an enlarged liver.

Vascular malformations produce hepatomegaly through several mechanisms, including hemorrhage into the liver or high-output cardiac failure with secondary vascular congestion, or through the size of the malformation itself.

## Biliary Obstruction

Biliary atresia occurs in approximately 1 of 8,000 births and is the most frequent reason for liver transplantation in children. The bile duct atresia may be extrahepatic, intrahepatic, or a combination thereof. The presence of jaundice, hepatomegaly, and acholic stools beginning during the first months of life in otherwise healthy-appearing infants is characteristic.[29] Extrahepatic atresia can be corrected surgically, and intrahepatic atresia can be treated using the hepatoportoenterostomy procedure of Kasai.[30] Nevertheless, many patients develop cirrhosis and portal hypertension requiring liver transplantation.[30]

Congenital hepatic fibrosis is an autosomal recessive disorder that occurs in childhood with hepatosplenomegaly, portal hypertension, and bleeding esophageal varices. Up to 75% of affected children have associated renal disease. Histologic analysis reveals diffuse periportal and perilobular fibrosis. Caroli disease is a congenital saccular dilation of intrahepatic bile ducts that is inherited in an autosomal recessive fashion. Symptoms are usually those of acute cholangitis manifesting in late childhood or young adulthood, with fever, icterus, abdominal pain, and a large, tender liver.

# ▶ EVALUATION

## *Relevant History and Physical Examination*

History and physical examination remain the cornerstone of establishing a prompt diagnosis in patients with hepatomegaly. A thorough history that explores not only gastrointestinal symptoms but also pulmonary and cardiac manifestations will often point in the right diagnostic direction. Physical examination of the liver should include an assessment of its size, consistency, texture, and tenderness. In addition, the liver should be auscultated with a stethoscope.

A firm and tender liver suggests an acute inflammatory disorder; a hard liver is often neoplastic. A smooth and exquisitely tender liver is found in conditions that cause vascular distention. Bruits are heard in arteriovenous malformations. Although a palpable liver may be a normal variant, the concomitant physical finding of an enlarged spleen usually suggests significant disease.

## *Laboratory Testing and Imaging*

Laboratory investigations should be directed at the suspected diagnosis. Liver function studies are usually necessary. The imaging study used most widely is ultrasonography, which is inexpensive, portable, reliable, and quickly obtainable in most settings. Liver masses detected on ultrasonography may be defined further by CT scanning or sulfur colloid scintigraphy. Hepatic angiography may be indicated in the evaluation of suspected vascular tumors. In patients with probable metabolic or genetic disorders, a percutaneous liver biopsy may be necessary to establish a diagnosis. In addition, the definitive diagnosis of a liver abscess can be made by ultrasound or CT-guided percutaneous liver aspiration.[31]

# ▶ MANAGEMENT

Treatment should be aimed at the underlying disease entity. Patients with inflammatory hepatitis require supportive care; those who have bacterial infections should receive appropriate antimicrobials. Surgical excision is the definitive treatment for liver tumors.

Chemotherapy may be a helpful adjunct in reducing tumor size either preoperatively or postoperatively.

The treatment of metabolic-genetic disorders includes dietary modifications and chelation therapy. Frequent small feedings of a high-protein, complex-carbohydrate diet, including continuous nighttime feeding via gastrostomy tubes, have been used successfully in managing glycogen storage disorders. Early treatment with D-penicillamine can prevent the progression of Wilson disease. In many cases, the use of zinc acetate has been approved by the US Food and Drug Administration (FDA) for maintenance therapy of patients with Wilson disease, even if presymptomatic.[32,33]

Exciting new developments have provided optimism for some disease entities for which no treatments were available in the past. For example, a synthetic enzyme, imiglucerase, has been highly effective in the treatment of Gaucher disease.[34] Other recombinant glucocerebrosidases, recently approved by the FDA or pending approval, include vela-glucerase alpha (Shire HGT, Cambridge, MA, USA) and taliglucerase alpha (Protalix Biotherapeutics, Carmiel, Israel; Pfizer, NY, USA). Both successfully completed phase III trials and were proved safe and clinically efficient in the treatment of Gaucher disease.[35,36] Although Indian childhood cirrhosis was previously thought to be uniformly fatal, chelation therapy with D-penicillamine has been shown to reduce mortality significantly if administered early in the disease.[37,38]

## When to Refer

- Hepatomegaly with concomitant splenomegaly
- Palpation of a hard liver
- Hepatomegaly with distended abdominal veins
- Audible bruit over the liver
- Suspicion of malignancy

## When to Admit

- Liver failure
- Impending liver failure

### REFERENCES


1. Reiff MI, Osborn LM. Clinical estimation of liver size in newborn infants. *Pediatrics.* 1983;71(1):46–48
2. Carpentieri U, Gustavson LP, Leach TM, Bunce H. Liver size in normal infants and children. *South Med J.* 1977;70(9):1096–1097
3. Lawson EE, Grand RJ, Neff RK, Cohen LF. Clinical estimation of liver span in infants and children. *Am J Dis Child.* 1978;132(5):474–476
4. Dhingra B, Sharma S, Mishra D, et al. Normal values of liver and spleen size by ultrasonography in Indian children. *Indian Pediatr.* 2010;47(6):487–492
5. Friis H, Ndhlovu P, Mduluza T, et al. Ultrasonographic organometry: liver and spleen dimensions among children in Zimbabwe. *Trop Med Int Health.* 1996;1(2):183–190
6. Johnson TN, Tucker GT, Tanner MS, Rostami-Hodjegan A. Changes in liver volume from birth to adulthood: a meta-analysis. *Liver Transpl.* 2005;11(12):1481–1493
7. Safak AA, Simsek E, Bahcebasi T. Sonographic assessment of the normal limits and percentile curves of liver, spleen, and kidney dimensions in healthy school-aged children. *J Ultrasound Med.* 2005;24(10):1359–1364

8. Konus OL, Ozdemir A, Akkaya A, et al. Normal liver, spleen, and kidney dimensions in neonates, infants, and children: evaluation with sonography. *AJR Am J Roentgenol.* 1998;171(6):1693–1698
9. Holmes J, Sundgren C, Ikle D, Finch J. A simple ultrasonic method for evaluating liver size. *J Clin Ultrasound.* 1977;5(2):89–91
10. Markisz JA, Treves ST, Davis RT. Normal hepatic and splenic size in children: scintigraphic determination. *Pediatr Radiol.* 1987;17(4):273–276
11. Niederau C, Sonnenberg A, Müller JE et al. Sonographic measurements of the normal liver, spleen, pancreas, and portal vein. *Radiology.* 1983;149(2):537–540
12. Noda T, Todani T, Watanabe Y, Yamamoto S. Liver volume in children measured by computed tomography. *Pediatr Radiol.* 1997;27(3):250–252
13. Mazonakis M, Damilakis J, Maris T, Prassopoulos P, Gourtsoyiannis N. Comparison of two volumetric techniques for estimating liver volume using magnetic resonance imaging. *J Magn Reson Imaging.* 2002;15(5):557–563
14. Hadler SC, Webster HM, Erben JJ, Swanson JE, Maynard JE. Hepatitis A in day-care centers. A community-wide assessment. *N Engl J Med.* 1980;302(22):1222–1227
15. Brook I, Frazier EH. Microbiology of liver and spleen abscesses. *J Med Microbiol.* 1998;47(12):1075–1080
16. Simeunovic E, Arnold M, Sidler D, Moore SW. Liver abscess in neonates. *Pediatr Surg Int.* 2009;25(2):153–156
17. Yang JG, Ma DQ, Peng Y, Song L, Li CL. Comparison of different diagnostic methods for differentiating biliary atresia from idiopathic neonatal hepatitis. *Clin Imaging.* 2009;33(6):439–446
18. Fishbein M, Mogren J, Mogren C, Cox S, Jennings R. Undetected hepatomegaly in obese children by primary care physicians: a pitfall in the diagnosis of pediatric nonalcoholic fatty liver disease. *Clin Pediatr (Phila).* 2005;44(2):135–141
19. Ozen H. Glycogen storage diseases: new perspectives. *World J Gastroenterol.* 2007;13(18):2541–2553
20. Baker A, Gormally S, Saxena R, et al. Copper-associated liver disease in childhood. *J Hepatol.* 1995;23(5):538–543
21. Pandit A, Bhave S. Present interpretation of the role of copper in Indian childhood cirrhosis. *Am J Clin Nutr.* 1996;63(5):830S–835S
22. Petrukhin K, Gilliam TC. Genetic disorders of copper metabolism. *Curr Opin Pediatr.* 1994;6(6):698–701
23. Prasad R, Kaur G, Nath R, Walia BN. Molecular basis of pathophysiology of Indian childhood cirrhosis: role of nuclear copper accumulation in liver. *Mol Cell Biochem.* 1996;156(1):25–30
24. Tanner MS. Role of copper in Indian childhood cirrhosis. *Am J Clin Nutr.* 1998;67(5 Suppl):1074S–1081S
25. Pankit AN, Bhave SA. Copper metabolic defects and liver disease: environmental aspects. *J Gastroenterol Hepatol.* 2002;17(Suppl 3):S403–S407
26. Bruha R, Marecek Z, Pospisilova L, et al. Long-term follow-up of Wilson disease: natural history, treatment, mutations analysis and phenotypic correlation. *Liver Int.* 2011;3(1):83–91
27. Schilsky ML. Wilson disease: current status and the future. *Biochimie.* 2009;91(10):1278–1281
28. Huster D. Wilson disease. *Best Pract Res Clin Gastroenterol.* 2010;24(5):531–539
29. Lee WS, Chai PF. Clinical features differentiating biliary atresia from other causes of neonatal cholestasis. *Ann Acad Med Singapore.* 2010;39(8):648–654
30. Khalil BA, Perera MT, Mirza DF. Clinical practice: management of biliary atresia. *Eur J Pediatr.* 2010;169(4):395–402
31. Men S, Akhan O, Köroglu M. Percutaneous drainage of abdominal abscess. *Eur J Radiol.* 2002;43(3):204–218
32. Marcellini M, Di Ciommo V, Callea F, et al. Treatment of Wilson's disease with zinc from the time of diagnosis in pediatric patients: a single-hospital, 10-year follow-up study. *J Lab Clin Med.* 2005;145(3):139–143
33. Wiggelinkhuizen M, Tilanus ME, Bollen CW, Houwen RH. Systematic review: clinical efficacy of chelator agents and zinc in the initial treatment of Wilson disease. *Aliment Pharmacol Ther.* 2009;29(9):947–958
34. Mistry P, Germain DP. Therapeutic goals in Gaucher disease. *Rev Med Interne.* 2006:27(Suppl 1):S30–S38
35. Goker-Alpan O. Optimal therapy in Gaucher disease. *Ther Clin Risk Manag.* 2010;6:315–323

36. Cox TM. Gaucher disease: clinical profile and therapeutic developments. *Biologics.* 2010;4:299–313
37. Bavdekar AR, Bhave SA, Pradhan AM, Pandit AN, Tanner MS. Long term survival in Indian childhood cirrhosis treated with D-penicillamine. *Arch Dis Child.* 1996;74(1):32–35
38. Pradhan AM, Bhave SA, Joshi VV, et al. Reversal of Indian childhood cirrhosis by D-penicillamine therapy. *J Pediatr Gastroenterol Nutr.* 1995;20(1):28–35

# Chapter 40

# High Blood Pressure

*Jayanthi Chandar, MD; Sarah E. Messiah, PhD, MPH; Gaston Zilleruelo, MD; Steven E. Lipshultz, MD*

Hypertension is a well-established cause of substantial morbidity and mortality in adults, particularly in the later years of life.[1,2] However, recent population-based studies have shown that during the past decade, mean blood pressure (BP) has increased among children and adolescents.[3,4] Furthermore, recent longitudinal cohort studies have revealed that elevated BP in childhood often continues into adulthood, predicting hypertension in young adulthood, and other studies have documented the familial nature of essential hypertension.[5-7]

Even mild to moderate elevations of BP in children almost certainly warrant close attention, lifestyle modifications, and possibly therapy. Mild and moderate levels of hypertension in childhood are generally not associated with marked symptoms, but routine screening will identify a fair number of children who have either primary or secondary hypertension. Definitive therapy can decrease later morbidity. All pediatricians should be familiar with the basic aspects of hypertension in children, including the diagnosis of normal and abnormal BP, the causes of high BP, and the treatment options.[2,8,9]

## ▶ DEFINITION OF HIGH BLOOD PRESSURE IN CHILDREN

The fourth report by the National Heart, Lung, and Blood Institute Task Force on Blood Pressure Control in Children based operational definitions of high BP in children on a combination of values found in healthy children, clinical experience, and consensus among leaders in the field.[2] In children and adolescents, hypertension is defined as an elevated BP that persists on repeated measurements at the 95th percentile or greater for age, height, and sex in a healthy population.[2,8] Stage 1 hypertension is defined as systolic and diastolic blood pressures that range from about the 95th percentile to 5 mm Hg above the 99th percentile, and stage 2 hypertension refers to systolic and diastolic blood pressures that are 5 mm Hg above the 99th percentile for age, height, and gender.[2] High-normal or prehypertensive BP is defined as a BP between the 90th and 95th percentiles (normal systolic and diastolic BPs are less than the 90th percentile). Severe hypertension (with the risk of end-organ injury) is defined as BP greater than the 99th percentile.[2,8]

Body size is the single most important determinant of BP in children and adolescents; thus, using accurate height percentiles is critical for correctly estimating BP percentiles (Figure 40-1 and Tables 40-1 and 40-2).

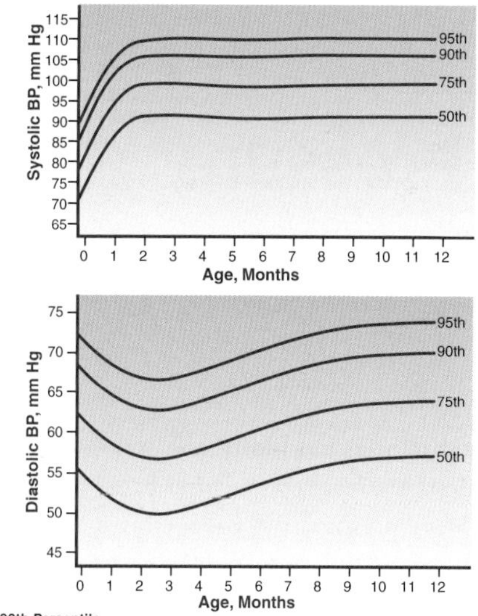


**90th Percentile**

| | | | | | | | | | | | | | |
|---|---|---|---|---|---|---|---|---|---|---|---|---|---|
| Systolic BP | 87 | 101 | 106 | 106 | 106 | 105 | 105 | 105 | 105 | 105 | 105 | 105 | 106 |
| Diastolic BP | 68 | 65 | 63 | 63 | 63 | 65 | 66 | 67 | 68 | 68 | 69 | 69 | 69 |
| Height (cm) | 51 | 58 | 63 | 66 | 68 | 70 | 72 | 73 | 74 | 76 | 77 | 78 | 80 |
| Weight (kg) | 4 | 4 | 5 | 5 | 6 | 7 | 8 | 9 | 9 | 10 | 10 | 11 | 11 |

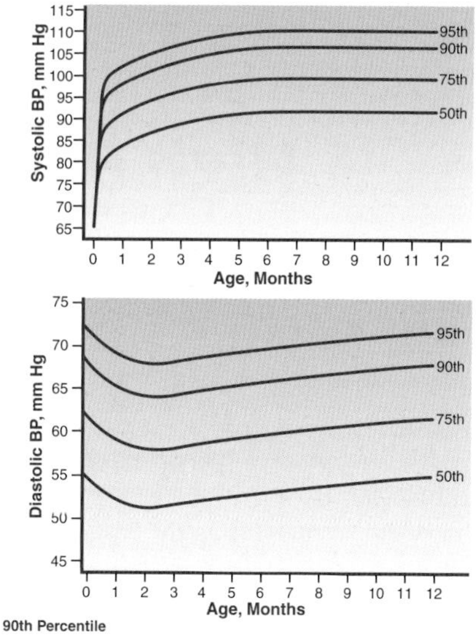


**90th Percentile**

| | | | | | | | | | | | | | |
|---|---|---|---|---|---|---|---|---|---|---|---|---|---|
| Systolic BP | 76 | 98 | 101 | 104 | 105 | 106 | 106 | 106 | 106 | 106 | 108 | 105 | 105 |
| Diastolic BP | 68 | 65 | 64 | 64 | 65 | 65 | 66 | 66 | 66 | 67 | 67 | 67 | 67 |
| Height (cm) | 54 | 55 | 56 | 58 | 61 | 63 | 66 | 68 | 70 | 72 | 74 | 75 | 77 |
| Weight (kg) | 4 | 4 | 4 | 5 | 5 | 6 | 7 | 8 | 9 | 9 | 10 | 10 | 11 |

**Figure 40-1**

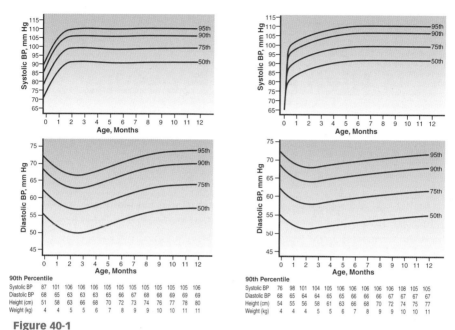

Age-, sex-, height-, and weight-specific percentiles of systolic and diastolic blood pressure in boys *(left)* and girls *(right)* from birth to 12 months of age.

## ▶ FACTORS INFLUENCING BLOOD PRESSURE IN CHILDREN

### *Age*

BP tends to increase throughout the first 2 decades of life.[10,11] The average systolic BP on the first day of life is 70 mm Hg, and it increases steadily for the next 2 months. It then tends to remain stable until 1 year of age, when it increases until adulthood. Diastolic BP increases slowly for the first week and then declines until 3 months of age. It then increases gradually until 1 year of age, when it returns to the level found in the first week. It again remains steady for the first 5 to 6 years, after which it begins to increase, along with systolic BP.[10,11] Children tend to maintain the same BP percentile rank relative to their peers as they grow, a pattern that continues through adolescence, supporting the idea that primary hypertension begins in childhood. Normative data have been derived in premature infants in whom the average systolic BP is lower and increases with gestational age.[12-14]

### *Body Size*

Body size is a major influence on BP in children.[15] As in adults, the relationship between BP and weight in the teenage years is particularly prominent.[16,17] Height is also related independently to BP at all ages.[2,10] However, chronic hypertension is becoming increasingly common in adolescents, primarily because of increases in the prevalence of overweight and obesity. During the past 3 decades, obesity rates have more than doubled for children ages 2 to 5 and 12 to 19 years, and the rates have more than tripled among children ages 6 to 11 years.[18] Presently in the United States, 9 million children older than 6 years are considered obese, with a body mass index (BMI) above the 95th percentile.[19,20]

### Table 40-1
## Blood Pressure and Height Percentiles for Boys by Age

| | | SYSTOLIC BP (mm Hg) | | | | | | | DIASTOLIC BP (mm Hg) | | | | | | |
|---|---|---|---|---|---|---|---|---|---|---|---|---|---|---|---|
| | | PERCENTILE OF HEIGHT | | | | | | | PERCENTILE OF HEIGHT | | | | | | |
| AGE (yr) | BP PERCENTILE* | 5 | 10 | 25 | 50 | 75 | 90 | 95 | 5 | 10 | 25 | 50 | 75 | 90 | 95 |
| 1 | 50 | 80 | 81 | 83 | 85 | 87 | 88 | 89 | 34 | 35 | 36 | 37 | 38 | 39 | 39 |
| | 90 | 94 | 95 | 97 | 99 | 100 | 102 | 103 | 49 | 50 | 51 | 52 | 53 | 53 | 54 |
| | 95 | 98 | 99 | 101 | 103 | 104 | 106 | 106 | 54 | 54 | 55 | 56 | 57 | 58 | 58 |
| | 99 | 105 | 106 | 108 | 110 | 112 | 113 | 114 | 61 | 62 | 63 | 64 | 65 | 66 | 66 |
| 2 | 50 | 84 | 85 | 87 | 88 | 90 | 92 | 92 | 39 | 40 | 41 | 42 | 43 | 44 | 44 |
| | 90 | 97 | 99 | 100 | 102 | 104 | 105 | 106 | 54 | 55 | 56 | 57 | 58 | 58 | 59 |
| | 95 | 101 | 102 | 104 | 106 | 108 | 109 | 110 | 59 | 59 | 60 | 61 | 62 | 63 | 63 |
| | 99 | 109 | 110 | 111 | 113 | 115 | 117 | 117 | 66 | 67 | 68 | 69 | 70 | 71 | 71 |
| 3 | 50 | 86 | 87 | 89 | 91 | 93 | 94 | 95 | 44 | 44 | 45 | 46 | 47 | 48 | 48 |
| | 90 | 100 | 101 | 103 | 105 | 107 | 108 | 109 | 59 | 59 | 60 | 61 | 62 | 63 | 63 |
| | 95 | 104 | 105 | 107 | 109 | 110 | 112 | 113 | 63 | 63 | 64 | 65 | 66 | 67 | 67 |
| | 99 | 111 | 112 | 114 | 116 | 118 | 119 | 120 | 71 | 71 | 72 | 73 | 74 | 75 | 75 |
| 4 | 50 | 88 | 89 | 91 | 93 | 95 | 96 | 97 | 47 | 48 | 49 | 50 | 51 | 51 | 52 |
| | 90 | 102 | 103 | 105 | 107 | 109 | 110 | 111 | 62 | 63 | 64 | 65 | 66 | 66 | 67 |
| | 95 | 106 | 107 | 109 | 111 | 112 | 114 | 115 | 66 | 67 | 68 | 69 | 70 | 71 | 71 |
| | 99 | 113 | 114 | 116 | 118 | 120 | 121 | 122 | 74 | 75 | 76 | 77 | 78 | 78 | 79 |
| 5 | 50 | 90 | 91 | 93 | 95 | 96 | 98 | 98 | 50 | 51 | 52 | 53 | 54 | 55 | 55 |
| | 90 | 104 | 105 | 106 | 108 | 110 | 111 | 112 | 65 | 66 | 67 | 68 | 69 | 69 | 70 |
| | 95 | 108 | 109 | 110 | 112 | 114 | 115 | 116 | 69 | 70 | 71 | 72 | 73 | 74 | 74 |

*Continued*

### Table 40-1
## Blood Pressure and Height Percentiles for Boys by Age—cont'd

| | | SYSTOLIC BP (mm Hg) | | | | | | | DIASTOLIC BP (mm Hg) | | | | | | |
|---|---|---|---|---|---|---|---|---|---|---|---|---|---|---|---|
| | | PERCENTILE OF HEIGHT | | | | | | | PERCENTILE OF HEIGHT | | | | | | |
| AGE (yr) | BP PERCENTILE* | 5 | 10 | 25 | 50 | 75 | 90 | 95 | 5 | 10 | 25 | 50 | 75 | 90 | 95 |
| | 99 | 115 | 116 | 118 | 120 | 121 | 123 | 123 | 77 | 78 | 79 | 80 | 81 | 81 | 82 |
| 6 | 50 | 91 | 92 | 94 | 96 | 98 | 99 | 100 | 53 | 53 | 54 | 55 | 56 | 57 | 57 |
| | 90 | 105 | 106 | 108 | 110 | 111 | 113 | 113 | 68 | 68 | 69 | 70 | 71 | 72 | 72 |
| | 95 | 109 | 110 | 112 | 114 | 115 | 117 | 117 | 72 | 72 | 73 | 74 | 75 | 76 | 76 |
| | 99 | 116 | 117 | 119 | 121 | 123 | 124 | 125 | 80 | 80 | 81 | 82 | 83 | 84 | 84 |
| 7 | 50 | 92 | 94 | 95 | 97 | 99 | 100 | 101 | 55 | 55 | 56 | 57 | 58 | 59 | 59 |
| | 90 | 106 | 107 | 109 | 111 | 113 | 114 | 115 | 70 | 70 | 71 | 72 | 73 | 74 | 74 |
| | 95 | 110 | 111 | 113 | 115 | 117 | 118 | 119 | 74 | 74 | 75 | 76 | 77 | 78 | 78 |
| | 99 | 117 | 118 | 120 | 122 | 124 | 125 | 126 | 82 | 82 | 83 | 84 | 85 | 86 | 86 |
| 8 | 50 | 94 | 95 | 97 | 99 | 100 | 102 | 102 | 56 | 57 | 58 | 59 | 60 | 60 | 61 |
| | 90 | 107 | 109 | 110 | 112 | 114 | 115 | 116 | 71 | 72 | 72 | 73 | 74 | 75 | 76 |
| | 95 | 111 | 112 | 114 | 116 | 118 | 119 | 120 | 75 | 76 | 77 | 78 | 79 | 79 | 80 |
| | 99 | 119 | 120 | 122 | 123 | 125 | 127 | 127 | 83 | 84 | 85 | 86 | 87 | 87 | 88 |
| 9 | 50 | 95 | 96 | 98 | 100 | 102 | 103 | 104 | 57 | 58 | 59 | 60 | 61 | 61 | 62 |
| | 90 | 109 | 110 | 112 | 114 | 115 | 117 | 118 | 72 | 73 | 74 | 75 | 76 | 76 | 77 |
| | 95 | 113 | 114 | 116 | 118 | 119 | 121 | 121 | 76 | 77 | 78 | 79 | 80 | 81 | 81 |
| | 99 | 120 | 121 | 123 | 125 | 127 | 128 | 129 | 84 | 85 | 86 | 87 | 88 | 88 | 89 |
| 10 | 50 | 97 | 98 | 100 | 102 | 103 | 105 | 106 | 58 | 59 | 60 | 61 | 61 | 62 | 63 |
| | 90 | 111 | 112 | 114 | 115 | 117 | 119 | 119 | 73 | 73 | 74 | 75 | 76 | 77 | 78 |

| | | | | | | | | | | | | | | | |
|---|---|---|---|---|---|---|---|---|---|---|---|---|---|---|---|
| | 95 | 115 | 116 | 117 | 119 | 121 | 122 | 123 | 77 | 78 | 79 | 80 | 81 | 81 | 82 |
| | 99 | 122 | 123 | 125 | 127 | 128 | 130 | 130 | 85 | 86 | 86 | 88 | 88 | 89 | 90 |
| 11 | 50 | 99 | 100 | 102 | 104 | 105 | 107 | 107 | 59 | 59 | 60 | 61 | 62 | 63 | 63 |
| | 90 | 113 | 114 | 115 | 117 | 119 | 120 | 121 | 74 | 74 | 75 | 76 | 77 | 78 | 78 |
| | 95 | 117 | 118 | 119 | 121 | 123 | 124 | 125 | 78 | 78 | 79 | 80 | 81 | 82 | 82 |
| | 99 | 124 | 125 | 127 | 129 | 130 | 132 | 132 | 86 | 86 | 87 | 88 | 89 | 90 | 90 |
| 12 | 50 | 101 | 102 | 104 | 106 | 108 | 109 | 110 | 59 | 60 | 61 | 62 | 63 | 63 | 64 |
| | 90 | 115 | 116 | 118 | 120 | 121 | 123 | 123 | 74 | 75 | 75 | 76 | 77 | 78 | 79 |
| | 95 | 119 | 120 | 122 | 123 | 125 | 127 | 127 | 78 | 79 | 80 | 81 | 82 | 82 | 83 |
| | 99 | 126 | 127 | 129 | 131 | 133 | 134 | 135 | 86 | 87 | 88 | 89 | 90 | 90 | 91 |
| 13 | 50 | 104 | 105 | 106 | 108 | 110 | 111 | 112 | 60 | 60 | 61 | 62 | 63 | 64 | 64 |
| | 90 | 117 | 118 | 120 | 122 | 124 | 125 | 126 | 75 | 75 | 76 | 77 | 78 | 79 | 79 |
| | 95 | 121 | 122 | 124 | 126 | 128 | 129 | 130 | 79 | 79 | 80 | 81 | 82 | 83 | 83 |
| | 99 | 128 | 130 | 131 | 133 | 135 | 136 | 137 | 87 | 87 | 88 | 89 | 90 | 91 | 91 |
| 14 | 50 | 106 | 107 | 109 | 111 | 113 | 114 | 115 | 60 | 61 | 62 | 63 | 64 | 65 | 65 |
| | 90 | 120 | 121 | 123 | 125 | 126 | 128 | 128 | 75 | 76 | 77 | 78 | 79 | 79 | 80 |
| | 95 | 124 | 125 | 127 | 128 | 130 | 132 | 132 | 80 | 80 | 81 | 82 | 83 | 84 | 84 |
| | 99 | 131 | 132 | 134 | 136 | 138 | 139 | 140 | 87 | 88 | 89 | 90 | 91 | 92 | 92 |
| 15 | 50 | 109 | 110 | 112 | 113 | 115 | 117 | 117 | 61 | 62 | 63 | 64 | 65 | 66 | 66 |
| | 90 | 122 | 124 | 125 | 127 | 129 | 130 | 131 | 76 | 77 | 78 | 79 | 80 | 80 | 81 |
| | 95 | 126 | 127 | 129 | 131 | 133 | 134 | 135 | 81 | 81 | 82 | 83 | 84 | 85 | 85 |
| | 99 | 134 | 135 | 136 | 138 | 140 | 142 | 142 | 88 | 89 | 90 | 91 | 92 | 93 | 93 |
| 16 | 50 | 111 | 112 | 114 | 116 | 118 | 119 | 120 | 63 | 63 | 64 | 65 | 66 | 67 | 67 |
| | 90 | 125 | 126 | 128 | 130 | 131 | 133 | 134 | 78 | 78 | 79 | 80 | 81 | 82 | 82 |

*Continued*

Table 40-1

## Blood Pressure and Height Percentiles for Boys by Age—cont'd

| | | SYSTOLIC BP (mm Hg) | | | | | | | DIASTOLIC BP (mm Hg) | | | | | | |
|---|---|---|---|---|---|---|---|---|---|---|---|---|---|---|---|
| | | PERCENTILE OF HEIGHT | | | | | | | PERCENTILE OF HEIGHT | | | | | | |
| AGE (yr) | BP PERCENTILE* | 5 | 10 | 25 | 50 | 75 | 90 | 95 | 5 | 10 | 25 | 50 | 75 | 90 | 95 |
| | 95 | 129 | 130 | 132 | 134 | 135 | 137 | 137 | 82 | 83 | 83 | 84 | 85 | 86 | 87 |
| | 99 | 136 | 137 | 139 | 141 | 143 | 144 | 145 | 90 | 90 | 91 | 92 | 93 | 94 | 94 |
| 17 | 50 | 114 | 115 | 116 | 118 | 120 | 121 | 122 | 65 | 66 | 66 | 67 | 68 | 69 | 70 |
| | 90 | 127 | 128 | 130 | 132 | 134 | 135 | 136 | 80 | 80 | 81 | 82 | 83 | 84 | 84 |
| | 95 | 131 | 132 | 134 | 136 | 138 | 139 | 140 | 84 | 85 | 86 | 87 | 87 | 88 | 89 |
| | 99 | 139 | 140 | 141 | 143 | 145 | 146 | 147 | 92 | 93 | 93 | 94 | 95 | 96 | 97 |

*BP,* blood pressure.

*The 90th, 95th, and 99th percentiles are 1.28, 1.645, and 2.326 standard deviations, respectively, above the mean.

From National High Blood Pressure Education Program Working Group on High Blood Pressure in Children and Adolescents. The fourth report on the diagnosis, evaluation, and treatment of high blood pressure in children and adolescents. *Pediatrics.* 2004;114(2):555–572.

**Table 40-2**
## Blood Pressure and Height Percentiles for Girls by Age

| | | SYSTOLIC BP (mm Hg) | | | | | | | DIASTOLIC BP (mm Hg) | | | | | | |
|---|---|---|---|---|---|---|---|---|---|---|---|---|---|---|---|
| | | PERCENTILE OF HEIGHT | | | | | | | PERCENTILE OF HEIGHT | | | | | | |
| AGE (yr) | BP PERCENTILE* | 5 | 10 | 25 | 50 | 75 | 90 | 95 | 5 | 10 | 25 | 50 | 75 | 90 | 95 |
| 1 | 50 | 83 | 84 | 85 | 86 | 88 | 89 | 90 | 38 | 39 | 39 | 40 | 41 | 41 | 42 |
| | 90 | 97 | 97 | 98 | 100 | 101 | 102 | 103 | 52 | 53 | 53 | 54 | 55 | 55 | 56 |
| | 95 | 100 | 101 | 102 | 104 | 105 | 106 | 107 | 56 | 57 | 57 | 58 | 59 | 59 | 60 |
| | 99 | 108 | 108 | 109 | 111 | 112 | 113 | 114 | 64 | 64 | 65 | 65 | 66 | 67 | 67 |
| 2 | 50 | 85 | 85 | 87 | 88 | 89 | 91 | 91 | 43 | 44 | 44 | 45 | 46 | 46 | 47 |
| | 90 | 98 | 99 | 100 | 101 | 103 | 104 | 105 | 57 | 58 | 58 | 59 | 60 | 61 | 61 |
| | 95 | 102 | 103 | 104 | 105 | 107 | 108 | 109 | 61 | 62 | 62 | 63 | 64 | 65 | 65 |
| | 99 | 109 | 110 | 111 | 112 | 114 | 115 | 116 | 69 | 69 | 70 | 70 | 71 | 72 | 72 |
| 3 | 50 | 86 | 87 | 88 | 89 | 91 | 92 | 93 | 47 | 48 | 48 | 49 | 50 | 50 | 51 |
| | 90 | 100 | 100 | 102 | 103 | 104 | 106 | 106 | 61 | 62 | 62 | 63 | 64 | 64 | 65 |
| | 95 | 104 | 104 | 105 | 107 | 108 | 109 | 110 | 65 | 66 | 66 | 67 | 68 | 68 | 69 |
| | 99 | 111 | 111 | 113 | 114 | 115 | 116 | 117 | 73 | 73 | 74 | 74 | 75 | 76 | 76 |
| 4 | 50 | 88 | 88 | 90 | 91 | 92 | 94 | 94 | 50 | 50 | 51 | 52 | 52 | 53 | 54 |
| | 90 | 101 | 102 | 103 | 104 | 106 | 107 | 108 | 64 | 64 | 65 | 66 | 67 | 67 | 68 |
| | 95 | 105 | 106 | 107 | 108 | 110 | 111 | 112 | 68 | 68 | 69 | 70 | 71 | 71 | 72 |
| | 99 | 112 | 113 | 114 | 115 | 117 | 118 | 119 | 76 | 76 | 76 | 77 | 78 | 79 | 79 |
| 5 | 50 | 89 | 90 | 91 | 93 | 94 | 95 | 96 | 52 | 53 | 53 | 54 | 55 | 55 | 56 |
| | 90 | 103 | 103 | 105 | 106 | 107 | 109 | 109 | 66 | 67 | 67 | 68 | 69 | 69 | 70 |
| | 95 | 107 | 107 | 108 | 110 | 111 | 112 | 113 | 70 | 71 | 71 | 72 | 73 | 73 | 74 |

*Continued*

**Table 40-2**
**Blood Pressure and Height Percentiles for Girls by Age—cont'd**

| | | SYSTOLIC BP (mm Hg) | | | | | | | DIASTOLIC BP (mm Hg) | | | | | | |
|---|---|---|---|---|---|---|---|---|---|---|---|---|---|---|---|
| | | PERCENTILE OF HEIGHT | | | | | | | PERCENTILE OF HEIGHT | | | | | | |
| AGE (yr) | BP PERCENTILE* | 5 | 10 | 25 | 50 | 75 | 90 | 95 | 5 | 10 | 25 | 50 | 75 | 90 | 95 |
| | 99 | 114 | 114 | 116 | 117 | 118 | 120 | 120 | 78 | 78 | 79 | 79 | 80 | 81 | 81 |
| 6 | 50 | 91 | 92 | 93 | 94 | 96 | 97 | 98 | 54 | 54 | 55 | 56 | 56 | 57 | 58 |
| | 90 | 104 | 105 | 106 | 108 | 109 | 110 | 111 | 68 | 68 | 69 | 70 | 70 | 71 | 72 |
| | 95 | 108 | 109 | 110 | 111 | 113 | 114 | 115 | 72 | 72 | 73 | 74 | 74 | 75 | 76 |
| | 99 | 115 | 116 | 117 | 119 | 120 | 121 | 122 | 80 | 80 | 80 | 81 | 82 | 83 | 83 |
| 7 | 50 | 93 | 93 | 95 | 96 | 97 | 99 | 99 | 55 | 56 | 56 | 57 | 58 | 58 | 59 |
| | 90 | 106 | 107 | 108 | 109 | 111 | 112 | 113 | 69 | 70 | 70 | 71 | 72 | 72 | 73 |
| | 95 | 110 | 111 | 112 | 113 | 115 | 116 | 116 | 73 | 74 | 74 | 75 | 76 | 76 | 77 |
| | 99 | 117 | 118 | 119 | 120 | 122 | 123 | 124 | 81 | 81 | 82 | 82 | 83 | 84 | 84 |
| 8 | 50 | 95 | 95 | 96 | 98 | 99 | 100 | 101 | 57 | 57 | 57 | 58 | 59 | 60 | 60 |
| | 90 | 108 | 109 | 110 | 111 | 113 | 114 | 114 | 71 | 71 | 71 | 72 | 73 | 74 | 74 |
| | 95 | 112 | 112 | 114 | 115 | 116 | 118 | 118 | 75 | 75 | 75 | 76 | 77 | 78 | 78 |
| | 99 | 119 | 120 | 121 | 122 | 123 | 125 | 125 | 82 | 82 | 83 | 83 | 84 | 85 | 86 |
| 9 | 50 | 96 | 97 | 98 | 100 | 101 | 102 | 103 | 58 | 58 | 58 | 59 | 60 | 61 | 61 |
| | 90 | 110 | 110 | 112 | 113 | 114 | 116 | 116 | 72 | 72 | 72 | 73 | 74 | 75 | 75 |
| | 95 | 114 | 114 | 115 | 117 | 118 | 119 | 120 | 76 | 76 | 76 | 77 | 78 | 79 | 79 |
| | 99 | 121 | 121 | 123 | 124 | 125 | 127 | 127 | 83 | 83 | 84 | 84 | 85 | 86 | 87 |
| 10 | 50 | 98 | 99 | 100 | 102 | 103 | 104 | 105 | 59 | 59 | 59 | 60 | 61 | 62 | 62 |
| | 90 | 112 | 112 | 114 | 115 | 116 | 118 | 118 | 73 | 73 | 73 | 74 | 75 | 76 | 76 |

| | | | | | | | | | | | | | | | |
|---|---|---|---|---|---|---|---|---|---|---|---|---|---|---|---|
| | 95 | 116 | 116 | 117 | 119 | 120 | 121 | 122 | 77 | 77 | 77 | 78 | 79 | 80 | 80 |
| | 99 | 123 | 123 | 125 | 126 | 127 | 129 | 129 | 84 | 84 | 85 | 86 | 86 | 87 | 88 |
| 11 | 50 | 100 | 101 | 102 | 103 | 105 | 106 | 107 | 60 | 60 | 60 | 61 | 62 | 63 | 63 |
| | 90 | 114 | 114 | 116 | 117 | 118 | 119 | 120 | 74 | 74 | 74 | 75 | 76 | 77 | 77 |
| | 95 | 118 | 118 | 119 | 121 | 122 | 123 | 124 | 78 | 78 | 78 | 79 | 80 | 81 | 81 |
| | 99 | 125 | 125 | 126 | 128 | 129 | 130 | 131 | 85 | 85 | 86 | 87 | 87 | 88 | 89 |
| 12 | 50 | 102 | 103 | 104 | 105 | 107 | 108 | 109 | 61 | 61 | 61 | 62 | 63 | 64 | 64 |
| | 90 | 116 | 116 | 117 | 119 | 120 | 121 | 122 | 75 | 75 | 75 | 76 | 77 | 78 | 78 |
| | 95 | 119 | 120 | 121 | 123 | 124 | 125 | 126 | 79 | 79 | 79 | 80 | 81 | 82 | 82 |
| | 99 | 127 | 127 | 128 | 130 | 131 | 132 | 133 | 86 | 86 | 87 | 88 | 88 | 89 | 90 |
| 13 | 50 | 104 | 105 | 106 | 107 | 109 | 110 | 110 | 62 | 62 | 62 | 63 | 64 | 65 | 65 |
| | 90 | 117 | 118 | 119 | 121 | 122 | 123 | 124 | 76 | 76 | 76 | 77 | 78 | 79 | 79 |
| | 95 | 121 | 122 | 123 | 124 | 126 | 127 | 128 | 80 | 80 | 80 | 81 | 82 | 83 | 83 |
| | 99 | 128 | 129 | 130 | 132 | 133 | 134 | 135 | 87 | 87 | 88 | 89 | 89 | 90 | 91 |
| 14 | 50 | 106 | 106 | 107 | 109 | 110 | 111 | 112 | 63 | 63 | 63 | 64 | 65 | 66 | 66 |
| | 90 | 119 | 120 | 121 | 122 | 124 | 125 | 125 | 77 | 77 | 77 | 78 | 79 | 80 | 80 |
| | 95 | 123 | 123 | 125 | 126 | 127 | 129 | 129 | 81 | 81 | 81 | 82 | 83 | 84 | 84 |
| | 99 | 130 | 131 | 132 | 133 | 135 | 136 | 136 | 88 | 88 | 89 | 90 | 90 | 91 | 92 |
| 15 | 50 | 107 | 108 | 109 | 110 | 111 | 113 | 113 | 64 | 64 | 64 | 65 | 66 | 67 | 67 |
| | 90 | 120 | 121 | 122 | 123 | 125 | 126 | 127 | 78 | 78 | 78 | 79 | 80 | 81 | 81 |
| | 95 | 124 | 125 | 126 | 127 | 129 | 130 | 131 | 82 | 82 | 82 | 83 | 84 | 85 | 85 |
| | 99 | 131 | 132 | 133 | 134 | 136 | 137 | 138 | 89 | 89 | 90 | 91 | 91 | 92 | 93 |
| 16 | 50 | 108 | 108 | 110 | 111 | 112 | 114 | 114 | 64 | 64 | 65 | 66 | 66 | 67 | 68 |
| | 90 | 121 | 122 | 123 | 124 | 126 | 127 | 128 | 78 | 78 | 79 | 80 | 81 | 81 | 82 |

*Continued*

### Table 40-2
## Blood Pressure and Height Percentiles for Girls by Age—cont'd

| | | SYSTOLIC BP (mm Hg) | | | | | | | DIASTOLIC BP (mm Hg) | | | | | | |
|---|---|---|---|---|---|---|---|---|---|---|---|---|---|---|---|
| | | PERCENTILE OF HEIGHT | | | | | | | PERCENTILE OF HEIGHT | | | | | | |
| AGE (yr) | BP PERCENTILE* | 5 | 10 | 25 | 50 | 75 | 90 | 95 | 5 | 10 | 25 | 50 | 75 | 90 | 95 |
| | 95 | 125 | 126 | 127 | 128 | 130 | 131 | 132 | 82 | 82 | 83 | 84 | 85 | 85 | 86 |
| | 99 | 132 | 133 | 134 | 135 | 137 | 138 | 139 | 90 | 90 | 90 | 91 | 92 | 93 | 93 |
| 17 | 50 | 108 | 109 | 110 | 111 | 113 | 114 | 115 | 64 | 65 | 65 | 66 | 67 | 67 | 68 |
| | 90 | 122 | 122 | 123 | 125 | 126 | 127 | 128 | 78 | 79 | 79 | 80 | 81 | 81 | 82 |
| | 95 | 125 | 126 | 127 | 129 | 130 | 131 | 132 | 82 | 83 | 83 | 84 | 85 | 85 | 86 |
| | 99 | 133 | 133 | 134 | 136 | 137 | 138 | 139 | 90 | 90 | 91 | 91 | 92 | 93 | 93 |

*BP,* blood pressure.

*The 90th, 95th, and 99th percentiles are 1.28, 1.645, and 2.326 standard deviations, respectively, above the mean.

From National High Blood Pressure Education Program Working Group on High Blood Pressure in Children and Adolescents. The fourth report on the diagnosis, evaluation, and treatment of high blood pressure in children and adolescents. *Pediatrics*. 2004;114(2):555–572.

### Metabolic Syndrome

Childhood obesity has been associated with a cluster of risk factors for cardiometabolic disease characterized by combinations of insulin resistance, dyslipidemia, and hypertension, which some have termed metabolic syndrome.[21] In turn, this syndrome is associated with the onset of type 2 diabetes and long-term atherosclerotic cardiovascular complications in both childhood and adulthood.[22] Although metabolic syndrome is not currently well-defined, it is increasingly being recognized as a serious complication of childhood obesity. Analysis of the 1999–2006 National Health and Nutrition Examination Surveys found that nearly 1 million US adolescents (about 4% of the total) aged 12 to 19 years have metabolic syndrome; among 8- to 11-year-olds, national prevalence estimates of the syndrome's components ranged from 2% to 9%; and among overweight adolescents, the prevalence of the syndrome is nearly 30%.[2,23] In addition, obstructive sleep apnea, an independent risk factor for resistant hypertension, is increasingly common in obese children.[15,24]

Identifying and treating children and adolescents at the earliest stages of chronic disease should be the goal of clinical practice, yet no clear guidelines have been developed for determining the risk for metabolic syndrome or appropriate thresholds for risk factors.

### Ethnicity

In the United States, mean BP in adults differs among racial and ethnic groups. Non-Hispanic black adults have the highest prevalence and incidence of hypertension. However, the age at which BP begins to differ across racial and ethnic groups is unclear. According to the National Heart, Lung, and Blood Institute Growth and Health Study, among other reports, BP is significantly higher for black girls than for white girls. The prevalence of primary hypertension in black adolescents is higher than that in their nonblack counterparts at lower ranges of BMI.[25] In addition, Mexican American children have a higher mean-adjusted BP than do non-Hispanic white children. In many instances, a higher BMI explains the difference in BP between different ethnic groups.[4] The increase in BMI in children in the United States has accounted for some of the increase in BP; however, other factors such as race contribute to higher BP levels.

### Genetics

Children from families with a history of hypertension tend to have higher BPs than do children from families without such a history, a relationship that generally supports the accepted conclusion that genes influence BP levels.[26,27] Other cardiovascular risk factors among parents, including disorders of lipid and glucose metabolism, hyperuricemia, poor nutrition, passive smoking, and physical inactivity, are also significantly correlated with the cardiovascular risk factors of their children.[28,29]

## ▶ CAUSES OF HIGH BLOOD PRESSURE IN CHILDREN

### Primary Hypertension

Primary hypertension (previously termed essential hypertension), long known to be the most common cause of hypertension in adults, used to be relatively uncommon in younger children. However, primary hypertension is now occurring more often in children, especially in adolescents. One recent study reported that about half of all children ($N = 159$) seen in a hypertension clinic, albeit a selected population, had primary hypertension, leading to the conclusion that the prevalence of primary hypertension in children is increasing. However, the findings of a tertiary care sample may not generalize to the rest of the population. In this study, the diagnosis of primary hypertension occurred in the presence of obesity (56%) and a positive family history of hypertension (86%).[30]

### Secondary Hypertension

Secondary hypertension is more common in children than in adults, and in most children, hypertension will be secondary to renal or renovascular causes (see Boxes 40-1 and 40-2).[2,10]

Severe hypertension can occur in neonates and has been reported in 3% of premature infants.[31] Hypertensive neonates often have evidence of congestive heart failure, respiratory distress, feeding difficulties, irritability, lethargy, coma, or seizures. In almost all cases, the hypertension is renal or renovascular in origin, most commonly from renal artery thrombi related to umbilical vessel catheterization.

Another common cause of high BP, especially from birth through the first year of life, is coarctation of the aorta.[32] Medical therapy for the hypertension is usually effective, and the long-term prognosis is surprisingly good.[3,12] High BP can also occur in infants who have bronchopulmonary dysplasia, patent ductus arteriosus, and increased intracranial pressure.[17] Hypertension has been described in neonates undergoing extracorporeal membrane oxygenation, possibly caused by volume overload.[33]

BOX 40-1

#### *Common Causes of Secondary Hypertension in Neonates and Infants*

- Renal artery thrombosis after umbilical artery catheterization
- Coarctation of the aorta
- Congenital renal parenchymal or structural disease
- Renal artery stenosis

BOX 40-2

#### *Common Causes of Secondary Hypertension in Children and Adolescents*

- Renal disease
- Renal artery stenosis
- Coarctation of the aorta
- Obstructive sleep apnea
- Prolonged treatment with steroids
- Amphetamines
- Mineralocorticoid excess
- Hyperthyroidism
- Pheochromocytoma
- Hypercalcemia
- Neurofibromatosis
- Neurogenic tumors
- Increased intracranial pressure
- Immobilization-induced essential hypertension

Renal parenchymal disease remains the most frequent cause of hypertension in older children and adolescents, accounting for 60% to 80% of cases.[2,17,34] Hypertension is evident at the initial diagnosis in almost 80% of all cases of acute poststreptococcal glomerulonephritis, and of those who are normotensive at diagnosis, nearly half will experience hypertension for a brief period during their illness. Hypertension is also associated with other forms of immune complex glomerulonephritis. It can be seen in membranoproliferative glomerulonephritis, systemic lupus erythematosus, diffuse proliferative glomerulonephritis, and immunoglobulin A nephropathy. Hemolytic uremic syndrome also is associated with hypertension, in proportion to the degree of arteriolar thrombosis. Nephrotic syndrome rarely leads to severe hypertension in children unless it is a manifestation of more serious renal disease. Reflux nephropathy, with 5% to 30% of affected children having high BP, is an important cause of hypertension.[35] Hypertension also occurs with polycystic kidney disease and Wilms tumor, but is less common with other renal structural malformations.[17]

Coarctation of the aorta is the most common nonrenal cause of hypertension in childhood, accounting for 5% to 15% of cases.[17] Hypertension can also occur immediately after repair of the coarctation and for years thereafter.[36,37] The risk for postoperative hypertension seems to be lower if the lesion is repaired before 5 years of age.[36,37] Renal artery stenosis, caused by fibromuscular dysplasia, Takayasu arteritis, Williams syndrome, or neurofibromatosis, constitutes 5% to 10% of childhood hypertension and may have marked symptoms caused by end-organ damage (congestive heart failure, left ventricular hypertrophy, retinal changes, and renal impairment).[38]

Endocrinopathies must be considered as potential causes of hypertension in children. The problem may be endogenous, arising from conditions such as hyperthyroidism, hypercalcemia, adrenal cortical hyperplasia, or increased catecholamine production caused by a pheochromocytoma. The problem can also be exogenous, arising from ingestion or abuse of glucocorticoids or other steroids. Because of its association with high BP, the use of oral contraceptives should always be considered as a possible cause of hypertension in adolescent girls.[17,34,39]

Various drugs can also be associated with hypertension, particularly sympathomimetics (cocaine, amphetamines, phenylephrine, and pseudoephedrine), and their use should be investigated in older children. Other drugs that can raise BP include nonsteroidal anti-inflammatory drugs, erythropoietin, and cyclosporine.[17,34,39]

## ▶ MEASURING BLOOD PRESSURE IN CHILDREN

Appropriate BP measurement techniques are important because false-positive readings are more likely when proper care is not taken.[10] All children older than 3 years should have their BP measured.[2,10] However, certain high-risk groups should have their BP measured before age 3 years (see Box 40-3).

BP should be taken with children and adolescents seated, and with infants supine. In addition, to obtain the most accurate measurements, the child should not have recently ingested stimulant drugs or food and should sit quietly for 5 minutes before the measurement, with his or her back supported and feet on the floor. The BP should preferably be measured in the right arm for consistency and comparison with standard tables. The right arm should be supported, with the elbow at the level of the heart.[2,10]

BOX 40-3

## *Conditions Under Which Children Younger Than 3 Years Should Have Their BP Measured*

- Prematurity, very low birth weight, history of neonatal hypertension or other neonatal complications requiring intensive care
- Congenital heart disease (repaired or nonrepaired)
- Recurrent urinary tract infections, hematuria, or proteinuria
- Renal disease or urologic malformations
- Family history of congenital renal disease
- Family history of moderate to severe hypertension
- Solid-organ transplantation
- Malignancy or bone marrow transplantation
- Treatment with drugs known to increase BP
- Other systemic illnesses associated with hypertension (eg, neurofibromatosis, tuberous sclerosis)
- Evidence of elevated intracranial pressure

Adapted from National High Blood Pressure Education Program Working Group on High Blood Pressure in Children and Adolescents. The fourth report on the diagnosis, evaluation, and treatment of high blood pressure in children and adolescents. *Pediatrics*. 2004;114(2):555–572.

An appropriately sized BP cuff should be used to take the measurement. The width of the cuff's bladder must be at least 40% of the circumference at the midpoint of the upper arm, and its length sufficient to cover at least 80% of the circumference of the arm.[2,10]

The cuff should be inflated to at least 30 mm Hg above the expected systolic BP, although too high a pressure in young children or infants may cause agitation. The stethoscope or Doppler crystal should be placed lightly over the brachial artery in the antecubital fossa, with the elbow remaining at the level of the heart.

Systolic BP is defined as the pressure at the onset of the first Korotkoff sound, and diastolic BP as the pressure at the fifth Korotkoff sound or at the disappearance or muffling of Korotkoff sounds. In some children, Korotkoff sounds can be heard until cuff pressure drops to 0 mm Hg. Measurements can be repeated with less pressure on the head of the stethoscope. If the fifth Korotkoff sound continues to identify very low pressures, the fourth sound can be recorded instead. BP should be measured twice at each visit, and the average systolic and average diastolic pressures should be recorded.[2,10]

Automated BP devices can provide serial, noninvasive BP measurements in newborns and infants, in whom auscultation is difficult, and in the intensive care unit, where frequent BP measurements are needed.[2,10] Automated measurements seem to correlate well with intraarterial readings.[40] These devices are relatively simple to use, and they minimize observer bias and terminal digit preference.[2,10] However, their reliability in the physician's office is less clear because they require frequent calibration and because reference standards have not been established.[2] These devices may overestimate BP and the incidence of hypertension. Elevated BP obtained on automated devices should be confirmed by auscultation. Thus, in general, auscultation is the recommended method of measuring BP in children.

Ambulatory monitoring has recently been used to help establish the diagnosis of hypertension and to track diurnal variations of BP in older children. The monitors are worn on the arm for 24 hours and measure BP regularly throughout the day and night. Ambulatory monitoring is helpful specifically in evaluating white-coat hypertension, the risk for hypertensive end-organ injury, and efficacy of treatment and drug resistance, and to diagnose masked hypertension and hypotension that may occur with the use of antihypertensive drugs.[41] In addition, ambulatory monitoring can be used to evaluate BP patterns in conditions such as episodic hypertension, chronic kidney disease, diabetes, and autonomic dysfunction. BP typically decreases by more than 10% during sleep, and the absence of this decrease is strongly associated with masked hypertension and end-organ damage. Systolic and diastolic BPs above the 95th percentile for age, sex, and height in more than 25% of ambulatory measurements are considered abnormal and require treatment. However, ambulatory BP monitoring of children and adolescents should only be used and interpreted by persons experienced in treating pediatric hypertension.[2]

## ▶ MECHANISMS OF BLOOD PRESSURE REGULATION

A complete discussion of the complex balance between hormonal and physical factors that regulate BP is beyond the scope of this chapter. Instead, the more important concepts are summarized here.

BP is the product of cardiac output and systemic resistance; therefore, anything that affects heart rate, stroke volume, blood volume, or peripheral resistance will alter BP. Peripheral resistance is affected not only by physical changes but also by the actions of various hormones on a given vascular bed. Angiotensin II, the major end product of the renin-angiotensin system, exerts the most hormonal control over BP. As a potent vasoconstrictor, it increases intravascular volume and is closely related to renal blood flow. Renin, the enzyme that stimulates the production of angiotensin II, is itself stimulated by volume depletion, hypotension, and salt depletion and is inhibited by volume expansion and salt loading.[42] Several other hormonal systems also affect renin release, such as circulating catecholamines, glucagon, and adrenocorticotropic and parathyroid hormones.[42] Angiotensin II provides feedback that inhibits renin release; mineralocorticoids and antidiuretic hormone do the same.

Drugs can also affect renin release. Vasodilators and diuretics stimulate renin release, whereas mineralocorticoids and beta blockers inhibit it. Other hormonal systems also help regulate BP. Catecholamine secretion increases BP, and in the presence of a pheochromocytoma or neuroblastoma, it can cause severe hypertension. Mineralocorticoids and glucocorticoids affect BP, and adrenal hypertrophy and tumors may lead to severe hypertension. Also, obesity is characterized by increased sympathetic nervous activity and insulin resistance, which result in sodium retention and in increased levels of renin, angiotensin II, and aldosterone.[43]

## ▶ DIAGNOSTIC EVALUATION

The first step in evaluating a child believed to have hypertension is to conduct a thorough history and physical examination. The medical history should include questions regarding all cardiovascular risk factors, symptoms suggestive of secondary hypertension, and possible target organ damage. In particular, attention should be paid to any history suggesting the recent onset of renal disease or of chronic urinary tract infections. In adolescents, the use of exogenous steroids, oral contraceptives, illicit drugs, tobacco, or alcohol should be specifically determined. A history of prematurity, patent ductus arteriosus, or bronchopulmonary dysplasia and a positive family history, including age of onset of essential hypertension, systemic disease, or endocrinopathy, may help direct further evaluations. A systems review that includes the details of diet, salt intake, and exercise will be helpful in eliciting reports of symptoms associated with specific diseases that can cause hypertension.

Critical in the physical examination is the careful measurement of BP, as described earlier, with special attention to using an appropriately sized cuff and good technique. BP should be measured in all 4 extremities, and the radial, brachial, and, most important, femoral pulses should be assessed. To identify any abnormalities, a complete examination should include an examination of the optic fundi; calculation of BMI (weight in kilograms divided by the square of height in meters); auscultation for carotid, abdominal, and femoral bruits; palpation of the thyroid gland; a thorough examination of the heart and lungs; examination of the abdomen for enlarged kidneys, masses, and abnormal aortic pulsation; palpation of the legs for edema and pulses; cutaneous examination for lesions associated with hypertension such as café au lait spots; and a neurologic assessment. These findings will further direct evaluation, which should be a stepwise investigation tailored to the age of the child and to the specific findings. For example, decreased femoral pulses may indicate coarctation of the aorta.[2]

Hypertension can be diagnosed and managed with an algorithm (Figure 40-2). Ideally, BP values should be an average of at least 2 separate measurements or, even better, of

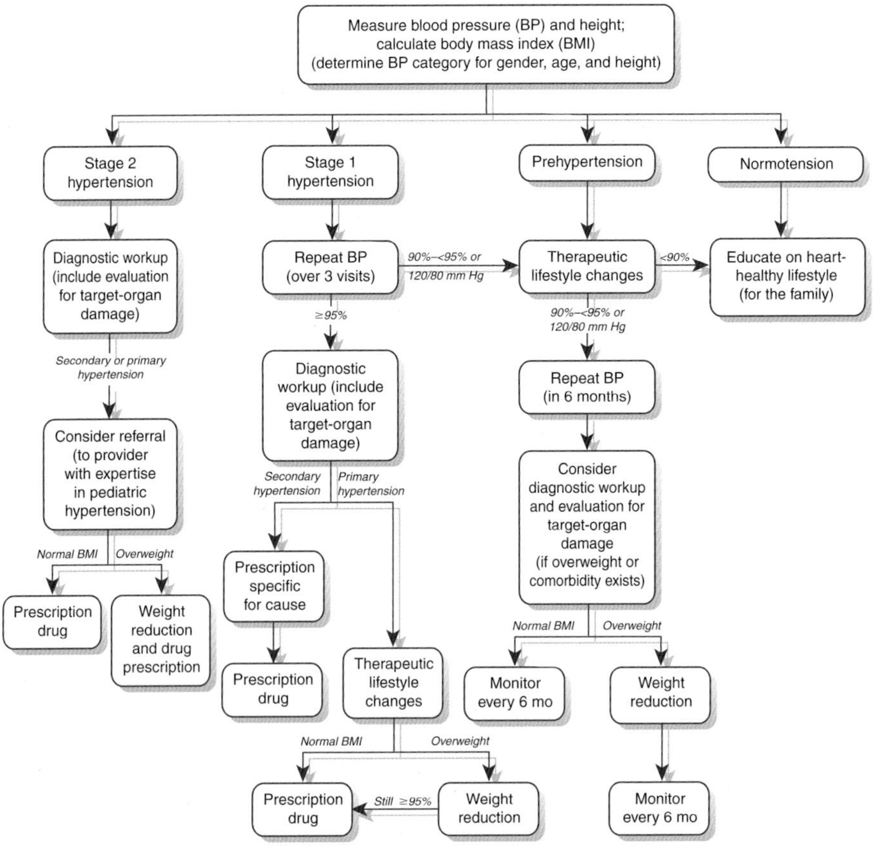


**Figure 40-2**

Algorithm for diagnosing high blood pressure in children. *(Modified from National High Blood Pressure Education Program Working Group on High Blood Pressure in Children and Adolescents. The fourth report on the diagnosis, evaluation, and treatment of high blood pressure in children and adolescents.* Pediatrics. *2004;114[2]:555–572.)*

measurements obtained on three separate occasions. All children should be screened for possible renal dysfunction by obtaining a urinalysis, complete blood count, serum urea nitrogen, creatinine, and serum electrolyte evaluation that includes glucose. A renal ultrasound may also be appropriate. If the family history is positive for essential hypertension, then a lipid profile that includes high- and low-density lipoprotein cholesterol and triglycerides will help assess cardiovascular risk (see Box 40-4).[2,10]

If hypertension is severe and the initial diagnostic tests are inconclusive, or if BP remains elevated after initial treatment, more intensive investigations are indicated. If a renal cause is suspected, further imaging of the genitourinary system may be necessary. A stepwise, age-appropriate approach is suggested for evaluation for renovascular hypertension. In the neonate, color Doppler ultrasound of the aorta and renal vessels is a relatively simple, safe, noninvasive, and quick way of detecting aortic, renal venous, and arterial thrombi. This can be performed in conjunction with a renal ultrasound, which is necessary to look for congenital and parenchymal abnormalities. Additional diagnostic tools such as measurement of resistive indices and peak systolic velocities in the renal arteries increase sensitivity and specificity for diagnosing renal artery stenosis.[44]

A negative Doppler study, however, does not exclude renovascular hypertension. Nuclear scintigraphy with angiotensin-converting enzyme (ACE) inhibition has moderate sensitivity and specificity. It can be useful to evaluate differential renal function and predict renal functional deterioration with the use of ACE inhibitors.[45]

Technical advances in recent years have improved the quality of images with high-resolution contrast-enhanced computed tomographic (CT) angiography, which can give 3-dimensional views of the renal arteries. The disadvantage is the exposure to radiation. Magnetic resonance angiography with gadolinium is also an alternative but requires sedation

**BOX 40-4**

## *Diagnostic Tests for Hypertension and Its Consequences*

### DIAGNOSTIC TESTS

- Urinalysis
- Complete blood cell count with platelets and blood smear
- Serum electrolytes, blood urea nitrogen, creatinine, calcium, phosphorus, albumin
- Antinuclear antibody, serum C3 complement
- Plasma renin and aldosterone
- Renal ultrasound with Doppler study of renal vessels
- Urinary metanephrine, norepinephrine, and epinephrine
- Thyroid function tests
- Urine toxicology

### TESTS FOR END-ORGAN DAMAGE

- Chest radiograph
- Electrocardiogram
- Echocardiogram
- Ophthalmologic examination

### ASSESSMENT OF ASSOCIATED RISK FACTORS

- Serum lipid profile
- Fasting insulin and glucose
- Serum uric acid

or general anesthesia and may not provide adequate spatial resolution compared with CT angiography. Both imaging modalities could still miss stenotic lesions of the renal arteries in small children. The gold standard for diagnosis of renovascular hypertension is digital subtraction angiography in which the visualization of blood vessels is enhanced by digitally subtracting images of background structures.[12,31,46]

Plasma renin activity can be used to screen for renovascular hypertension and mineralocorticoid disease. Thyroid function or serum catecholamine tests may be helpful if hyperthyroidism or pheochromocytoma is suspected.

Cardiac evaluation is an important part of the examination.[2,39] In addition to a thorough physical examination that includes feeling the femoral pulse, electrocardiography and echocardiography may identify coarctation of the aorta and will provide information about left ventricular mass. Left ventricular hypertrophy is the most prominent evidence of target-organ damage. Thus, in children with established hypertension, left ventricular mass should be assessed at diagnosis and periodically thereafter.[2] Formal stress testing can help assess normal and abnormal BP responses to exercise, which might be especially informative in young athletes.[2,39] Ambulatory BP measurements can help detect hypertension and determine the amount of time each day that BP is elevated.

## ▶ THERAPY FOR HIGH BLOOD PRESSURE

The justification for treating children who have marked hypertension comes from the results of adult trials showing that reducing BP has positive effects on cardiovascular status and reduces the risk for target-organ damage. Pediatric studies showing beneficial effects on cardiovascular status are few.[12,47]

Therapeutic lifestyle changes are generally recommended for children with mild or moderate hypertension. Initiating a low-salt or no-added-salt diet is reasonable because many patients will be salt sensitive. In addition, the intake of fresh vegetables, fruits, fiber, and low-fat dairy products should be increased.[48]

Body size is a major determinant of BP, and weight loss is often associated with reduced systolic and diastolic pressures. Maintaining a normal weight in childhood reduces the likelihood of high BP in adulthood. Weight loss also is associated with decreased BP sensitivity to salt and decreases in other risk factors, such as dyslipidemia and insulin resistance.

Exercise as an adjunct to weight loss often reduces BP even more than weight loss alone. Increasing regular physical activity and decreasing sedentary activities are important in preventing hypertension in childhood and adolescence. Lifestyle modifications are recommended for all stages of hypertension because exercise reduces BP in all individuals regardless of body mass index. When children and adolescents do not respond to lifestyle modifications or have conditions such as stage 2 systemic hypertension, secondary hypertension, or established hypertensive target-organ damage, medications are indicated. Because the long-term effects of antihypertensive therapy in children are not well studied, a definite indication for drug therapy is needed before starting treatment (see Table 40-3).[2]

All classes of antihypertensive drugs lower BP in children; therefore, the choice of therapy depends on the underlying etiology. It is useful to determine whether hypertension is renin mediated or non–renin mediated. Volume-dependent hypertension as seen in poststreptococcal glomerulonephritis is responsive to diuretics. Diuretics are not desirable in active athletes because of the risk for hypovolemia and hypokalemia.[33] ACE inhibitors and receptor blockers

**Table 40–3**
**Antihypertensive Drugs Commonly Used to Manage Chronic Hypertension in Children**

| DRUG | INITIAL DOSE (mg/kg/day) | MAXIMAL DOSE | INTERVAL (TIMES/DAY) |
|---|---|---|---|
| **ACE INHIBITORS** | | | |
| Benazepril[a] | 0.2 | 40 mg | 1 |
| Captopril[b] | 0.15–0.5 | 6 mg/kg/day | 3–4 |
| Enalapril[b] | 0.08–0.5 | 40 mg | 1–2 |
| Fosinopril[a] | 0.1–0.6 | 40 mg | 1 |
| Lisinopril[a] | 0.07 | 40 mg | 1 |
| **ANGIOTENSIN RECEPTOR BLOCKERS** | | | |
| Irbesartan[a] | | | |
| 6–12 yr | 2 | 75–150 mg | 1–2 |
| ≥13 yr | 2 | 150–300 mg | 1–2 |
| Losartan | 0.7 | 100 mg | 1–2 |
| Candesartan | 0.05–0.4 | 32 mg | 1–2 |
| Valsartan | 1.3 | 160 mg | 1 |
| **ALPHA AND BETA BLOCKERS** | | | |
| Labetalol | 1–4 | 1,200 mg | 2 |
| Atenolol | 0.5–1.2 | 100 mg | 1 |
| Bisoprolol/HCTZ[a] | 2.5/6.25 mg/day | 10/6.25 mg | 1 |
| Metoprolol | 1–2 | 200 mg | 1–2 |
| Propranolol | 1–4 | 640 mg | 2–4 |
| **CALCIUM CHANNEL BLOCKERS** | | | |
| Amlodipine | 0.1–0.6 | 20 mg | 1–2 |
| Felodipine[a] | 2.5 mg/day | 10 mg | 1 |
| Isradipine | 0.15–0.2/dose | 20 mg | 2–4 |
| Extended-release nifedipine | 0.25–0.5 | 120 mg | 1 |
| **CENTRAL ALPHA–AGONIST** | | | |
| Clonidine (≥12 yr) | 0.05–0.2 mg/day | 2.4 mg | 2–4 |
| **DIURETICS** | | | |
| HCTZ | 1–4 | 200 mg | 1–2 |
| Furosemide | 0.5–2 | 6 mg/kg/dose | 2–4 |
| Spironolactone | 1–3.3 | 200 mg | 2–4 |
| Amiloride | 0.4–0.625 | 20 mg | 1 |
| **VASODILATORS** | | | |
| Hydralazine | 0.75–1 | 200 mg | 2–4 |
| Minoxidil | 0.1–0.5 mg/kg/dose | 20 mg | 2 |

*ACE,* angiotensin–converting enzyme; *HCTZ,* hydrochlorothiazide.
[a]Not recommended before age 6 years.
[b]The lowest effective dose of these drugs is used in neonates because it can cause acute deterioration in renal function.

are useful in proteinuric renal disease for controlling hypertension, reducing proteinuria, and slowing progression of kidney disease. They have to be used with caution in female adolescents because of the risk for ACE inhibitor fetopathy. Beta blockers and calcium channel blockers can be used in children with hypertension and migraine.[12] Beta blockers should not be used in active athletes because they decrease cardiac contractility, heart rate, and maximum oxygen uptake.[49]

The noncardioselective beta blockers can cause hypoglycemia after intense exercise.[12] They can be problematic for patients who have reactive airway disease or diabetes. Angiotensin blockers and calcium channel blockers have the least adverse effects in the physically active adolescent.

The basic medication strategy is to start with a single drug and assess the response. Additional drugs should be added one at a time, always attempting to target a different mechanism. In primary hypertension, the drug of first choice is usually an ACE inhibitor or a calcium channel blocker. The α-agonists are generally considered to be second-line drugs. For children who have chronic primary hypertension but no hypertensive target-organ damage, the goal of drug therapy should be to reduce BP to below the 95th percentile for sex, age, and height. For children with chronic renal disease, diabetes, or hypertensive target-organ damage, the goal of therapy should be to reduce BP to below the 90th percentile for sex, age, and height.[2] Patients with stage 1 hypertension can be monitored every 3 to 6 months. Patients with stage 2 hypertension should be monitored more closely depending on the degree of control. Hypertension should be treated judiciously in patients with elevated intracranial pressure.

Note that ACE inhibitors and angiotensin receptor blockers are teratogenic. Avoidance of pregnancy is suggested in sexually active females.

## ▶ ATHLETIC PARTICIPATION BY CHILDREN WITH HYPERTENSION

Children should be encouraged to participate in noncompetitive physical activity because regular aerobic exercise reduces both systolic and diastolic BP. Dynamic exercise greatly increases systolic BP and decreases diastolic BP, whereas isometric exercise increases both. Children with stage 2 hypertension need to be cautious about participating in competitive sports with highly static components (see Figure 40-3 and Table 40-4).[50–52]

The dynamic component is the estimated percentage of maximal oxygen uptake (max $O_2$). Higher uptake increases cardiac output. The static component is the percentage of maximal voluntary contraction. Higher contractions increase blood pressure.

## ▶ HYPERTENSIVE EMERGENCY AND URGENCY

A hypertensive emergency or malignant hypertension is defined as a sudden elevation in blood pressure posing an immediate threat to the integrity of the cardiovascular system, kidneys, or central nervous system. Permanent neurologic damage, blindness, and chronic renal failure are some of the long-term consequences of malignant hypertension. Hypertensive emergency or crisis may occur in individuals previously not known to have hypertension or in those known to have chronic hypertension or kidney disease. Initial treatment should focus on reducing BP to alleviate acute symptoms, not necessarily to make the patient normotensive. Hypertensive emergencies should be treated with an intravenous antihypertensive

| Increasing Static Component → | A. Low (<40% max $O_2$) | B. Moderate (40%–70% max $O_2$) | C. High (>70% max $O_2$) |
|---|---|---|---|
| III. High (>50% MVC) | Bobsledding/luge,[a,b] field events (throwing), gymnastics,[a,b] martial arts,[a] sailing, sport climbing, water skiing,[a,b] weight lifting,[a,b] | Body building,[a,b] downhill skiing,[a,b] skateboarding,[a,b] snowboarding,[a,b] wrestling[a,b] | Boxing,[a,c] canoeing/kayaking, cycling,[a,b] decathalon, rowing, speed-skating,[a,b] triathlon[a,b] |
| II. Moderate (20%–50% MVC) | Archery, auto racing,[a,b] diving,[a,b] equestrian,[a,b] motorcycling[a,b] | American football,[a] field events (jumping), figure skating,[a] rodeoing,[a,b] rugby,[a] running (sprint), surfing,[a,b] synchronized swimming[b] | Basketball,[a] ice hockey,[a] cross-country skiing (skating technique), lacrosse,[a] running (middle distance), swimming, team handball |
| I. Low (<20% MVC) | Billiards, bowling, cricket,[d] curling, golf, riflery | Baseball/softball,[a] fencing, table tennis, volleyball | Badminton, cross-country skiing (classic technique), field hockey,[a] orienteering, race walking, racquetball/ squash, running (long distance), soccer,[a] tennis |

Increasing Dynamic Component →

**Figure 40-3**

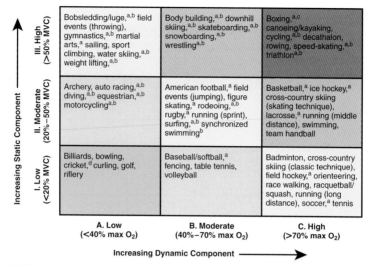

Classification of sports. This classification is based on peak static and dynamic components achieved during competition. It should be noted, however, that higher values may be reached during training. The increasing dynamic component is defined in terms of the estimated percent of maximal oxygen uptake (max $O_2$) achieved and results in an increasing cardiac output. The increasing static component is related to the estimated percent of maximal voluntary contraction (MVC) reached and results in an increasing blood pressure load. The lowest total cardiovascular demands (cardiac output and blood pressure) are shown in **green** and the highest in **red. Blue, yellow, and orange** depict low moderate, moderate, and high moderate total cardiovascular demands. [a]Danger of bodily collision. [b]Increased risk if syncope occurs. [c]Participation is not recommended by the American Academy of Pediatrics. [d]The American Academy of Pediatrics classifies cricket as a low-static, moderate dynamic sport. *(Adapted with permission from Mitchell JH, Haskell W, Snell P, et al. Task force 8: classification of sports.* J Am Coll Cardiol. *2005;45(8):1364–1367.)*

**Table 40-4**
## Exercise Guidelines for Adolescents With Hypertension, by Intervention or Evaluation

| | INTERVENTION | EXERCISE |
|---|---|---|
| Prehypertension | Daily physical activity<br>Well-balanced diet<br>Weight management<br>Caffeine, drugs, tobacco, and stimulant use to be reviewed<br>BP check every 6 months | No restriction<br>Can participate in competitive athletic sports<br>Encourage aerobic exercises |
| Stage 1 hypertension | Evaluation for end-organ damage<br>Lifestyle modifications as with prehypertension | No restriction<br>Can participate in competitive athletic sports if no end-organ damage<br>Encourage aerobic exercises |
| Stage 2 hypertension | Evaluation for end-organ damage<br>Evaluation by medical specialist<br>Lifestyle modifications as with prehypertension<br>Pharmacologic treatment | Restriction from high static sports<br>Eligibility for competitive sports depends on extent of cardiac disease<br>Encourage aerobic exercises, with intensity determined by extent of cardiac disease |

**Table 40–5**
**Drugs Used to Treat Hypertensive Emergencies and Hypertensive Urgencies**

| HYPERTENSIVE EMERGENCY | ROUTE | DOSE | ADVERSE EFFECTS |
|---|---|---|---|
| Sodium nitroprusside | IV | 0.5–0.8 mcg/kg/min | Thiocyanate toxicity with decreased renal function |
| Nicardipine | IV | 1–3 mcg/kg/min | Headache; increased intracranial pressure |
| Labetalol | IV: infusion-bolus | 0.25–1.5 mg/kg/hr; 0.2–1 mg/kg/dose Maximum, 20 mg/dose | Use with caution in hyperkalemia and congestive heart failure |
| Fenoldopam | IV | 0.8–3.0 mcg/kg/min | Tachycardia; increased intracranial pressure |
| Enalaprilat | IV | 0.005–0.01 mg/kg/day | Acute renal failure and hyperkalemia |
| Hydralazine | IV | 0.1–0.5 mg/kg/dose q4–6hr | Tachycardia, flushing, lupus-like syndrome |
| Nifedipine | Sublingual | 0.1–0.25 mg/kg/dose | Precipitous drop in blood pressure; tachycardia; headache |
| Esmolol | IV | Bolus 100–500 mcg over 1 min; 25–100 mcg/kg/min; can increase to 500 mcg/kg/min | Can cause congestive heart failure, bradycardia, and bronchospasm; contraindicated in cocaine toxicity |
| Clevidipine | IV | 0.5–3.5 mcg/kg/min | Contraindicated in lipid disorders, egg and soy allergy |
| Phentolamine | IV | 0.1–0.2 mg/kg/dose | Orthostatic hypotension, tachycardia, gastrointestinal disturbances |
| **Hypertensive Urgency** | | | |
| Furosemide | IV/PO | 1–2 mg/kg/dose | Electrolyte disturbances |
| Clonidine | PO | 0.05–0.3 mg | Rebound hypertension; sedation |
| Minoxidil | PO | 0.1–2 mg/kg/dose | Pericardial effusion |

*IV,* intravenous; *PO,* by mouth.

medication that can steadily reduce BP, decreasing the pressure by no more than 25% over the first 8 hours and then gradually reducing it to normal over the next 24 to 48 hours (see Table 40-5). In contrast, hypertensive urgency is severe hypertension with no acute (or minimal) end-organ damage. It produces less serious symptoms, such as severe headache or vomiting. Urgencies can be treated by either intravenous or oral antihypertensives.[53]

## ▶ CONCLUSION

Evidence of a link between the onset of hypertension in childhood and adult morbidity and mortality from end-organ damage is increasing. As pediatricians become more aware of the importance of monitoring BP in childhood and diagnosing hypertension earlier, they have the opportunity to decrease its long-term adverse cardiovascular effects. Even small reductions in BP can improve the health of children and their cardiovascular status later in life. Of equal importance for physicians is the need to educate parents and children about the health dangers of obesity because this condition has become increasingly prevalent.

## When to Refer

- Stage 1 hypertension
- Stage 2 hypertension

Specific conditions requiring referral

- Symptomatic essential hypertension
- Secondary hypertension
- Hypertension with diabetes
- Evidence of target-organ damage (left ventricular hypertrophy)
- Neonatal hypertension

## When to Admit

- Hypertensive emergencies (associated with manifestations in other organs)
- Hypertensive urgencies (severe BP elevation without other organ involvement)
- Acute glomerular diseases
- Poststreptococcal glomerulonephritis
- Hemolytic uremic syndrome
- Renal artery stenosis
- Fibromuscular dysplasia
- Previous umbilical artery catheter
- Neurofibromatosis
- Pheochromocytoma
- Coarctation of aorta
- Noncompliance with current antihypertensive medication
- Cocaine toxicity
- Dialysis patients with excessive volume expansion

## *TOOLS FOR PRACTICE*

### Engaging Patient and Family

- *High Blood Pressure in Children* (fact sheet), American Academy of Pediatrics (www.healthychildren.org/English/health-issues/conditions/heart/Pages/High-Blood-Pressure-in-Children.aspx)

### Medical Decision Support

- *The Fourth Report on the Diagnosis, Evaluation, and Treatment of High Blood pressure in Children and Adolescents* (Web page), National Heart, Lung, and Blood Institute (www.nhlbi.nih.gov/files/docs/resources/heart/hbp_ped.pdf)

## AAP POLICY STATEMENTS

National High Blood Pressure Education Program Working Group on High Blood Pressure in Children and Adolescents. The fourth report on the diagnosis, evaluation, and treatment of high blood pressure in children and adolescents. *Pediatrics.* 2004;114(2):555–576 (AAP endorsed) (pediatrics.aappublications.org/content/114/Supplement_2/555.full)

Demorest RA, Washington RL; American Academy of Pediatrics Council on Sports Medicine and Fitness. Athletic participation by children and adolescents who have systemic hypertension. *Pediatrics.* 2010;125(6):1287–1294. Reaffirmed May 2013 (pediatrics.aappublications.org/content/125/6/1287.full)

## REFERENCES


1. World Health Organization. World health report 2002. Reducing risks, promoting healthy life, 2002. Geneva, Switzerland. Available at www.who.int/whr/2002. Accessed October 16, 2014
2. National High Blood Pressure Education Program Working Group on High Blood Pressure in Children and Adolescents. The fourth report on the diagnosis, evaluation, and treatment of high blood pressure in children and adolescents. *Pediatrics.* 2004;114:555–576
3. Cook S, Weitzman M, Auinger P, Nguyen M, Dietz WH. Prevalence of a metabolic syndrome phenotype in adolescents: findings from the third National Health and Nutrition Examination Survey, 1988-1994. *Arch Pediatr Adolesc Med.* 2003;157:821–827
4. Muntner P, He J, Cutler JA, Wildman RP, Whelton PK. Trends in blood pressure among children and adolescents. *JAMA.* 2004;291:2107–2113
5. Chen W, Srinivasan SR, Li S, Xu J, Berenson GS. Metabolic syndrome variables at low levels in childhood are beneficially associated with adulthood cardiovascular risk: the Bogalusa Heart Study. *Diabetes Care.* 2005;28:126–131
6. Cook NR, Gillman MW, Rosner BA, Taylor JO, Hennekens CH. Combining annual blood pressure measurements in childhood to improve prediction of young adult blood pressure. *Stat Med.* 2000;19:2625–2640
7. Zinner SH, Rosner B, Oh W, Kass EH. Significance of blood pressure in infancy. Familial aggregation and predictive effect on later blood pressure. *Hypertension.* 1985;7:411–416
8. Chobanian AV, Bakris GL, Black HR, et al. Seventh report of the Joint National Committee on Prevention, Detection, Evaluation, and Treatment of High Blood Pressure. *Hypertension.* 2003;42:1206–1252
9. Sinaiko AR. Treatment of hypertension in children. *Pediatr Nephrol.* 1994;8:603–609
10. Report of the Second Task Force on Blood Pressure Control in Children—1987. Task Force on Blood Pressure Control in Children. National Heart, Lung, and Blood Institute, Bethesda, Maryland. *Pediatrics.* 1987;79:1–25
11. Sinaiko AR. Hypertension in children. *N Engl J Med.* 1996;335:1968–1973
12. Adelman RD. Neonatal hypertension. *Pediatr Clin North Am.* 1978;25:99–110
13. Zubrow AB, Hulman S, Kushner H, Falkner B. Determinants of blood pressure in infants admitted to neonatal intensive care units: a prospective multicenter study. Philadelphia Neonatal Blood Pressure Study Group. *J Perinatol.* 1995;15:470–479
14. Dionne JM, Abitbol CL, Flynn JT. Hypertension in infancy: diagnosis, management and outcome. *Pediatr Nephrol.* 2012;27:17–32
15. Arens R, Muzumdar H. Childhood obesity and obstructive sleep apnea syndrome. *J Appl Physiol.* 2010;108:436–444
16. Lauer RM, Clarke WR. Childhood risk factors for high adult blood pressure: the Muscatine Study. *Pediatrics.* 1984;84:633
17. Sharma A, Sinaiko AR. Systemic hypertension. In: Emmanouilides GC, ed. *Moss and Adams Heart Disease in Infants, Children and Adolescents.* 5th ed. Baltimore, MD: Williams and Wilkins; 1995
18. Institute of Medicine. *Preventing Childhood Obesity: Health in the Balance.* Washington, DC: National Academy Press; 2004
19. Centers for Disease Control and Prevention. Overweight and Obesity. www.cdc.gov/nccdphp/dnpa/obesity/index.htm. Accessed October 16, 2014

20. Sorof JM, Lai D, Turner J, Poffenbarger T, Portman RJ. Overweight, ethnicity, and the prevalence of hypertension in school-aged children. *Pediatrics.* 2004;113:475–482
21. Steinberger J, Daniels SR, Eckel RH, et al. Progress and challenges in metabolic syndrome in children and adolescents: a scientific statement from the American Heart Association Atherosclerosis, Hypertension, and Obesity in the Young Committee of the Council on Cardiovascular Disease in the Young; Council on Cardiovascular Nursing; and Council on Nutrition, Physical Activity, and Metabolism. *Circulation.* 2009;119:628–647
22. Morrison JA, Friedman LA, Gray-McGuire C. Metabolic syndrome in childhood predicts adult cardiovascular disease 25 years later: the Princeton Lipid Research Clinics Follow-up Study. *Pediatrics.* 2007;120:340–345
23. Messiah SE, Arheart KL, Luke B, Lipshultz SE, Miller TL. Relationship between body mass index and metabolic syndrome risk factors among US 8- to 14-year-olds, 1999 to 2002. *J Pediatr.* 2008;153:215–221
24. Wolf J, Hering D, Narkiewicz K. Non-dipping pattern of hypertension and obstructive sleep apnea syndrome. *Hypertens Res.* 2010;33:867–871
25. Brady TM, Fivush B, Parekh RS, Flynn JT. Racial differences among children with primary hypertension. *Pediatrics.* 2010;126:931–937
26. Munger RG, Prineas RJ, Gomez-Marin O. Persistent elevation of blood pressure among children with a family history of hypertension: the Minneapolis Children's Blood Pressure Study. *J Hypertens.* 1988;6:647–653
27. Shear CL, Burke GL, Freedman DS, et al. Values of childhood blood pressure measurements and family history in predicting future blood pressure status: results from eight years of follow-up in the Bogalusa Heart Study. *Pediatrics.* 1996;77:862–869
28. Gordon T, Kannel WB, eds. An epidemiological investigation of cardiovascular disease: the Framingham Study. *US DHEW.* 1972;1:271968–1972
29. Shurtleff D. Some characteristics related to the incidence of cardiovascular disease and death: the Framingham Study, 18-year follow-up. *US DHEW.* 1974;74:599
30. Flynn JT, Alderman MH. Characteristics of children with primary hypertension seen at a referral center. *Pediatr Nephrol.* 2005;20:961–966
31. Adelman RD. Long-term follow-up of neonatal renovascular hypertension. *Pediatr Nephrol.* 1987; 1:35–41
32. Varda NM, Gregoric A. A diagnostic approach for the child with hypertension. *Pediatr Nephrol.* 2005;20:499–506
33. Boedy RF, Goldberg AK, Howell CG Jr, et al. Incidence of hypertension in infants on extracorporeal membrane oxygenation. *J Pediatr Surg.* 1990;25:258–261
34. Peters RM, Flack JM. Diagnosis and treatment of hypertension in children and adolescents. *J Am Acad Nurse Pract.* 2003;15:56–63
35. Lerner GR, Fleischmann LE, Perlmutter AD. Reflux nephropathy. *Pediatr Clin North Am.* 1987;34:747–770
36. Liberthson RR, Pennington DG, Jacobs ML, Daggett WM. Coarctation of the aorta: review of 234 patients and clarification of management problems. *Am J Cardiol.* 1979;43:835–840
37. Sealy WC. Paradoxical hypertension after repair of coarctation of the aorta: a review of its causes. *Ann Thorac Surg.* 1990;50:323–329
38. Deal JE, Snell MF, Barratt TM, Dillon MJ. Renovascular disease in childhood. *J Pediatr.* 1992; 121:378–384
39. Hackman AM, Bricker JT. Preventive cardiology, hypertension and dyslipidemia. In: Garson A Jr, ed. *The Science and Practice of Pediatric Cardiology.* 2nd ed. Baltimore, MD: Williams and Wilkins; 1998
40. Colan SD, Fujii A, Borow KM, MacPherson D, Sanders SP. Noninvasive determination of systolic, diastolic and end-systolic blood pressure in neonates, infants and young children: comparison with central aortic pressure measurements. *Am J Cardiol.* 1983;52:867–870

41. Urbina E, Alpert B, Flynn J, et al. Ambulatory blood pressure monitoring in children and adolescents: recommendations for standard assessment: a scientific statement from the American Heart Association Atherosclerosis, Hypertension, and Obesity in Youth Committee of the Council on Cardiovascular Disease in the Young and the Council for High Blood Pressure Research. *Hypertension.* 2008;52:433–451
42. Ingelfinger JR. The renin-angiotensin system and other hormonal systems in the control of blood pressure. In: Ingelfinger JR. *Pediatric Hypertension.* Philadelphia, PA: WB Saunders; 1982
43. Lambert GW, Straznicky NE, Lambert EA, Dixon JB, Schlaich MP. Sympathetic nervous activation in obesity and the metabolic syndrome—causes, consequences and therapeutic implications. *Pharmacol Ther.* 2010;126:159–172
44. Krumme B, Blum U, Schwertfeger E, et al. Diagnosis of renovascular disease by intra- and extrarenal Doppler scanning. *Kidney Int.* 1996;50:1288–1292
45. Chandar JJ, Sfakianakis GN, Zilleruelo GE, et al. ACE inhibition scintigraphy in the management of hypertension in children. *Pediatr Nephrol.* 1999;13:493–500
46. Marks SD, Tullus K. Update on imaging for suspected renovascular hypertension in children and adolescents. *Curr Hypertens Rep.* 2012;14:591–595
47. Sladowska-Kozłowska J, Litwin M, Niemirska A, et al. Change in left ventricular geometry during antihypertensive treatment in children with primary hypertension. *Pediatr Nephrol.* 2011;26: 2201–2209
48. Sacks FM, Svetkey LP, Vollmer WM, et al. Effects on blood pressure of reduced dietary sodium and the dietary approaches to stop hypertension (DASH) diet. DASH-Sodium Collaborative Research Group. *N Engl J Med.* 2001;344:3–10
49. Chick TW, Halperin AK, Gacek EM. The effect of antihypertensive medications on exercise performance: a review. *Med Sci Sports Exerc.* 1988;20:447–454
50. Rice SG, American Academy of Pediatrics Council on Sports Medicine and Fitness. Medical conditions affecting sports participation. *Pediatrics.* 2008;121:841–848
51. McCambridge TM, Benjamin HJ, Brenner JS, et al. Athletic participation by children and adolescents who have systemic hypertension. *Pediatrics.* 2010;125:1287–1294
52. Mitchell JH, Haskell W, Snell P, Van Camp SP. Task Force 8: classification of sports. *J Am Coll Cardiol.* 2005;45:1364–1367
53. Chandar J, Zilleruelo G. Hypertensive crisis in children. *Pediatr Nephrol.* 2012;27:741–751
54. Adelman RD. Management of hypertensive emergencies. In: Portman RJ, Sorof JM, Ingelfinger JR, eds. *Pediatric Hypertension.* Totowa, NJ: Human Press; 2004
55. Burg FD, Ingelfinger JR, Polin RA, et al. *Current Pediatric Therapy.* 18th ed. Philadelphia, PA: Saunders Elsevier; 2006
56. Frohlich ED, Apstein C, Chobanian AV, et al. The heart in hypertension. *N Engl J Med.* 1992;327: 998–1008
57. Portman R, Sorof J, Ingelfinger J, eds. *Pediatric Hypertension.* Totowa, NJ: Humana Press; 2004
58. Sadowski RH, Falkner B. Hypertension in pediatric patients. *Am J Kidney Dis.* 1996;3:305–315
59. Update on the 1987 Task Force Report on High Blood Pressure in Children and Adolescents: a working group report from the National High Blood Pressure Education Program. National High Blood Pressure Education Program Working Group on Hypertension Control in Children and Adolescents. *Pediatrics.* 1996;98:649–658
60. de Ferranti SD, Gauvreau K, Ludwig DS, et al. Prevalence of the metabolic syndrome in American adolescents: findings from the Third National Health and Nutrition Examination Survey. *Circulation.* 2004;110:2494–2497

# Hirsutism, Hypertrichosis, and Precocious Sexual Hair Development

*Genna W. Klein, MD; Mariam Gangat, MD*

## ▶ INTRODUCTION

The extent, distribution, and character of body hair depend on age, sex, ethnicity, and genetics. When evaluating a child or adolescent for the presence of body hair, understanding the history, physiology of the hair follicle, and hair development is essential in determining if the appearance of hair warrants immediate investigation, expectant management, or reassurance.

## ▶ BACKGROUND

### Definitions

*Hirsutism* is the presence of excessive terminal hair in androgen dependent and male pattern areas (especially in females). *Hypertrichosis* is excess hair growth, not limited to androgen-sensitive areas, and can be generalized or localized.[1]

*Virilization* (or masculinization) is a result of (usually pathologic) androgen overproduction, with signs including clitoral or phallic enlargement, masculine body habitus, and deepening of the voice. *Pubarche* and *adrenarche*, although at times used interchangeably, more precisely refer to the onset of sexual hair noted on clinical examination and the biochemical rise of adrenal androgens, respectively. *Hyperandrogenism* is the presence of elevated androgens, manifested either clinically by hirsutism, virilization, acne, male-patterned baldness, or biochemically with elevated androgen levels.

### The Hair Follicle

The human body is covered by 5 million hair follicles. The only areas free of hair are the lips, palms, and soles. There are 3 main types of human hair, which are present at different times and at different locations in the human life cycle: lanugo, vellus, and terminal hair types. Lanugo hair sheds during fetal life, and is followed postnatally by vellus hair. Vellus hair (fine, short, and usually lightly pigmented or nonpigmented), is normally seen over the face and arms of children. Terminal hair (thicker, longer and pigmented), is normally found on the scalp, eyebrows, and eyelashes from the time of birth.[2] Hair growth involves 3 asynchronous cycles: growth (anagen phase), rapid involution (catagen phase), and resting

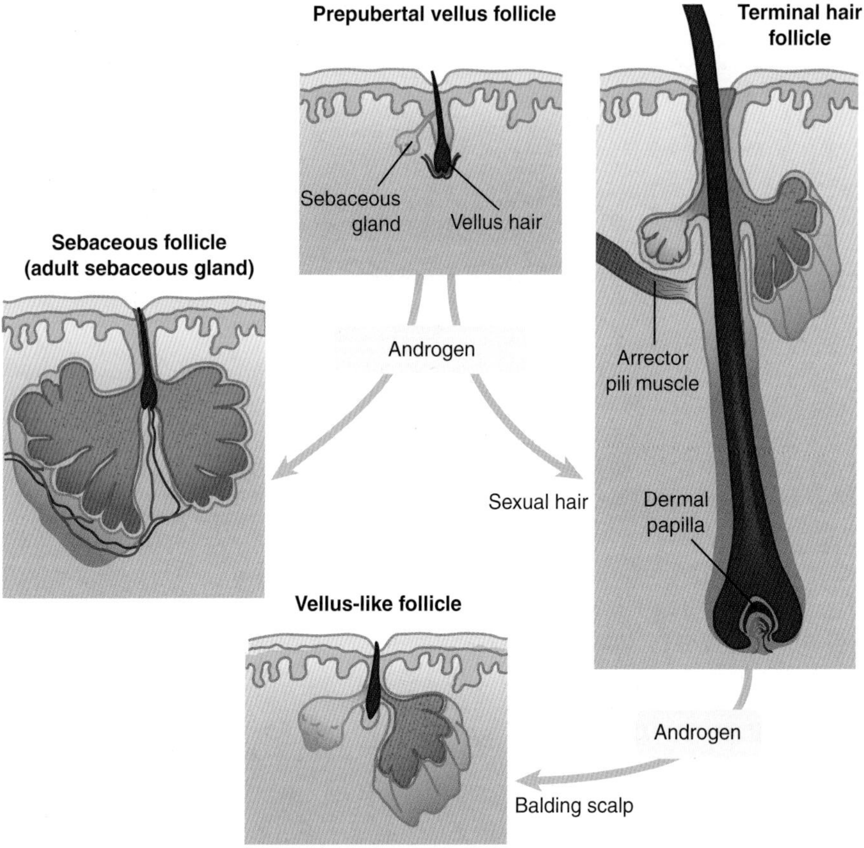


**Figure 41-1**
Depending on location and androgen level, the prepubertal vellus hair follicle is transformed into a terminal hair follicle or adult sebaceous hair follicle. Scalp terminal hair follicles under androgen exposure can transform back to a vellus type hair follicle. *(Reprinted with permission from Rosenfield RL. Hirsutism.* N Engl J Med. *2005;353:2578–2588.)*

(telogen phase). The anagen phase comprises 8% to 85% of the cycle and determines the length and diameter of hair.

Androgens are the primary hormones involved in hair growth, regulating the prolongation of the anagen phase and transformation of vellus to terminal hairs. This occurs first during puberty in androgen-sensitive areas. Paradoxically, the same androgens cause miniaturization or the transformation of terminal hair to vellus hair on specific areas of the scalp in genetically susceptible individuals, causing male-pattern alopecia (Figure 41-1).[3]

The primary androgen affecting hair growth is testosterone. In normal pubertal females, up to 50% of testosterone production is from the ovaries and adrenal glands. The remainder is derived from peripheral conversion of weaker androgens to testosterone in adipose tissue and skin.[4] Most of the testosterone in the circulation is bound to albumin (lower affinity) or sex hormone binding globulin (SHBG) (higher affinity); SHBG is therefore the primary regulator of free testosterone activity. Within hair follicles, type II 5α-reductase regulates the

BOX 41-1

## *Essential Elements in the History and Physical Examination for Complaint of Excess Hair*

**HISTORY**

- General
  - Current age
  - Ethnicity
  - History of weight change
  - Height acceleration
- Hair Growth Description
  - Age of onset
  - Progression of hair growth
  - Location/distribution of hair
- Presence of Other Premature/Abnormal Pubertal Features (Body Odor, Irregular Menses)
- Medical Problems
  - Neurologic conditions
  - Developmental history
- Medications
  - Exposure to exogenous sources of androgens
- Birth History
  - Birth weight/length
  - Perinatal problems
- Family History
  - Maternal polycystic ovary syndrome (PCOS)
  - Early infant demise
  - Hirsute or infertile female relatives

**PHYSICAL EXAMINATION**

- General
  - Blood pressure
  - Anthropometric measurements
  - Dysmorphology
  - Masculinization
- Skin
  - Acne, oily skin
  - Café au lait spots, striae
- Hair
  - Type (lanugo, vellus, terminal)
  - Amount/severity
  - Location/pattern (androgen-dependent areas vs generalized)
- Thyroid enlargement
- Puberty
  - Tanner stage pubic hair
  - Females: breast Tanner staging, areolar hair, clitoromegaly, vaginal mucosa (estrogenization)
  - Males: testicular volume, phallic enlargement

conversion of testosterone to dihydrotestosterone (DHT), a more potent androgen because of its higher affinity for the nuclear androgen receptor.

## ▶ INITIAL EVALUATION OF HAIR GROWTH

The evaluation of a patient with complaints of excess hair begins with a careful history and physical examination with specific points relevant to the chief complaint (Box 41-1).

In a preadolescent child, the chief complaint is usually that of body hair or odor. In an adolescent patient, the primary complaint depends on sex. Females typically complain of menstrual irregularities or dermatological manifestations of hyperandrogenism, including severe acne, hirsutism, or androgenic alopecia. Adolescent males come to attention much less frequently unless virilization is rapidly progressive or clinical signs such as alopecia or acne are excessive.

## ▶ HYPERTRICHOSIS

### *Presentation*

The initial task on examination is to differentiate between true sexual hair and hypertrichosis. The former will be dark, coarse, terminal hair that is limited to androgen-dependent regions, while hypertrichosis refers to excess hair growth relative to persons of the same age, sex, and ethnicity but excluding androgen-induced hair growth.[5] If true sexual hair is abnormally present, androgen levels should be measured and, if elevated, the source of hyperandrogenism should be investigated (see Hyperandrogenism).

## Classification

Hypertrichosis is described based on type of hair (lanugo, vellus, or terminal), age of onset (congenital or acquired), distribution (generalized or circumscribed), and location (forehead, ear, neck, back).[5] Although hypertrichosis is uncommon in children, there are many causes and associated conditions, some of which are listed in Box 41-2.

Classification of the different forms of congenital generalized hypertrichosis is difficult given its rarity and overlap of features. For example, *universal congenital hypertrichosis* is often used interchangeably with *Ambras syndrome*, characterized by extremely long vellus hair growth over the entire body (except palms, soles, and mucosae).[1,2,4,5] Other experts think that Ambras syndrome is a separate entity.[2] A careful examination with attention to the hair type and distribution is critical in classification. The mode of inheritance in most cases is autosomal dominant, although families with apparent X-linked transmission have been described.[5] In a separate form, *congenital hypertrichosis lanuginose*, affected infants present at birth with generalized homogeneous lanugo hair, which progressively sheds over the first year of life.[5] The mode of inheritance is autosomal dominant although sporadic cases have been reported.[6]

While the above types are rare, an interesting more common form of hypertrichosis is *prepubertal hypertrichosis*, in which the hair is noted at birth and progresses, with a predilection for (terminal) hair growth on the forehead, eyebrows, upper back, and upper limbs.[7] Circumscribed forms of hypertrichosis also exist. An example of such is *lumbosacral hypertrichosis*, which, if seen on the newborn examination, should prompt an expeditious evaluation for an occult spinal dysraphism. Of note, hypertrichosis can be an early manifestation of pubarche, so the prepubertal patient should be observed for progression of the hair development specific to androgen-dependent areas.

**BOX 41-2**

### *Causes of Hypertrichosis and Associated Conditions*

**CONGENITAL/GENETIC DISORDERS**

- Congenital hypertrichosis lanuginose
- Universal congenital hypertrichosis/Ambras syndrome
- Mucopolysaccharidosis
- Cornelia de Lange syndrome
- Trisomy 18
- Fetal hydantoin syndrome
- Fetal alcohol syndrome

**SYSTEMIC ILLNESS**

- Anorexia nervosa
- Hypothyroidism
- Malnutrition
- Malignancies

**MEDICATIONS**

- Corticosteroids
- Diazoxide
- Phenytoin
- Cyclosporine
- Streptomycin
- Minoxidil

### Treatment

Hypertrichosis can be a source of embarrassment for affected children and adolescents. Patients should be counseled that different treatment options are favored for different ages, types of hair, and body locations, but that all treatments have their limitations, pros, and cons. Treatments can be divided into different categories: physical cosmetic interventions (bleaching, waxing, plucking, trimming, shaving, chemical depilatories, electrolysis); light sources and lasers (of which there are different types); and pharmacological treatment.[1,5] Further discussion on treatment modalities can be found in the discussion on *hirsutism* below. It is important to consider, however, that since hypertrichosis is androgen independent, antiandrogen therapies are not indicated for its treatment.

## ▶ HYPERANDROGENISM

When the history and physical examination are consistent with increased production of androgens, hormonal levels should be drawn to help determine the source. Causes can be broadly divided into the location of hormone production: adrenal, gonadal, tumor, or exogenous. Exogenous sources include androgenic medications and anabolic steroids.

### Adrenal Hyperandrogenism

#### Adrenal Anatomy and Adrenarche

The adrenal cortex comprises 3 zones, each responsible for a different hormone pathway. The zona glomerulosa synthesizes aldosterone under regulation of the renin-angiotensin system. The zona fasiculata (glucocorticoid synthesis) and the zona reticularis (androgen synthesis) are regulated by the hypothalamic-pituitary-adrenal (HPA) axis. Corticotropin-releasing hormone (CRH) from the hypothalamus stimulates secretion of adrenocorticotropic hormone (ACTH) from the pituitary gland, which in turn stimulates the adrenal gland. *Adrenarche* is characterized by the maturation of the zona reticularis, leading to increased androgen production and the appearance of pubic hair (*pubarche*). The main androgens derived from the adrenal glands are dehydroepiandrosterone (DHEA), dehydroepiandrosterone sulfate (DHEAS), androstenedione, and testosterone. Adrenarche has a role in sexual maturation; however, it occurs independently from gonadotropin-dependent puberty.

#### Premature Adrenarche

*Premature adrenarche* refers to the earlier than normal timing of this process: before age 8 years in girls and age 9 in boys. However, there is racial and ethnic variation in the age at which puberty begins in normal children. Premature adrenarche is seen more commonly in females and black children.[8,9] It has also been associated with fetal growth restriction, as seen in small for gestational age (SGA) babies and in prematurity.[10] The concept of fetal programming and the association of pre- and post-natal weight gain with premature adrenarche, the development of obesity, metabolic syndrome, and PCOS offers attractive, yet incompletely understood mechanisms whereby nutritional, hormonal (GH-IGF system and insulin, for example) and epigenetic phenomena might link early processes with subsequent disease.[11,12]

**PRESENTATION AND DIFFERENTIAL DIAGNOSES.** These children usually present with pubic hair, initially noted perilabially in girls and at the base of the penis in boys.

Associated findings can include axillary hair and odor, oily skin, or mild acne. Signs of virilization are absent. Transient height acceleration and advancement of bone age may be present; however, final adult height is usually unaffected in cases in which the premature adrenarche is deemed benign (once other causes of premature hair development are excluded). Exposure to an exogenous hormone or drug must be ruled out because premature adrenarche caused by exogenous sources is reversible with removal of the source. Examples of exogenous causes include a family member who is using a testosterone gel without taking proper precautions for close contacts. Of more concern, premature adrenarche may be the first sign of a serious underlying disorder such as an androgen-secreting adrenal tumor or congenital adrenal hyperplasia (CAH). In these conditions, signs of virilization can be present and the bone age is significantly advanced.

**CONGENITAL ADRENAL HYPERPLASIA.** Congential adrenal hyperplasia represents a group of autosomal recessive disorders involving a deficiency in 1 of the enzymes in adrenal steroid synthesis, leading to impaired cortisol production and increased ACTH production. Shunting of precursors proximal to the enzymatic block results in increased androgen production. The disease manifestations vary clinically and biochemically with each specific enzyme deficiency. The most common cause is 21-hydroxylase deficiency (mutations in the CYP21B gene located on chromosome 6) leading to decreased aldosterone and cortisol and increased production of androstenedione and testosterone. Although the classic form is usually diagnosed in infancy with salt-wasting in boys and ambiguous genitalia plus salt wasting in girls, a *non-classic 21-hydroxylase deficiency* typically presents later in life, with premature adrenarche, hirsutism, or menstrual abnormalities.

## Evaluation and Treatment

If the findings are consistent with sexual hair development (with or without axillary hair, axillary odor, or acne) without any rapid progression, signs of virilization, or signs of true puberty (testicular enlargement in boys and breast development in girls), close follow-up is recommended. Baseline adrenal hormone levels (DHEA, DHEAS, androstenedione, testosterone, 17-hydroxyprogesterone) as well as a bone age (radiograph of left hand and wrist) may be performed. In children with premature adrenarche, androgen levels are in the early-pubertal range and the bone age is usually within 2 standard deviations of chronologic age.

If progression of pubic hair is rapid, signs of virilization are present, or there is moderate elevation of androgen levels or advancement of bone age, an ACTH stimulation test is warranted to rule out nonclassical (or late-onset) CAH. Markedly elevated androgen levels or significant advancement of bone age suggests an androgen-producing adrenal or gonadal tumor. If a tumor is suspected, ultrasound or MRI for localization is necessary. Further, if there are signs of true pubertal development, other baseline or stimulation tests to evaluate the hypothalamic-pituitary-gonadal (HPG) axis as well as hypothalamic-pituitary imaging may be necessary. The evaluation and treatment of true precocious puberty will be discussed briefly below and in Chapter 62, Puberty: Normal and Abnormal.

Once a careful evaluation excludes these other conditions, reassurance and continued follow-up of growth and pubertal progression is necessary to make sure that the initial complaints and investigations do not herald a more serious condition. No specific medical treatment is indicated for premature adrenarche. Although premature adrenarche has been characterized as a benign condition (with many sources referring to it as *benign premature adrenarche),* studies in girls have shown associations with conditions such as PCOS and metabolic syndrome.[13,14] Obesity and acanthosis nigricans are more common in patients with premature adrenarche. Offspring of women with PCOS are at higher risk for premature adrenarche, and brothers of women with PCOS have been found to have higher levels of DHEAS than brothers of unaffected women, suggesting a common cause or risk factor.[15] These findings also lend support to a role for both adrenal and ovarian hyperandrogenism in PCOS, as opposed to it being merely an ovarian process (see section on PCOS). Although these associations among pre- and postnatal growth patterns, obesity, adrenarche, hyperandrogenism, metabolic derangements, and PCOS phenotypes have led to numerous hypotheses regarding common underlying hormonal mechanisms, a single cause remains elusive.[12,16]

### Gonadal Hyperandrogenism

The differential diagnosis of premature pubarche is age-dependent and may be the presenting sign of a more serious underlying endocrinopathy.[17]

#### Precocious Puberty

Precocious puberty can be generally divided into gonadotropin-dependent or gonadotropin-independent precocity.

*Gonadotropin-dependent,* also referred to as *central* or *true* precocious puberty, results from abnormalities of the central nervous system that disrupt the balance between inhibitory and stimulatory factors. These abnormalities include congenital malformations, tumors, and acquired causes such as trauma, infection, surgery, radiation, or chemotherapy. A unique congenital malformation is hypothalamic hamartoma, which is ectopically located neural tissue containing gonadotropin-releasing hormone (GnRH) secretory neurons. For most affected females, no specific cause of central precocious puberty can be identified, and precocity is therefore classified as idiopathic. GnRH agonists are the mainstay of treatment for central precocious puberty. The increased potency and continuous stimulation desensitizes the pituitary to stimulation from endogenous GnRH, thus halting further progression of puberty.

*Gonadotropin-independent* precocious puberty can be caused by gonadal tumors, McCune-Albright syndrome, and in males by familial testotoxicosis—a disorder caused by a missense mutation of the luteinizing hormone (LH) receptor. Peripheral precocious puberty can induce maturation of the HPG axis, and secondarily lead to true central precocity.

#### Infancy

In the neonatal period, there is activation of the HPG axis, leading to androgen production. Peak testosterone production between 1 to 3 months of age coupled with a transient increase in the sensitivity of sexual hair follicles is thought to cause the appearance of pubic hair in the first few months of life. The pubic hair tends to occur in atypical locations—on the mons pubis in girls and on the scrotum in boys; it generally regresses spontaneously.[18]

## Young Child

While generally not the presenting sign of normal central puberty, sexual hair can precede the initial signs of true puberty in up to 20% of normal boys and girls. Therefore, *premature adrenarche* may be the presenting sign of *premature central precocious puberty* (CPP), defined as occurring before age 8 years in girls and 9 years in boys. Chapter 62, Puberty: Normal and Abnormal, reviews pubertal development in normal and abnormal states. Briefly, puberty is the process of physical changes leading to sexual maturity, reproductive capability, and completion of skeletal growth. The process is initiated by *gonadarche* or reactivation of the HPG axis. The HPG axis is regulated by central inhibitory and stimulatory neurotransmitters, as well as peripheral factors such as nutrition and body mass composition. Increased pulsatile release of GnRH from the arcuate nucleus of the hypothalamus acts on the pituitary to stimulate LH and follicle-stimulating hormone (FSH) production. In females, LH acts on the ovarian theca cells and stimulates androgen production. Testosterone diffuses to the nearby granulosa cells where FSH stimulates aromatase conversion of testosterone to estrogen. In males, LH acts on the Leydig cells to stimulate testosterone production while FSH acts on the Sertoli cells to initiate and maintain spermatogenesis.

In girls, breast bud development (*thelarche*) is typically the initial physical change in puberty, which is then followed by the appearance of pubic hair. Height acceleration or growth spurt occurs early in girls, always preceding menarche. In boys, testicular enlargement (>3 mL in volume) is generally the first sign of puberty, followed by penile enlargement, and development of pubic hair. The growth spurt occurs later in boys. A careful physical examination at the time of initial consultation, as well as continued follow-up for the development of other pubertal signs is crucial in determining if the child has isolated adrenarche or the evolution of CPP.

## Adolescent Female

In the adolescent female presenting with signs of hyperandrogenism, the differential diagnosis includes PCOS, idiopathic hirsutism, nonclassical CAH, exogenous exposure, or tumor. The diagnostics of the latter 3 conditions have been discussed previously.

**POLYCYSTIC OVARY SYNDROME.** Polycystic ovary syndrome (PCOS) was first described by Stein and Leventhal in 1935.[19] It is the most common endocrine disorder affecting adolescent females and women of childbearing age. Although a single cause continues to elude scientists, much has been discovered regarding contributing factors and comorbidities. The diagnostic criteria have been adjusted and remain variable given different expert panel consensus statements. This, as well as imprecision with androgen assays, has made determination of true prevalence difficult.[20,21] Most endocrinologists accept menstrual irregularities as the symptom of anovulation, combined with either biochemical or clinical evidence of ovarian hyperandrogenism as the pillars of diagnosis of PCOS. Although polycystic ovaries can support the diagnosis of PCOS, their absence does not rule out the diagnosis.[22] As with the workup of the younger child for premature pubarche, it is imperative to exclude other causes of hyperandrogenism, such as exogenous exposure, tumor, and congenital adrenal hyperplasia, among others, prior to diagnosing a patient with PCOS. Further, other endocrinopathies can masquerade as PCOS, such as severe hypothyroidism and hypercortisolism.

PCOS in adolescence can manifest differently than in adult women. Whereas the chief complaint bringing the adult woman to medical attention may be menstrual irregularity or infertility, adolescent females might be more troubled by excess hair, acne, male-pattern alopecia, or menstrual irregularities, including even primary amenorrhea in some. Further, adolescent females with menstrual irregularities or weight gain and acne might be falsely led to believe that these findings are merely physiologic changes associated with pubertal development. This can lead to a delay in medical attention, evaluation, and treatment, as well as a negative effect on self-esteem.

PCOS is likely a polygenic, multifactorial condition. Multiple associated symptoms and biochemical derangements have been regarded as common to most females with PCOS. While obesity and insulin resistance, for example, play a role in many patients, there are lean women with PCOS as well. Fetal origins of PCOS have been studied, with attention to exposures in utero and the subsequent development of of insulin resistance and hyperandrogenism, as in the child with premature adrenarche.[23] Further, children born SGA have an increased risk for PCOS.[24] Ovarian hyperandrogenism is a feature in PCOS, with the contribution of adrenal hyperandrogenism as well. The ovarian theca cells produce weak androgens in response to stimulation by LH by the pituitary gland. In nonpathological states, the granulosa cells, under control of FSH, aromatize the androgens to estrogens. In PCOS an imbalance of LH/FSH leads to a decreased ability to aromatize excess androgen, and failure of the establishment of a dominant follicle, thus resulting in anovulation.

Although insulin resistance is a fundamental component of PCOS, it is unknown whether it causes, exacerbates, or functions as a marker for the condition. Females with PCOS are more insulin resistant than weight-matched females without PCOS. Whereas the liver, muscle, and adipose tissues are resistant to insulin in predisposed hosts, the ovary and adrenal glands maintain sensitivity to insulin. This results in enhanced ovarian hyperandrogenemia. Hyperinsulinism also decreases the level of sex hormone binding globulin (SHBG), which in turn increases the level of available free testosterone.

The manifestation of PCOS is variable across ages and ethnicities, and even within the individual. As mentioned, menstrual irregularities implying anovulation and clinical or biochemical hyperandrogenism are cardinal features. It is important to note that some girls and women with menstrual irregularity do ovulate, and conversely, some girls and women who bleed regularly are not experiencing ovulatory cycles. Most often, however, the presentation related to menses is oligomenorrhea or secondary amenorrhea, although primary amenorrhea and dysfunctional uterine bleeding are possible complaints as well.

The evaluation of a female suspected of having PCOS begins with a careful history and physical examination. Family history of hormonal disorders, infertility, hirsutism, or unexplained newborn demise (unrecognized congenital adrenal hyperplasia with adrenal crisis) should be explored. A complete past medical history, including birth data (for SGA), medications, and exposures is important, along with the timing of puberty and menstrual history. The presence of other findings related to the differential diagnosis of menstrual irregularities should be sought: disordered eating, large weight fluctuations, pregnancy, symptoms of thyroid disease, galactorrhea, and so on. The tempo of physical changes, including menstrual irregularities, and dermatological or other manifestations of hyperandrogenemia, if present, is crucial to determine if the process is gradual as opposed to sudden and rapidly progressive. The latter is more consistent with an exposure or an androgen-secreting tumor, and may be accompanied by more significant signs of virilization, including voice deepening and clitoromegaly, which are only rarely seen in PCOS.

A complete physical examination is warranted to evaluate a female with menstrual irregularities, including a blood pressure check, body mass index measurement, careful inspection of optic discs for papilledema, skin for acanthosis nigricans, palpation of the thyroid, and breast examination for galactorrhea. Furthermore, specific attention should be given to the dermatological signs of hyperandrogenism, including acne (severity, location, extent), alopecia, and hirsutism. The modified Ferriman-Gallwey score is a widely accepted method of quantifying hirsutism.[3,25] This system estimates the amount of terminal hair in 9 areas: upper lip, chin, arms, thighs, chest, and upper and lower abdomen and back. Each area is assigned a score of 0 (absent) to 4 (extensive hair growth visible); therefore, the total score can range from 0 to 36. A score of 8 or greater indiciates hirsutism; 8 to 15 indicates moderate hirsutism and greater than 15 indicates severe hirsutism (Figure 41-2).

Although widely used, this system has several limitations including the subjective nature of the assessment, inability to account for focal hirsutism, and lack of population based data that take into account racial and ethnic differences in body hair. Examination of the genitalia for clitoromegaly as well as the presence of estrogenized vaginal mucosa also should be done.

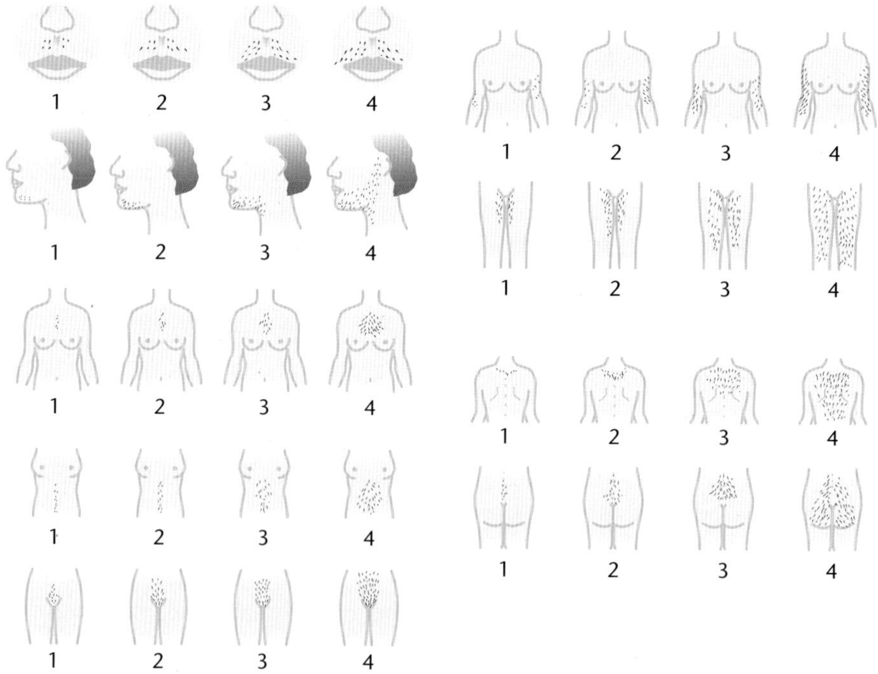

**Figure 41-2**

Modified Ferriman-Gallwey (F-G) hirsutism scoring system. The F-G score should be used during clinical examination of a woman with hirsutism. *(Reprinted with permission from Yildiz BO, Bolour S, Woods K, Moore A, Azziz R. Visually scoring hirsutism.* Hum Reprod Update. *2009;16[1]:51–64.)*

The laboratory evaluation of a woman suspected of having PCOS will be driven by the physician's index of suspicion and whether a previous workup for menstrual irregularities has been performed. If the patient has not been evaluated in the past, the full complement of studies may include a complete blood count and metabolic profile, LH, FSH, prolactin, thyroid function tests, pregnancy test, estradiol, and chromosomal analysis. Free testosterone is the single most helpful test in the diagnosis of PCOS. Alternatively, a total testosterone test with SHBG level can be done. Testosterone assays have been notorious for lack of standardization and precision, especially in the lower concentrations that are expected in women. Tandem mass spectrometry is available through commercial laboratories, and should be used if possible.[22,26] DHEAS and androstenedione levels are often elevated in females with PCOS as well. Insulin resistance with hyperinsulinism is seen in many patients with PCOS, more commonly when the patient is obese. Because PCOS is associated with metabolic syndrome, affected females should be screened for glucose abnormalities. Appropriate evaluations could include a hemoglobin A1c, fasting glucose, and a 2-hour oral glucose tolerance test, along with fasting lipid panel and complete metabolic profile. The increased risk of obstructive sleep apnea in women with PCOS has been attributed to hyperandrogenism, rather than to obesity alone.[27]

**IDIOPATHIC HIRSUTISM.** Idiopathic hirsutism is a diagnosis of exclusion, defined as hirsutism with regular ovulation and normal androgen levels. Many mechanisms have been implicated, including minor ovarian or adrenal functional hyperandrogenism, increased peripheral conversion of testosterone to DHT, or abnormalities in the androgen receptor leading to increased sensitivity of hair follicles to normal androgen levels.[28] A careful history, including a complete menstrual history as well as details of the onset and progression of the hair growth, and physical examination are important to exclude other diagnoses. Of note, menstrual regularity does not preclude an anovulatory state. Thus it is recommended to obtain an early-morning free testosterone level in the following patients: women with moderate or severe hirsutism, women with hirsutism of any degree with sudden onset or rapid progression, or women with accompanying signs or symptoms suggesting malignancy or PCOS.[26]

## Treatment

Treatment options for hirsutism can be divided into pharmacological therapy and cosmetic management. Education about reasonable expectations is crucial: the effects of pharmacological therapy do not become evident before 6 to 12 months of treatment because of the long duration of the anagen phase of the hair cycle. The choice of treatment depends on patient preference, the extent to which the area of hirsutism is amenable to cosmetic hair removal, and cost of treatment.

In PCOS, there are 4 levels of treatment: restoration of menstrual regularity; treatment of hirsutism, which is typically the most distressing symptom of androgen excess in adolescents; treatment of obesity and metabolic abnormalities if they exist; and improvement of psychological impairment that may be associated with any of the above.

The first line of pharmacological treatment for both idiopathic hirsutism and hirsutism in PCOS is oral contraceptive pills (OCPs), which inhibit ovarian androgen biosynthesis in 2 ways: suppression of gonadotropin secretion and increased hepatic SHBG production (thereby decreasing free androgen concentrations). OCPs usually combine a synthetic estrogen and progestin. Products that contain low-androgenic progestins, such as drosperinone or norgestimate, should be used. In addition to decreasing hirsutism, OCPs regulate menstrual cycles and protect the endometrium which is beneficial in PCOS. Side effects include breast tenderness, gastrointestinal discomfort, and worsening of headaches in a patient with migraines. The most serious side effect is the risk of venous thromboembolism, which is increased in women older than 35, with a history of cigarette smoking, and with a personal or family history of a clotting disorder. A careful assessment of these risks is warranted. Drosperinone has been implicated in imparting an even higher risk of thromboembolism than other progestins, but it is not clear if that risk is clinically significant.[29,30] The long-term effect of OCPs on metabolic risks (lipid abnormalities and glucose tolerance) have not been closely studied, and should be kept in mind when choosing a regimen.[31,32]

If hirsutism persists after 6 months of treatment with an OCP, or if the use of an OCP is contraindicated or not desired, an antiandrogen can be used. In women of child-bearing potential, antiandrogen medications should not be used without adequate birth control measures because feminization of the male fetus can theoretically occur. Spironolactone, the most widely prescribed antiandrogen, is also an aldosterone antagonist and so should not be used in patients with renal failure, hyperkalemia or in conjunction with other medications that cause hyperkalemia. Spironolactone is a competitive inhibitor of the androgen receptor and also inhibits 5α-reductase activity, thus demonstrating properties of both flutamide and finasteride, other antiandrogens which have been used in the treatment of hirsutism. A study comparing these 3 agents demonstrated similar efficacies in the treatment of hirsutism after 6 months.[33] The long-term use of pharmacological therapy for hirsutism in adolescent females has not been studied.[31]

Cosmetic forms of hair removal include both temporary and permanent methods. Temporary treatments include hair removal from the skin surface (depilation) and those that extract hairs from above the bulb (epilation). Depilation methods include shaving and the use of chemical depilatory agents. Shaving is the least expensive method. Contrary to common belief, shaving does not increase the diameter of the hair follicle or affect the rate of hair growth; however, shaving can cause irritation and folliculitis. Depilatory agents dissolve hair by reducing the disulfide bonds and peptides of hair keratin at the skin surface. They can cause irritant dermatitis. Bleaching, although not a method of hair removal, can camouflage dark hair. Epilation methods include plucking and waxing. Plucking can be painful and time-consuming, making it useful only in small areas such as the face.

Electrolysis and photoepilation are methods of permanent hair reduction, not removal. Electrolysis involves placing a fine needle in the hair follicle and applying an electrical current. Because each follicle is treated individually, the process is time-consuming and difficult if large areas need treatment. Photoepilation uses lasers and other light sources such as IPL to damage hair follicles without damaging the surrounding tissues. It is most effective in patients with light skin complexion and dark hair. Although hair follicles are destroyed, vellus hair follicles can remain, and in patients with hyperandrogenism these follicles can convert to terminal hair resulting in hair regrowth. Photoepilation requires multiple treatments, is expensive, and can cause dyspigmentation and scarring.

Eflornithine hydrochloride cream, which has been approved for the treatment of facial hirsutism, irreversibly inhibits ornithine decarboxylase (ODC) in hair follicles. Essential in hair growth, ODC catalyzes the synthesis of polyamines, small cationic molecules that play a role in cell proliferation in hair follicle development and growth. The cream can be added to photoepilation therapy for a more rapid initial response.

In adolescents with PCOS who have abnormalities of glucose or significant hyperinsulinism, treatment should be aimed at managing metabolic abnormalities in conjunction with the above measures. Dietary and exercise changes should be the first-line treatment for obesity and dyslipidemia. Although these measures can be extremely challenging, it should be emphasized to the patient that as little as a 5% to 10% weight loss can have significant clinical outcomes, including improvement in biochemical hyperandrogenism, menstrual regularity, and glycemic profiles.[32,34] Lifestyle changes with small achievable goals should be set. The current evidence suggests that multiple dietary strategies can be successful as long as they are nutritionally adequate and can be sustained. Goals for exercise should focus on overall health improvement, not weight loss.

Glucophage, a biguanide insulin sensitizing agent, is the single oral antihyperglycemic drug approved for use in children as young as 10 years of age. It inhibits hepatic glucose production and increases insulin sensitivity in peripheral tissues. The common side effects of nausea and diarrhea can be minimized by starting at a low dose, titrating upward as tolerated, and taking it with meals. Long-term treatment with glucophage has been associated with malabsorption of $B_{12}$.[35] The most serious, although rare, complication is lactic acidosis. Glucophage is contraindicated with renal or hepatic impairment, severe congestive heart failure, or a history of alcohol abuse. It is used along with OCPs in the treatment of PCOS, especially in patients with diabetes or impaired glucose tolerance. In patients in whom OCPs are contraindicated or not desired, glucophage has been used as monotherapy.

Although the treatment of infertility is not a common issue in adolescence, the implication of PCOS on future fertility should be discussed with affected young women. At the time when fertility is desired, referral to a reproductive endocrinologist is appropriate.

## ▶ SUMMARY

Abnormal or excessive hair development is a common presenting complaint in the pediatric population. A thorough history and physical examination will guide further evaluation and separate benign conditions from more serious pathology. Premature adrenarche and PCOS may be manifestations of the same disease process, which may have origins in fetal life.

### When to Refer

- Signs of adrenarche (pubic hair, axillary hair, and/or odor) prior to age 8 in girls and 9 in boys
- Signs of virilization (clitoromegaly, masculine body habitus) in girls at any age
- Signs of virilization (penile enlargement, deepening of the voice) in boys prior to age 9 or rapid virilization at any age
- Signs of puberty in girls (breast development, menarche) prior to age 8
- Signs of puberty in boys (testicular enlargement) prior to age 9
- Symptoms of PCOS (hirsutism, menstrual irregularities) in girls
- Metabolic syndrome (obesity, hypertension, insulin resistance or type 2 diabetes mellitus, dyslipidemia)

## When to Admit

- Hypertension secondary to suspected mineralocorticoid excess (congenital adrenal tumor [CAH]–C-11 hydroxylase deficiency)
- Central nervous system (CNS) symptoms (headaches, visual changes) secondary to CNS lesions
- Severe abdominal and/or pelvic pain secondary to suspected mass
- Marked hyperglycemia requiring insulin treatment

## TOOLS FOR PRACTICE

### Engaging Patient and Family

- *Puberty—Ready or Not, Expect Some Changes* (handout), American Academy of Pediatrics (patiented.solutions.aap.org)
- *What Is a Pediatric Endocrinologist?* (fact sheet), American Academy of Pediatrics (www.healthychildren.org/English/family-life/health-management/pediatric-specialists/pages/What-is-a-Pediatric-Endocrinologist.aspx)

## AAP POLICY STATEMENT

American Academy of Pediatrics Committee on Adolescence, American College of Obstetricians and Gynecologists, Committee on Adolescent Health Care. Menstruation in girls and adolescents: using the menstrual cycle as a vital sign. *Pediatrics.* 2006;118(5):2245–2250 (pediatrics.aappublications.org/content/118/5/2245.full)

## REFERENCES


1. Kunte C, Wolff H, Gottschaller C, Hohenleutner U. Therapy of hypertrichosis. *J Dtsch Dermatol Ges.* 2007;5:807–810
2. Rashid RM, White LE. A hairy development in hypertrichosis: a brief review of Ambras syndrome. *Dermatol Online J.* 2007;13:8
3. Rosenfield RL. Clinical practice. Hirsutism. *N Engl J Med.* 2005;353:2578–2588
4. Abdel-Rahman MY, Hurd WW. Androgen excess. Medscape. January 2011. emedicine.medscape.com/article/273153-overview. Accessed October 16, 2014
5. Trüeb RM. Causes and management of hypertrichosis. *Am J Clin Dermatol.* 2002;3:617–627
6. Mendiratta V, Harjai B, Gupta T. Hypertrichosis lanuginosa congenita. *Pediatr Dermatol.* 2008;25:483–484
7. Barth JH, Wilkinson JD, Dawber RP. Prepubertal hypertrichosis: normal or abnormal? *Arch Dis Child.* 1988;63:666–668
8. Dorn LD, Rotenstein D. Early puberty in girls: the case of premature adrenarche. *Womens Health Issues.* 2004;14:177–183
9. Banerjee S, Raghavan S, Wasserman EJ, et al. Hormonal findings in African-American and Caribbean Hispanic girls with premature adrenarche: implications for polycystic ovarian syndrome. *Pediatrics.* 1998;102:E36
10. Neville KA, Walker JL. Precocious pubarche is associated with SGA, prematurity, weight gain, and obesity. *Arch Dis Child.* 2005;90:258–261
11. Xita N, Tsatsoulis A. Fetal origins of the metabolic syndrome. *Ann N Y Acad Sci.* 2010;1205:148–155
12. Belgorosky A, Baquedano MS, Guercio G, Rivarola MA. Adrenarche: postnatal adrenal zonation and hormonal and metabolic regulation. *Horm Res.* 2008;70:257–267
13. Ibáñez L, Dimartino-Nardi J, Potau N, Saenger P. Premature adrenarche—normal variant or forerunner of adult disease? *Endocr Rev.* 2000;21:671–696
14. Kousta E. Premature adrenarche leads to polycystic ovary syndrome? Long-term consequences. *Ann N Y Acad Sci.* 2006;1092:148–157

15. Legro RS, Kunselman AR, Demers L, et al. Elevated dehydroepiandrosterone sulfate levels as the reproductive phenotype in the brothers of women with polycystic ovary syndrome. *J Clin Endocrinol Metab.* 2002;87:2134–2138
16. Vuguin P, Linder B, Rosenfeld RG, Saenger P, DiMartino-Nardi J. The roles of insulin sensitivity, insulin-like growth factor I (IGF-I), and IGF-binding protein-1 and -3 in the hyperandrogenism of African-American and Caribbean Hispanic girls with premature adrenarche. *J Clin Endocrinol Metab.* 1999;84:2037–2042
17. Leung AK, Robson WL. Premature adrenarche. *J Pediatr Health Care.* 2008;22:230–233
18. Nebesio TD, Eugster EA. Pubic hair of infancy: endocrinopathy or enigma? *Pediatrics.* 2006;117:951–954
19. Stein I, Leventhal M. Amenorrhea associated with bilateral polycystic ovaries. *Am J Obstet Gynecol.* 1935;29:181–185
20. Legro RS, Schlaff WD, Diamond MP, et al. Total testosterone assays in women with polycystic ovary syndrome: precision and correlation with hirsutism. *J Clin Endocrinol Metab.* 2010;95(12):5305–5313
21. March WA, Moore VM, Willson KJ, et al. The prevalence of polycystic ovary syndrome in a community sample assessed under contrasting diagnostic criteria. *Hum Reprod.* 2010;25:544–551
22. Azziz R, Carmina E, Dewailly D, et al. The Androgen Excess and PCOS Society criteria for the polycystic ovary syndrome: the complete task force report. *Fertil Steril.* 2009;91:456–488
23. Utriainen P, Jääskeläinen J, Romppanen J, Voutilainen R. Childhood metabolic syndrome and its components in premature adrenarche. *J Clin Endocrinol Metab.* 2007;92(11):4282–4285
24. Rosenfield RL. Clinical review: identifying children at risk for polycystic ovary syndrome. *J Clin Endocrinol Metab.* 2007;92:787–796
25. Yildiz BO, Bolour S, Woods K, Moore A, Azziz R. Visually scoring hirsutism. *Hum Reprod Update.* 2010;16:51–64
26. Martin KA, Chang RJ, Ehrmann DA, et al. Evaluation and treatment of hirsutism in premenopausal women: an Endocrine Society clinical practice guideline. *J Clin Endocrinol Metab.* 2008;93(4):1105–1120
27. Tasali E, Van Cauter E, Ehrmann DA. Polycystic ovary syndrome and obstructive sleep apnea. *Sleep Med Clin.* 2008;3:37–46
28. Harrison S, Somani N, Bergfeld WF. Update on the management of hirsutism. *Cleve Clin J Med.* 2010;77:388–398
29. van Grootheest K, Vrieling T. Thromboembolism associated with the new contraceptive Yasmin. *BMJ.* 2003;326:257
30. van Hylckama Vlieg A, Helmerhorst FM, Vandenbroucke JP, Doggen CJ, Rosendaal FR. The venous thrombotic risk of oral contraceptives, effects of oestrogen dose and progestogen type: results of the MEGA case-control study. *BMJ.* 2009;339:b2921
31. Ojaniemi M, Tapanainen P, Morin-Papunen L. Management of polycystic ovary syndrome in childhood and adolescence. *Horm Res Paediatr.* 2010;74(5):372–375
32. Diamanti-Kandarakis E. PCOS in adolescents. *Best Pract Res Clin Obstet Gynaecol.* 2010;24:173–183
33. Moghetti P, Tosi F, Tosti A, et al. Comparison of spironolactone, flutamide, and finasteride efficacy in the treatment of hirsutism: a randomized, double blind, placebo-controlled trial. *J Clin Endocrinol Metab.* 2000;85:89–94
34. Moran LJ, Pasquali R, Teede HJ, Hoeger KM, Norman RJ. Treatment of obesity in polycystic ovary syndrome: a position statement of the Androgen Excess and Polycystic Ovary Syndrome Society. *Fertil Steril.* 2009;92:1966–1982
35. de Jager J, Kooy A, Lehert P, et al. Long term treatment with metformin in patients with type 2 diabetes and risk of vitamin B-12 deficiency: randomised placebo controlled trial. *BMJ.* 2010;340:c2181

Box 42-1

## *Differential Diagnosis of Pediatric Hoarseness by Category*

### CONGENITAL

- Laryngeal anomalies
  - Laryngomalacia
  - Glottic webs
  - Subglottic stenosis
  - Laryngeal cleft
- Cystic lesions
  - Laryngocele
  - Saccular cyst
  - Thyroglossal duct cyst
  - Cervical bronchogenic cyst
- Angiomas
  - Lymphatic malformation
  - Hemangioma
  - Arteriovenous malformation
- Cri du chat syndrome

### NEUROGENIC (CONGENITAL AND ACQUIRED)

- Supranuclear (eg, hydrocephalus)
- Nuclear (Arnold-Chiari malformation, Guillain-Barré syndrome)
- Peripheral (eg, myasthenia gravis, cardiovascular anomalies, recurrent laryngeal nerve trauma)
- Psychogenic hoarseness

### VOCAL FOLD ABUSE

- Vocal fold nodules
- Vocal fold polyps

### NEOPLASIA

- Papilloma
- Squamous cell carcinoma

### PHYSICAL VOICE CHANGE OF PUBERTY

### INFLAMMATORY

- Infectious
  - Viral laryngopharyngitis (upper respiratory tract infection)
  - Viral laryngotracheitis (croup)
  - Bacterial supraglottitis (epiglottitis)
  - Rare infections: (*Candida,* diptheria, tuberculosis, leprosy)
- Noninfectious
  - Laryngopharyngeal reflux
  - Allergic laryngitis
  - Foreign body
  - Angioedema
  - Rheumatoid arthritis
  - Relapsing polychondritis
  - Chemical irritation (smoking, secondhand smoke, toxic fumes, inhaled medications)

### TRAUMATIC

- Hematoma
- Laryngeal cartilage fracture
- Impacted foreign body
- Postintubation
  - Arytenoid dislocation
  - Fold avulsion
  - Granuloma
  - Acquired glottic web
  - Subglottic stenosis
- Recurrent laryngeal nerve injury
  - Thyroidectomy
  - Tracheotomy
  - Cardiac surgery
  - Tracheoesophageal fistula repair
  - Tracheal resection
  - Penetrating neck wound

Adapted with permission from Friedberg J, El-Hakim H. Hoarseness. In: Bluestone CD, Stool SE, Kenna MA, eds. *Pediatric Otolaryngology.* 4th ed. Philadelphia, PA: WB Saunders; 2003.

Box 42-2

## *Differential Diagnosis of Pediatric Hoarseness by Age*

**0 TO 6 MONTHS**

- Traumatic intubation
- Iatrogenic: surgical
- Neurogenic: central or peripheral
- Neoplastic: hemangioma
- Congenital: web, cleft, cyst

**6 MONTHS TO 5 YEARS**

- Traumatic: foreign bodies, intubation
- Infectious: URI
- Neoplastic: papillomas
- Behavioral, traumatic: nodules
- Inflammatory: allergy, LPR

**5 TO 13 YEARS**

- Behavioral, traumatic: nodules
- Infectious: URI
- Inflammatory: allergy, LPR
- Neoplastic

**13 TO 18 YEARS**

- Infectious: URI
- Inflammatory: allergy, LPR
- Behavioral, traumatic:
  - Male: mutational or transitional voice
  - Female: nodules
- Functional: muscle tension dysphonia

*LPR,* laryngopharyngeal reflux; *URI,* upper respiratory infection.
Adapted and modified with permission from Smith ME, Gray SD. Voice. In: Bluestone CD, Stool SE, Kenna MA, eds. *Pediatric Otolaryngology.* 4th ed. Philadelphia, with permission PA: WB Saunders; 2003.

be associated with aphonia, stridor, and respiratory distress. Laryngeal webs vary from thin slips of tissue between the anterior areas of the vocal folds to complete laryngeal atresia, which is incompatible with life unless recognized immediately. Atresia or near-total atresia has been referred to as congenital high airway obstruction syndrome.[7] Laryngeal saccular cysts are characterized by symptoms of airway obstruction and dysphagia. Saccular cysts are filled with mucinous fluid and arise as a result of an abnormal dilation of the saccule of the larynx secondary to secretory outflow obstruction.

Posterior laryngeal clefts are an uncommon laryngeal anomaly that result in an abnormal opening in the posterior larynx. Clefts can simply involve the posterior laryngeal commissure, but may extend through the cricoid inferiorly through the tracheoesophageal septum. Symptoms depend on the extent of the cleft; at birth, clefts typically cause aspiration, stridor, respiratory distress, and weak cry.

Subglottic hemangiomas classically occur between the first and sixth month of life, with varying degrees of respiratory distress, stridor, cough, dysphagia, and hoarseness.[8] The natural history of hemangiomas is that of proliferation followed by involution. Subglottic hemangiomas can be unilateral, bilateral, or circumferential, and are more common in girls than in boys. Cutaneous hemangiomas of the head and neck are found concurrently in approximately 50% of cases of subglottic hemangioma.

A relationship may exist between pediatric and adult laryngeal disease and reflux.[9,10] Whereas gastroesophageal reflux (GER) refers to the backflow of stomach contents into the esophagus, laryngopharyngeal reflux (LPR) refers to the backflow of stomach contents into the throat, or laryngopharynx. Gastroesophageal reflux disease commonly produces emesis, dysphagia, sleep disturbance, and failure to thrive.[11] The association among GER,

LPR, and various neonatal laryngeal disorders such as hoarseness, posterior laryngitis, and silent aspiration, however, is an area of intense study that remains complicated and controversial.[12–14]

### Older Child

Older children and adolescents are subject to many of the same sources of hoarseness as adults. Infectious, inflammatory, traumatic, and neoplastic conditions such as laryngitis, LPR, vocal nodules, and respiratory papillomata are the leading causes of hoarseness among older children.[14]

Hoarseness of childhood from infectious disorders such as infective laryngitis, supraglottitis, and laryngotracheobronchitis rarely present a diagnostic challenge; however, concern over the airway should always take precedence. For example, hoarse voice may be an early indicator of the impending airway compromise seen in epiglottitis.

Although debate continues as to the specific role of LPR in the development of laryngeal lesions and hoarseness in children, infrequent reflux events have been shown to cause hoarseness in adults.[15] LPR has also been found in association with pediatric laryngeal manifestations such as vocal fold nodules, posterior laryngitis, false vocal fold edema, vocal fold granulomas, functional voice disorders, and hoarseness.[10,16,17] In addition, animal studies have shown that subglottic stenosis results when gastric acid is applied to the subglottic mucosa of dogs.[18]

Vocal nodules arise from phonotrauma or voice abuse and are more common in boys than in girls.[19] Symptoms may fluctuate based on aggravation by vocal abuse and respiratory tract infections. Sudden worsening of symptoms is sometimes seen when polyps swell from internal hemorrhage with excessive vocal trauma. Children with vocal nodules may share symptoms with other members of the immediate family who have similar vocal traits.

Airway trauma is also a potential cause of hoarseness in the older child and adolescent. Sources include blunt or penetrating injuries and intubation trauma.

Hoarseness of a progressive and unrelenting nature suggests a possible neoplastic cause. Ninety-eight percent of pediatric laryngeal neoplasms are benign, and recurrent respiratory papillomatosis (RRP) is by far the most common lesion.[13] RRP may be found on upper aerodigestive tract mucosal surfaces other than that of the larynx and have a characteristic cluster-of-grapes appearance. RRP may, however, be indistinguishable from the rare but ominous laryngeal squamous cell carcinoma of childhood.

Hoarseness in the adolescent years may also be of behavioral or psychogenic etiology. Mutational voice disorder occurs in male adolescents and results in hoarseness and high pitch during the stress of physiologic pubertal voice change. Paradoxical vocal fold dysfunction (seen more often in girls) is a disorder of psychogenic origin often misdiagnosed as asthma, which can produce episodic stridor or hoarseness.[20]

## ▶ EVALUATION

### Relevant History

A thorough history is an essential part of the investigation of hoarseness. The age of the child is a critical factor in the development of an appropriate differential diagnosis, as is information on the quality of the voice with speech or crying, exacerbating or alleviating factors, and associated symptoms. Neurologic and congenital fixed anatomic lesions typically occur at birth, whereas inflammatory, neoplastic, traumatic, or iatrogenic causes of hoarseness occur later. The onset and course of dysphonia should be considered. Intermittent dysphonia may be related to infectious or inflammatory causes such as laryngitis, whereas persistent dysphonia may suggest a fixed anatomic lesion. A progressive, unremitting hoarse voice may suggest an enlarging neoplasm.

A review of medical and surgical history is also helpful. Patients with hoarseness who have symptoms such as regurgitation or vomiting, feeding difficulties, throat clearing, foreign body sensation, and cough may have underlying reflux.

Stridor that accompanies hoarseness should be investigated and treated expeditiously, because turbulent airflow resulting from airway obstruction may be life threatening.

### Physical Examination

A thorough physical examination, including a complete head and neck examination, should be part of the evaluation of pediatric hoarseness. Inspection of cranial nerve function and for craniofacial anomalies may reveal the underlying cause of a patient's hoarseness. Cutaneous head and neck hemangiomas, for example, may suggest a potential laryngeal hemangioma. Signs of aspiration during deglutition may be suggestive of sensorimotor causes of dysphonia such as vocal fold paralysis.

### Laryngoscopy

An essential part of the otolaryngologic physical examination is visualization of the larynx. Flexible nasopharyngolaryngoscopy, indirect mirror laryngoscopy, and rigid videostroboscopy are all methods for visualizing the larynx that can provide useful, if not diagnostic, clues as to the source of a patient's hoarseness.

Indirect laryngoscopy using a mirror can be performed on cooperative children and can allow the physician to visualize gross disease and inflammatory changes in the larynx. This technique has largely been replaced by flexible fiberoptic nasopharyngolaryngoscopy, which provides clear views of laryngeal anatomy and function. Flexible endoscopy can be performed on virtually all age groups, although toddlers and patients who are developmentally delayed pose the greatest challenge to the examiner. Topical anesthesia can be used with topical decongestants to facilitate the examination. The flexible endoscope is gently passed through the nose or mouth. Examination in a nonmonitored setting, however, is not advisable if the patient has a tenuous airway or severe congenital cardiac anomalies.

Videostroboscopy uses a rigid, angled telescope placed gently into the oropharynx for dynamic examination of laryngeal anatomy and function. Examination requires a cooperative child. Videostroboscopy uses rapidly pulsed light to examine the vibratory characteristics of the vocal fold mucosa. Examinations are recorded on video to allow for repeated assessments viewed at different speeds to enhance visualization of the vibratory quality of the laryngeal mucosa. Vocal nodules or other lesions on the surface of the vocal fold will dampen the mucosal wave.

### Imaging

The role of diagnostic imaging in the workup of the hoarse child is of prime importance when the physician suspects CNS disease, external compression, malignancy, or external trauma.

Chest and neck plain-film radiographs may demonstrate mediastinal masses, cardiovascular anomalies, or abnormalities in the air column, suggesting possible infectious or obstructive diseases.

Computed tomography and virtual bronchoscopy are excellent methods for specifically defining the caliber of the airway and for delineating the site and extent of pathologic changes in airway caliber.[21,22] Indications for laryngeal or neck computed tomography include congenital cysts, solid neoplasms, and external trauma.

Magnetic resonance imaging is helpful when suspicion exists of CNS disease such as the Arnold-Chiari malformation, and when evaluating possible airway hemangiomas or vascular malformations.

### Reflux Testing

Symptomatic or overt GER and LPR in the hoarse child may not necessitate expensive or invasive diagnostic studies. In the absence of identifiable disease in the hoarse child, however, investigation into LPR may be warranted. Although consensus on the role of LPR as it relates to various otolaryngologic manifestations is lacking, at least 1 study has used pH monitoring to suggest an association between pediatric reflux and hoarse voice in a cohort of children.[17,23] Several diagnostic modalities exist for the workup of LPR, including pH monitoring, impedance testing, nuclear medicine scintiscan, barium esophagoscopy, and direct laryngoscopy with or without biopsy.

Ambulatory 24-hour single-electrode pH monitoring remains the gold standard for the diagnosis of GER in infants and children.[24] The double-electrode pH probe, with distal esophageal and pharyngeal electrodes, however, is thought to be the best method for diagnosing LPR and the otolaryngologic manifestations of GER.[25,26]

Although pH-monitoring studies remain the gold standard for diagnosis of GER and LPR, they do not detect episodes of nonacidic reflux. Multichannel intraluminal impedance monitoring and nuclear medicine scintigraphy can measure both acidic and nonacidic episodes of reflux, which may play a role in such serious events as apnea, apparent life-threatening events, aspiration, and sleep disturbance.[27,28] Nuclear medicine scintiscans have specificity between 83% and 100%, but they have been shown to be only 15% to 59% sensitive and lack a standardized technique, limiting the usefulness of comparisons between studies.[17] Impedance monitoring evaluates the pH-independent change in intraluminal electrical resistance that occurs with the movement (anterograde or retrograde) of a bolus of food, liquid, or gas within the esophagus.[29] This technique may be a reliable tool for evaluating the association between GER-related symptoms and nonacidic reflux events, and it may ultimately replace pH monitoring as the standard tool for detecting LPR in infants and children.[22,30]

Barium esophagram has variable sensitivity and specificity for the diagnosis of LPR. It is useful mainly for detecting anatomic abnormalities such as hiatal hernia.[31]

Laryngoscopy with biopsy may be the most specific test for LPR, but at least 1 study has failed to show a correlation between laryngoscopy and upper pH probe findings with significant laryngeal histopathologic inflammatory findings.[32]

## ▶ MANAGEMENT

### Congenital Lesions

Management of hoarse voice resulting from unilateral or bilateral vocal fold paralysis is usually secondary to stabilization of the airway and management of dysphagia and aspiration.

Tracheotomy is sometimes required in patients with bilateral vocal fold paralysis, but conservative management in select patients has been advocated.[33] However, patients with congenital or acquired unilateral vocal fold paralysis often recover normal vocal quality by spontaneous resolution of the paralysis or by compensatory movement of the unaffected fold over time. Recovery has been noted up to 11 years after paralysis.[34] In cases of persistent unilateral fold paralysis with persistent hoarseness, the treatment of choice remains speech therapy, although reports have surfaced of successful surgical vocal fold medialization techniques in the children.[33,35]

Laryngeal webs are managed surgically, either endoscopically or via more extensive open laryngotracheal reconstruction techniques. The type of operation depends primarily on the location and extent of the lesion, with thin webs being more amenable to endoscopic management.

Saccular cysts of the larynx are often managed endoscopically with excellent results via aspiration and marsupialization by sharp dissection or with the carbon dioxide ($CO_2$) laser. Cyst recurrence, however, is well documented following endoscopic management, and open resection of the cyst may be necessary in these cases.

Posterior laryngeal clefts vary greatly in their extent and symptoms. Extensive or symptomatic clefts must be repaired as early as possible. Although endoscopic repair is possible in small clefts limited to the larynx and upper trachea, more extensive open techniques are used for larger clefts. Tracheotomy may also be placed in cases in which staged reconstruction of the cleft is necessary, and a gastrostomy tube is often needed to limit aspiration and protect the operative site following surgical repair of the cleft.

### Neoplasia

Subglottic hemangioma is a complicated airway anomaly without a universally accepted treatment. Numerous management options exist, including close observation, systemic or intralesional steroids, laser ablation, open surgical excision, and tracheotomy.

Recurrent respiratory papillomatosis associated with human papilloma virus (HPV), represents another airway tumor with a large number of accepted primary and adjuvant therapeutic modalities. $CO_2$ laser excision was developed as a treatment for RRP in the 1970s and remains a popular method for removing laryngeal papilloma, although it is associated with potentially severe sequelae such as airway fire, scarring, chronic laryngeal edema with airway compromise, vocal fold scarring, and poor voice. Nonlaser therapies such as cold dissection and powered débridement have also been used successfully for excision of RRP with comparable outcomes. Several adjuvant therapies, such as intralesional cidofovir, $\alpha$-interferon, indole-3-carbinol, bevacizumab, and heat-shock protein E7, have been used with varying degrees of efficacy and safety.[36] There is hope that with the introduction of HPV vaccines there may be a future generational shift in the reduction of RRP.

### Inflammation and Infection

Behavioral and lifestyle modifications; pharmacotherapy using $H_2$ antagonists, proton-pump inhibitors, prokinetic agents, and antacids; and surgical therapy with fundoplication are acceptable for the management of GER and LPR in infants and children.

Viral laryngitis and laryngotracheobronchitis are generally treated conservatively, but they may require airway protection or intravenous steroids in severe cases. Bacterial infections such as epiglottitis and membranous laryngotracheobronchitis, though now rare, necessitate early airway protection and intravenous antibiotics directed against *Staphylococcus aureus* and *Haemophilus influenzae,* unless culture results direct differently.

### *Trauma*

The management of vocal fold nodules resulting from phonotrauma primarily relies on behavioral modification and speech therapy aimed at maximizing vocal hygiene. Only in rare circumstances is surgical excision indicated, because failure to correct the underlying voice misuse is likely to result in nodule recurrence.

Arytenoid dislocation resulting from intubation trauma can be adequately treated if recognized and reduced early under anesthesia with microlaryngoscopy.

Blunt laryngeal trauma resulting in hoarseness necessitates close observation and may require the use of systemic corticosteroids and tracheotomy in cases of severe laryngeal injury and edema. In adolescents with laryngeal fracture, open reduction and fixation may be required.

For patients with hoarseness related to iatrogenic unilateral vocal fold immobility, injection or external vocal fold medialization have been showed to be effective. Recurrent laryngeal nerve reinnervation procedures are also emerging as promising therapeutic options for long-term improvement.

## ▶ SUMMARY

Most cases of pediatric hoarseness result from benign, reversible, and self-limited disease; however, some causes of hoarseness are progressive, malignant, and potentially life-threatening. Thorough evaluation, precise diagnosis, and appropriate intervention are therefore essential.

### When to Refer

- Recognized cardiac, esophageal, or neurologic disease
- Progressive hoarseness
- Presence of cutaneous hemangioma
- Hoarseness after external trauma or uneventful intubation
- Poor speech intelligibility or psychosocial sequelae
- Hoarseness that has been present since birth

### When to Admit

- Presence of respiratory distress, stridor, tachypnea, or tachycardia
- Hoarseness following external trauma

### *TOOLS FOR PRACTICE*

**Engaging Patient and Family**

- *Hoarseness* (fact sheet), American Academy of Otolaryngology—Head and Neck Surgery (www.entnet.org/content/hoarseness)

## Medical Decision Support

- *Clinical Practice Guideline: Hoarseness (Dysphonia)* (guideline), American Academy of Otolaryngology—Head and Neck Surgery (www.entnet.org/content/clinical-practice-guideline-hoarseness-dysphonia)

## *REFERENCES*


1. Leeper HA, Leonard JE, Iverson RL. Otorhinolaryngologic screening of children with vocal quality disturbances. *Int J Pediatr Otorhinolaryngol.* 1980;2:123–131
2. Carding PN, Roulstone S, Northstone K; ALSPAC Study Team. The prevalence of childhood dysphonia: a cross-sectional study. *J Voice.* 2006;20:623–630
3. Friedberg J, El-Hakim H. Hoarseness. In: Bluestone CD, Stool SE, Kenna MA, eds. *Pediatric Otolaryngology.* 4th ed. Philadelphia, PA: WB Saunders; 2003
4. de Jong AL, Kuppersmith RB, Sulek M, Friedman EM. Vocal cord paralysis in infants and children. *Otolaryngol Clin North Am.* 2000;33:131–149
5. Wiatrak BJ. Congenital anomalies of the larynx and trachea. *Otolaryngol Clin North Am.* 2000;33:91–110
6. Holinger PH, Brown WT. Congenital webs, cysts, laryngoceles and other anomalies of the larynx. *Ann Otol Rhinol Laryngol.* 1967;76:744–752
7. Lim FY, Crombleholme TM, Hedrick HL, et al. Congenital high airway obstruction syndrome: natural history and management. *J Pediatr Surg.* 2003;38:940–945
8. Shikhani AH, Jones MM, Marsh BR, Holliday MJ. Infantile subglottic hemangiomas. An update. *Ann Otol Rhinol Laryngol.* 1986;95:336–347
9. Kalach N, Gumpert L, Contencin P, Dupont C. Dual-probe pH monitoring for the assessment of gastroesophageal reflux in the course of chronic hoarseness in children. *Turk J Pediatr.* 2000;42:186–191
10. Kuhn J, Toohill RJ, Ulualp SO, et al. Pharyngeal acid reflux events in patients with vocal cord nodules. *Laryngoscope.* 1998;108:1146–1149
11. A standardized protocol for the methodology of esophageal pH monitoring and interpretation of the data for the diagnosis of gastroesophageal reflux. Working Group of the European Society of Pediatric Gastroenterology and Nutrition. *J Pediatr Gastroenterol Nutr.* 1992;14:467–471
12. Mandell DL, Kay DJ, Dohar JE, Yellon RF. Lack of association between esophageal biopsy, bronchoalveolar lavage, and endoscopy findings in hoarse children. *Arch Otolaryngol Head Neck Surg.* 2004;130:1293–1297
13. Koufman JA, Amin MR, Panetti M. Prevalence of reflux in 113 consecutive patients with laryngeal and voice disorders. *Otolaryngol Head Neck Surg.* 2000;123:385–388
14. Zalzal GH, Tran LP. Pediatric gastroesophageal reflux and laryngopharyngeal reflux. *Otolaryngol Clin North Am.* 2000;33:151–161
15. Koufman J, Sataloff RT, Toohill R. Laryngopharyngeal reflux: consensus conference report. *J Voice.* 1996;10(3):215–216
16. Bach KK, McGuirt WF Jr, Postma GN. Pediatric laryngopharyngeal reflux. *Ear Nose Throat J.* 2002;81 (9 suppl 2):27–31
17. Gumpert L, Kalach N, Dupont C, Contencin P. Hoarseness and gastroesophageal reflux in children. *J Laryngol Otol.* 1998;112:49–54
18. Little FB, Koufman JA, Kohut RI, Marshall RB. Effect of gastric acid on the pathogenesis of subglottic stenosis. *Ann Otol Rhinol Laryngol.* 1985;94:516–519
19. McMurray JS. Medical and surgical treatment of pediatric dysphonia. *Otolaryngol Clin North Am.* 2000;33:1111–1126
20. Tilles SA. Vocal cord dysfunction in children and adolescents. *Curr Allergy Astma Rep.* 2003;3(6):467–472
21. Liu P, Daneman A. Computed tomography of intrinsic laryngeal and tracheal abnormalities in children. *J Comput Assisted Tomogr.* 1984;8(4):662–669
22. Burke AJ, Vining DJ, McGuirt WF, Postma G, Browne JD. Evaluation of airway obstruction using virtual endoscopy. *Laryngoscope.* 2000;110:23–29

23. Stavroulaki P. Diagnostic and management problems of laryngopharyngeal reflux disease in children. *Int J Pediatr Otorhinolaryngol.* 2006;70:579–590
24. Rudolph CD, Mazur LJ, Liptak GS, et al. Guidelines for evaluation and treatment of gastroesophageal reflux in infants and children: recommendations of the North American Society for Pediatric Gastroenterology and Nutrition. *J Pediatr Gastroenterol Nutr.* 2001;32(Suppl 2):S1–S31
25. Koufman JA, Aviv JE, Casiano RR, Shaw GY. Laryngopharyngeal reflux: position statement of the committee on speech, voice, and swallowing disorders of the American Academy of Otolaryngology-Head and Neck Surgery. *Otolaryngol Head Neck Surg.* 2002;127:32–35
26. Contencin P, Narcy P. Nasopharyngeal pH monitoring in infants and children with chronic rhinopharyngitis. *Int J Pediatr Otorhinolaryngol.* 1991;22:249–256
27. Ruth M, Carlsson S, Månsson I, Bengtsson U, Sandberg N. Scintigraphic detection of gastro-pulmonary aspiration in patients with respiratory disorders. *Clin Physiol.* 1993;13:19–33
28. Orenstein SR. An overview of reflux-associated disorders in infants: apnea, laryngospasm, and aspiration. *Am J Med.* 2001;111(Suppl 8A):60S–63S
29. Wenzl TG, Moroder C, Trachterna M, et al. Esophageal pH monitoring and impedance measurement: a comparison of two diagnostic tests for gastroesophageal reflux. *J Pediatr Gastroenterol Nutr.* 2002;34:519–523
30. Wenzl TG. Evaluation of gastroesophageal reflux events in children using multichannel intraluminal electrical impedance. *Am J Med.* 2003;115(Suppl 3A):161S–165S
31. McGuirt WF. Gastroesophageal reflux and the upper airway. *Pediatr Clin North Am.* 2003;50:487–502
32. McMurray JS, Gerber M, Stern Y, et al. Role of laryngoscopy, dual pH probe monitoring, and laryngeal mucosal biopsy in the diagnosis of pharyngoesophageal reflux. *Ann Otol Rhinol Laryngol.* 2001;110:299–304
33. Miyamoto RC, Parikh SR, Gellad W, Licameli GR. Bilateral congenital vocal cord paralysis: a 16-year institutional review. *Otolaryngol Head Neck Surg.* 2005;133:241–245
34. Parikh SR. Pediatric unilateral vocal fold immobility. *Otolaryngol Clin North Am.* 2004;37:203–215
35. Tucker HM. Vocal cord paralysis in small children: principles in management. *Ann Otol Rhinol Laryngol.* 1986;95:618–621
36. Andrus JG, Shapshay SM. Contemporary management of laryngeal papilloma in adults and children. *Otolaryngol Clin North Am.* 2006;39:135–158

# Chapter 43

# Hyperhidrosis

*Nancy K. Barnett, MD*

When excessive (beyond the norm for thermoregulation) localized sweating occurs in childhood, the child or the family usually expresses concern because the sweating is either odiferous or so intense that it interferes with hand functions (eg, holding a pencil) or foot functions. Axillary hyperhidrosis usually becomes more of a problem in adolescence because of the embarrassment of the sweat ring on clothing and the odor associated with bacterial degradation of apocrine sweat. The apocrine glands are stimulated at puberty by androgenic hormones. Palmar and plantar hyperhidrosis caused by eccrine sweat production may occur at any age. Eccrine sweat glands controlling thermoregulation are most numerous on the palms, soles, and axillae.

Palmoplantar hyperhidrosis is thought to be stimulated by anxiety, whereas axillary hyperhidrosis is probably stimulated by both heat and emotion. Both stop during sleep.[1] Researchers have postulated that emotions and the temperature of the blood perfusing the hypothalamus stimulate the secretion of the hormones that regulate the autonomic nervous system's control of perspiration such that cholinergic sympathetic fibers hyperstimulate eccrine and apoeccrine sweat glands.[2]

## ▶ EVALUATION

Excessive sweating that is not limited to the palms, soles, and axillae may be caused by and indicate a systemic disorder, such as infection, hypoglycemia, drug withdrawal, lymphoma, thyrotoxicosis, pheochromocytoma, or Riley-Day syndrome. These disorders should be considered in the presence of generalized increased perspiring.

## ▶ MANAGEMENT

Systemic anticholinergic agents may block acetylcholine, the sympathetic innervation terminal neurotransmitter to eccrine glands, and help hyperhidrosis, but the side effects of cholinergic blockage preclude their long-term use. The application of prescription 20% aluminum chloride (eg, Drysol) every other day has been an effective treatment for palmar sweating. Plantar hyperhidrosis also responds to aluminum salts, and absorbent powders (eg, Zeasorb) are used more easily here than on the palms. Some authors report successful control of palmar and plantar hyperhidrosis with tap-water iontophoresis.[3]

Palmar and plantar hyperhidrosis can be controlled by inhibiting sweat production with subepidermal injections of botulinum A toxin, which purportedly blocks the presynaptic acetylcholine release and is effective for as long as 12 months. Patients as young as 14 years have been treated in this manner, but temporary or, rarely, permanent muscle and nerve injury from the injections limits the toxin's usefulness in these locations.[3,4]

For bromhidrosis (malodorous hyperhidrosis) of the soles, cleansing frequently with drying deodorant soaps and applying topical antibiotics (erythromycin or clindamycin) may help. The patient should go barefoot whenever possible.

Axillary hyperhidrosis is troublesome because continual sweating makes maintaining an effective antiperspirant in contact with the axillary skin difficult. One approach is to apply prescription 20% solution of aluminum chloride in anhydrous ethanol to the axillary vault.[5] A problematic side effect of this treatment can be an irritant contact dermatitis, uncomfortable enough to require hydrocortisone cream for relief of inflammation. For individuals who have axillary hyperhidrosis and bromhidrosis, frequent clothing changes may be necessary, as may the use of topical antibiotics and deodorant powders. Propranolol and anxiolytics are options to reduce emotional stress.

Successful axillary sweat gland chemodenervation with intradermal botulinum toxin injections is being increasingly used and is an approved indication for the toxin.[3,6] In extreme cases, when these measures fail and the patient is desperate for relief, local axillary skin can be excised or glands removed by less scarring curettage or liposuction techniques with reasonable expectation of success. Because of its attendant complications, ganglion sympathectomy cannot be recommended for most patients who have axillary hyperhidrosis.[3] Hyperhidrosis is often life altering, and data exist to support management, even with significant measures like axillary suction curettage, because it improves quality of life.[2]

Management of primary palmoplantar and axillary hyperhidrosis may have the secondary benefit of decreasing the significant risk for associated infections such as warts, dermatophytosis, and pitted keratolysis as well as eczematous dermatitis, which can coexist.[7]

## When to Refer

- Hyperhidrosis that interferes with the function of a body part (eg, hand so slippery wet that the child cannot hold a pencil)
- Generalized excessive sweating
- Socially isolating hyperhidrosis as a result of odor or excessive drenching of clothing

### *REFERENCES*

1. Hamberger J, Grimes K, Naumann M, et al. Recognition, diagnosis and treatment of primary focal hyperhidrosis. *J Am Acad Dermatol.* 2004;51:274–286
2. Bechara FG, Gambichler T, Bader A, et al. Assessment of quality of life in patients with primary axillary hyperhidrosis before and after suction-curettage. *J Am Acad Dermatol.* 2007;57:207–212
3. Jacobs AA, Desai A, Markus R. Don't sweat hyperhidrosis: a review of current treatment. *Cosmetic Dermatol.* 2005;18:725–731
4. Shelley WB, Talanin NY, Shelley ED. Botulinum toxin therapy for palmar hyperhidrosis. *J Am Acad Dermatol.* 1998;38:227–229
5. Shelley WB, Hurley HJ Jr. Studies on topical antiperspirant control of axillary hyperhidrosis. *Acta Derm Vener* (Stockh). 1975;55:241–260
6. Heckmann M, Ceballos-Baumann AO, Plewig G; Hyperhidrosis Study Group. Botulinum toxin A for axillary hyperhidrosis (excessive sweating). *N Engl J Med.* 2001;344:488–493
7. Walling HW. Primary hyperhidrosis increases the risk of cutaneous infection: a case-control study of 387 patients. *J Am Acad Dermatol.* 2009;61:242–246

# Chapter 44

# Hypotonia

*Alfred J. Spiro, MD*

Hypotonia indicates diminished resistance to passive movement around the range of motion of a joint. The commonly used term *floppy* refers to hypotonia, or weakness, or both. No readily administered, accurate test exists to quantify hypotonicity. Furthermore, tone, especially in a young infant, may vary greatly during the day or even during the examination. Hypotonia is not a diagnosis in itself; however, the origin of a neonate's floppiness may be obvious in, for example, overwhelming sepsis, meningitis, or marked hyperbilirubinemia. Central nervous system (CNS) abnormalities are commonly associated with hypotonia. Generally, central hypotonia involves diminished tone without appreciably diminished strength coupled with preserved or hyperactive deep tendon reflexes. In disorders of the motor unit (lesions of the anterior horn cell, peripheral nerve, myoneural junction, or muscle), strength is usually diminished, and tone may be reduced as a result. Hypotonia that is not associated with a motor unit disorder is more common than hypotonia caused by an underlying motor unit disorder. Testing of strength in infants and young children is difficult, even for experienced examiners; it can usually be done by observation of how strong a baby's kicking and pushing are, for example, or by functional testing.

## ▶ HYPOTONIA NOT CAUSED BY MOTOR UNIT DISORDERS

Disorders virtually anywhere in the brain may be associated with hypotonia. Global developmental delay is a common, but not universal, accompanying feature, as is microcephaly. Magnetic resonance imaging (MRI) of the brain may be helpful in documenting the lesion in some cases. In many instances, a specific diagnosis cannot be made. As infants who have hypotonicity get older, the abnormal tone may evolve into spasticity and the diagnosis of spastic quadriplegia, spastic diplegia, or other form of cerebral palsy becomes evident. A common misconception is that cerebral palsy is caused by obstetrical trauma; in most instances, the cause of cerebral palsy remains unknown.[1,2] Nevertheless, a review of birth records, drug administration, and factors surrounding prematurity is indicated. On examination, deep-tendon reflexes are usually but not always hyperactive. Abnormalities of tone in patients with cerebral palsy are usually global; that is, both proximal and distal. Treatment of various types of cerebral palsy is supportive and symptomatic and usually requires a multidisciplinary team effort.

Several genetic syndromes, Down syndrome among the most common, are associated with hypotonia; the diagnosis can be made on clinical grounds and with appropriate genetic studies. Newborns and young infants with Prader-Willi syndrome may be extremely hypotonic and demonstrate a diminished level of consciousness. As these babies get older, tone may improve, and they may become obese. They have characteristic almond-shaped eyes, short stature, and some degree of intellectual disability and hypogonadism; some have severe eating disorders and scoliosis, but these features are usually not present until school age. The clinical features coupled with analysis showing a deletion in the chromosome 15q11-13 region can generally establish the diagnosis.

Several of the Ehlers-Danlos syndromes[3] may simulate hypotonicity, but the major feature of this group of connective tissue disorders is hyperlaxity of joints. Weakness is not a prominent feature.

Hypothyroidism and other metabolic disorders may be accompanied by hypotonia. Neonatal screening generally includes a test for hypothyroidism. If the diagnosis is not obvious on physical examination, then appropriate thyroid function studies can be done.

## ▶ HYPOTONIA CAUSED BY MOTOR UNIT DISORDERS

### History

In taking the history, the primary care physician should note whether hypotonia was present at birth or was recognized later. Parents of first children may have no basis for comparison and may not recognize an abnormality. Occasionally, photographs or family videos can be extremely useful in revealing abnormalities denied or not noted by parents. Breech presentation is common in babies who are subsequently diagnosed as having a motor unit disorder, but the reason for this has not been established. Congenital hip dislocation may be present in children who have central core disease, a congenital myopathy.[4]

Thorough questioning can usually determine whether the hypotonia is improving or worsening or if weakness is periodic, as observed in hyperkalemic periodic paralysis (a rare autosomal-dominant disorder with onset usually in infancy or early childhood). The distribution of weakness, whether it is predominantly proximal, distal, or global, can also be identified with questions such as whether the baby or child moves the fingers and toes better than the large muscles of the pelvic and shoulder girdles. Details of the child's developmental milestones also can provide a clue to the nature of the lesion. For example, language development is normal in infantile progressive spinal muscular atrophy (SMA)[5] and impaired in myotonic dystrophy.[6]

Facial muscle weakness, observed in some congenital myopathies, can be considered if the parents state that the child sleeps with the eyelids partially open. Extraocular muscles, in addition to facial muscles, are abnormal in myotubular myopathy.[7] Acquired autoimmune myasthenia gravis[8] and myasthenic syndromes[9] can occur in young children and may cause ptosis, extraocular muscle weakness, and, in some cases, generalized weakness and respiratory distress. Less severely affected patients may have only limited abnormal findings at the time of examination. Family videos taken at the times of the patient's maximal clinical involvement can be useful to document signs not seen in the examining room. Physicians should inquire about swallowing and sucking difficulties.

Details of the family history can be helpful because many of the motor unit disorders are genetic. The presence of consanguinity suggests an autosomal-recessive entity. Examining parents and siblings can sometimes be revealing because some genetic disorders may be expressed quite subtly in family members and often are overlooked. Facial muscle weakness is a common example; patients do not seek medical attention if they cannot puff up their cheeks, whistle, or squeeze their eyelids closed completely, all features seen in certain congenital myopathies or facioscapulohumeral muscular dystrophy.[10] If early-onset myotonic dystrophy type 1 is thought to exist, then the child's mother and other family members should be examined for myotonia (slowed relaxation after a voluntary or induced muscle contraction) because neither percussion nor electrical myotonia is observed in infants or very young children.

### Physical Examination

The physician should conduct a thorough search for systemic disorders. Dysmorphic features such as high-arched palate and dental malocclusion are observed in some congenital myopathies, such as nemaline myopathy. An enlarged heart and congestive heart failure are observed in glycogen storage disease caused by acid maltase deficiency. Clubfoot deformity is commonly seen in the infantile form of myotonic dystrophy. Joint abnormalities and scoliosis are common in several motor unit disorders.

A striking paucity of spontaneous movement is observed in infantile progressive SMA[11]; paradoxical respiration, in which the chest wall moves inward during inspiration instead of expanding, is also observed often.

In infants and in children younger than 5 years, manual muscle testing generally cannot be accomplished reliably, making observation of spontaneous movement and functional testing, such as the ability to hold the head erect, sit, roll over, and stand, and walk on heels and toes, mandatory. Assessing cranial nerve function should emphasize identifying facial and extraocular muscle weakness, as well as fasciculation and atrophy of the tongue. Fasciculation of the tongue, observed in infantile progressive SMA,[11] should be assessed with the tongue not protruded and with the child not crying. Tremulousness of the outstretched fingers (minipolymyoclonus[12]) is seen almost exclusively in SMA with a protracted course and in some hereditary sensorimotor neuropathies. Generally, deep-tendon reflexes are reduced or absent in motor unit disorders but preserved in most cases of myasthenia gravis. With hypotonia of central origin, reflexes are preserved or hyperactive; however, many exceptions to this rule can be found. The presence or absence of extensor plantar responses is also often difficult to assess in young children; these responses may normally be present at up to a year or more of age.

### Laboratory Studies

Laboratory studies include blood testing, neurophysiologic evaluation, and histologic examination of muscle. Laboratory studies should be goal directed and performed in an orderly manner. Serum muscle enzyme levels, particularly creatine kinase, are always markedly elevated in Duchenne and Becker muscular dystrophy but are not always increased in congenital myopathies. They are generally normal or only minimally increased in spinal muscular atrophy. DNA studies for diagnostic purposes are readily available in many commercial and research laboratories (see Gene Tests or OMIM in the Tools for Practice section at the end of this chapter) for several motor unit disorders, including infantile progressive SMA, myotonic dystrophy, various hereditary sensorimotor neuropathies, selected mitochondrial myopathies, and Duchenne and Becker muscular dystrophy. When these disorders are thought to exist on clinical grounds, an appropriate DNA study may be all that is needed to document the diagnosis. Thus, a child who has classic infantile progressive SMA can be spared many painful studies when the DNA study is conclusive.[13] Other noninvasive studies, such as computed tomography, MRI, or sonographic imaging of muscles, can assess muscle mass accurately; in the presence of very small muscles, imaging is indicated if a muscle biopsy is contemplated. Electromyographic studies can be useful in the diagnosis of motor unit disorders,[14] but because of the pain involved and the need for sedation in some cases, they should be used with discretion when DNA studies are not helpful. Nerve conduction studies can be extremely useful in distinguishing the various types of peripheral neuropathies seen in infants and children. Repetitive stimulation studies are very helpful in diagnosing disorders of the myoneural junction, including infantile botulism, but testing can be quite painful. Physicians who are experienced in the particular technical and other problems encountered in this age group should perform all electrodiagnostic studies in young children.

Muscle biopsies, performed either with a special needle or surgically, are most useful in myopathies such as congenital myopathies,[4] congenital muscular dystrophy, metabolic myopathies, and mitochondrial disorders.[15] Many specialized analytical studies are available when needed. In virtually all instances when a biopsy is performed, sections should be taken for histochemical, biochemical, ultrastructural, and genetic studies, although not all of these studies are used in every case.

## Selected Motor Unit Disorders

### Anterior Horn Cell Disease

Given the near elimination of paralytic poliomyelitis in the United States, the various types of infantile progressive SMA constitute the major disease in this category. Eponyms have been applied to these disorders, including Werdnig-Hoffmann disease, but these terms may be misleading and confusing. Now, a much more useful operational classification of SMA (Table 44-1) is commonly used.[11]

In all types of infantile progressive SMA, cognition is normal, as are extraocular muscles. Weakness and muscle wasting are proximal more than distal and are more pronounced in the legs than in the arms. Fasciculation of the tongue and minipolymyoclonus[12] (in types I and II, respectively) are observed often, and areflexia and normal sensation are the rule. Joint contractures and scoliosis may develop, especially in type II. All forms are autosomal recessive, with the responsible gene having been located at 5q11-q13. A deletion of the survival motor neuron gene has been identified in most patients, making this situation useful for diagnostic purposes and for prenatal diagnosis.[16] Recent advances in understanding the molecular basis of this disorder have made phenotype-genotype correlation possible.

**Table 44-1**
**Spinal Muscular Atrophy**

| Type | Age of Onset | Course |
|---|---|---|
| I | Birth to 6 mo | Never sits independently, even when placed; progressive; demise <2 y |
| II | 6–18 mo | Sits independently when placed; life expectancy into the 20s or later |
| III | >18 mo | Weakness after having learned to walk; normal life expectancy |

Treatment generally is supportive and includes physical therapy and, when needed, respiratory and nutritional support and genetic counseling. Scoliosis is common in type II and must be addressed appropriately with a body jacket, molded back support, or surgery. Most children who have type II can use a motorized wheelchair at approximately 2 to 3 years of age. Life expectancy in type II can be well into adulthood.

## Peripheral Nerve Disorders

Peripheral nerve disorders are rare in infancy and very early childhood. Hypomyelinating neuropathy[17] can produce severe weakness, hypotonia, and areflexia in a neonate or young infant. The diagnosis can be anticipated when extremely abnormal nerve conduction studies are encountered and can be confirmed with DNA studies or with a nerve biopsy. Hereditary sensorimotor neuropathies, with the many variants of Charcot-Marie-Tooth disease, are the most common cause of childhood peripheral nerve disorders and may cause both gait abnormalities from weakness of the anterior tibialis muscles and deformities of the foot.[18] Ankle jerks are often diminished or absent, but all reflexes may be preserved in the early phases of peripheral neuropathies. Nerve conduction studies can be extremely useful in separating axonal from demyelinating neuropathies. DNA studies can be diagnostic in selected hereditary neuropathies, especially the demyelinating and the X-linked varieties. Treatment addresses symptoms; some children who have foot drop may require bracing.

Several CNS disorders may have a demyelinating form of peripheral nerve involvement in addition to abnormalities in the cerebral white matter; these include metachromatic leukodystrophy, Krabbe disease, and adrenoleukodystrophy.

## Myoneural Junction Disorders

Several disorders of the myoneural junction[8,9] affect children and infants: passively acquired autoimmune myasthenia gravis, also known as transient neonatal myasthenia; acquired autoimmune myasthenia gravis, also known as juvenile or childhood myasthenia; nonautoimmune myasthenic syndromes, also known as congenital myasthenia gravis; and infantile botulism.[19]

Passively acquired autoimmune myasthenia gravis occurs in approximately 20% of infants born to mothers who have myasthenia gravis. All newborns of seropositive mothers have acetylcholine receptor antibodies, but only a small portion are symptomatic, most mildly, but some more severely, with hypotonia, a weak cry, swallowing and sucking difficulty, facial diapiresis, respiratory distress, external ophthalmoparesis, and ptosis. The diagnosis can be made quickly when, after administering intravenous edrophonium, the abnormal findings subside. When the newborns are symptomatic, pyridostigmine can be given orally until symptoms are no longer present. The dose is then tapered, usually over a period of 1 to 2 weeks. These infants do not have clinical features of myasthenia gravis after the initial involvement. If weakness does not occur by 1 week of age, then it is highly unlikely to develop.

Major features of acquired autoimmune myasthenia include fatigability and fluctuating weakness of extraocular, facial, and lingual muscles, and, in some instances, mild or severe generalized weakness and hypotonicity of the limbs. An acute fulminating onset may be encountered in young children. The diagnosis can be made by using the edrophonium test and confirmed with the acetylcholine receptor antibody test, although the latter is not necessarily positive in milder cases and is less useful in children than in older individuals. Electrodiagnostic studies can be used in selected instances in children but are generally less useful than in adults. The mediastinum should be radiographed to assess thymic size, and thyroid function studies should be obtained to exclude associated hypo- or hyperthyroidism. Treatment includes judicious use of anticholinesterase drugs and, when needed, immunosuppressive treatment, intravenous gamma globulin, corticosteroids, and thymectomy.

Nonautoimmune myasthenic syndromes[9] may be associated with ocular, bulbar, or respiratory involvement and, in some instances, with progressive weakness and hypotonicity. Some disorders may be genetic; patients are seronegative. Specialized electrodiagnostic and ultrastructural studies are required to establish an exact diagnosis, which is important in selecting appropriate therapy. For the moment, genetic studies for diagnosis are available only within a research setting. Some patients respond to anticholinesterase inhibitors or corticosteroids; others require diaminopyridine or other specific medications.

Infantile botulism[19] is characterized by onset at an average age of slightly more than 3 months that produces weakness and hypotonia, poor feeding, constipation, and diminished activity. The onset may be rapid, developing over 2 to 3 days. The diagnosis is confirmed when the toxin is documented in the stool or when the organism is isolated from culture, but repetitive stimulation studies can by extremely useful in establishing the diagnosis quickly. Treatment is supportive; specific immune globulin may prove to be therapeutic.

## Myopathies

Myopathies constitute a diverse group of genetic, inflammatory, and metabolic disorders that involve muscle and, in many cases, other organ systems, including the brain and heart. Inflammatory myopathies (dermatomyositis) are seen only rarely in very young children and generally produce subacute weakness, not hypotonia. Patients with Duchenne muscular dystrophy (among the most common muscular disorders) do not have hypotonia in infancy. In the infantile form of myotonic dystrophy–type 1[15] hypotonia can be severe at birth. Obtundation, difficulty with sucking and swallowing, weakness of facial muscles, clubfeet, and areflexia may be present. Myotonia will not be present either clinically or electrically until patients are older than 5 years. A neonate who survives will gain strength and tone and will eventually walk. Until strength and tone improve, assisted ventilation and gastrostomy tube feedings are often needed. Myotonic dystrophy–type 1 is an autosomal-dominant disorder; however, when it occurs in the neonatal period, it is virtually always the mother who transmitted the gene. She should be examined for the characteristic features of the disease, which include reflex and percussion myotonia, weakness of the neck flexor muscles, smallness of the sternocleidomastoid muscles, weakness of the wrist extensors and anterior tibialis muscles and facial muscles, and, often, intellectual disability. For children who first exhibit myotonic dystrophy beyond infancy, either parent may have transmitted the gene, which is located on 19q13. DNA studies can be done to document the diagnosis and predict the prognosis. This condition is an expanded trinucleotide repeat disorder, with correlation between the severity and the number of repeats. Family members should be provided with genetic counseling, given that prenatal diagnosis is available. Treatment is supportive.

Several congenital myopathies have been identified[4] and are generally diagnosed on muscle biopsy by their characteristic morphologic mechanism. These myopathies, typified by nemaline myopathy, are often hereditary and are associated with varying degrees of hypotonia and weakness and sometimes with respiratory and sucking problems early in life. Some have rather characteristic clinical features. For example, in X-linked myotubular myopathy of very early onset,[7] the extraocular and facial muscles are weak, in addition to generalized hypotonia and weakness. Central core disease is associated with congenital hip dislocation and a propensity for malignant hyperpyrexia. In some congenital myopathies, the gene location has been identified, but DNA testing is not yet available for establishing the diagnosis.

The congenital muscular dystrophies comprise a diverse group of diseases in which varying degrees of weakness and hypotonia are present early in life. Muscle biopsy shows characteristic, but not specific, pathologic findings, and more refined studies are required. The serum muscle enzymes (creatine kinase) are generally elevated, and, in some forms of this disorder, merosin is absent on the biopsy specimen.[20] The merosin-deficient type of congenital muscular dystrophy is often associated with intellectual disability, seizures, and white matter brain abnormalities. In Japan, Fukuyama-type congenital muscular dystrophy[21] is common and is also associated with severe CNS abnormalities.

Facioscapulohumeral muscular dystrophy[10] usually occurs in older children but, at times, will produce severe facial weakness in early childhood. Although sometimes sporadic, most cases are autosomal-dominant and parents of affected children should be examined for involvement that may be very mild and go unnoticed, such as facial muscular weakness, scapular winging, and a round-shouldered stance. This disease is genetically linked to high-frequency hearing deficits. Treatment is symptomatic, and it is appropriate to offer genetic counseling. DNA studies are available to document the diagnosis when this disorder is thought to exist, making electrodiagnostic testing and muscle biopsy unnecessary.

Glycogen storage disease caused by deficient acid maltase,[22] in addition to its neuromuscular manifestations (hypotonia and weakness), is associated with a markedly enlarged heart and congestive heart failure. The diagnosis can be made readily by specific blood tests. Enzyme replacement therapy has recently become available; without this treatment, the prognosis is dismal. This condition is an autosomal-recessive disorder with the responsible gene located at 17q23.

An increasing number of mitochondrial encephalomyopathies[15] are being reported that have varying CNS and muscle involvement. Lactic acidemia is common, but specialized genetic and other studies on muscle mitochondria are needed to provide a specific diagnosis if DNA studies are unrevealing. Treatment addresses symptoms.

Congenital hypotonia with favorable outcome[23] or benign congenital hypotonia is a retrospective diagnosis used to denote infants who have hypotonia of early onset with a benign course. This relatively unclear disorder is often associated with joint hyperlaxity, sometimes also noted in parents or other relatives. In many instances, by 5 years of age, the children are indistinguishable from other children their age.

## When to Refer

- Persistent lack of normal motor development
- Regression of motor development
- Sudden or precipitous worsening of tone or strength
- Swallowing dysfunction
- New onset of neurologic signs

## *TOOLS FOR PRACTICE*

### Medical Decision Support

- *Online Mendelian Inheritance in Man* (online database), Johns Hopkins University (omim.org)
- *Gene Tests* (Web site), (www.genetests.org)
- *Core Signs of Weakness* (videos), National Task Force for Early Identification of Childhood Neuromuscular Disorders (www.childmuscleweakness.org/index.php/videos)
- *Motor Delays: Early Identification and Referral* (article), *Pediatrics*, Vol 131, Issue 6, 2013 (pediatrics.aappublications.org/content/131/6/e2016.full)

## *REFERENCES*


1. Kuban KCK, Leviton A. Cerebral palsy. *N Engl J Med.* 1994;330:188–195
2. Perlman JM. Intrapartum hypoxic-ischemic cerebral injury and subsequent cerebral palsy: medicolegal issues. *Pediatrics.* 1997;99:851–859
3. Grahame R. Joint hypermobility and genetic collagen disorders: are they related? *Arch Dis Child.* 1999;80:188–191
4. Goebel HH. Congenital myopathies: the current status. *J Child Neurol.* 1999;14:30–31
5. Anhuf D, Eggermann T, Rudnik-Schöneborn S, Zerres K. Determination of SMN1 and SMN2 copy number using TaqMan technology. *Hum Mutat.* 2003;22:74–78
6. Harper PS. *Myotonic Dystrophy.* 3rd ed. London, UK: WB Saunders; 2001
7. Barth PG, Dubowitz V. X-linked myotubular myopathy—a long-term follow-up study. *Eur J Paeditr Neurol.* 1998;2:49–56
8. Spiro AJ. Disorders of the myoneural junction. In: Berg BO, ed. *Principles of Child Neurology.* New York, NY: McGraw-Hill; 1996
9. Kraner S, Laufenberg I, Strassburg HM, Sieb JP, Steinlein OK. Congenital myasthenic syndrome with episodic apnea in patients homozygous for a CHAT missense mutation. *Arch Neurol.* 2003;60:761–763
10. Okinaga A, Matsuoka T, Umeda J, et al. Early-onset facioscapulohumeral muscular dystrophy: two case reports. *Brain Dev.* 1997;19:563–567
11. Prasad AS, Prasad C. The floppy infant: contribution of genetic and metabolic disorders. *Brain Dev.* 2003;27:457–476
12. Spiro AJ. Minipolymyoclonus: a neglected sign in childhood spinal muscular atrophy. *Neurology.* 1970;20:1124–1126
13. Lefebvre S, Bürglen L, Reboullet S, et al. Identification and characterization of a spinal muscular atrophy-determining gene. *Cell.* 1995;80:155–165
14. Russell JW, Afifi AK, Ross MA. Predictive value of electromyography in diagnosis and prognosis of the hypotonic infant. *J Child Neurol.* 1992;7:387–391
15. Shoubridge EA. Mitochondrial encephalomyopathies. *Curr Opin Neurol.* 1998;11:491–496
16. Lefebvre S, Bürglen L, Frézal J, Munnich A, Melki J. The role of the SMN gene in proximal spinal muscular atrophy. *Hum Mol Genet.* 1998;7:1531–1536
17. Mandich P, Mancardi GL, Varese A, et al. Congenital hypomyelination due to myelin protein zero Q215X mutation. *Ann Neurol.* 1999;45:676–678
18. Ouvrier RA. *Peripheral Neuropathy in Childhood.* 2nd ed. New York, NY: Raven Press; 2002
19. McMaster P, Piper S, Schell D, Gillis J, Chong A. A taste of honey. *J Paediatr Child Health.* 2000;36:596–597
20. Jones KJ, Morgan G, Johnston H, et al. The expanding phenotype of laminin alpha2 chain (merosin) abnormalities: case series and review. *J Med Genet.* 2001;38:649–657
21. Hayashi YK, Ogawa M, Tagawa K, et al. Selective deficiency of alpha-dystroglycan in Fukuyama-type congenital muscular dystrophy. *Neurology.* 2001;57:115–121
22. Amalfitano A, Bengur AR, Morse RP, et al. Recombinant human acid alpha-glucosidase enzyme therapy for infantile glycogen storage disease type II: results of a phase I/II clinical trial. *Genet Med.* 2001;3:132–138
23. Carboni P, Pisani F, Crescenzi A, Villani C. Congenital hypotonia with favorable outcome. *Pediatr Neurol.* 2002;26:383–386

# Chapter 45

# Inattention and Impulsivity

*Lawrence S. Wissow, MD, MPH*

## ▶ INTRODUCTION

Symptoms of inattention and impulsivity affect many children, including a large number whose symptoms do not rise to the level of a disorder. Attention-deficit/hyperactivity disorder (ADHD) occurs in about 8% of children and youth,[1] who experience significant impairment in their functioning as a result of their symptoms. As part of their condition, individuals with ADHD often have deficits in social skills, impairing their abilities to function well in school and social settings.[2] ADHD is frequently comorbid with learning difficulties, and the 2 conditions can mimic each other in school or during cognitive tasks outside of school (including time devoted to doing homework). Thus, ADHD can result in significant adverse consequences. Follow-up studies have found that children with ADHD, particularly those untreated, are at greater risk for school failure, underemployment, difficulty with legal authorities, substance abuse, and morbidity from risky behaviors including motor vehicle crashes and sexually transmitted infections.[3]

The guidance in this chapter applies to the care of children presenting with undifferentiated symptoms of inattention and impulsivity in pediatric clinical settings.

This chapter is based on the work of the World Health Organization, whose recommendations may be updated annually. The most up-to-date information can be found at www.who.int.

## ▶ FINDINGS SUGGESTING INATTENTION AND IMPULSIVITY

Inattention and impulsivity occur commonly during childhood. When these symptoms occur more persistently and to a greater degree than is seen in a child's peers, there may be cause for concern. Often, the child's teacher is the first to observe the symptoms or to encourage medical attention for them. A summary of the symptoms and clinical findings that suggest inattention and impulsivity can be found in Box 45-1. These symptoms may be elicited from parents, teachers, or youth. Because observers often disagree about behavioral and emotional symptoms, collecting information from all 3 sources can be helpful, and the process of reconciling differences can itself be therapeutic.

BOX 45-1

## *Indications in History From Youth or Parent*

- Excitability, impatience, angry outbursts (more than is seen in peers)
- Wandering attention (greater than is seen in peers)
- Difficulties with behavior at home and in the classroom
- Academic difficulties
- Parents and teachers presuming diagnosis of ADHD or seeking diagnosis of ADHD

## ▶ TOOLS TO ASSIST WITH IDENTIFICATION

Since many children do not spontaneously disclose their symptoms, standardized wide-range psychosocial screening instruments may be used to identify children with emotional and behavioral difficulties that may include symptoms of inattention and impulsivity. Diagnostic criteria for ADHD require presence of symptoms in more than 1 setting; therefore, collateral reports from the school or child care center, as well as the parent(s), are critical elements in the identification process. Several instruments have versions to collect information from the youth, parents, and teachers. Table 45-1 provides an overview of general psychosocial screening tools available in the public domain, along with results raising concerns in the areas of inattention and impulsivity. Use of additional instruments, such as the Vanderbilt ADHD Rating Scales, can then help to confirm findings of the initial screening, corroborate a concern raised by a teacher or parent, and serve as a benchmark to track treatment progress. Use of a functional assessment tool such as the Impact Supplement of the Strengths and Difficulties Questionnaire (SDQ) or the Columbia Impairment Scale (CIS) will assist in determining whether the child is significantly impaired by the symptoms. Use of a tool to assess the effect of the child's problem on other members of the family may also be helpful; the Caregiver Strain Questionnaire (CGSQ) is an example of such a tool.

## ▶ ASSESSMENT

Assessment begins by differentiating the child's symptoms from normal behavior. All children may be inattentive or impulsive at times, but, for some children, inattention and impulsivity limit their adaptability to normal peer and family situations and interfere with learning. Inattention and impulsivity are typical characteristics of preschool children, but extremes of these behaviors warrant further evaluation (eg, concern that the behavior is harming family or peer relationships, interfering with learning, or putting the child at risk for expulsion from child care or school because of behavior). Boisterousness or dreaminess can be normal behavior patterns in older children. Children with limited social experiences and those whose environment is relatively less structured may seem impulsive and inattentive compared to their peers, especially when entering highly structured situations such as a classroom or organized group activities.

**Table 45-1**
**General Psychosocial Screening/Results Suggesting Inattention and Impulsivity**

| SCREENING INSTRUMENT | SCORE |
|---|---|
| Pediatric Symptom Checklist (PSC)-35 | • Total score ≥24 for children 5 years and younger.<br>• ≥28 for those 6–16 years.<br>• ≥30 for those 17 years and older.<br>AND<br>• Further discussion of items related to attention and impulse control confirms a concern in that area. |
| PSC-17 | • Attention subscale is ≥7.<br>AND<br>• Further discussion of items related to attention and impulse control confirms a concern in that area. |
| Strengths and Difficulties Questionnaire (SDQ) | • Total symptom score of >19.<br>• Hyperactivity scale score of 7–10 (see instructions at www.sdqinfo.com).<br>• Impact scale (back of form) score of 1 (medium impairment) or ≥2 (high impairment).<br>AND<br>• Further discussion of items related to attention and impulse control confirms a concern in that area. |

Table 45-2 provides a summary of conditions, such as hearing or vision problems, receptive and expressive language problems, learning disorders, and sleep deprivation, which may mimic or co-occur with inattention and impulsivity problems.

## ▶ PLAN OF CARE FOR CHILDREN WITH INATTENTION AND IMPULSIVITY

The care of a child experiencing symptoms of inattention and impulsivity can begin in the primary care setting from the time symptoms are recognized, even if the child's symptoms do not rise to the level of a disorder or referral to a mental health specialist is ultimately part of the care plan.

### *Engage Child and Family in Care*

Without engagement, most families will not seek or persist in care. The process may require multiple primary care visits.[4]

Reinforce strengths of the child and family (eg, good relationships with at least 1 parent or important adult, prosocial peers, concerned or caring family, help-seeking, connection to positive organizations) as a method of engagement, and identify any barriers to addressing the problem (eg, stigma, family conflict, resistance to treatment). Use "common factors" techniques[5] to build trust and optimism, reach agreement on incremental next steps, develop a plan of care, and collaboratively determine the role of the primary care physician. A key step is to reach agreement that there is a reason to consider intervention, and, ideally, that there are concrete problems that the family would like to see addressed. Regardless of other

**Table 45-2**
**Conditions That May Mimic or Co-occur With Inattention and Impulsivity**

| CONDITION | RATIONALE |
|---|---|
| Hearing or vision problems | All children who seem inattentive should be screened for sensory deficits. |
| Sleep deprivation | Sleep problems can cause inattention and irritability. Attention-deficit/hyperactivity disorder (ADHD) may contribute to difficulty sleeping. |
| ADHD | Diagnosis requires that a child have a persistent pattern of inattention and/or hyperactivity-impulsivity that interferes with functioning or development. These patterns are characterized as 6 or more symptoms of inattention (eg, careless with detail; fails to sustain attention; seems not to listen; does not finish instructed tasks; poor self-organization; avoids tasks requiring sustained mental effort; loses things; easily distracted; and seems forgetful) or hyperactivity [eg, fidgets; leaves seat when should be seated; runs or climbs excessively and inappropriately; noisy in play; persistent motor activity unmodified by social context (but this is seen less in teens); talks excessively; blurts out answers before question completed; fails to wait turn; and interrupts others' conversation or games] for at least 6 months. Further features necessary to make this diagnosis include the following:<br>• These symptoms were present prior to age 12 years.<br>• These symptoms are present in at least 2 types of settings (eg, home and school).<br>• The symptoms cause significant distress or impaired functioning.<br>• The symptoms are not better explained by another psychiatric disorder. |
| Learning problems or disabilities | If symptoms of inattention and impulsivity are associated with problems of school performance, the child may be experiencing learning difficulties. See Chapter 49, Learning Difficulty, to explore this possibility. |
| Developmental problems | Children with overall intellectual or social limitations may seem less able to control their impulses and to focus and maintain their attention than their age-mates. |
| Language impairment or disorder | Children with receptive or expressive language impairment may be frustrated and inattentive at least in part because of difficulty understanding what others say or being able to express themselves. Similar problems can arise when children are learning a new language and cannot yet fully function at the level of their peers or teachers. |
| Depression | May co-occur with ADHD. Marked sleep disturbance, disturbed appetite, low mood, or tearfulness could indicate that a child is depressed as well as having attention difficulties. See Chapter 14, Depression. |
| Exposure to adverse childhood experiences (ACE) | Children who have experienced or witnessed trauma; violence; a natural disaster; separation from a parent; parental divorce or separation; parental substance use; neglect; or physical, emotional, or sexual abuse are at high risk of developing symptoms suggesting inattention and impulsivity. These symptoms may mask or be expressions of emotional difficulties such as adjustment disorder or posttraumatic stress disorder (PTSD). Some symptoms of PTSD may resemble symptoms of ADHD (eg, hypervigilance may mimic hyperactivity, or dissociation may mimic inattention). These children may also manifest other forms of anxiety. Inquiring about previous trauma in a confidential setting is important. See Chapter 6, Anxiety. |
| Anxiety | Anxious children may experience difficulty concentrating. See Chapter 6, Anxiety. |

**Table 45-2**
**Conditions That May Mimic or Co-occur With Inattention and Impulsivity—cont'd**

| CONDITION | RATIONALE |
|---|---|
| Bereavement | Most children will experience the death of a family member or friend sometime in their childhood. Other losses may also trigger grief responses—separation or divorce of parents, relocation, change of school, deployment of a parent in military service, breakup with a girlfriend or boyfriend, or remarriage of parent. Such losses are traumatic. They may result in such symptoms as sadness, anxiety, difficulty concentrating, poor impulse control, or academic decline immediately following the loss and, in some instances, more persistently. See also Chapter 14, Depression and the discussion of PTSD in Chapter 6, Anxiety. |
| Physical illness | Medical issues that can mimic or provoke symptoms of inattention and impulsivity include thyroid disease, hypoglycemia, hyperglycemia, side effects of medications (eg, bronchodilators), and endocrine tumors (eg, rarely pheochromocytoma). |
| Substance use | Children with symptoms of inattention and impulsivity may self-medicate with alcohol, nicotine, or other drugs. Conversely, children using substances may manifest inattention, impulsivity, and deteriorating school performance. |
| Conduct or oppositional disorders | See Chapter 16, Disruptive Behavior and Aggression, to differentiate these symptoms from problems of inattention and impulsivity and ADHD. |
| Tourette syndrome | Children with repetitive movements (tics) should be identified. In children with Tourette syndrome, ADHD symptoms may precede onset of tics. Stimulant medication may worsen tics. It is important to tailor treatment to the child's most pressing symptoms before deciding the risks and benefits of using stimulants in children with both problems. |

Derived from American Psychiatric Association. *Diagnostic and Statistical Manual of Mental Disorders.* 5th ed. Arlington, VA: American Psychiatric Association; 2013

roles, the primary care physician can encourage a positive view of treatment on the part of the child and family.

## Offer Psychoeducation About ADHD, the Differential Diagnosis, and the Process of Arriving at a Diagnosis

Parents have likely heard about ADHD from other sources; their knowledge and concerns about the conditions may vary widely. They may have worries about being coerced into labeling their child with the condition by demands from the pediatrician or schools. The clinician can ask about what they know and what questions they may have. She can explain the process of making a provisional diagnosis and investigating alternatives, including language and learning problems, anxiety, and normal variation in development and temperament. Perhaps most importantly, the clinician can assure parents that she will not be jumping to a diagnosis, but rather will work with them to collect relevant information, make a plan of treatment, and then reevaluate the situation as time goes on. At some point, parents will also want to know more about the natural history of the condition and the implications it may have for their child's future. It is reasonable to say that these sorts of problems are common and highly amenable to treatment of various kinds, and, while sometimes persistent, tend to be more easily managed as the child gets older.

### Encourage Healthy Habits

Regular exercise and outdoor play are beneficial to all children and may be particularly helpful to inattentive and impulsive children. These children may also benefit from participation in structured sports activities, which offer exercise as well as the opportunity to build social skills such as taking turns, following rules, and handling success and disappointment. Also important are regular sleep habits, special time with parents, praise for good behavior, and reinforcement of the child's strengths. Limiting media exposure may be particularly important for these children. Television programs, movies, and computer games can be overstimulating; long hours in these activities can produce irritability. Unrestricted access to a television or computer, especially in the child's bedroom, can contribute to loss of sleep, failure to do homework, and the risk of seeing programming that contributes to increased activity.

### Reduce Stress

Consider the child's social environment (eg, family social history, parental depression screening, results of any family assessment tools administered, reports from child care or school). Symptoms of inattention and hyperactivity will generally worsen in stressful settings. The physician can guide parents in providing a safe, structured environment and coach parents in working constructively with the child's school. The physician can also address stresses on family members—if they have problems with mood or irritability, they will have more difficulty adapting to and moderating the child's behavior.

### Offer Initial Intervention(s)

The strategies described in the following text are common elements of evidence-based and evidence-informed psychosocial interventions for management of children's behavior. They are applicable to the care of children with mild or emerging symptoms of inattention and impulsivity and to those with impairing symptoms that do not rise to the level of a disorder. They can also be used along with other specific interventions for ADHD.

*Guide parents in managing the child's behavior.* Good practices include the following:

- **Tangible rewards:** Rewards or privileges contingent on performance of routine tasks (eg, TV or computer time contingent on attaining a realistic goal). These rewards are most effective when coupled with a system for helping the child be aware of his or her own level of functioning, including charts that monitor events such as completion of homework without a reminder, staying "on-task" in school for a prearranged time before taking a break, carrying out chores at home before being asked.
- **Parent praise:** Conscious effort by parent to identify and comment on positive aspects of child's behavior (eg, compliment child, especially when desired action is spontaneous).
- **Parent monitoring:** Use of some systematic means to rate the child's burden of specific ADHD symptoms and overall social, emotional, and academic function (eg, weekly use of Vanderbilt scales or a customized checklist, often with simultaneous teacher ratings). Monitoring helps the parent advocate for the child and can help take pressure off the child by giving short-term, objective measures of progress.
- **Time-out:** Avoiding reinforcement of undesired behavior through arguing or allowing the behavior to continue (eg, child is required to sit without attention or activity for a brief period as a consequence for an undesired behavior).

Box 45-2

## *Strategies for Working Constructively With a Child's School*

- Obtain consent for the clinician to exchange information with the child's teacher.
- Establish constructive 3-way (parent, teacher, pediatrician) communication with the school.
- Ask if testing has been requested and taken place to detect special educational needs.
- Monitor academic progress, helping to reinforce successes and identify particular subjects or educational settings where more support is needed.
- Advocate for appropriate classroom strategies.
  - o Have the child sit at the front of the class.
  - o If possible, engage the child in active learning, (eg, have the child go to the blackboard to write answers to questions).
  - o Give extra time to stay organized (eg, write down assignments, make sure that all needed materials are taken home or gathered for a project, have the child repeat back what he or she is to do).
  - o Break longer assignments into shorter pieces (also helpful for homework).
  - o Coordinate reports of behavior with home—consider a daily report card of behavior and subsequent rewards or consequences.

- **Commands/limit setting:** Use of clear, simple commands that ideally give the child a warning of impending expected behavior, an opportunity to perform it, a warning of consequences for nonperformance, and a consistent consequence (eg, "You can do 1 more puzzle and then we have to go…now it's time to go…if you don't put the puzzle away now, you can't chose the music we listen to in the car.").

*If there are battles over homework, offer guidelines.* Box 45-2 provides suggestions for parents to consider in addressing homework issues.

*If child meets diagnostic criteria for ADHD, consider specific therapy.* The course of treatment depends on the child's age and should be noted in the overall care plan.

For preschool-aged children (4–5 years of age), evidence-based, parent- or teacher-administered behavior therapy is considered the first line of treatment. Use of medications may be considered—ideally with specialist consultation—if behavioral treatment does not provide sufficient improvement or if evidence-based treatment is not available.

For elementary school–aged children (6–11 years of age), US Food and Drug Administration–approved medications for ADHD and/or evidence-based parent- and/or teacher-administered behavior therapy is considered first-line treatment for ADHD, preferably both. The evidence is particularly strong for stimulant medications and sufficient but less strong for atomoxetine, extended-release guanfacine, and extended-release clonidine (in that order).

For adolescents (12–18 years of age), Food and Drug Administration–approved medications for ADHD with the assent of the adolescent along with behavior therapy are considered treatment for ADHD.[6]

### Provide Resources

Families may find support and resources from organizations such as Children and Adults With Attention-Deficit/Hyperactivity Disorder (www.chadd.org). Helpful publications are included in Tools for Practice: Engaging Patient and Family at the end of this chapter. Provide the family with contact numbers and resources in case of emergency.

### Monitor the Child's Progress Toward Therapeutic Goals

Child care, preschool, or school reports can be helpful in monitoring progress. The Vanderbilt scales (parent and teacher), SDQ (parent, teacher), and Pediatric Symptom Checklist (PSC) can be helpful in monitoring progress with symptoms and functioning. Both medications and behavioral treatments need careful titration to achieve their desired effects without the development of side effects. The need for higher-than-recommended doses of medication could be a sign of difficulties with adherence or a need to switch to a different medication. Behavioral treatments can be difficult to implement and maintain. Physicians can work with families to adapt behavioral suggestions to family circumstances and to explore barriers to other aspects of treatment, including effective engagement with schools.

It is important for the clinician to help the family understand that it is not uncommon for treatment to be successful for a period and then seem to lose effectiveness. This can happen when there are new stresses or demands, or when, after a period of success, there has been a letup on treatment. If modifying existing treatment and exploring ways of dealing with new stresses do not help get function back to baseline, then new treatments, or new diagnoses, need to be considered. In particular, as school demands increase, learning issues may need to be considered even if they were not seen as contributing problems in the past.

### Involve Specialist(s)

*Involve specialist(s) if the child does not respond to initial interventions or if the following clinical circumstances exist:*

- Child has severe functional impairment.
- Child has severely disruptive behavior or aggression.
- Child has comorbid depression or posttraumatic stress disorder, or if problems with mood, behavior, and development seem more prominent than difficulties with attention or impulsivity.
- Symptoms are threatening school performance or the achievement of other developmentally important goals (eg, developing and sustaining friendships).
- The child or parent is very distressed by the symptom(s).
- There are co-occurring behavior problems. (The combination of shyness, anxiety, and behavior problems is thought to be particularly risky for future behavior problems of a more serious nature.)
- The child's symptoms were preceded by serious trauma.
- The child has ADHD and contraindications to stimulants or marked side effects with stimulants.
- The child's problems are occurring in the context of other family emotional or behavioral problems that have not been alleviated with primary care interventions.

*When specialty care is needed, ensure that it is evidence-informed and assist the family in accessing it.* Pharmacologic interventions and a number of evidence-based and evidence-informed psychosocial interventions are available for the treatment of ADHD in children and adolescents. Ideally, those referred for care in the mental health specialty system would

Box 45-3

## *American Academy of Pediatrics Recommendations for Treatment of Attention-deficit/Hyperactivity Disorder*

- Recommendations for treatment of children and youth with ADHD vary depending on the patient's age.
  - For *preschool-aged children (4–5 years of age)*, the primary care clinician should prescribe evidence-based parent- and/or teacher-administered behavior therapy as the first line of treatment (quality of evidence A/strong recommendation) and may prescribe methylphenidate if the behavior interventions do not provide significant improvement and there is moderate-to-severe continuing disturbance in the child's function. In areas in which evidence-based behavioral treatments are not available, the clinician needs to weigh the risks of starting medication at an early age against the harm of delaying diagnosis and treatment (quality of evidence B/recommendation).
  - For *elementary school-aged children (6–11 years of age)*, the primary care clinician should prescribe FDA-approved medications for ADHD (quality of evidence A/strong recommendation) and/or evidence-based parent- and/or teacher-administered behavior therapy as treatment for ADHD, preferably both (quality of evidence B/strong recommendation). The evidence is particularly strong for stimulant medications and sufficient but less strong for atomoxetine, extended-release guanfacine, and extended-release clonidine (in that order) (quality of evidence A/strong recommendation). The school environment, program, or placement is a part of any treatment plan.
  - For *adolescents (12–18 years of age)*, the primary care clinician should prescribe FDA-approved medications for ADHD with the assent of the adolescent (quality of evidence A/strong recommendation) and may prescribe behavior therapy as treatment for ADHD (quality of evidence C/recommendation), preferably both.
- Primary care clinicians should titrate doses of medication for ADHD to achieve maximum benefit with minimum adverse effects (quality of evidence B/strong recommendation).

For more information, see American Academy of Pediatrics Subcommittee on Attention-Deficit/Hyperactivity Disorder, Steering Committee on Quality Improvement. ADHD: clinical practice guideline for the diagnosis, evaluation, and treatment of attention-deficit/hyperactivity disorder in children and adolescents. *Pediatrics*. 2011;128(5):1007–1022 (pediatrics.aappublications.org/content/128/5/1007.full).
Adapted from *Caring for Children With ADHD: A Resource Toolkit for Clinicians*. Copyright 2011 American Academy of Pediatrics.

have access to the safest and most effective treatments. Box 45-3 provides a summary of these interventions. Youth referred for mental health specialty care complete the referral process only 61% of the time, and a significantly smaller number persist in care.[7]

Note that not all evidence-based interventions may be available in every community. If a particular intervention is not available, this becomes an opportunity to collaborate with others in the community to advocate on behalf of children. Increasingly, states offer both telepsychiatry services and consultation/referral support "warmlines" that help physicians provide initial treatment and locate resources. The availability of the latter form of help is tracked at the National Network of Child Psychiatry Access Programs (www.nncpap.org).

*Reach agreement on respective roles in the child's care.* If the child is referred to mental health specialty care, the physician may be responsible for initiating medication or adjusting doses; monitoring response to treatment; monitoring adverse effects; engaging and encouraging the child's and family's positive view of treatment; and coordinating care provided by parents, school, medical home, and specialists. In fact, the child may improve just knowing that the clinician is involved and interested. Resources available to help clinicians in these roles are provided in Tools for Practice: Medical Decision Support.

## ACKNOWLEDGMENT

The author and editor wish to acknowledge the contributions of Linda Paul, MPH, manager of the AAP Mental Health Leadership Work Group.

## TOOLS FOR PRACTICE

### Engaging Patient and Family

- *ADHD: What Every Parent Needs to Know* (book), Reiff MI, American Academy of Pediatrics (shop.aap.org)
- *Addressing ADD Naturally* (book), Xlibris Corporation, 2010

### Medical Decision Support

- *Caring for Children with ADHD: A Resource Toolkit for Clinicians* (toolkit), American Academy of Pediatrics (shop.aap.org)
- *NICHQ Vanderbilt Assessment Scale* (scale), National Institute for Children's Health Quality (www.nichq.org/childrens-health/adhd/resources/vanderbilt-assessment-scales)
- *Pediatric Symptom Checklist* (screen), Massachusetts General Hospital (www.massgeneral.org/psychiatry/services/psc_forms.aspx)
- *Strengths & Difficulties Questionnaire* (screen), Youth in Mind, Ltd. (www.sdqinfo.com)

## AAP POLICY STATEMENTS

American Academy of Pediatrics Subcommittee on Attention-Deficit/Hyperactivity Disorder, Steering Committee on Quality Improvement and Management. ADHD: clinical practice guideline for the diagnosis, evaluation, and treatment of attention-deficit/hyperactivity disorder in children and adolescents. *Pediatrics.* 2011;128(5):1007–1022 (pediatrics.aappublications.org/content/128/5/1007)

## REFERENCES

1. Visser SN, Lesesne CA, Perou R. National estimates and factors associated with medication treatment for childhood attention-deficit/hyperactivity disorder. *Pediatrics.* 2007;119(Suppl 1):S99–S106
2. McQuade JD, Hoza B. Peer problems in attention deficit hyperactivity disorder: current status and future directions. *Dev Disabil Res Rev.* 2008;14:320–324
3. Wolraich ML, Wibbelsman CJ, Brown TE, et al. Attention-deficit/hyperactivity disorder among adolescents: a review of the diagnosis, treatment, and clinical implications. *Pediatrics.* 2005;115:1734–1746
4. Foy JM; American Academy of Pediatrics Task Force on Mental Health. Enhancing pediatric mental health care: algorithms for primary care. *Pediatrics.* 2010;125(Suppl 3):S109–S125
5. Kemper KJ, Wissow L, Foy JM, Shore SE. *Core Communication Skills for Primary Clinicians.* Wake Forest School of Medicine. nwahec.org/45737. Accessed January 9, 2015
6. American Academy of Pediatrics Subcommittee on Attention-Deficit/Hyperactivity Disorder, Steering Committee on Quality Improvement and Management. ADHD: clinical practice guideline for the diagnosis, evaluation, and treatment of attention-deficit/hyperactivity disorder in children and adolescents. *Pediatrics.* 2011;128:1007–1022
7. Rushton J, Bruckman D, Kelleher K. Primary care referral of children with psychosocial problems. *Arch Pediatr Adolesc Med.* 2002;156:592–598

# Chapter 46

# Irritability and Fussiness

*Diana King, MD; Waseem Hafeez, MBBS*

Irritability, "a condition in which a person, organ, or a part responds excessively to a stimulus,"[1] is a common complaint in children, especially in neonates and infants. Although experienced physicians can recognize irritability in a child, a concise definition is difficult because some subjectivity exists in the use of the term. Although it is not a quantifiable symptom, irritability includes episodes of crying or fussiness despite attempts at comforting the infant. While it is not a symptom of any specific illness, most parents recognize that something might be wrong with the child even though other symptoms may not yet exist.

Irritability results from lack of vital nutrients (eg, oxygen, glucose), the presence of noxious stimuli (eg, pain, toxins), or an emotional state (eg, anger, frustration). It may have different causes and manifestations in infants, children, and adolescents. Whereas older children and adolescents may offer explanations that help clarify their complaint, an infant or preverbal child is unable to provide such information. Acute irritability may be associated with life-threatening illnesses requiring urgent intervention and stabilization before a search for the cause begins. A parent who seeks care for an infant who is fussier than usual may arrive with the child in shock, in respiratory distress, or having a seizure. An organized approach to the differential diagnosis minimizes unnecessary testing. If the child does not have an immediately life-threatening condition, then a complete history and thorough physical examination are the first steps in the evaluation of irritability and, in many cases, will reveal the cause of the symptom. Many common infectious, traumatic, toxic, allergic, and inflammatory conditions can be diagnosed by history and physical examination alone. Laboratory or radiologic procedures may confirm a clinical suspicion. An algorithm to differentiate some life-threatening conditions from less serious causes of irritability is presented in Figure 46-1.

## ▶ ACUTE IRRITABILITY IN THE ILL-APPEARING CHILD

### *Central Nervous System*

Children younger than 2 years have a high risk for significant brain injury after both accidental and nonaccidental traumatic brain injury (TBI). In data collected between 2002 and 2006, the National Center for Injury Prevention and Control found that children aged 0 to 4 years had the highest rate of TBI-related emergency department visits (1,256 per 100,000 population), with falls, motor vehicle crash, and inflicted trauma as the leading causes.[2] The incidence of intracranial injury was 13% in infants 0 to 2 months of age, 6% in infants 3 to 11 months of age, and 2% in infants 12 months or older. The American Academy of

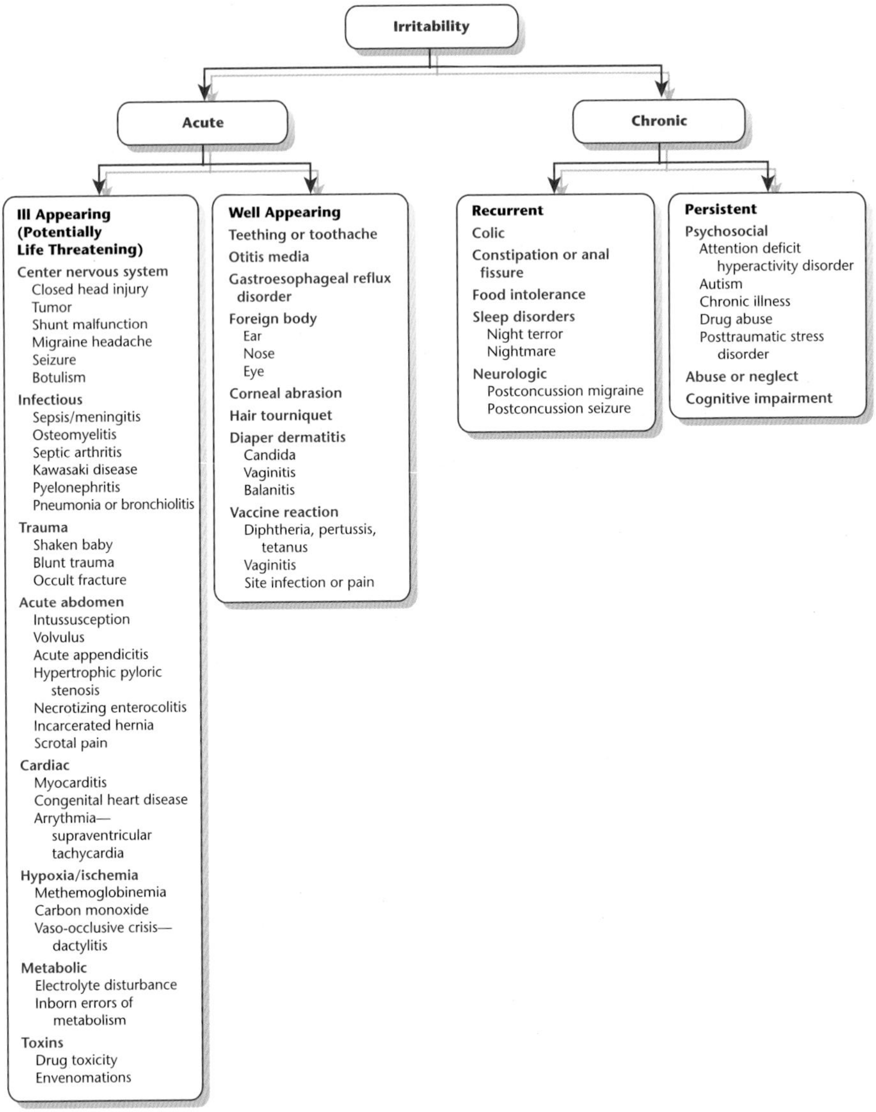


**Figure 46-1**
Algorithm for evaluation of the irritable infant.

Pediatrics has recommended guidelines for evaluation and management of head injury in this age group.[3] A history of a fall from the bed, infant-walker, stairs, or bicycle can often be obtained. To determine the need for computed tomography scan in clinically important TBI, prediction rules have been identified which include in children younger than 2 years abnormal mental status, loss of consciousness, scalp hematoma except frontal, palpable skull fracture, severe mechanism of injury, and not acting normally according to the parents. In addition to these findings, the prediction rule for children aged 2 years and older also includes vomiting, severe headache, and signs of basilar skull fracture.[4]

A special concern is for children who sustain concussions from sports-related injuries. The American Academy of Neurology defines concussion as "a trauma-induced alteration in mental status that may or may not involve loss of consciousness." The term *post-concussive syndrome* refers to the constellation of acute symptoms, which can be somatic (headache, dizziness, blurriness), emotional (irritability, anxiety), and cognitive (concentration and memory difficulties). The term *second impact syndrome* has been proposed for an athlete who has sustained a concussion, sustains a second head injury before symptoms associated with the first have fully cleared, and is at risk for a catastrophic outcome such as permanent disability or death.[5] To manage these injuries, a concussion grading scale has been developed with return-to-play guidelines that include physical and cognitive rest and rehabilitation.[6]

Increased intracranial pressure (ICP) from a brain tumor may produce acute irritability and altered behavior without the usual preceding symptoms such as headache or loss of coordination and ataxia. Primary brain tumors in the posterior fossa are the most common solid malignancies in infants and children younger than 7 years. In young children, the diagnosis of a brain tumor may be delayed because their symptoms are subtle (headache, irritability, or drowsiness) or similar to those of more common illnesses, such as gastrointestinal disorders (vomiting). Hydrocephalus, another cause of raised ICP, often occurs in infancy with irritability, vomiting, a tense or bulging fontanel, and an increasing head circumference that crosses percentile lines. Older children usually complain of headaches. Neuroimaging shows congenital malformation (myelomeningocele, Chiari syndrome, Dandy Walker malformation, aqueductal stenosis, arteriovenous malformation) or germinal matrix intraventricular hemorrhage of prematurity. Hydrocephalus is treated by the introduction of ventriculoperitoneal shunts to reduce the ICP. The ventriculoperitoneal shunt may become obstructed or infected, or it may malfunction, causing overdrainage or underdrainage, initially causing irritability, headache, vomiting, or lethargy.

Undiagnosed migraine headache may manifest itself in the preverbal child with irritability. Headaches attributable to migraine occur in 8% to 12% of children younger than 3 years.[7] There seems to be an association of infantile colic with excessive crying and irritability with later diagnosis of migraine.[8] Children with seizures, especially unwitnessed, may seem irritable during an aura or the postictal phase. Neonatal seizures, more commonly seen in preterm infants than term infants, may have only subtle symptoms such as ocular or pedaling movements, lip smacking, or apnea. Nonconvulsive status epilepticus, which includes absence and partial complex seizures, is a relatively rare cause of abnormal behavior resulting from continuous or intermittent seizure activity in the absence of any motor component. The hallmark of nonconvulsive status epilepticus is a diagnostic electroencephalogram associated with irritability and a change in behavior or mental status.[9]

Infant botulism, most commonly foodborne, may initially cause difficulty in feeding, irritability, lethargy, weak cry, and constipation. As the disease progresses, drooling, dysphagia, loss of head control, respiratory distress, and flaccid paralysis may occur from progressive bulbar involvement.

### Infections

The primary care physician should suspect a bacterial infection in a child with fever and irritability. Infants with meningitis may have irritability, lethargy, and poor feeding. If the fontanel is still open, then it may be bulging. Lumbar puncture is diagnostic, and treatment with intravenous antibiotics should not be delayed. The introduction of vaccines against *Haemophilus influenzae* type B and *Streptococcus pneumoniae* has changed the epidemiology of bacterial meningitis in children. Infants younger than 3 months of age are most commonly infected with Group B streptococci and gram-negative bacilli.[10] Encephalitis from herpes simplex virus should also be considered.[11] In children older than 3 months, the most common pathogens are *Streptococcus pneumoniae* and *Neisseria meningitidis*.[12]

Irritability and decreased movement of a limb should raise concern for osteomyelitis. Swelling and erythema of the soft tissue overlying the bone may exist, often with a history of preceding trauma. Joint pain, fever, irritability, and a limp should raise concern for septic arthritis. Examination will reveal erythema, swelling, or warmth over the affected joint, with restricted movement. With septic arthritis of the hip, swelling and redness may not be visible, and the pain may be referred to the knee. Blood should be analyzed for culture, complete blood count, and C-reactive protein to help establish a diagnosis. An orthopedist should be consulted for possible surgical drainage.[13]

Irritability is one of the most common associated symptoms in children with Kawasaki disease. The principal clinical manifestations of this systemic vasculitis are fever, rash, conjunctival injection, erythema of lips and mouth, cervical adenopathy, and changes in the extremities. Bacteremia and urinary tract infections can also produce irritability, along with fever in an ill-appearing infant.[14]

### Trauma

A systematic search for injuries should be performed on any child with a history of trauma. Inflicted injuries are more difficult to diagnose because the signs may be subtle and the history is often misleading. Abusive head trauma is the leading cause of traumatic death in children younger than 2 years. The rotational forces sustained during shaking cause movement of the brain within the subdural space and tearing of the bridging veins, resulting in subdural hematoma. The shearing forces can also cause diffuse axonal injury. Clinical signs of abusive head trauma may be poor feeding, vomiting, lethargy, or irritability. More severe central nervous system dysfunction can result in death.[15]

In infants and young children, the pressure of the lap belt of a restraint system in a motor vehicle crash or other blunt abdominal trauma can lead to intra-abdominal bleeding, initially displayed as irritability from tissue hypoperfusion and pain. Many traumatic causes of irritability that are not life threatening may be apparent on initial physical examination and include fractures and dislocations.

### Acute Abdomen

Intussusception is seen most often between the ages of 3 months and 5 years, with a peak incidence at 6 to 11 months. The child seems colicky, cries, and may draw the knees toward the chest; this episode may last a few minutes and then subside. The child often looks better between episodes, but the irritability gradually increases and vomiting becomes more frequent and sometimes bilious. Mandeville et al[16] found the classic triad of intermittent colicky abdominal pain, vomiting, and bloody stools was present in more than 65% of patients; and in patients younger than 12 months, irritability was an important clinical predictor.

Appendicitis is the most common condition requiring emergency surgery in children. Abdominal pain in a young child may first manifest as irritability, before the appearance of nausea, vomiting, fever, and right lower quadrant tenderness. Perforation rates for appendicitis are higher in children than in adults (30%–65%), and, given that the omentum is less developed in children, perforations are less likely to be walled off or localized.[17]

Hypertrophic pyloric stenosis may become symptomatic as early as the first week of life and as late as the fifth month. Symptoms begin with nonbilious vomiting after feeding, and as the disease progresses the vomiting becomes projectile. The baby may initially seem normal, but hunger makes the infant irritable, and signs of dehydration eventually become apparent. The finding of an olive shaped mass in the right upper quadrant of the abdomen is diagnostic, and confirmed by ultrasound.

Malrotation with midgut volvulus peaks during the first month of life but can occur any time in childhood. The neonate will be irritable initially; as the bowel becomes obstructed and necrotic, bilious vomiting and shock may result from perforation.

Necrotizing enterocolitis is typically seen in premature infants in their first few weeks of life.[18] It may rarely be seen in full term infants, within the first 2 weeks after birth, particularly with a stressor such as infection or anoxic event. Infants are ill appearing, irritable, and lethargic, with distended abdomen and bloody stools. Abdominal plain-film finding of pneumatosis intestinalis, caused by gas in the submucosal intestinal wall, is diagnostic of necrotizing enterocolitis with ultrasound becoming increasingly used to make the diagnosis while avoiding radiation. Because of a high mortality rate, management includes early surgical consultation and aggressive fluid resuscitation, bowel rest, and broad-spectrum antibiotic coverage.

Sixty percent of incarcerated inguinal hernias occur during the first year of life, especially in infants born preterm, with symptoms of irritability, vomiting, and pain in the groin and abdomen. A testicular examination is imperative in all male patients with irritability or abdominal pain. On examination a nonfluctuant tender mass is present in the inguinal region and may extend down into the scrotum. With the onset of ischemia of the involved bowel the pain becomes more intense and localized to the scrotum, and the infant may have bilious vomiting with the presence of bloody stools. An attempt should be made to reduce the incarcerated hernia manually by gentle compression. Sedation or analgesia, elevation of the lower torso, and an ice pack may be helpful. If reduction is unsuccessful or the child shows signs of small bowel obstruction, then operative reduction of the incarcerated hernia should be performed. Irritability with scrotal pain may also result from epididymitis, torsion of the testis, or torsion of the appendix testis.

## Cardiac System

Acute myocarditis can be a challenging diagnosis to make because the clinical presentation can vary. The diagnosis should be considered in an irritable child with resting tachycardia and respiratory symptoms. An electrocardiogram may reveal sinus tachycardia, ventricular hypertrophy, and ST and T wave changes. Low voltage QRS complexes, or an abnormal QRS axis, may be present. Chest radiograph may reveal cardiomegaly, pulmonary edema, or pleural effusion. Elevated C-reactive protein, serum troponin, and aspartate aminotransferase levels will support the diagnosis, and an echocardiogram will show reduced ventricular function.

Cardiac magnetic resonance is a noninvasive method to confirm the diagnosis, but the gold standard is an endomyocardial biopsy.[19] The presence of immune complexes indicates an immune-mediated process, and immunosuppressive therapy may be indicated. Treatment includes inotropic support, diuretics, and afterload reducers in a critical care setting.[20]

Anomalous left coronary artery originating from the pulmonary artery (ALCAPA) is a congenital abnormality that can present in early infancy with irritability, poor feeding, and difficulty breathing.[21] The electrocardiogram may reveal abnormal Q waves in leads $V_4$-$V_6$, I and aVL, or an abnormal R wave progression.[22]

An infant with supraventricular tachycardia may present with irritability, poor feeding, vomiting, cyanosis, or pallor. Physical examination will reveal a rapid, regular rhythm; electrocardiogram is diagnostic.[23]

## Hypoxic or Ischemic Events

Carbon monoxide (CO) poisoning and methemoglobinemia cause irritability by producing hypoxia. CO binds to hemoglobin with an affinity more than 200 times that of oxygen, whereas methemoglobin is unable to bind to oxygen. Both actions result in a leftward shift of the oxygen-hemoglobin dissociation curve and decreased oxygen delivery to the tissues. A history of smoke inhalation and exposure to an indoor gas stove or to automobile exhaust fumes may not be forthcoming without prompting. Early findings with CO poisoning are similar to influenza-like symptoms of headache, irritability, and dizziness, whereas prolonged exposure may result in altered mental status. Arterial measurement of carboxyhemoglobin is diagnostic.

Methemoglobinemia in infancy may be either hereditary or related to hypoxic events, medication use (sulfonamides, topical anesthetics, metoclopramide), products containing nitrites and nitrates (contaminated well water or foods with naturally occurring nitrates such as spinach, green beans, carrots, and squash), or to diarrhea, probably from the nitrite-forming bacteria in the gut.[24] Hereditary methemoglobinemia is usually mild, whereas the acquired disease can be life threatening. The hallmarks of methemoglobinemia are characteristic blue-gray cyanosis that is not improved with oxygen despite normal arterial oxygen tension and chocolate brown appearance of arterial blood. Pulse oximetry will not be reliable as high levels of methemoglobin will tend to cause a pulse oximeter reading of about 85% regardless of the true level of oxygen saturation. Treatment of the patient begins with 100% supplemental oxygen by nonrebreather mask and aggressive supportive care. In CO poisoning, hyperbaric oxygen therapy may be indicated in certain clinical conditions; methylene blue is an effective treatment for methemoglobinemia.

In children with sickle cell anemia, ischemia may cause painful vaso-occlusive crisis. The first presentation in infants and younger children is usually irritability and dactylitis (painful swelling of the hands and feet) as a result of vascular stasis and ischemia. Treatment includes analgesia, hydration, and rest.

## Metabolic System

Hypoglycemia, hypo- or hypernatremia, hypo- or hypercalcemia, hypomagnesemia, and inborn errors of metabolism can all cause irritability.[25] Hypoglycemia is defined as a glucose level of 40 mg/dL or less and can be a primary process or caused by sepsis, ingestion, or cardiac or respiratory failure.[26] Rapid detection and treatment of hypoglycemia can prevent irreversible neurologic damage. Hyponatremia can result from gastrointestinal losses or water intoxication, whereas hypernatremia is seen with diarrhea in which the water losses exceed salt loss, when replacement fluid has too high a sodium content, or with improper preparation of infant formula. Hypocalcemia in the newborn period may cause irritability, poor feeding, and lethargy; later in infancy and during childhood, hypocalcemia is seen with rickets. Hypercalcemia is a rare electrolyte disturbance resulting from hyperparathyroidism, vitamin D intoxication, or idiopathic causes. Hypomagnesemia is found with hypocalcemia.

The inborn errors of metabolism that cause irritability are those in which a toxic intermediate accumulates. Organic and aminoacidemias and urea cycle disorders result in metabolic acidosis or hyperammonemia. They are symptomatic in the first few weeks of life, with vomiting, poor feeding, irritability, and lethargy. When a milder degree of enzyme dysfunction is present, clinical disease may be triggered by a bacterial or viral illness.[27]

### Toxins and Drugs

Life-threatening intoxication may result from heavy metals such as lead and mercury, drugs of abuse such as cocaine and alcohol, envenomation by scorpions and snakes, overdoses of or idiosyncratic reactions to medications, and contact with agricultural, industrial, or household chemicals. Thorough questioning about recent use of lawn chemicals, pesticides, and cleaning products may be the only clues to these factors as a cause of irritability because many of these chemicals will not be detected by standard toxicologic screenings of blood and urine. Prescribed or over-the-counter medications such as beta-agonists, antiepileptics, decongestants, antihistamines, antitussives, and various cold preparations may cause irritability even when used as directed and certainly when overused. Cocaine, alcohol, phencyclidine hydrochloride, inhalants, and other drugs of abuse are known to cause irritability. Infants and children may be exposed to these substances by passive means transplacentally,[28] by ingestion of breast milk,[29] or by inhalation. They may accidentally ingest alcohol, cigarettes, or other substances left within reach. A positive history may be difficult to elicit, and a toxicologic screen may not always be helpful; thus a strong index of suspicion is needed. Substance use or withdrawal should be considered in the differential diagnosis of any adolescent with chronic persistent irritability. In rare instances, intentional poisoning may be the cause of a child's distress.

### Malignancy

Many physicians remember at least 1 child who has had complaints of irritability and intermittent fever in whom leukemia with bone pain was diagnosed. Malignancies of all sorts may have a component of irritability among their symptoms and must be considered carefully when no other diagnosis is forthcoming.

## ▶ ACUTE IRRITABILITY IN THE WELL-APPEARING CHILD

Irritability in infants has been attributed to a variety of causes of pain or discomfort that may become obvious during the evaluation. Dental caries and teething may cause an infant to be fussy or irritable. In addition to irritability, teething may be accompanied by loose stools but not fever.[30] Cold teething rings may provide some relief, but numbing gels with benzocaine are less helpful and may be harmful as they have been associated with methemoglobinemia.

Acute otitis media is a common cause of irritability, with or without fever, in children younger than 2 years and in those attending child care. Also common, particularly in the first year of life, is gastroesophageal reflux, which may be asymptomatic or reveal itself with postprandial irritability, recurrent vomiting, and inadequate weight gain.

Other sources of irritability and nonspecific crying episodes may be related to a foreign body in the ear or nose, a corneal abrasion, hair wrapped around a digit or penis, diaper rash, nonspecific vaginitis, balanitis, insect and spider bites or stings, and pain from the site of a vaccination. A thorough head-to-toe examination, including special attention to the eyes, ears, digits, and genitalia, is essential to establish a diagnosis.

A foreign body in the ear or nose, if present for a prolonged period, results in foul-smelling discharge. If visible, the object may be removed with forceps, by gentle irrigation, or by suction; otherwise removal should be done under sedation or general anesthesia. Disk batteries need to be removed emergently because they may leak and can cause tissue destruction. An insect in the ear canal can make a child very irritable and may be removed after first killing the insect with mineral oil or lidocaine.

Foreign bodies under the eyelid, inward turned eyelashes, or a baby scratching the eyes may cause corneal abrasion. The child may be irritable, with increased tearing, conjunctival injection, and photophobia. Diagnosis is made by Wood lamp examination after instillation of fluorescein into the eye. A foreign body may be removed by a moistened cotton-tipped applicator or by irrigation.

A hair tourniquet around a child's digit or genitals can cause irritability and pain. A thorough examination in the creases of the digits is essential because prolonged constricting bands may compromise distal circulation.

In some instances the source of a child's irritability will be found only on thorough examination of the genitalia, which may reveal evidence of vaginitis, balanitis, or an anal fissure. Diaper dermatitis, common after a diarrheal illness, with *Candida* infection or as an allergic reaction to the diaper material, is another potential cause of irritability in infants.

Infants can certainly be irritable after the administration of a vaccine, with local erythema, swelling, and tenderness at the injection site. Persistent, inconsolable crying lasting 3 hours or more within 48 hours of receiving whole-cell pertussis DTP vaccine have been reported but is significantly lower with the newer acellular-pertussis DTaP vaccine.[31]

## ▶ CHRONIC IRRITABILITY

Chronic irritability may be recurrent or persistent in a child and challenges both the parents'[32] and the physician's skills. Psychosocial causes may top the list, but toxic, neurologic, metabolic, and miscellaneous causes must be considered and are shown in Figure 46-1. Irritability as a chronic feature of a child's behavior may indicate significant problems with familial relationships and the ability to master the environment. Infants may be irritable because of parental-infant temperament mismatches, maternal depression,[33] or stress within the family from, for example, the birth of a new child. Abuse and neglect of a child may provoke irritable behavior or outbursts. An older child or adolescent who has a psychiatric condition such as depression, psychosis, autism, post-traumatic stress disorder, or substance abuse may be described as irritable by parents and others. The investigation and treatment of irritability in these situations may require a multidisciplinary and long-term approach.

### *Chronic Recurrent Irritability*

Colic is characterized by paroxysms of irritability or crying that begin and resolve without apparent cause in infants younger than 5 months of age. Criteria for the diagnosis are episodes of crying lasting 3 or more hours per day, occurring 3 or more days per week for at least 1 week. Colic typically peaks at 6 weeks and abates by 3 to 4 months. The physical examination is normal, and growth and development are not affected.[34]

Constipation in the older infant or child, another common cause of recurrent irritability, is associated with inadequate fluid intake, low-fiber diet, dietary changes, and toilet training. The passage of large, hard stools can result in anal fissures, which make the situation worse as the child becomes even more reluctant to defecate because of the pain.

Food allergy affects approximately 6% to 8% of infants and young children and approximately 3.5% to 4% of adults.[35] The most common food allergens include cow's milk, eggs, peanuts, wheat, and shellfish. Milk protein allergy is usually seen in the first few months of life: children are irritable and have blood-streaked stools, although they are otherwise healthy. Treatment involves switching to hypoallergenic formulas derived from cow's milk then gradually advancing to an unrestricted diet by 9 to 12 months of age.

Night terrors, typically occurring between 2 and 4 years of age during nonrapid eye movement sleep, usually begin with sudden and prolonged periods of inconsolable crying and end spontaneously, with the child rapidly returning to sleep. A nightmare occurs during rapid eye movement sleep, characterized by a frightening dream, which fully awakens the child, and return to sleep is delayed. Vivid recollection of the dream occurs, appropriate to the child's developmental and maturational stage. (See Chapter 71, Sleep Disturbances, Nonspecific.)

Neurologic disorders, such as brain tumors, migraine headaches, seizures, and postconcussion syndrome, are causes of chronic or recurrent irritability among older children and adolescents. Postconcussion syndrome is particularly distressing to families because the head injury may have occurred months or years before and may even have seemed minor, yet the irritability and behavior changes may be a persistent and major complaint.[36]

### *Chronic Persistent Irritability*

#### Psychosocial Disorders

Attention-deficit/hyperactivity disorder is the most commonly diagnosed biological-behavioral disorder of childhood, occurring in approximately 8% to 10% of school-aged children. The children may have coexisting externalizing disorders (conduct disorder and oppositional defiant disorder) and internalizing disorders (depression and anxiety disorders).[37] A common presentation in infants and young children may be irritability from frustration as a result of family and peer relationships, propensity to accidental injury, and difficulty with academic work.

Autism spectrum disorder usually first manifests itself in children younger than 3 years. Early symptoms include irritability, deficits in verbal and social interaction, repetitive behaviors, failure to participate within groups, and hours spent in solitary play.

Children with a chronic condition face stressors beyond their illness itself, such as altered physical development and appearance, high absenteeism, and inability of their peer groups to accept their disease.[38] The investigation and treatment of irritability in this context may require a multidisciplinary and long-term approach.

### Children With Cognitive Impairments

Children with severe intellectual disabilities are unable to verbalize what they are experiencing and are left to endure pain more often than healthy children. Although their caregivers are usually adept at reading their child's body language and behaviors to know when the child is in pain, the parent is not always able to identify the specific cause. These children are likely to experience pain from the same sources as unimpaired children (teething, sore throat, headache, minor trauma) but are also at risk for additional sources of pain and discomfort. Muscle spasms, gastroesophageal reflux, constipation, and urinary tract infections are frequent causes of irritability. In children with spastic quadriplegia, pathologic fractures often occur as a result of decreased bone density, limb rigidity, and joint contractures. Children with intellectual disabilities often require treatment for seizures, respiratory conditions, and constipation with drugs that have a high incidence of behavioral side effects (irritability, aggression, and hyperactivity).[39,40]

A wide variety of chronic disorders have irritability as a prominent or sole component. Hormonal effects associated with adolescence in both boys and girls can cause moodiness and irritability.[41,42]

## ▶ SUMMARY

Irritability has a variety of causes and can be indicative of life-threatening or relatively trivial or transient disorders, which is why it elicits a high degree of concern. In an ill-appearing infant or child the initial task is stabilization followed by a thorough search for a cause. In a well-appearing infant or child an organized approach is needed to determine the source of the irritability. A complete history and thorough physical examination can most often determine the cause. In puzzling cases, serial examinations and staged laboratory investigations may be necessary.

### *TOOLS FOR PRACTICE*

#### Engaging Patient and Family

- *Prevent Shaken Baby Syndrome* (handout), American Academy of Pediatrics (patiented.solutions.aap.org)
- *Returning to Learning Following a Concussion* (article), *Pediatrics*, Vol 132, Issue 5, 2013 (pediatrics.aappublications.org/content/132/5/948.full)

#### Medical Decision Support

- *Guidelines for Pediatric Concussion* (guideline), Ontario Neurotrauma Foundation (onf.org/documents/guidelines-for-pediatric-concussion)

### *AAP POLICY STATEMENTS*

Christian CW, Block R; American Academy of Pediatrics Committee on Child Abuse and Neglect. Abusive head trauma in infants and children. *Pediatrics*. 2009;123(5):1409–1411. Reaffirmed March 2013 (pediatrics.aappublications.org/content/123/5/1409)

American Academy of Pediatrics Section on Orthopaedics, Committee on Pediatric Emergency Medicine, Section on Critical Care, Section on Surgery, Section on Transport Medicine, Committee on Pediatric Emergency Medicine, and Pediatric Orthopedic Society of North America. Management of pediatric trauma. *Pediatrics.* 2008;121(4):849–854. Reaffirmed April 2013 (pediatrics.aappublications.org/content/121/4/849)

## REFERENCES


1. Greenes DS, Schutzman SA. Clinical indicators of intracranial injury in head injured children. *Pediatrics.* 1999;104:861–867
2. Faul M, Xu L, Wald MM, Coronaddo VG. *Traumatic Brain Injury in the United Stages: Emergency Department Visits, Hospitalizations, and Deaths 2002–2006.* Atlanta, GA: Centers for Disease Control and Prevention, National Center for Injury Prevention and Control; 2010
3. American Academy of Pediatrics Committee on Quality Improvement, American Academy of Family Physicians Commission on Clinical Policies and Research. The management of minor closed head injury in children. *Pediatrics.* 1999;104:1407–1415
4. Kuppermann N, Holmes JF, Dayan PS, et al. Identification of children at very low risk of clinically-important brain injuries after head trauma: a prospective cohort study. *Lancet.* 2009;374:1160–1170
5. Cantu RC. Second-impact syndrome. *Clin Sports Med.* 1998;17:37–44
6. Halstead ME, Walter KD; American Academy of Pediatrics Council on Sports Medicine and Fitness. Sport-related concussion in children and adolescents. *Pediatrics.* 2010;126:597–615
7. Zuckerman B, Stevenson J, Bailey V. Stomachaches and headaches in a community sample of preschool children. *Pediatrics.* 1987;79:667–682
8. Romanello S, Spiri D, Marcuzzi E, et al. Association between childhood migraine and history of infantile colic. *JAMA.* 2013;309:1607–1612
9. Riggio S. Nonconvulsive status epilepticus: clinical features and diagnostic challenges. *Psychiatr Clin North Am.* 2005;28:653–664
10. Nigrovic LE, Malley R, Kupperman N. Cerebrospinal fluid pleocytosis in children in the era of bacterial conjugate vaccines. *Pediatr Emer Care.* 2009;25:112–120
11. Pinnintis S, Kimberlin DW. Neonatal herpes simplex virus infections. *Pediatr Clin North Am.* 2013; 60:351–365
12. Greenhow TL, Hung Y-Y, Herz AM. Changing epidemiology of bacteremia in infants aged 1 week to 3 months. *Pediatrics* 2012;129:e590–e596
13. Paakkonen M, Peltola H. Bone and joint infections. *Pediatr Clin North Am.* 2013;60:425–436
14. Baker AL, Lu M, Minch L, et al. Associated symptoms in the ten days before diagnosis of Kawasaki disease. *J Pediatr.* 2009;154:592–595
15. Herman BE, Makoroff KL, Corneli HM. Abusive head trauma. *Pediatr Emer Care.* 2011;27:65–69
16. Mandeville K, Chien M, Willyerd FA, et al. Intussusception: clinical presentations and imaging characteristics. *Pediatr Emerg Care.* 2012;28:842–844
17. McCollough M, Sharieff GQ. Abdominal pain in children. *Pediatr Clin North Am.* 2006;53:107–137, vi
18. Yee WH, Soraisham AS, Shah VS, et al. Incidence and timing of presentation of necrotizing enterocolitis in preterm infants. *Pediatrics.* 2012;129:e298–e304
19. Freedman SB, Haladyn JK, Floh A, et al. Pediatric myocarditis: emergency department clinical findings and diagnostic evaluation. *Pediatrics.* 2007;120:1278–1285
20. May LJ, Patton DJ, Fruitman DS. The evolvoing approach to paediatric myocarditis: a review of the current literature. *Cardiol Young.* 2011;21:241–251
21. Tuo G, Marasini M, Brunelli C, et al. Incidence and clinical relevance of primary congential anomalies of the coronary arteries in children and adults. *Cardiol Young.* 2013;23:381–386
22. Hoffman JIE. Electrocardiogram of anomalous left coronary artery from the pulmonary artery in infants. *Pediatr Cardiol.* 2013;34:489–491
23. Salerno JC, Seslar SP. Supraventricular tachycardia. *Arch Pediatr Adolesc Med.* 2009;163:268–274
24. Guay J. Methemoglobinemia related to local anesthetics: a summary of 242 episodes. *Anesth Analg.* 2009;108:837–845

25. Claudius I, Fluharty C, Boles R. The emergency department approach to newborn and childhood metabolic crisis. *Emerg Med Clin North Am.* 2005;23:843–883, x
26. Losek JD. Hypoglycemia and the ABC'S (sugar) of pediatric resuscitation. *Ann Emerg Med.* 2000; 35:43–46
27. Kamboj M. Clinical approach to the diagnosis of inborn errors of metabolism. *Pediatr Clin North Am.* 2008;55:1113–1127
28. Levy M, Spino M. Neonatal withdrawal syndrome: associated drugs and pharmacologic management. *Pharmacotherapy.* 1993;3:202–211
29. Chasnoff IJ, Lewis DE, Squires L. Cocaine intoxication in a breast-fed infant. *Pediatrics.* 1987;80: 836–838
30. Wake M, Hesketh K, Lucas J. Teething and tooth eruption in infants: a cohort study. *Pediatrics.* 2000;106:1374–1379
31. American Academy of Pediatrics. *Red Book: 2010 Report of the Committee on Infectious Diseases.* Pickering LK, ed. 29th ed. Elk Grove Village, IL: American Academy of Pediatrics; 2012:553–566
32. Keefe MR, Froese-Fretz A. Living with an irritable infant: maternal perspectives. *Am J Child Nurs.* 1991;16:255–259
33. Currie ML, Rademacher R. The pediatrician's role in recognizing and intervening in postpartum depression. *Pediatr Clin North Am.* 2004;51:785–801, xi
34. Hyman PE, Milla PJ, Benninga MA, et al. Childhood functional gastrointestinal disorders: neonate/ toddler. *Gastroenterology.* 2006;130:1519–1526
35. Sampson HA. Food allergy. *J Allergy Clin Immunol.* 2003;111:540–547
36. Hou R, Moss-Morris R, Peveler R, et al. When a minor head injury results in enduring symptoms: a prospective investigation of risk factors for postconcussional syndrome after mild traumatic brain injury. *J Neurol Neurosurg Psychiatry.* 2012;83:217–223
37. American Academy of Pediatrics Subcommittee on Attention-Deficit/Hyperactivity Disorder, Steering Committee on Quality Improvement and Management. ADHD: clinical practice guideline for the diagnosis, evaluation, and treatment of attention-deficit/hyperactivity disorder in children and adolescents. *Pediatrics.* 2011;128:1007–1022
38. Goldson E. The behavioral aspects of chronic illness. In: Greydanus DE, Wolraich ML, eds. *Behavioral Pediatrics.* New York, NY: Springer-Verlag; 1992
39. Massaro M, Pastore S, Ventura A, Barbi E. Pain in cognitively impaired children: a focus for general pediatricians. *Eur J Pediatr.* 2013;172:9–14
40. Hauer J. Identifying and managing sources of pain and distress in children with neurological impairment. *Pediatr Ann.* 2010;39:198–205
41. Buchanan CM, Eccles JS, Becker JB. Are adolescents the victims of raging hormones: evidence for activational effects of hormones on moods and behavior at adolescence. *Psychol Bull.* 1992;111:62–107
42. Mortola JF. Issues in the diagnosis and research of premenstrual syndrome. *Clin Obstet Gynecol.* 1992;35:587–598

# Chapter 47

# Jaundice

*Debra H. Pan, MD; Yolanda Rivas, MD*

*Jaundice* is a yellowish discoloration of the skin, sclerae, and mucous membranes resulting from deposition of the bile pigment bilirubin. The presence of jaundice on clinical examination indicates *hyperbilirubinemia,* which is defined as a total serum bilirubin greater than 1.5 mg/dL. In general, jaundice becomes evident at serum bilirubin concentrations greater than 3 mg/dL in older children and greater than 5 mg/dL in newborns.[1]

Hyperbilirubinemia is typically characterized by the fraction of bilirubin that is increased, unconjugated (indirect), or conjugated (direct). Elevation of either of these fractions results in jaundice. Conjugated hyperbilirubinemia refers to a direct bilirubin greater than 2 mg/dL or greater than 20% of the total bilirubin concentration. The presence of conjugated hyperbilirubinemia suggests hepatobiliary tract conditions.

## ▶ BILIRUBIN METABOLISM

To identify the cause of jaundice, the pediatrician or other physician must be familiar with the normal metabolism of bilirubin, which is the end product of heme degradation.[2] Heme is produced from the breakdown of hemoglobin (70%–80%) and other hemoproteins (20%–30%). The conversion from heme to bilirubin follows a 2-step process that occurs mainly in the reticuloendothelial cells of the spleen, liver, and bone marrow. Heme is converted to biliverdin by the microsomal enzyme heme oxygenase and then to bilirubin by the cytosolic enzyme biliverdin reductase. This unconjugated bilirubin is a hydrophobic compound that is tightly bound to serum albumin and is transported to the liver for conjugation and clearance.

The metabolism of bilirubin follows 4 distinct steps: (1) The bilirubin is taken up across the sinusoidal (basolateral) membrane of the hepatocyte by a membrane receptor carrier. (2) Once inside the hepatocyte, the bilirubin binds to cytosolic glutathione S-transferase, historically known as ligandin.[3] It is then conjugated with glucuronic acid by the enzyme bilirubin UDP-glucuronosyl transferase (BUGT) in the endoplasmic reticulum to form bilirubin monoglucuronides and diglucuronides.[4] (3) Water-soluble bilirubin glucuronides are excreted into the bile through the apical canalicular membrane. This process is mediated by adenosine triphosphate–dependent transporters. Almost all the bilirubin in adult human bile is of the conjugated form, with bilirubin monoglucuronides accounting for 15% and diglucuronides accounting for 85%. In contrast, neonates have a higher concentration of bilirubin monoglucuronides in their bile because of a lower BUGT activity. The monoglucuronides are easily deconjugated and reabsorbed in the intestine. (4) The excreted bilirubin is further metabolized by bacterial flora to form urobilinoids, which are then eliminated in the feces, thus preventing the intestinal absorption of bilirubin.[5]

Bilirubin glucuronides can also be deconjugated by bacteria or tissue β-glucuronidase in the intestine and then reabsorbed in the terminal ileum, a process known as *enterohepatic circulation.*[6] Newborns are at high risk for bilirubin absorption from the intestine because of the high concentration of bilirubin monoglucuronides in their bile, the lack of intestinal bacterial flora to efficiently produce urobilinoids, and the high content of bilirubin and β-glucuronidase in meconium. Conditions that delay the passage of meconium can result in neonatal hyperbilirubinemia.

## ▶ SERUM BILIRUBIN

Serum bilirubin is conventionally measured by spectrophotometry based on the Van den Bergh (diazo) reaction.[7] Conjugated (direct) bilirubin reacts rapidly and unconjugated (indirect) bilirubin reacts slowly with diazo reagents. Indirect bilirubin is calculated as the difference between the total bilirubin and the direct bilirubin fraction. Although the terms *direct* and *conjugated* bilirubin are used interchangeably, direct bilirubin actually consists of 2 components: conjugated bilirubin and δ-bilirubin. In hepatobiliary obstruction, bilirubin glucuronides are not excreted properly from the hepatocyte into the bile. Under these circumstances, bilirubin glucuronides can reflux back into the systemic circulation and covalently bind to albumin. This conjugated bilirubin-albumin compound is known as δ-bilirubin.[8] Methods such as high-performance liquid chromatography can measure δ-bilirubin as well as α-, β-, and γ-bilirubin that corresponds to the unconjugated, monoconjugated, and diconjugated forms, respectively.[9] Because of the long half-life of albumin, δ-bilirubin accounts for the prolonged direct hyperbilirubinemia occasionally observed after restoration of normal bile flow.

## ▶ DIFFERENTIAL DIAGNOSIS

When discussing the differential diagnosis in a patient with jaundice, one should first categorize hyperbilirubinemia as either unconjugated or conjugated. It is helpful then to discuss each category separately in 2 different age groups: (1) newborns and young infants (infants <6 months), and (2) older infants (infants >6 months) and children. In general, unconjugated hyperbilirubinemia is common in neonates but relatively rare thereafter. Neonatal unconjugated hyperbilirubinemia is usually transient and benign, but marked increases of bilirubin can be toxic to the central nervous system. On the other hand, conjugated hyperbilirubinemia is always pathologic. When present in young infants, it is often related to primary hepatobiliary disorders, systemic or metabolic diseases, or genetic defects in bilirubin and bile acid metabolism or transport. In older children, viral hepatitis and drug- or toxin-induced liver damage are more prevalent.

## ▶ JAUNDICE IN NEWBORNS AND YOUNG INFANTS

A brief list of the causes of jaundice in newborns and young infants is presented in Box 47-1.

### *Unconjugated Hyperbilirubinemia*

The transition from intrauterine to extrauterine life is commonly associated with hyperbilirubinemia. Newborns have a total bilirubin level greater than the adults' normal limit of

BOX 47-1

## *Differential Diagnosis of Jaundice in Newborns and Young Infants*[a]

**UNCONJUGATED HYPERBILIRUBINEMIA**

***Increased production of bilirubin***

- Hemolysis (ABO-Rh incompatibility, erythrocyte defects, erythrocyte enzyme defects, disseminated intravascular coagulopathy)
- Polycythemia
- Cephalohematoma resorption

***Decreased hepatocellular uptake or conjugation***

- Prematurity
- Congenital hypothyroidism
- Physiologic jaundice of the newborn
- Breast milk jaundice
- Drug toxicity
- Gilbert syndrome, Crigler-Najjar syndrome

**CONJUGATED HYPERBILIRUBINEMIA**

***Liver diseases***

- Acute liver damage (ischemia, hypoxia, acidosis)
- Infection (sepsis, TORCH [toxoplasmosis, other agents, rubella, cytomegalovirus, herpes simplex])
- Viral or other hepatitis
- Parenteral nutrition associated liver disease
- Metabolic liver disease (galactosemia, neonatal hemochromatosis, $\alpha_1$-antitrypsin deficiency, tyrosinemia, mitochondrial defects)
- Hormones and drugs

***Obstruction of biliary system***

- Congenital anomalies (biliary atresia, choledochal cyst)

***Defects of bilirubin metabolism or transport***

- Progressive familial intrahepatic cholestasis
- Dubin-Johnson syndrome, Rotor syndrome

[a]Young infants defined as infants younger than 6 months.

1.5 mg/dL. More than half of newborns develop clinical jaundice in the first week of life, with most of them having unconjugated hyperbilirubinemia.

## Increased Production of Bilirubin

Nonphysiologic jaundice should always be considered part of the differential diagnosis in neonatal jaundice. When evaluating patients with jaundice, factors such as early onset, rapid progression, and persistence of jaundice beyond 2 weeks of life always suggest a pathologic cause. In most instances, pathologic unconjugated hyperbilirubinemia results from either excessive production or abnormal hepatic clearance of bilirubin.

Hemolysis is the most common cause of excessive bilirubin production in neonates and is usually observed within the first 24 hours of life. Hemolysis is often seen in association with maternal–fetal blood type incompatibility. ABO and Rh incompatibility are the 2 most common types leading to hemolytic disease of the newborn. ABO incompatibility occurs in approximately 15% of all pregnancies but results in hemolytic disease in only 3% of newborns, with less than 0.1% of infants needing exchange transfusion.[10] Hemolysis caused by ABO incompatibility is usually seen in newborns with blood type A or B born to blood type O mothers. Laboratory findings include a weakly positive direct Coombs test, high reticulocyte count, spherocytes on blood smear, and high levels of unconjugated bilirubin. Hemolytic disease in Rh incompatibility usually develops when an Rh-negative mother has become sensitized after exposure to Rh-positive fetal blood during a previous pregnancy. Rh incompatibility is less common and usually more severe than ABO incompatibility.[11] In the United States, the prevalence of the Rh-negative genotype is approximately 15% in whites, 5% in blacks, and less than 1% in Asians.[12] Rh incompatibility occurs in approximately 1.06 per 1,000 live births.[13] Affected infants usually develop jaundice in the first hours of life. Anemia and hepatosplenomegaly are common features. In severe cases, fetal hydrops from intrauterine hemolysis may be present at birth. Laboratory findings include a positive direct Coombs test, high reticulocyte count, anemia, and high unconjugated bilirubin levels. The prophylactic use of RhoGAM (anti-D gammaglobulin) in Rh-negative mothers has greatly decreased the incidence of this type of hemolytic disease of the newborn.[14]

Other causes of hemolysis leading to unconjugated hyperbilirubinemia in the neonate include hemoglobinopathies such as α-thalassemia, red blood cell enzyme defects, and neonatal polycythemia. α-Thalassemia should be suspected in newborns with jaundice and a moderate hypochromic, microcytic, hemolytic anemia.[15] Erythrocyte enzyme defects such as glucose-6-phosphate dehydrogenase (G6PD) or pyruvate kinase deficiency may cause hemolysis at any age. Neonatal polycythemia can cause an increase in bilirubin production as a result of an absolute increase in red blood cell mass. Unconjugated hyperbilirubinemia occurs in 2% to 22% of newborns with polycythemia.[16] Cephalohematomas also can lead to an increased bilirubin production from rapid breakdown of red blood cells in the extravascular space.

## Decreased Hepatocellular Uptake or Conjugation of Bilirubin

Drugs such as aspirin, cephalosporins, and sulfonamides can impair bilirubin transport by altering bilirubin–albumin binding.[17] Rifampin has been demonstrated to competitively inhibit hepatocellular uptake of bilirubin.[18] Unconjugated hyperbilirubinemia is associated with a decreased BUGT activity in conditions such as physiologic jaundice of the newborn and breast milk jaundice, and with a delayed maturation of BUGT in hypothyroidism.

Crigler-Najjar and Gilbert syndromes are 2 types of familial unconjugated hyperbilirubinemia caused by several mutations in the gene encoding for BUGT.[19] *Crigler-Najjar syndrome* is a rare familial form of unconjugated hyperbilirubinemia caused by mutations in the gene encoding BUGT1, leading to either absent (type 1) or decreased (type 2) BUGT activity. Crigler-Najjar syndrome type 1 is an autosomal recessive disease, which presents with severe nonhemolytic jaundice in the first hours of life. Crigler-Najjar syndrome type 2 is an autosomal dominant disease. Jaundice is usually less severe in type 2 and may improve with phenobarbital treatment. *Gilbert syndrome* is rarely diagnosed in this age group, and is further discussed in the Jaundice in Older Infants and Children section.

### Conjugated Hyperbilirubinemia

Conjugated hyperbilirubinemia, also known as *cholestatic jaundice,* is always pathologic. It can occur as a result of impaired bile formation by the hepatocyte or from obstruction to bile flow through the intrahepatic or extrahepatic biliary system. Conditions associated with conjugated hyperbilirubinemia include primary hepatobiliary disorders, genetic or metabolic diseases, systemic infections, and drug toxicity. *Neonatal cholestasis* refers to infants younger than 3 months who have cholestatic jaundice regardless of the cause. With the availability of new diagnostic techniques, the number of patients with an identified specific cause has increased.[20]

## Systemic Illnesses

Congenital TORCH (toxoplasmosis, other agents, rubella, cytomegalovirus, herpes simplex) infections have been associated with conjugated hyperbilirubinemia.[21] Infants with TORCH infections often have a low birth weight, hepatosplenomegaly, and cutaneous manifestations, as well as ophthalmologic and central nervous system involvement. Common laboratory findings include anemia, thrombocytopenia, increased transaminases, and cholestasis. Other infections, such as HIV and hepatitis B and C, may also be associated with conjugated hyperbilirubinemia in newborns or young infants. However, these infections have decreased with improved prenatal screening.

Patients with sepsis may develop jaundice and hepatocellular dysfunction.[22] The most frequent bacterial organisms associated with conjugated hyperbilirubinemia in neonates are *Escherichia coli, Streptococcus* group B, and *Listeria monocytogenes.* Conjugated hyperbilirubinemia may also develop in newborns and young infants with urinary tract infections.[23]

Critically ill patients, including young infants with no previous underlying liver disease, may develop jaundice with other signs of hepatic dysfunction, such as increased transaminases.[24] Conditions such as cardiopulmonary arrest, shock, and severe metabolic acidosis may cause an acute ischemic insult to the liver resulting in hepatocyte necrosis. Affected patients will have a marked increase in serum transaminase levels and direct hyperbilirubinemia developing within 24 to 48 hours after the insult. In most cases, the liver function will normalize once the initial insult is corrected; rarely, patients may develop acute liver failure.

Liver disease associated with parenteral nutrition (PN) is often seen in patients who receive PN for more than 2 weeks.[25] There is growing literature suggesting that soybean-based lipid emulsions are the major factor accounting for PN-associated liver disease. Recent data have demonstrated that using lipid emulsions based on fish oil can reverse or prevent PN cholestasis.[26] Similar results have been achieved by limiting the soybean-based lipid emulsions to 1 g/kg/day or less.[27]

## Metabolic Disorders

Metabolic liver diseases usually manifest during early infancy and should always be considered in the differential diagnosis in a newborn or young infant with cholestasis, especially when associated with hypoglycemia, hyperammonemia, or lactic acidosis.[28,29]

*Galactosemia* is an inborn error of galactose metabolism inherited as an autosomal recessive trait, with an estimated occurrence of 1 in 60,000. The classic transferase-deficiency galactosemia can affect multiple organs, including the liver, kidneys, brain, eyes, intestines, and gonads. The hepatocellular damage in galactosemia is caused by accumulation of toxic metabolites of galactose-1-phosphate and galactitol in the liver. The clinical presentation varies from mild liver disease to fulminant liver failure in the neonatal period. Patients often have vomiting, diarrhea, and poor feeding. They can also present with *E coli* sepsis. Jaundice can also be found in patients with other inborn errors of carbohydrate metabolism, such as hereditary fructose intolerance and certain types of glycogen storage diseases. In these conditions, the onset of symptoms rarely occurs during early infancy.

*Neonatal hemochromatosis* is a rare and severe liver disease in newborns. The typical pathologic finding is excessive iron deposition in extrahepatic sites. It has been recently hypothesized that this condition is caused by maternal alloimmunity directed at the fetal liver.[30] Infants with neonatal hemochromatosis usually experience intrauterine growth restriction and are born prematurely. In most cases, signs and symptoms of acute liver failure are present at birth or develop soon thereafter. The clinical presentation includes hypoglycemia, cholestatic jaundice, hypoalbuminemia, and profound coagulopathy. Transaminases can be slightly increased or even normal. Typical laboratory findings include increased ferritin and transferrin saturation and a relatively low transferrin level. Neonatal hemochromatosis should be strongly considered in all newborns with acute liver failure. Diagnosis can be aided by punch biopsy of the lip mucosa; the tissue sample is analyzed for iron deposition in the salivary glands. New treatment modalities include the use of intravenous immunoglobulin and exchange transfusions.[31]

*$\alpha_1$-Antitrypsin deficiency* is a relatively common genetic disorder, with the homozygous *PiZZ* genotype found in 1 in 1,600 to 2,000 live births. Only 10% of patients with $\alpha_1$-antitrypsin deficiency will develop signs and symptoms of liver disease.[32] This disorder typically manifests in the first few months of life with jaundice, although the onset of liver disease can occur later in life. Liver injury results from the hepatotoxic effect of retained mutant $\alpha_1$ *ATZZ* molecules in the endoplasmic reticulum of the hepatocyte.

*Tyrosinemia type 1,* also known as *hepatorenal tyrosinemia,* is a rare disorder that affects multiple organs, including the liver, kidneys, and peripheral nerves.[33] The deficiency of fumarylacetoacetate hydrolase, an enzyme involved in tyrosine degradation, results in tissue accumulation of tyrosine and other intermediate metabolites. Clinical findings range from severe liver disease or acute liver failure in early infancy to chronic liver disease in older children. The striking laboratory finding is a markedly increased $\alpha$-fetoprotein level. Patients with this condition may develop hepatocellular carcinoma early in life. The presence of succinylacetone in urine or blood is pathognomonic for tyrosinemia. Early diagnosis is important because specific medical therapy will improve quality of life and delay disease progression.

Primary mitochondrial hepatopathies are caused by a variety of defects, including mitochondrial DNA depletion, respiratory chain defects, fatty acid oxidation defects,[34,35] and mitochondrial membrane enzyme defects. In addition to having signs and symptoms of liver disease, affected patients have neuromuscular problems. Marked lactic acidosis is a relatively common feature. Symptoms usually develop within the first few months of life.

## Obstructive Jaundice

*Extrahepatic biliary atresia* (EHBA) is an idiopathic, destructive, inflammatory process of both the extrahepatic and intrahepatic bile ducts.[36,37] Affected infants typically develop jaundice and acholic stools at around 2 weeks of age; however, in early stages, the stools may still have bile pigment. Infants with cholestatic jaundice need prompt referral and evaluation for EHBA because the prognosis can be improved by early diagnosis and timely surgery. Abdominal sonography is a useful screening tool. The absence of gallbladder or the appearance of a *triangular cord sign* at the hilar region is suggestive of EHBA. However, the presence of a gallbladder on sonography does not exclude this condition. Abdominal sonography can also exclude other causes of cholestasis, such as choledochal cysts, gallstones, or biliary sludge. Liver biopsy is usually performed when evaluating patients with suspected EHBA, although the histologic findings are not always conclusive. The diagnosis is confirmed at the time of endoscopic retrograde cholangiopancreatography (ERCP) with cholangiogram or intraoperative cholangiogram.[38] Once the diagnosis is made, a hepatoportoenterostomy or Kasai procedure is then performed in an effort to reestablish bile flow.

*Choledochal cysts* are rare congenital anomalies of the biliary tract characterized by varying degrees of cystic dilation of the biliary tree. Choledochal cysts may be detected at any age; 18% of cases are diagnosed during the first year of life. The classic presentation of jaundice, abdominal pain, and right epigastric mass is rarely observed in infants and young children.[39]

*Alagille syndrome,* also known as *arteriohepatic dysplasia,* is inherited as an autosomal dominant condition with variable penetrance.[40] It is characterized by paucity of the intrahepatic bile ducts, peripheral pulmonary stenosis, butterfly vertebrae, posterior embryotoxon, and peculiar facies. Jaundice and pruritus are often present as the main clinical features during infancy. Mutations in the Jagged 1 (*JAG1*) gene are identified in most patients.[41] The diagnosis is confirmed by genetic testing.

### Isolated Bile Acid Metabolism Defects

Progressive familial intrahepatic cholestasis (PFIC) has been identified as a distinct group of conditions involving intrahepatic cholestasis from bile acid transport defects leading to impairment of bile excretion.[42] Three distinct gene mutations have been identified, accounting for the 3 major subtypes of this condition, including *PFIC1, PFIC2,* and *PFIC3.* Genetic testing is available to detect these mutations. Affected patients often develop jaundice in the first few months of life. In addition, they may also have severe pruritus, growth failure, fat-soluble vitamin deficiency, abnormal coagulation profile, and increased serum bile acids. The disease usually progresses to cirrhosis and liver failure early in life.

## ▶ JAUNDICE IN OLDER INFANTS AND CHILDREN

A brief list of the differential diagnosis of jaundice in older infants and children is presented in Box 47-2. In this age group, jaundice is an unusual sign and may suggest a serious clinical condition.

### *Unconjugated Hyperbilirubinemia*

Unconjugated hyperbilirubinemia is seen in older infants and children usually associated with underlying hemolytic diseases such as sickle cell anemia, G6PD deficiency, or hereditary spherocytosis. Mild unconjugated hyperbilirubinemia may also result from nonhemolytic conditions such as *Gilbert syndrome*, a benign disorder that affects 7% of the general population. It is inherited as an autosomal dominant trait, although an autosomal recessive pattern has been described.[43] An insertional mutation of the *UGT1A1* gene results in a reduced level of expression of the gene. Jaundice does not typically develop until after puberty and is usually seen during prolonged fasting or in association with acute viral illnesses. Patients usually have mild indirect hyperbilirubinemia with otherwise normal liver tests and no evidence of ongoing hemolysis.

BOX 47-2

## Differential Diagnosis of Jaundice in Older Infants[a] and Children

**UNCONJUGATED HYPERBILIRUBINEMIA**

- Hemolysis: erythrocyte defects, erythrocyte enzyme defect (glucose-6-phosphate dehydrogenase), disseminated intravascular coagulopathy
- Gilbert syndrome

**CONJUGATED HYPERBILIRUBINEMIA**

***Liver disease***

- Viral hepatitis (hepatitis A, B, C, E)
- Hepatitis caused by other viruses (herpes simplex virus, Epstein-Barr virus, cytomegalovirus)
- Toxins and drugs (ethanol, acetaminophen, isoniazid, phenytoin)
- Autoimmune hepatitis
- Metabolic liver disease ($\alpha_1$-antitrypsin deficiency, tyrosinemia, Wilson disease, mitochondrial defects)
- Nonalcoholic fatty liver disease
- Acute liver damage: ischemia, hypoxia, acidosis
- Parenteral nutrition–associated liver disease
- Pregnancy related (acute fatty liver of pregnancy, preeclampsia)
- Malignancy

***Obstruction of the biliary system***

- Choledochal cyst
- Cholelithiasis or choledocholithiasis
- Cholecystitis
- Diseases of the bile ducts (primary sclerosing cholangitis, AIDS cholangiopathy)

***Bilirubin metabolism or transport defects***

- Progressive familial intrahepatic cholestasis
- Dubin-Johnson syndrome, Rotor syndrome

[a]Older infants defined as infants older than 6 months.

## Conjugated Hyperbilirubinemia

### Liver Disease

Jaundice can develop as a result of acute or chronic viral hepatitis, autoimmune hepatitis, and drug- or toxin-induced hepatic injury. Metabolic liver diseases are much less common in older children, with the exception of Wilson disease. Infiltrative malignancies can also cause jaundice at any age. The incidence of acute viral hepatitis A has decreased in the United States with the use of vaccination. Children younger than 5 years with acute hepatitis A infection tend to be anicteric. The disease rarely causes fulminant liver failure. Hepatitis E infection has been increasingly recognized recently and has a clinical course similar to that of hepatitis A.[44] Hepatitis B or C infection is usually anicteric and chronic in children. Other viruses. such as Epstein-Barr virus, cytomegalovirus, adenovirus, and enterovirus, can also cause acute hepatitis, although jaundice is not always present.

*Autoimmune hepatitis* (AIH) is a progressive inflammatory condition of the liver of unknown etiology, which can progress to cirrhosis if not promptly diagnosed and treated.[45] AIH should always be considered in the differential diagnosis in a patient with increased transaminases. Jaundice is present in more than one-half of patients with AIH. Hyperglobulinemia is often evident, and autoantibodies such as antinuclear antibody, anti–smooth muscle antibody, and anti–liver-kidney microsomal antibody may be positive or negative. A positive liver–kidney microsomal antibody categorizes the disease as AIH type 2, which may have a more fulminant course and can present as acute liver failure.[46] AIH type 1 is more common, with onset likely before adolescence.

*Drug-induced liver injury* is initially suspected based on circumstantial evidence.[47] It can be classified into 3 types—(1) hepatic, (2) cholestatic, or (3) mixed hepatic-cholestatic—according to different clinical features. Cholestasis is more prominent when damage to bile duct epithelial cells occurs, resulting in an impaired bile flow. Cholestatic jaundice can be caused by many different drugs, including estrogen or oral contraceptive pills, erythromycin, cyclosporine, and haloperidol.[48] Acetaminophen overdose can cause acute hepatitis with zone 3 hepatocyte necrosis. Most cases of drug-induced liver damage spontaneously resolve once the drug responsible for the injury is withdrawn.

*Wilson disease* is an autosomal recessive disorder of human copper metabolism, with clinical onset usually after 5 years of age.[49] Mutations in the *ATP7B* gene lead to impaired biliary excretion of copper, which results in a progressive accumulation of copper in the liver and subsequently in other organs and tissues. Hemolytic anemia, Kayser-Fleischer rings in the eyes, and neuropsychiatric symptoms are classic features of the disease. Copper deposition in the liver can result in acute or chronic hepatitis, cirrhosis, or even fulminant liver failure with severe cholestatic jaundice.

### Biliary Obstruction

*Cholelithiasis* is the most common cause of biliary obstruction in children and is often associated with obesity, dyslipidemia, or an underlying hemolytic disease. Children usually present with vomiting and right upper quadrant abdominal pain, with or without jaundice.[50] Primary sclerosing cholangitis is characterized by stenosis, dilation, and fibrosis involving the intrahepatic or extrahepatic biliary tree, or both. It is the most common form of chronic liver disease in children with inflammatory bowel disease. Cholestatic jaundice is seen in less than one-half of affected patients.[51]

### Hepatic Bilirubin Transport Defects

Dubin-Johnson syndrome and Rotor syndrome are both inherited as autosomal recessive disorders. Dubin-Johnson syndrome is caused by mutations in the canalicular transporter gene, which result in an impaired secretion of conjugated bilirubin, whereas Rotor syndrome involves an impaired intracellular storage capacity of the liver for binding anions.[52,53] In both syndromes, conjugated hyperbilirubinemia is present without abnormalities in other liver tests. The striking characteristic in Dubin-Johnson syndrome is a brown to black discoloration of the liver, which results from pigment deposition in the lysosomes. The liver histology is otherwise normal in both syndromes.

## ▶ EVALUATION

### *History*

A detailed history is essential when evaluating a patient with jaundice because the information obtained may help to identify the cause. Special attention should be paid to the presence of signs and symptoms, such as a viral prodrome, abdominal pain or distention, acholic stools, dark urine, or pruritus. In neonates, the prenatal and birth history may help identify potential risk factors. In older children, the patient's age at the time of onset of jaundice, associated signs and symptoms, and exposure to hepatotoxic agents are of paramount importance. A detailed family history should include information about the presence of persistent jaundice, chronic liver diseases, hemolysis, and metabolic diseases. Distinguishing among acute and chronic liver diseases, intrahepatic processes and extrahepatic biliary tract obstruction, or primary liver diseases and systemic diseases is the major goal at the time of the initial evaluation. This approach may guide the physician in selecting appropriate laboratory tests and imaging studies that can lead to a definitive diagnosis.

## Physical Examination

In general, patients with jaundice from unconjugated hyperbilirubinemia have bright-yellow skin, whereas patients with jaundice from conjugated hyperbilirubinemia have dark green–yellow skin. Patients should undergo a complete physical examination with special focus on general appearance, growth, and development; signs of cardiovascular dysfunction; neurologic signs; and organomegaly. The size and the character of the liver should be carefully determined. The newborn or infant liver is a large organ relative to body size. In newborns, the mean liver span is 5.9 cm along the midclavicular line, calculated by measuring the distance between the percussed upper and palpated lower liver edges.[54] The healthy infant's liver may be palpable and is typically less than 2 cm below the right costal margin.[55] The consistency and character of the liver edge may help determine the nature of underlying liver disease. An enlarged liver resulting from an acute intrahepatic process is usually tender but soft. A cirrhotic liver may have a hard and irregular edge; however, its edge is not always palpable.

A thorough abdominal examination should be performed to identify the presence of an enlarged spleen or any other abdominal masses, areas of tenderness, and ascites, as well as the abdominal cutaneous venous pattern. The tip of the spleen can normally be palpated below the left costal margin in newborns and infants. Splenomegaly in a patient with underlying liver disease implies portal hypertension, especially in the presence of ascites and a prominent abdominal cutaneous venous pattern. Other physical findings may indicate a particular cause, such as xanthomas in primary biliary cirrhosis, Kayser-Fleischer rings in Wilson disease, and characteristic facial features and posterior embryotoxon in Alagille syndrome.

## Laboratory Tests

Initial laboratory studies include a complete blood cell count (CBC), liver tests, and a coagulation profile. Isolated hyperbilirubinemia with otherwise normal liver tests suggests the possibility of hemolytic disease or bilirubin metabolism defects. A CBC is useful in detecting hemolysis, indicated by the presence of anemia with fragmented red blood cells (schistocytes) and increased reticulocytes on the smear. Thrombocytopenia is typically seen in patients with portal hypertension and hypersplenism.

Aspartate aminotransferase (AST) and alanine aminotransferase (ALT) levels are the most frequently used markers of hepatocellular injury.[56] ALT is a more specific indicator of hepatocyte injury because AST also increases with hemolysis and myocardial or skeletal muscle injury. In general, a marked increase in AST and ALT occurs in severe viral hepatitis, acute toxin- or drug-induced hepatic necrosis, or ischemia.[57] A mild increase of AST and ALT is seen in nonalcoholic fatty liver disease, chronic viral hepatitis, and drug toxicity. Declining AST and ALT levels usually indicate hepatocyte recovery. However, in the course of fulminant liver failure, if seen in association with a worsening liver synthetic function, falling AST and ALT levels may be an ominous sign of massive hepatic necrosis, with few viable hepatocytes remaining to further release these enzymes.[58] AST and ALT levels are less useful in patients with chronic end-stage liver disease because they can be normal or only slightly increased in the presence of marked fibrosis of the liver.

Alkaline phosphatase and γ-glutamyltransferase (GGT) are useful markers for intrahepatic and extrahepatic cholestasis. In most hepatobiliary diseases, both alkaline phosphatase and GGT are increased. However, in progressive familiar intrahepatic cholestasis (types 1 and 2), a normal or low GGT is observed in the presence of a high alkaline phosphatase. Isolated increase of alkaline phosphatase may be seen in patients with nonhepatobiliary diseases such as bone disorders.[59] Normal GGT values in newborns may be 5 to 8 times greater than those in adults.[60]

Prothrombin time (PT) and albumin are used to evaluate hepatic synthetic function. An abnormal PT results from an impaired hepatic synthesis of coagulation factors I, II, V, VII, and X or deficiency of vitamin K (or both). Parenteral administration of vitamin K generally normalizes a prolonged PT in patients with vitamin K deficiency associated with cholestatic jaundice, but not in patients with hepatocellular disease. In acute liver injury, a markedly increased PT suggests the possibility of fulminant liver failure. Hypoalbuminemia may be seen in patients with acute and chronic liver diseases. In the early stages of acute liver injury, the serum albumin may not be a reliable indicator of hepatic synthetic function because it has a long half-life of approximately 21 days.

Based on the clinical information obtained and results of the initial laboratory tests, further evaluation including imaging studies may be warranted, including blood and urine cultures, viral serologic studies, toxin and drug screen, autoimmune markers, $\alpha_1$-antitrypsin phenotype, ceruloplasmin, urine succinyl acetone, and serum bile acids. In newborns or young infants with jaundice and abnormal liver tests, TORCH titers should also be obtained.

## Imaging Studies

Ultrasonography is the most useful initial imaging modality in the assessment of the intrahepatic and extrahepatic biliary system in patients with jaundice.[61] This noninvasive study may help identify abnormalities such as biliary atresia, choledochal cyst, hepatic cystic lesions, and cholelithiasis. Computed tomographic scans may be preferred when general anatomic information of the hepatobiliary system is desired or a noncystic hepatic lesion is suspected. Nuclear scintigraphy is a useful study when considering the diagnosis of acute cholecystitis or chronic acalculous cholecystitis.[62] Magnetic resonance cholangiopancreatography (MRCP) is a noninvasive study that identifies abnormalities of the intrahepatic and extrahepatic biliary system. ERCP provides similar information to that of the MRCP, but it allows the possibility of therapeutic interventions such as sphincterotomy, biliary stone extraction, or stent placement.[63]

Liver biopsy provides information on the histology and architecture of the liver and has become an invaluable diagnostic tool in the evaluation of patients with liver disease; it is also helpful in assessing disease progression. Liver biopsy is most commonly performed in patients with persistently abnormal liver tests, especially when conventional laboratory and imaging studies do not lead to a specific diagnosis. The use of liver biopsy in the diagnosis of acute liver injury is limited because of the nonspecific histologic changes commonly found.

## ▶ MANAGEMENT

The treatment of newborns with unconjugated hyperbilirubinemia is based on the revised guideline published by the American Academy of Pediatrics.[64] This guideline provides a framework for detecting neonatal hyperbilirubinemia and preventing kernicterus in term and near-term newborn infants. It also emphasizes the importance of a systematic assessment of the risks of severe hyperbilirubinemia, close follow-up, and prompt intervention when necessary.

The management of patients with direct hyperbilirubinemia should focus on correcting the underlying cause, optimizing nutrition, and controlling pruritus. Malabsorption of fat and fat-soluble vitamins is commonly seen in patients with cholestasis because they have an impaired bile secretion. Unlike long-chain triglycerides, which require bile acid micelles for solubilization, medium-chain triglycerides (MCTs) are relatively water soluble and directly absorbed into the portal system. Therefore, a diet high in MCTs should be used to promote growth in children with chronic cholestasis. Formulas with a relatively high MCT concentration are often used in patients with cholestasis. Supplementation of fat-soluble vitamins A, D, E, and K is essential. Serum vitamin levels should be routinely followed to monitor adequate supplementation.

In the attempt to control cholestasis-associated pruritus, several different therapeutic agents have been used with very little success. Ursodeoxycholic acid has been shown to lower serum bile acid levels by increasing bile flow.[65] Other agents, such as cholestyramine, a bile acid–binding resin, and rifampin, an antibiotic used in the treatment of tuberculosis, have also been used.[66,67]

Liver transplantation in children is now an accepted therapy for many life-threatening liver diseases.[68] Current survival rates for children after liver transplantation are 90% at 1 year and 85% at 3 years.[69] EHBA is the most common indication for liver transplantation in children; other indications include $\alpha_1$-antitrypsin deficiency, fulminant liver failure, chronic hepatitis, metabolic liver disease, and cirrhosis of unknown origin. Early referral and transfer to a liver transplantation center are important to assure a good outcome.

### When to Refer

- Unexplained jaundice
- Direct hyperbilirubinemia at any age
- Persistence of abnormal liver tests
- Hepatomegaly or splenomegaly

### When to Admit

- Jaundice in an ill patient
- Feeding intolerance and dehydration
- Inpatient management of underlying conditions
- Impending acute liver failure

## TOOLS FOR PRACTICE

### Engaging Patient and Family

- *Jaundice* (fact sheet), American Academy of Pediatrics (healthychildren.org/English/ages-stages/baby/Pages/Jaundice.aspx)
- *Jaundice and Your Newborn* (handout), American Academy of Pediatrics (patiented.solutions.aap.org)

### Medical Decision Support

- *BilliTool* (interactive tool), Tony Burgos, MD, et al (bilitool.org)
- *Jaundice/Kernicterus* (Web page), Centers for Disease Control and Prevention (www.cdc.gov/ncbddd/jaundice/index.html)

## AAP POLICY STATEMENTS

Bhutani VK; American Academy of Pediatrics Committee on Fetus and Newborn. Phototherapy to prevent severe neonatal hyperbilirubinemia in the newborn infant 35 weeks or more of gestation. *Pediatrics.* 2011;128(4):e1046–e1052 (pediatrics.aappublications.org/content/128/4/e1046.full)

North American Society for Pediatric, Gastroenterology, Hepatology, and Nutrition. Guideline for the evaluation of cholestatic jaundice in infants: recommendations of the North American Society for Pediatric Gastroenterology, Hepatology, and Nutrition. *J Pediatr Gastroenterol Nutr.* 2004;39:115–128 (AAP endorsed)

## REFERENCES


1. Reiser DJ. Neonatal jaundice: physiologic variation or pathologic process. *Crit Care Nurs Clin North Am.* 2004;16(2):257–269
2. Ostrow JD, Jandl JH, Schmid R. The formation of bilirubin from hemoglobin in vivo. *J Clin Invest.* 1962;41:1628–1637
3. Wolkoff AW, Goresky CA, Sellin J, Gatmaitan Z, Arias IM. Role of ligandin in transfer of bilirubin from plasma into liver. *Am J Physiol.* 1979;236:E638–E648
4. Dutton G. *The Biosynthesis of Glucuronides.* London, UK: Academic Press; 1966
5. Vítek L, Carey MC. Enterohepatic cycling of bilirubin as a cause of 'black' pigment gallstones in adult life. *Eur J Clin Invest.* 2003;33:799–810
6. Poland RL, Odell GB. Physiologic jaundice: the enterohepatic circulation of bilirubin. *N Engl J Med.* 1971;284:1–6
7. Van Den Bergh HAA. Uber ein direkte und indirekte diazoreaktion auf bilirubin. *Biochem Zeitshrift.* 1916;77
8. Brett EM, Hicks JM, Powers DM, Rand RN. Delta bilirubin in serum of pediatric patients: correlations with age and disease. *Clin Chem.* 1984;30:1561–1564
9. Weiss JS, Gautam A, Lauff JJ, et al. The clinical importance of a protein-bound fraction of serum bilirubin in patients with hyperbilirubinemia. *N Engl J Med.* 1983;309:147–150
10. Zipursky A. Isoimmune hemolytic disease. In: Nathan DG, Oski FA, eds. *Hematology of Infancy and Childhood.* 4th ed. Philadelphia, PA: WB Saunders; 1994
11. Blanchette VS, Zipursky A. Assessment of anemia in newborn infants. *Clin Perinatol.* 1984;11:489–510
12. Prokop UG. Rhesus blood groups. In: Prokop O, Uhlenbruck G, eds. *Human Blood and Serum Groups.* New York, NY: Wiley Interscience; 1969
13. Chávez GF, Mulinare J, Edmonds LD. Epidemiology of Rh hemolytic disease of the newborn in the United States. *JAMA.* 1991;265:3270–3274
14. Mayne S, Parker JH, Harden TA, Dodds SD, Beale JA. Rate of RhD sensitisation before and after implementation of a community based antenatal prophylaxis programme. *BMJ.* 1997;315:1588
15. Luchtman-Jones L, Wilson DB. Disorders of the fetus and infant. In: Fanaroff AA, Martin RJ, eds. *Neonatal-Perinatal Medicine: Disorders of the Fetus and Infant.* 7th ed. St Louis, MO: Mosby; 2002

16. Wiswell TE, Cornish JD, Northam RS. Neonatal polycythemia: frequency of clinical manifestations and other associated findings. *Pediatrics.* 1986;78:26–30
17. Brodersen R, Robertson A. Ceftriaxone binding to human serum albumin: competition with bilirubin. *Mol Pharmacol.* 1989;36:478–483
18. Zilly W, Breimer DD, Richter E. Pharmacokinetic interactions with rifampicin. *Clin Pharmacokinet.* 1977;2:61–70
19. Kadakol A, Ghosh SS, Sappal BS, et al. Genetic lesions of bilirubin uridine-diphosphoglucuronate glucuronosyltransferase (UGT1A1) causing Crigler-Najjar and Gilbert syndromes: correlation of genotype to phenotype. *Hum Mutat.* 2000;16:297–306
20. Balistreri WF, Bezerra JA. Whatever happened to "neonatal hepatitis"? *Clin Liver Dis.* 2006;10:27–53
21. Jorio Benkhraba M, El Harim Roudies L, El Malki Tazi A. [Infectious jaundice of the newborn infant]. *Maroc Med.* 1983;5:150–156
22. Kluska V, Kania V, Váchalová V. [Jaundice, sepsis, and pyuria in the newborn and in small infants]. *Cesk Pediatr.* 1968;23:678–684
23. Seeler RA, Hahn K. Jaundice in urinary tract infection in infancy. *Am J Dis Child.* 1969;118:553–558
24. Askin DF, Diehl-Jones WL. The neonatal liver: part III: pathophysiology of liver dysfunction. *Neonatal Netw.* 2003;22:5–15
25. Bell RL, Ferry GD, Smith EO, et al. Total parenteral nutrition-related cholestasis in infants. *JPEN J Parenter Enteral Nutr.* 1986;10:356–359
26. Goulet O, Joly F, Corriol O, Colomb-Jung V. Some new insights in intestinal failure-associated liver disease. *Curr Opin Organ Transplant.* 2009;14:256–261
27. Cowles RA, Ventura KA, Martinez M, et al. Reversal of intestinal failure-associated liver disease in infants and children on parenteral nutrition: experience with 93 patients at a referral center for intestinal rehabilitation. *J Pediatr Surg.* 2010;45:84–87
28. Saudubray JM, Nassogne MC, de Lonlay P, Touati G. Clinical approach to inherited metabolic disorders in neonates: an overview. *Semin Neonatol.* 2002;7:3–15
29. Moyer V, Freese DK, Whitington PF, et al. Guideline for the evaluation of cholestatic jaundice in infants: recommendations of the North American Society for Pediatric Gastroenterology, Hepatology and Nutrition. *J Pediatr Gastroenterol Nutr.* 2004;39:115–128
30. Knisely AS, Mieli-Vergani G, Whitington PF. Neonatal hemochromatosis. *Gastroenterol Clin North Am.* 2003;32:877–889
31. Rand EB, Karpen SJ, Kelly S, et al. Treatment of neonatal hemochromatosis with exchange transfusion and intravenous immunoglobulin. *J Pediatr.* 2009;155(4):566–571
32. Perlmutter DH. Alpha-1-antitrypsin deficiency: diagnosis and treatment. *Clin Liver Dis.* 2004;8:839–859
33. Russo PA, Mitchell GA, Tanguay RM. Tyrosinemia: a review. *Pediatr Dev Pathol.* 2001;4:212–221
34. Bioulac-Sage P, Parrot-Roulaud F, Mazat JP, et al. Fatal neonatal liver failure and mitochondrial cytopathy (oxidative phosphorylation deficiency): a light and electron microscopic study of the liver. *Hepatology.* 1993;18:839–846
35. Brivet M, Boutron A, Slama A, et al. Defects in activation and transport of fatty acids. *J Inherit Metab Dis.* 1999;22:428–441
36. Davenport M. Biliary atresia. *Semin Pediatr Surg.* 2005;14:42–48
37. Kobayashi H, Stringer MD. Biliary atresia. *Semin Neonatol.* 2003;8:383–391
38. Ohnuma N, Takahashi T, Tanabe M, Yoshida H, Iwai J. The role of ERCP in biliary atresia. *Gastrointest Endosc.* 1997;45:365–370
39. Miyano T, Yamataka A. Choledochal cysts. *Curr Opin Pediatr.* 1997;9:283–288
40. Alagille D, Estrada A, Hadchouel M, et al. Syndromic paucity of interlobular bile ducts (Alagille syndrome or arteriohepatic dysplasia): review of 80 cases. *J Pediatr.* 1987;110:195–200
41. Oda T, Elkahloun AG, Pike BL, et al. Mutations in the human Jagged1 gene are responsible for Alagille syndrome. *Nat Genet.* 1997;16:235–242
42. Pratt DS. Cholestasis and cholestatic syndromes. *Curr Opin Gastroenterol.* 2005;21(3):270–274
43. Bosma P, Chowdhury JR, Jansen PH. Genetic inheritance of Gilbert's syndrome. *Lancet.* 1995;346:314–315

44. Dalton HR, Bendall R, Ijaz S, Banks M. Hepatitis E: an emerging infection in developed countries. *Lancet Infect Dis*. 2008;8:698–709
45. Oettinger R, Brunnberg A, Gerner P, et al. Clinical features and biochemical data of Caucasian children at diagnosis of autoimmune hepatitis. *J Autoimmun*. 2005;24:79–84
46. Squires RH. Autoimmune hepatitis in children. *Curr Gastroenterol Rep*. 2004;6:225–230
47. Maddrey WC. Drug-induced hepatotoxicity: 2005. *J Clin Gastroenterol*. 2005;39:S83–S89
48. Plaa GL, Priestly BG. Intrahepatic cholestasis induced by drugs and chemicals. *Pharmacol Rev*. 1976;28:207–273
49. Kitzberger R, Madl C, Ferenci P. Wilson disease. *Metab Brain Dis*. 2005;20:295–302
50. Friesen CA, Roberts CC. Cholelithiasis. Clinical characteristics in children. Case analysis and literature review. *Clin Pediatr (Phila)*. 1989;28:294–298
51. Wilschanski M, Chait P, Wade JA, et al. Primary sclerosing cholangitis in 32 children: clinical, laboratory, and radiographic features, with survival analysis. *Hepatology*. 1995;22:1415–1422
52. Paulusma CC, Kool M, Bosma PJ, et al. A mutation in the human canalicular multispecific organic anion transporter gene causes the Dubin-Johnson syndrome. *Hepatology*. 1997;25:1539–1542
53. Zimniak P. Dubin-Johnson and Rotor syndromes: molecular basis and pathogenesis. *Semin Liver Dis*. 1993;13:248–260
54. Reiff MI, Osborn LM. Clinical estimation of liver size in newborn infants. *Pediatrics*. 1983;71:46–48
55. Walker WA, Mathis RK. Hepatomegaly. An approach to differential diagnosis. *Pediatr Clin North Am*. 1975;22:929–942
56. Ellis G, Goldberg DM, Spooner RJ, Ward AM. Serum enzyme tests in diseases of the liver and biliary tree. *Am J Clin Pathol*. 1978;70:248–258
57. De Ritis F, Coltorti M, Giusti G. Serum-transaminase activities in liver disease. *Lancet*. 1972;1:685–687
58. Chopra S, Griffin PH. Laboratory tests and diagnostic procedures in evaluation of liver disease. *Am J Med*. 1985;79:221–230
59. Knight JA, Haymond RE. gamma-Glutamyltransferase and alkaline phosphatase activities compared in serum of normal children and children with liver disease. *Clin Chem*. 1981;27:48–51
60. Priolisi A, Didato M, Fazio M, Gioeli RA. [Changes of serum gamma-glutamyltranspeptidase activity in full-term and pre-term newborn infants during the first 2 weeks of life]. *Minerva Pediatr*. 1980;32:291–296
61. Lai MW, Chang MH, Hsu SC, et al. Differential diagnosis of extrahepatic biliary atresia from neonatal hepatitis: a prospective study. *J Pediatr Gastroenterol Nutr*. 1994;18:121–127
62. Ziessman HA. Scintigraphy in the gastrointestinal tract. *Curr Opin Radiol*. 1992;4:105–116
63. Fox VL, Werlin SL, Heyman MB. Endoscopic retrograde cholangiopancreatography in children. Subcommittee on Endoscopy and Procedures of the Patient Care Committee of the North American Society for Pediatric Gastroenterology and Nutrition. *J Pediatr Gastroenterol Nutr*. 2000;30:335–342
64. American Academy of Pediatrics Subcommittee on Hyperbilirubinemia. Management of hyperbilirubinemia in the newborn infant 35 or more weeks of gestation. *Pediatrics*. 2004;114:297–316
65. Alagille D. Management of chronic cholestasis in childhood. *Semin Liver Dis*. 1985;5:254–262
66. Datta DV, Sherlock S. Cholestyramine for long term relief of the pruritus complicating intrahepatic cholestasis. *Gastroenterology*. 1966;50:323–332
67. Cynamon HA, Andres JM, Iafrate RP. Rifampin relieves pruritus in children with cholestatic liver disease. *Gastroenterology*. 1990;98:1013–1016
68. Tiao G, Ryckman FC. Pediatric liver transplantation. *Clin Liver Dis*. 2006;10:169–197
69. Martin SR, Atkison P, Anand R, Lindblad AS; SPLIT Research Group. Studies of pediatric liver transplantation 2002: patient and graft survival and rejection in pediatric recipients of a first liver transplant in the United States and Canada. *Pediatr Transplant*. 2004;8:273–283

# Chapter 48

# Joint Pain

*David M. Siegel, MD, MPH; Bethany Marston, MD*

Pediatricians are often faced with clinical situations involving musculoskeletal aches and pains, and within this group of symptoms lies the subset of joint pain. In fact, 1 of every 6 to 10 pediatric outpatient visits includes a musculoskeletal complaint.[1] Discomfort in a joint can result from a wide variety of causes, and the possibilities must be considered to allow appropriate evaluation and management. A systematic approach to patients who experience pain or swelling in 1 or more joints helps physicians arrive at an accurate diagnosis and course of therapy.

## ▶ DEFINITIONS

Joint pain, or arthralgia, is the subjective experience of pain referable to a bony articulation. In a young child, this might be inferred from the patient's refusal to move an extremity. The term *arthralgia* should only be used if the discomfort originates in the joint itself; it is important to distinguish arthralgia from myalgia, or muscle pain, and from other types of pain that may involve the limbs but not the joints. The term *arthritis* should be used only when there is evidence of inflammation in the joint; findings of swelling, tenderness, warmth, or erythema should be demonstrable, along with pain with motion. In the joint, inflammation is also accompanied by stiffness or loss of motion. *Arthropathy* is a term that can be used to describe any disease of a joint, regardless of its cause.

## ▶ ETIOLOGY

Inflammatory causes of musculoskeletal pain are typically subacute or chronic, and are characterized by swelling, loss of motion, and a subjective sense of stiffness that is often prolonged after periods of inactivity. A relatively rapid onset of joint symptoms in the setting of fever, rash, lymphadenopathy, or other systemic complaints should raise concern for an infectious process or a systemic inflammatory disease. Traumatic causes of musculoskeletal pain can typically be identified by the sudden onset of symptoms following a fall, a blow, or other injury. Repetitive stress injuries, hypermobility arthralgias, and other mechanical noninflammatory syndromes can be subacute or chronic in onset, but are characterized by exacerbation of pain and stiffness after activity or at the end of a vigorous day, rather than upon awakening or after periods of inactivity.

## ▶ DIFFERENTIAL DIAGNOSIS

The differential diagnosis of joint pain should begin by determining whether the disease is inflammatory or noninflammatory. Inflammatory joint disease can result from rheumatic or nonrheumatic causes. Noninflammatory diseases may result from trauma, repetitive stress, congenital or developmental anomalies, or other mechanical causes.

### Rheumatic Diseases

The most common rheumatic disease of childhood is juvenile idiopathic arthritis (JIA), previously referred to as *juvenile rheumatoid arthritis*, which occurs in up to 1 in 1,000 children worldwide.[2] Onset can be from the second year of life through late adolescence. The oligoarticular subtype is characterized by involvement of 4 or fewer joints, typically large joints with asymmetric distribution. This subtype has a good long-term prognosis, but can cause growth abnormalities, and especially in patients with a positive antinuclear antibody it carries an increased risk of eye involvement with iridocyclitis. When more than 4 joints are involved, JIA is subtyped as polyarticular, and this form is more likely to involve small as well as larger joints. A subset of patients with polyarticular JIA have serum IgM rheumatoid factor and typically more symmetric joint disease. Systemic onset juvenile arthritis (sometimes called *Still disease*)[3] is marked by high, spiking fevers; an evanescent, salmon-pink, maculopapular rash; lymph node, spleen, and liver enlargement; anemia; leukocytosis; and other laboratory evidence of pronounced inflammation. Arthritis may not be present at the onset of systemic findings, but should be present for 6 weeks or longer to establish the diagnosis of any form of JIA.[4] Evaluation and management of JIA depends on the subtype present.

Juvenile forms of ankylosing spondylitis or spondyloarthropathy can start with involvement in the large joints of the lower extremities or in the entheses (insertion of a tendon or ligament into a bone); at onset, there may be no axial disease. Small joint involvement is often asymmetric when present, and dactylitis (sausage digits) can occur if several joints and intervening soft tissues in a single finger or toe are swollen. The classic presentation of ankylosing spondylitis includes sacroiliac involvement in late adolescence, and further axial disease can progress in adulthood. Severe disease leads to the radiographic finding of *bamboo spine*, which is caused by diffuse paravertebral fusions resulting in very limited back and neck movement. The human leukocyte antigen (HLA)-B27 is seen in about 90% of patients with ankylosing spondylitis.[5] Spondylarthropathies are more common in boys than girls, unlike many other forms of juvenile arthritis. A similar pattern of asymmetric large joint and sacroiliac disease can be seen in patients with inflammatory bowel disease. Children with psoriasis, or with a first degree relative with psoriasis, may also have a similar presentation, with a predisposition for large joints, sacroiliac disease, and occasionally dactylitis.

Several other systemic inflammatory diseases may cause or be associated with arthritis. Systemic lupus erythematosus, more common in girls than boys and infrequently seen before adolescence, is a multisystem disease that can involve almost any organ in the body. Arthralgias and sometimes arthritis are not uncommon, and may be the presenting symptom. Juvenile dermatomyositis is characterized more by skin rashes and muscle inflammation and weakness than joint disease, but can also be accompanied by joint pain or swelling in some cases. Sjögren syndrome, scleroderma, and mixed connective tissue disease are other connective tissue diseases occasionally seen in children that can cause joint symptoms. Systemic autoinflammatory syndromes, often referred to as *periodic fever syndromes*, including familial Mediterranean fever, tumor necrosis factor receptor-associated periodic syndrome, hyperimmunoglobulin D syndrome, and cryopyrinopathies, are genetic diseases that may be associated with arthritis in addition to recurrent fevers. Kawasaki disease and Henoch-Schönlein purpura, along with other types of vasculitis, are also systemic inflammatory diseases that can cause arthritis. Many other inflammatory conditions cause arthritis in adults, including sarcoidosis and crystalline arthritis, but these are quite rare in children.

## Infectious and Postinfectious Arthritis

Acute bacterial infection of the joint, or *septic arthritis*, is foremost among this group and represents a medical emergency. The usual manifestation is the rapid onset of pain in a joint, typically accompanied by fever. The joint itself is red, warm, swollen, and exquisitely tender to palpation or with movement. This clinical situation demands immediate arthrocentesis for diagnosis and therapy. Analysis of the fluid for appearance (opaque), viscosity (usually low), mucin clot (friable), cell count (>100,000 white blood cells/$mm^3$ with at least 80% polymorphonuclear cells), glucose (usually low, much less than serum), and protein (high) helps establish the diagnosis. Most important, a portion of the fluid must be Gram stained to assess for bacterial organisms. Cultures can direct definitive antimicrobial therapy. In the past, for a child younger than 4 years, *Haemophilus influenzae* was the most commonly responsible organism; but with the institution of regular immunization, these bacteria are no longer a major consideration in septic arthritis. *Staphylococcus aureus* and *Streptococcus* species now are more likely to be the causative organisms.[6] In addition to joint fluid cultures, blood cultures may also yield growth of the organism, occasionally in the absence of a positive joint fluid culture.

*Osteomyelitis* is an acute infection of the bone. However, when one of the long bones next to a joint (eg, the distal femur and knee) is infected, the patient may describe pain in the joint, and a sterile effusion may even be present.[7] Although unusual, the bacterial infection can directly invade the adjacent joint space from the bone, particularly in young children.

Systemic bacterial infections, notably those caused by *Neisseria meningitidis* and *Neisseria gonorrhoeae*, also can produce arthritis, although the organism is usually not isolated from the joint in these cases. After joint aspiration and establishment of at least a strong suspicion of a purulent arthritis, the child should be hospitalized and appropriate intravenous antibiotic therapy initiated. Prompt, aggressive therapy usually brings about recovery without adverse side effects, although some foci, such as the hip joint, can remain persistent problems. Because of the tenuous blood supply to the femoral capital epiphysis, purulent arthritis of the hip can lead to chronic problems despite timely intervention.

Diskitis, a disorder characterized by back pain and tenderness over the spinous process contiguous to the involved disk space, causes joint pain, sometimes with low-grade fever, but often with none. *Staphylococcus aureus* has been isolated from the blood and disk space in some instances, but often no culture-proven cause can be found. The presentation can involve sensory and motor complications resulting from nerve root impingement, and an epidural abscess must be considered in the differential diagnosis.

*Borrelia burgdorferi* is a tick-borne spirochete responsible for Lyme disease.[8] The syndrome, which was first described in Old Lyme, Connecticut,[9] is characterized by an initial tick bite that often (but not always) causes a large, circular, spreading, erythematous lesion known as *erythema migrans*. Meningoencephalitis, neuritis, and carditis also may occur. The arthritis occurs later in the course as recurrent attacks of inflammation of the large joints (85%–90% of cases involve the knee),[10] with each recurrence usually lasting no more than 1 or 2 weeks. Occasionally, symptoms may persist for several months, and chronic, persistent arthritis of the knee has been reported.[10] A short course of high-dose amoxicillin therapy seems to shorten the course of the rash and perhaps attenuates the arthritis, and nonsteroidal anti-inflammatory drug (NSAID) therapy relieves the symptoms. Specific antibiotic regimens are suggested for different stages of disease and ages of patients.[11] Although a vaccine against *B burgdorferi* was developed and distributed, it was taken off the market in 2002 and is no longer available.[11]

In addition to bacteria, other infectious organisms can cause joint disease. Viruses, including rubella, mumps, varicella, parvovirus, adenovirus, the Epstein-Barr virus, and HIV, all can affect synovial tissue. Manifestations of the viral syndrome (rash, fever, mucous membrane involvement) usually precede joint involvement. Infectious hepatitis, on the other hand, can cause arthritis before overt hepatic involvement. Rubella immunization is associated with arthralgia and arthritis in as many as 3% of children who receive the vaccine, although rarely, if ever, with any sequelae.[12] Other less common infections that can involve the joints include brucellosis, leptospirosis, tularemia, Rocky Mountain spotted fever, and rat-bite fever. Mycobacteria can cause arthritis, as can various fungal agents, particularly in immunocompromised individuals.

Reactive arthritis, previously referred to as *Reiter syndrome*—a triad of urethritis, conjunctivitis, and arthritis—may appear in children and adolescents. In children, it is often triggered by an episode of enteritis.[13] Reactive arthritis is more common in boys than in girls, and making the diagnosis depends on excluding direct infectious causes of the inflammation. The arthritis predominantly occurs in large joints; again, it is often but not exclusively associated with the HLA-B27 class 1 major histocompatibility locus. The disorder is treated initially with anti-inflammatory drugs. Most children recover within a few months, although some follow a more chronic and relapsing course and can progress to ankylosing spondylitis. Transient synovitis of the hip, previously called *toxic synovitis*, also can cause arthralgia, arthritis, or both. This generally occurs in preschool or young school-aged children, and has a good prognosis. Etiology is unclear, but it may be viral or postviral in nature.[14]

Acute rheumatic fever is less common than it once was, but is still an important consideration in a child with the acute onset of arthritis or arthralgia. This follows an infection with group A streptococcus, usually pharyngitis, usually and typically by about 2 or 3 weeks. Diagnosis is made using the Jones criteria, which include migratory arthritis or arthralgias as well as fever, carditis, rash (erythema marginatum), central nervous system involvement, subcutaneous nodules, elevated acute phase reactants and prolonged PR interval. A distinct condition called *poststreptococcal reactive arthritis* may occur after a streptococcal infection, in the absence of other findings.[15] The arthritis may be more severe, and this may occur sooner after the preceding illness than is the case with rheumatic fever.

## Noninflammatory Causes of Joint Pain

Trauma causing fractures, dislocations, cartilage, ligamentous, or tendon injury, or other soft tissue damage are common in children and can cause joint pain, depending on the location of the injury. A careful history can usually provide information about the mechanism of the event. Physical abuse (non-accidental trauma) should be considered whenever signs of trauma are evident, and accidents that represent neglect on the part of parents or guardians need to be recognized and pursued. Any suspicious history or circumstance demands complete investigation.

Other more chronic mechanical stressors can lead to subacute arthralgia. Patellofemoral pain syndrome, also called *chondromalacia patellae*, is a common cause of anterior knee pain in children and adolescents, and is often bilateral. Knee pain is usually related to activity, and the child may report symptoms of "locking" with prolonged sitting, or "giving way" with extended standing. Exercises that strengthen the quadriceps femoris and adductor muscles can produce marked improvement. Repetitive activities can lead to chronic tendonitis or bursitis in periarticular areas, and are common in athletes, dancers, musicians, and other children who practice or perform repetitive movements. Stress fractures are uncommon in children but should be considered in an athlete with chronic bone or joint pain. Some injuries are specific to a developmental stage, such as Osgood-Schlatter disease, Sever disease, and other forms of apophysitis. These occur only in skeletally immature individuals who have either a repetitive or acute injury to the apophysis, which is a secondary ossification center to which a tendon attaches, and which is the weakest point of the biomechanical unit. These are treated by activity modification, rehabilitation, and analgesia as needed. Slipped capital femoral epiphysis is another condition seen only in skeletally immature children, in which the capital femoral epiphysis is displaced from the femoral neck. This may manifest as hip or sometimes thigh or knee pain, and is seen typically in overweight adolescents, and is diagnosed by imaging.

Some children experience arthralgias in the lower extremities, termed *growing pains*, which tend to be worse at night. These are not associated with warmth, swelling, or limitation of movement of the affected joints. Imaging will be normal. These children rarely have pain in the mornings, and have normal daytime activities. Symptoms can often be alleviated with a bedtime dose of NSAID or acetaminophen. Children with hypermobility syndrome often have a similar pattern of pain, worse after activity and improved by rest. Children with this disorder have increased joint laxity, and can be diagnosed by the presence of at least 3 of the following signs: hyperflexion of the wrist, bringing the thumb in contact with the volar surface of the forearm; hyperextension of the fingers to parallel with the forearm; hyperextension of the elbow to at least −10 degrees; hyperextension of the knee to at least −10 degrees; and hyperflexion of the spine such that with forward flexion, the palms can be placed flat on the ground with the feet together and without flexing the knees.[16] Some genetic disorders of connective tissue, including Marfan syndrome and Ehlers-Danlos syndrome, can cause pronounced hypermobility.

In an adolescent with chronic diffuse pain and fatigue without evidence of rheumatic disease on examination or laboratory studies, juvenile primary fibromyalgia syndrome should be considered. Multiple sets of diagnostic criteria have been published, but these generally include widespread pain for several months, presence of specific tender points on examination, and the presence of severe fatigue and nonrestorative sleep.[17,18] These children often also have headaches, depression or anxiety, a sense of cognitive impairment, numbness or tingling or stiffness in the limbs, irritable bowel symptoms, or other complaints. Treatment should be multidisciplinary, and should include patient and family education, exercise, and psychological interventions such as cognitive behavioral therapy. Some patients benefit from medications including non-narcotic analgesics, low-dose tricyclic antidepressants, other antidepressants, and γ-aminobutyric acid agonists such as gabapentin or pregabalin.

Children who present with localized limb pain, sometimes after an injury but out of proportion to examination findings, may have complex regional pain syndrome (CRPS). The affected area should also demonstrate some evidence of autonomic dysfunction such as localized edema, increased sweating, or change in temperature or color. As with juvenile fibromyalgia, onset is most common in adolescent girls, and concurrent sleep disruption and psychological conditions are also common. Treatment consists of aggressive physical and occupational therapy,[19] psychological and behavioral therapies, and sometimes pharmacotherapy or localized interventions such as nerve blocks.

### Other Causes

Hematologic disorders that have articular manifestations include hemophilia and sickle cell disease. In the latter disorder, the hand-foot syndrome type of vaso-occlusive crisis is a common initial presentation in children between 1 and 4 years of age.

Bone pain can also occur in patients with osteoid osteomas, which are benign bone tumors most often seen in older children and teens. Pigmented villonodular synovitis is a benign neoplasm of the synovium which can present with joint pain and swelling. Leukemia is the most common malignant condition to present with bone or joint pain, although lymphoma, neuroblastoma, and Ewing and other sarcomas can also cause these symptoms.

## ▶ EVALUATION

A complete history is indispensable in the initial assessment of a child with joint pain. The physical examination can then substantiate or alleviate suspicions raised during the interview. Distinguishing among arthritis, arthralgia, periarticular pain, and myalgia is essential. Further testing, including appropriate imaging, can confirm or further clarify the nature of bony or soft tissue abnormalities suspected based on the history and examination findings. In some cases, the diagnosis can be reinforced by laboratory testing. Markers of inflammation, including erythrocyte sedimentation rate, C-reactive protein, and others, are often abnormal in inflammatory conditions. In some cases, appropriate specific tests or cultures can confirm a specific rheumatic or infectious diagnosis.

## ▶ TREATMENT

Management of joint pain that is secondary to an inflammatory arthritis focuses on subduing inflammation and preserving normal range of motion, strength, and function. NSAIDs are often used as initial therapy. In patients with oligoarticular disease, especially those with a single persistently active joint, intraarticular corticosteroids can be effective. Systemic corticosteroids occasionally have a place in therapy of other JIA subtypes, although they are used much less often than in the past, and with a goal of limited duration. Methotrexate has come to play a central role in the medical management of children with JIA and some other inflammatory conditions who require therapy beyond NSAIDs. Other immunomodulatory agents, such as sulfasalazine, leflunomide, and hydroxychloroquine may also be used in some patients. Many patients who have resistant joint inflammation or high-risk phenotypes benefit from biologic agents, including antitumor necrosis factor alpha agents, IL-1 or IL-6 antagonists, and others.[20]

Any child with a bacterial infection of the joint space or bone should be promptly identified and treated with intravenous antibiotics. Other infectious causes of arthritis may also require treatment, such as those caused by Lyme disease or *Neisseria* infection. Others, such as parvovirus, will generally resolve spontaneously, so treatment is supportive.

In patients with joint pain resulting from trauma, therapy includes rest, ice, NSAIDs, or other analgesics, though any unstable injury should be promptly evaluated by an orthopedist to determine the need for external or surgical stabilization. There may also be a role for surgical treatment of longstanding joint damage resulting from chronic or severe inflammatory arthritis or mechanical derangements, and sometimes surgical interventions are necessary for establishing a clear diagnosis, as in synovial biopsy for atypical infections or bone biopsy for osteomyelitis.

After arriving at a diagnosis and plan of therapy, the physician must also offer management for the psychological aspects of joint disease. In children with ongoing joint problems, issues related to chronic pediatric disease must be addressed. The child may be unable to keep up with peers in physical activity and may be faced with having to make many health care visits, resulting in school absences. Many physicians think that environmental stress, in addition to the stress caused by the disease, can exacerbate various chronic conditions, and such may occur in children with JIA.

Children faced with hospitalization for an acute problem, such as septic arthritis, are exposed to all the complications of being taken out of their family and school environment, as well as having to deal with an institutional setting. Children with ongoing joint disease, even those with only a mild disability, should be provided with the services of a specialized social worker, counselor, or psychologist. Family resources (both emotional and financial) need to be assessed and support provided when needed. Discussion groups or support groups composed of these children and their families can be helpful because they offer an opportunity to compare experiences and coping mechanisms. Attention to the physical dimension alone does not provide adequate care in these diseases. A functionally minor disability can cause major problems of body image and feelings of lack of independence that must be dealt with appropriately. As with other chronic physical disorders of childhood and adolescence, long-term psychosocial sequelae also may develop.[21]

## When to Refer

Orthopaedics
- Fracture
- Ligamentous or cartilage injury to joint
- Continuous pain in a joint with deformity

Rheumatology
- Suspicion of juvenile arthritis or other rheumatologic disorder

Infectious diseases
- Septic arthritis
- Lyme disease; other spirochetal infection
- Osteomyelitis

Hematology
- Sickle cell disease
- Hemophilia

Gastroenterology
- Joint symptoms associated with inflammatory bowel disease

Occupational or physical therapy
- Joint disease complicated by contractures, weakness, poor function
- Hypermobility syndrome
- Pain amplification syndromes (eg, fibromyalgia, CRPS)

Mental health
- Suspicion of somatization or conversion disorder

## When to Admit

- Fracture requiring open fixation or traction
- Systemic onset juvenile arthritis with macrophage activation syndrome
- Septic arthritis
- Osteomyelitis
- Severe sickle cell pain crisis
- Admit to rehabilitation if inadequate response to outpatient occupational or physical therapy

## TOOLS FOR PRACTICE

### Engaging Patient and Family

- *What is a Pediatric Rheumatologist?* (fact sheet), American Academy of Pediatrics (www.healthychildren.org/English/family-life/health-management/pediatric-specialists/Pages/What-is-a-Pediatric-Rheumatologist.aspx)

### Medical Decision Support

- *Red Book: 2012 Report of the Committee on Infectious Diseases,* 29th ed (book), American Academy of Pediatrics (shop.aap.org)

## REFERENCES

1. De Inocencio J. Epidemiology of musculoskeletal pain in primary care. *Arch Dis Child.* 2004;89:431–434
2. Oen KG, Cheang M. Epidemiology of chronic arthritis in childhood. *Semin Arthritis Rheum.* 1996;26:575–591
3. Still GF. On a form of chronic joint disease in children. *Med Chir Trans.* 1897;80:47–59
4. Petty RE, Southwood TR, Manners P, et al. International League of Associations for Rheumatology classification of juvenile idiopathic arthritis: second revision, Edmonton, 2001. *J Rheumatol.* 2004;31:390–392
5. Jaakkola E, Herzberg I, Laiho K, et al. Finnish HLA studies confirm the increased risk conferred by HLA-B27 homozygosity in ankylosing spondylitis. *Ann Rheum Dis.* 2006;65:775–780
6. Luhmann JD, Luhmann SJ. Etiology of septic arthritis in children: an update for the 1990s. *Pediatr Emerg Care.* 1999;15:40–42
7. Perlman MH, Patzakis MJ, Kumar PJ, Holtom P. The incidence of joint involvement with adjacent osteomyelitis in pediatric patients. *J Pediatr Orthop.* 2000;20:40–43
8. Taccetti G, Trapani S, Ermini M, Falcini F. Reactive arthritis triggered by Yersinia enterocolitica: a review of 18 pediatric cases. *Clin Exp Rheumatol.* 1994;12:681–684
9. Steere AC, Malawista SE, Snydman DR, et al. Lyme arthritis: an epidemic of oligoarticular arthritis in children and adults in three Connecticut communities. *Arthritis Rheum.* 1977;20:7–17

10. Gerber MA, Zemel LS, Shapiro ED. Lyme arthritis in children: clinical epidemiology and long-term outcomes. *Pediatrics.* 1998;102:905–908
11. American Academy of Pediatrics. Lyme disease (lyme borreliosis, *Borrelia burgdorferi* infection). In: Pickering LK, Baker CJ, Kimberlin DW, Long SS, eds. *Red Book: 2012 Report of the Committee on Infectious Diseases.* Elk Grove Village, IL: American Academy of Pediatrics; 2012:474–479
12. Phillips PE. Viral arthritis in children. *Arthritis Rheum.* 1977;20:584–589
13. Hannu T. Reactive arthritis. *Best Pract Res Clin Rheumatol.* 2011;25:347–357
14. Nouri A, Walmsley D, Pruszczynski B, Synder M. Transient synovitis of the hip: a comprehensive review. *J Pediatr Orthop B.* 2014;23(1):32–36
15. Barash J, Mashiach E, Navon-Elkan P, et al. Differentiation of post-streptococcal reactive arthritis from acute rheumatic fever. *J Pediatr.* 2008;153:696–699
16. Biro F, Gewanter HL, Baum J. The hypermobility syndrome. *Pediatrics.* 1983;72:701–706
17. Wolfe F, Smythe HA, Yunus MB, et al. The American College of Rheumatology 1990 criteria for the classification of fibromyalgia. Report of the Multicenter Criteria Committee. *Arthritis Rheum.* 1990;33:160–172
18. Wolfe F, Clauw DJ, Fitzcharles MA, et al. The American College of Rheumatology preliminary diagnostic criteria for fibromyalgia and measurement of symptom severity. *Arthritis Care Res (Hoboken).* 2010;62:600–610
19. Sherry DD, Wallace CA, Kelley C, Kidder M, Sapp L. Short- and long-term outcomes of children with complex regional pain syndrome type I treated with exercise therapy. *Clin J Pain.* 1999;15:218–223
20. Beukelman T, Patkar NM, Saag KG, et al. 2011 American College of Rheumatology recommendations for the treatment of juvenile idiopathic arthritis: initiation and safety monitoring of therapeutic agents for the treatment of arthritis and systemic features. *Arthritis Care Res (Hoboken).* 2011;63:465–482
21. LeBovidge JS, Lavigne JV, Donenberg GR, Miller ML. Psychological adjustment of children and adolescents with chronic arthritis: a meta-analytic review. *J Pediatr Psychol.* 2003;28:29–39

# Chapter 49

# Learning Difficulty

*Barbara L. Frankowski, MD, MPH*

## ▶ BACKGROUND AND SIGNIFICANCE

Learning difficulties can occur at any age and for a variety of reasons. They invariably cause frustration for the child or adolescent, which can lead to or compound behavior problems and emotional distress. The effects of learning difficulties, whatever their cause, can be profound, with economic and emotional consequences far into adult life. Children who do not receive timely intervention are at risk not only for academic failure, but also for the psychosocial morbidities that accompany limited academic achievement, such as substance abuse and juvenile delinquency.[1] Some children with learning difficulties are among the 7%[2] of US 15- through 24-year-olds who drop out of school, leading to chronic unemployment, poverty, and higher risk of health problems throughout adulthood. The drop-out rate is higher among minority populations of black non-Hispanics (8%) and Hispanics (22.5%) than white children.[2] Clearly, learning difficulties are an important concern for primary care physicians providing services to children and adolescents.

## ▶ PRIMARY CARE PHYSICIAN'S ROLE

It is the primary care physician's role to recognize that a child is experiencing difficulty in learning, to help the family sort out the cause of the child's learning difficulties, to identify referral sources for psychological and educational assessment, to ensure that the child receives the educational resources he or she needs and is entitled to, to address any medical or mental health problems that may be associated with the child's learning difficulties, and to guide the family in advocating and providing a supportive environment for the child.

## ▶ RECOGNITION OF CHILDREN WITH LEARNING DIFFICULTIES

The primary care physician has opportunities at routine health supervision visits to elicit parental concerns, to monitor children's developmental progress and functioning, and to screen for developmental delays and symptoms of social and emotional problems. The physician may also receive referrals from childcare or school personnel who have observed that the child has difficulty learning compared with his or her peers or is experiencing behavioral problems in the classroom. There may be a family history of learning problems, compounding concerns about the child's progress in learning. Box 49-1 and Table 49-1 for signs and symptoms that a child is experiencing learning difficulties.

Box 49-1

## *Symptoms and Clinical Findings Suggesting Learning Difficulties*

**INDICATIONS FROM YOUTH'S OR PARENT'S HISTORY**

- Child has experienced a delay in language development or has difficulty understanding language despite normal hearing and vision.
- Child has difficulty following directions.
- Child has difficulty learning letters, numbers, and colors.
- Child has struggled to read, grasp math concepts, or write in comparison with her peers.
- Letter reversals (b/d), inversions (m/w), transpositions (felt/left), substitutions (house/home), or confusion of arithmetic signs persist past peers.
- Child avoids reading aloud, writing, or homework.
- Child or parent is frustrated with the child's academic performance.
- Parent perceives child is "lazy" in school.
- Child is perceived as an "underachiever."
- Classroom behavior or inattention has become a problem.
- Other family members have experienced learning difficulties or did not complete high school.

Table 49-1

**Findings Suggesting Learning Difficulty**

| MEASUREMENT | SCORE |
|---|---|
| End-of-grade test scores or achievement test scores | Percentiles are low (≤15%) or markedly scattered, or the child is performing considerably less well than would be expected for his or her intelligence. |
| Report cards | Grades are low or markedly scattered. |
| Intelligence tests | Percentiles are within the normal range or significantly higher than measures of academic achievement. |

## ▶ CAUSES OF LEARNING DIFFICULTIES

### *Lack of School Readiness*

Some young children experience difficulties in learning because they are not yet ready for the school experience, socially, emotionally, or physically; because they do not have language and literacy skills comparable with their peers; or because their family or culture does not value their education. Box 49-2 outlines the specific traits a child should ideally possess in order to be ready for school, and Box 49-3 identifies key family and community supports for preparing a child for school.

Finally, many schools are not prepared to educate children with the full range of abilities and disabilities. Measurement of children's readiness for kindergarten should be used to assess the effectiveness of community-based programs and to prepare schools to meet the child's ongoing needs, rather than to exclude or delay children from their formal educational experience.[3] Box 49-4 highlights key elements of schools that are ready for children.

**Box 49-2**

### *Traits for School Readiness*

- Physical well-being and motor development: good health status and alertness; any physical disabilities identified and accommodated
- Social and emotional development: turn-taking, cooperation, empathy, and the ability to express his or her own emotions
- Approaches to learning: enthusiasm, curiosity, family and cultural values supportive of learning
- Language development: skills in understanding and speaking the language spoken in the classroom; adequate vocabulary and other literacy skills, including print awareness, story sense, and writing and drawing processes
- General knowledge and cognition: sound-letter association, awareness of spatial relations, and number concepts

**Box 49-3**

### *Preparing the Child for School: Key Elements*

- At least a high school education or equivalent for parents
- High-quality prenatal health care for the mother
- Optimal nutrition for mother and child
- Comprehensive health care for the child
- Daily physical activity
- Daily time with parent in learning activities (eg, reading, conversation, family meals)
- Access to high-quality preschool for children in impoverished environments
- Access to programs for children and parents who speak English as a second language

**Box 49-4**

### *Preparing the School for the Child: Key Elements*

- High-quality preschools for children in impoverished environments
- Programs and teacher training for children of all ability levels
- Preschool screening of children aimed at measuring the outcome of their preschool programs and at identifying and addressing students' needs (not at excluding children or delaying their school entry)

## *Medical, Mental Health, and Developmental Problems*

Learning difficulties may also be caused by cognitive limitations, a language or learning disorder; vision or hearing impairment; behavioral and emotional problems; a chronic disease that affects the child's concentration, interpersonal relationships, or school attendance; sleep deprivation; or medication affecting concentration or alertness. See Table 49-2 for a listing of problems that can cause or co-occur with learning difficulties.

**Table 49-2**
**Conditions That May Cause Poor School Performance or Co-occur With Learning Difficulties**

| CONDITION | RATIONALE |
|---|---|
| Hearing or vision problems | All children who are experiencing learning difficulties should be screened for sensory deficits. |
| Sleep deprivation | Sleep problems can cause inattention and irritability and contribute to poor school performance; conversely, poor school performance and homework struggles may contribute to difficulty sleeping. |
| Developmental problems | Children with overall intellectual or social limitations will learn more slowly than their age-mates. Children with low achievement and low intellectual levels often have the same problems as children with learning disabilities. |
| Attention-deficit/hyperactivity disorder (ADHD) | Children who are inattentive or impulsive may manifest poor academic performance. They may have problems with getting the work completed and turned in, rather than skill deficits. Conversely, children experiencing academic difficulties may seem restless and inattentive. See Chapter 45, Inattention and Impulsivity. |
| Exposure to adverse childhood experiences (ACE) | Children who have experienced or witnessed trauma, violence, a natural disaster, separation from a parent, parental divorce or separation, parental substance use, neglect, or physical, emotional, or sexual abuse are at high risk of developing emotional difficulties such as adjustment disorder or post-traumatic stress disorder (PTSD). Children with PTSD can manifest poor concentration, memory problems, school refusal, and academic decline. These children may also manifest other forms of anxiety. Physicians may want to consider speaking separately and confidentially with the youth and parents to explore this possibility. Parents are often unaware of exposures that children may have had at school or in the community. There may be major traumas in the family (eg, serious illness in a parent, maltreatment of the child, death or incarceration of a loved one) that are similarly not discussed or disclosed. The 3 hallmark symptom clusters of PTSD are reexperiencing, avoidance of memories or situations that recall the trauma, and hypervigilance (ie, increased worry about safety, startling or anxiousness at unexpected sounds or events). See also Chapter 6, Anxiety. |
| Anxiety | Anxious children may experience difficulty concentrating and perform poorly on tests. See Chapter 6, Anxiety. |
| Bereavement | Most children will experience the death of a family member or friend sometime in their childhood. Other losses may also trigger grief responses—separation or divorce of parents, relocation, change of school, deployment of a parent in military service, breakup with a girlfriend or boyfriend, or remarriage of parent. Such losses are traumatic. They may result in such symptoms as sadness, anxiety, difficulty concentrating, poor impulse control, or academic decline immediately following the loss and in some instances, more persistently. See also Chapter 14, Depression, and the discussion of PTSD in Chapter 6, Anxiety. |
| Depression | Depression may cause a decline in school performance, result from poor school performance, or simply coexist with learning disabilities. Marked sleep disturbance, disturbed appetite, low mood, or tearfulness could indicate that a child (or more commonly, an adolescent) is depressed. See Chapter 14, Depression. |

**Table 49-2**
**Conditions That May Cause Poor School Performance or Co-occur With Learning Difficulties—cont'd**

| CONDITION | RATIONALE |
|---|---|
| Physical illness | Medical issues that may have an effect on school performance include all illnesses that may interfere with the child's attendance. Some illnesses (or symptoms caused by the illnesses) can affect attention in the classroom (eg, hypo- or hyperthyroidism, neurologic disorders, post-traumatic brain injury, undiagnosed diabetes), as can side effects of medications such as bronchodilators or anticonvulsants. |
| Substance use | Children frustrated with their school performance may use substances such as alcohol, nicotine, or other drugs to alleviate their frustrations, or self-medicate with caffeine or cocaine. Conversely, children using substances may manifest inattention, impulsivity, and deteriorating school performance. See Chapter 75, Substance Use: Initial Approach in Primary Care. |
| Conduct or oppositional disorders | These disorders may cause poor academic performance, and frustration with poor academic performance can exacerbate conduct or oppositional problems. See Chapter 16, Disruptive Behavior and Aggression. |
| Autism spectrum disorders including high-functioning autism, which was formerly known as pervasive development disorder, and Asperger syndrome | Children who have these difficulties also have problems with social relatedness (eg, poor eye contact, preference for solitary activities, language [often stilted], and range of interests [persistent and intense interest in a particular activity or subject]). They often will have very rigid expectations for routine and become anxious or angry if these expectations are not met. As such, these children may manifest difficulties in the classroom and many of the symptoms associated with learning disorders. |

### *Learning Disabilities*

Rarely diagnosed before a child enters school, learning disabilities (LDs) represent a broad array of specific learning challenges that significantly impede a child's ability to perform at the expected grade level. They generally occur in the context of normal sensory functioning and otherwise normal cognitive capabilities and, by definition, are not the result of a primary emotional disorder or lack of opportunity (although frustration and low self-esteem associated with LDs may contribute to development of problems such as anxiety, depression, or oppositionality). Learning disabilities are clearly familial, with genetics contributing substantially to a child's risk.[4] It is estimated that between 5% and 17.5% of individuals meet diagnostic criteria for LDs and approximately 2 million US schoolchildren aged 6 to 11 years are affected.[5] Eighty percent of those identified have dyslexia or a reading disorder.

## ▶ ASSESSMENT OF CHILDREN WITH LEARNING DIFFICULTIES

Assessment begins by differentiating the child's symptoms from normal behavior. Children learn at different rates. Typically developing children younger than 7 years may reverse and transpose letters and experience some frustration with new learning tasks, particularly if the child has had limited preschool experience or other children in the classroom have had more exposure to formal school experiences. Many children will have 1 or more of the symptoms in Box 49-1 from time to time. Children who have missed school for an illness, changed schools, or experienced a significant loss may experience transient problems with school functioning. Some parents have unrealistic expectations, based on their own learning experiences or that of older siblings or children of friends.

It is important to explore sources of stress in the family, school, or community, as any of these can cause inattentiveness and distraction in the child.

A full physical and psychosocial assessment of the child will serve to identify conditions that can cause or co-occur with learning difficulties (Table 49-2).

Two categories of medical risk deserve special attention: prematurity and cyanotic congenital heart disease. Premature infants are at significantly higher risk for global developmental delays and for LDs.[6] In particular, children born at less than 32 weeks' gestation or who experience perinatal and postnatal complications such as prolonged ventilation, intracranial hemorrhage, sepsis, seizures, prolonged acidosis, or hypoglycemia are at higher risk for neurodevelopmental sequellae. Similarly, children surviving severe congenital cardiac anomalies are at high risk for LDs.[7] Several genetic disorders have been linked to risk for various forms of LD. In particular, children with Klinefelter syndrome, Turner syndrome, velocardiofacial syndrome, and spina bifida with shunted hydrocephalus have all been shown to be at significant risk for LDs.[8] When 1 of these risk factors is identified, the physician should have a low threshold to refer for psychological and educational assessment.

Adolescents who present with learning difficulties are a particular challenge for the primary care physician. An adolescent who has been progressing normally with academics may suddenly develop learning difficulties. It is possible that the adolescent may have a mild learning disability for which he or she has compensated in lower grades, but which is now causing difficulty in meeting the more rigorous demands of middle or high school. Together or separately, the adolescent may have mild attentional problems that have not required any special intervention up until this point. However, it is also possible that the adolescent has other problems causing or contributing to learning difficulties, such as inadequate amounts of sleep, poor nutrition, inadequate physical activity, anxiety, depression, or substance abuse. The adolescent could also, or alternatively, be struggling with issues of sexual orientation or bullying that cause stress in the school environment. It is important to consider all these possibilities when assessing an adolescent with learning difficulties.

To further the assessment of any child or adolescent with learning difficulties, the physician can communicate with school personnel (eg, guidance counselor, classroom teacher, school psychologist) to request data and observations such as the following:

- **Intelligence testing:** School personnel may be willing to administer a cognitive screening test or, if there are apparent discrepancies between intelligence and academic achievement, a full battery of psychological tests.
- **Achievement testing:** School personnel can provide a screening test or reports of achievement or end-of-grade tests.
- **Full psychoeducational evaluation:** School psychologist or community psychologist may provide, by referral.
- **School placement and special services.**

- **Individualized Educational Program (IEP) or 504 plan,** if in place.
- **History of academic progress, behavior and discipline, and peer interactions.**

Use of additional instruments such as the Vanderbilt ADHD Rating Scale (see Tools for Practice) and general psychosocial screens [Pediatric Symptom Checklist (PSC)-35, PSC-17, Strengths and Difficulties Questionnaire (SDQ)] can be used to identify children who may have psychosocial problems contributing to their learning difficulties.

## ▶ PLAN OF CARE FOR CHILDREN WITH LEARNING DIFFICULTIES

The care of a child experiencing learning difficulties can begin in the primary care setting from the time symptoms are recognized, even if the child's problems do not rise to the level of a disorder or referral to the school or to a mental health specialist is ultimately part of the care plan.

### *Engage Child and Family in Care*

Without engagement, most families will not seek or persist in care. The process may require multiple primary care visits.

Reinforce strengths of the youth and family as a method of engagement and identify any barriers to addressing the problem (eg, stigma, family conflict, resistance to academic testing or special education). Use "common factors" techniques[9] to build trust and optimism, reach agreement on incremental next steps, develop a plan of care, and collaboratively determine the role of the primary care physician. Regardless of other roles, the primary care physician can encourage a positive view of treatment on the part of the youth and family.

### *Encourage Healthy Habits*

Encourage exercise, outdoor play, balanced and consistent diet, sleep (critically important to mental health), avoidance of exposure to frightening or violent media, limitation of screen time to less than 1 to 2 hours per day, special time with parents, acknowledgment of child's strengths, and special efforts to support the child and help him or her to feel competent, special, positive, and appreciated.

### *Reduce Stress*

Consider the child's social environment (eg, family social history, parental depression screening, results of any family assessment tools administered, reports from child care or school). Questions to raise might include the following:

*Is the parent punitive or critical?* If parents' psychosocial problems are affecting their relationship with the child, explore their readiness to address these problems as part of helping their child. Encourage praise for their child's efforts. Urge parents to avoid comparisons with siblings or peers and to keep up the child's self-esteem. Urge parents to nurture the child's nonacademic gifts, such as art or music, and encourage participation in extracurricular activities that provide social experiences uncomplicated by academic performance and competition (eg, scouts, faith-based youth group, boys' or girls' club).

*Are there battles over homework?* Advise parents that the child is not lazy. Provide guidance about helping with homework (and requesting modified assignments, as appropriate). See Box 49-5 on Guidelines for Homework Battles.

Box 49-5

## *Guidelines for Homework Battles*

- Establish a routine (not waiting until evening to get started).
- Identify another student your child can call to clarify homework assignments.
- Limit distractions (eg, TV, computer, phone).
- Assist child in dividing assignments into small, manageable segments (especially important for long-range assignments and large projects).
- Assist child in getting started (eg, read directions together, watch child complete first items).
- Monitor without taking over.
- Praise good effort and completion of tasks.
- Do not insist on perfection.
- Offer incentives ("When you've finished, we can…").
- Help child study for tests.
- Do not force child to spend excessive time on homework; write a note to the teacher if the child put forth good effort but was not able to complete it.
- If child fails to turn in completed work, develop a system with the teacher to collect it on arrival.
- If unable to provide homework supervision and assistance, or if homework battles are adversely affecting the parent-child relationship, ask the teacher for help finding a tutor.

*Is the child exposed to criticism or teasing at school? Is the child's teacher supportive and patient?* Provide strategies for communication between school personnel and home; coach them to praise progress and effort, not just outcomes, and to address teasing or bullying.

*Are school authorities proceeding with assessment in accordance with the child's rights?* Inform parents about the child's rights under the Individuals with Disabilities Education Act (IDEA) and Section 504 of the Rehabilitation Act. It is important to obtain information about how these 2 acts are specifically implemented in your state and school districts. If a child has a learning disability, he or she qualifies for specialized educational services, and IDEA requires that the school develop an Individual Education Plan (IEP). The IEP documents the child's current level of functioning, establishes goals, and delineates the services needed to meet those goals in the least restrictive environment possible. The parent is entitled to meet with school personnel to review and approve the IEP. If the child does not qualify for specialized educational services but has minor challenges that can be helped by minor classroom modifications (eg, preferential seating, homework modifications), the school may develop a 504 plan for the child. If the parent is dissatisfied with the school's response to the child's needs, there is an appeal process within the school system.

If the school is not adequately addressing the child's needs, the physician may offer referral to a community mental health professional such as a psychologist or developmental-behavioral pediatrician, or an educational tutor. Results of this assessment may provide support for the parent's advocacy efforts in the school system or may guide the family in developing tutorial assistance for the child.

Whatever interventions are planned, it is important to acknowledge and reinforce protective factors (eg, good relationships with at least 1 parent or important adult, pro-social peers, concerned or caring family, help-seeking, and connection to positive organization[s]).

### Offer Initial Interventions

The strategies described below are applicable to the care of children with mild or emerging learning difficulties, as well as diagnosed learning disorders. They can also be used as initial primary care management of children with learning difficulties while readying children for further assessment or educational services or awaiting access to evaluation and treatment.

*Address comorbid conditions.*

*If there are battles over homework, offer guidelines to parents.* Box 49-5 provides guidelines for parents to address homework battles.

### Provide Resources

Families may find the National Center for Learning Disabilities (www.ncld.org) a helpful source for information and support. Parents with questions about special education law may wish to consult a dedicated resource like Wrightslaw (www.wrightslaw.com). Helpful brochures, publications, and Web sites are included in Tools for Practice: Engaging Patient and Family.

### Monitor the Child's Progress Toward Educational Goals

School reports can be helpful in monitoring progress. Screening instruments that gather information from multiple reporters (youth, parent, teacher), such as the SDQ, can be helpful in monitoring progress with symptoms and functioning.

### Involve Specialist(s)

*Involve education or mental health specialist(s) if child does not respond to initial interventions or if indicated by the following clinical circumstances:*

- The child or parent is very distressed by the symptom(s).
- There are co-occurring behavior problems not responsive to primary care management.
- School evaluation is incomplete or untimely.
- Parent's relationship with school is adversarial.
- Child and family have conflicts not responsive to primary care management.
- Parent is very negative toward child or unresponsive to primary care guidance.

*Consider seeing a geneticist* for a diagnostic genetic workup if there are persistent concerns that interventions are not producing results.

*Reach agreement on respective roles in the child's care.* The primary care physician may be responsible for advising the family about the child's rights under IDEA; reducing stresses on the child while awaiting further assessment and treatment; engaging and encouraging the child's positive view of his or her evaluation and specialized instruction; monitoring academic progress; observing for and addressing any comorbidities; and coordinating care provided by parents, school, medical home, and specialists. Resources available to help physicians in this role are provided in Tools for Practice. The primary care physician may also review with the family whether the child's school interventions are evidence-based ones, or refer to a developmental-behavioral pediatrician who is more knowledgeable in this area.

### TOOLS FOR PRACTICE

#### Engaging Patient and Family

- *Individualized Education Program (IEP) Meeting Checklist* (handout), American Academy of Pediatrics (www.brightfutures.org/mentalhealth/pdf/families/mc/iep.pdf)

- *Learning Disabilities: What Parents Need to Know* (handout), American Academy of Pediatrics (www.healthychildren.org/English/health-issues/conditions/learning-disabilities/Pages/Learning-Disabilities-What-Parents-Need-To-Know.aspx)
- *Reading for Children: Grades 1–6* (handout), American Academy of Pediatrics (www.brightfutures.org/mentalhealth/pdf/families/mc/grades.pdf)
- *Your Child's Mental Health: When to Seek Help and Where to Get Help* (handout), American Academy of Pediatrics (patiented.solutions.aap.org)

### Medical Decision Support

- *The LD Navigator* (Web site), National Center for Learning Disabilities (ldnavigator.ncld.org)
- *Practice Parameters* (Web page), American Academy of Child & Adolescent Psychiatry (www.aacap.org/cs/root/member_information/practice_information/practice_parameters/practice_parameters)
- *Vanderbilt ADHD Rating Scale* (scale), (www.brightfutures.org/mentalhealth/pdf/professionals/bridges/adhd.pdf)

## AAP POLICY STATEMENTS

Adams RC, Tapia C; American Academy of Pediatrics Council on Children With Disabilities. Clinical report: early intervention, IDEA Part C services, and the medical home: collaboration for best practices and best outcomes. *Pediatrics.* 2013;132(4):e1073–e1088 (pediatrics.aappublications.org/content/132/4/e1073)

American Academy of Pediatrics Section on Ophthalmology, Council on Children with Disabilities; American Academy of Ophthalmology; American Association for Pediatric Ophthalmology and Strabismus; American Association of Certified Orthoptists. Joint statement: learning disabilities, dyslexia, and vision. *Pediatrics.* 2009;124(2):837–844. Reaffirmed July 2014 (pediatrics.aappublications.org/content/124/2/837)

American Academy of Pediatrics Council on Children With Disabilities, Medical Home Implementation Project Advisory Committee. Patient- and family-centered care coordination: a framework for integrating care for children and youth across multiple systems. *Pediatrics.* 2014;133(5):e1451–e1460 (pediatrics.aappublications.org/content/133/5/e1451)

American Academy of Pediatrics Council on Children With Disabilities. Provision of educationally related services for children and adolescents with chronic diseases and disabling conditions. *Pediatrics.* 2007;119(6):1218–1223 (pediatrics.aappublications.org/content/119/6/1218)

Handler SM, Fierson WM; American Academy of Pediatrics Section on Ophthalmology and Council on Children With Disabilities, American Academy of Ophthalmology, American Association for Pediatric Ophthalmology and Strabismus, American Association of Certified Orthoptists. Joint technical report: learning disabilities, dyslexia, and vision. *Pediatrics.* 2011;127(3):e818–e856 (pediatrics.aappublications.org/content/127/3/e818)

Moeschler JB, Shevell M; American Academy of Pediatrics Committee on Genetics. Clinical report: comprehensive evaluation of the child with intellectual disability or global developmental delays. *Pediatrics.* 2014;134(3):e903–e918 (pediatrics.aappublications.org/content/134/3/e903)

## REFERENCES

1. Esser G, Schmidt MH. Children with specific reading retardation—early determinants and long-term outcome. *Acta Paedopsychiatr.* 1994;56:229–237
2. US Census Bureau. School Enrollment–Social and Economic Characteristic of Students: October 2005. Detailed Tables. Table 1. http://www.census.gov/population/www/socdemo/school/cps2005.html. Accessed February 24, 2010
3. High PC; American Academy of Pediatrics Committee on Early Childhood, Adoption, and Dependent Care and Council on School Health. School readiness. *Pediatrics.* 2008;121:e1008–e1015

4. Pennington BF. Genetics of learning disabilities. *J Child Neurol.* 1995;10(Suppl 1):S69–S77
5. American Academy of Pediatrics Section on Ophthalmology, Council on Children with Disabilities; American Academy of Ophthalmology; American Association for Pediatric Ophthalmology and Strabismus; American Association of Certified Orthoptists. Joint statement: learning disabilities, dyslexia, and vision. *Pediatrics.* 2009;124:837–844
6. Rais-Bahrami K, Short BL. Premature and small-for-dates infants. In: Batshaw ML, Pellegrino L, Roizen NJ, eds. *Children with Disabilities.* 6th ed. Baltimore, MD: Paul H. Brookes Publishing; 2007:107–122
7. Bellinger DC, Wypij D, duPlessis AJ, et al. Neurodevelopmental status at eight years in children with dextro-transposition of the great arteries: the Boston Circulatory Arrest Trial. *J Thorac Cardiovasc Surg.* 2003;126:1385–1396
8. Rourke BP, Ahmad SA, Collins DW, Hayman-Abekki BA, Hayman-Abello SE, Warriner EM. Child clinical/pediatric neuropsychology: some recent advances. *Ann Rev Psychol.* 2002;53:309–339
9. Kemper KJ, Wissow L, Foy JM, Shore SE. *Core Communication Skills for Primary Clinicians.* Wake Forest School of Medicine. nwahec.org/45737. Accessed January 9, 2015

# Chapter 50

# Limp

*Ginger Janow, MD; Norman T. Ilowite, MD*

Limp is a common presenting complaint in both pediatric primary care offices and emergency departments. While the most common cause of limp is trauma, there are many other etiologies, ranging in severity from benign to life-threatening. Limp is defined as an abnormal gait pattern. Distinguishing a limp in a young child can be particularly challenging as the mature gait cycle does not fully develop until after 7 years of age.[1]

## ▶ DIFFERENTIAL DIAGNOSIS

### *General*

The differential diagnosis of a limp is broad, and is best considered as 7 categories: trauma, vascular, infectious, malignancy or tumor, skeletal anomalies, inflammatory diseases, and neuromuscular disorders.

### *Trauma*

The most common cause of limp is trauma. If the history and physical examination suggest a fracture, ligament damage, or tendon damage, the patient should be referred to an orthopedist. Otherwise, rest, ice, compression, elevation, and analgesics are the mainstays of therapy. Radiographic evaluation should be guided by the history and physical examination.

### *Vascular*

**Legg-Calvé-Perthes disease** is characterized by avascular necrosis of the femoral head. Most often seen in the 5- to 10-year-old age group, it is more common in boys than girls. Patients generally present with groin or referred knee pain and an antalgic limp, with increased pain on activity. On examination, they generally have pain and limitation upon internal hip rotation. Early in the course, plain radiographs may be normal or may show increased density of the femoral head on the affected side, but later will show subchondral lucency, and ultimately, collapse and destruction of the femoral epiphysis (Figure 50-1). Once the diagnosis is suspected, pediatric orthopedics should be consulted for further workup and management.

**Osteochondritis dissecans** is the result of ischemia of the subchondral bone and can occur in multiple joints, although the knee is the most common. It generally occurs in adolescents, and most often presents with knee pain, swelling, and the sensation of the knee giving way. On physical examination, there is often joint swelling and pain on motion. Plain radiographs reveal a radiolucent zone separating the osteochondral fragment from the rest of the bone.

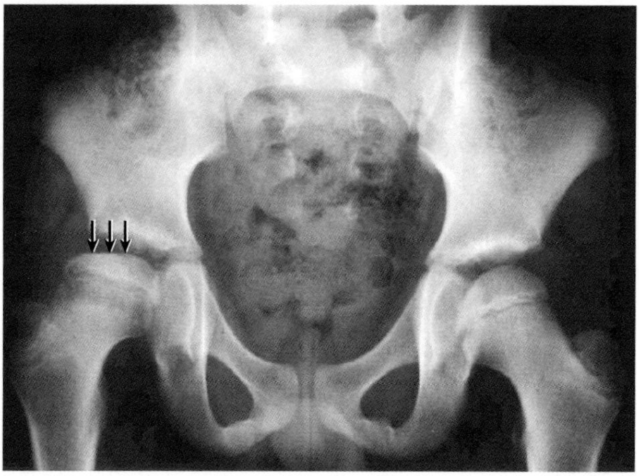

**Figure 50-1**
AP pelvis in an 8-year-old boy with right hip pain and limp. Right femoral head epiphysis shows loss of height and mixed sclerotic and lytic appearance *(arrows)* of Legg-Calvé-Perthes disease. *(From Barkin RM, Barkin SZ, Barkin AZ. The limping child.* J Emerg Med. *2000;18[3]:331–339. Copyright © 2000, Elsevier, with permission.)*

## Infectious

**Septic arthritis**, or infection within the joint space, is among the most emergent causes of a limp, requiring rapid identification and treatment to avoid long-term damage and disability. The 2 peaks in incidence are in the toddler years and in adolescence. In most cases, the onset of pain is rapid and is accompanied by a fever and refusal to bear weight. On physical examination, the joint is generally swollen, warm, tender, and extremely painful with range of motion. If a septic joint is suspected, laboratory evaluation should include evaluation of synovial fluid (with Gram stain, culture, and cell count), blood culture, complete blood count (CBC), sedimentation rate (ESR) and C-reactive protein (CRP). Plain radiographs may reveal a joint effusion. An ESR of less than 20 mm/hr or a normal CRP lowers the likelihood of a serious infectious cause but does not exclude the diagnosis of skeletal infection.[2] Etiologic agents are isolated in the blood or synovial fluid in 34% to 82% of cases.[3] Synovial fluid generally reveals an elevated white blood cell count with increased segmented neutrophils (Table 50-1).

In the toddler age group, the most common organisms are *Staphylococcus aureus, Kingella kingae,* and in young infants. *Haemophilus influenzae* type b (Hib) previously accounted for 70% of cases of septic arthritis in children from 2 months to 2 years of age, but this pathogen has been virtually eradicated following universal Hib vaccine implementation. Group B streptococcus is the most common cause of invasive bacterial infection in infants less than 2 months of age, and both bone and joint infection can occur. In the adolescent age group, *S aureus* is still the most common pathogen, but gonococcal arthritis should be considered in the sexually active teen. If septic arthritis is suspected, orthopedics should be consulted for joint aspiration and drainage should be promptly performed in cases of hip or shoulder infection. Gram stain and culture, when positive, should guide antibiotic management.

**Table 50-1**
**Characteristics of Synovial Fluid**

| GROUP AND CONDITION | COLOR AND CLARITY | VISCOSITY | WBC COUNT | PMN (%) |
|---|---|---|---|---|
| ***Noninflammatory*** | | | | |
| Normal | Yelllow and clear | Very high | <200 | <25 |
| Traumatic arthritis | Xanthochromic and turbid | High | <2,000 | <25 |
| Osteoarthritis | Yellow and clear | High | 1,000 | <25 |
| ***Inflammatory*** | | | | |
| Systemic lupus erythematosus | Yellow and clear | Normal | 5,000 | 10 |
| Rhematic fever | Yellow and cloudy | ↓ | 5,000 | 10–50 |
| Chronic arthritis | Yellow and cloudy | ↓ | 15,000–20,000 | 75 |
| Reactive arthritis | Yellow and opaque | ↓ | 20,000 | 80 |
| ***Pyogenic*** | | | | |
| Tuberculosis arthritis | Yellow-white and cloudy | ↓ | 25,000 | 50–60 |
| Septic arthritis | Serosanguineous and turbid | ↓ | 50,000–300,000 | >75 |

From Petty RE, Cassidy JT. Chronic arthritis in childhood. In: Cassidy JT, Laxer RM, Petty RE, Lindsley CB. *Textbook of Pediatric Rheumatology.* 6th ed. Philadelphia, PA: Elsevier Saunders; 2011, with permission.

**Osteomyelitis** is most common in the toddler age group but can be seen in all age groups, and is usually caused by the same organisms responsible for septic arthritis. The pathogenesis of infection is generally hematogenous seeding, but osteomyelitis may follow penetrating trauma or deep contiguous infection as may occur with decubitus ulcers. Involvement of long bones is most common; femur or tibia are the 2 most common sites reported. Patients often present with fever, pain in the affected extremity and limp, and may report preceding trauma. Physical examination findings are dependent upon the location of the infection, but point tenderness over the bony metaphysis is highly suggestive of osteomyelitis in the child with limp. Plain radiographs are often negative upon presentation, but generally show abnormalities 10 to 21 days after onset. Magnetic resonance imaging (MRI) scan may be diagnostic and should be used to guide surgical drainage if subperiosteal abscess is suspected. Laboratory evaluation is similar to that for septic arthritis. An orthopedist must be involved in the management, and input from an infectious diseases specialist is often helpful in the choice of antibiotic treatment. *S aureus* is far and away the most common pathogen associated with hematogenous osteomyelitis in children. *Pseudomonas aeruginosa* is a notable pathogen following nail puncture wounds involving the foot. Of note, children with sickle cell disease are especially at risk for osteomyelitis, and *Salmonella* is more often the responsible agent than *Staphylococcus*.

**Diskitis**, a relatively rare infection of the disk space, is most common in toddlers. Patients usually have a limp, or refuse to walk, sit, or perform any motion that requires range of motion of the affected region of the spine. Physical examination reveals pain over the involved disc space and decreased range of motion of the spine. The child generally does not seem ill or febrile, but may have increased inflammatory markers. The causative organism is usually *Staphylococcus aureus*, and treatment includes antibiotics and rest.[4]

## Malignancy or Tumor

**Leukemia** presents with musculoskeletal pain in 15% to 30% of cases, and is most common in the 2- to 5-year-old age group.[5] The limp is usually accompanied by systemic symptoms, including fever, pallor, and fatigue. History will often reveal pain that wakes the patient from sleep and is generally out of proportion to findings on clinical examination.[6] On physical examination, the child may have frank arthritis, bone tenderness, or bone pain. Laboratory evaluation will often show an abnormally high or low WBC count with anemia and thrombocytopenia. Thrombocytopenia and night waking can help differentiate malignancy from systemic juvenile idiopathic arthritis, which can also manifest as joint pain with systemic symptoms.[6] Plain radiographs may reveal leukemic lines, which appear as metaphyseal sclerotic bands, and osteopenia.

**Osteosarcoma** is a malignant tumor seen primarily in adolescents. Patients often report night waking with pain and have tenderness at the affected site. Plain films generally show an abnormality in the bone, most often in the metaphyses of long bones. Once osteosarcoma is suspected, the patient should be immediately referred to a pediatric oncologist.

**Osteoid osteoma** is a benign tumor seen throughout childhood and adolescence. Patients typically have localized pain that is worse in the evenings and responds dramatically to nonsteroidal anti-inflammatory drugs. If left untreated, the tumor can cause asymmetric limb growth. Plain radiographs typically reveal cortical thickening and sclerosis with a less than 1 cm radiolucent nidus (Figure 50-2). However, the nidus is not visible on plain radiographs in 15% of cases.[7] Therefore, if the index of suspicion is high, computed tomography (CT), MRI, or bone scan should be pursued to establish the diagnosis.

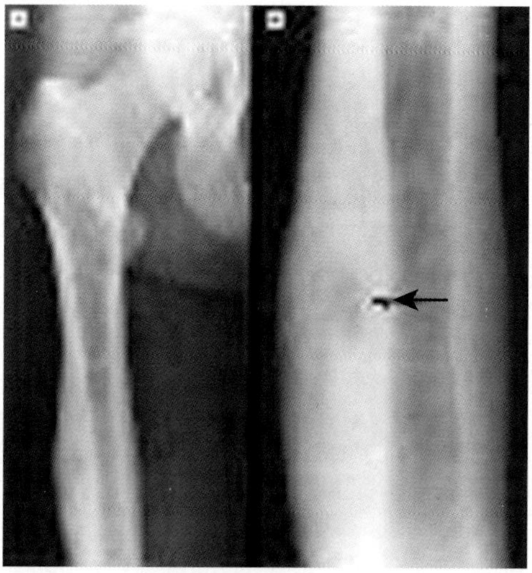

**Figure 50-2**

**Osteoid osteoma.** Views of the midshaft of the femur demonstrate a dense sclerotic lesion with cortical thickening containing a small oval lucent nidus (arrow). *(From Eisenberg RL.* An Atlas of Differential Diagnosis. *4th ed. Philadelphia, PA: Lippincott Williams & Wilkins; 2003. Copyright © 2003 Lippincott Williams & Wilkins.)*

## Skeletal Anomalies

**Congenital hip dysplasia** is most commonly diagnosed in infancy but can manifest as a delay in walking or as an abnormal gait in the toddler age group. On physical examination, there is typically decreased abduction and extension of the affected hip with 1-sided toe walking to compensate for an apparent leg-length discrepancy. Beyond infancy, the anomaly is visible on standing radiograph (Figure 50-3). In the newborn period an ultrasound is generally diagnostic. Treatment after the newborn period generally requires surgical intervention, and referral to a pediatric orthopedist is necessary.

**Discoid meniscus** is a condition most commonly seen in school-aged children, in which the lateral meniscus is discoid rather than crescent-shaped. Patients often report pain with activity. On physical examination, the physician may notice swelling of the knee or the inability to fully extend the knee, as well as tenderness along the lateral joint line. Plain radiographs are normal and MRI is required for diagnosis.

**Tarsal coalition**, or abnormal ossification between the talus or navicular and calcaneus, generally occurs in adolescents and is often associated with foot pain. The physical examination reveals a stiff, flat foot in eversion with contracture of the peroneal muscles. Tarsal coalition can often be diagnosed on oblique radiographs of the ankle joint; however, if the plain radiograph is negative but there is a high index of suspicion, CT may be diagnostic.[8] Management initially involves rest but may involve surgery in severe cases.

**Slipped capital femoral epiphysis (SCFE)** most commonly occurs in the 10 to 16 year age group and is more common in black than Hispanic children, and more common in Hispanic than white children. Obese adolescent males have a higher rate of SCFE as do children with hypothyroidism, low growth hormone level, pituitary tumors, craniopharyngioma, Down syndrome, renal osteodystrophy, and adiposogenital syndrome. It occurs when the femoral

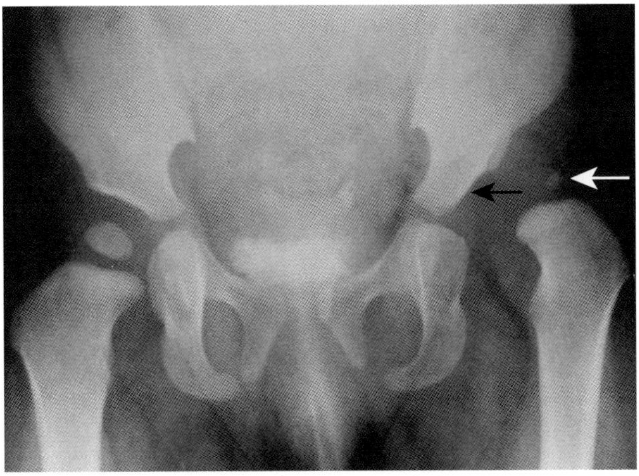

**Figure 50-3**

AP pelvis in a 14-month-old girl with an abnormal gait and difficulty walking. The left proximal femur is displaced superolaterally. The white arrow shows a small capital femoral epiphysis. The black arrow shows a steep acetabular roof. The patient had previously unrecognized developmental dysplasia of the left hip. Contrast in the bladder is from a voiding cystourethrogram. *(From Barkin RM, Barkin SZ, Barkin AZ. The limping child.* J Emerg Med. *2000;18[3]:331–339. Copyright © 2000, Elsevier, with permission.)*

epiphysis slides posteriorly, resulting in limited internal rotation of the hip. Symptom onset can be acute or insidious with weeks to months of intermittent vague symptoms before the patient seeks medical attention. Plain radiographs in the frog-leg position are generally diagnostic (Figure 50-4). Patients suspected of having SCFE should be referred to a pediatric orthopedist for surgical management.

### *Inflammatory Diseases*

**Juvenile idiopathic arthritis (JIA)** is the general term used to describe arthritis lasting for greater than 6 weeks in a child 16 years or younger with no known cause. The specific subtype of JIA is determined by the number of joints and specific joints involved, associated systemic symptoms, and HLA-B27 positivity. The age of onset varies by subtype. Symptoms at onset include joint pain and swelling, limp, morning preponderance of pain, and morning stiffness. With systemic JIA, patients may also report fever and rash. Physical examination reveals arthritis in 1 or more joints, most often the knee. Arthritis manifests as swelling, limitation of motion, warmth, with pain on motion and/or tenderness. If present, leg-length discrepancy and muscle atrophy of the affected extremity suggest a chronic process. Laboratory evaluation should be performed to rule out other causes of arthritis and to assess inflammatory markers. Lyme serology (only in those from or who visited endemic areas), antistreptolysin O titer, and parvovirus should be sent in the appropriate clinical setting as well as a CBC, ESR, and CRP. Once the diagnosis of JIA is made, additional laboratory tests including rheumatoid factor, anticyclic citrullinated peptide antibody, antinuclear antibody, and HLA-B27 typing can help clarify subtype. Plain radiographs may reveal a joint effusion or joint-space narrowing and erosions, but are often normal. If JIA is suspected, the patient should be referred to a pediatric rheumatologist for further workup and treatment.

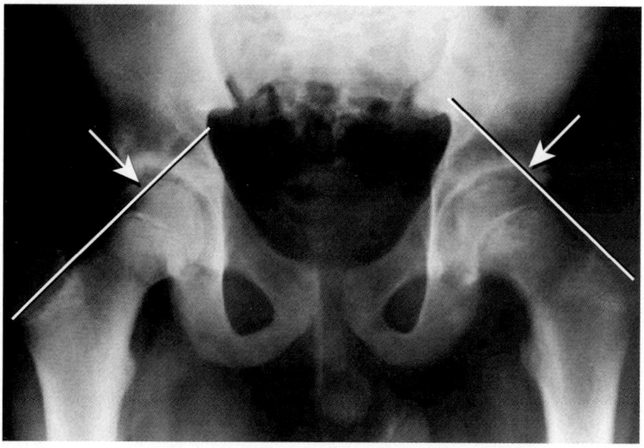

**Figure 50-4**

AP pelvis in a 13-year-old boy complaining of left hip pain and limp. A Klein line is drawn along the superolateral cortex of the femoral neck. The arrow shows posteromedial slippage of the left femoral epiphysis and widening of the physis, consistent with SCFE. *(From Barkin RM, Barkin SZ, Barkin AZ. The limping child.* J Emerg Med. *2000;18[3]:331–339. Copyright © 2000, Elsevier, with permission.)*

**Systemic lupus erythematosus** is a chronic autoimmune disease affecting multiple organs associated with antinuclear antibodies. It is more common in black, Asian, and Hispanic females. One of the many symptoms associated with lupus is a nonerosive arthritis which can present with a limp. If there are other symptoms of lupus present and the index of suspicion is high, laboratory workup should include an antinuclear antibody, CBC, and a urinalysis, as well as the work up mentioned above to rule out infectious causes of arthritis. If lupus is suspected, the patient should be referred to a pediatric rheumatologist for further workup and treatment.

**Transient synovitis** most often presents as hip arthritis in children between the ages of 3 and 8 years. It may be preceded by a viral infection. It is generally less symptomatic than septic arthritis, without associated fever, and inflammatory markers may be normal or only mildly elevated. Transient synovitis generally lasts for 7 to 10 days.[9] The patient often presents with a limp but is not ill-appearing. Physical examination commonly reveals pain on motion of the hip with mild limitation. Treatment generally includes rest and nonsteroidal anti-inflammatory medication, and symptoms generally resolve spontaneously.

**Juvenile dermatomyositis (JDM)** is a chronic autoimmune inflammatory myopathy and vasculopathy typically presenting with a heliotrope rash, Gottron papules (violet-colored inflammatory lesions over the knuckles) and proximal muscle weakness. Arthritis can also occur. Laboratory evaluation reveals elevated muscle enzymes, and noncontrast fat-suppressed MRI shows proximal muscle edema. Patients suspected of having JDM should be referred to a pediatric rheumatologist.

### *Neuromuscular Disorders*

**Cerebral Palsy (CP)**, a nonprogressive motor disorder that develops in the first 3 years of life, is the most common neurologic cause of limp in a child. The disease itself is highly variable. Physical examination may reveal spasticity of the knee or ankle joint with hyperreflexia and clonus. Patients with CP often benefit from evaluation by a pediatric neurologist and a pediatric physiatrist.

**Muscular dystrophy (MD)**, most often the X-linked Duchenne type, typically affects children between the ages of 2 and 5 years and often first manifests as delayed ambulation. The patient may demonstrate toe walking and a positive Gower sign (inability to rise from the floor without leaning on his legs with his hands), as well as proximal muscle weakness. On laboratory examination, the serum creatine phosphokinase is elevated. Patients suspected of having MD should be referred to a pediatric neurologist.

## ▶ EVALUATION

### *History*

The history is crucial in narrowing the differential diagnosis of a limp. The physician should first rule out any known trauma. If the mechanism of injury described by the parent or child does not correlate with the physical findings, nonaccidental trauma should be considered. Careful details regarding the duration of symptoms, exact location (asking the child to point with 1 finger may be helpful), acuity of onset, time of day of symptoms, quality of pain, and severity are often important for making a diagnosis.

**Duration**: An acute-onset limp is more likely to result from a mechanical problem, specific hip disorder, or a transient infectious process. Limp that lasts for longer than 6 weeks is more consistent with chronic causes such as JIA or malignancy.

**Location**: While asking for a specific location of the pain is important, consider that some pain in the lower extremity is referred. Hip pathology is generally reported as groin pain, but can also be referred to the knee. Pain over the greater trochanter is less likely from pathology of the hip itself and may represent inflammation of the trochanteric bursa (rare in children) or enthesitis. Pain specific to the shaft of the bone outside the setting of trauma is more concerning for malignancy or focal lesions and less consistent with joint pathology.

**Timing of symptoms**: Limp that occurs in the morning and resolves as the day goes on is characteristic of inflammatory joint pain, as seen in arthritis. Pain or limp that worsens with activity is more likely to be from biomechanical factors secondary to trauma or overuse. Unilateral pain that wakes the child at night is worrisome for malignancy or osteoid osteoma.

**Severity**: Pain that is severe or limits activity or function is concerning.

**Systemic symptoms**: Fever or weight loss is more suggestive of an infectious, oncologic, or inflammatory cause. Rash may give helpful clues to the diagnosis, as in the case of Lyme arthritis, parvovirus-associated arthritis, Henoch-Schönlein purpura, or systemic-onset JIA.

### *Physical Examination*

The extent and focus of the physical examination should be tailored to the individual based on the history obtained. If any indication of systemic illness exists, then a complete examination should be conducted. In the absence of systemic signs, most of the examination can be directed toward the back and lower extremities. Complaints of thigh or knee pain may be referred from a hip process and require thorough evaluation of the hip joint. Particularly with younger children, a great deal of useful information may be gained by opportunistic observation of the child before entering the examination room or when engaged in other activities.

### *Gait Examination*

A normal, mature, synchronous gait consists of a stance phase (weight-bearing phase), which begins with the heel-strike and plantar-flexion and ends with toe-off. This leads into the swing phase which starts with toe-off and finishes with heel-strike. This phase requires forward rotation, pelvic tilt, and lumbar spine stability to ensure a coordinated gait. Determining the phase of gait affected can help elucidate the cause (Table 50-2).

### *Joints and Musculoskeletal Examination*

General inspection of the lower extremities for evidence of skin breakdown, ecchymosis, erythema, or swelling may help localize the problem, using the nonaffected limb for comparison. A side-to-side disparity in leg length or muscle bulk suggests chronicity. Leg length can be measured from the anterior superior iliac spine to the distal end of the ipsilateral medial malleolus. Palpation of the extremity along all surfaces can also help localize focal pathology.

Each joint of the lower extremity should be evaluated independently for evidence of trauma or inflammation. Range of motion, size and contour should be symmetric, emphasizing the importance of side-to-side comparison. If joint involvement is suspected, the joints of the upper extremities and spine should be fully evaluated as well.

**Table 50-2**
**Gait Abnormalities and Associated Pathology**

| TYPE OF GAIT ABNORMALITY | CAUSE | DESCRIPTION | ASSOCIATED PATHOLOGY |
|---|---|---|---|
| Antalgic | Pain on weight bearing | Shortened stance on affected leg with shortened swing phase on contralateral side | Soft-tissue or skeletal trauma, chondromalacia patellae, arthritis, osteomyelitis, inguinal lymphadenitis, abdominal infection, Legg-Calvé-Perthes disease, slipped capital femoral epiphysis, bone neoplasia, rickets, tarsal coalitions |
| Vaulting | Joint pain or muscle weakness | Straight-legged walking (locking of knee causes the child to "vault" over leg) | Arthritis, skeletal dysplasias, congenital short femur, neurologic and neuromuscular disease, soft-tissue infection (dependent on affected joint/site) |
| Steppage | Peroneal nerve injury or weakness of the tibialis anterior muscle | Foot drop | Congenital talipes equinovarus, chronic pain syndromes |
| Trendelenburg | Hip abductor weakness or hip joint instability | Hip girdle drops on affected side, trunk moves over affected side to maintain balance | Hip arthritis, myositis, osteomyelitis, soft-tissue infection, abdominal infection (including psoas abscess, appendicitis, peritonitis), Legg-Calvé-Perthes disease, slipped capital femoral epiphysis, developmental dysplasia of the hip, neurologic disease, dermatomyositis and neuromuscular disease |

**Sacroiliac (SI) joint**. The sacroiliac joint is where the sacrum attaches to the ilium. On physical examination, the joint can be palpated directly under the dimples of Venus. The Gaenslen maneuver, in which the patient hangs 1 leg off the table and pulls the opposite knee towards the chest, is a test for inflammation of the sacroiliac joint (Figure 50-5). The test is considered positive if the patient has pain in the buttock opposite the knee that is being held. The SI joint is often involved in 1 of the subtypes of JIA, enthesitis-related JIA; alternatively, insidious infection of the SI joint can occur.

**Hip joint**. Children with hip pathology tend to hold the joint in a flexed, abducted, and externally rotated position, taking pressure off of the joint.[10] The hip joint can be isolated on physical examination using a maneuver called the logroll. The examiner places a hand on the mid-thigh and mid-shin of the patient and gently rolls the hip internally and externally, taking care not to simultaneously manipulate the knee joint.

**Knee joint**. The knee should be compared to the contralateral knee to assess for swelling, which often manifests as a loss of bony landmarks. The knee should be assessed for warmth and tenderness, as well as pain on motion or limitation of motion with either flexion or extension. Patellofemoral syndrome (formerly known as chondromalacea patella) can be assessed with the patellar inhibition test, whereby the examiner applies pressure to the patellar tendon proximal to the patella, and asks the patient to tense the quadriceps muscles. If this reproduces the patient's pain, it is considered a positive test. Anterior cruciate

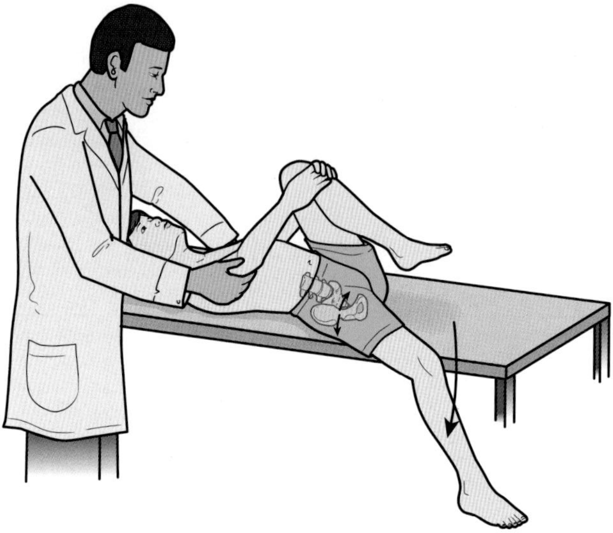

**Figure 50-5**
Pain with this maneuver is indicative of pathology within the sacroiliac joint.

ligamentous (ACL) injury can be assessed using the anterior drawer test: with the patient lying flat and the knee bent at 90 degrees, the examiner pulls the calf forward. If the tibial excursion is greater than normal, the test is considered positive and is suggestive of loss of ACL integrity. A Lachman maneuver is an appropriate substitute to evaluate the integrity of the ACL: the knee is placed at 30 degrees of flexion, and while the femur is stabilized with 1 of the examiner's hands the tibia is pulled anteriorly with the other hand (Figure 50-6). If there is no clear end point of anterior movement, or absence of a "clunk," the test is considered positive. The posterior drawer test is used to assess for injury to the posterior cruciate ligament (PCL), and is performed similarly to the anterior drawer test, but the shin is pushed posteriorly; excessive posterior movement is suggestive of PCL injury. Injury to the lateral collateral ligament (LCL) and medial collateral ligament (MCL) can be assessed by placing the patient flat on the back with the knee held at 30 degrees of flexion; the shin is shifted from side to side to test the integrity of the LCL (varus stress) and MCL (valgus stress). To assess for meniscal injuries, first palpate over the joint line for tenderness. The McMurray test examines the integrity of the medial and lateral menisci. To test the medial meniscus, the patient lies in the supine position with the knee in full flexion; with 1 hand, the examiner stabilizes the joint, applying pressure to the lateral aspect of the joint providing valgus stress, while with the opposite hand the examiner holds the heel of the patient and laterally rotates the tibia while extending the knee. To assess lateral meniscal integrity, the medial meniscus is stabilized by 1 hand while the tibia is rotated medially and the knee is extended by the other hand.[11] If the patient has pain or the examiner feels a snap or click, the test is positive.

**Ankle.** The ankle is comprised of 2 joints, the tibiotalar joint and the subtalar joint. The tibiotaler joint is responsible for dorsiflexion and plantar flexion, and the subtalar joint is responsible for inversion and eversion. Pain over the Achilles tendon or at the sites of

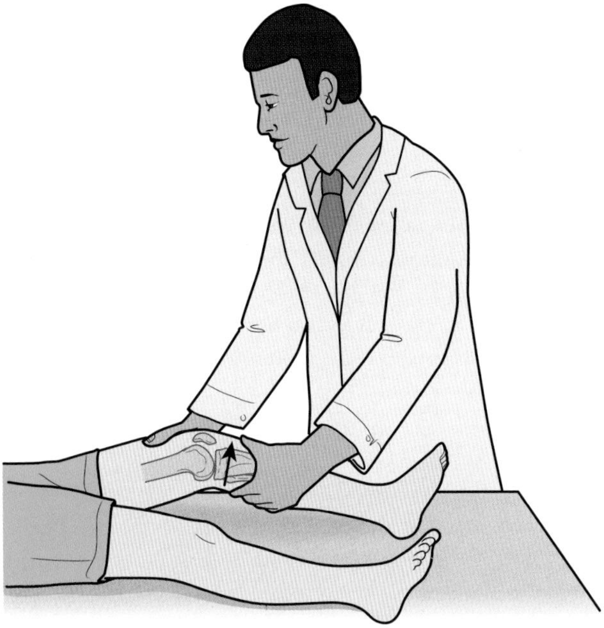

**Figure 50-6**
With one hand stabilizing the femur, the proximal tibia is moved forward with the other hand. The absence of a distinct endpoint of forward tibial movement is suggestive of ACL injury.

attachment of the plantar fascia may be suggestive of a tendonitis, or in the setting of chronic pain, may be associated with enthesitis related to JIA.

### General Examination

On initial examination, the most important determination is whether or not the patient is ill-appearing, as this may be associated with more urgent problems such as a septic joint or a systemic disease. The patient should be assessed for any rashes or lesions suggestive of specific disorders. A thorough neurologic assessment should be performed, including an evaluation of muscle strength and function, sensation, and reflexes.

### Laboratory Testing

In cases of known trauma, blood testing is often not necessary. A CBC and measure of acute phase reactants are useful if inflammatory or infectious causes are suspected (see Differential Diagnosis for specific laboratory abnormalities by disease). If a septic joint is likely, joint aspiration should be performed and blood cultures should be obtained prior to initiation of antibiotics. Antinuclear antibody (ANA) testing in the absence of objective evidence of arthritis is not necessary unless there are additional clinical findings suggestive of autoimmune disease (vasculitic/malar rash, palatal ulcers, hair loss, serositis, renal or CNS disease). In the setting of chronic arthritis, the ANA is useful to delineate risk of developing uveitis, but it is not diagnostic. Approximately 20% of healthy children have a positive ANA without any underlying disease. If arthritis is seen on physical examination and the history is suggestive of the associated diseases, Lyme titers, gonococcal cultures, parvovirus IgG and IgM, anti-DNASE B and antistreptolysin O titers may be warranted.

### *Imaging*

#### Radiographs

Plain-film radiographs remain an important tool in the evaluation of limp, particularly in diagnosing fractures, hip disease, spinal abnormalities, and foot disease (eg, tarsal coalition). Obtaining at least 2 views of the affected area is essential; with suspected hip disease, the 2 views should be the anteroposterior (AP) and frog-leg lateral (Lauenstein) views of the pelvis. Diagnosis-specific radiographic findings are reviewed in the Differential Diagnosis section.

#### Ultrasound

Ultrasound can be used to assess musculoskeletal pathology. Joint effusions, synovial thickening, and increased blood flow seen by power Doppler are suggestive of underlying inflammation. While the cause of inflammation cannot be determined by this method, it may be a useful adjuvant to the history and physical examination.[12]

#### Bone Scintigraphy

Bone scintigraphy measures the uptake of technetium-99m, which is increased at sites of high bone turnover. It is therefore most useful in the diagnosis of osteomyelitis, diskitis, stress fractures, osteoid osteomas, Legg-Calvé-Perthes disease, and neoplasm, especially if the location of the pathology is difficult to identify.[13] However, MRI is often preferred to bone scintigraphy to spare children radiation exposure and to provide more specific information.

#### Computed Tomography

Computed tomography is most useful for evaluating boney pathology, including tarsal coalition, spondylolisthesis, spondylolysis, or osteoid osteoma. However, it exposes the patient to a high dose of radiation and its use should therefore be limited to situations where other imaging modalities are inadequate or unavailable.

#### Magnetic Resonance Imaging

Magnetic resonance imaging offers information about bone formation and inflammation as well as soft tissues without exposing the child to radiation, and is therefore the imaging modality of choice for clarifying difficult diagnoses. In cases of arthritis, osteomyelitis, diskitis, stress fractures, osteoid osteomas, Legg-Calvé-Perthes disease, and neoplasm, MRI is often crucial to diagnosis.

## When to Refer

Limp is a common presenting complaint in pediatric emergency departments and primary care offices. History and physical examination are crucial to diagnosing the cause of a limp, and imaging is an important adjuvant to the physical examination. There are very few emergent causes of limp, but they do occur, and suspicion of any of the following causes does warrant referral:

- Septic joint
- Malignancy
- Surgical cause (eg, appendicitis, psoas abscess)
- Serious fracture

Once these emergent causes of limp have been excluded, if the workup is negative, an observation period of 1 to 2 weeks may be appropriate. Following the observation period, if the diagnosis is still unclear, referral to an orthopedist, rheumatologist, or neurologist may be necessary depending on the clinical scenario.

## REFERENCES


1. Perry DC, Bruce C. Evaluating the child who presents with an acute limp. *BMJ.* 2010;341:c4250
2. Huttenlocher A, Newman TB. Evaluation of the erythrocyte sedimentation rate in children presenting with limp, fever, or abdominal pain. *Clin Pediatr (Phila).* 1997;36:339–344
3. Kang SN, Sanghera T, Mangwani J, Paterson JM, Ramachandran M. The management of septic arthritis in children: systematic review of the English language literature. *J Bone Joint Surg Br.* 2009;91:1127–1133
4. Gouliouris T, Aliyu SH, Brown NM. Spondylodiscitis: update on diagnosis and management. *J Antimicrob Chemother.* 2010;65(Suppl 3):iii11–iii24
5. Marwaha RK, Kulkarni KP, Bansal D, Trehan A. Acute lymphoblastic leukemia masquerading as juvenile rheumatoid arthritis: diagnostic pitfall and association with survival. *Ann Hematol.* 2010;89: 249–254
6. Jones OY, Spencer CH, Bowyer SL, et al. A multicenter case-control study on predictive factors distinguishing childhood leukemia from juvenile rheumatoid arthritis. *Pediatrics.* 2006;117:e840–e844
7. Lee EH, Shafi M, Hui JH. Osteoid osteoma: a current review. *J Pediatr Orthop.* 2006;26: 695–700
8. Bohne WH. Tarsal coalition. *Curr Opin Pediatr.* 2001;13:29–35
9. Caird MS, Flynn JM, Leung YL, et al. Factors distinguishing septic arthritis from transient synovitis of the hip in children. A prospective study. *J Bone Joint Surg Am.* 2006;88:1251–1257
10. Renshaw TS. The child who has a limp. *Pediatr Rev.* 1995;16:458–465
11. Magee DJ. Knee. In: Magee DJ, ed. *Orthopedic Physical Assessment.* 5th ed. St. Louis, MO: Saunders; 2008:727–843
12. Jacobson JA. Musculoskeletal ultrasound and MRI: which do I choose? *Semin Musculoskelet Radiol.* 2005;9:135–149
13. Myers MT, Thompson GH. Imaging the child with a limp. *Pediatr Clin North Am.* 1997;44:637–658

# Chapter 51

# Loss of Appetite

*Nancy McGreal, MD; Martin H. Ulshen, MD*

Loss of appetite (anorexia) is a common symptom in children. Acute illness in childhood is often associated with transient loss of appetite. Prolonged loss of appetite associated with poor weight gain or loss of weight usually signifies a serious chronic illness, either organic or psychogenic.

## ▶ PATHOPHYSIOLOGIC FEATURES

The mechanisms that regulate hunger and satiety are complex and redundant, remaining incompletely understood.[1,2] Appetite is regulated by multiple nuclei and signaling pathways in the hypothalamus, now known to be much more complex than the previously described *satiety center* in the ventromedial hypothalamus and the *feeding center* in the lateral hypothalamus. The hypothalamus detects peripheral signals, including gut hormones and blood-borne nutrients. Vagal nerve afferents from the gastrointestinal (GI) tract and hepatoportal region terminate in the brainstem, and information is conveyed to the hypothalamus. Both appetite-stimulating and appetite-suppressing neuropeptides are secreted in the hypothalamus. Central control of appetite is influenced by anticipation of a pleasurable meal, visual and taste sensations, ambient temperature, and changes in blood levels of glucose or other nutrients, as well as by limbic signals from higher central nervous system (CNS) regions. Initiators of satiety include vagal input from gastric distention, cholecystokinin from the intestine and CNS, and other humoral factors, including insulin, glucagon-like peptide-1, pancreatic polypeptides, and endorphins. Each individual may have a set point for body fat content. Deviations may cause alterations in diet intake, a process apparently mediated by the interaction of the hormones leptin, produced in adipose cells, and ghrelin, produced by endocrine cells in the stomach and GI tract, with receptors in the hypothalamus.[3,4] Leptin suppresses and ghrelin stimulates appetite. Changes in the levels of these hormones influence the release of CNS neuropeptides, including neuropeptide Y, melanocyte-stimulating hormone, and the orexins.

Cytokines are key mediators of the appetite suppression that occurs with acute and chronic illnesses.[5,6] Interleukin-1β, interleukin-6, and tumor necrosis factor-α, for example, have been shown to induce anorexia by acting directly on the hypothalamus.[7] Effects on the peripheral nervous system and on hormone levels occur as well.

## ▶ DIFFERENTIAL DIAGNOSIS

When considering anorexia, the physician must first separate complaints based on unrealistic parental dietary expectations from justified parental concern over a child's diminished nutritional intake. In the former situation, the child is typically growing well and appropriately thriving. Although significant GI disease commonly leads to poor appetite, anorexia may be the result of disease that is distant from the bowel. In the newborn period, poor oral intake by an infant who is developmentally capable of feeding may be the first indication of a major disorder, such as sepsis, meningitis, urinary tract infection, congenital viral infection, a GI anomaly, CNS disease, renal failure, or an inborn error of metabolism.

During infancy, a wide spectrum of causes can account for inadequate caloric intake. An acute infectious disease is a common cause of transient anorexia in infants. If no obvious explanation exists for poor feeding, then the pediatrician should always consider the possibility of an oral disease (eg, thrush), gastroesophageal reflux disease, eosinophilic esophagitis, renal tubular acidosis, dietary protein intolerance, or a neurologic disorder. Occasionally, an infant will lack interest in feeding from the first days of life but in every other respect will appear normal; such an infant may well need enteral feeding supplementation.[8] Emotional deprivation is a common cause of failure to thrive; a thorough social history is essential to the evaluation. Early observation of parent–infant interaction in the hospital, including feeding techniques, may be helpful. An infant who has not received oral feedings for a prolonged period because of medical problems (eg, esophageal disease, short bowel syndrome) may not be interested when feedings are introduced by mouth. The mother and infant may require training (typically provided by an occupational therapist, physical therapist, or speech pathologist) and gradual advancement of an oral diet.

Box 51-1 presents a list of causes of loss of appetite that are applicable to both infants and children. Generally, the best approach to anorexia is to treat the underlying condition.

## ▶ EVALUATION

In formula-fed infants, a state of chronically inadequate caloric intake can be identified objectively by computing the total calories ingested, most of which come from formula, and comparing this total with the estimated caloric requirements for weight. Such computation is more difficult with breastfed infants, although intake may be established by weighing the infant before and after feedings. If the nursing infant has a reduced intake, the physician must establish whether maternal milk production is inadequate or the infant is too weak or disinterested to nurse.

In older children and adolescents, an adequate evaluation of nutritional intake requires careful calorie counts. If the possibility of malabsorption is a concern, a calorie count and 72-hour stool collection for fat analysis may be ordered. Separating children who have poor appetites from children who do not eat for fear of worsening their symptoms is important from the outset. Children with abdominal pain from chronic inflammatory bowel disease or chronic constipation may not eat because doing so increases their pain. Similarly, children with chronic diarrhea may find that eating less leads to less frequent stooling. These children may actually not have anorexia, and treatment aimed at improving the other symptoms may result in rapid improvement in oral intake.

## ▶ TREATMENT

Enlisting the help of a dietitian to plan diets can be useful for maximizing nutritional intake in older children. Nutritional supplements may be indicated, either high-calorie milkshakes or commercial high-calorie supplements. Several medications, including cyproheptadine

BOX 51-1

## *Causes of Decreased Appetite in Infants and Children*

### ORGANIC DISEASE

- Infections (acute or chronic)
- Neurologic causes
  - Cerebral palsy
  - Congenital degenerative disease (eg, neurodegenerative disorders, spino-muscular atrophy, muscular dystrophy)
  - Hypothalamic lesion
  - Increased intracranial pressure, including a brain tumor
  - Static encephalopathy
- GI causes
  - Oral or esophageal lesions (eg, thrush, herpes simplex, dental caries, ankyloglossia)
  - Gastroesophageal reflux
  - Eosinophilic esophagitis
  - Dietary protein intolerance
  - Bowel obstruction (especially with gastric or intestinal distention)
  - Inflammatory bowel disease
  - Celiac disease
  - Constipation
  - Esophageal motility disorder (eg, cricopharyngeal dysfunction, achalasia, connective tissue disorder)
- Cardiac causes
  - Congestive heart failure or cyanotic heart disease
- Metabolic causes
  - Renal failure, renal tubular acidosis, or both
  - Liver failure
  - Inborn errors of metabolism
  - Lead poisoning
- Nutritional causes
  - Marasmus
  - Iron deficiency
  - Zinc deficiency
- Drugs
  - Morphine
  - Digitalis
  - Antimetabolites
  - Methylphenidate
  - Amphetamines
  - Topiramate
- Prolonged restriction of oral feedings, beginning in the neonatal period
- Tumor
- Chronic febrile conditions (eg, rheumatoid arthritis, rheumatic fever)

### PSYCHOLOGICAL FACTORS

- Anxiety, fear, depression, mania (limbic influence on the hypothalamus)
- Avoidance of symptoms associated with meals (abdominal pain, nausea, diarrhea, bloating, urgency, dumping syndrome)
- Anorexia nervosa
- Excessive weight loss and food aversion in athletes, simulating anorexia nervosa

and megestrol acetate, have been shown to stimulate appetite. Although cyproheptadine does not seem to affect appetite in all children treated, when successful, the response is dramatic.[9] Megestrol acetate,[6] a progesterone derivative, has been administered for cancer-related anorexia, primarily in adults. Its potential side effects on the endocrine system include adrenal insufficiency. Weight gained with megestrol acetate may be, to a large extent, from increased fat mass. Eicosapenteanoic acid, an omega-3 fatty acid, has been evaluated in the treatment of adult and pediatric cancer-associated anorexia with equivocal results.[10] In some disorders, such as congenital heart disease, initial nasogastric or nasoduodenal infusion of nutrients may be necessary to promote growth.[11] If prolonged supplementation proves necessary, a gastrostomy tube can be placed. Parenteral nutrition may be indicated in specific situations. However, expertise with this modality and close supervision are required, and caretakers need special training if the parenteral nutrition is to be provided at home. Refeeding after severe malnutrition requires careful consideration of potential cardiac and metabolic complications.[12]

## When to Refer

- Loss of appetite without an obvious explanation, especially in association with weight loss or failure to thrive
- Anorexia nervosa

## When to Admit

- Weight loss or lack of weight gain that is unresponsive to outpatient management
- Requirement to initiate enteral or parenteral feeding because of inadequate oral intake

### REFERENCES


1. Plata-Salaman C. Regulation of hunger and satiety in man. *Dig Dis Sci.* 1991;9(5):253–268
2. Zac-Varghese S, Tan T, Bloom SR. Hormonal interactions between gut and brain. *Discov Med.* 2010;10(55):543–552
3. Auwerx J, Staels B. Leptin. *Lancet.* 1998;351(9104):737–742
4. Zigman JM, Elmquist JK. Minireview: From anorexia to obesity—the yin and yang of body weight control. *Endocrinology.* 2003;144(9):3749–3756
5. Konsman JP, Dantzer R. How the immune and nervous systems interact during disease-associated anorexia. *Nutrition.* 2001;17(7–8):664–668
6. Plata-Salaman CR. Cytokines and anorexia: a brief overview. *Semin Oncol.* 1998;25(1 Suppl 1): 64–72
7. Deboer MD, Marks DL. Cachexia: lessons from melanocortin antagonism. *Trends Endocrinol Metab.* 2006;17(5):199–204
8. Lichtman SN, Maynor A, Rhoads JM. Failure to imbibe in otherwise normal infants. *J Pediatr Gastroenterol Nutr.* 2000;30(4):467–470
9. Homnick DN, Marks JH, Hare KL, Bonnema SK. Long-term trial of cyproheptadine as an appetite stimulant in cystic fibrosis. *Pediatr Pulmonol.* 2005;40(3):251–256
10. Dewey A, Baughan C, Dean T, Higgins B, Johnson I. Eicosapentaenoic acid (EPA, an omega-3 fatty acid from fish oils) for the treatment of cancer cachexia. *Cochrane Database Syst Rev.* 2007;24(1):CD004597
11. Vanderhoof JA , Hofschire PJ, Baluff MA, et al. Continuous enteral feedings. An important adjunct to the management of complex congenital heart disease. *Am J Dis Child.* 1982;136(9):825–827
12. Solomon SM, Kirby DF. The refeeding syndrome: a review. *J Parenter Enteral Nutr.* 1990; 14(1):90–97

# Chapter 52

# Lymphadenopathy

*Geoffrey A. Weinberg, MD; George B. Segel, MD; Caroline Breese Hall, MD*[†]

Enlargement of 1 or more lymph nodes is a common finding in childhood. Lymphadenopathy may be defined as any lymph node enlargement; all lymph nodes that are palpable are technically considered enlarged. However, nodes in the cervical chain, occipital, and inguinal areas drain regions that are commonly infected in childhood and are often mildly enlarged (<1 cm in diameter) in children who are otherwise healthy.

The clinically relevant problems in assessing lymphadenopathy are whether any lymph node or lymph node aggregate or chain is abnormal and requires further assessment; if abnormal, whether the nodes are benign, primarily inflammatory, or malignant; and what the appropriate evaluation, diagnosis, and management should be.

## ▶ CHARACTERISTICS OF LYMPH NODE ENLARGEMENT

### *Components of the Lymphatic System*

The lymphatic system includes not only lymph nodes but also the spleen, thymus, tonsils, Waldeyer ring, appendix, and Peyer patches in the intestine. Potentially palpable lymph node groups and their drainage areas are listed in Table 52-1. The location of the lymphatics of the head and neck and lymph node drainage are shown in Figure 52-1 and may serve as a guide to palpation of these superficial nodes.

### *Lymph Node Features*

Abnormalities of the palpable lymph nodes are assessed by noting the node's size, location, mobility, tenderness, erythema (inflammatory reaction), and consistency and whether it is matted. Nodes smaller than 1 cm are often found in the cervical chain and in the femoral areas. They are often somewhat larger in the inguinal areas. Similarly, nodes smaller than 0.5 cm may be palpated in the occipital, postauricular (mastoid), and axillary chains. Small occipital and postauricular nodes are common in infants but not older children, whereas cervical and inguinal nodes are common after age 2 years. The distribution by age is shown in Table 52-2. In the submental or submaxillary regions, intraoral or facial infections may enlarge the nodes to more than 1 cm. However, finding lymph nodes of any size in the supraclavicular or epitrochlear areas is unusual. Thus, lymph nodes of the same size observed in 2 different regions may have markedly different implications. For example, a 1-cm node in the cervical region of a 5-year-old child is very likely benign, whereas a 1-cm supraclavicular node requires a biopsy because it is unlikely to result from superficial inflammatory disease and may reflect intrathoracic or intraabdominal malignancy. Noninflammatory nodes greater than 2 to 2.5 cm require biopsy.

[†]Deceased

**Table 52-1**
**Correlations Between Lymph Node Locations and Disease Origin**

| LYMPH NODE GROUPS | AREA OF DRAINAGE |
|---|---|
| Occipital | Posterior scalp, neck |
| Anterior auricular, parotid | Lateral pinna, frontotemporal, eyelids |
| Posterior auricular | Mastoid area and pinna |
| Superior (anterior) cervical | Posterior scalp and neck, tongue, pharynx, larynx |
| Inferior (posterior) cervical | Posterior scalp, neck, pectorals, and arm |
| Submental | Apex of tongue and lower lip |
| Submaxillary | Tongue, buccal cavity, lips, and cheek |
| Supraclavicular | *Right:* Inferior neck and mediastinum<br>*Left:* Inferior neck, mediastinum, and upper abdomen |
| Mediastinal, hilar | *Anterior:* Thymus, pericardium<br>*Posterior:* Esophagus, pericardium, liver surface<br>*Hilar:* Lungs |
| Axillary | Greater part of arm and shoulder; superficial, anterior, and lateral thoracic and upper abdominal wall |
| Epitrochlear | Hand, forearm, and elbow |
| Abdominal | Abdominal organs to various mesenteric nodes and to retroperitoneal nodes |
| Inguinal, femoral | Leg and genitalia |

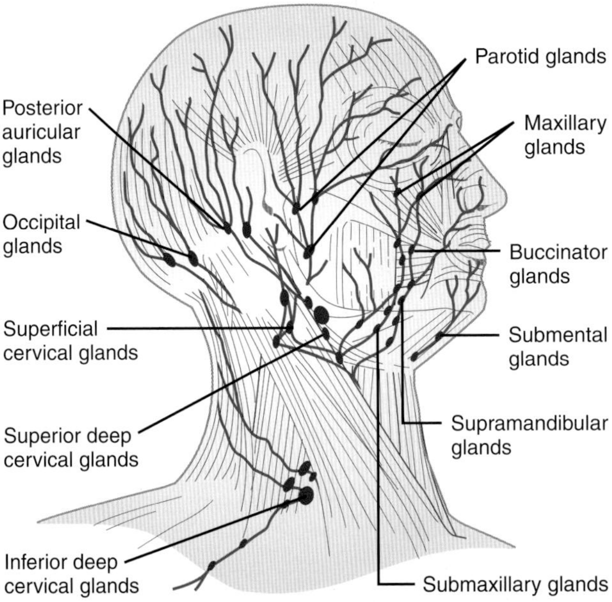


**Figure 52-1**
Lymph nodes and lymphatics of the head and neck. The nodes in the region below the mandible are designated *submaxillary*. (*Reproduced from* Anatomy of the Human Body by Henry Gray, *20th edition, with permission from Bartleby.com, Inc.*)

**Table 52–2**
**Prevalence of Lymphadenopathy by Age**

| | | PALPABLE NODES | | | | | | | | | |
|---|---|---|---|---|---|---|---|---|---|---|---|
| | | OCCIPITAL | | POSTAURICULAR | | SUBMANDIBULAR | | CERVICAL | | NO PALPABLE NODES | |
| AGE | NUMBER OF PATIENTS | NUMBER | (%) | NUMBER | (%) | NUMBER | (%) | NUMBER | (%) | NUMBER | (%) |
| 0–6 mo | 52 | 17 | (32) | 7 | (13) | 1 | (2) | 1 | (2) | 32 | (62) |
| 7–12 mo | 31 | 8 | (26) | 4 | (13) | 1 | (3) | 8 | (26) | 16 | (52) |
| 13–23 mo | 39 | 4 | (10) | 3 | (7) | 7 | (18) | 11 | (28) | 20 | (52) |
| 2 years | 35 | 3 | (8) | 2 | (6) | 7 | (20) | 16 | (45) | 11 | (32) |
| 3 years | 27 | 2 | (7) | 0 | (0) | 7 | (26) | 9 | (33) | 11 | (41) |
| 4 years | 20 | 0 | (0) | 0 | (0) | 5 | (25) | 11 | (55) | 7 | (35) |
| 5 years | 19 | 0 | (0) | 1 | (5) | 4 | (21) | 12 | (63) | 5 | (26) |
| **Total** | **223** | **34** | **(15)** | **17** | **(8)** | **32** | **(14)** | **68** | **(30)** | **102** | **(45)** |

Reproduced with permission from Herzog LW. Prevalence of lymphadenopathy of the head and neck in infants and children. *Clin Pediatr.* 1983;22:485–487.

Fluctuance and signs of inflammation surrounding a group of enlarged lymph nodes are helpful in reaching a diagnosis, particularly if an infectious source is found distal to the node area. These findings strongly suggest an infectious, primarily bacterial cause (Table 52-3), usually requiring systemic antibiotic therapy. If no inflammation is found, the consistency is firm, and the nodes are not mobile, then an underlying malignancy may be present, such as a lymphoma, sarcoma, or neuroblastoma. Hard, fixed nodes are seen more often in adults who have metastatic carcinoma. The nodes of Hodgkin disease and lymphoma are more matted than hard, although nodes associated with neuroblastoma, rhabdomyosarcoma, and other childhood malignancies may mimic the findings in adults.

## ▶ DIFFERENTIAL DIAGNOSIS

The major differential diagnostic categories for enlarged lymph nodes include infectious (inflammatory), neoplastic, immunologic, storage, and other diseases. Table 52-3 provides a summary of the common and unusual conditions associated with lymphadenopathy.

### *Infections*

Infectious problems may be localized or systemic. If localized, the primary site of infection draining to the involved lymph node area should be identified (see Table 52-1). Lymph nodes enlarge most often in reaction to a localized or generalized infection, but a node can itself become intrinsically infected, resulting in lymphadenitis.

The common pyogenic bacteria (*Staphylococus aureus* and *Streptococcus pyogenes*), atypical mycobacteria, and *Bartonella henselae* (cat-scratch disease) are most likely to cause localized adenopathy. Generalized adenopathy or regional adenopathy associated with adenopathy

**Table 52-3**
**Entities Associated With Lymphadenopathy[a]**

| | GENERALIZED | CERVICAL | OTHER REGIONAL |
|---|---|---|---|
| **INFECTIONS** | | | |
| ***Viral*** | | | |
| Respiratory viruses (adenoviruses, picornaviruses, respiratory syncytial virus [RSV], parainfluenza, influenza, coronaviruses) | | 1–3+ | |
| Epstein-Barr virus (EBV) | 2–3+ | 3+ | + |
| Cytomegalovirus (CMV) | 2+ | 2+ | |
| Primary human herpesvirus type 6 (HHV-6) | | + | 2–3+ (postoccipital) |
| Parvovirus B19 | 1–2+ | | 2+ |
| Human immunodeficiency virus (HIV) | 2–3+ | + | + |
| Rubella | 2+ | 3+ | + |
| Rubeola | 1–2+ | 3+ | |
| Varicella zoster | 1–2+ | + | + |

**Table 52-3**
**Entities Associated With Lymphadenopathy—cont'd**

| | GENERALIZED | CERVICAL | OTHER REGIONAL |
|---|---|---|---|
| Herpes simplex virus (HSV) | | 3+ | 1–2+ (genital infection) |
| HHV-8 | 2–3+ | 2–3+ | + |
| Hepatitis A | + | 2+ | |
| **Bacterial** | | | |
| *Staphylococcus aureus* | | 3+ | 2–3+ |
| *Streptococcus pyogenes* | + | 3+ | 2–3+ |
| *Bartonella henselae* (cat-scratch disease) | + | | 2–3+ |
| *Bartonella bacilliformis* (Oroya fever, verruga peruana) | 3+ | 3+ | 3+ |
| *Yersinia enterocolitica* | + | | 3+ |
| *Salmonella typhi* | 2–3+ | | 2+ |
| Tularemia | + | 3+ | 2+ |
| Brucellosis | 2–3+ | + | + |
| Dental, gingival infections | | 2–3+ | 2–3+ |
| Postanginal sepsis *(Fusobacterium)* | | 2–3+ | |
| *Mycobacterium tuberculosis* | + | 2–3+ | 2–3+ |
| Atypical mycobacteria | | 2–3+ | 2–3+ |
| Syphilis | 2–3+ | + | + |
| Lyme disease | | | + |
| Leptospirosis | 3+ | + | + |
| **Rickettsia/Chlamydia** | | | |
| Lymphogranuloma venereum | | | 3+ |
| Ehrlichiosis | 2–3+ | | |
| *Rickettsia tsutsugamushi* | 3+ | 2–3+ | 3+ |
| **Protozoan** | | | |
| Toxoplasmosis | + | 3+ | + |
| Malaria | + | | |
| **Parasitic** *(Toxocara canis, Toxocara cati, Baylisascaris procyonis, Trichinella spiralis,* filariaris*)* | 1–2+ | + | 1–2+ |
| Myiasis | | + | 1–2+ |
| **Fungal** | | | |
| Histoplasmosis | 1–3+ | + | 1–2+ |
| Coccidioidomycosis | 1–3+ | + | 1–2+ |
| Tinea capitis | | | 2–3+ |
| **IMMUNIZATIONS** | | | |
| Viral | + | | + |
| Typhoid | + | | + |
| Bacille Calmette-Guérin (BCG) | | | 1–3+ |

*Continued*

**Table 52-3**
**Entities Associated With Lymphadenopathy—cont'd**

| | GENERALIZED | CERVICAL | OTHER REGIONAL |
|---|---|---|---|
| **NEOPLASTIC** | | | |
| Leukemia | 1–2+ | | |
| Lymphoma | 1–3+ | 2–3+ | 2–3+ |
| Hodgkin disease | | 2–3+ | 2–3+ |
| Metastatic, solid tumors (neuroblastoma, Wilms tumor, Ewing sarcoma, rhabdomyosarcoma) | 1–2+ | | 1–2+ |
| **HISTIOCYTOSES** | | | |
| Langerhans cell histiocytosis | | 1–3+ | |
| Malignant histiocytosis | | 1–2+ | 1–2+ |
| Sinus histiocytosis (Rosai-Dorfman disease) | | 3+ | |
| Hemophagocytic syndromes | 1–2+ | 2+ | |
| **IMMUNOLOGIC** | | | |
| Deficiency syndromes | 1–2+ | 1–2+ | 2–3+ |
| Autoimmune lymphoproliferative syndrome (ALPS) | 2–3+ | | |
| Serum sickness | 2+ | + | + |
| Ommen syndrome | 1–2+ | + | + |
| Juvenile idiopathic arthritis | 1–2+ | + | + |
| Atopic disease, eczema | 2–3+ | 2+ | 2–3+ |
| Castleman disease | 1–3+ | 3+ | 2–3+ |
| **MEDICATIONS (Phenytoin and others)** | **1–2+** | | |
| **STORAGE DISEASES (Gaucher disease, Niemann-Pick disease)** | **2–3+** | | **1–3+** |
| **GRANULOCYTE DEFECTS** | | | |
| Chronic granulomatous disease | + | 1–2+ | 2–3+ |
| Leukocyte adhesion deficiencies | | 1–3+ | 1–3+ |
| Chédiak-Higashi anomaly | | 1–3+ | 1–3+ |
| **OTHER** | | | |
| Kawasaki disease | | 2–3+ | |
| Hemoglobinopathic conditions | + | 1–2+ | |
| Hemophilia with HIV | 2–3+ | + | + |
| Sarcoidosis | 2–3+ | + | 1–2+ |
| Gianotti-Crosti syndrome | 3+ | + | + |
| Necrotizing lymphadenitis (Kikuchi-Fujimoto disease) | + | 2–3+ | 2–3+ |
| Insect bites | | + | + |
| Kimura disease | | 2–3+ | 1–2+ |
| Addison disease | 1–2+ | | |
| Hyperthyroidism | 1–3+ | | |

[a]Numbers represent relative prominence and incidence of lymphadenopathy.

BOX 52-1

## *Anatomic Locations of Mediastinal Masses*

**ANTERIOR MEDIASTINUM**

- Lymphoma
- Thymoma
- Malignant germ cell tumor
- Benign teratoma
- Substernal goiter
- Thymic hyperplasia
- Thymic cyst
- Mesenchymal tumors

**MIDDLE MEDIASTINUM**

- Lymphoma
- Tuberculosis
- Sarcoidosis
- Histoplasmosis
- Castleman disease
- Bronchogenic cyst
- Sarcoma

**POSTERIOR MEDIASTINUM**

- Neuroblastoma
- Ganglioneuroma
- Neurofibroma
- Primitive neuroectodermal tumor
- Sarcoma
- Germ cell tumor
- Schwannoma
- Duplication cyst

elsewhere is more likely caused by infections from viruses, spirochetes, or, sometimes, *Toxoplasma* spp. *Mycobacterium tuberculosis* may produce localized or multiple sites of adenitis. Fungal infections, such as histoplasmosis, occasionally cause generalized lymphadenopathy when disseminated, but most fungal infections, if associated with adenopathy at all, produce regional enlargement.

### *Neoplastic Diseases*

Primary neoplastic diseases are the other major consideration in both localized and generalized adenopathy. Included in this category are lymphomas, leukemia, histiocytosis, and metastases from solid tumors such as neuroblastoma, Wilms tumor, Ewing sarcoma, and rhabdomyosarcoma. If a mediastinal mass is identified, then the diagnostic considerations vary with the anatomic location within the mediastinum (Box 52-1).

### *Immunologic and Inflammatory Diseases*

Generalized lymphadenopathy also may be associated with chronic inflammatory conditions, such as juvenile idiopathic arthritis, other autoimmune diseases, and sarcoidosis; with reactions to certain drugs, such as phenytoin and isoniazid; or with serum sickness. Unusual causes, such as hyperthyroidism and Addison disease, also should be included in the differential diagnosis of generalized adenopathy.

## ▶ ASSESSMENT

The evaluation of lymphadenopathy is summarized in Table 52-4 and discussed in detail below.

### *History, Physical Examination, and Chest Imaging*

The history and physical examination may reveal a source of a localized infection, such as a dental abscess, mastoiditis, scalp infection, insect bite, or cat scratch. Alternatively, systemic diseases, such as infectious mononucleosis, juvenile idiopathic arthritis, and infection

**Table 52-4**
**Evaluation of Lymphadenopathy**

| | | |
|---|---|---|
| **History** | Exposures (animals, foods, travel)<br>Medications<br>Weight loss<br>Fevers<br>Night sweats<br>Bone pain | |
| **Physical examination** | Palpable node areas<br>Tonsils<br>Spleen and liver | |
| **Imaging** | Chest radiograph<br>Ultrasound—abdomen and pelvis<br>Possibly computed tomography, magnetic resonance imaging, nucleotide or positron emission tomographic scanning | |
| **Laboratory** | ***Neoplasia***<br>CBC with differential count and blood smear<br>Sedimentation rate, C-reactive protein<br>Uric acid, phosphate, lactate dehydrogenase<br>Catecholamines, vanillylmandelic acid, homovanillic acid<br>***Infections (common)***<br>**General**<br>CBC with differential count<br>Sedimentation rate, C-reactive protein<br>Gram stain of exudate<br>**Specific** | |
| | Viral, respiratory<br>Epstein-Barr virus (EBV)<br>Cytomegalovirus (CMV)<br>Human immunodeficiency virus (HIV)<br>Cat-scratch disease | Rapid antigen screening, polymerase chain reaction, histochemical, serology, and culture |
| | Bacterial<br>*Staphylococcus aureus*<br>Anaerobes<br>*Streptococcus* (group A)<br>Mycobacteria (purified protein derivative [PPD] or interferon-$\gamma$ release assay [IGRA])<br>Atypical mycobacteria (PPD) | Skin test, rapid antigen screening, histochemical, serology, and culture |
| | ***Autoimmune***<br>Antinuclear antibody<br>Anti–double-stranded DNA<br>Serum ferritin | |
| **Surgery** | ***Biopsy***[a]<br>Histology, cytochemistry, flow cytometry, DNA studies, chromosomes<br>***Needle aspiration***<br>Reserved for surgically inaccessible nodes<br>Requires skilled cytopathologist | |

*CBC,* complete blood count.
[a]Requires the availability of pediatric pathology.

with the human immunodeficiency virus, may be suggested by other characteristic historical and physical findings. The physical examination should include all the palpable nodes (see Table 52-1). Furthermore, assessment of enlarged lymph nodes that have no obvious inflammatory explanation requires a chest radiograph or computed tomography (CT) scan to determine whether enlarged mediastinal or hilar nodes are present. The chest radiograph is the study most commonly omitted in evaluating patients who have lymphadenopathy; the identification of mediastinal or hilar adenopathy would preclude trials of antibiotics, which often delay a diagnostic biopsy.

### *Imaging*

The abdominal lymph nodes, including retroperitoneal, periportal, and celiac nodes, as well as the nodes of the splenic hilum, are difficult to evaluate without sophisticated imaging techniques. The spleen, which is primarily lymphoid tissue, may be enlarged in infectious, immunologic, and neoplastic disorders and may be delineated by ultrasound or CT examination. Abdominal and pelvic lymph nodes may be visualized by ultrasonography or may require techniques such as CT and magnetic resonance imaging. The sensitivity and specificity of methods to define chest (mediastinal or hilar) lymphadenopathy are variable. In one study of patients thought to have tuberculosis, the chest radiograph was 67% sensitive and 59% specific compared with spiral chest CT with contrast. Newer techniques include positron emission tomography and scintigraphy.

### *Complete Blood Cell Count and Acute Phase Reactants*

A complete blood cell count may reveal the reactive lymphocytes of infectious mononucleosis or a granulocytosis with a shift to the left, suggesting systemic bacterial infection. Bicytopenia (eg, anemia, granulocytopenia, thrombocytopenia) would be a red flag that a hematologic malignancy, such as leukemia or lymphoma, or a metastatic disease involving the bone marrow, such as neuroblastoma, may underlie the lymphadenopathy. The finding of nucleated erythrocytes and immature granulocytes (leukoerythroblastic blood picture) on the blood film is an ominous sign suggesting bone marrow irritation, with premature release of blood cell precursors. This finding may be seen in metastatic diseases such as neuroblastoma and rhabdomyosarcoma, with immunologic vasculitis and with granulomas (mycobacteria) in the marrow. Isolated leukopenia and neutropenia may also be seen with viral infections or severe bacterial infections (particularly in infants). Other studies may be useful in assessing lymphadenopathy, including C-reactive protein and erythrocyte sedimentation rate, that detect a systemic inflammatory reaction and may reflect infection, vasculitis, or neoplasm.

### *Infectious Evaluation*

The diagnostic workup of potential infectious lymphadenopathy is diverse and depends on the history, the patient's age, the location of the nodes (whether cervical, localized, or generalized), and the signs of inflammation accompanying the adenopathy. The cause of acute, inflamed, and localized adenopathy is often infectious and likely to be bacterial. A purified protein derivative or interferon-$\gamma$ release assay is indicated when tuberculosis is a possibility. Material should be obtained for culture and histologic or pathologic examination when possible, particularly in patients who do not respond to initial therapy. In children who have acute cervical adenitis, needle aspiration of an acutely inflamed, sometimes fluctuant, node demonstrates the infecting organism in two-thirds or more of cases. In certain cases, a biopsy may be required. If tuberculosis or atypical mycobacterial infection is thought to be present (eg, young children with subacute lymphadenopathy in the submandibular or submental regions), then needle aspiration should be avoided to prevent spread of the infection; excisional biopsy is required. The material obtained from biopsy or aspiration should be cultured aerobically and anaerobically and examined histologically, including special stains such as that for cat-scratch disease (Warthin-Starry silver stain). Specific diagnosis by serologic assessment, antigen detection, polymerase chain reaction, and culture is available for most of the common agents causing lymphadenopathy in children (most prominently serology for *B. Henselae* [cat-scratch disease]). The erythrocyte sedimentation rate or the C-reactive protein may be useful in assessing underlying inflammation, but both may be elevated in immunologic and neoplastic diseases as well.

After initial evaluation by history, physical examination, chest radiograph, and preliminary laboratory studies, the physician may not yet have an obvious explanation for the node enlargement. If a bacterial source for localized adenopathy (eg, pharyngitis, cervical nodes) is suggested, then a limited course of 7 to 10 days of antibiotic therapy may be tried. However, if the nodes have not regressed significantly, then prompt further evaluation is necessary. At this time, a chest radiograph should be obtained if it has not already been performed. Hilar or mediastinal adenopathy requires prompt assessment of neoplastic or granulomatous causes. Even in the absence of mediastinal or hilar adenopathy, prompt biopsy of significantly enlarged, unexplained lymph nodes should permit institution of appropriate therapy.

## Biopsy

Biopsy of significant adenopathy should be performed early if no evidence of infection or other cause exists and particularly if mediastinal or hilar nodes are enlarged. The biopsy should encompass the central mass of the enlarged nodes so that a misdiagnosis of reactive inflammation in adjacent nodes can be avoided. This circumstance is particularly common in Hodgkin disease, in which an adjacent smaller lymph node may be more accessible and technically easier to biopsy but may not demonstrate the presence of Reed-Sternberg cells. Fine-needle aspiration is not recommended for biopsy of superficial, accessible nodes, although it might be useful for intrathoracic nodes to avoid thoracotomy. Appropriate expertise is required for interpretation, and negative findings are not definitive. For subacute, submandibular, or submental lymphadenopathy in which atypical mycobacteria are suspected, complete excisional biopsy provides both diagnosis and therapy.

Mediastinal adenopathy may be associated with airway or vascular obstruction (superior vena cava syndrome), presenting a critical risk if anesthesia or sedation is administered and a major dilemma in establishing a diagnosis.

Any biopsy should be performed at a medical center that specializes in the care of children so that all appropriate touch preparations, cultures, special cytochemical or immunologic stains, flow cytometry, and biochemical, cytogenetic, and DNA studies are obtained. The pathology of Hodgkin disease, lymphoma, and other similar round-cell tumors may be difficult to establish and requires the assessment of a pediatric pathologist who has experience in these diseases. Immunophenotyping, cytogenetic analysis, molecular studies of gene rearrangement, and electron microscopy may be required for precise diagnosis. These studies, in conjunction with the histopathologic assessment, are central to the assessment and subsequent management, which may involve complex treatment with surgery, radiation, chemotherapy, or immunotherapy.

## ▶ TREATMENT

### *Infectious Diseases (Details of Treatment—See Specific Organism)*

Therapy of lymphadenitis depends on determining its cause or the most likely cause. Acute adenitis, particularly of the cervical area in young children, is frequently associated with infection from group A β-hemolytic streptococci or *Staphylococcus aureus*. The latter is particularly likely in adenitis that progresses to fluctuance. In the neonate and rarely in older children, group B streptococci may cause localized adenitis with or without cellulitis. In children beyond the neonatal period who have acute localized adenitis, particularly cervical adenitis, therapy should be initiated with an antibiotic directed at group A streptococci and penicillinase-producing strains of *S aureus* (eg, amoxicillin-clavulanic acid or cephalexin). Recently, infections with community-acquired methicillin-resistant *S aureus* in some areas have increased dramatically in children with skin and localized infections. In such circumstances, treatment should include an antibiotic to cover methicillin-resistant *S aureus* (eg, clindamycin or trimethoprim-sulfamethoxazole).[1] For most patients, oral therapy is adequate.

The usual course of therapy is 10 to 14 days, but therapy should be continued for at least 5 days after the signs of acute inflammation have subsided. For patients who have suppurative adenitis from these organisms, drainage is not only diagnostic (by culturing the exudate obtained), but also therapeutic. A few patients may not respond to oral therapy, even with a drug to which the organism is sensitive. Parenteral antibiotic therapy then is required.

If an anaerobic infection is thought to be present, then therapy depends, in part, on the location of the adenitis, the type of organism, and the severity of the illness. Most anaerobic infections of the cervical and submental areas are serious infections associated with mouth flora, requiring inpatient therapy with clindamycin or metronidazole, possibly in combination with third-generation cephalosporins.

Both *M tuberculosis* and atypical mycobacteria can cause adenitis, with the latter being more frequent in children. Differentiating these may be difficult but is important because many strains of atypical mycobacteria are resistant to the usual antitubercular chemotherapy, and excisional biopsy may be required. If tubercular infection is thought to be present, then appropriate therapy for *M tuberculosis* should be initiated while awaiting identification and sensitivities of the organism. Adenitis that is thought to be tubercular should not be incised or drained.

Cat-scratch adenitis is usually self-limited and generally requires no specific therapy. The discovery of *Bartonella* species, especially *B henselae*, as the prime cause of cat-scratch disease has raised the possibility for specific antibiotic therapy, and some antibiotics alone or combined, including azithromycin, rifampin, and doxycycline, may be of clinical benefit.[2-4] If nodes become markedly enlarged, tender, and fluctuant, then aspiration may help relieve symptoms; incision and drainage, however, should be avoided.[2-4]

For the unusual case of severe primary herpes simplex virus infection with localized adenitis, treatment with oral acyclovir has shortened the clinical course.[5,6]

### Neoplastic Disease

The treatment of neoplastic diseases today is, in most instances, oriented toward cure, with the effectiveness of therapy for lymphocytic and myelocytic leukemia, lymphomas, and Wilms and other tumors having improved markedly. The specific treatment of childhood cancer often involves combinations of chemotherapy, radiation therapy, and surgery, all of which depend on the individual diagnosis and are beyond the scope of this presentation. However, prompt, accurate diagnosis is essential for instituting specific treatment and optimal care of these patients.

## When to Refer

- History and physical examination do not suggest an infectious cause.
- Potentially infectious nodes have not responded to a course of antibiotics.
- Supraclavicular, mediastinal, or hilar adenopathy is present.
- A biopsy is considered; biopsies should be performed only at a center specializing in the care of children.

## When to Admit

- Biopsy requires hospitalization—for example, supraclavicular, mediastinal, or hilar biopsy.
- Biopsy results require inpatient treatment or further evaluation.
- An infection requires intravenous therapy.

### REFERENCES


1. Treatment of community-associated MRSA infections. *Med Lett Drugs Ther*. 2006;48:13–14
2. Batts S, Demers DM. Spectrum and treatment of cat-scratch disease. *Pediatr Infect Dis J*. 2004;23: 1161–1162
3. American Academy of Pediatrics. Cat-scratch disease. In: Pickering LK, Baker CJ, Kimberlin DW, Long SS, eds. *Red Book: 2012 Report of the Committee on Infectious Diseases*. 29th ed. Elk Grove Village, IL: American Academy of Pediatrics; 2012:269–271
4. Bass JW, Freitas BC, Freitas AD, et al. Prospective randomized double blind placebo-controlled evaluation of azithromycin for treatment of cat-scratch disease. *Pediatr Infect Dis J*. 1998;17:447–452
5. Amir J, Harel L, Smetana Z, Varsano I. Treatment of herpes simplex gingivostomatitis with aciclovir in children: a randomised double blind placebo controlled study. *BMJ*. 1997;314:1800–1803
6. American Academy of Pediatrics. Herpes simplex. In: Pickering LK, Baker CJ, Kimberlin DW, Long SS, eds. *Red Book: 2012 Report of the Committee on Infectious Diseases*. 29th ed. Elk Grove Village, IL: American Academy of Pediatrics; 2012:398–408

# Chapter 53

# Macrocephaly

*Oscar H. Purugganan, MD, MPH*

## ▶ DEFINITION

Macrocephaly is defined as a head circumference of more than 2 standard deviations above the mean (about the 97th percentile) based on age and gender. Head circumference values should be plotted in appropriate head circumference charts (see Chapter 55, Microcephaly), such as the Centers for Disease Control and Prevention (CDC) growth charts (for children 0–3 years). For children older than 3 years, the Nellhaus charts had been used previously,[1] although new age- and sex-appropriate US charts were published in 2010.[2]

## ▶ DIFFERENTIAL DIAGNOSES

Head size is influenced by the different components that make up the cranial cavity. Among the causes of a large head in children are hydrocephalus, an enlarged brain *(megalencephaly)*, a thickened skull, and space-occupying lesions. These conditions are not mutually exclusive, and some children may have more than 1 underlying factor (Box 53-1).

### *Hydrocephalus*

Hydrocephalus, an enlargement of the ventricular system, may be congenital or acquired. The clinical presentation is influenced by the age of onset and the underlying condition causing the hydrocephalus. An enlarging head circumference is the most obvious finding in an infant whose cranial sutures have not fused. In the older child whose sutures have fused, significant head enlargement does not occur, but other signs and symptoms of increased intracranial pressure, such as headaches, vomiting, and papilledema, may occur.

Conventionally, hydrocephalus has been classified as either communicating or noncommunicating, depending on whether the connection between the ventricular system and the subarachnoid space is intact. Communicating hydrocephalus results from either the impaired absorption of cerebrospinal fluid by the arachnoid villi (from meningeal irritation caused by meningitis, trauma, or malignant infiltration) or less commonly with overproduction of cerebrospinal fluid from a choroid plexus papilloma. Noncommunicating or obstructive hydrocephalus is marked by enlargement of the ventricular system proximal to the site of an obstruction. The obstruction may be an anatomic defect, such as aqueductal stenosis, or the result of a tumor, infection, or infiltrate. In many cases, however, the classification of hydrocephalus as either communicating or noncommunicating may not be clear-cut; common causes of hydrocephalus, such as intraventricular hemorrhage and intrauterine infections, may lead to both communicating and noncommunicating hydrocephalus.

BOX 53-1

## *Causes of Macrocephaly*

### HYDROCEPHALUS

- Intraventricular hemorrhage
- Meningomyelocele
- Dandy Walker malformation
- Aqueductal stenosis
- Malignancy
- Intrauterine infections
- Meningitis
- Space-occupying lesions
- Benign accumulation of extracranial fluid

### MEGALENCEPHALY

#### *Megalencephaly—metabolic*
- Mucopolysaccharidoses
- Leukodystrophies
  - Canavan disease
  - Alexander disease
- Glutaric aciduria

#### *Megalencephaly—anatomic*
- Overgrowth syndromes
- Neurocutaneous syndromes
- Achondroplasia
- Autism
- Fragile X syndrome
- Various other genetic syndromes (OMIM)

#### *Megalencephaly—idiopathic (benign)*

### SKULL THICKENING AND SKULL ABNORMALITIES

- Thalassemia
- Cleidocranial dysostosis and other skeletal disorders

### SPACE-OCCUPYING LESIONS

- Vascular malformations
- Intracranial tumors
- Subdural effusion
- Subdural hematoma

Intraventricular hemorrhage occurs in about 15% of premature infants with birth weight less than 1,500 g.[3] The severity of hemorrhage is graded as follows:
- Grade I: subependymal hemorrhage
- Grade II: intraventricular hemorrhage without ventricular dilation
- Grade III: intraventricular hemorrhage with ventricular dilation
- Grade IV: intraventricular and intraparenchymal hemorrhage[4]

Although subtle changes in head circumference may be present, macrocephaly is not always evident in an infant with intraventricular hemorrhage. Grade III and IV hemorrhages are associated with poorer neurodevelopmental outcomes than grades I and II, with an estimated 35% and 90% of affected children, respectively, showing neurologic sequelae.[3]

Hydrocephalus with Chiari type II defect is present in 80% of children with myelomeningocele.[5] Macrocephaly is commonly the first manifestation of the Dandy Walker malformation, a cystic dilation of the fourth ventricle, with hypoplasia of the cerebellar vermis and a variety of other cranial malformations.[6] Head size may be normal at birth, but acceleration in head growth is noted in most children by 1 year of age, sometimes with prominence of the posterior part of the skull.[4]

Congenital aqueductal stenosis, which may occur sporadically or be transmitted by X-linked inheritance, causes severe hydrocephalus that may complicate labor and delivery with cephalopelvic disproportion and lead to signs and symptoms of increased intracranial pressure after birth.

A condition characterized by a benign accumulation of extracranial fluid, probably subarachnoid, is identified in many children with macrocephaly who have an unremarkable neurologic examination. The exact nature of the extracranial collection has not been clearly established, leading to problems with nomenclature; the condition is variously referred to, whether accurately or inaccurately, as benign macrocephaly, external hydrocephalus, benign extracerebral fluid collections, benign subdural collections, and benign enlargement of the subarachnoid space.[7-9] Neuroimaging reveals an extracerebral fluid collection most evident in the prefrontal area and, in some cases, mild nonprogressive dilation of the ventricular system. The size of the brain is normal. Affected children may have normal or large head circumferences at birth. In the succeeding months, the head circumference grows to greater than the 98th percentile and then generally parallels the normal growth curves. The large head size is an isolated feature, and the affected child has an otherwise normal neurologic examination and age-appropriate development, although transient early developmental delays, especially in the first year of life, may be observed. The condition seems to be self-limited, with normalization of computed tomography scan findings usually by 2½ years of age.[10] The relationship of this condition to benign megalencephaly, wherein the brain is large but no extracranial fluid accumulation is present in a child who is also neurologically intact, has not been established and is not fully understood.[10,11] More recently, an association with subdural hematoma in infancy has been suggested.[12,13]

## Megalencephaly

Another common cause of macrocephaly is an enlargement of the brain. Traditionally, megalencephaly is classified as metabolic or anatomic. In metabolic megalencephaly, enlargement of the brain is caused by an inborn error of metabolism that leads to the abnormal deposition of some substrate in the brain. The head circumference is usually normal at birth and then enlarges and may cross percentiles over time.[4] It coincides with significant developmental delays and psychomotor regression. Most of these inborn errors are autosomal recessive disorders. The mucopolysaccharidoses, leukodystrophies such as Canavan disease and Alexander disease, are examples of metabolic conditions causing macrocephaly. In Hurler syndrome, the most severe form of mucopolysaccharidosis resulting from a deficiency of α-L-iduronidase, an enlarging head may be noted to cross percentiles during infancy. Coarse facial features, frontal bossing, and corneal clouding are characteristic findings of the syndrome.[14] In the infantile form of Canavan disease, a leukodystrophy that predominantly affects Ashkenazi Jews from a deficiency of aspartoacylase, macrocephaly is associated with irritability, poor visual fixation, head lag, and motor delay, which are noted in the first few months of life.[15] Alexander disease is a rare, mostly sporadic condition characterized by abundant accumulation of glial fibrillary acidic protein in Rosenthal fibers. Affected infants exhibit macrocephaly, seizures, spasticity, and developmental regression.[16]

In anatomic megalencephaly, the large head size is usually present at birth[17] and is often associated with neurodevelopmental impairment. The brain is abnormally large because of an increase in the size and number of its cells.[4] The Online Mendelian Inheritance in Man (OMIM) provides a comprehensive list of syndromes associated with macrocephaly and megalencephaly.[18] In overgrowth syndromes, macrocephaly is usually present at birth as part of a generalized increase in body size. An example is Sotos syndrome, which is associated with facial dysmorphism, neurodevelopmental deficits such as poor coordination and cognitive and behavioral problems, and macrocephaly that may result from a combination of megalencephaly, ventricular enlargement, and midline anomalies.[19] It has been reported that about 90% of clinical cases of Sotos syndrome have mutations or deletions involving the *NSD1* gene in chromosome 5q35.[20] Neurocutaneous syndromes such as neurofibromatosis, tuberous sclerosis, and hypomelanosis of Ito are associated with megalencephaly in addition to characteristic skin findings, intracranial conditions, and neurodevelopmental problems.[14] In achondroplasia, megalencephaly is present in a child with short stature, shortened proximal arms and legs (rhizomelia), and dysmorphic facial features. Affected individuals usually have normal intelligence but are at risk for hydrocephalus, obstructive sleep apnea or central apnea, and spine and joint problems.[21,22] Compared with the general population, a disproportionately large number of autistic children have enlarged head circumferences.[23-28] The pattern of brain growth in some autistic children seems to be abnormal, with acceleration of head growth in early childhood,[23] hyperplasia in cerebral gray matter and cerebral and cerebellar white matter,[24] and a slight decrease in brain volume during adolescence.[25] Whether this acceleration in head growth in early childhood relates to the behavioral and developmental features of autism remains unclear. Mutations in the phosphatase and tensin homolog *(PTEN)* gene, which have been associated with a spectrum of disorders with a predisposition to hamartomas and certain cancers such as Cowden syndrome, Bannayan-Riley-Ruvalcaba syndrome, and Proteus syndrome, have been identified in some autistic children with severe macrocephaly.[29,30] Fragile X syndrome is associated with a constellation of physical findings, including macrocephaly, a longish face with prominent ears, joint hyperextensibility, and enlarged testes.[14] A family history on the mother's side of intellectual disability, developmental and behavioral problems, and autistic behaviors suggests the possibility of this X-linked disorder.

A child with a large head who has no significant collection of extraventricular or intraventricular fluid, a normal neurologic examination and developmental history, no signs of raised intracranial pressure, and a family history of large head sizes in normal adults can be considered to have benign or idiopathic megalencephaly.[5,31,32] Although these individuals have been thought to develop normally, recent evidence suggests they may exhibit mild neurodevelopmental dysfunction such as incoordination and visual-motor weaknesses.[11]

### Other Causes of Macrocephaly

Thickening of the skull is a rare cause of macrocephaly. Children with a hemolytic anemia, such as β-thalassemia, may exhibit frontal bossing attributable to extracranial hematopoiesis in their skull bones. Cleidocranial dysostosis is an autosomal disorder of abnormal bone formation characterized by delayed closure of fontanelles, widening of the head circumference, and other skeletal abnormalities.[33] Space-occupying lesions, such as an arteriovenous malformation or a brain tumor, may also produce macrocephaly. Although usually asymptomatic, subdural effusion is a complication of bacterial meningitis that may produce an enlarging head circumference, bulging anterior fontanelle, and signs of increased intracranial pressure in infants.[34] Subdural hematoma may present with macrocephaly in infants but is usually associated with other symptoms as well.

## ▶ EVALUATION

### Relevant History

A review of previously measured head circumferences can ascertain whether a child has had any change in the pattern or percentiles of head circumference over time. A large head circumference at birth presupposes a cause of prenatal origin, necessitates a detailed prenatal history, and may indicate anatomic megalencephaly. Conditions that may cause congenital macrocephaly include X-linked aqueductal stenosis and the overgrowth syndromes. An abnormally enlarging head postnatally in a child with neurodevelopmental problems is a clue to an acquired condition, such as acquired hydrocephalus or a possible metabolic disorder. The history should explore delays in the developmental milestones; regression in motor, language, and social skills; seizures; and signs of increased intracranial pressure such as lethargy, vomiting, and behavioral changes. A family history of any genetic, neurologic, and developmental condition may be a red flag for similar disorders, whereas a history of otherwise normal parents and siblings with large heads can be reassuring.

## Physical Examination

The physical examination of the child with macrocephaly should focus on the specific issues listed in Box 53-2.

Monitoring of head size must be performed periodically during health care maintenance visits. In the presence of a rapid enlargement in head circumference, more frequent monitoring, at the very least, is necessary. Measurements should be plotted on the appropriate head circumference charts. A disproportionately enlarged head in relation to height and weight may indicate a primary neurologic disorder. Measuring the size of the fontanelles and palpating sutures are important. Significant hydrocephalus in infants may produce a bulging anterior fontanelle and separation of cranial sutures, which are uncommon in anatomic megalencephaly. A vein of Galen arteriovenous malformation may produce a cranial bruit on auscultation. Because macrocephaly is a feature of many genetic syndromes, dysmorphic features and other organ involvement should be noted. Examination of the skin may reveal café au lait spots, axillary freckling, ash-leaf spots, and a whorled pattern of pigmentation that may indicate a neurocutaneous disorder. Careful neurologic examination is critical and may reveal abnormalities in muscle tone and posture, asymmetries, persistence of primitive reflexes, and hyperreflexia. Developmental assessment may reveal cognitive impairment, autistic features, learning disabilities, or behavioral difficulties. It is also important to measure the head circumference of the parents and make note of any dysmorphic features they may have.

**BOX 53-2**

### *Physical Examination of a Child With Macrocephaly*

- Accurate measurement of the head circumference and assessment of the pattern of head growth
- Inspection and palpation of the skull
- Comparison of the head circumference with other growth parameters
- Presence or absence of dysmorphic features
- Presence or absence of congenital abnormalities involving other organ systems
- Thorough neurologic and developmental assessment, including a check for signs of increased intracranial pressure
- Skin examination using Wood lamp

## Laboratory Testing

Metabolic testing is available to identify many of the storage diseases and is recommended in a child exhibiting developmental regression. Genetic testing should be done as appropriate for the clinical assessment.

## Imaging

Neuroimaging is the procedure of choice in evaluating macrocephaly. For infants with open fontanelles, head ultrasound is useful in identifying intraventricular hemorrhage, hydrocephalus, and intracranial tumors. This procedure is especially useful in infants because it eliminates the need for sedation. Computed tomography can identify hydrocephalus, intracranial calcifications, and hemorrhages. Magnetic resonance imaging (MRI) is most informative, especially in identifying gray and white matter disease (eg, leukodystrophy), migration defects, hydrocephalus, and posterior fossa lesions. MRI is also helpful in studying the subtleties in subdural and subarachnoid hemorrhages.[35] Consultation with a neurologist or radiologist may be helpful in deciding which procedure would be most appropriate. MRI is generally not indicated in patients with autism and macrocephaly unless there are other concerns not explained by autism (eg, focal neurologic findings, cranial nerve dysfunction, severe headache).[36] A skeletal survey may reveal bone age abnormalities in the overgrowth syndromes and radiologic abnormalities that may be present in the mucopolysaccharidoses, bone dysplasias, or trauma.

## Management

The management of macrocephaly depends on its cause. Shunting procedures are the treatment of choice for significant and progressive hydrocephalus; however, shunt infection, obstruction, and malfunction are not rare and continue to be challenges in the care of these children. In premature infants, the risk for complications is even greater; medical management with pharmacologic agents (carbonic anhydrase inhibitors or other diuretics) and serial lumbar punctures may be used as initial therapy.[37] Medical management is also used in asymptomatic or minimally symptomatic patients with slowly progressive hydrocephalus. For Dandy Walker cysts, shunting has been recommended to drain the hydrocephalus or the posterior fossa cyst, or both.[4] Children in whom inborn errors of metabolism are suspected should be referred for genetic evaluation, treatment, and counseling. Although the treatment for these conditions is mainly supportive and symptomatic, bone marrow transplantation and enzyme replacement therapy are promising interventions for certain disorders. Although no specific treatment is available for anatomic megalencephaly, pediatricians should be aware of the association with developmental and cognitive problems, which warrant early intervention and special education services. The presence of subdural hematoma requires further evaluation (eg, skeletal survey, retinal examination) and may include referral to a child abuse expert. Serial measurement of the head circumference and clinical assessments are generally all that are needed for benign accumulation of extracranial fluid and idiopathic megalencephaly.

## When to Refer

- Head circumference of more than 2 standard deviations above the mean (especially 3 standard deviations above the mean)

- Head circumference that is crossing percentiles or rapidly growing
- Dysmorphic features
- Abnormal neurologic examination
- Regression in developmental skills or significant developmental delay
- Suspected child abuse

## When to Admit

- Signs of increased intracranial pressure or mental status change
- Shunt infection or malfunction

## *TOOLS FOR PRACTICE*

### Medical Decision Support

- *Growth Charts* (charts), Centers for Disease Control and Prevention (www.cdc.gov/growthcharts)
- *CDC Growth Charts: United States* (article), National Center for Health Statistics (www.cdc.gov/nchs/data/ad/ad314.pdf)
- *Online Mendelian Inheritance in Man* (online database), Johns Hopkins University (omim.org)
- *United States head circumference growth reference charts: birth to 21 years* (article), *The Journal of Pediatrics,* Vol 156, Issue 6, 2010 (www.jpeds.com/article/S0022-3476%2810%2900020-X/abstract)

## *REFERENCES*

1. Nellhaus G. Head circumference from birth to eighteen years. Practical composite international and interracial graphs. *Pediatrics.* 1968;41:106–114
2. Rollins JD, Collins JS, Holden KR. United States head circumference growth reference charts: birth to 21 years. *J Pediatr.* 2010;156:907–913
3. Volpe JJ. Intracranial hemorrhage: germinal matrix—intraventricular hemorrhage of the premature infant. In: Volpe JJ. *Neurology of the Newborn.* 4th ed. Philadelphia, PA: WB Saunders; 2001
4. Fenichel GM. Disorders of cranial volume and shape. In: Fenichel GM. *Clinical Pediatric Neurology: A Signs and Symptoms Approach.* Philadelphia, PA: Elsevier Saunders; 2009
5. DeMyer W. Microcephaly, microencephaly, megalocephaly and megalencephaly. In: Swaiman KE, Ashwal S, eds. *Pediatric Neurology: Principles and Practice.* 3rd ed. St Louis, MO: Mosby; 1999
6. Has R, Ermiş H, Yüksel A, et al. Dandy-Walker malformation: a review of 78 cases diagnosed by prenatal sonography. *Fetal Diagn Ther.* 2004;19:342–347
7. Hamza M, Bodensteiner JB, Noorani PA, Barnes PD. Benign extracerebral fluid collections: a cause of macrocrania in infancy. *Pediatr Neurol.* 1987;3:218–221
8. Alper G, Ekinci G, Yilmaz Y, et al. Magnetic resonance imaging characteristics of benign macrocephaly in children. *J Child Neurol.* 1999;14:678–682
9. Bodensteiner JB. Benign macrocephaly: a common cause of big heads in the first year. *J Child Neurol.* 1999;14(10):678–682
10. Alvarez LA, Maytal J, Shinnar S. Idiopathic external hydrocephalus: natural history and relationship to benign familial macrocephaly. *Pediatrics.* 1986;77:901–907
11. Sandler AD, Knudsen MW, Brown TT, Christian RM Jr. Neurodevelopmental dysfunction among nonreferred children with idiopathic megalencephaly. *J Pediatr.* 1997;131:320–324
12. Ghosh PS, Ghosh D. Subdural hematoma in infants without accidental or nonaccidental injury: benign external hydrocephalus, a risk factor. *Clin Pediatr (Phila).* 2011;50:897–903

13. Ravid S, Maytal J. External hydrocephalus: a probable cause for subdural hematoma in infancy. *Pediatr Neurol.* 2003;28:139–141
14. Jones KL. *Smith's Recognizable Patterns of Human Malformation.* 6th ed. Philadelphia, PA: Elsevier Saunders; 2006
15. Traeger EC, Rapin I. The clinical course of Canavan disease. *Pediatr Neurol.* 1998;18:207–212
16. Gordon N. Alexander disease. *Eur Paediatr Neurol.* 2003;7:395–399
17. Olney AH. Macrocephaly syndromes. *Semin Pediatr Neurol.* 2007;14:128–135
18. OMIM—Online Mendelian Inheritance in Man. McKusick-Nathans Institute for Genetic Medicine, Johns Hopkins University (Baltimore, MD), and National Center for Biotechnology Information, National Library of Medicine (Bethesda, MD), 2000. Available at: www.ncbi.nlm.nih.gov/omim. Accessed October 23, 2014
19. Cohen MM. Mental deficiency, alterations in performance, and CNS abnormalities in overgrowth syndromes. *Am J Med Genet.* 2003;117(1):49–56
20. Tatton-Brown K, Douglas J, Coleman K, et al. Genotype-phenotype associations in Sotos syndrome: an analysis of 266 individuals with NSD1 aberrations. *Am J Hum Genet.* 2005;77:193–204
21. Castiglia PT. Achondroplasia. *J Pediatr Health Care.* 1996;10:180–182
22. Gordon N. The neurological complications of achondroplasia. *Brain Dev.* 2000;22:3–7
23. Courchesne E, Carper R, Akshoomoff N. Evidence of brain overgrowth in the first year of life in autism. *JAMA.* 2003;290:337–344
24. Courchesne E, Karns CM, Davis HR, et al. Unusual brain growth patterns in early life in patients with autistic disorder: an MRI study. *Neurology.* 2001;57:245–254
25. Aylward EH, Minshew NJ, Field K, Sparks BF, Singh N. Effects of age on brain volume and head circumference in autism. *Neurology.* 2002;59:175–183
26. Bolton PF, Roobol M, Allsopp L, Pickles A. Association between idiopathic infantile macrocephaly and autism spectrum disorders. *Lancet.* 2001;358:726–727
27. Fidler DJ, Bailey JN, Smalley SL. Macrocephaly in autism and other pervasive developmental disorders. *Dev Med Child Neurol.* 2000;42:737–740
28. Dementieva YA, Vance DD, Donnelly SL, et al. Accelerated head growth in early development of individuals with autism. *Pediatr Neurol.* 2005;32:102–108
29. Varga EA, Pastore M, Prior T, Herman GE, McBride KL. The prevalence of PTEN mutations in a clinical pediatric cohort with autism spectrum disorders, developmental delay, and macrocephaly. *Genet Med.* 2009;11:111–117
30. Buxbaum JD, Cai G, Chaste P, et al. Mutation screening of the PTEN gene in patients with autism spectrum disorders and macrocephaly. *Am J Med Genet B Neuropsychiatr Genet.* 2007;144B:484–491
31. Day RE, Schutt WH. Normal children with large heads—benign familial megalencephaly. *Arch Dis Child.* 1979;54:512–517
32. Asch AJ, Myers GJ. Benign familial macrocephaly: report of a family and review of the literature. *Pediatrics.* 1976;57:535–539
33. Glass RBJ, Fernbach SK, Norton KI, et al. The infant skull: a vault of information. *Radiographics.* 2004;24:507–522
34. Behrman R, Kliegman R, Jenson H. eds. *Nelson Textbook of Pediatrics.* 17th ed. Philadelphia, PA: Saunders; 2000
35. Stoodley N. Neuroimaging in non-accidental head injury: if, when, why and how. *Clin Radiol.* 2005; 60:22–30
36. Filipek PA, Accardo PJ, Baranek GT, et al. The screening and diagnosis of autistic spectrum disorders. *J Autism Dev Disord.* 1999;29:439–484
37. Garton HJ, Piatt JH. Hydrocephalus. *Pediatr Clin North Am.* 2004;51:305–325
38. Zahl SM, Wester K. Routine measurement of head circumference as a tool for detecting intracranial expansion in infants: what is the gain? A nationwide survey. *Pediatrics.* 2008;121:e416–e420

# Chapter 54

# Medically Unexplained Symptoms

*Rebecca Baum, MD; John Campo, MD*

## ▶ BACKGROUND

Medically unexplained symptoms (MUS) can present significant challenges and frustrations to the children affected by them, their families, and the physicians involved in their care. While medically unexplained physical symptoms are often associated with mental health issues, children with MUS often present in primary care and general medical settings rather than the mental health setting. Patients with MUS often present for multiple office visits and are at risk for potentially dangerous and unnecessary evaluations, laboratory tests, and procedures.[1] Patients and families may be frustrated and confused by the physician's judgment that "nothing is wrong" despite continued pain and impairment. MUS are thus an important entity for physicians to recognize to help facilitate accurate assessment and intervention.

Historically, physicians have been trained in the biomedical model that explains the presence of physical symptoms with a diagnosis based on the presence of pathology consistent with a specific disease.[2] In this model, unexplained symptoms may not be presumed to be real, or may be considered representative of a mental disorder. This dichotomous approach, termed *dualism*, distinguishes between physical and mental disorders by virtue of whether there is evidence of a biomedical explanation. It is increasingly being recognized that such dualistic thinking is inadequate to address the entity of MUS. Using this model, physicians may complicate care, or even put patients at risk, in an attempt to avoid "missing" explanatory physical disease. Families and patients may feel stigmatized, misunderstood, and lacking in an explanation for their symptoms.

Our current understanding of pain suggests that it is an unpleasant sensory and emotional experience representative of physiologic changes and tissue damage. This suggests that pain is a derivative of demonstrable tissue pathology, yet pain can also be experienced subjectively in the absence of demonstrable pathology. Similarly, the level of pain experienced in association with a given degree of tissue damage may also vary. Rather than focusing on false dichotomies between physical and psychological health, it is preferable to recognize the connection between psychology and physiology.[3] The term *somatization* is used to reflect the experience of the individual, including his subjective experience, distress, and desire to seek medical care, in the setting of MUS.[4]

## ▶ EPIDEMIOLOGY

Medically unexplained symptoms are often encountered across childhood and adolescence, with pain and fatigue being especially common in all age groups. It is also important to remember that the presence of 1 type of MUS typically predicts the presence of other MUS. In preschool children, abdominal pain is a common manifestation.[5] Among children and adolescents, headache and abdominal pain are the most prevalent symptoms,[6,7] though other types of pain, such as limb and chest pain, are often reported.[8] Fatigue is a particularly common complaint in teens.[9] Other symptoms include urinary, cardiovascular, rheumatologic, and gastrointestinal complaints. MUS suggesting neurologic or sensory impairment, often referred to as "conversion" symptoms, are relatively unusual in community settings yet more common in specialty settings. A study of teens in the Ontario Child Health Study suggested a prevalence of recurrent somatic symptoms in the primary care setting of 4% for boys and 11% for girls.[10] Other studies report that between 2% and 20% of children in primary care present with MUS.[8] Boys and girls may have different clinical presentations, with some studies suggesting that girls report more somatic symptoms than boys and more frequently report symptoms of headache or abdominal pain than boys, particularly with increasing age into adolescence.[9–11] All types of MUS can be associated with significant impairment for patients and their families. This includes missed school days, increased health care utilization, distress, patient suffering, limitation of activities, impaired peer interactions, and significant effect on family functioning.[12]

The precise etiology of MUS is unknown. Certain associations and risk factors have been identified (Box 54-1). In general, children with emotional and behavioral problems are more likely to experience MUS than otherwise healthy children. In a primary care sample, children identified as somatizers had a higher frequency of emotional/behavioral problems, including internalizing symptoms such as worrying, fear of new situations, and problems with separation.[12] Children with diagnosed mental health disorders such as anxiety, depression, and disruptive behavior disorders have also been found to exhibit more somatic symptoms, including headache, abdominal pain, and musculoskeletal pain.[9,11]

**Box 54-1**

### *Risk Factors for the Development of Medically Unexplained Symptoms*

- Genetics
- Modeling
- Physical illness
- School stressors
- Family stressors
- High-achieving families
- Parental overprotection
- Secondary gain[a]
- Impaired or limited coping mechanisms
- Difficulty identifying/expressing feelings
- Difficulty with transitions
- Psychiatric comorbidity
- Trauma

[a]Secondary gain refers to the social and familial reinforcement of the symptom.

Derived from Ibeziako P, Bujoreanu S. Approach to psychosomatic illness in adolescents. *Curr Opin Pediatr*. 2011;23: 384–389.

## ▶ CLASSIFICATION

Definitions for conditions characterized by chronic pain and physical suffering are detailed in the *Diagnostic and Statistical Manual of Mental Disorders, Fifth Edition (DSM-5),* under the category of Somatic Symptom and Related Disorders. This category replaces that of Somatoform Disorders in *DSM-IV.* These disorders are characterized by pain or other somatic symptoms in association with impairment in functioning and significant individual distress. Somatic Symptom Disorder (SSD) is the diagnosis applied in the presence of distressing or impairing somatic symptoms along with excessive, maladaptive, or disproportionate thoughts or feelings about the physical symptoms. See Table 54-1 for additional disorders in this category, including Illness Anxiety Disorder, which replaces hypochondriasis, Conversion Disorder, and Psychological Factors Affecting Medical Condition. Factitious Disorder, defined by the intentional falsification of symptoms with the apparent goal of achieving behavioral and social benefits associated with the sick role, is now included in this category as well. Historically, these disorders were considered when a medical explanation could not be found, although, in many cases, it can be difficult and counterproductive to fully exclude an exhaustive list of potential medical conditions. In *DSM-5,* the key compenent of these disorders is the presence of somatic symptoms *and* the way they are interpreted by the patient, rather than solely by the lack of medical explanation. Children with these disorders experience significant impairment across 1 or several domains, including relationships with peers or parents, school functioning, and participation in extracurricular activities. Table 54-1 describes the categories of somatic symptom and related disorders according to *DSM-5,* with the same criteria applied to both adults and children.

When considering the presence of a somatic disorder, it is important to assess for physical disorders that may be causing or contributing to the child's symptoms. However, the physician is cautioned to avoid unnecessary testing once it can be reasonably assumed that a medical disorder has been excluded, which can present a challenge for physicians.[13] It is recommended that somatic disorders be included in the differential diagnosis rather than relegated to a diagnosis of exclusion. Other conditions to include in the differential diagnosis

**Table 54-1**
**Classification of Somatic Symptom and Related Disorders**

| DISORDER | DESCRIPTION |
|---|---|
| Somatic Symptom Disorder | • Presence of ≥1 somatic symptoms that are distressing or result in signficant disruption of daily life.<br>• Excessive thoughts, feelings, or behaviors related to the somatic symptoms.<br>• Symptoms must be persistent (usually >6 months). |
| Illness Anxiety Disorder | • Preoccupation with having a serious illness (≥6 months).<br>• If a medical condition or strong family history is present, worry is out of proportion to the likelihood of severe illness; somatic symptoms, if present, are mild.<br>• High degree of anxiety about one's health.<br>• Excessive engagement in health-related behavior or avoidance of necessary health care. |

*Continued*

**Table 54-1**
**Classification of Somatic Symptom and Related Disorders—cont'd**

| DISORDER | DESCRIPTION |
|---|---|
| Conversion Disorder | • Presence of ≥1 symptoms of altered voluntary motor or sensory function that result in significant distress or impairment.<br>• Evaluation suggests that symptoms are incompatible with recognized medical conditions. |
| Psychological Factors Affecting Other Medical Conditions | • Presence of psychological or behavioral factors that result in delayed recovery or added health risk, interfere with treatment, or escalate the need for medical treatment.<br>• An underlying medical condition must be present. |
| Facititious Disorder (Imposed on Self or Imposed on Another) | • Intentional falsification of physical or psychological signs or symptoms or infliction of injury.<br>• Deceptive behavior is present. |
| Other Specified Somatic Symptom and Related Disorder | • Presence of somatic symptoms that cause significant distress or impairment but do not meet full criteria for another category of somatic symptom and related disorders.<br>• May be used when symptoms are brief (eg, 6 months) or just below the diagnostic criteria. |
| Unspecified Somatic Symptom and Related Disorder | • Presence of somatic symptoms that cause significant distress or impairment but do not meet full criteria for another category of somatic symptom and related disorders.<br>• Used only in unusual situations when there is insufficient information to make a more specific diagnosis. |

Derived from American Psychiatric Association. *Diagnostic and Statistical Manual of Mental Disorders.* 5th ed. Arlington, VA: American Psychiatric Association; 2013.

of MUS include Psychological Factors Affecting Other Medical Conditions, which describes the presence of psychological factors and symptoms associated with an underlying medical condition. Conditions such as anxiety and depression may also result in pain and fatigue and thus should be considered the primary diagnosis in those circumstances.

## ▶ ASSESSMENT

An empathetic and collaborative approach is recommended when considering MUS. Children affected by MUS and their families may be frustrated by frequent office visits, multiple laboratory tests, and being told that "nothing is wrong" despite patient suffering. While the approach to each child should be individualized, general principles can help guide successful assessment. Important aspects to consider during the assessment process are presented in Box 54-2. MUS should be approached just as any other symptom in the pediatric history, with a review of symptom characteristics including duration, frequency, intensity, and moderating factors. Special attention should be paid to environmental stressors, opportunities for secondary gain, and emotional factors such as anxiety, depression, or other psychological symptoms.

Box 54-2

## *Important Principles in the Assessment of Children With Medically Unexplained Symptoms*

- Acknowledge symptoms, patient experience, and family concerns.
- Review past evaluations and treatment.
- Investigate fears related to symptoms.
- Remain alert to unrecognized medical diagnosis.
- Avoid unnecessary tests.
- Avoid diagnosis by exclusion.
- Understand symptom timing, context, and characteristics.

Adapted from Campo JV, Fritz G. A management model for pediatric somatization. *Psychosomatics.* 2001;42:467–476.

In addition to a careful history, standardized tools can be helpful in the assessment process. The Children's Somatization Inventory (CSI) can be used to assess for the presence of multiple somatic symptoms. It has been revised to a 24-item questionnaire that includes parent and child (age $\geq$7) versions and is available in the public domain.[14] The Functional Disability Inventory is a 15-item questionnaire with parent and child (age $\geq$8) versions that can be used to assess health status across multiple domains.[15]

## ▶ MANAGEMENT

Collaborative care in the management of MUS requires communicating diagnostic impressions to the family in a clear and honest manner.[16] Families may benefit from a discussion of the interplay between physiologic and emotional factors, with reassurance that the absence of diagnosable medical disease does not minimize the child's suffering or negate the reality of the problem. Physicians should be mindful of the stigma associated with mental health conditions and avoid the mind-body dualism that may characterize MUS as being "all in your head."[13] The use of placebo and other forms of deception in attempts to achieve diagnosis or reduce symptoms is discouraged.[13]

Once diagnostic impressions are communicated and questions are discussed, the physician must then attempt to shift the family's focus from the cause of symptoms to improving the child's functioning and reducing suffering.[17] The physician should facilitate the development of a treatment plan that addresses physical pain, stress reduction, and reduction of stigma while fostering hope that the child will improve. Goals should be developed collaboratively and should be meaningful to the child and family. In many cases, treatment will involve an interprofessional approach involving medical, mental health, and allied health disciplines. Clear communication across disciplines is essential.

A number of interventions have been proposed for the treatment of somatic disorders, and thus MUS (Table 54-2). Treatments may be delivered independently or in combination, although medication is rarely successful if used without supportive therapies.

**Table 54-2**
**Interventions for Children With Somatic Disorders**

| INTERVENTION | CHARACTERISTICS |
|---|---|
| Cognitive behavioral therapy | May involve a combination of<br>• Cognitive restructuring (eg, "I realize I have some pain today, but I can still go for a walk with my friends.")<br>• Relaxation<br>• Graded exposure to unpleasant experiences[a] |
| Rehabilitative approach | Focus on coping and improving health status |
| Behavioral intervention | Approaches include<br>• Reinforcement of healthy behaviors<br>• Minimization of secondary gain |
| Self-management | Possible techniques include mindfulness, hypnosis, imagery, and relaxation. |
| Family intervention | Involves work with the family system that may inadvertently reinforce the sick role |
| Maximal treatment of psychiatric comorbidities | Important to consider given the high prevalence of mental health conditions in children with medically unexplained symptoms |
| Medication management | Should be considered for<br>• The treatment of underlying mental health conditions<br>• Somatic symptoms that accompany mental health conditions |

[a]Masia Warner C, Reigada LC, Fisher PH, et al. CBT for anxiety and associated somatic complaints in pediatric medical settings: an open pilot study. *J Clin Psychol Med Settings*. 2009;16(2):169–177.
Derived from Dell ML, Campo JV. Somatoform disorders in children and adolescents. *Psychiatr Clin North Am*. 2011;34:643–660.

A substantial portion of the child's treatment may occur outside the realm of primary care. In these circumstances, an important role for the pediatrician is one of care coordination, hope, and support. Pediatricians may be especially helpful in recognizing MUS as a possiblility and making timely referrals to mental health professionals as indicated. In situations where symptoms are less intense or impairing, primary care management may be appropriate. In either case, pediatricians can play a key role in supporting families through the assessment and treatment process, which includes conveying an understanding that their concerns will be taken seriously and addressing parental anxiety, if present. Physicians in underserved areas may find themselves providing more direct care given challenges related to mental health and specialty care access. The psychiatric literature contains excellent resources for pediatricians who are interested in the assessment and initial management of MUS. In addition, a number of states are implementing psychiatric consultation resources for physicians that can provide guidance, education, and, in some cases, facilitated referrals provided by Child and Adolescent Psychiatry.[18,19] More information about these programs can be accessed through the National Network of Child Psychiatry Access Programs.[20] Pediatricians should also be aware of their own frustration, as somatic disorders may present signficant challenges in the primary care setting. Seeking advice and support from colleagues and specialists can be helpful in alleviating this frustration.

## ▶ PROGNOSIS

In general, the prognosis for children presenting with MUS is favorable, but proper symptom recognition and intervention are essential.[3] An association has been documented between MUS in children and subsequent anxiety or depression in adulthood, as well as between anxiety and depression in childhood and subsequent impairing somatic symptoms in adulthood.[21] Further studies will be needed to determine if identification and intervention in childhood can mitigate the development of lifelong symptoms. Meanwhile, it is clear that pediatricians play a key role in the initial management of the child with MUS, as well as in family support and care coordination. This type of approach can reduce child and family frustration, lead to improved outcomes, and be a rewarding experience for the physician who is able to help guide families through this complex process.

### *TOOLS FOR PRACTICE*

#### Medical Decision Support

- *Pediatric Symptom Checklist* (screen), Massachusetts General Hospital (www.massgeneral.org/psychiatry/services/psc_forms.aspx)
- *Strengths & Difficulties Questionnaires* (screen), Youth in Mind, Ltd (www.sdqinfo.com)
- *Children's Somatization Inventory* (screen), (sitemason.vanderbilt.edu/site/jnsciA/Questionnaires)
- *Functional Disability Inventory* (screen), (sitemason.vanderbilt.edu/site/jnsciA/Questionnaires)

### *REFERENCES*


1. Sumathipala A, Siribaddana S, Hewege S, et al. Understanding the explanatory model of the patient on their medically unexplained symptoms and its implication on treatment development research: a Sri Lanka Study. *BMC Psychiatry*. 2008;8:54
2. Chambers TL. Semeiology—a well established and challenging paediatric speciality. *Arch Dis Child.* 2003;88:281–282
3. Ibeziako P, Bujoreanu S. Approach to psychosomatic illness in adolescents. *Curr Opin Pediatr.* 2011;23:384–389
4. Lipowski ZJ. Somatization: the concept and its clinical application. *Am J Psychiatry*. 1988;145:1358–1368
5. Domènech-Llaberia E, Jané C, Canals J, et al. Parental reports of somatic symptoms in preschool children: prevalence and associations in a Spanish sample. *J Am Acad Child Adolesc Psychiatry*. 2004;43:598–604
6. Egger HL, Angold A, Costello EJ. Headaches and psychopathology in children and adolescents. *J Am Acad Child Adolesc Psychiatry*. 1998;37:951–958
7. Hyams JS, Burke G, Davis PM, Rzepski B, Andrulonis PA. Abdominal pain and irritable bowel syndrome in adolescents: a community-based study. *J Pediatr*. 1996;129:220–226
8. Goodman JE, McGrath PJ. The epidemiology of pain in children and adolescents: a review. *Pain*. 1991;46:247–264
9. Larsson BS. Somatic complaints and their relationship to depressive symptoms in Swedish adolescents. *J Child Psychol Psychiatry*. 1991;32:821–832
10. Offord DR, Boyle MH, Szatmari P, et al. Ontario Child Health Study. II. Six-month prevalence of disorder and rates of service utilization. *Arch Gen Psychiatry*. 1987;44:832–836
11. Egger HL, Costello EJ, Erkanli A, Angold A. Somatic complaints and psychopathology in children and adolescents: stomach aches, musculoskeletal pains, and headaches. *J Am Acad Child Adolesc Psychiatry*. 1999;38:852–860
12. Campo JV, Jansen-McWilliams L, Comer DM, Kelleher KJ. Somatization in pediatric primary care: association with psychopathology, functional impairment, and use of services. *J Am Acad Child Adolesc Psychiatry*. 1999;38:1093–1101

13. Campo JV, Fritz G. A management model for pediatric somatization. *Psychosomatics*. 2001;42:467–476
14. Walker LS, Beck JE, Garber J, Lambert W. Children's Somatization Inventory: psychometric properties of the revised form (CSI-24). *J Pediatr Psychol*. 2009;34:430–440
15. Claar RL, Walker LS. Functional assessment of pediatric pain patients: psychometric properties of the functional disability inventory. *Pain*. 2006;121:77–84
16. Dell ML, Campo JV. Somatoform disorders in children and adolescents. *Psychiatr Clin North Am*. 2011;34:643–660
17. Griffin A, Christie D. Taking the psycho out of psychosomatic: using systemic approaches in a paediatric setting for the treatment of adolescents with unexplained physical symptoms. *Clin Child Psychol Psychiatry*. 2008;13:531–542
18. Sarvet B, Gold J, Bostic JQ, et al. Improving access to mental health care for children: the Massachusetts Child Psychiatry Access Project. *Pediatrics*. 2010;126:1191–1200
19. Pediatric Psychiatry Network Web site. ppn.mh.ohio.gov/default.aspx. Accessed January 15, 2015
20. National Network of Child Psychiatry Access Programs Web site. www.nncpap.org/existing-programs.html. Accessed January 15, 2015
21. Campo JV. Annual research review: functional somatic symptoms and associated anxiety and depression—developmental psychopathology in pediatric practice. *J Child Psychol Psychiatry*. 2012;53:575–592

# Chapter 55

# Microcephaly

*Oscar H. Purugganan, MD, MPH*

## ▶ DEFINITION OF TERMS

Microcephaly refers to a head size that is 2 standard deviations below the mean (about the third percentile) based on age and gender. In itself, microcephaly means a small head; *micrencephaly* is the accurate term for a small brain. Because the forces of brain growth generally determine ultimate cranium size, a small brain leads to a small head. Without further brain growth, secondary closure of the sutures of the skull will ensue before the expected time, which should be differentiated from *craniosynostosis* in which primary and premature closure of sutures occurs with a normally growing brain.[1]

## ▶ MEASUREMENT AND USE OF GROWTH CHARTS

Measuring the head circumference is an important element of the pediatric physical examination and should be performed at each well-child visit, especially in the first 3 years of life.[2] Accurate measurements are critical and should be plotted on standardized charts. In the United States, the Centers for Disease Control and Prevention (CDC) released the latest growth charts in 2000.[3,4] These charts, which include head circumference charts, were based on 5 national health surveys from 1963 to 1994 and have been updated from the 1977 growth charts. A new feature of these updated charts is the inclusion of curves for 3rd and 97th percentiles, which are important cutoffs in the measurements of head circumference. The World Health Organization (WHO) released new international growth charts for children up to 5 years of age in 2006.[5] These charts represent growth standards derived from healthy children growing under optimal conditions from 6 sites worldwide. Their applicability in various clinical settings (including the US) and their potential effect on clinical practice are currently being investigated.[6,7] Head circumferences of children older than 3 years have traditionally been plotted on the growth curves developed by Nellhaus[8]; newer US-normed head circumference charts from birth to 21 years were published in 2010.[9] Charts are available for special populations with disturbances in growth, such as Down syndrome,[10] Williams syndrome,[11] achondroplasia,[12] and very low birth weight.[13]

Head circumference is measured by using a flexible, nonstretchable tape, running along the head above the supraorbital ridges and across the most prominent part of the occiput.[14] This measurement is known as the occipitofrontal circumference and has been shown to correlate with brain volume.[15] More instructive than a single measurement is a series of measurements over time, which can identify head circumferences that may be crossing percentiles while still falling within the normal range. Brain growth is maximal during the last few weeks of gestation to the first 2 years of life. Boys average a slightly larger head size than girls; the average head size at birth for boys in the United States is about 36 centimeters, and for girls about 35 centimeters.[3]

## ▶ DIFFERENTIAL DIAGNOSIS

Microcephaly is a physical finding and not a diagnosis. A multitude of conditions exist that can lead to a small brain. These conditions can be either genetic or environmental (see Box 55-1). They can be syndromic or nonsyndromic.

Clinically, a useful approach to the evaluation of microcephaly is to determine whether the small head circumference is noted at birth (congenital microcephaly) or whether the head circumference does not grow as expected after birth (acquired microcephaly).

Congenital microcephaly (noted at birth) can be either from genetic or environmental causes.

Genetic microcephaly is almost always present at birth; Rett syndrome (see below) is a notable exception. In these conditions, the brain structure may be either normal or abnormal.

In microcephaly vera, or true microcephaly, the brain is very small, usually 3 standard deviations below the mean, but the brain architecture is grossly normal.[16,17] Patients almost always have intellectual disability (ID) but have an otherwise unremarkable neurologic examination. A sloping forehead and prominent ears are usually the only dysmorphic features. Transmission is mainly autosomal recessive, although autosomal-dominant and X-linked forms also exist. Three genes that cause microcephaly vera have been identified: microcephalin *(MCPH)*, abnormal spindle in microcephaly[18,19] *(ASPM)*, and deoxynucleotide carrier *(DNC)* protein, which is implicated in Amish microcephaly.[20]

**BOX 55-1**

### *Causes of Microcephaly*

**GENETIC CAUSES**

- Microcephaly vera (isolated microcephaly with grossly normal brain architecture)
- Microcephaly with abnormal brain architecture (eg, lissencephaly, polymicrogyria)
- Genetic syndromes
  - o Miller-Dieker lissencephaly
  - o Seckel syndrome
  - o Rubinstein-Taybi syndrome
  - o Trisomy 21 syndrome
  - o Trisomy 13 syndrome
  - o de Lange syndrome
  - o Rett syndrome
- Metabolic disorders
  - o Aminoacidopathies
  - o Mitochondrial
- Asymptomatic familial

**ENVIRONMENTAL CAUSES**

- Teratogens
  - o Alcohol
  - o Maternal phenylketonuria
  - o Intrauterine irradiation
  - o Other teratogenic drugs (eg, hydantoin)
- Intrauterine infections
- Maternal health problems
- Hypoxic-ischemic encephalopathy
- Traumatic brain injury
- Meningitis
- Malnutrition

More common than microcephaly vera is a microcephalic child who has severe neurologic impairment such as seizures, spasticity, and global developmental delays. Neuroimaging may identify abnormal brain architecture such as defective prosencephalization (eg, holoprosencephaly), migration disorders (eg, lissencephaly, schizencephaly, pachygyri, polymicrogyri, heterotopias), and midline defects (eg, agenesis of corpus callosum).[16,17]

Microcephaly may be associated with other clinical findings that collectively represent a genetic syndrome. Miller-Dieker syndrome, which is caused by a deletion on the short arm of chromosome 17, is characterized by a small, smooth brain or lissencephaly (the most extreme of migration defects), facial dysmorphism, and severe ID. In Seckel syndrome, a rare autosomal-recessive disorder that has been mapped to loci in chromosomes 3 and 18, central nervous system (CNS) anomalies that suggest an underlying neuronal migration disorder[21] are present together with growth retardation, intellectual disability, and a *bird-headed* facial appearance.[22] Children with Rubinstein-Taybi syndrome have microcephaly, significant developmental problems, facial abnormalities, and broad thumbs and toes. Microdeletions of the cyclic adenosine monophosphate response element–binding protein gene on chromosome 16 have been implicated in this disorder.[22,23] Trisomies account for some cases of microcephaly. A classic example is Down syndrome (trisomy 21 syndrome) in which microcephaly is part of the characteristic phenotype that includes distinct facial features, congenital heart anomalies, and growth retardation. In de Lange syndrome, affected children have growth retardation, microcephaly, hirsutism, and unusual facial features such as synophrys and low anterior hairline. Most cases are sporadic, but an autosomal dominant inheritance has been suggested. *Smith's Recognizable Patterns of Human Malformation* and the online reference Online Mendelian Inheritance in Man (OMIM) provide comprehensive lists of conditions that are associated with abnormalities in head size.[22,24]

Based on the definition of microcephaly, it follows that about 2.5% of all children would be classified as microcephalic, and, most certainly, some of these children will be neurologically normal, especially those with head sizes immediately below 2 standard deviations from the mean (head circumference >3 standard deviations below the mean is almost always associated with some degree of neurologic impairment).[25] In individuals with isolated microcephaly who are neurologically intact and have normal intelligence, measuring the head circumferences of the parents and siblings is important. A family history of small head size in the context of normal development and neurologic examination describes asymptomatic familial microcephaly.[26]

Prenatal environmental factors may also lead to congenital microcephaly. A small head circumference at birth often reflects a condition of early prenatal origin. Intrauterine infections such as cytomegalovirus, toxoplasmosis, and rubella have been implicated in the development of microcephaly, and may also produce intrauterine growth retardation, hepatosplenomegaly, cardiac defects, retinopathy, cataracts, and hearing loss. Prenatal toxins that may lead to microcephaly in the newborn are alcohol,[27] drugs of abuse such as cocaine,[28] and irradiation. These environmental insults affect other organ systems as well, and microcephaly may be observed as a part of a syndrome. Prenatal exposure to alcohol may lead to intrauterine growth retardation, including microcephaly, facial features such as small palpebral fissures, smooth philtrum and thin upper lip, heart and eye defects, and behavioral and cognitive deficits, in a spectrum of disorders that range from alcohol-related neurodevelopmental disorder to fetal alcohol syndrome (FAS).[27,29] Untreated maternal phenylketonuria and hyperphenylalaninemia produce findings very similar to those of FAS: microcephaly (the most consistent finding), ID, facial dysmorphism, and cardiac defects.[30]

Head size that is not increasing as expected is a clue to an acquired microcephaly[31] (also called postnatal-onset microcephaly), and investigation as to possible environmental and genetic causes should be initiated. Microcephaly from these causes is usually apparent by 2 years of age.[25] A recent study classified 5 causal groups for acquired macrocephaly: idiopathic, or no identifiable cause; familial; syndromic, with associated anomalies; symptomatic, following a pathogenic event; and mixed.[32]

A genetic cause of microcephaly that does not usually present at birth is Rett syndrome, a condition exhibited almost exclusively in girls that is associated with a deceleration in head growth toward the second year of life leading to microcephaly, developmental regression, autistic features, and unusual hand mannerisms (hand-wringing and hand-washing movements). This genetic disorder has been mapped to the X chromosome and linked to a deletion of the *MeCP2* gene. Most cases are sporadic.[22] Genetic causes also include metabolic disorders that may lead to a deceleration of head growth in the first year of life; these conditions should be considered, especially if there is a history of parental consanguinity, episodic symptoms such as vomiting and encephalopathy, and developmental regression.[25,31]

Severe perinatal asphyxia is an important environmental cause of acquired microcephaly. The asphyxiated newborn has a normal head circumference at birth, but head growth decelerates, and microcephaly and suboptimal head growth may be observed by 12 months of age,[33] although acquired microcephaly can sometimes be detected as early as 6 weeks of age in infants who have had severe asphyxia.[34] These children go on to develop significant neuromotor and cognitive deficits. Other environmental causes of acquired microcephaly are meningitis, malnutrition, traumatic brain injury, and abusive head trauma.

With multiple suture craniosynostosis, primarily a problem of the skull rather than the brain, the head circumference may be small at birth, or head growth may abruptly cease during infancy. The shape of the skull is asymmetrical, and evidence exists of bony ridging in the area of the fused sutures. Signs of increased intracranial pressure may be present. These characteristics clearly differentiate the microcephaly associated with craniosynostosis from *micren*cephaly in which the small head is round, symmetrical, smooth, and devoid of bony ridging in the area of the sutures.[1] Premature closure of sutures may be an isolated feature or a part of a syndrome. Single-suture synostoses are not likely to cause microcephaly.

## ▶ EVALUATION

### *Relevant History*

Congenital microcephaly necessitates a thorough review of the prenatal history. Any potential exposure to toxins must be explored, such as the use of alcohol or other drugs of abuse. Poor maternal health during the pregnancy, intrauterine infections, and conditions causing placental insufficiency contribute to a suboptimal uterine environment that may lead to congenital microcephaly and intrauterine growth retardation. So, too, do psychosocial factors, as marked by lack of prenatal care and low levels of maternal education.[35] A pedigree analysis can help identify a family history of genetic syndromes, miscarriages, or microcephaly. Taking note of the head sizes of the parents and siblings is an important component of the evaluation. A review of systems may identify medical problems such as feeding difficulties, seizures, and previous infections such as meningitis. The history should also include a chronology of developmental milestones, as well as a description of the child's current function and behavior, with close attention to possible developmental regression.

## Physical Examination

The physical examination of the microcephalic child should focus on the following:

1. Accurate measurement of the head circumference and assessment of the pattern of head growth and the onset of microcephaly if previous measurements are available
2. Inspection and palpation of the skull, looking for asymmetry and bony ridging
3. Comparison of the head circumference with other growth parameters
4. Presence or absence of dysmorphic features
5. Presence or absence of congenital abnormalities involving other organ systems
6. Careful examination of the skin
7. Careful neurologic and developmental assessment

Accurate measurement and plotting on appropriate charts are critical (see earlier discussion). Head circumference of premature infants is adjusted for the degree of prematurity until about 2 years of age. For infants with birth weight of less than 1,000 g, corrected age is often used until 3 years or when growth has caught up based on normal growth curves.[14] Inspection and palpation of the skull may reveal an asymmetrical skull and face and bony ridging that are suggestive of craniosynostosis, the presence of which leads the pediatrician to a different approach in evaluation and management. A head circumference that is disproportionately small in relation to the child's weight and height is a likely indicator of a CNS condition. When microcephaly is part of generalized growth retardation, or when it is associated with dysmorphic facial features and multiple–organ system involvement, the search for conditions that may have a more systemic effect on the child should be investigated, such as chromosomal disorders, intrauterine infections, or exposure to toxins. Children with congenital microcephaly seem to have a higher frequency of major malformations when compared with normocephalic infants.[36] Examination of the skin may reveal the rash of an intrauterine infection. A thorough neurologic examination should assess for asymmetries, abnormalities in muscle tone, posture, strength, and reflexes. A developmental assessment may reveal generalized psychomotor retardation and motor delays, as well as speech/language and cognitive impairments.

## Laboratory Testing

The laboratory evaluation should be guided by the differential diagnoses. Children who are thought to have intrauterine infections must be tested for prenatal infections (toxoplasmosis, rubella, cytomegalovirus, syphilis, human immunodeficiency virus, herpes) and have ophthalmologic and audiologic evaluations. A microcephalic newborn with other congenital anomalies and atypical facial features should have a genetic consultation and evaluation. Genetic testing is available for many disorders, including chromosomal disorders, Miller-Dieker syndrome, and Rett syndrome. For children with microcephaly and dysmorphic features, the availability of array comparative genomic hybridization (aCGH) testing has enhanced the likelihood of a genetic diagnosis.[37] Metabolic testing is usually not recommended in the evaluation of an asymptomatic newborn with microcephaly; however, it should be considered in cases of postnatal-onset microcephaly, especially with a history of parental consanguinity, episodic symptoms, or developmental delays or regression.[25,37]

### Imaging

In the evaluation of a child with microcephaly, several neuroimaging modalities are available to identify abnormalities in brain structure. The yield is significantly higher in cases of severe microcephaly (>3 standard deviations below the mean) compared with mild microcephaly (2–3 standard deviations below the mean).[25] Magnetic resonance imaging (MRI) is most suitable for identifying gray and white matter disease and migration defects such as lissencephaly, pachygyria, and polymicrogyria. However, MRI is limited in its ability to study bone and calcifications. Computed tomography is useful to identify intracranial calcifications that may result from intrauterine infections, the skull abnormalities seen with premature fusion of cranial sutures, and ventricular system abnormalities. In infants with open fontanelles, ultrasonography of the head can be helpful in delineating cranial abnormalities. A skull radiograph can demonstrate intracranial calcifications and the characteristic bone findings in craniosynostosis but cannot detect abnormalities in brain structure. Consultation with a neuroradiologist may be helpful in determining which procedure, if any, is appropriate for a given child.

Practice parameters for the evaluation of the child with microcephaly have been developed by the Quality Standards Subcommittee of the American Academy of Neurology and the Practice Committee of the Child Neurology Society.[25]

## ▶ MANAGEMENT

The management of microcephaly is largely symptomatic and preventive. Appropriate prenatal care, maternal education and nutrition, avoidance of teratogenic substances, screening for intrauterine infections, and management of maternal health conditions may minimize the number of preventable cases of microcephaly. Because many children with microcephaly may have other medical issues (eg, cerebral palsy, seizures, ophthalmologic disorders), the pediatrician should monitor for these conditions and initiate the provision of interventions as needed.[25] Children with microcephaly require close follow-up for developmental issues and can benefit from early intervention and special education services as needed. Genetic counseling must be offered to parents who have offspring with genetic disorders. Children suspected to have craniosynostosis require neurosurgical consultation.

### When to Refer

- Consider for head circumference of more than 2 standard deviations below the mean (especially >3 standard deviations)
- Head circumference deceleration or poor head growth
- Dysmorphic features
- Abnormal neurologic examination and development
- Regression in motor, language, and social skills
- Seizures
- Suspected craniosynostosis

### When to Admit

- Signs of increased intracranial pressure
- Mental status change

### *TOOLS FOR PRACTICE*

## Medical Decision Support

- *Growth Charts*, Centers for Disease Control and Prevention (www.cdc.gov/growthcharts)
- *Online Mendelian Inheritance in Man* (online database), Johns Hopkins University (omim.org)
- *United States Head Circumference Growth Reference Charts: Birth to 21 Years* (article), *Journal of Pediatrics*, Vol 156, Issue 6, 2010

### *REFERENCES*


1. Cohen MM. Editorial: perspectives on craniosynostosis. *Am J Med Genet A*. 2005;136A:313–326
2. Green M, Palfrey JS, eds. *Bright Futures: Guidelines for Health Supervision of Infants, Children, and Adolescents*. 2nd ed. rev. Arlington, VA: National Center for Education in Maternal and Child Health; 2002
3. Kuczmarski RJ, Ogden CL, Grummer-Strawn LM, et al. *CDC Growth Charts: United States. Advance Data From Vital and Health Statistics; no. 314*. Hyattsville, MD: National Center for Health Statistics; 2000
4. Centers for Disease Control and Prevention, National Center for Health Statistics. 2000 CDC Growth Charts: United States. www.cdc.gov/growthcharts. Accessed October 23, 2014
5. World Health Organization. Child Growth Standards. http://www.who.int/childgrowth/standards/en. Accessed October 23, 2014
6. Daymont C, Hwang WT, Feudtner C, Rubin D. Head-circumference distribution in a large primary care network differs from CDC and WHO curves. *Pediatrics*. 2010;126:e836–e842
7. Júlíusson PB, Roelants M, Hoppenbrouwers K, Hauspie R, Bjerknes R. Growth of Belgian and Norwegian children compared to the WHO growth standards: prevalence below -2 and above +2 SD and the effect of breastfeeding. *Arch Dis Child*. 2011;96:916–921
8. Nellhaus G. Head circumference from birth to eighteen years. Practical composite international and interracial graphs. *Pediatrics*. 1968;41:106–114
9. Rollins JD, Collins JS, Holden KR. United States head circumference growth reference charts: birth to 21 years. *J Pediatr*. 2010;156:907–913
10. Cronk C, Crocker AC, Pueschel SM, et al. Growth charts for children with Down syndrome: 1 month to 18 years of age. *Pediatrics*. 1988;81:102–110
11. Williams Syndrome Association. Doctors resources for Williams syndrome. Available at: www.williams-syndrome.org. Accessed October 23, 2014
12. Horton WA, Rotter JI, Rimoin DL, Scott CI, Hall JG. Standard growth curves for achondroplasia. *J Pediatr*. 1978;93:435–438
13. Sherry B, Mei Z, Grummer-Strawn L, Dietz WH. Evaluation of and recommendations for growth references for very low birth weight (< or =1500 grams) infants in the United States. *Pediatrics*. 2003;111:750–758
14. US Department of Health and Human Services, Health Resources and Services Administration, Maternal and Child Health Bureau. MCHB training module: interpreting growth in head circumference. Available at: www.mchb.hrsa.gov. Accessed October 23, 2014
15. Bray PF, Shields WD, Wolcott GJ, Madsen JA. Occipitofrontal head circumference—an accurate measure of intracranial volume. *J Pediatr*. 1969;75:303–305
16. Volpe JJ. Overview: normal and abnormal human brain development. *Ment Retard Dev Disabil Res Rev*. 2000;6:1–5
17. Mochida GH, Walsh CA. Molecular genetics of human microcephaly. *Curr Opin Neurol*. 2001;14:151–156
18. Woods CG. Human microcephaly. *Curr Opin Neurobiol*. 2004;14:112–117
19. Suri M. What's new in neurogenetics? Focus on "primary microcephaly." *Eur J Paediatr Neurol*. 2003;7:389–392
20. Korf BR. What's new in neurogenetics? Amish microcephaly. *Eur J Paediatr Neurol*. 2003;7:393–394

21. Shanske A, Caride DG, Menasse-Palmer L, Bogdanow A, Marion RW. Central nervous system anomalies in Seckel syndrome: report of a new family and review of the literature. *Am J Med Genet.* 1997;70:155–158
22. OMIM—Online Mendelian Inheritance in Man. McKusick-Nathans Institute for Genetic Medicine, Johns Hopkins University (Baltimore, MD), and National Center for Biotechnology Information, National Library of Medicine (Bethesda, MD), 2000. www.ncbi.nlm.nih.gov/omim. Accessed October 23, 2014
23. Breuning MH, Dauwerse HG, Fugazza G, et al. Rubinstein-Taybi syndrome caused by submicroscopic deletions within 16p13.3. *Am J Hum Genet.* 1993;52:249–254
24. Jones KL. *Smith's Recognizable Patterns of Human Malformation.* 6th ed. Philadelphia, PA: Elsevier Saunders; 2006
25. Ashwal S, Michelson D, Plawner L, et al. Practice parameter: evaluation of the child with microcephaly (an evidence-based review): report of the Quality Standards Subcommittee of the American Academy of Neurology and the Practice Committee of the Child Neurology Society. *Neurology.* 2009;73:887–897
26. DeMyer W. Microcephaly, micrencephaly, megalocephaly and megalencephaly. In: Swaiman KE, Ashwal S, eds. *Pediatric Neurology: Principles and Practice.* 3rd ed. St Louis, MO: Mosby; 1999
27. Kvigne VL, Leonardson GR, Neff-Smith M, et al. Characteristics of children who have full or incomplete fetal alcohol syndrome. *J Pediatr.* 2004;145:635–640
28. Singer LT, Salvator A, Arendt R, et al. Effects of cocaine/polydrug exposure and maternal psychological distress on infant birth outcomes. *Neurotoxicol Teratol.* 2002;24:127–135
29. Paintner A, Williams AD, Burd L. Fetal alcohol spectrum disorders—implications for child neurology, part 2: diagnosis and management. *J Child Neurol.* 2012;27:355–362
30. Levy HL, Ghavami M. Maternal phenylketonuria: a metabolic teratogen. *Teratology.* 1996;53: 176–184
31. Rosman NP, Tarquinio DC, Datseris M, et al. Postnatal-onset microcephaly: pathogenesis, patterns of growth, and prediction of outcome. *Pediatrics.* 2011;127:665–671
32. Baxter PS, Rigby AS, Rotsaert MH, Wright I. Acquired microcephaly: causes, patterns, motor and IQ effects, and associated growth changes. *Pediatrics.* 2009;124:590–595
33. Mercuri E, Ricci D, Cowan FM, et al. Head growth in infants with hypoxic-ischemic encephalopathy: correlation with neonatal magnetic resonance imaging. *Pediatrics.* 2000;106:235–243
34. Ellis M, Manandhar D, Costello A. Head growth and cranial assessment at neurological examination in infancy. *Dev Med Child Neurol.* 2003;45:427
35. Krauss MJ, Morrissey AE, Winn HN, Amon E, Leet TL. Microcephaly: an epidemiologic analysis. *Am J Obstet Gynecol.* 2003;188:1484–1489
36. Vargas JE, Allred EN, Leviton A, Holmes LB. Congenital microcephaly: phenotypic features in a consecutive sample of newborn infants. *J Pediatr.* 2001;139:210–214
37. Abuelo D. Microcephaly syndromes. *Semin Pediatr Neurol.* 2007;14:118–127

# Chapter 56

# Nonconvulsive Periodic Disorders

*Sarah M. Roddy, MD*

A variety of paroxysmal nonepileptic disorders occur in children.[1] These disorders have a wide range of clinical features that mimic seizures, and distinguishing them from seizures is important so that the child is not treated inappropriately with anticonvulsants. A thorough history is often all that is needed to make the diagnosis, although a few patients may require a more extensive evaluation.

## ▶ BREATH-HOLDING SPELLS

Breath-holding spells, or infantile syncope, occur in approximately 5% of children. Most children who have breath-holding spells begin having episodes between 6 and 18 months of age, although spells may begin in the first few weeks of life. The frequency of episodes ranges from once a year to several times daily. The history of the episode and the surrounding events is the most important part of the evaluation of a child who has such spells. Because the familial incidence of breath-holding spells is high, the parents should be questioned about episodes in other family members.

Two types of breath-holding spells occur: cyanotic and pallid. The cyanotic type is more common than the pallid form and is usually precipitated by frustration or anger. During such spells, children cry vigorously and then hold their breath in expiration. Apnea is followed by cyanosis, with opisthotonic posturing and loss of consciousness. Recovery is usually quick, with return of respiration and consciousness within 1 minute. Evaluation of children who have severe cyanotic breath-holding spells has shown an underlying autonomic system dysregulation that may contribute to the pathophysiologic features of the episodes.[2-4] Pallid breath-holding episodes are usually provoked by sudden fright or minor injuries, especially falling and hitting the occiput. The child gasps or cries briefly and then abruptly becomes quiet, loses consciousness, has pallor, and becomes limp. The child may then develop clonic jerks. Pallid breath-holding spells are a vasovagal phenomenon. The precipitating event induces a vagally mediated asystole, leading to cerebral ischemia. Ocular compression during simultaneous electroencephalographic and electrocardiographic tracing in children who have pallid breath-holding spells has shown asystole with flattening of the electroencephalogram without electrical seizure activity.[1] The clonic jerks are caused by cerebral hypoxia rather than by epileptiform discharges from the brain.

The prognosis for children who have either type of breath-holding is excellent; most outgrow the episodes by school age. Children who have pallid breath-holding spells may later develop syncope.[1] Treatment is directed mainly at reassuring the family of the benign nature of the episodes. The pediatrician or other physician should emphasize that the episodes are not seizures and that they do not lead to intellectual disability or epilepsy. Because cyanotic episodes are often precipitated by temper tantrums, anger, and frustration, advice about behavior management may be helpful. Anemia has been described as a contributing factor in breath-holding spells, and treating it may reduce the incidence of the episodes.[6,7] Atropine is effective for pallid breath-holding episodes, but its use is rarely warranted. Anticonvulsants should not be used because they are not effective in treating either type of breath-holding spell (see Chapter 78, Temper Tantrums and Breath-Holding Spells).

## ▶ SYNCOPE

Syncope, or fainting, is an acute and transient loss of consciousness caused by reduced cerebral perfusion. Episodes are relatively common, particularly among teenagers.[8] Postural hypotension, which may occur after a sudden change from a sitting or reclining position to a standing position, can precipitate an episode. Emotional upset, fright, and overheating are also common provoking stimuli. Cardiac disorders, including arrhythmias, aortic stenosis, and severe cyanotic heart disease, may cause syncope by reducing cardiac output and causing cerebral hypoxia. In rare cases, episodes of syncope have been reported with swallowing, coughing, urinating, and defecating.[9]

Patients have presyncopal symptoms that may include light-headedness, anxiety, sweating, nausea, generalized numbness, and visual changes described as constriction or darkening of vision. Observers notice marked pallor and clammy skin. These symptoms are followed by loss of consciousness and slumping to the floor. Once the patient is recumbent and cerebral perfusion is restored, consciousness returns within a few seconds. If the patient is held with the head above the body and cerebral perfusion is not restored, clonic movements may occur. As with pallid breath-holding spells, these movements occur as a result of cerebral ischemia rather than epileptiform discharges from the brain. Patients are not disoriented or confused after an episode of syncope, although they may be tired.

The history is important in diagnosing syncope and should include a description of the event by the patient and an observer. Although laboratory evaluation is seldom needed, if atypical elements are involved, such as absence of a precipitating factor or confusion after the episode, an electroencephalogram or a cardiac evaluation, including Holter monitoring, may be appropriate. Evaluation with tilt-table testing can be helpful for children who have unexplained syncope.[10] Treatment consists of teaching the patient and family about managing an episode. Because patients have presyncopal symptoms, they should be instructed to sit or lie down as soon as the symptoms begin, thereby preventing progression to loss of consciousness. If the patient loses consciousness, the parent should place the child in a recumbent position with the head lower than the trunk. Parents often pick up a child who has fainted; they should be cautioned against this action because they may prolong the period of unconsciousness (see Chapter 77, Syncope, for a more detailed discussion of syncope and its causes).

## ▶ BENIGN PAROXYSMAL VERTIGO

Benign paroxysmal vertigo of childhood is a disorder characterized by brief attacks of vertigo. Symptoms usually appear within the first 3 or 4 years of life, although they may begin later. Episodes are characterized by abrupt onset, with the child appearing fearful and unable to maintain normal posture and gait. The child may seek support and clutch the parent or abruptly sit down or fall. In severe cases, the child may be limp and incapable of using the extremities. Pallor and diaphoresis are usually apparent, and vomiting and nystagmus sometimes occur. An episode typically lasts less than 30 seconds or, in rare cases, a few minutes. A brief period of postural instability may follow the episode; but within a few minutes, the instability resolves. Consciousness is not altered during the episode, and only rarely does the child feel sleepy after it. The frequency of episodes varies from as many as several weekly to 1 episode every few months. Audiograms are normal. Oculovestibular testing with cold-water calorics is difficult to perform in young children, and results vary. When properly done, testing shows no abnormalities in vestibular function.[11] The results of radiographic studies of the temporal bone and electroencephalographic recordings are also normal. Included in the differential diagnosis of vertigo in childhood are brainstem lesions, posterior fossa tumors, and epilepsy. The history and physical examination usually differentiate benign paroxysmal vertigo from these more serious disorders. In most cases, no treatment is necessary, and anticonvulsants are not effective. Antihistamines such as dimenhydrinate have been used in some patients who have frequent episodes, with an apparent reduction in the number of episodes. Because the frequency of attacks varies, assessing the effect of therapy accurately is difficult. Attacks of vertigo usually stop spontaneously over a period of a few years. Some children with benign paroxysmal vertigo later develop migraine headaches[12] (see Chapter 17, Dizziness and Vertigo).

## ▶ SHUDDERING ATTACKS

Shuddering or shivering episodes are a benign movement disorder that probably occurs in many children at one time or another. The episodes are brief and characterized by paroxysmal rapid tremors involving primarily the head and arms. Some episodes may involve flexion of the head, elbow, trunk, and knees, with adduction of the elbows and knees.[13] Consciousness is not altered during the episodes. The frequency varies, with some children having more than 100 episodes daily. Emotional factors, including excitement, fear, anger, and frustration, may precipitate episodes. Shuddering episodes may start as early as a few months of age or not until later in childhood. The number of episodes usually declines gradually. The pathophysiologic mechanism of the episodes is unclear, although the attacks have been postulated to be an expression of an essential tremor.[13,14] Electroencephalographic monitoring has shown that the episodes are not epileptiform in nature.[15] In most cases, no treatment is necessary. If episodes are severe and interfere with activities, treatment with propranolol may be helpful.[16] Anticonvulsants are ineffective and should not be used.

## ▶ BENIGN NEONATAL SLEEP MYOCLONUS

Sudden brief jerks of the extremities are normal in children and adults when falling asleep. Sleep-related myoclonus in neonates is called *benign neonatal sleep myoclonus.* The myoclonic jerks begin in the first month of life, often within the first day, and are present only during sleep, disappearing when the infant awakens.[17] The jerking movements may start in one extremity and then progress to involve the other extremities, or they may begin bilaterally. The upper extremities are involved more often than the lower extremities. Jerks occur every 2 to 3 seconds for several minutes, although they have been reported to last up to 12 hours.[18] Rocking the crib and repetitive sounds may provoke the myoclonus.[19] Development is normal, and no neurologic deficits are present. Electroencephalographic results are normal, with no epileptiform discharges associated with the myoclonus.[18] The major differential diagnosis of neonatal sleep myoclonus is a seizure disorder. A history of episodes only during sleep and a normal electroencephalogram help differentiate this benign disorder from seizures. The myoclonus usually diminishes gradually during the first 6 months of life, although it has rarely lasted until 3 years.[20] No treatment is necessary. The infants do not subsequently develop epilepsy or cognitive delay.[21]

## ▶ NIGHT TERRORS

Night terrors or sleep terrors are a sleep disorder with some features that mimic partial complex seizures. They occur in up to 6% of children, with a peak incidence in late preschool-aged and early school-aged children.[22] Affected children often have a family history of either night terrors or another sleep disorder. The episodes usually occur during the first 2 hours after falling asleep. The child sits up in bed abruptly and screams or talks unintelligibly. If the child's eyes are open, they have a glazed look. During the episode, the child appears to be hallucinating and does not respond to the parents. Tachycardia and diaphoresis result from activation of the sympathetic nervous system. In some cases, the child may sleepwalk. Night terrors usually last approximately 10 minutes, with the child then relaxing and abruptly falling back to sleep. On awakening, the child does not remember the episode. Night terrors are caused by a rapid partial arousal from deep, slow-wave sleep. Febrile illness and sleep deprivation may trigger night terrors.[23]

Electroencephalography does not show seizure activity during the episodes. It is important to differentiate night terrors from nightmares, which occur later in the sleep cycle, during rapid eye movement (REM) sleep, and are associated with easy arousal and recall of the content, or at least the occurrence, of the nightmare. Night terrors usually occur less often as the child gets older, although episodes may continue into adolescence and adulthood. The nature of the episodes should be explained to the parents. Although parents tend to try to wake and reassure the child, they should be told that the child is not aware of their presence, and attempts to awaken the child are not helpful and may increase agitation. If the child is sleep deprived, parents should take steps to increase the amount of sleep the child is getting. If night terrors persist despite adequate sleep, a sleep study may be needed to evaluate for obstructive sleep apnea, which can trigger night terrors.[24] In most cases, no medication is indicated. However, if episodes are frequent or severe, a benzodiazepine, imipramine, or L-5-hydroxytryptophan may be helpful.[23,25]

## ▶ NARCOLEPSY

Narcolepsy is a sleep–wake disorder characterized by excessive and inappropriate periods of sleep during the day. The daytime sleepiness interrupts activities and does not diminish in response to adequate amounts of sleep at night. Naps may last from a few minutes to longer than an hour. In addition to the excessive daytime sleep, patients often have cataplexy, sleep paralysis, and hypnagogic hallucinations. Cataplexy is a transient partial or complete loss of tone, often triggered by an emotional reaction such as laughter or fright. The individual does not lose consciousness. Sleep paralysis occurs as the patient falls asleep or awakens and is characterized by the inability to move or speak. Hypnagogic hallucinations occur while falling asleep, can be auditory or visual, and may be very frightening to a child.

The estimated prevalence of narcolepsy is 0.02% to 0.05%.[26] Onset usually occurs in the second decade, although it has been reported in toddlers. Sleep studies in patients who have narcolepsy show extremely short sleep onset latency. In narcolepsy, REM sleep occurs within 15 minutes of sleep onset; in healthy patients, 90 minutes of non-REM sleep precede the first REM period. A strong association exists between narcolepsy and the human leukocyte class II antigen DQB1*0602.[27] Human leukocyte antigen typing may be helpful but is not diagnostic. The hypocretin peptides that are important for maintaining wakefulness may be absent on cerebrospinal fluid studies, especially in cases involving cataplexy.[28] Sleep studies are important in diagnosing narcolepsy. Included in the differential diagnosis of excessive daytime sleepiness are chronic illness, sleep apnea, hypothyroidism, depression, and seizures.

Narcolepsy is a lifelong condition, but central nervous system stimulants such as methylphenidate and modafinil help reduce the frequency of naps. Tricyclic medications such as imipramine are used to treat cataplexy and the other associated symptoms.[29]

## When to Refer

- Diagnosis cannot be made by history and physical examination
- Need exists for subspecialty expertise

## When to Admit

- Child needs video electroencephalographic monitoring to evaluate an episode

### REFERENCES

1. Lombroso CT, Lerman P. Breathholding spells (cyanotic and pallid infantile syncope). *Pediatrics.* 1967;39(4):563–581
2. DiMario FJ, Burleson JA. Autonomic nervous system function in severe breath-holding spells. *Pediatr Neurol.* 1993;9(4):268–274
3. DiMario FJ, Bauer L, Baxter D. Respiratory sinus arrhythmia in children with severe cyanotic and pallid breath-holding spells. *J Child Neurol.* 1998;13(9):440–442
4. Akalin F, Turan S, Güran T, Ayabakan C, Yilmaz Y. Increased QT dispersion in breath-holding spells. *Acta Paediatr.* 2004;93(6):770–774
5. Orii KE, Kato Z, Osamu F, et al. Changes of autonomic nervous system function in patients with breath-holding spells treated with iron. *J Child Neurol.* 2002;17(5):337–340
6. Colina KF, Abelson HT. Resolution of breath-holding spells with treatment of concomitant anemia. *J Pediatr.* 1995;126(3):395–397
7. Daoud AS, Batieha A, al-Sheyyab M, Abuekteish F, Hijazi S. Effectiveness of iron therapy on breath-holding spells. *J Pediatr.* 1997;130(4):547–550
8. Driscoll DJ, Jacobsen SJ, Porter CJ, Wollan PC. Syncope in children and adolescents. *J Am Coll Cardiol.* 1997;29:1039–1045
9. Hannon DW, Knilans TK. Syncope in children and adolescents. *Curr Probl Pediatr.* 1993;23(9): 358–384
10. Samoil D, Grubb BP, Kip K, Kosinski DJ. Head-upright tilt table testing in children with unexplained syncope. *Pediatrics.* 1993;92(3):426–430
11. Finkelhor BK, Harker LA. Benign paroxysmal vertigo of childhood. *Laryngoscope.* 1987;97(10): 1161–1163
12. Lanzi G, Balottin U, Fazzi E, et al. Benign paroxysmal vertigo of childhood: a long-term follow-up. *Cephalagia.* 1994;14:458–460

13. Vanasse M, Bedard P, Andermann F. Shuddering attacks in children: an early clinical manifestation of essential tremor. *Neurology.* 1976;26(11):1027–1030
14. Kanazawa O. Shuddering attacks-report of four children. *Pediatr Neurol.* 2000;23(5):421–424
15. Holmes GL, Russman BS. Shuddering attacks: evaluation using electroencephalographic frequency modulation radiotelemetry and videotape monitoring. *Am J Dis Child.* 1985;140:72–73
16. Barron TF, Younkin DP. Propranolol therapy for shuddering attacks. *Neurology.* 1992;42(1): 258–259
17. Di Capua M, Fusco L, Ricci S, Vigevano F. Benign neonatal sleep myoclonus: clinical features and video-polygraphic recordings. *Mov Disord.* 1993;8(2):191–194
18. Turanli G, Senbil N, Altunbasak S, Topcu M. Benign neonatal sleep myoclonus mimicking status epilepticus. *J Child Neurol.* 2004;19(1):62–63
19. Alfonso I, Papazian O, Alcardi J, Jeffries HE. A simple maneuver to provoke benign neonatal sleep myoclonus. *Pediatrics.* 1995;96(6):1161–1163
20. Egger J, Grossman G, Auchterlonie IA. Benign sleep myoclonus in infancy mistaken for epilepsy. *BJM.* 2003;326(7396):975–976
21. Vaccerio ML, Valenti MA, Carullo A, et al. Benign neonatal sleep myoclonus: case report and follow-up of four members of an affected family. *Clin Electroencephalogr.* 2003;34(1):15–17
22. DiMario FJ Jr, Emery S III. The natural history of night terrors. *Clin Pediatr.* 1987;26(10): 505–511
23. Mason TB 2nd, Pack AI. Sleep terrors in childhood. *J Pediatr.* 2005;147(3):388–392
24. Guilleminault C, Palombini L, Pelayo R, et al. Sleepwalking and sleep terrors in prepubertal children: what triggers them? *Pediatrics.* 2003;111(1):e17–e25
25. Bruni O, Ferri R, Miano S, Verrillo E. L-5-Hydroxytryptophan treatment of sleep terrors in children. *Eur J Pediatr.* 2004;163(7):402–407
26. Hublin C, Kaprio J, Partinen M, et al. The prevalence of narcolepsy: an epidemiological study of the Finnish Twin Cohort. *Ann Neurol.* 1994;35(6):709–716
27. Mignot E, Hayduk R, Black J, Grumet FC, Guilleminault C. HLA DQB1*0602 is associated with cataplexy in 509 narcoleptic patients. *Sleep.* 1997;20(11):1012–1020
28. Mignot E, Lammers GJ, Ripley B, et al. The role of cerebrospinal fluid hypocretin measurement in the diagnosis of narcolepsy and other hypersomnias. *Arch Neurol.* 2002;59(10):1553–1562
29. Dyken ME, Yamada T. Narcolepsy and disorders of excessive somnolence. *Prim Care Clin Office Pract.* 2005;32(2):389–413

# Chapter 57

# Odor (Unusual Urine and Body)

*Erik Langenau, DO, MS*

Unusual odors in children may be a chief complaint, symptom, or sign. The odors may emanate from the breath, urine, skin, sputum, vomitus, stool, or vagina,[1] and they can provide helpful clues in the diagnosis of many specific conditions.

## ▶ DEFINITION OF TERMS

Although unusual odors can be caused by many different conditions, bromhidrosis and halitosis require careful attention.

Bromhidroisis, a condition in which sweat is malodorous and offensive, is caused by decomposition of products from the apocrine, eccrine, and sebaceous glands.[2] Apocrine bromhidrosis, which begins after puberty with a characteristic acrid or sweaty odor, results from a combination of short-chain fatty acids, ammonia, androgenic steroids, hexanoic acid, and saturated ketones and indoles.[2] Eccrine bromhidrosis results from bacterial interaction with moist keratin and is caused by hyperhidrosis, obesity, intertrigo, and diabetes mellitus; it is aggravated by hot weather and occurs primarily in the soles, palms, and intertriginous areas.[2]

Halitosis is an offensive odor emanating from the mouth or air-filled cavities such as the nose, sinuses, or pharynx[3]; it may be physiologic or pathologic, with numerous causes, such as xerostomia (dry mouth), periodontitis, sinusitis, tonsillitis, or gastroesophageal reflux.[4]

## ▶ EVALUATION OF UNUSUAL ODORS

The differential diagnosis of unusual odors is extensive and includes numerous systemic, metabolic, toxic, and infectious diseases. The physician may inquire about the presence or absence of an odor when evaluating a child with a particular infection, dermatologic condition, metabolic disease, or ingestion.[1,5–7] After a thorough history and physical examination is conducted, the differential diagnosis of an unusual odor can become more focused.

### *Chief Complaint*

If an unusual body odor is the chief complaint, a thorough history of the present illness helps narrow the differential diagnosis. Relevant questions may include the following:
When did you first notice the odor?
What does it smell like?

Does it smell like anything familiar?
What is the quality?
What is the intensity?
Does it seem to come from a certain part of the body?
Does bathing or cleaning make it better?
Are there any other associated symptoms, such as vomiting, weight loss, lethargy?
Do other members of the family have similar odors?
Do any family members have metabolic or infectious diseases?
Have you seen any insertion of a foreign body in the nose, ear, anus, or vagina?
Has your child taken any oral or topical medications, vitamins, herbal supplements, or toxins?
How has the odor affected the child and family?

## Physical Examination

In assessing an odor, the examiner should note the character of the odor, determine the patient's age (and stage of pubertal development), check for any other signs or symptoms during a complete examination with the child unclothed, and attempt to localize the odor to a particular body site.

In a routine medical encounter, an odor may be the first observation when the patient enters the examining room. Odors are often difficult to describe because of insufficient standards for classifying, qualifying, quantifying, and teaching about them.[8,9] Historically and practically, odors have been compared with others for which physicians have common experience, and odor strength is characterized by such adjectives as strong or faint. In addition, individuals differ in their ability to detect at least some odors and in their assessments of whether certain odors are offensive. Gas-liquid chromatography and enhanced odor classification systems now allow more precise identification of odors.[10] Artificial nose technology, which can sense a wide range of volatile chemicals and be trained in pattern recognition, may soon become a tool to supplement the physician's own nose.[11,12] Artificial noses or bioelectronic noses have already been used to detect diseases such as tuberculosis, urinary tract infections, *Helicobacter pylori* infection,[13] gastroesophageal reflux disease,[14] bacterial vaginosis,[15] diabetes,[16] and a number of cancers.[17]

If a patient reports an intermittent unusual odor that is never detected by others, then the possibility of temporal lobe epilepsy with olfactory manifestations should be entertained.[18] On the other hand, if the physician notices a clearly offensive body odor, but the patient or parent does not, then anosmia should be considered. Causes of impaired olfaction may include various endocrinopathies such as Kallmann syndrome, diabetes, Turner syndrome, and hypothyroidism; neuropsychiatric conditions such as schizophrenia; infections such as rhinitis and sinusitis; autoimmune diseases such as Sjögren syndrome, granulomatosis with polyangiitis (formerly known as Wegener granulomatosis) and multiple sclerosis; or medications including metronidazole, tetracycline, captopril, and amphetamines.[8,19–22]

Physicians should also be aware that odor recognition involves complicated molecular and genetic mechanisms.[23] Sex, age, and genetic variation may lead to differences in abilities and thresholds for detecting odors.[8,21,24] Physicians and patients may therefore vary in their ability to detect certain odors.

## ▶ DIFFERENTIAL DIAGNOSIS OF UNUSUAL ODORS

An array of odors can be associated with the human body and clothing, and subtle differences in odor can be found among people as well. Therefore the first task may be to decide whether a particular odor truly is peculiar and whether it emanates from the body. The odor may be simply a normal body odor that draws attention because of its intensity or because the complainant is unusually sensitive to or concerned about it.

### *Normal Body Odor*

Normal body odors derive from secretions of the sweat and apocrine glands, vagina, cervix, respiratory tract, urine, feces, breath, and flatus.[5] Odor may be produced or modified by the action of normal or abnormal microbial flora.

In Western culture, people often minimize body odors by frequently changing their clothing, bathing, and using deodorants, antiperspirants, mouthwashes, douches, or scents applied to the skin. If one of these artificial odors is too strong, then the physician may wonder what the patient is trying to hide. On the other hand, if a patient does not practice these customs, then the physician may detect an odor that is offensive and then must decide why the patient is not complying with social expectations.

Body odor changes with puberty, and a characteristic adult odor may prompt a child (or the child's parents) to seek medical attention.

### *Axillary Odor*

Axillary odor, which varies in intensity from person to person, is often the strongest odor associated with adolescents and adults.[5] Its pungency has long been attributed to the action of aerobic diphtheroids on apocrine secretions. Recent work has identified odor-binding proteins that originate in the apocrine glands. The most abundant of the smelly compounds may be (E)-3-methyl-2-hexenoic acid.[25] Bacterial decomposition of androsterone is another possible cause of axillary odor.[26] Axillary hair seems to retain or spread odor.[27]

Some adolescents and adults have axillary odor that is unusually strong, a condition called osmidrosis axillae or axillary apocrine bromhidrosis. The odor emanates from the apocrine glands. Possible explanations include specific features of apocrine androgen metabolism,[28] bacterial alteration of sweat,[29] and abnormally large and numerous apocrine glands.[30] A variety of topical interventions, as well as surgical excisions, have been used to treat this condition.

### *Vaginal Odor*

The odor of postpubertal vaginal secretions varies among individuals and with the menstrual cycle. Vulvar secretions, vaginal wall transudates, exfoliated cells, cervical mucus, fluids from the endometrium and uterine tubes, and metabolic products of the vaginal microflora all contribute.[31] Some people characterize the resulting odor as unpleasant, even in the absence of vaginitis. Odor during menses is usually rated as the most offensive.[31] Some individuals may be concerned about these normal odors. The rotten fish smell of the vaginal discharge associated with bacterial vaginosis is caused by trimethylamine.[32]

### *Mouth Odor*

The odor of a healthy mouth is assumed to be inoffensive in childhood; however, *bad breath* is not uncommon, even in an otherwise well child. Halitosis in the absence of disease is thought to be caused by volatile sulfur compounds (hydrogen sulfide and methyl mercaptan), which are formed when the oral flora metabolize proteins that are found in the saliva or adhering to the teeth, tongue, or gums.[4] Halitosis is exacerbated by infrequent eating and drinking, which ordinarily have a flushing action. Acutely, halitosis may accompany a variety of childhood respiratory tract and gastrointestinal infections. Persistent halitosis should prompt evaluation for dental or gingival disease, a nasal foreign body, lung disease, or gastroesophageal reflux.[4]

Simple oral hygiene can temporarily modify mouth odor. Brushing the teeth and the dorsoposterior surface of the tongue and then rinsing with water or a mouthwash may well reduce both the concentrations of volatile sulfur compounds and the offensive odor.[4]

### Foot Odor

Eccrine bromhidrosis, tinea pedis (athlete's foot), and pitted keratolysis have been associated with increased foot odor. Each of these conditions may be exacerbated by occlusive footwear (eg, boots) and a hot, humid climate. The odor from eccrine bromhidrosis of the feet is thought to result from the breakdown of keratin and lipids by diphtheroids; fatty acid metabolites may be the agents responsible for the odor.[2] Pitted keratolysis (plantar keratolysis puncta) is characterized by white plaques and shallow pits on the plantar surface. Various gram-positive bacteria and dermatophytes have been identified in affected patients. The odor is thought to be related to the breakdown products (such as thiols and thioesters) of these microorganisms within the stratum corneum.[2] Conditions associated with foot odor may respond to a combination of moisture control, topical antibiotics, and antifungal agents.

### Metabolic Abnormalities

Certain metabolic defects are associated with an unusual odor of the urine,[33] sweat, and other body fluids because of accumulation of odoriferous metabolic precursors or byproducts. These metabolic disorders and associated odors are listed in Table 57-1. Metabolic disorders should be suspected if an infant has an unusual body odor, especially if the patient is ill appearing, malnourished, or ketotic. Recognizing the odor in a compatible clinical situation may lead to early diagnosis, and prompt treatment may prevent progressive brain damage or death. A specialist in metabolic diseases should be consulted, and an appropriate diet should be started while a more thorough metabolic evaluation is being completed. The odor itself may lead to embarrassment, low self-esteem, and psychosocial problems. In some conditions, dietary manipulation may reduce the malodor as well as other symptoms.[34]

### Foreign Bodies

Retention of a foreign body in an orifice may lead to a focal foul smell. Retained foreign bodies within the vagina (eg, tampons, diaphragms), auditory canals, and nostrils are common causes of local foul odor. A retained foreign body may also be related to a generalized body odor because odoriferous substances are absorbed and secreted in sweat.[52] Nasal foreign bodies are the most commonly associated with this condition.[53,54]

### Inhalation, Poisoning, and Ingestion

When inhalation or ingestion of a toxic substance is suspected, odor may provide a clue to the substance involved. Common associations are listed in Table 57-2. When puzzled, the physician should consult a poison control center.

**Table 57-1**
**Metabolic Abnormalities Associated With Unusual Odor**

| DISEASE | DESCRIPTION OF ODOR | CLINICAL FEATURES | METABOLIC DEFECT |
|---|---|---|---|
| 3-hydroxy-3-methylglutaryl-CoA lyase deficiency | Cat urine | Malaise, hypoglycemia, hepatomegaly, transaminitis, mild acidosis | 3-hydroxy-3-methylglutaryl-CoA lyase |
| Glutaric aciduria type II (multiple acyl-CoA dehydrogenase deficiency) | Sweaty feet, acrid, stale | Hypoglycemia, hypotonia, hepatomegaly, respiratory distress, death | Electron transfer flavoprotein (ETF) or ETF:ubiquinone oxidoreductase (ETF:QO) |
| Hawkinsinuria | Swimming pool | Failure to thrive, hepatomegaly, anemia, irritability | 4-hydroxyphenylpyruvate dioxygenase |
| Hypermethioninemia | Boiled cabbage | Usually asymptomatic. Some develop intellectual disability, dystonia. | Methionine adenosyltransferase |
| Isovaleric acidemia | Sweaty feet, acrid | Acidosis, vomiting, dehydration, coma, mild-to-moderate intellectual disability, aversion to protein foods | Isovaleric acid CoA dehydrogenase |
| Ketoacidosis | Fruity, acetone-like, decomposing apples | Vomiting, dehydration, altered mental status, lethargy | Ketoacidosis (eg, from starvation or insulin deficiency) |
| Maple syrup urine disease | Maple syrup, burnt sugar, curry, malt, caramel, fenugreek beans | Severe form: feeding difficulty, vomiting, lethargy, acidosis, seizures, coma leading to death in first months of life | Mitochondrial branched-chain alpha–keto dehydrogenase complex |
| | | Intermediate form: mild acidosis, intellectual disability, developmental delay, ophthalmoplegia | |
| | | Intermittent form: episodic ataxia and lethargy that may progress to coma | |
| | | Thiamine-responsive form: respond to supplementation | |
| | | E3-deficient form: variable expression | |
| Multiple carboxylase deficiency | Tomcat urine | Failure to thrive, hypotonia, vomiting, seizures, rash | Holocarboxylase synthetase |
| Oasthouse urine disease (methionine malabsorption syndrome; Smith-Strang disease) | Dried celery, malt, hops, yeast, beer | Diarrhea, intellectual disability, spasticity, attacks of hyperpnea, fever, edema | Kidney and intestinal transport of methionine, branched-chain amino acids, tyrosine, and phenylalanine |
| Phenylketonuria | Musty; similar to a mouse, horse, wolf, or barn | Vomiting, progressive mental retardation, microcephaly, eczema, decreasing pigmentation, seizures, spasticity | Phenylalanine hydroxylase |

*Continued*

**Table 57-1**
**Metabolic Abnormalities Associated With Unusual Odor—cont'd**

| DISEASE | DESCRIPTION OF ODOR | CLINICAL FEATURES | METABOLIC DEFECT |
|---|---|---|---|
| Trimethylaminuria (fish odor syndrome) | Dead or rotting fish | Usually asymptomatic with isolated finding. Fish odor of urine and body. | Trimethylamine oxidase |
| Tyrosinemia | Boiled cabbage, rancid butter | Liver failure, death | Fumarylacetoacetate hydrolase deficiency |

Data derived from multiple sources.[1,2,34–51]

**Table 57-2**
**Inhalations, Poisonings, and Ingestions Associated With Recognizable Odors**

| ODOR | SITE | SUBSTANCE IMPLICATED |
|---|---|---|
| Bitter almond | Breath | Cyanide (chokecherry, apricot pits), jetberry bush |
| Burned rope | Breath | Marijuana |
| Camphor | Breath | Naphthalene (mothballs) |
| Carrots | Breath | Water hemlock (cicutoxin) |
| Coal gas | Breath | Coal gas (associated with odorless but toxic carbon monoxide) |
| Disinfectant | Breath | Phenol, creosote |
| Fishy | Breath | Zinc or aluminum phosphide |
| Fruity, acetone or decomposing apples | Breath | Lacquer, salicylates, chloroform |
| Fruity, alcohol | Breath | Alcohol (ethanol, isopropyl alcohol), phenol, acetone, amyl nitrites *(poppers)* |
| Fruity, pearlike | Breath | Chloral hydrate, paraldehyde |
| Garlic | Breath, vomitus, stool | Arsenic |
| | Breath, vomitus | Phosphorus, tellurium, parathion, malathion, dimethyl sulfoxide, selenium |
| Glue | Breath, vomitus | Toluene, solvents *(huffing)* |
| Hydrocarbon | Breath, vomitus | Hydrocarbons |
| Medicinal, musty | Urine | Penicillins, cephalosporins |
| Metallic | Breath | Iodine |
| | Stool | Arsenic |
| | Vomitus | Arsenic, phosphorus |
| Rotten eggs | Breath | Hydrogen sulfide mercaptans, disulfiram, dimethyl sulfate, N-acetylcysteine |
| Severe bad breath | Breath | Amphetamines |
| Shoe polish | Breath | Nitrobenzene |
| Stale tobacco | Breath | Nicotine |
| Sulfides or amines | Skin | War gases |
| Violets | Urine, vomitus | Turpentine |
| Wintergreen | Breath | Methyl salicylate |

Data derived from multiple sources.[1,2,6,55,56]

Penicillin and cephalosporins give the urine a medicinal or musty smell.[2] Topical benzoyl peroxide has been implicated in at least 1 case of persistent body odor.[57] Thiourea compounds give the breath a sweet smell, resembling that of decaying vegetables.[58] Newborns have smelled spicy when their mothers ate particular curries before labor.[59]

### Other Diseases

Odor may suggest either the presence of an infection (Table 57-3) or other acquired medical conditions (Table 57-4).

**Table 57-3**
**Odor as a Clue to Infection**

| INFECTION | ODOR |
|---|---|
| ***Respiratory and Ear, Nose, and Throat Infections*** | |
| Candidiasis | Sweet, fruity |
| Diphtheria | Sweet |
| Intranasal foreign body | Foul and putrid |
| Lung abscess, empyema, bronchiectasis, fetid bronchitis | Foul, putrid breath or sputum |
| *Pseudomonas* infection, otitis externa | Foul cerumen |
| Rubella | Fresh-plucked feathers |
| Trench mouth, tonsillitis, gingivitis | Severe halitosis |
| Tuberculous lymphadenitis (scrofula) | Stale beer |
| Typhoid fever | Fresh-baked brown bread |
| Yellow fever | Butcher shop |
| ***Skin Infections*** | |
| *Candida* (skin) | Heavily sweet |
| Decubitus ulcer | Foul |
| Diphtheria (skin) | Sweet |
| Erythroderma | Rancid |
| Hidradenitis suppurativa | Lingering, pungent |
| Pitted keratolysis (gram-positive bacteria and dermatophytes) | Cheesy, sweaty, rotten smell from feet |
| *Pseudomonas* skin infection (burns) | Musty, fruity, grapelike, wet corn tortillas |
| Syphilis (condyloma latum) | Foul |
| Tinea capitis | Mousy, mouse urine–like |
| ***Genitourinary Infections*** | |
| Bacterial vaginosis | Amine, fishy vaginal discharge |
| Genital warts (condyloma acuminatum) | Foul |
| Urinary tract infection with urea-splitting bacteria | Ammoniacal urine |
| Vaginal foreign body, vaginitis | Foul vaginal discharge |

*Continued*

**Table 57-3**
**Odor as a Clue to Infection—cont'd**

| INFECTION | ODOR |
|---|---|
| ***Gastrointestinal Infections*** | |
| Rotavirus gastroenteritis | Full |
| Shigellosis | Rancid stool |
| ***Neurologic Infections*** | |
| *Cryptococcus* meningitis | Alcohol smell to cerebrospinal fluid |
| ***Miscellaneous Infections*** | |
| Chorioamnionitis | Foul-smelling amniotic fluid |
| ***Infectious Etiologic Agents*** | |
| Anaerobic bacteria | Foul-smelling wound, rotten apples |
| *Candida* infection | Sweet, fruity, beer odor in peritoneal dialysate |
| Clostridium gas gangrene | Rotten apples |
| Proteolytic bacteria | Pus that smells similar to feces or overripe cheese |
| Proteus infection | Mousy |
| *Pseudomonas aeruginosa* | Musty, fruity, grapelike, wet corn tortillas |

Data derived from multiple sources.[1,2,4,6,13,32,60–63]

**Table 57-4**
**Other Conditions Associated With Specific Odors**

| DISEASE | ODOR |
|---|---|
| ***Systemic Diseases*** | |
| Hepatic failure | Breath: musty fish, raw liver, feces, rotten eggs, or newly mown clover *(Fetor hepaticus)* (caused by mercaptans such as dimethyl sulfide) |
| Ketoacidosis (diabetes or starvation) | Breath: fruity, acetone-like, decomposing apples (caused by ketones) |
| Uremia | Urine: fishy (caused by dimethylamine and trimethylamine) |
| | Breath: ammoniac (caused by ammonia) |
| ***Vitamin Deficiencies*** | |
| Pellagra (niacin deficiency) | Sour or musty bread |
| Scurvy (vitamin C deficiency) | Putrid |
| ***Dermatologic Conditions*** | |
| Psoriasis (pustular) | Skin: heavy |
| Skin diseases with protein breakdown (pemphigus) | Skin: foul, unpleasant |
| ***Gastrointestinal Conditions*** | |
| Malabsorption | Feces: foul |
| Melena (gastrointestinal bleeding) | Feces: foul |
| ***Surgical Conditions*** | |
| Esophageal diverticulum | Breath: feculent, foul |

*Continued*

**Table 57-4**
**Other Conditions Associated With Specific Odors—cont'd**

| DISEASE | ODOR |
|---|---|
| ***Surgical Conditions*** **cont'd** | |
| Intestinal obstruction | Breath: feculent, foul |
| | Vomitus: feculent |
| Nasal foreign body | Skin and nasal cavity: fetid, putrid |
| Peritonitis | Vomitus: fecal |
| Portacaval shunt, portal vein thrombosis | Breath: sweet |
| ***Miscellaneous*** | |
| Acute tubular necrosis | Urine: stale water |
| Trans-3-methyl-2-hexanoic acid, which may or may not be elevated in patients with schizophrenia[64,65] | Sweat and skin: unpleasant, pungent, heavy[1,66] |

Data derived from multiple sources.[1,2,4,6,64–68]

## ▶ SUMMARY

Once an odor is identified and evaluated, a proper diagnostic and treatment plan can begin. Identification of odors can be impeded by poor association between odors and names and failure to retrieve the name of an odor.[69] Physicians can be trained to improve their sense of odor recognition with the aid of educational materials (study guides), simulations with volatile samples on rounds,[70] surgical simulators,[71] and sniffing bar test tubes.[56]

Odor is imprecise. Not surprisingly, with many other diagnostic aids at hand, today's physicians have minimized olfactory cues.[52] However, odor should not be neglected; it may be the patient's primary concern, causing severe psychosocial distress. Odor identification may provide diagnostic clues that may aid in the detection and treatment of an underlying disease process.

*The author would like to acknowledge the valuable contribution of Modena H. Wilson, MD, MPH, to this chapter.*

### REFERENCES

1. Hayden GF. Olfactory diagnosis in medicine. *Postgrad Med J.* 1980;67:110–118
2. Senol M, Fireman P. Body odor in dermatologic diagnosis. *Cutis.* 1999;63:107–111
3. Ayers KM, Colquhoun AN. Halitosis: causes, diagnosis, and treatment. *N Z Dent J.* 1998;94:156–160
4. Messadi DV, Younai FS. Halitosis. *Dermatol Clin.* 2003;21:147–155, viii
5. Liddell K. Smell as a diagnostic marker. *Postgrad Med J.* 1976;52:136–138
6. Smith M, Smith LG, Levinson B. The use of smell in differential diagnosis. *Lancet.* 1982;2:1452–1453
7. Simmons TL. What's that smell? A 10-year-old female with a strong odor. *Pediatr Nurs.* 2013;39:37–38
8. Stitt WZ, Goldsmith A. Scratch and sniff. The dynamic duo. *Arch Dermatol.* 1995;131:997–999
9. Yeshurun Y, Sobel N. An odor is not worth a thousand words: from multidimensional odors to unidimensional odor objects. *Annu Rev Psychol.* 2010;61:219–241, C1–C5
10. Kaeppler K, Mueller F. Odor classification: a review of factors influencing perception-based odor arrangements. *Chem Senses.* 2013;38:189–209

11. Stitzel SE, Aernecke MJ, Walt DR. Artificial noses. *Annu Rev Biomed Eng.* 2011;13:1–25
12. Oh EH, Song HS, Park TH. Recent advances in electronic and bioelectronic noses and their biomedical applications. *Enzyme Microb Technol.* 2011;48:427–437
13. Pavlou AK, Turner AP. Sniffing out the truth: clinical diagnosis using the electronic nose. *Clin Chem Lab Med.* 2000;38:99–112
14. Timms C, Thomas PS, Yates DH. Detection of gastro-oesophageal reflux disease (GORD) in patients with obstructive lung disease using exhaled breath profiling. *J Breath Res.* 2012;6:016003
15. Chandoik S, Crawley BA, Oppenheim BA, et al. Screening for bacterial vaginosis: a novel application of artificial nose technology. *J Clin Pathol.* 1997;50:790–791
16. Wang P, Tan Y, Xie H, Shen F. A novel method for diabetes diagnosis based on electronic nose. *Biosens Bioelectron.* 1997;12:1031–1036
17. Bijland LR, Bomers MK, Smulders YM. Smelling the diagnosis: a review on the use of scent in diagnosing disease. *Neth J Med.* 2013;71:300–307
18. Chen C, Shih YH, Yen DJ, et al. Olfactory auras in patients with temporal lobe epilepsy. *Epilepsia.* 2003;44:257–260
19. Schiffman SS. Taste and smell in disease. *N Eng J Med.* 1983;308:1275–1279
20. Kamath V, Turetsky BI, Seligman SC, et al. The influence of semantic processing on odor identification ability in schizophrenia. *Arch Clin Neuropsychol.* 2013;28:254–261
21. Malaspina D, Goetz R, Keller A, et al. Olfactory processing, sex effects and heterogeneity in schizophrenia. *Schizophr Res.* 2012;135:144–151
22. Schecklmann M, Schwenck C, Taurines R, et al. A systematic review on olfaction in child and adolescent psychiatric disorders. *J Neural Transm.* 2013;120:121–130
23. Lancet D. Olfaction. Exclusive receptors. *Nature.* 1994;372:321–322
24. Joussain P, Thevenet M, Rouby C, Bensafi M. Effect of aging on hedonic appreciation of pleasant and unpleasant odors. *PLoS One.* 2013;8:e61376
25. Spielman AI, Sunavala G, Harmony JA, et al. Identification and immunohistochemical localization of protein precursors to human axillary odors in apocrine glands and secretions. *Arch Dermatol.* 1998;134:813–818
26. Gower DB, Mallet AI, Watkins WJ, et al. Transformations of steroid sulphates by human axillary bacteria: a mechanism for human odour formation? *Biochem Soc Trans.* 1997;25:16S
27. Leyden JJ, McGinley KJ, Hölzle E, Labows JN, Kligman AM. The microbiology of the human axilla and its relationship to axillary odor. *J Invest Dermatol.* 1981;77:413–416
28. Sato T, Sonoda T, Itami S, Takayasu S. Predominance of type I 5alpha-reductase in apocrine sweat glands of patients with excessive or abnormal odour derived from apocrine sweat (osmidrosis). *Br J Dermatol.* 1998;139:806–810
29. Tung TC, Wei FC. Excision of subcutaneous tissue for the treatment of axillary osmidrosis. *Br J Plast Surg.* 1997;50:61–66
30. Bang YH, Kim JH, Paik SW, et al. Histopathology of apocrine bromhidrosis. *Plast Reconstr Surg.* 1996;98:288–292
31. Huggins GR, Preti G. Vaginal odors and secretions. *Clin Obstet Gynecol.* 1981;24:355–377
32. Brand JM, Galask RP. Trimethylamine: the substance mainly responsible for the fishy odor often associated with bacterial vaginosis. *Obstet Gynecol.* 1986;68:682–685
33. Burke DG, Halpern B, Malegan D, et al. Profiles of urinary volatiles from metabolic disorders characterized by unusual odors. *Clin Chem.* 1983;29:1834–1838
34. Boustead C. Fish-odour syndrome: dealing with offensive body odour. *Nurs Times.* 1996;92:30–31
35. Budd MA, Tanaka K, Holmes LB, et al. Isovaleric acidemia. Clinical features of a new genetic defect of leucine metabolism. *N Engl J Med.* 1967;277:321–327
36. Chhabria S, Tomasi LG, Wong PW. Ophthalmoplegia and bulbar palsy in variant form of maple syrup urine disease. *Ann Neurol.* 1979;6:71–72
37. Chuang DT, Shih VE. Maple syrup urine disease (branched-chain ketoaciduria). In: Scriver CR, Beaudet AL, Sly WS, et al, eds. *The Metabolic and Molecular Bases of Inherited Disease.* 8th ed. Vol II. New York, NY: McGraw-Hill; 2001

38. Dusheiko G, Kew MC, Joffe BI, et al. Recurrent hypoglycemia associated with glutaric aciduria type II in an adult. *N Engl J Med.* 1979;301:1405–1409
39. Mace JW, Goodman SI, Centerwall WR, et al. The child with an unusual odor. *Clin Pediatr.* 1976;15:57–62
40. McCandless SE. A primer on expanded newborn screening by tandem mass spectroscopy. Primary care. *Clin Off Pract.* 2004;31:583–604
41. Monastiri K, Limame K, Kaabachi N, et al. Fenugreek odour in maple syrup urine disease. *J Inherit Metab Dis.* 1997;20:614–615
42. Morris MD, Lewis BD, Doolan PD, Harper HA. Clinical and biochemical observations on an apparently nonfatal variant of branched-chain ketoaciduria (maple syrup urine disease). *Pediatrics.* 1961;28:918–923
43. Niederwieser A, Steinmann B, Exner U, et al. Multiple acyl-Co A dehydrogenation deficiency (MADD) in a boy with nonketotic hypoglycemia, hepatomegaly, muscle hypotonia and cardiomyopathy. Detection of N-isovalerylglutamic acid and its monoamide. *Helv Paediatr Acta.* 1983;38:9–26
44. Rezvani I. An approach to inborn errors of metabolism. In: Behrman RE, Kliegman RM, Jenson HB, eds. *Nelson Textbook of Pediatrics.* 17th ed. Philadelphia, PA: Saunders; 2004
45. Robinson BH, Oei J, Sherwood WG, et al. Hydroxymethylglutaryl CoA lyase deficiency: features resembling Reye syndrome. *Neurology.* 1980;30:714–718
46. Schulman JD, Lustberg TJ, Kennedy JL, Museles M, Seegmiller JE. A new variant of maple syrup urine disease (branched chain ketoaciduria). Clinical and biochemical evaluation. *Am J Med.* 1970;49:118–124
47. Sciver CR, MacKenzie S, Clow CL, et al. Thiamine-responsive maple-syrup-urine disease. *Lancet.* 1971;1:310–312
48. Shevell MI, Didomenicantonio G, Sylvain M, et al. Glutaric acidemia type II: neuroimaging and spectroscopy evidence for developmental encephalomyopathy. *Pediatr Neurol.* 1995;12:350–353
49. Sidbury JB, Smith EK, Harlan W. An inborn error of short-chain fatty acid metabolism. The odor-of-sweaty-feet syndrome. *J Pediatr.* 1967;70:8–15
50. Smith AJ, Strang LB. An inborn error of metabolism with the urinary excretion of alpha-hydroxy-butyric acid and phenylpyruvic acid. *Arch Dis Child.* 1958;33:109–113
51. Wilcken B, Hammond JW, Howard N, et al. Hawkinsinuria: a dominantly inherited defect of tyrosine metabolism with severe effects in infancy. *N Engl J Med.* 1981;305:865–868
52. Feinstein RJ. Nasal foreign bodies and bromidrosis. *JAMA.* 1979;242:1031
53. Katz HP, Katz JR, Bernstein M, Marcin J. Unusual presentation of nasal foreign bodies in children. *JAMA.* 1979;241:1496
54. Moriarty RA. Nasal foreign body presenting as an unusual odor. *Am J Dis Child.* 1978;132:97–98
55. Anderson CE, Loomis GA. Recognition and prevention of inhalant abuse. *Am Fam Physician.* 2003;68:869–874
56. Goldfrank L, Weisman R, Flomenbaum N. Teaching the recognition of odors. *Ann Emerg Med.* 1982;11:684–686
57. Molberg P. Body odor from topical benzoyl peroxide. *N Engl J Med.* 1981;304:1366
58. Stewart WK, Fleming LW. Use your nose (letter). *Lancet.* 1983;1:426
59. Hauser GJ, Chitayat D, Berns L, Braver D, Muhlbauer B. Peculiar odours in newborns and maternal prenatal ingestion of spicy food. *Eur J Pediatr.* 1985;144:403
60. Kavic SM, Cohn SM. Infection based on odor. *J Trauma.* 1996;41:1077
61. Newton ER. Preterm labor, preterm premature rupture of membranes, and chorioamnionitis. *Clin Perinatol.* 2005;32:571–600
62. Poulton J, Tarlow MJ. Diagnosis of rotavirus gastroenteritis by smell. *Arch Dis Child.* 1987;62:851–852
63. Turney JH. Use your nose (letter). *Lancet.* 1983;1:426
64. Gordon SG, Smith K, Rabinowitz JL, Vagelos PR. Studies of trans-3-methyl-2-hexenoic acid in normal and schizophrenic humans. *J Lipid Res.* 1973;14:495–503
65. Fireman P. Response letter to the editor. *Cutis.* 2002;69:316
66. Smith K, Thompson GF, Koster HD. Sweat in schizophrenic patients: identification of the odorous substance. *Science.* 1969;166:398–399

67. Najarian JS. The diagnostic importance of the odor of urine. *N Engl J Med.* 1980;303:1128
68. Rockey DC. Gastrointestinal bleeding. *Gastroenterol Clin.* 2005;34:699–718
69. Cain WS. To know with the nose: keys to odor identification. *Science.* 1979;203:467–470
70. Lukas T, Berner ES, Kanakis C. Diagnosis by smell? *J Med Educ.* 1977;52:349–350
71. Spencer BS. Incorporating the sense of smell into haptic surgical simulators. *Stud Health Technol Inform.* 2005;114:54–62

# Chapter 58

# Petechiae and Purpura

*Lisa Figueiredo, MD; Adam S. Levy, MD*

## ▶ INTRODUCTION

Petechiae and purpura result from a wide variety of underlying disorders and may occur at any age. Petechiae are small (1–3 mm), red, nonblanching macular lesions caused by intradermal capillary bleeding (Figure 58-1). Purpura are larger, typically raised lesions resulting from bleeding within the skin (Figures 58-2 and 58-3). Purpura can vary somewhat in color based on the age of the lesion as the blood within the skin is metabolized and fades. Similar to petechiae, purpura do not blanch and may occur anywhere on the body.

## ▶ EVALUATION

The evaluation of a patient with petechiae or purpura begins with a complete history that can readily eliminate most disorders from the differential diagnosis. Special attention must be paid to recent trauma, bleeding history, medication use, and symptoms consistent with infection, malignancy, and autoimmune, vasculitic, connective tissue, or rheumatologic

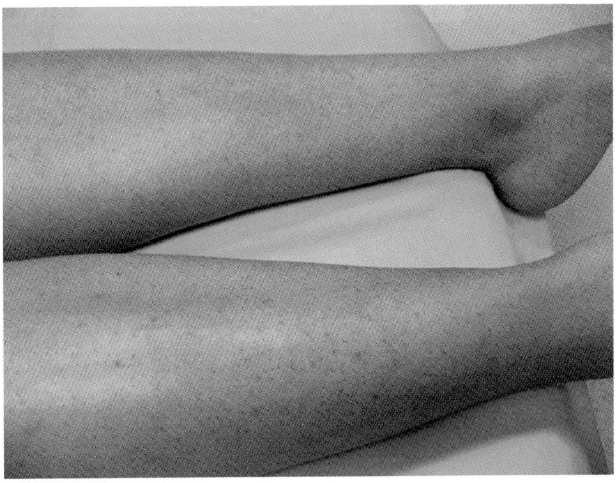

**Figure 58-1**
Cutaneous petechiae on the shins and ankles: nonblanching, erythematous macules, often less than 3 mm in size.

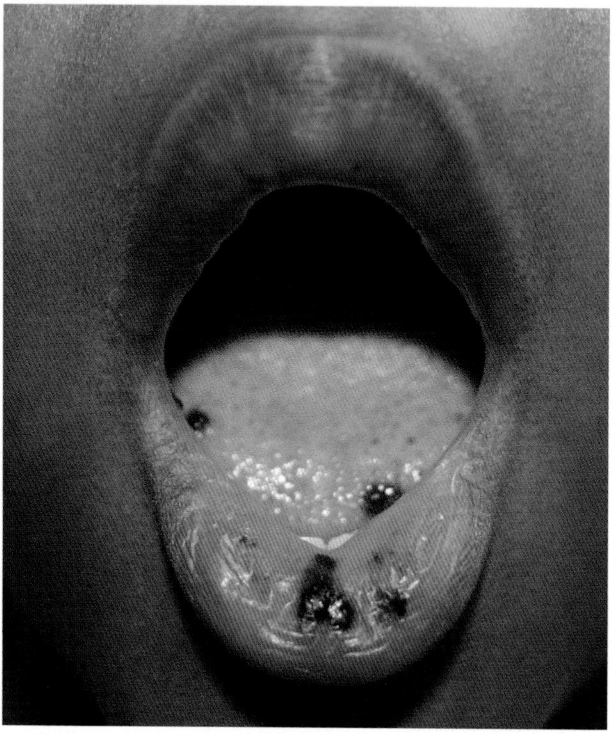

**Figure 58-2**
Occasional petechiae on the face and large, bullous hemorrhages on the buccal mucosa.

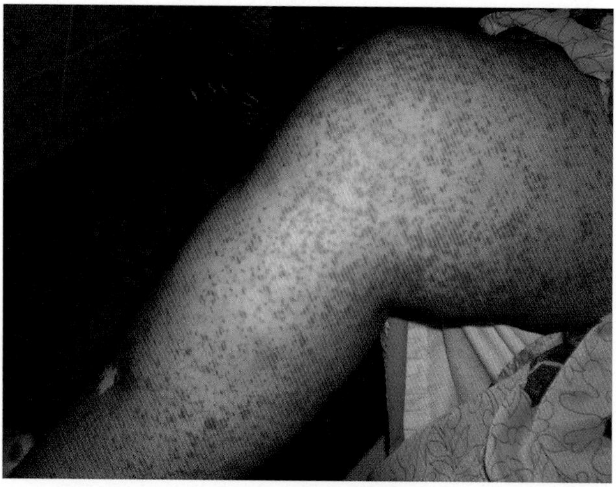

**Figure 58-3**
Palpable purpura of the lower extremity: erythematous, nonblanching papules that often measure more than 3 mm in size.

disorders. Physical examination should determine whether the skin findings are isolated or evidence that a more generalized process is present. Particular physical findings to evaluate include hepatosplenomegaly, lymphadenopathy, arthritis, arthralgias, or findings that are consistent with an acute viral syndrome. The history and physical examination will dictate the appropriate laboratory evaluations, but at a minimum, a complete blood count with platelets and differential count, as well as assessing prothrombin time and partial thromboplastin time, are typically indicated. Likely diagnoses are detailed here, and the complete evaluation indicated will be discussed.

## ▶ DIFFERENTIAL DIAGNOSIS—GENERAL CONSIDERATIONS

Neither petechiae nor purpura are pathognomonic of a specific disorder. The physician must entertain a broad differential diagnosis and consider disorders of hemostasis as well as infection, autoimmune disorders, trauma, malignancy, and other rare causes (eg, vasculitis, connective tissue disorders). The age at presentation, overall appearance, and the extent of the lesions may help define the underlying pathophysiologic mechanism. For example, scant petechiae on the face of a well-seeming newborn would not be particularly concerning after a vaginal delivery because these lesions are likely caused by the trauma of passing through the birth canal. However, a newborn with diffuse petechiae warrants further evaluation.[1,2] If the child seems ill, then sepsis must be strongly considered; if the child seems well, then a platelet disorder should be considered. Thus, petechiae and purpura must be evaluated in the overall context of the patient, severity and extent of the lesions, and history and age of the patient.

With petechiae or purpura, the possibility of a hemostatic defect is always a concern. For isolated petechiae, the physician must consider a primary platelet disorder (ie, low platelet number, platelet dysfunction). Purpura may result from a platelet disorder or other coagulation defect, which can be classified as primary or as a secondary phenomenon from an underlying disease. Platelet disorders can also be classified into disorders of platelet production, disorders of platelet survival (destruction), or disorders of platelet function. In the case of connective tissue disorders, easy bruising is not secondary to a hemostatic defect, but rather is caused by the fragility of the capillaries and the perivascular connective tissues. As such, easy bruising and bleeding may be characteristic manifestations of disorders unrelated to the commonly considered clotting and platelet disorders.[3] In general, however, when presented with a patient with petechiae and purpura, the physician must consider thrombocytopenia as the proximate cause.

The normal platelet count is between 150,000 and 450,000/mm.[4] Patients with a platelet count greater than 80,000 will be hemostatically normal as long as platelet function is not altered. With a platelet count between 50,000 and 80,000, increased bleeding with trauma is likely, but spontaneous bleeding would be unusual. Between 20,000 and 50,000, a mild bleeding diathesis is expected. With a count of less than 20,000, spontaneous mucosal bleeding can occur, and a count of less than 10,000 is concerning for spontaneous severe bleeding.

### *Infectious Causes of Petechiae and Purpura*

The mechanism by which a variety of viruses cause thrombocytopenia is not clear and may involve decreased platelet production or immune-mediated destruction.

Live virus vaccinations, notably varicella and measles, can cause moderate thrombocytopenia.[4] Cytomegalovirus has been implicated in thrombocytopenia, but treatment of cytomegalovirus has not affected the outcome of patients monitored for chronic thrombocytopenia.[5] Parvovirus has been associated both with isolated thrombocytopenia and with pancytopenia.[6–8] Dengue fever and other viral hemorrhagic fevers are known to cause thrombocytopenia, and patients may develop petechiae and purpura as a result.[9,10] Rickettsial diseases such as Rocky Mountain spotted fever may produce a petechial rash. Alterations of the endothelial lining of blood vessels cause thrombi formation and platelet destruction. Thrombocytopenia and disseminated intravascular coagulation (DIC) may develop.[11] Malaria can also cause either mild or profound thrombocytopenia through mechanisms that are not well defined.[12–14] HIV has been associated with thrombocytopenia resulting from bone marrow suppression (ie, poor production) and immune-mediated destruction.[15]

Platelet consumption is common in children with bacteremia and sepsis even before frank DIC has developed. In an ill-appearing child with petechiae or purpura, infectious causes must be considered and appropriate antibiotics administered based on likely pathogens. Bacterial meningitis in particular must be considered for the febrile ill child with petechiae or purpura.

Purpura fulminans has been associated with viral infections, as well as *Streptococcus* and *Meningococcus* species. Microscopic thromboses in arterioles result in purpura and infarction and bleeding within the skin and subcutaneous tissue. These lesions may coalesce and become necrotic, and patients typically develop full DIC.

## Disorders of Platelet Production: Malignancy and Bone Marrow Failure Syndrome

Although most patients with petechiae or purpura have a benign process, perhaps the greatest concern for the physician and parents is malignancy. As such the history must rule out the classic signs and symptoms of malignancy, including fevers, night sweats, weight loss, lymphadenopathy or other masses, pallor, malaise, bone pain, and anorexia. Of course, many of these symptoms overlap with those seen in infectious and autoimmune processes; thus the physical examination will help the physician greatly. Petechiae or purpura in the setting of hepatosplenomegaly or impressive lymphadenopathy would put leukemia high on the differential diagnosis. Other marrow-infiltrating malignancies must also be considered. If the history or physical examination is consistent with a malignancy, then in addition to a complete blood count and screening coagulation studies, a comprehensive metabolic panel, liver function tests, lactate dehydrogenase, and uric acid should be immediately obtained. A manual differential count of the peripheral blood should be performed as well. An important point to note is that the absence of leukemic blasts on a peripheral blood smear does *not* rule out leukemia. The diagnosis of leukemia can be made if peripheral blasts are present; however, having few or no peripheral blasts seen on routine microscopy is not uncommon for patients with leukemia.

Isolated profound thrombocytopenia is not likely to result from a malignancy; however, when more than 1 cell line on a blood count is abnormal, a bone marrow process must be considered. Laboratory findings consistent with malignancy include elevated lactate dehydrogenase, and an elevated uric acid and abnormal serum electrolytes may result from tumor lysis even before therapy is started. A chest radiograph should be obtained immediately because patients may have occult but massive mediastinal lymphadenopathy.

Petechiae and purpura may be the presenting signs in patients with bone marrow failure secondary to nonmalignant processes. Abnormal hematopoiesis usually causes alteration of more than 1 cell line or all cell lines (pancytopenia). Bone marrow failure may occur secondary to infectious processes (viral, bacterial with sepsis), medication use (notably a variety of antibiotics and anticonvulsants), profound nutritional deficits, or rare bone marrow failure syndromes (eg, Fanconi anemia, myelodysplastic disease, Wiskott-Aldrich syndrome). Bone marrow aspiration and biopsy are usually indicated to rule out malignancy and define the abnormal hematopoiesis.

### Disorders of Platelet Function: Primary Platelet Disorders

Petechiae and purpura may result from a primary platelet disorder, either qualitative or quantitative. The qualitative disorders result from platelet dysfunction; that is, the absolute platelet number is normal, but the platelets lose normal hemostatic function. In most instances, platelet dysfunction is acquired and results from medication use. The classic example is aspirin, which causes the irreversible inhibition of cyclooxygenase within platelets. Other causes of acquired platelet dysfunction include uremia and liver disease, although the mechanisms of poor platelet function in these settings are not clear.[16]

Although von Willebrand disease is not a primary platelet disorder, patients commonly present with painless mucocutaneous bleeding. For this reason it should be considered in patients who have petechiae and purpura with a normal platelet count and no other obvious systemic disease.[17] Von Willebrand disease is the most common bleeding disorder and affects approximately 1% of the population. It results from a qualitative or quantitative deficiency of von Willebrand factor, a protein required for platelet adhesion. Coagulation screening along with factor VIII and von Willebrand factor assays can establish the diagnosis.

A variety of platelet function disorders can be considered in patients with a normal to near-normal platelet number but who are bleeding and have petechiae or purpura. These disorders, which are rare, can be diagnosed by a hematologist with specialized platelet aggregation studies or morphologic study of platelets. Such disorders include Glanzmann thrombasthenia, Hermansky-Pudlak syndrome, and Chédiak-Higashi syndrome. Bernard-Soulier syndrome, an inherited platelet disorder, is characterized by variable thrombocytopenia and large defective platelets.[18]

### Disorders of Platelet Survival (Destruction)

Isolated thrombocytopenia in an otherwise well child may lead to petechiae or purpura as the chief complaint. Idiopathic (or immune) thrombocytopenic purpura is a diagnosis of exclusion that produces profound isolated thrombocytopenia and petechiae or purpura but few other findings on physical examination. The laboratory workup should be normal except for thrombocytopenia. No other blood cell line is affected, and microscopic review of the blood reveals platelets that are too few in number but large in size, indicating that they are young. Idiopathic thrombocytopenic purpura is a disorder in which the platelet lifespan is reduced to minutes or hours rather than the normal several days. The incidence is highest in children between 2 and 8 years of age. Although physicians performed bone marrow aspirates in the past to rule out malignancy or other bone marrow failure syndromes, most now think that the diagnosis can be made clinically, and bone marrow studies are rarely indicated.[19–21]

Typically, one-third of the total body platelet mass is sequestered within the spleen at any time. Whatever the cause of increased spleen size, mild thrombocytopenia may result. Common causes of hypersplenism include liver disease, a variety of infections (including Epstein-Barr virus and malaria, among others), and metabolic diseases (eg, Gaucher disease).[22] Hypersplenism alone does not typically cause platelet counts below 50,000. Alternative explanations should be considered for patients with moderate-severe thrombocytopenia.

Henoch-Schönlein purpura is an autoimmune vasculitic disorder that often presents with palpable purpura. The classic distribution of purpura is on the buttocks and legs, but purpura may be more disseminated. Laboratory evaluations fail to reveal an identifiable coagulopathy, nor is there a defect in the quality or quantity of their platelets. The etiology of the palpable purpura is thought to be secondary to the vasculitis resulting in inflammation and weakening of the vessel walls. Other findings in Henoch-Schönlein purpura may include arthritis, arthralgias, abdominal pain, and renal impairment.[23–25]

Hemolytic uremic syndrome (HUS) produces a constellation of findings, including thrombocytopenia, hemolytic anemia, and renal failure, and has been associated with a variety of infections, most notably *Escherichia coli* O157:H7.[26]

Thrombotic thrombocytopenic purpura (TTP) shares some clinical features with HUS but is a distinct syndrome related to either inherited or acquired loss of function in the ADAMTS13 protease that cleaves von Willebrand factor. TTP, rarely seen in children, is characterized by purpura, thrombocytopenia, DIC, hemolytic anemia, thrombotic strokes, and elevated lactate dehydrogenase.[27]

Giant vascular malformations may cause intravascular destruction of platelets. Kasabach-Merritt syndrome is the classic example of a giant hemangioma causing severe thrombocytopenia secondary to platelet destruction. These lesions are generally readily apparent; however, multiple smaller vascular malformations that are more difficult to define may cause platelet destruction as well. Although laboratory evaluation often fails to reveal a coagulopathy, thrombocytopenia or altered hemostasis may be associated with rare vascular disorders and connective tissue syndromes such as the hereditary telangiectasias, Ehlers-Danlos syndrome, Marfan syndrome, and osteogenesis imperfecta.

## ▶ SUMMARY

Petechiae and purpura may result from a variety of mechanisms requiring the physician to obtain a complete history and perform a thorough physical examination. Both primary hematologic disorders and systemic disorders are in the differential diagnosis. Prompt referral to a pediatric hematologist may be indicated to rule out malignancy or help manage altered hemostasis.

## When to Refer

- Platelet count less than 100,000/mm$^3$
- Diffuse petechiae or purpura
- Focal petechiae or purpura not clearly associated with trauma
- Evidence of more than 1 cell line abnormality on complete blood count

## When to Admit

- Patient with toxic appearance
- Moderate to severe bleeding
- Concern for poor adherence

### *REFERENCES*


1. Roberts I, Murray NA. Neonatal thrombocytopenia: causes and management. *Arch Dis Child Fetal Neonatal Ed.* 2003;88:F359–F364
2. Thomas AE. The bleeding child; is it NAI? *Arch Dis Child.* 2004;89:1163–1167
3. De Paepe A, Malfait F. Bleeding and bruising in patients with Ehlers-Danlos syndrome and other collagen vascular disorders. *Br J Haematol.* 2004;127:491–500
4. Johnson CM, de Alarcon P. Evaluation of a child with thrombocytopenia in platelet dysfunction. In: Sills RH, ed. *Practical Algorithms in Pediatric Hematology and Oncology.* Basel, Switzerland: Karger; 2003
5. Levy AS, Bussel J. Immune thrombocytopenic purpura: investigation of the role of cytomegalovirus infection. *Br J Haematol.* 2004;126:622–623
6. Heegaard ED, Rosthøj S, Petersen BL, et al. Role of parvovirus B19 infection in childhood idiopathic thrombocytopenic purpura. *Acta Paediatr.* 1999;88:614–617
7. Aktepe OC, Yetgin S, Olcay L, Ozbek N. Human parvovirus B19 associated with idiopathic thrombocytopenic purpura. *Pediatr Hematol Oncol.* 2004;21:421–426
8. McNeely M, Friedman J, Pope E. Generalized petechial eruption induced by parvovirus B19 infection. *J Am Acad Dermatol.* 2005;52:S109–S113
9. Schexneider KI, Reedy EA. Thrombocytopenia in dengue fever. *Curr Hematol Rep.* 2005;4:145–148
10. Halstead SB. Other viral hemorrhagic fevers. In: *Nelson's Textbook of Pediatrics.* 14th ed. Philadelphia, PA: WB Saunders; 1992
11. Clements ML. Rickettsiae. In: *Nelson's Textbook of Pediatrics.* 14th ed. Philadelphia, PA: WB Saunders; 1992
12. Rodríguez-Morales AJ, Sánchez E, Vargas M, et al. Occurrence of thrombocytopenia in Plasmodium vivax malaria. *Clin Infect Dis.* 2005;41:130–131
13. Magill AJ. Malaria: diagnosis and treatment of falciparum malaria in travelers during and after travel. *Curr Infect Dis Rep.* 2006;8:35–42
14. Rodríguez-Morales AJ, Sánchez E, Vargas M, et al. Anemia and thrombocytopenia in children with Plasmodium vivax malaria. *J Trop Pediatr.* 2006;52:49–51
15. Scaradavou A. HIV-related thrombocytopenia. *Blood Rev.* 2002;16:73–76
16. Dunsmore K, de Alarcon P. Platelet dysfunction. In: Sills RH, ed. *Practical Algorithms in Pediatric Hematology and Oncology.* Basel, Switzerland: Karger; 2003
17. Favaloro EJ, Lillicrap D, Lazzari MA, et al. von Willebrand disease: laboratory aspects of diagnosis and treatment. *Haemophilia.* 2004;10(Suppl 4):164–168
18. Nurden AT, Freson K, Seligsohn U. Inherited platelet disorders. *Haemophilia.* 2012;18(Suppl 4):154–160
19. Calpin C, Dick P, Poon A, Feldman W. Is bone marrow aspiration needed in acute childhood idiopathic thrombocytopenic purpura to rule out leukemia? *Arch Pediatr Adolesc Med.* 1998;152:345–347
20. Cines DB, Blanchette VS. Immune thrombocytopenic purpura. *N Engl J Med.* 2002;346:995–1008
21. Nugent DJ. Childhood immune thrombocytopenic purpura. *Blood Rev.* 2002;16:27–29

22. Johnson CM, de Alarcon P. Evaluation of a child with thrombocytopenia. In: Sills RH, ed. *Practical Algorithms in Pediatric Hematology and Oncology*. Basel, Switzerland: Karger; 2003
23. Wilson DB. Acquired platelet defects. In: *Nathan and Oski's Hematology of Infancy and Childhood*. 6th ed. Philadelphia, PA: WB Saunders; 2003
24. Ting TV, Hashkeș PJ. Update on childhood vasculitides. *Curr Opin Rheumatol.* 2004;16:560–565
25. Ballinger S. Henoch-Schonlein purpura. *Curr Opin Rheumatol.* 2003;15:591–594
26. Trapani S, Micheli A, Grisolia F, et al. Henoch Schonlein purpura in childhood: epidemiological and clinical analysis of 150 cases over a 5-year period and review of literature. *Semin Arthritis Rheum.* 2005;35:143–153
27. Siegler R, Oakes R. Hemolytic uremic syndrome; pathogenesis, treatment, and outcome. *Curr Opin Pediatr.* 2005;17:200–204

Chapter 59

# Polyuria

*Ryan S. Miller, MD; Samuel M. Libber, MD; Leslie Plotnick, MD*

Polyuria, or excessive urinary volume, is a symptom common to many pediatric disorders. It may be defined clinically as urine production of more than 2 $L/m^2/24$ hours or functionally as inappropriately high urine output relative to circulating volume and osmolality[1] (Table 59-1). Although polyuria is often associated with polydipsia, frequent urination, and nocturia, these features may occur with normal urine output. Differentiating polyuria from other conditions depends on total urine output. In situations in which the exact daily urinary volume is unknown, a detailed history of fluid intake and urinary habits may help delineate the primary symptom.

With an older child, the parent may perceive an increase in fluid intake to be more prominent than polyuria. However, infants with polyuria, because they do not have independent access to fluids, are more likely to fall into negative water balance, with weight loss, dehydration, and electrolyte disturbances. Chronic or recurrent electrolyte disturbances in unrecognized diabetes insipidus (DI) may result in growth failure and central nervous system (CNS) injury.

## ▶ PATHOPHYSIOLOGIC FEATURES

Normal serum osmolality and water balance are maintained primarily by release of arginine vasopressin (antidiuretic hormone [ADH]), thirst, and kidney function. Serum osmolality is tightly regulated—an increase in osmolality as small as 1% stimulates measurable release of vasopressin from the posterior pituitary.[2] Vasopressin binds the V2 receptor of the renal tubules, resulting in insertion of aquaporin-2 protein at the apical surface of cortical cells and allowing water to enter the cell. Under normal conditions, plasma osmolality is maintained within a narrow range—about 285 to 290 mOsm/kg. Vasopressin levels rise as plasma osmolality increases above this range. However, maximal antidiuresis is reached at a plasma vasopressin concentration of 4 pmol/L, at which point urine cannot be further concentrated (Figure 59-1).

**Table 59-1**
**Normal Urine Volume**

| AGE RANGE | DAILY OUTPUT (24 hr) |
|---|---|
| Newborn | 150 mL/kg |
| Infant | 110 mL/kg |
| Older child | 40 mL/kg |

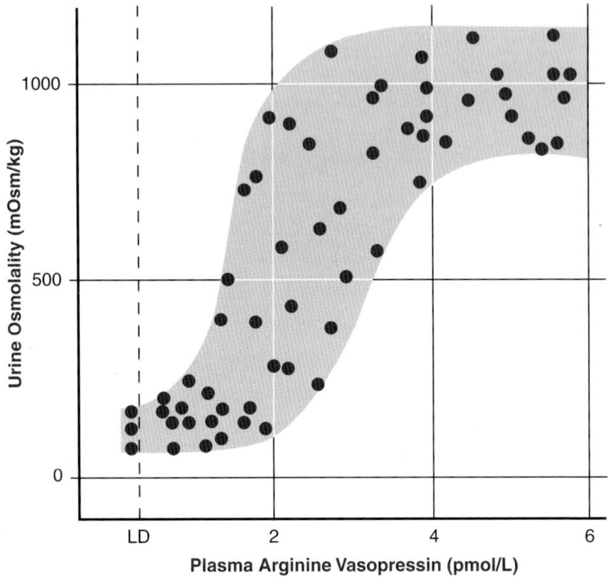


**Figure 59-1**
Relation between urine osmolality and plasma arginine vasopressin under various states of hydration. The stippled area is the normal reference range. *LD* represents the limit of detection of the assay (0.3 pmol/L). *(From Baylis PH, Cheetham T. Diabetes insipidus.* Arch Dis Child. *1998;79(1):84–89, with permission.)*

Vasopressin alone cannot restore fluid balance and osmolality; fluid replenishment is also required. Small increases in osmolality have been shown experimentally to stimulate thirst by increasing the concentration of solutes such as sodium chloride and sucrose (solutes that do not readily cross nerve cell membranes).[3] This action results in intracellular dehydration, activating osmoreceptors in the brain that initiate neural mechanisms and resulting in generation of thirst. The osmolality at which thirst is experienced is likely higher than the point at which vasopressin production rises.

## ▶ DIFFERENTIAL DIAGNOSIS

Polyuria can be caused by any one of several conditions that play a role in water balance, each of which leads to the excretion of large volumes of dilute urine. Disorders of water balance fall into 4 major categories: central DI, nephrogenic DI, excessive fluid intake, and osmotic diuresis. DI is characterized by polyuria, polydipsia, dilute urine, dehydration, and hypernatremia. Central DI results from a deficiency in vasopressin secretion, whereas nephrogenic DI is the result of reduced renal sensitivity to circulating vasopressin. Polyuria can also be a manifestation of excessive persistent fluid intake (primary polydipsia) or osmotic (solute) diuresis, as in uncontrolled diabetes mellitus (DM). In reaching a diagnosis in a patient who has polyuria, the physician must consider the systems involved in maintaining normal serum osmolality and water balance (Box 59-1).

### Central Diabetes Insipidus

Central or neurogenic DI is a condition in which secretion of vasopressin by the posterior lobe of the pituitary gland is inadequate to maintain normal serum osmolality, resulting in

**BOX 59-1**

## *Differential Diagnosis of Polyuria in Childhood*

1. Neurogenic vasopressin deficiency
   a. Familial
   b. Idiopathic
   c. Congenital malformations (septo-optic dysplasia, holoprosencephaly, encephalocele)
   d. Acquired
      i. Head trauma
      ii. Vascular event (thrombosis or hemorrhage)
      iii. Postinfection (meningitis, encephalitis, congenital cytomegalovirus, toxoplasmosis)
      iv. Tumor (craniopharyngioma, germinoma, optic glioma)
      v. Systemic infiltrative diseases (histiocytosis, syphilis, tuberculosis, sarcoidosis)
      vi. Inflammatory (lymphocytic hypophysitis)
      vii. Guillain-Barré syndrome
      viii. Autoimmune disorders
2. Renal vasopressin insensitivity
   a. Familial nephrogenic diabetes insipidus
      i. V2 receptor gene defect (X-linked)
      ii. Aquaporin-2 gene defect (autosomal recessive)
   b. Acquired
      i. Postobstructive
      ii. Drug-induced (lithium, amphotericin B)
      iii. Associated with systemic disease (sickle cell disease, sarcoidosis, amyloidosis)
      iv. Metabolic (hypercalcemia, hypokalemia)
3. Other renal disorders
   a. Renal tubular defects (cystinosis, distal renal tubular acidosis, Bartter syndrome, renal Fanconi syndrome, ARC syndrome)
   b. Nephronopthisis
4. Excessive fluid intake
   a. Primary polydipsia
   b. Water intoxication
5. Osmotic diuresis
   a. Diet-induced
   b. Drug-induced
   c. Diabetes mellitus (type 1 or 2)

*ARC,* arthrogryposis, renal tubular dysfunction, and cholestasis.

diuresis of varying degrees of severity. Of the known causes of central DI, nearly one-half of all cases result from a primary brain tumor, and about 18% are from histiocytosis or infiltrative processes. About 25% of cases are considered idiopathic. Familial vasopressin deficiency, also known as familial neurohypophyseal diabetes insipidus (FNHDI), is typically an autosomal dominant disorder and is rare, accounting for about 5% of all cases of DI. Although many mutations have been reported in the arginine vasopressin *(AVP)* gene, most cases involve mutations in the gene for neurophysin II *(NPII),* the carrier protein for AVP.[4] In FNHDI, symptoms typically do not appear until 5 to 10 years of age.[5] The syndrome consisting of DI, DM, optic atrophy, and deafness (DIDMOAD syndrome) typically presents in early childhood.[6] Vasopressin deficiency is associated with certain congenital malformations (eg, septo-optic dysplasia, holoprosencephaly) and can result from CNS injury or tumor resection. After head trauma or surgery, patients may have a period of antidiuresis after transient polyuria, followed by persistent central DI (triple-phase response).[7]

In recent years, fewer cases of DI have been diagnosed as idiopathic, and a higher proportion have been diagnosed as occurring secondary to CNS infection or intracranial birth defects.[8] Autoantibodies to hypothalamic vasopressin cells have been detected in some children previously thought to have idiopathic DI. Interestingly, about 50% of the patients who have histiocytosis also have vasopressin cell autoantibodies.[9] In adolescents with acquired lymphocytic or granulomatous hypophysitis, hyperprolactinemia and other anterior pituitary dysfunction may accompany the DI.[10] The physician must search diligently for an underlying lesion that may not be evident at the initial evaluation.

### Nephrogenic Diabetes Insipidus

Renal disorders, both congenital and acquired, may be associated with polyuria because of a complete or partial inability of the renal tubule to concentrate urine despite normal or elevated circulating levels of vasopressin. Inherited forms of nephrogenic DI are rare, and symptoms of profound polyuria—vomiting, fever, failure to thrive, and hypernatremic dehydration—typically occur within the first weeks of life. Breastfed infants may show signs later than those who are bottle fed because of the lower osmotic load in human milk. The condition can be associated with damage to the CNS or even death if the infant develops recurrent hypernatremic dehydration. Older children and adults may be able to adjust their oral fluid intake to maintain serum osmolality. Mutations in the vasopressin V2 receptors of the distal convoluted tubule and collecting duct have been reported in affected members of kindreds with nephrogenic DI.[11,12] A rare form of autosomal recessive nephrogenic DI has been described in patients with mutations in the gene for the water-channel protein aquaporin-2.[13]

Besides the hereditary form of nephrogenic DI, the physician must consider other renal tubular defects in which vasopressin resistance has been observed. Patients who have cystinosis, distal renal tubular acidosis, renal Fanconi syndrome, or Bartter syndrome may have polyuria. An association between nephrogenic DI and the syndrome consisting of arthrogryposis, renal tubular dysfunction, and cholestasis (ARC syndrome) has been recognized; affected children are prone to severe growth impairment, as well as to intellectual disability and deafness.[14] Structural abnormalities of the kidney leading to polyuria include congenital abnormalities such as renal dysplasia, familial juvenile nephronophthisis–medullary cystic disease, and oligomeganephronia, as well as acquired lesions caused by chronic pyelonephritis or obstructive uropathy.

In a systematic review of causes of nephrogenic DI, the most frequently reported risk factors for reversible vasopressin insensitivity were lithium, antibiotics, antifungals, antineoplastic agents, and antivirals.[15] Longer duration of treatment with lithium correlated with increased risk for irreversible DI. Metabolic disturbances can also result in reversible vasopressin resistance. Hypercalcemia and hypokalemia each may be associated with a nephropathy in which tubular ability to conserve water is lost. Certain systemic disorders, such as sickle cell disease, sarcoidosis, and amyloidosis, also may cause renal tubular dysfunction and result in polyuria.

### Excess Water Intake

Polyuria is sometimes a consequence rather than a cause of excessive fluid intake. The ailment has a gradual onset, unlike the more abrupt onset typical of central DI. Primary polydipsia is a rare cause of polyuria in childhood.[16] In primary polydipsia, excess fluid intake can alter the renal medullary concentration gradient, leading to a relatively hypo-osmolar state. Primary polydipsia is diagnosed after excluding other possible causes of excessive water intake. However, as recently demonstrated in a child who was found to have a mutation in the *AVP* gene, an individual with evolving central DI can have a normal water deprivation test early in the disease course.[17]

The term *psychogenic polydipsia* has been used to characterize excessive water drinking in institutionalized psychiatric patients and is most commonly associated with schizophrenia.[18,19] Although some investigators believe this disorder is caused by a primary psychiatric disturbance, a study of adult patients with polydipsia and hyponatremia showed evidence of a defect in water excretion, osmoregulation of water intake, and vasopressin secretion.[20] Although typical antipsychotic drugs such as haloperidol have been associated with worsening of polydipsia, clozapine has been reported to significantly reduce excessive water intake in limited studies.[19,21]

### *Osmotic Diuresis*

Some patients have polyuria with renal water loss resulting from an osmotic diuresis. Glycosuria is frequently found to be the cause of sudden onset of polyuria in children with uncontrolled DM. In both type 1 and type 2 DM, diminished carbohydrate use results in hyperglycemia and glycosuria. When present in the urine at high concentrations, glucose acts as an osmotic diuretic, resulting in polyuria. Chronic hyperglycemia may also cause a form of partial nephrogenic DI.[22] Osmotic diuresis may also be provoked by mannitol, radiologic contrast agents, or high-protein feedings (in which urea acts as the osmotic agent), or after the relief of bilateral urinary tract obstruction.[23] Treatment with large volumes of dextrose-containing intravenous fluids can also result in hyperglycemia and polyuria. In contrast, renal glycosuria is characterized by a defect in renal tubular reabsorption of glucose, resulting in glycosuria without hyperglycemia or polyuria.

## ▶ EVALUATION

A detailed history often reveals the cause of polyuria. Age at onset, pattern of fluid intake, and rate of onset of polyuria are informative. A thorough feeding history can help identify infants who have water intoxication. New onset of nocturia is often the first manifestation of loss of concentrating ability. Young children with DI can have irritability as a result of hypernatremia and dehydration. Family history is important, given that familial forms of both central and nephrogenic DI exist. In most cases of familial nephrogenic DI, severe polyuria occurs within the first weeks of life. Growth failure is a feature common to both nephrogenic and central DI.

A 24-hour measurement of fluid intake and output is helpful to confirm polyuria before ordering laboratory tests. Urine specific gravity on a first-voided morning specimen is helpful but can be affected by the presence of glycosuria, proteinuria, or radiocontrast material. Both types of DI and primary polydipsia result in relatively dilute urine. Patients with disorders resulting in renal tubular damage, such as sickle cell disease, are more likely to have isosthenuria with specific gravities in the neighborhood of 1.010. Urinalysis with microscopy performed on a first-voided morning specimen also provides valuable information. Protein, casts, or formed blood elements in the urine suggest a renal disorder. Glycosuria with ketonuria strongly suggests DM. Other baseline studies include serum electrolytes, glucose, urea, phosphate, creatinine, calcium, osmolality, liver function tests, and complete blood count (Table 59-2).

**Table 59-2**
**Interpretation of Baseline Values**

| CLINICAL SITUATION | SERUM SODIUM (mEq/L) | SERUM OSMOLALITY (mOsm/kg) | URINE OSMOLALITY | PLASMA VASOPRESSIN |
|---|---|---|---|---|
| Normal | 135–145 | 280–290 | 50–1200 | Normal |
| Central diabetes insipidus | Normal or elevated | Normal or elevated | <200 | Low |
| Nephrogenic diabetes insipidus | Normal or elevated | Normal or elevated | <300 | Normal or elevated |
| Primary polydipsia | Low normal | Normal or low | <200 | Low |

Adapted from Saborio P, Tipton G, Chan J. Diabetes insipidus. *Pediatr Rev.* 2000;21:122–129.

Urine osmolality is best interpreted with a concomitant serum sample. A hyperosmolar state would suggest vasopressin deficiency or insensitivity, provided that the serum glucose concentration is normal. Low serum osmolality with hyponatremia suggests either primary polydipsia or water intoxication as the most likely diagnosis. Serum sodium level is usually normal in DI as long as free access to fluids exists and the thirst mechanism is intact. Hypernatremia is commonly seen in infants with DI or when a central lesion exists that also impairs thirst.[24] Blood chemistries will detect causes of nephrogenic DI, such as hypercalcemia and renal impairment.

In polyuric children with low urine specific gravity and no glycosuria, the next step in evaluation is referral to a specialist for a formal water deprivation test to determine whether a defect exists in vasopressin production or renal responsiveness.[25] In the case of patients with very low urine osmolality who are strongly suspected of having nephrogenic DI, the response to exogenous ADH can be determined without the need for prior fluid deprivation. Water deprivation testing should be undertaken with great caution in younger children and should not be performed in newborns. Because of the possibility of volume depletion, the study should be carried out during the day when supervision is optimum and should follow a 24-hour period of free access to fluids.

At baseline, the physician should record vital signs and weight and obtain blood and urine for osmolality, urine specific gravity, serum sodium concentration, serum urea nitrogen level, and hematocrit. Blood should also be obtained at the beginning and conclusion of fluid deprivation to determine plasma ADH levels, which may be helpful if the response to the water deprivation test is equivocal. Fluid intake is restricted for up to 8 hours, during which time the patient must be supervised closely to avoid surreptitious drinking. The patient should be weighed and have vital signs recorded every 2 hours for the first 4 hours, then hourly. Blood and urine should be collected after 4 hours, then every 2 hours for osmolality, serum sodium, and urine specific gravity measurements. The test should be terminated when 1 of the following endpoints is reached: (1) the patient has lost 5% or more of body weight, (2) urine specific gravity is greater than 1.020, (3) urine osmolality exceeds 600 mOsm/kg, (4) plasma osmolality exceeds 300 mOsm/kg, or (5) serum sodium exceeds 147 mEq/L. At the conclusion of the test, weight and vital signs should be recorded and blood and urine collected for osmolality, serum sodium, and urine specific gravity.

**Table 59-3**
**Interpretation of Water Deprivation Test and Vasopressin Administration**

| CLINICAL SITUATION | PLASMA VASOPRESSIN | URINE OSMOLALITY | URINE SPECIFIC GRAVITY AFTER VASOPRESSIN |
|---|---|---|---|
| Normal | Increased | >800 | Increased |
| Central diabetes insipidus | Low | <300 | Increased |
| Nephrogenic diabetes insipidus | High | <200 | Unchanged |
| Primary polydipsia | Unchanged | 500–600 | Unchanged or increased |

Adapted from Saborio P, Tipton G, Chan J. Diabetes insipidus. *Pediatr Rev.* 2000;21:122–129.

In healthy children, and in most children with primary polydipsia, the weight remains constant, the urine specific gravity rises, and the urine volume decreases. Concentrating ability is frequently impaired in primary polydipsia, resulting in a maximal urine osmolality of 500 to 600 mOsm/kg, compared with greater than 800 mOsm/kg in healthy individuals. This difference likely results from a reduction in the osmotic gradient across the distal renal tubule, with reduced renal sensitivity to vasopressin (Table 59-3).[26]

In the setting of continued diuresis, dehydration, weight loss, and hyperosmolality, the physician should suspect a diagnosis of DI. A small rise in urine osmolality may occur in both forms of DI from either partial vasopressin deficiency (central) or partial vasopressin resistance (nephrogenic). Administration of exogenous ADH may help differentiate between the 2 disorders (see Table 59-3). In an older child, the test can be performed after a water deprivation test or at a subsequent visit. Extreme caution is required when performing this test on infants or small children because of the danger of fluid overload and hyponatremia.[27] The patient is given free access to water after administration of desmopressin acetate (DDAVP), a synthetic derivative of vasopressin. Subsequently, intake, output, and urine specific gravity are recorded every 30 to 60 minutes.

In a patient with complete vasopressin deficiency, the urine output will fall, and urine osmolality will increase significantly. Distinguishing between patients with partial central DI and primary polydipsia may be difficult. Individuals with partial DI may have an exaggerated response to the submaximal rise in vasopressin induced by fluid deprivation.[28] Urine may be maximally concentrated when plasma osmolality is greater than 295 mOsm/kg. In this situation, there may be no further response to administration of exogenous ADH, a pattern suggestive of primary polydipsia. Patients who have primary polydipsia will have an increase in urine osmolality but no response to exogenous ADH because endogenous release is intact. Patients with complete nephrogenic DI do not increase urine osmolality in response to exogenous ADH administration. In patients with partial nephrogenic DI, urine osmolality may increase but will still be significantly lower than 300 mOsm/kg. In contrast, patients with partial vasopressin deficiency typically achieve a urine osmolality greater than 300 mOsm/kg after fluid deprivation.

Patients with vasopressin deficiency are best referred to an endocrinologist or neurologist so that the cause of the DI can be determined. A full investigation of other pituitary functions, visual-field examination, and magnetic resonance imaging of the brain will likely be the next steps in evaluation. Patients should be allowed free access to fluids, and their serum and urine osmolality should be monitored closely. When a diagnosis of central DI has been made, studies must be undertaken to ascertain the cause. Although many cases are idiopathic, a thorough evaluation for an underlying organic lesion must be conducted. The tumor markers human chorionic gonadotropin and a-fetoprotein should be measured, and magnetic resonance imaging of the pituitary and hypothalamus should be performed to assess for pituitary masses, craniopharyngioma, pinealoma, or pituitary stalk abnormalities. Up to 70% of patients with central DI will lose the normal hyperintense signal of the posterior pituitary.[29]

## ▶ MANAGEMENT

Management of polyuria depends largely on the underlying diagnosis and must be individualized carefully. In most cases, the results are gratifying, but patients are often found to have a chronic disease that requires close, long-term surveillance.

In a severely ill patient with central DI, aqueous vasopressin (0.1–0.2 U/kg) may be given subcutaneously every 4 to 6 hours. Vasopressin may also be given by continuous intravenous infusion. Reported starting doses vary from 0.5 to 4.6 mU/kg/hr; these doses should be increased or decreased as needed.[30,31] Vasopressin is a potent vasoconstrictor and may cause tissue ischemia and severe lactic acidosis, particularly at high infusion rates. Once the child's condition has stabilized, management consists of desmopressin acetate, which can be administered orally in tablet form or instilled intranasally and should be given at the lowest dose that produces antidiuretic effect. When given intranasally, the total daily dose may range from 5 mcg in infants to 40 mcg in older children divided into 2 or 3 doses as needed. Children receiving dose multiples of 10 mcg may use the nasal spray; those receiving smaller or intermediate doses must use the rhinal tube. Desmopressin may also be administered effectively and safely orally.[32,33] Therapeutic doses of oral desmopressin are generally 15 to 20 times larger than intranasal doses, and greater variability exists in the effective dose. Consequently, response to treatment must be monitored closely if changing route of administration.

Treatment of small children and infants with central DI can be difficult, with rapid changes in serum osmolality potentially leading to complications. The parents must carefully monitor fluid intake and output in the younger child. Because young infants are exclusively fed liquids and have high fluid requirements, the addition of vasopressin can greatly increase the risk for severe hyponatremia. These children are best managed with fluid therapy alone. Small doses of desmopressin may be required if adequate fluid intake is difficult to maintain or if caloric intake is inadequate because of excessive fluid consumption. The risk for hyponatremia can be reduced by allowing escape from the antidiuretic effect for 1 hour before the next dose. A child with adipsia or hypodipsia is best managed by fixing the desmopressin dose and fluid intake. Daily weights and frequent sodium levels are useful in assessing fluid status at home.[34]

In patients who have primary polydipsia, after a neurogenic lesion or gene mutation has been ruled out, medical therapy is not indicated. Psychiatric evaluation, however, may be useful in addressing the origin of the polydipsia.

Patients who have structural renal diseases leading to polyuria should be referred to a pediatric nephrologist. Children with nephrogenic DI should be allowed free access to fluids; parents of infants who have this disorder need to offer frequent water feedings to allow their infants to maintain osmotic homeostasis. A low-salt diet has been helpful in reducing urine output; thiazide diuretics can reduce polyuria further by reducing the amount of urine delivered to the distal tubule. Indomethacin[35] and amiloride,[36] when given concurrently with a thiazide, have each been found effective at reducing urine output.

Osmotic diuresis induced by drugs or diet generally is self-limited. In DM, polyuria secondary to hyperglycemia and glycosuria resolves with treatment of the underlying condition.

## When to Refer

- Hypotonic polyuria (confirmed by 24-hour urine and urine osmolality <300 mOsm). Perform water deprivation test.
- Polyuria after neurosurgery
- Polyuria and polydipsia secondary to DM

## When to Admit

- Polyuria and dehydration
- Diabetic ketoacidosis
- Severe hypernatremia
- Suspected diabetes insipidus in an infant
- Hypernatremia with MRI or neurologic findings suggestive of a brain tumor

### *REFERENCES*


1. Leung A, Robson W, Halperin M. Polyuria in childhood. *Clin Pediatr.* 1991;30:634
2. Robertson GL, Shelton RL, Athar S. The osmoregulation of vasopressin. *Kidney Int.* 1976;10:25–37
3. McKinley MJ, Johnson AK. The physiological regulation of thirst and fluid intake. *News Physiol Sci.* 2004;19:1–6
4. Arima H, Oiso Y. Mechanisms underlying progressive polyuria in familial neurohypophysial diabetes insipidus. *J Neuroendocrinol.* 2010;22:754–757
5. McLeod JF, Kovács L, Gaskill MB, et al. Familial neurohypophyseal diabetes insipidus associated with a signal peptide mutation. *J Clin Endocrinol Metab.* 1993;77:599A–599G
6. Rötig A, Cormier V, Chatelain P, et al. Deletion of mitochondrial DNA in a case of early-onset diabetes mellitus, optic atrophy and deafness (DIDMOAD, Wolfram syndrome). *J Inherit Metab Dis.* 1993;16:527–530
7. Lindsay RS, Seckl JR, Padfield PL. The triple-phase response—problems of water balance after pituitary surgery. *Postgrad Med J.* 1995;71:439–441
8. Greger NG, Kirkland RT, Clayton GW, Kirkland JL, et al. Central diabetes insipidus. 22 years' experience. *Am J Dis Child.* 1986;140:551–554
9. Scherbaum WA. Autoimmune hypothalamic diabetes insipidus ("autoimmune hypothalamitis"). *Prog Brain Res.* 1992;93:283–292
10. Heinze HJ, Bercu BB. Acquired hypophysitis in adolescence. *J Pediatr Endocrinol Metab.* 1997;10:315–321
11. Bichet DG, Birnbaumer M, Lonergan M, et al. Nature and recurrence of AVPR2 mutations in X-linked nephrogenic diabetes insipidus. *Am J Hum Genet.* 1994;55:278–286
12. Merendino JJ, Speigel AM, Crawford JD, et al. Brief report: a mutation in the vasopressin V2-receptor gene in a kindred with X-linked nephrogenic diabetes insipidus. *N Engl J Med.* 1993;328:1538–1541
13. Deen PM, Verdijk MA, Knoers NV, et al. Requirement of human renal water channel aquaporin-2 for vasopressin-dependent concentration of urine. *Science.* 1994;264:92–95
14. Coleman RA, Van Hove JL, Morris CR, Rhoads JM, Summar ML. Cerebral defects and nephrogenic diabetes insipidus with the ARC syndrome: additional findings or a new syndrome (ARCC-NDI)? *Am J Med Genet.* 1997;72:335–338
15. Garofeanu CG, Weir M, Rosas-Arellano MP, et al. Causes of reversible nephrogenic diabetes insipidus: a systematic review. *Am J Kidney Dis.* 2005;45:626–637

16. Kohn B, Norman ME, Feldman H, Their SO, Singer I. Hysterical polydipsia (compulsive water drinking) in children. *Am J Dis Child.* 1976;130:210–212
17. Stephen MD, Fenwick RG, Brosnan PG. Polyuria and polydipsia in a young child: diagnostic considerations and identification of novel mutation causing familial neurohypophyseal diabetes insipidus. *Pituitary.* 2012;15(Suppl 1):S1–S5
18. de Leon J, Verghese C, Tracy JI, Josiassen RC, Simpson GM. Polydipsia and water intoxication in psychiatric patients: a review of the epidemiological literature. *Biol Psychiatry.* 1994;35:408–419
19. Illowsky BP, Kirch DG. Polydipsia and hyponatremia in psychiatric patients. *Am J Psychiatry.* 1988;145:675–683
20. Goldman MB, Luchins DJ, Robertson GL. Mechanisms of altered water metabolism in psychotic patients with polydipsia and hyponatremia. *N Engl J Med.* 1988;318:397–403
21. Spears NM, Leadbetter RA, Shutty MS Jr. Clozapine treatment in polydipsia and intermittent hyponatremia. *J Clin Psychiatry.* 1996;57:123–128
22. McKenna K, Morris AD, Ryan M, et al. Renal resistance to vasopressin in poorly controlled type 1 diabetes mellitus. *Am J Physiol Endocrinol Metab.* 2000;279:E155–E160
23. Bishop MC. Diuresis and renal functional recovery in chronic retention. *Br J Urol.* 1985;57:1–5
24. McIver B, Connacher A, Whittle I, et al. Adipsic hypothalamic diabetes insipidus after clipping of anterior communicating artery aneurism. *Br Med J.* 1991;303:1465–1467
25. Dashe AM, Cramm RE, Crist CA, Habener JF, Solomon DH. A water deprivation test for the differential diagnosis of polyuria. *JAMA.* 1963;185:699–703
26. Cheetham T, Baylis PH. Diabetes insipidus in children: pathophysiology, diagnosis and management. *Paediatr Drugs.* 2002;4(12):785–796
27. Koskimies O, Pylkkänen J, Vilska J. Water intoxication in infants caused by the urine concentration test with vasopressin analogue (DDAVP). *Acta Paediatr Scand.* 1984;73:131–132
28. Miller M, Dalakos T, Moses AM, Fellerman H, Streeten DH. Recognition of partial defects in antidiuretic hormone secretion. *Ann Intern Med.* 1970;73:721–729
29. Sato N, Ishizaka H, Yagi H, Matsumoto M, Endo K. Posterior lobe of the pituitary in diabetes insipidus: dynamic MR imaging. *Radiology.* 1993;186(2):357–360
30. McDonald JA, Martha PM, Kerrigan J, et al. Treatment of the young child with postoperative central diabetes insipidus. *Am J Dis Child.* 1988;143:201–204
31. Rogers MC, Helfaer MA. *Handbook of Pediatric Intensive Care.* 2nd ed. Baltimore, MD: Williams and Wilkins; 1995
32. Boulgourdjian EM, Martinez AS, Ropelato MG, et al. Oral desmopressin treatment of central diabetes insipidus in children. *Acta Paediatr.* 1997;86(11):1261–1262
33. Fjellestad-Paulsen A, Paulsen O, d'Agay-Abensour L, Lundin S, Czernichow P. Central diabetes insipidus: oral treatment with dDAVP. *Regul Pept.* 1993;45:303–307
34. Ball SG, Vaidja B, Baylis PH. Hypothalamic adipsic syndrome: diagnosis and management. *Clin Endocrinol.* 1997;47:405–409
35. Libber S, Harrison H, Spector D. Treatment of nephrogenic diabetes insipidus with prostaglandin synthesis inhibitors. *J Pediatr.* 1986;108:305–311
36. Knoers N, Monnens LA. Amiloride-hydrochlorothiazide versus indomethacin-hydrochlorothiazide in the treatment of nephrogenic diabetes insipidus. *J Pediatr.* 1990;117:499–502
37. Decaux G, Soupart A, Vassart G. Non-peptide arginine-vasopressin antagonists: the vaptans. *Lancet.* 2008;371:1624–1632
38. Keating JP, Schears GJ, Dodge PR. Oral water intoxication in infants. An American epidemic. *Am J Dis Child.* 1991;145:985–990
39. Moritz ML, Ayus JC. New aspects in the pathogenesis, prevention, and treatment of hyponatremic encephalopathy in children. *Pediatr Nephrol.* 2010;25:1225–1238
40. Nzerue CM, Baffoe-Bonnie H, You W, Falana B, Dai S. Predictors of outcome in hospitalized patients with severe hyponatremia. *J Natl Med Assoc.* 2003;95:335–343

# Chapter 60

# Proteinuria

*Robert P. Woroniecki, MD, MS; Pamela S. Singer, MD*

In adults, *proteinuria* is defined as a urinary protein excretion exceeding 150 mg/day. In children, protein excretion exceeding 4 mg/m$^2$/hour is considered abnormal. Proteinuria may indicate the presence of renal injury and predict progressive renal disease[1–4]; in adults, proteinuria is also an established independent risk factor for cardiovascular disease.[5] Large losses of protein through the urine lead to hypercholesterolemia and hypertriglyceridemia, both of which, if sustained for a long time, increase cardiovascular mortality.[6] Medications that reduce proteinuria provide important long-term benefits for adult patients with chronic kidney disease and this beneficial effect has been extrapolated to children.[7]

## ▶ PATHOPHYSIOLOGIC FEATURES

Under physiologic conditions, the glomerular filtration barrier, composed of podocytes and vascular endothelium separated by the glomerular basement membrane, limits the passage of macromolecules from blood into urine based on both molecular size and electrical charge. The size barrier for filtration consists of pores with a diameter of approximately 40 Å in the slit diaphragm located between foot processes that is similar or smaller than the size of albumin (69 kDa).[8] In addition, the glomerular capillary wall contains heparan sulfate and proteoglycans, which are negatively charged and thus repel macromolecules with the same electrical charge, such as albumin.[9] Most inflammatory glomerular diseases lead to morphologic alteration of the size barrier and loss of negative charges, leading to proteinuria. Another factor that affects protein movement across glomerular capillary walls is glomerular hemodynamics (ie, glomerular plasma flow rate, hydrostatic and oncotic forces). A reduction in the number of functioning nephrons leads to hyperfiltration in the remaining nephrons and to proteinuria.[10]

Low–molecular-weight proteins, such as $\beta_2$-microglobulin, retinol-binding protein, and $\beta_1$-microglobulin, are freely filtered through the glomerulus and are subsequently reabsorbed by the proximal tubule. Tubular injury results in impaired ability to reabsorb these proteins and their loss in the urine.[11] Some proteins, such as the Tamm-Horsfall mucoprotein (uromodulin), a major constituent of urinary casts, are formed by the cells of the thick ascending loop of Henle.[12]

## ▶ LABORATORY EVALUATION OF PROTEINURIA

The diagnosis of proteinuria depends on laboratory assessment of the level of protein in the urine. The 3 ways urine is tested are the dipstick test, assessment of a timed urine sample, and assessment of the urine protein-creatinine (P/Cr) ratio from an untimed urine sample.

### Dipstick Test

The most commonly performed urine screening method for protein is the dipstick test. Tetrabromophenol on the reagent strip reacts with the amino group of the protein and changes the color of the strip. The test reports findings as negative, trace, and 1+ (30 mg/dL), 2+ (100 mg/dL), 3+ (300 mg/dL), and 4+ (2,000 mg/dL).

The dipstick test primarily detects albumin and is less sensitive to low–molecular-weight proteins and β-globulins. Because the test measures the concentration of protein, false-negative results may occur with highly dilute urine. Conversely, false-positive results may occur with concentrated urine. Generally, a result of 1+ or more in a specimen with a specific gravity of less than 1.015 indicates abnormal protein loss.[13]

The detection of protein depends on pH: extremely alkaline urine may yield a false-positive reading. Other causes of false-positive readings are prolonged immersion of the strip; hematuria, pyuria, or bacteriuria; presence of detergents and contaminating antiseptics, such as chlorhexidine and benzalkonium chloride; presence of antibiotics, such as penicillins, cephalosporins, sulfonamides, and tolbutamide; or presence of radiographic contrast materials.[13,14] An alternative office procedure to measure urinary protein is precipitation with sulfosalicylic acid. This measurement is a more accurate estimate of the total urinary proteins, including those of low molecular weight.[14] False-positive results can occur in the previously mentioned conditions.

A positive dipstick result should be confirmed by urinalysis, and urine P/Cr ratio preferably performed on the first urine voided in the morning.

### Timed Urine Sample

The traditional and most accurate way of quantifying urinary protein excretion is to measure protein in a timed sample collected over a 24-hour period. The patient is instructed to void right after waking in the morning. This first urine is discarded, and all subsequent urines are collected. The last urine sample added to the collection should be 24 hours after the first one.

In adults, a protein excretion of less than 150 mg in 24 hours is considered normal. In children, an excretion rate of less than 4 mg/m$^2$/hour is considered normal, 4 to 40 mg/m$^2$/hour is abnormal, and more than 40 mg/m$^2$/hour is considered nephrotic-range proteinuria. The adequacy of the sample can be determined by measuring the creatinine excretion in the sample. Steady-state daily creatinine excretion is 20 mg/kg/day in children from 1 to 12 years of age and 22 to 25 mg/kg in older children, and may be lower in females or children with reduced muscle mass. However, this method is cumbersome, can be impractical in children, and is fraught with error from under- and over-collection.[15]

### Urine Protein-Creatinine Ratio

Measurement of the P/Cr ratio in an untimed (spot) urine sample offers a reliable method for classification of proteinuria. This method is easier than a 24-hour urine collection.[16] Studies in adults and children have shown a strong correlation between untimed urine P/Cr ratio and 24-hour urine collection.[16,17] A ratio of more than 3.5:1 indicates nephrotic-range proteinuria, and ratios of less than 0.2:1 in patients aged 2 and older and less than 0.5:1 in children aged between 6 and 24 months are considered normal.[18]

## ▶ PREVALENCE

Finding proteinuria in a single urine specimen in children and adolescents is relatively common. However, the presence of persistent and not orthostatic proteinuria, also called *fixed proteinuria,* on repeat testing indicates renal disease until proven otherwise.[19] The prevalence of proteinuria, both fixed and orthostatic, is generally between 5% and 15%.[12] Prevalence of orthostatic proteinuria seems to rise with age, peaking in adolescence, with subsequent decline and a nadir in adulthood. For boys, prevalence peaks at age 16 years; for girls, the peak is at 13 years.[20]

## ▶ ETIOLOGY

The basic evaluation of proteinuria should address the following issues: pathological or nonpathological cause; presence or absence of symptoms; amount of protein loss; presence or absence of associated findings, such as hematuria, hypertension, azotemia; and other urinary or systemic abnormalities.

### Nonpathological Proteinuria

*Nonpathological proteinuria* results from the adjustment of the kidney to extraneous physiologic conditions (ie, growth, exercise, fever, systemic illness). The level of proteinuria is generally less than 1 g/day and is not associated with edema.[21]

### Postural or Orthostatic Proteinuria

*Orthostatic proteinuria* accounts for 60% of all cases of asymptomatic proteinuria in children, with a higher incidence in adolescents.[22] Children with this condition have normal urinary protein excretion in the supine position but spill abnormal amounts of protein in the upright position. The proteinuria decreases to normal range or disappears when they have been recumbent for a few hours, as in overnight sleep. These children are asymptomatic; proteinuria is usually found on a routine urinalysis. The cause of orthostatic proteinuria is unknown.[23] It has been postulated that orthostatic proteinuria might result from higher than normal release of norepinephrine and angiotensin II upon standing, or transient compression of the left renal vein in the fork between the superior mesenteric artery and the aorta (renal nutcracker).[24–26] Edema, hypertension, and hematuria are absent, and creatinine clearance and complements are normal. Renal ultrasound and histopathological tests are also normal, although these tests are not usually performed in the evaluation process.

Children with asymptomatic proteinuria should be assessed for postural (orthostatic) proteinuria. The standard method is to collect a first-morning urine and if it is negative for protein on the dipstick, or if the measured P/Cr ratio is less than 0.2:1, the patient has orthostatic proteinuria. The more formal (although not currently used) orthostatic test for postural proteinuria includes 2 separate collections, one in the supine position and the other in the upright position. At bedtime, the child goes to bed immediately after voiding (the urine is discarded). The child is then allowed to sleep. All urine passed during the night, including the first specimen voided the next morning, is collected in a jar (specimen 1), and the time of the first-morning voiding is recorded. Then the child goes about daily activities but collects all urine in a second jar (specimen 2) for approximately the next 12 hours. This collection is the upright collection, which ends at bedtime, when the time is again recorded.

In patients with orthostatic proteinuria, the sample obtained in the supine position will be free of protein or will contain a normal amount of protein; however, the sample obtained in upright position will contain an abnormal amount of protein. Children with orthostatic proteinuria generally excrete less than 1 g of protein in 24 hours.[14]

The diagnosis of postural proteinuria can also be made by assessing the first-morning urine. If this sample has no protein, or if it has a P/Cr ratio less than 0.2:1, then a presumptive diagnosis of orthostatic proteinuria can be made. Long-term follow-up studies in adults have documented the benign nature of orthostatic proteinuria, although rare cases of glomerulosclerosis have been identified later in life in patients who were initially found to have proteinuria with an orthostatic component.[27–29] Therefore, long-term follow-up of children is necessary unless the proteinuria resolves. Signs to anticipate include appearance of hematuria, hypertension, increase in serum creatinine concentration, or proteinuria exceeding 1 g/day.[21]

### Transient Proteinuria

As many as 30% to 50% of children with proteinuria may have *transient, nonfixed proteinuria.* It can accompany fever, exercise, stress, dehydration, congestive heart failure, or seizures.[30] Transient proteinuria may be found in children having a temperature of 38.3°C or higher.[31] It usually does not exceed 2+ on the dipstick test and resolves when the fever abates.

Proteinuria associated with vigorous exercise rarely exceeds 2+ on the dipstick test. Transient proteinuria seems to be related to intensity of exercise rather than duration.[32] It may be explained by an increased glomerular filtration barrier permeability and a partial inhibition of tubular reabsorption of protein.[33] The effect of exercise increases with age.[34] Transient proteinuria is considered benign if proteinuria resolves after 48 hours of rest.

## *Pathological Proteinuria*

### Persistent or Fixed Asymptomatic Proteinuria

Patients with a positive dipstick test (1+ or greater) should undergo a more accurate test, such as P/Cr ratio or a quantitative measurement of protein excretion. Orthostatic proteinuria should be excluded by repeat measurements on a first-morning void if the initial sample was taken at random. In the absence of other abnormalities, patients with 2 or more positive semiquantitative or quantitative tests, 1 to 2 weeks apart, are diagnosed as having fixed proteinuria.[35] The prevalence in school-aged children may be as high as 6%.[19,36] Various causes are listed in Table 60-1.

*Pathological proteinuria* can be classified as either glomerular or tubular. Glomerular proteinuria, which is the more common of the 2 forms, is associated with increased permeability of glomerular filtration barrier. Glomerular proteinuria may be selective (plasma proteins with molecular weights up to and including albumin), as in minimal change disease, or nonselective (albumin and large–molecular-weight proteins, such as immunoglobulin G), as in most forms of glomerulonephritis. *Tubular proteinuria* results from decreased tubular protein reabsorption that results from tubular dysfunction (see Table 60-1).

**Table 60-1**
**Classification of Pathological Proteinuria**

| GLOMERULAR | TUBULAR |
|---|---|
| **Nephrotic Syndrome** | **Genetic** |
| Idiopathic | Polycystic kidney disease |
| Minimal change | Cystinosis |
| Mesangial proliferation | Wilson disease |
| Focal segmental glomerulosclerosis | Lowe syndrome |
| Membranous nephropathy | Galactosemia |
| **Glomerulonephritis** | Renal tubular acidosis |
| Postinfectious | Dent disease |
| Immunoglobulin A nephropathy | **Acquired** |
| Membranoproliferative glomerulonephritis | Interstitial nephritis |
| **Systemic disease** | Acute tubular necrosis |
| **Systemic lupus erythematosus** | Heavy metal poisoning |
| **Vasculitis** | Drugs or toxins |
| **Tumor** | |
| **Subacute bacterial endocarditis** | |
| **Infection (HIV, hepatitis)** | |
| **Drugs or toxins** | |
| **Obesity** | |
| **Other** | |

## Symptomatic Proteinuria

Symptomatic proteinuria associated with gravity-dependent edema, hypoalbuminemia, and hyperlipidemia is defined as a nephrotic syndrome. However, some children with nephrotic-range proteinuria and hypoalbuminemia remain completely asymptomatic. Edema in nephrotic syndrome results from multiple factors acting in concert, including increased distal nephron sodium reabsorption, increased capillary permeability, and low plasma oncotic pressure associated with hypoalbuminemic states.[37]

Proteinuria may be associated with other abnormalities, including hematuria, hypertension, and azotemia, as seen in glomerulonephritis. Patients with a combination of nephritis and nephrotic syndrome pose a clinical challenge even to the most experienced nephrologist.

# ▶ EVALUATION

## *History*

The first step in evaluating a child with proteinuria is obtaining a thorough history. History should include questions about recent illnesses, fever, rash, and arthralgias; change in urine output and color; symptoms of chronic disease (eg, weight loss, fatigue); and duration and severity of symptoms. History of urinary tract infections and family history of urinary reflux, hypertension, and deafness are important.

## *Physical Examination*

Physical examination should include measurements of growth parameters, blood pressure, and identification of edema, ascites, and pallor, as well as documentation of the presence or absence of any joint or skin lesions.

### Laboratory Evaluation

The presence of proteinuria should be confirmed by a urine P/Cr ratio on a first-morning urine sample. Once confirmed, fixed proteinuria should be quantified by a 24-hour urine collection for measurement of protein and creatinine (to determine adequacy of the sample). Serum electrolytes, blood urea nitrogen, and creatinine help determine the level of kidney function. Serum albumin, cholesterol, and triglycerides guide the determination of the severity of metabolic changes that occur as a result of urine protein loss. Complement levels, anti–streptolysin O titers, hepatitis serologic testing, and HIV testing may be indicated based on the child's history. Renal ultrasound may be performed to assess for structural abnormalities. The patient should be referred to a pediatric nephrologist if any abnormalities are found during the initial workup. Some of the other warning signs of proteinuria are listed in Box 60-1.

The steps in evaluating proteinuria are illustrated in Figure 60-1.

Asymptomatic children with proteinuria should be tested to determine its etiology.[14]

Assessment of total protein is appropriate in children to identify both albuminuria and low–molecular-weight proteinuria. Patients with a positive dipstick test of 1+ or greater should undergo confirmation by assessment of the P/Cr ratio within 3 months. Under most circumstances, first-morning spot urine protein and creatinine samples should be used to detect and monitor proteinuria in children.

Orthostatic proteinuria must be excluded by measuring P/Cr ratio in a first-morning urine sample. Patients with 2 or more positive first-morning P/Cr tests, obtained at 1- to 2-week intervals, should be diagnosed as having persistent or fixed proteinuria. Monitoring proteinuria in patients with chronic kidney disease should be performed by quantitative methods.

## ▶ MANAGEMENT

If orthostatic proteinuria is diagnosed, the child should be monitored with annual office visits and check of first-morning urine P/Cr ratio. Renal biopsy should be considered in certain situations with persistent proteinuria (see Box 60-2).

If isolated fixed proteinuria less than 1 g/day is detected (urine P/Cr ratio ), restrictions on the child's lifestyle and physical activity are not necessary. Children with proteinuria should receive the recommended daily allowance of protein for their age.[38,39]

**Box 60-1**

### *Warning Signs of Proteinuria*

- Persistent, fixed, nonorthostatic proteinuria
- Proteinuria associated with other urinary abnormalities, such as hematuria, or urinary casts
- Proteinuria associated with renal insufficiency, anemia, or hypertension
- Family history of renal disease, kidney stones, dialysis, deafness, or autoimmune conditions
- Proteinuria associated with comorbidities such as prematurity, congenital anomalies of other organ systems, hypertension, diabetes, and obesity

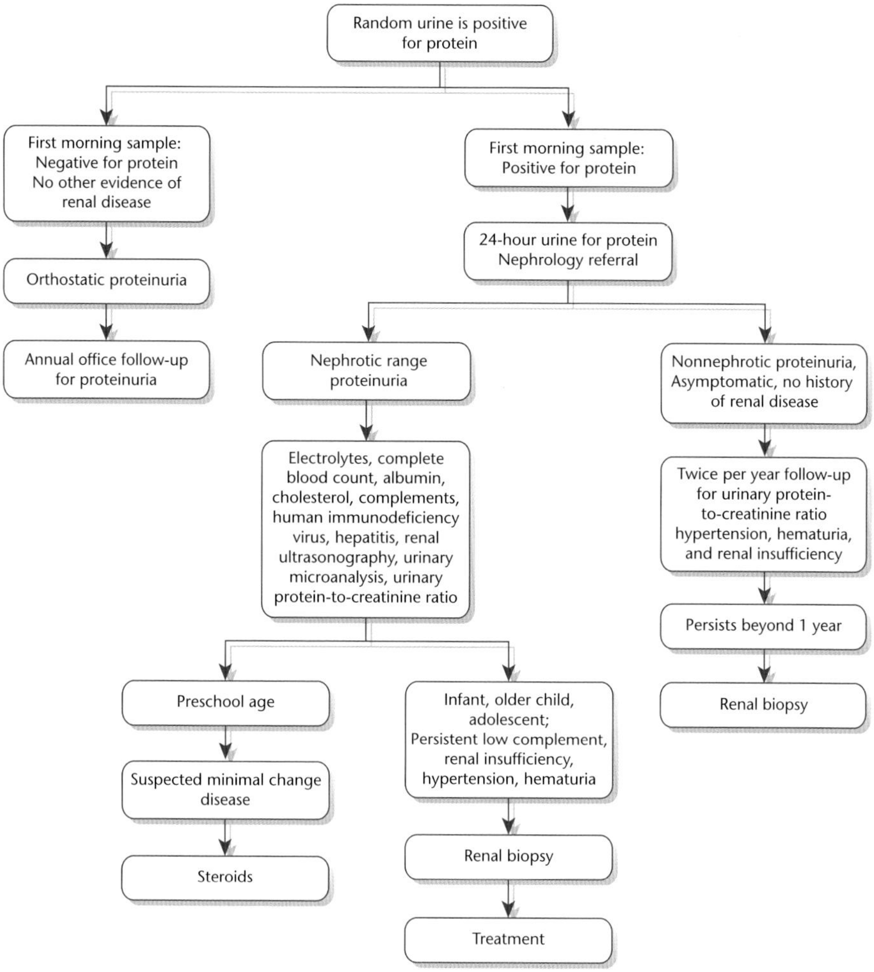


**Figure 60–1**
Diagnostic approach in a patient with proteinuria.

**Box 60-2**

## *Indications for Renal Biopsy in Persistent Proteinuria*

- Fixed, asymptomatic, isolated proteinuria >1 g/day
- Persistent hematuria and cellular casts
- Renal insufficiency
- Persistently low complement levels
- Hypertension
- Systemic symptoms such as recurrent rashes, joint pains, or fever
- Systemic lupus erythematosus
- Family history of kidney disease or autoimmune disease
- Corticosteroid-resistant nephrotic syndrome

## When to Refer

- Persistent, fixed, nonorthostatic proteinuria
- Proteinuria associated with other urinary abnormalities, such as hematuria
- Proteinuria associated with renal insufficiency, anemia, or hypertension
- Family history of renal disease, deafness, or autoimmune condition
- Proteinuria associated with comorbidities such as prematurity, congenital anomalies of other organ systems, hypertension, diabetes, and obesity

## When to Admit

- Anasarca resistant to outpatient management
- Proteinuria associated with significant renal insufficiency
- Proteinuria associated with significant hypertension

## *TOOLS FOR PRACTICE*

### Engaging Patient and Family

- *Proteinuria* (fact sheet), American Academy of Pediatrics (www.healthychildren.org/English/health-issues/conditions/genitourinary-tract/Pages/Proteinuria.aspx)
- *Proteinuria* (fact sheet), National Kidney and Urologic Diseases Information Clearinghouse, National Institute of Diabetes and Digestive and Kidney Diseases, and National Institutes of Health (kidney.niddk.nih.gov/KUDiseases/pubs/proteinuria/index.aspx)

### Medical Decision Support

- *Pathologic Proteinuria Calculator* (interactive tool), (www.metrohealthresearch.org/schelling)

## *REFERENCES*


1. Williams JD, Coles GA. Proteinuria–a direct cause of renal morbidity? *Kidney Int.* 1994;45:443–450
2. Ruggenenti P, Perna A, Mosconi L, Pisoni R, Remuzzi G. Urinary protein excretion rate is the best independent predictor of ESRF in non-diabetic proteinuric chronic nephropathies. "Gruppo Italiano di Studi Epidemiologici in Nefrologia" (GISEN). *Kidney Int.* 1998;53:1209–1216
3. Keane WF, Eknoyan G. Proteinuria, albuminuria, risk, assessment, detection, elimination (PARADE): a position paper of the National Kidney Foundation. *Am J Kidney Dis.* 1999;33:1004–1010
4. Eddy AA. Proteinuria and interstitial injury. *Nephrol Dial Transplant.* 2004;19:277–281
5. Kannel WB, Stampfer MJ, Castelli WP, Verter J. The prognostic significance of proteinuria: the Framingham study. *Am Heart J.* 1984;108:1347–1352
6. Sytkowski PA, Kannel WB, D'Agostino RB. Changes in risk factors and the decline in mortality from cardiovascular disease. The Framingham Heart Study. *N Engl J Med.* 1990;322:1635–1641
7. Remuzzi G, Chiurchiu C, Ruggenenti P. Proteinuria predicting outcome in renal disease: nondiabetic nephropathies (REIN). *Kidney Int Suppl.* 2004;(92):S90–S96
8. Wartiovaara J, Ofverstedt LG, Khoshnoodi J, et al. Nephrin strands contribute to a porous slit diaphragm scaffold as revealed by electron tomography. *J Clin Invest.* 2004;114:1475–1483
9. Kanwar YS, Farquhar MG. Presence of heparan sulfate in the glomerular basement membrane. *Proc Natl Acad Sci U S A.* 1979;76:1303–1307
10. Kriz W, LeHir M. Pathways to nephron loss starting from glomerular diseases-insights from animal models. *Kidney Int.* 2005;67:404–419
11. Tomlinson PA. Low molecular weight proteins in children with renal disease. *Pediatr Nephrol.* 1992;6:565–571
12. Mckenzie Jk, Patel R, Mcqueen Eg. The excretion rate of Tamm-Horsfall urinary mucoprotein in normals and in patients with renal disease. *Australas Ann Med.* 1964;13:32–39

13. Ettenger RB. The evaluation of the child with proteinuria. *Pediatr Ann.* 1994;23:486–494
14. Hogg RJ, Portman RJ, Milliner D, et al. Evaluation and management of proteinuria and nephrotic syndrome in children: recommendations from a pediatric nephrology panel established at the National Kidney Foundation conference on proteinuria, albuminuria, risk, assessment, detection, and elimination (PARADE). *Pediatrics.* 2000;105:1242–1249
15. Abitbol C, Zilleruelo G, Freundlich M, Strauss J. Quantitation of proteinuria with urinary protein/creatinine ratios and random testing with dipsticks in nephrotic children. *J Pediatr.* 1990;116:243–247
16. Price CP, Newall RG, Boyd JC. Use of protein:creatinine ratio measurements on random urine samples for prediction of significant proteinuria: a systematic review. *Clin Chem.* 2005;51:1577–1586
17. Tsai WS, Tsau YK, Chen CH, Sheu JN. Correlation between total urinary protein quantitation and random urine sample protein/creatinine ratio in children. *J Formos Med Assoc.* 1991;90:760–763
18. Ginsberg JM, Chang BS, Matarese RA, Garella S. Use of single voided urine samples to estimate quantitative proteinuria. *N Engl J Med.* 1983;309:1543–1546
19. Vehaskari VM, Rapola J. Isolated proteinuria: analysis of a school-age population. *J Pediatr.* 1982;101:661–668
20. Wagner MG, Smith FG, Tinglof BO, Cornberg E. Epidemiology of proteinuria. A study of 4,807 schoolchildren. *J Pediatr.* 1968;73:825–832
21. Bergstein JM. A practical approach to proteinuria. *Pediatr Nephrol.* 1999;13:697–700
22. Norman ME. An office approach to hematuria and proteinuria. *Pediatr Clin North Am.* 1987;34:545–560
23. Devarajan P. Mechanisms of orthostatic proteinuria: lessons from a transplant donor. *J Am Soc Nephrol.* 1993;4:36–39
24. Brandt JR, Jacobs A, Raissy HH, et al. Orthostatic proteinuria and the spectrum of diurnal variability of urinary protein excretion in healthy children. *Pediatr Nephrol.* 2010;25:1131–1137
25. Nathan H. Observations on aberrant renal arteries curving around and compressing the renal vein; possible relationship to orthostatic proteinuria and to orthostatic hypertension. *Circulation.* 1958;18:1131–1134
26. Mazzoni MB, Kottanatu L, Simonetti GD, et al. Renal vein obstruction and orthostatic proteinuria: a review. *Nephrol Dial Transplant.* 2011;26:562–565
27. Springberg PD, Garrett LE, Thompson AL, et al. Fixed and reproducible orthostatic proteinuria: results of a 20-year follow-up study. *Ann Intern Med.* 1982;97:516–519
28. Rytand DA, Spreiter S. Prognosis in postural (orthostatic) proteinuria: forty to fifty-year follow-up of six patients after diagnosis by Thomas Addis. *N Engl J Med.* 1981;305:618–621
29. Berns JS, McDonald B, Gaudio KM, Siegel NJ. Progression of orthostatic proteinuria to focal and segmental glomerulosclerosis. *Clin Pediatr (Phila).* 1986;25(3):165–166
30. Houser M. Assessment of proteinuria using random urine samples. *J Pediatr.* 1984;104:845–848
31. Marks MI, McLaine PN, Drummond KN. Proteinuria in children with febrile illnesses. *Arch Dis Child.* 1970;45:250–253
32. Poortmans JR. Postexercise proteinuria in humans. Facts and mechanisms. *JAMA.* 1985;253:236–240
33. Poortmans JR. Renal response to exercise in healthy and diseased patients. *Nephrologie.* 1995;16:317–324
34. Poortmans JR, Geudvert C, Schorokoff K, De Plaen P. Postexercise proteinuria in childhood and adolescence. *Int J Sports Med.* 1996;17:448–451
35. National Kidney Foundation. K/DOQI clinical practice guidelines for chronic kidney disease: evaluation, classification, and stratification. *Am J Kidney Dis.* 2002;39:S1–S266
36. Yoshikawa N, Kitagawa K, Ohta K, Tanaka R, Nakamura H. Asymptomatic constant isolated proteinuria in children. *J Pediatr.* 1991;119:375–379
37. Svenningsen P, Bistrup C, Friis UG, et al. Plasmin in nephrotic urine activates the epithelial sodium channel. *J Am Soc Nephrol.* 2009;20:299–310
38. Wingen AM, Fabian-Bach C, Schaefer F, Mehls O. Randomised multicentre study of a low-protein diet on the progression of chronic renal failure in children. European Study Group of Nutritional Treatment of Chronic Renal Failure in Childhood. *Lancet.* 1997;349:1117–1123
39. Uauy RD, Hogg RJ, Brewer ED, et al. Dietary protein and growth in infants with chronic renal insufficiency: a report from the Southwest Pediatric Nephrology Study Group and the University of California, San Francisco. *Pediatr Nephrol.* 1994;8:45–50

# Chapter 61

# Pruritus

*Nancy K. Barnett, MD*

Pruritus, or itch, is the subjective perception of a cutaneous disturbance that is relieved by scratching or rubbing. It is usually not brought to the primary care physician's attention unless it is generalized, chronic, or associated with an eruption. In such instances, however, pruritus must be treated with great respect because severe itching can be incapacitating. In addition, scratching or rubbing the itch can produce extensive disfigurement in the form of linear excoriations or lichenified plaques and can predispose the patient to cutaneous infections. Constant scratching can even cause social isolation because, at times, people view the child with pruritus as being contagious or unclean.

## ▶ DEFINITION OF TERMS

Because itch is a subjective sensation, objective evaluation to delineate its pathophysiologic characteristics has been difficult. However, current thinking implicates nonspecific itch receptors. Thought to be free, fine nerve endings at the dermoepidermal junction, these receptors transmit the pruritic sensation along dedicated, slow-conduction velocity, unmyelinated C fibers.[1] The exact mediators and their release triggers are unknown. Mast cell histamine has elicited itch fairly consistently in experimental settings[2] and appears to be active in human disease, as may be other local mediators such as substance P and interleukin.[3] Other experimental triggers that have produced itch are physical pressure, heat, and electric shock. Researchers believe that the nerve impulses from the intraepithelial histamine-sensitive, unmyelinated C fibers ascend to the lamina I in the dorsal horn of the spinal cord and travel along the contralateral spinothalamic tract to the thalamus. They are then transferred to multiple areas of the cortex and are interpreted as itch. A subsequent desire to scratch arises in the cortex.[4] The dorsolateral prefrontal cortex and contralateral caudate nucleus and putamen areas in atopic patients and the anterior cingulate cortex have been identified as activated when histamine-induced itch and scratch are traced. In contrast, the primary motor and sensorimotor cortices and superior parietal lobe are activated in healthy controls.[5] Itch is not a mild form of pain; the pathways are different, and aspirin alone does not relieve itch.

Certain circumstances alter the interpretation of the degree of pruritus. For example, the itch threshold in and around areas of active dermatitis can be lowered by psychic stress, decreased skin hydration, or increased skin temperature, and during the night.[2,6] Pain can inhibit the itch sensation, and scratching can stimulate pain receptors.

## ▶ DIFFERENTIAL DIAGNOSIS

In children, local cutaneous disease rather than systemic disease is by far the most common cause of generalized pruritus. Pruritogenic itch arising in the skin is the focus of this chapter, and discussing neuropathic, neurogenic, and psychogenic itch[7] is beyond the scope. The major differential diagnoses of generalized pruritus with skin lesions in children are infestation (scabies, pediculosis, insect bites, and papular urticaria), atopic dermatitis, miliaria, contact dermatitis, and acute or chronic urticaria.

Children may also itch with cutaneous diseases such as psoriasis, lichen planus, and linear immunoglobulin A bullous disease of childhood. These children should be referred to a dermatologist for evaluation and management, as should a child with pruritus who is otherwise healthy and does not have bites, eczema, heat rash, contact dermatitis, or hives. The child who has pruritus, from whatever cause, is at risk for psychological damage, infection secondary to impetiginization, and scarification.

Systemic causes of itch in the child who has pruritus but no skin lesions are hyperthyroidism and hypothyroidism, leukemia or lymphoma, chronic renal failure, obstructive biliary disease, and xerosis (generalized dry skin).

## ▶ EVALUATION AND MANAGEMENT

Most of the common cutaneous diseases associated with generalized pruritus can be diagnosed based on a thorough history and physical examination. The answers to the following questions may help diagnose infestation of one sort or another and direct therapy toward topical steroids, long clothes, and repellents:

Are any individual pruritic papules found with a central punctum?

If so, are they on exposed or nonexposed areas?

Does anyone else in the family have similar lesions? A family history of allergy, asthma, or eczema in a child who has a chronic eczematous dermatitis over extensor surfaces in infancy and flexural areas in childhood suggests atopic dermatitis. Hydration and emollients will reduce the pruritus and should be the mainstay of therapy, although mid- and low-potency topical steroids for inflammation, antibiotics for secondary infection, and cool compresses may also be required to bring the scratch-itch cycle under control. Short courses (<8 weeks) of topical immunomodulators such as tacrolimus and pimecrolimus may be helpful in relieving atopic itch on facial skin and thin areas such as the axillae, but these medications should not be prescribed as chronic therapy. A tolerable (nonsoporific) dose of an antihistamine may relieve itch and should be given about 1 hour before bedtime because the itch threshold is lower at night than it is during the daytime. Hydroxyzine seems to be the most effective agent.[8] Data conflict about the use of nonsedating antihistamines for controlling itch.[9] Pinpoint crystalline or erythematous papules in areas of occlusion and sweating—that is, miliaria crystallina and miliaria rubra (heat rash)—can be controlled by simple measures such as applying dusting powders, avoiding tight clothing, and reducing exposure to high ambient temperatures.

In most instances, contact dermatitis is readily recognizable because of a linear array of papulovesicular erythematous lesions and sharp borders that conform to the shape of the contactant.

Acute urticaria, usually from exposure to a drug or other ingestant, produces intensely pruritic, erythematous, and edematous plaques and papules. Thorough historical and environmental sleuthing may reveal the cause of a contact allergic or contact irritant dermatitis, but the cause of 90% of acute urticaria cases remains a mystery. If the patient has not used any new drug or food, and if the hives persist despite regular use of antihistamines for several days, then a reasonable course of action would be to obtain a throat culture and a complete blood count with differential and to screen for mycoplasmal disease and infectious mononucleosis to rule out occult streptococcal, mycoplasmal, and viral infections. On rare occasions, a skin biopsy may be helpful. Physical urticarias should demonstrate dermatographism, which can be a helpful diagnostic tool.

For the child who has pruritus with no primary skin disorder, a complete blood count with differential count, complete chemistry panel, thyroid function tests (thyroid-stimulating hormone/free $T_4$), urinalysis, and chest radiograph should be obtained to assess for possible systemic causes, especially before suggesting a psychogenic cause for the itching.

To relieve itching and prevent scarring (both mental and physical), the scratch-itch cycle must be broken. Itching provokes scratching, and when the scratching stops, the itching returns. To control itching, the following steps can be helpful:

- Keep the patient's fingernails short to prevent damage from scratching.
- Keep the child fully clothed except when applying medications.
- Apply bland emollient creams frequently, especially after bathing. Overwashing, especially without sealing in the water with an occlusive cream, may dry out the skin and worsen itch. A home humidifier may increase the relative humidity in the air and lessen dry skin itch.
- Apply cool compresses to relieve intense pruritus and to remove crusts and debris.
- Apply topical steroids for short periods (generally <2 weeks) to control inflammation.
- Increase the dose of antihistamine until the scratching stops or marked drowsiness occurs, and then reduce the dose to a level that controls the scratching but does not cause drowsiness.
- Advise the family to avoid stress, heat, and irritants (eg, wool, pet danders).
- See the patient frequently to provide support.
- If the child is old enough to understand, explain why these methods are being used.

Topical capsaicin, menthol, phenol, doxepin, and pramoxine may be indicated for localized use in some cases, but the potential for contact irritation and systemic absorption limits their prolonged or widespread use.[10] Referral to the dermatologist is generally indicated in such a circumstance. Ultraviolet B light therapy may be helpful for generalized pruritus such as occurs in biliary cirrhosis or severe chronic atopic dermatitis.[11] Chronic localized and intractable itch may respond to neurologic "sensor resetting," in which the brain is fooled into believing the affected area is normal by mirror treatment, because we have come to understand that the sensation of itch results more from central perception than local reception.[12]

## When to Refer

- Pruritus with uncommon disease (eg, psoriasis, bullae)
- Chronic pruritus without cutaneous disease to evaluate for systemic cause
- Pruritus uncontrolled by usual topical steroids and antihistamines

## TOOLS FOR PRACTICE

### Engaging Patients and Family

- *What is a Pediatric Dermatologist?* (fact sheet), American Academy of Pediatrics (www.healthychildren.org/English/family-life/health-management/pediatric-specialists/Pages/What-is-a-Pediatric-Dermatologist.aspx)

### Medical Decision Support

- *Pediatric Dermatology: A Quick Reference Guide* (book), American Academy of Pediatrics (shop.aap.org)
- *Dermatology Course Series—Skin Infections* (online course), American Academy of Pediatrics (pedialink.aap.org)

## REFERENCES

1. Yosipovitch G, Greaves MW, Schmelz M. Itch. *Lancet.* 2003;361:690–694
2. Cormia FE. Experimental histamine pruritus. I. Influence of physical and psychological factors on threshold reactivity. *J Invest Dermatol.* 1952;19:21–34
3. Greaves MW, Wall PD. Pathophysiology of itching. *Lancet.* 1996;348:938–940
4. Wallengren J. Neuroanatomy and neurophysiology of itch. *Dermatol Ther.* 2005;18:292–303
5. Ishiuji Y, Coghill RC, Patel TS, et al. Distinct patterns of brain activity evoked by histamine-induced itch reveal an association with itch intensity and disease severity in atopic dermatitis. *Br J Dermatol.* 2009;161:1072–1080
6. Edwards AE, Shellow WV, Wright ET, Dignam TF. Pruritic skin diseases, psychological stress, and the itch sensation. A reliable method for the induction of experimental pruritus. *Arch Dermatol.* 1976;112:339–343
7. Fazio SB, Ship AN. Abnormal uterine bleeding. *South Med J.* 2007;100:376–382
8. Rhoades RB, Leifer KN, Cohan R, Wittig HJ. Suppression of histamine-induced pruritus by three antihistaminic drugs. *J Allergy Clin Immunol.* 1975;55:180–185
9. O'Donoghue M, Tharp MD. Antihistamines and their role as antipruritics. *Dermatol Ther.* 2005;18:333–340
10. Krishnan A, Koo J. Psyche, opioids, and itch: therapeutic consequences. *Dermatol Ther.* 2005;18:314–322
11. Rivard J, Lim HW. Ultraviolet phototherapy for pruritus. *Dermatol Ther.* 2005;18:344–354
12. Gwande A. The itch. In: *The New Yorker.* June 30, 2008

# Chapter 62

# Puberty: Normal and Abnormal

*Robert K. Kritzler, MD; Dominique Long, MD; Leslie Plotnick, MD*

Disorders of pubertal development constitute one of the most frequent referrals to pediatric endocrinology clinics. In many cases, no endocrine problem is found. A referral may be avoided by a careful evaluation, including family history, and a few simple laboratory procedures. The availability of pediatric endocrinology consultation and the pediatrician or other physician's level of comfort in diagnosing and treating disorders of puberty heavily influence the decision to refer.

## ▶ NORMAL PUBERTY

During puberty, a series of complex hormonal changes takes place. The hypothalamus secretes pulses of gonadotropin-releasing hormone (GnRH), which stimulates pituitary gonadotropin production of luteinizing hormone (LH) and follicle-stimulating hormone (FSH). Concomitantly, the previously very sensitive hypothalamic-pituitary-gonadal feedback loop becomes less sensitive to the negative effect of gonadal steroids. As a result, gonadotropin levels rise, stimulating the secretion of greater amounts of sex steroids, either testosterone or estradiol, depending on the gender of the child, leading to the physical changes of puberty. This process is called *gonadarche*. The hypothalamic-pituitary-gonadal axis is active during fetal life and infancy until it enters an inactive state during the prepubertal years. Genetic factors determine 50% to 80% of the variation in pubertal timing.[1] Environmental influences also play a role, particularly nutritional status. It has also been suggested that environmental chemicals capable of disrupting endocrine activity may affect pubertal timing. Leptin, which is secreted by adipocytes and regulates appetite and metabolism through the hypothalamus, is thought to play a permissive role in regulating the timing of puberty.[2] Adrenarche is a separate process that refers to an increase in the secretion of adrenal androgens during puberty and is associated with the development of pubic hair, axillary hair, body odor, and acne. The mechanism that triggers the maturation of the adrenal cortex at puberty remains poorly understood.

In most girls, puberty begins between 8 and 13 years of age, with breast development (thelarche) usually the first sign. Menarche follows the onset of breast development by approximately 2 years. A growth spurt accompanies the changes, usually peaking before menarche. The range of normal variation, however, is quite wide, and differences have been reported between ethnic groups. A secular trend toward earlier puberty has taken place: the most recent data from the National Health and Nutrition Examination Survey (NHANES) 1992–2002 show a decline in the overall average age at menarche to 12.34 years (12.06 years, 12.52 years, and 12.09 years in non-Hispanic black girls, non-Hispanic white girls, and Mexican American girls, respectively).[3] Although an association exists between earlier sexual maturation in girls and increasing levels of adiposity, it remains unclear from existing data whether this relationship is causal. The average age at menarche declined by 2.3 months between NHANES III (1988–1994) and NHANES 1999–2002. Significantly, NHANES 1999–2002 had more girls with body mass index greater than the 85th or 95th percentile and had a different racial and ethnic composition.[3] Although the overall age at menarche decreased, the changes within racial and ethnic groups was much smaller, indicating that the overall decrease in age at menarche may be because of changes in the population distribution of race and ethnicity and relative weight.

The mean ages for onset of breast development according to NHANES III data were 10.25, 11.05, and 10.70 years in non-Hispanic black girls, non-Hispanic white girls, and Mexican American girls, respectively. Similarly, the mean ages for onset of sexual hair in girls were 10.25, 10.96, and 11.17 years.[4] A recent multicenter study suggests that there continues to be a modest decrease in mean age of breast development, especially in black and Hispanic girls.

In most boys, puberty begins between 9 and 14 years of age. Testicular enlargement is usually the first sign of puberty. NHANES III data found the mean ages of genital development in boys to be 10.79, 11.08, and 11.09 years for non-Hispanic black boys, non-Hispanic white boys, and Mexican American boys, respectively. Similarly, the mean ages for onset of sexual hair were 11.48, 11.81, and 12.20 years.[5] Peak height velocity for boys is typically 2 years later than it is for girls and usually occurs during mid to late puberty (see Table 62-1 for summary of pubertal milestones by age).

The time of puberty is one of profound change, both physical and psychological. Problems of sexual identity, body image, adolescent independence, and peer acceptance are frequent. Because the ranges of age of normal puberty are wide, children of similar chronologic age may have markedly different physical maturity. When pubertal development is precocious or delayed, many of these problems are compounded.

**Table 62-1**
**Onset of Pubertal Milestones (Years)[a,b]**

| | NON-HISPANIC WHITES | NON-HISPANIC BLACKS | MEXICAN AMERICANS |
|---|---|---|---|
| **GIRLS** | | | |
| Thelarche | 11.05 (9.7)[c] | 10.25 (8.8)[c] | 10.7 (9.3)[c] |
| Sexual hair development | 10.96 | 10.25 | 11.17 |
| Menarche | 12.52 | 12.06 | 12.09 |
| **BOYS** | | | |
| Testicular enlargement | 11.08 | 10.79 | 11.09 |
| Sexual hair development | 11.81 | 11.48 | 12.20 |

[a]Note: All ages are expressed as means.
[b]From National Health and Nutrition Examination Survey III (1988–1994) and National Health and Nutrition Examination Survey (1999–2002).
[c]Biro FM, Greenspan LC, Galvez MP, et al. Onset of breast development in a longitudinal cohort. *Pediatrics.* 2013;132:1019–1027

## ▶ GYNECOMASTIA

Pubertal gynecomastia occurs in approximately 40% of healthy boys and usually resolves within 2 years. Clinical presentation may include breast tenderness and asymmetry. The mean age of occurrence is between 14 and 15.5 years and usually occurs after Tanner stage 3. Pubertal gynecomastia is thought to result from an increase in the ratio of estrogen to androgen. Treatment in most cases is reassurance; however, gynecomastia that does not resolve after 2 years or that develops rapidly may require a referral. Initial screening blood work includes levels of testosterone, estradiol, LH, FSH, prolactin, and a β-human chorionic gonadotropin as well as liver function tests. Medical therapy with clomiphene (antiestrogen), tamoxifen (estrogen antagonist), testolactone (peripheral aromatase inhibitor), and danazol (synthetic derivative of testosterone) has been reported to be successful; however, no randomized controlled trials have been conducted. Surgical intervention remains the mainstay of treatment. Whereas most pubertal gynecomastia is benign, pathologic causes include Klinefelter syndrome, partial androgen insensitivity syndrome, hyperprolactinemia, liver disorders, adrenal carcinoma, biosynthetic defects in testosterone production, androgen receptor defects, increased activity of peripheral aromatase, and certain drugs. Drugs that have an estrogen-like effect (diethylstilbestrol, oral contraceptive pills, digitalis, estrogen-containing cosmetics), that increase estrogen formation (gonadotropins, clomiphene), or that inhibit testosterone action (ketoconazole, spironolactone, cimetidine, isoniazid, methyldopa, captopril, tricyclic antidepressants, diazepam, marijuana, phenothiazines) have been associated with gynecomastia.

## ▶ DELAYED PUBERTY

Few matters are of greater concern to the adolescent than remaining short in stature or sexually underdeveloped. Delayed development demands the immediate attention of the physician.

Puberty is considered delayed in girls who have no breast development by 13 years of age or in boys who have no testicular enlargement by 14 years of age. In girls, a delay of longer than 4 to 5 years from onset of puberty to menarche is also cause for concern. Similarly, maturation arrest in boys warrants evaluation.

Constitutional delay, a slow maturation with appropriate hormonal levels and delayed bone age, accounts for most cases of delayed pubertal development. This problem is identified more frequently in boys than in girls, perhaps because of general societal and peer group reaction to short and sexually underdeveloped boys. The delay is frequently familial. In many instances, early signs of puberty are found on thorough examination, which permits the physician to reassure the child and the parents. Affected children should be followed closely. The presence of chronic systemic diseases that can lead to delayed puberty may be difficult to differentiate from constitutional delay as a cause for the delay.

The remainder of the differential diagnosis of delayed development relates to failure at either the hypothalamic-pituitary level, shown by low serum gonadotropins (hypogonadotropic hypogonadism), or the gonadal level, shown by elevated gonadotropins (hypergonadotropic hypogonadism). Either of these conditions may result from genetic disorders or acquired illnesses (see Box 62-1). The workup of the patient is directed toward identifying the specific cause. Common initial screening tests are shown in Box 62-2 and include a

BOX 62-1

## *Causes of Delayed Puberty*

1. Constitutional delay
2. Deficiency of gonadotropin-releasing hormone secretion by the hypothalamus
   a. Genetic and molecular causes
      i. Isolated deficiency
      ii. Kallmann syndrome
      iii. Laurence-Moon-Bardet-Biedl syndrome
      iv. Prader-Willi syndrome
   b. Acquired causes
      i. Infection
      ii. Neoplasm
      iii. Infiltrative disease
      iv. Trauma
3. Deficiency of gonadotropin secretion by the pituitary
   a. Genetic
      i. Panhypopituitarism (including transcription factor mutations in *PROP1, HESX1*, and *LHX3*)
      ii. Isolated deficiency
      iii. Fertile eunuch (normal follicle-stimulating hormone, low luteinizing hormone)
      iv. Leptin or leptin-receptor deficiency
   b. Acquired
      i. Infection
      ii. Tumor
      iii. Excess prolactin secretion, adenoma
      iv. Trauma
4. Gonadal disorders
   a. Genetic and molecular
      i. Turner syndrome (45,X or structural X abnormalities or mosaicism)
      ii. Klinefelter syndrome (47,XXY)
      iii. Noonan syndrome
      iv. Syndromes of complete androgen insensitivity (no sexual hair)
      v. del Castillo syndrome (Sertoli cells only)
      vi. Pure gonadal dysgenesis
      vii. Myotonic dystrophy
      viii. Receptor mutations
   b. Acquired
      i. Infections
         (1) Gonorrhea (male)
         (2) Virus (mumps, coxsackie)
         (3) Tuberculosis (male)
      ii. After radiation or chemotherapy
      iii. Mechanical causes
         (1) Torsion
         (2) Surgery
         (3) Congenital anorchia (vanishing testes syndrome)
         (4) Autoimmune
5. Adrenal and gonadal steroid enzyme deficiencies
6. Excessive exercise, malnutrition
7. Chronic systemic diseases
   a. Congenital heart disease
   b. Chronic pulmonary disease
   c. Inflammatory bowel disease, celiac disease
   d. Chronic renal failure and renal tubular acidosis
   e. Hypothyroidism
   f. Poorly controlled diabetes mellitus
   g. Sickle cell anemia, thalassemia
   h. Collagen-vascular disease
   i. Anorexia nervosa
   j. HIV infection

thorough history, physical examination, and assessment of growth velocity. A bone age assessment is often helpful. For delayed development to be the result of an undiagnosed systemic illness is relatively uncommon, but if the history or physical examination suggests a systemic illness, then specific screening may include a complete blood count, electrolytes, renal and liver function tests, erythrocyte sedimentation rate and C-reactive protein, inflammatory bowel disease panel, and celiac disease panel. A screen for endocrinopathies should include thyroid-stimulating hormone and thyroid hormone levels, gonadotropins (LH, FSH), testosterone, estradiol, and insulin-like growth factor I. Other tests that a specialist may order include insulin-like growth factor–binding protein 3, prolactin, karyotype, brain

BOX 62-2

## Evaluation for Delayed Puberty

**INITIAL SCREENING TESTS (AS INDICATED)**

- Thorough history, physical examination, and calculation of growth velocity
- Bone age
- Luteinizing hormone, follicle-stimulating hormone
- Testosterone or estrogen, depending on gender
- Thyroid-stimulating hormone, thyroid hormone

*If systemic disease is thought to exist*

- Complete blood count
- Erythrocyte sedimentation rate, C-reactive protein
- Comprehensive panel (electrolytes; renal and liver function tests)
- Insulin-like growth factor I, insulin-like growth factor–binding protein 3
- Urinalysis
- Celiac disease panel (antiendomysial immunoglobulin A [IgA] antibody or tissue transglutaminase IgA and total IgA levels)
- Inflammatory bowel disease panel
- Prolactin

**OTHER TESTS (IF INDICATED)**

- Karyotype
- Brain magnetic resonance imaging
- Pelvic ultrasound
- Gonadotropin-releasing hormone (GnRH) or GnRH analog stimulation test

magnetic resonance imaging (MRI), pelvic ultrasound, and GnRH testing assessing for signs of central puberty.

Treatment should be directed toward the cause of the delayed development. If sex steroid secretion is deficient as a result of either gonadal failure or gonadotropin deficiency, then treatment focuses on replacing the appropriate sex steroid. In constitutional delay, waiting may be the best course. In boys, however, a short course of low-dose injectable testosterone (eg, 50–100 mg monthly for 4 doses) may be indicated if the delayed development is affecting the boy's psychological well-being. In girls, cosmetic treatment, such as the use of a padded bra, is helpful. Estrogen therapy is necessary only occasionally. In patients who have GnRH or gonadotropin deficiency, fertility may be induced with GnRH or gonadotropin therapy. In any case, strong psychological support must be provided to the adolescent and sometimes to the family. If the problem is difficult diagnostically, or if hormonal therapy is desired, then referral should be made to a pediatric endocrinologist.

## ▶ PRECOCIOUS PUBERTY

Classically, precocious puberty is the appearance of secondary sexual characteristics before 8 years of age in girls and 9 years in boys. But a substantial number of girls, 27.2% of black girls and 6.7% of white girls, have breast or sexual hair development by 7 years of age.[6] As a result of these data, the Drug and Therapeutics and Executive Committees of the Pediatric Endocrine Society published recommendations proposing that the age cutoff for precocious puberty should be decreased to 7 years in white girls and 6 years in black girls unless the tempo of puberty is abnormal, the bone age is advanced more than 2 years, the predicted height is less than 150 cm (59 inches), focal neurologic deficits are present, headaches are present, or the family's or the child's emotional state is affected adversely.[7] These recommendations are controversial, and although extensive evaluation in 6- to 8-year-old girls is usually not revealing of pathologic abnormality, each child must be considered individually.

Early stimulation of the hypothalamic-pituitary axis, with resultant gonadotropin secretion and sex steroid secretion, is termed *central precocious puberty*. Sex steroid secretion that is independent of pituitary gonadotropin secretion may be termed *peripheral* or *pseudoprecocious puberty*. Box 62-3 lists the causes of these 2 conditions. Precocity may be isosexual (appropriate for phenotype) or heterosexual (appropriate for opposite gender phenotype) and is significantly more common in girls than it is in boys. Box 62-4 lists the causes of heterosexual precocious puberty. In girls, idiopathic precocious puberty is the single most common diagnosis and accounts for 85% of central precocious puberty, whereas 60% of precocious puberty in boys has a pathologic cause.[1] Girls adopted from developing countries may be at particular risk for precocious puberty.[8] Internationally adopted girls have shown a trend toward early and rapidly progressing puberty that may be related to the increased metabolic activity exhibited if catch-up growth occurs after adoption.[9] Precocious puberty can significantly reduce adult height and can, in some cases, have an adverse effect on a child's and a family's emotional state.

## ▶ VARIATIONS OF PUBERTY

Two entities not requiring treatment are isolated premature breast development (thelarche) and isolated premature development of sexual hair (adrenarche). Premature thelarche occurs in girls between 6 months and 3 years of age. Breast development is usually moderate, often regresses, and is seen without other signs of precocious puberty. Specifically, estrogen or gonadotropin levels do not increase significantly, and statural and skeletal maturation accelerate only mildly, if at all. Premature thelarche does not progress to complete precocious puberty. Premature adrenarche usually occurs between 5 and 7 to 8 years of age.

**BOX 62-3**

### *Causes of Isosexual Precocious Puberty*

1. Central (with pituitary gonadotropin secretion)
   a. Idiopathic
   b. Central nervous system abnormalities
      i. Congenital anomalies (hydrocephalus)
      ii. Tumors (hypothalamic, pineal, other)
      iii. Hamartoma
      iv. Postinflammatory condition
      v. Trauma
      vi. Syndromes
         (1) Neurofibromatosis
         (2) Tuberous sclerosis
   c. Hypothyroidism (severe)
2. Peripheral
   a. Exogenous sex steroids
   b. Gonadal tumors or cysts
   c. Adrenal hyperplasia or tumor
   d. Ectopic gonadotropin–secreting tumors (chorioepithelioma, hepatoblastoma, teratoma)
   e. Familial Leydig cell hyperplasia, receptor mutation
   f. McCune-Albright syndrome, G-protein mutation

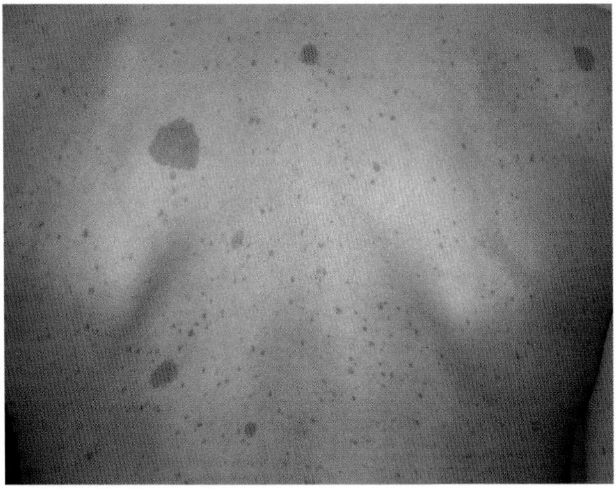

**Figure 63-1**
Café au lait macules in a patient who has neurofibromatosis type 1.

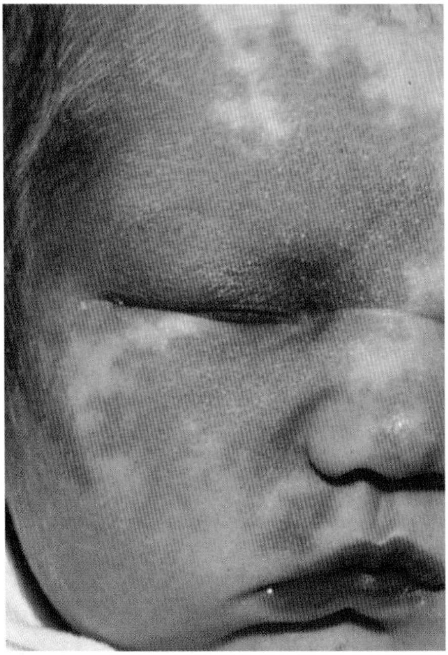

**Figure 63-2**
A port-wine stain is an example of an erythematous patch.

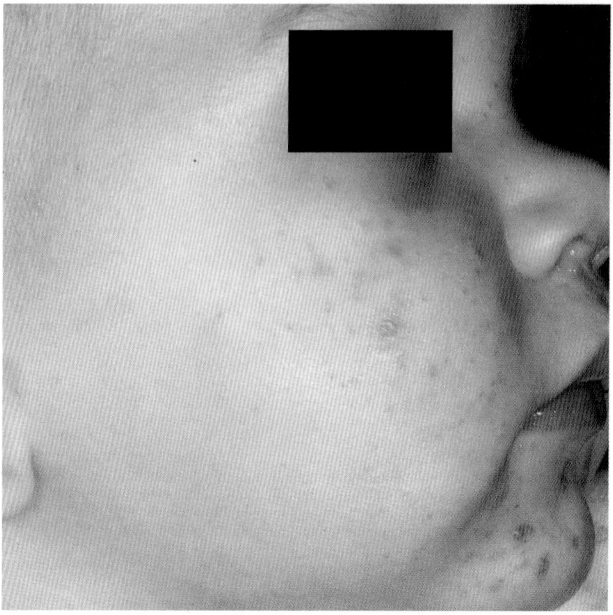

**Figure 63-3**
Neonatal acne is composed of erythematous papules and papulopustules.

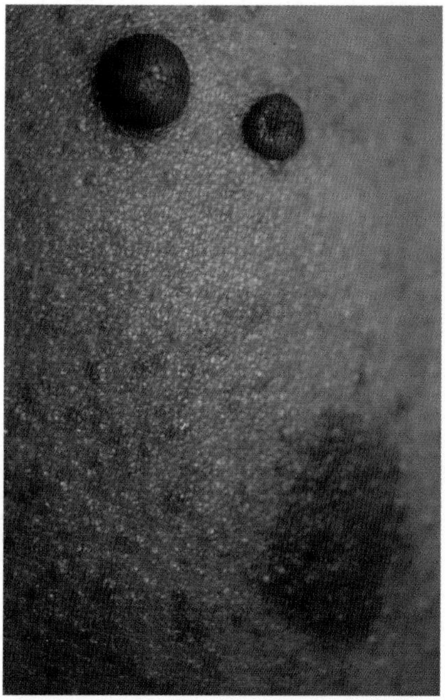

**Figure 63-4**
Nodules representing neurofibromas in a patient who has neurofibromatosis type 1.

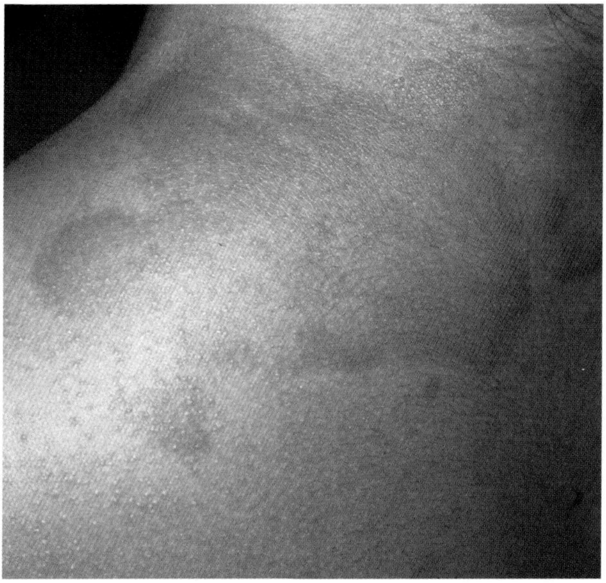

**Figure 63-5**
Pink wheals in a patient who has urticaria.

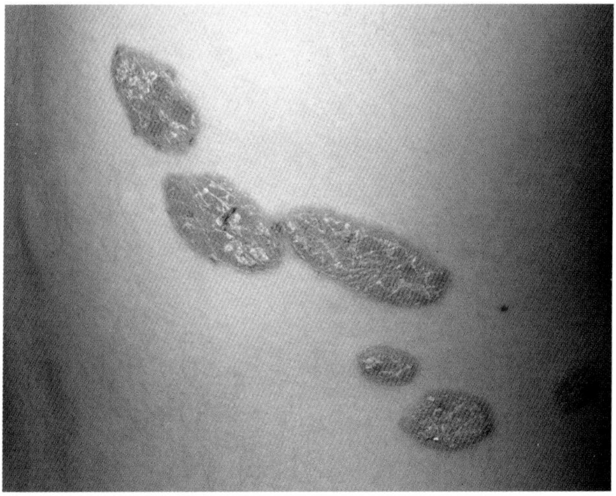

**Figure 63-6**
Scaling plaques, plateau-like lesions, are observed in psoriasis.

that represent sacs containing fluid or semisolid material) (Figure 63-7, Figure 63-8, and Figure 63-9). A depressed lesion may be an *erosion* (a superficial loss of epidermis with a moist base) or an *ulcer* (a deeper lesion extending into or below the dermis) (Figure 63-10).

## Distribution

Given that certain disorders have unique patterns of distribution, noting the parts of the body involved may provide an important clue to diagnosis. For example, seborrheic dermatitis

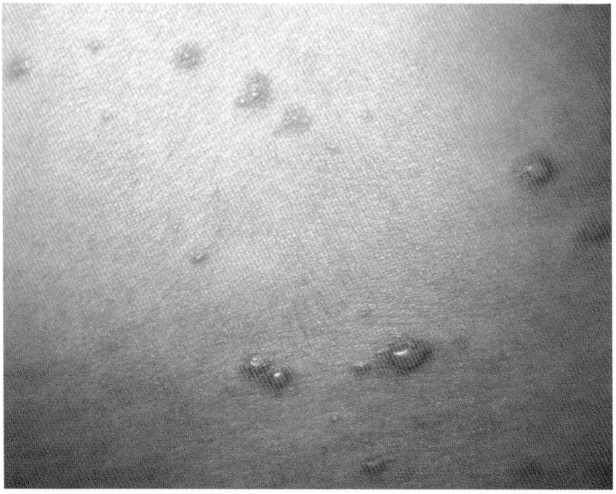

**Figure 63-7**
Vesicles, as seen here in varicella, are filled with clear or serous fluid.

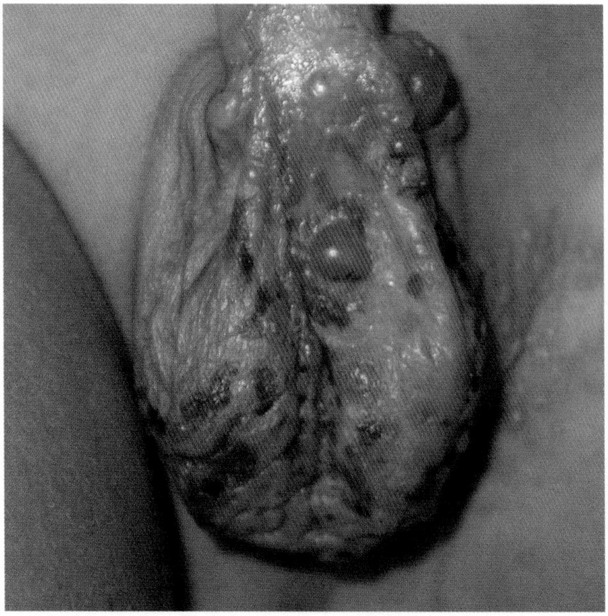

**Figure 63-8**
Bullae, filled with clear fluid, are observed in chronic bullous disease of childhood.

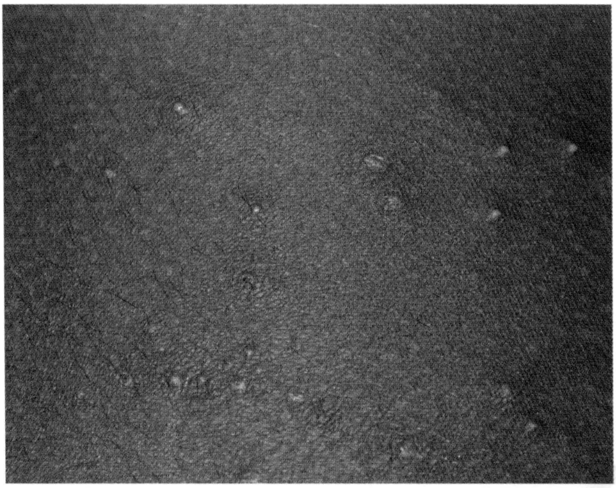

**Figure 63-9**
Pustules are filled with purulent material. This patient has folliculitis.

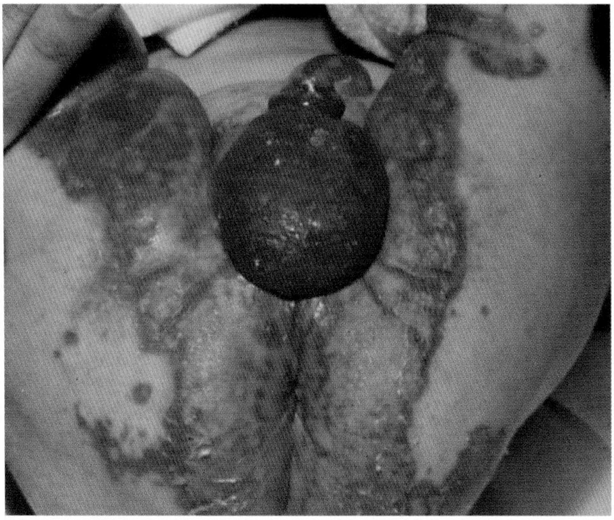

**Figure 63-10**
Erosions, as seen in this infant who has acrodermatitis enteropathica, represent a superficial loss of epidermis.

commonly involves not only the scalp but also the eyebrows and nasolabial folds. Psoriasis also affects the scalp, but lesions are often seen in areas that are traumatized, such as the elbows and knees. Acne is limited to the face, back, and chest, sites of the highest concentrations of pilosebaceous follicles.

## *Arrangement*

Lesions may appear in lines (eg, vesicles in contact dermatitis from poison ivy), be grouped or clustered (eg, vesicles in herpes simplex virus infection), follow a dermatome (eg, vesicles in herpes zoster), or form an annulus or ring (eg, papules in granuloma annulare or a patch in erythema migrans) (Figure 63-11, Figure 63-12, Figure 63-13, and Figure 63-14).

## Color

Although the color of a lesion may be obvious, descriptive terms that can be helpful include *skin colored*, *erythematous* (pink or red), *hyperpigmented* (tan, brown, or black), *hypopigmented* (the amount of pigment is decreased but not entirely absent), *depigmented* (all pigment is absent, as occurs in vitiligo), or *violaceous*. When erythematous lesions are observed, the examiner should note whether they blanch. The red color in skin depends on hemoglobin within red blood cells. If the red cells are within vessels (as occurs in urticaria, for example), compression of the skin forces the cells into deeper vessels, and blanching occurs. However, if the cells are outside vessels, as occurs in forms of vasculitis, blanching will not occur; nonblanching lesions are termed *petechiae*, *purpura*, and *ecchymoses*.

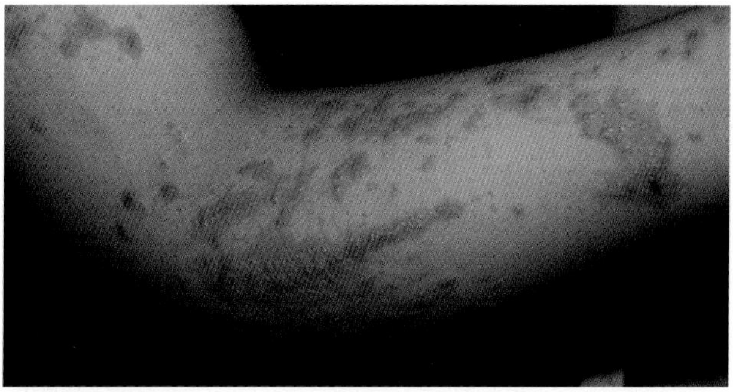

**Figure 63-11**
A linear arrangement of papules or vesicle often occurs in contact dermatitis caused by poison ivy.

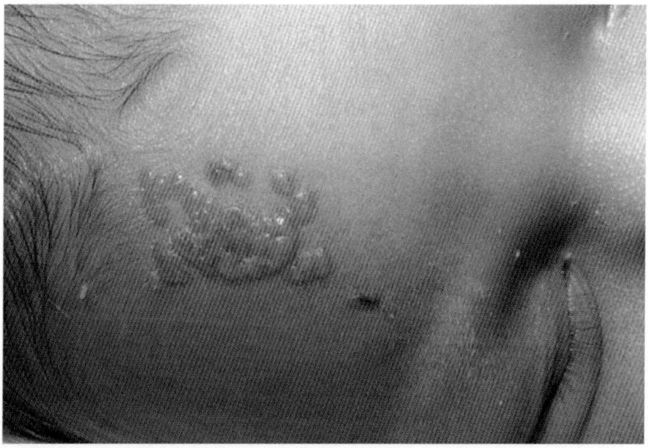

**Figure 63-12**
Grouped vesicles are characteristic of herpes simplex virus infection on the skin.

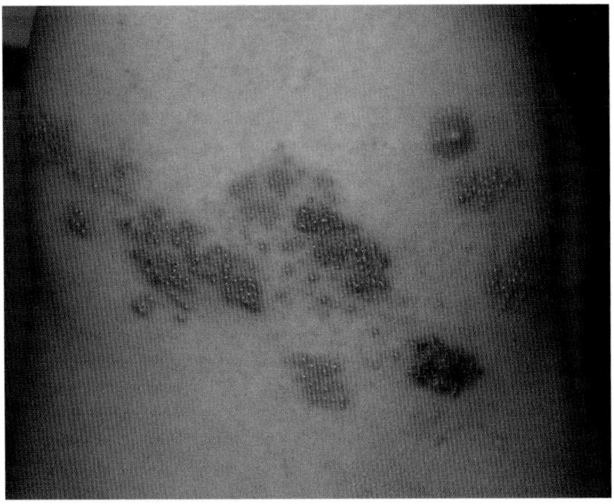

**Figure 63-13**
Herpes zoster is characterized by grouped vesicles on erythematous bases distributed along a dermatome.

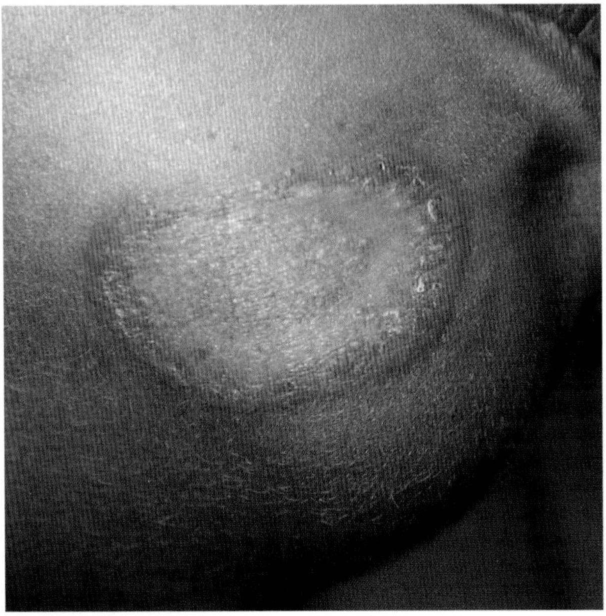

**Figure 63-14**
An annulus (ie, ring-shaped lesion) is typical of tinea corporis.

## Secondary Changes

Secondary changes are alterations in the skin that may accompany primary lesions. These changes, too, can be valuable in differential diagnosis. *Crusting* represents dried fluid; it is commonly seen after the rupture of vesicles or bullae, as occurs with the honey-colored crust of impetigo. In contrast, *scaling* represents epidermal fragments that are characteristic of several disorders, among which are fungal infections (eg, tinea corporis) and psoriasis. *Atrophy* is an area of surface depression from absence of the dermis or subcutaneous fat. Atrophic skin often appears thin and wrinkled. *Lichenification* is a thickening of the skin that results from chronic rubbing or scratching (as occurs in atopic dermatitis, for example); as a result, skin markings (ie, creases) appear more prominent.

## ▶ DIAGNOSIS

Once the primary lesions are identified, along with their distribution, arrangement, color, and secondary changes, these observations should be formulated into 1 or 2 sentences. For example, "Located on the extensor surfaces of the extremities are erythematous, scaling papules, and plaques. Scaling of the scalp and pitting of the nails are evident." Such formulations assist in differential diagnosis. Identifying scaling papules and plaques, as in the previous example, places the patient's condition into the category of papulosquamous (elevated and scaling) diseases and eliminates countless other disorders from consideration. In children, the most common papulosquamous disorders are chronic atopic or contact dermatitis, tinea corporis, and pityriasis rosea; less common conditions are psoriasis, secondary syphilis, lichen planus, dermatomyositis, and lupus erythematosus. Given the location of the lesions on extensor surfaces and involvement of the scalp and nails, psoriasis becomes a primary consideration.

Boxes 63-1 and Box 63-2 assist in differential diagnosis based on the morphology of lesions. Notably, however, these tables are not exhaustive; rather, they list the most commonly

**Box 63-1**

### *Differential Diagnosis of Rashes in Neonates*

**ELEVATED LESIONS**

***Papules***

**Common**

- Erythematous
  - Erythema toxicum
  - Miliaria rubra
  - Acne
  - Candidiasis
  - Scabies
- White
  - Milia
- Yellow
  - Sebaceous gland hypertrophy
- Skin colored
  - Epidermal nevus
  - Skin tags

**Uncommon**

- Yellow
  - Juvenile xanthogranuloma
- Yellow/tan
  - Mastocytosis

***Nodules***

**Common**

- Erythematous
  - Hemangioma

**Uncommon**

- Skin colored
  - Condylomata acuminata
  - Dermoid cyst
- Yellow
  - Mastocytosis

***Plaques***

**Common**

- Skin colored or yellow
  - Nevus sebaceus
- Skin colored
  - Epidermal nevus

***Vesicles or bullae***

**Common**

- Erythema toxicum
- Miliaria crystallina

Box 63-1

## *Differential Diagnosis of Rashes in Neonates—cont'd*

- Sucking blisters
- Bullous impetigo
- Herpes simplex virus infection

**Uncommon**

- Incontinentia pigmenti
- Aplasia cutis congenita
- Varicella
- Epidermolysis bullosa
- Epidermolytic icthyosis

***Pustules***

**Common**

- Erythema toxicum
- Transient neonatal pustular melanosis
- Miliaria pustulosa
- Herpes simplex virus infection
- Folliculitis
- Acne
- Candidiasis
- Scabies

**Uncommon**

- Acropustulosis of infancy

### FLAT LESIONS

***Macules***

**Common**

- Hypopigmented
  - Prehemangioma
  - Postinflammatory hypopigmentation
- Hyperpigmented
  - Transient neonatal pustular melanosis
  - Café au lait macule
  - Postinflammatory hyperpigmentation
  - Congenital melanocytic nevus

**Uncommon**

- Hypopigmented
  - Ash leaf macule

***Patches***

**Common**

- Erythematous
  - Salmon patch (nevus simplex)
  - Hemangioma (early)
  - Port-wine stain
  - Atopic dermatitis
  - Seborrheic dermatitis
  - Diaper dermatitis (irritant or seborrheic)
- Hyperpigmented
  - Dermal melanosis
  - Lentigo

**Uncommon**

- Erythematous
  - Acrodermatitis enteropathica
- Hyperpigmented
  - Pigment mosaicism
- Hypopigmented
  - Pigment mosaicism
  - Nevus depigmentosus

### DEPRESSED LESIONS

***Erosions***

**Common**

- Bullous impetigo (after bullae rupture)
- Neonatal herpes simplex virus infection (after vesicles rupture)
- Staphylococcal scalded skin syndrome

**Uncommon**

- Aplasia cutis congenita
- Acrodermatitis enteropathica
- Epidermolysis bullosa
- Epidermolytic icthyosis

Box 63-2

## *Differential Diagnosis of Rashes in Older Infants, Children, and Adolescents*

### ELEVATED LESIONS

#### *Papules Without Scaling*

**Common**

- Erythematous
  - Viral exanthems (Many exanthems have a papular as well as macular component.)
  - Scarlet fever
  - Insect bites
  - Scabies
  - Urticaria
  - Papular urticaria
  - Acne
  - Early lesions of guttate psoriasis
  - Erythema multiforme
- Skin colored
  - Keratosis pilaris
  - Molluscum contagiosum
  - Flat warts
- Hyperpigmented
  - Nevus (intradermal)

**Uncommon**

- Yellow/tan
  - Mastocytosis

#### *Plaques Without Scaling*

**Common**

- Skin colored
  - Nevus sebaceus
  - Epidermal nevus
- Hyperpigmented
  - Congenital melanocytic nevus

#### *Papules or Plaques With Scaling (Papulosquamous Diseases)*

**Common**

- Tinea corporis
- Pityriasis rosea
- Chronic atopic or contact dermatitis
- Psoriasis

**Uncommon**

- Dermatomyositis
- Lupus erythematosus
- Lichen planus

#### *Nodules*

**Common**

- Erythematous
  - Pyogenic granuloma
- Skin colored
  - Wart
  - Callus
  - Corn
  - Epidermal cyst
  - Granuloma annulare

**Uncommon**

- Erythematous
  - Angiofibroma (ie, adenoma sebaceum)
- Skin colored
  - Neurofibroma
- Yellow/tan
  - Mastocytosis

#### *Vesicles or Bullae*

**Common**

- Contact dermatitis
- Bullous impetigo
- Varicella
- Herpes simplex virus infection
- Hand-foot-and-mouth disease
- Erythema multiforme

**Uncommon**

- Polymorphous light eruption
- Linear immunoglobulin A dermatosis

#### *Pustules*

**Common**

- Folliculitis
- Scabies
- Acne
- Periorificial dermatitis

**Uncommon**

- Associated with systemic bacterial infection (eg, disseminated gonococcal infection)

### FLAT LESIONS

#### *Macules*

**Common**

- Erythematous
  - Viral exanthems
  - Drug eruptions

Box 63-2

## *Differential Diagnosis of Rashes in Older Infants, Children, and Adolescents—cont'd*

- Hypopigmented
  - Pityriasis alba (postinflammatory hypopigmentation)
  - Tinea versicolor
  - Vitiligo
  - Halo nevus
- Hyperpigmented
  - Freckles
  - Postinflammatory hyperpigmentation
  - Tinea versicolor
  - Café au lait macules
  - Melanocytic nevus

**Uncommon**
- Hypopigmented
  - Lichen sclerosus et atrophicus
  - Scleroderma
  - Ash leaf macule
  - Piebaldism

***Patches***
**Common**
- Erythematous
  - Salmon patch (nevus simplex)
  - Port-wine stain
  - Atopic dermatitis
- Hyperpigmented
  - Dermal melanosis
  - Becker nevus
  - Lentigo

**Uncommon**
- Erythematous
  - Toxic shock syndrome (diffuse macular ["sunburn-like"] erythema)
- Hyperpigmented
  - Pigment mosaicism
  - Incontinentia pigmenti

**DEPRESSED LESIONS**

***Erosions***
**Common**
- Bullous impetigo (after bullae rupture)
- Herpes simplex virus infection (after vesicles rupture)
- Staphylococcal scalded skin syndrome

**Uncommon**
- Epidermolysis bullosa

**HAIR LOSS**

***Congenital***
- Localized
  - Nevus sebaceus
  - Epidermal nevus
  - Aplasia cutis congenita
- Diffuse
  - Hair shaft abnormalities
  - Hypothyroidism

***Acquired***
- Localized
  - Friction alopecia
  - Tinea capitis
  - Traction alopecia
  - Trichotillomania
  - Alopecia areata
  - Psoriasis
  - Secondary syphilis
  - Scleroderma
- Diffuse
  - Telogen effluvium
  - Chemotherapy
  - Hypothyroidism
  - Acrodermatitis enteropathica

encountered disorders and a few less common ones to consider. Formulating a dermatologic differential diagnosis rests not only on the primary lesion but also on other information, such as the distribution, arrangement, and color of lesions and the presence of any secondary change. When the patient's physical findings do not immediately make the diagnosis clear, a textbook or atlas of dermatology, consultant, or other resource can provide assistance.

## *SUGGESTED READINGS*

Cohen BA. *Pediatric Dermatology.* 4th ed. St. Louis, MO: Elsevier Saunders; 2013

Krowchuk DP, Mancini AM, eds. *Pediatric Dermatology: A Quick Reference Guide.* Elk Grove Village, IL: American Academy of Pediatrics; 2007

Paller AS, Mancini AJ. *Hurwitz Clinical Pediatric Dermatology.* 3rd ed. Philadelphia, PA: Elsevier Saunders; 2006

# Chapter 64

# Recurrent Infections

*David L. Goldman, MD*

Pediatric primary care physicians frequently encounter children who have recurrent infections, most of whom are otherwise healthy. Reassuring the parents of these children that no underlying abnormality exists is particularly important. Much less commonly, recurrent infections are a sign of an underlying, possibly immunologic, disorder. Early identification of these children is critical because prompt intervention can decrease morbidity and mortality.

## NORMAL PATTERN OF INFECTIONS IN CHILDHOOD

Generally, healthy children experience 6 to 8 upper respiratory tract infections per year in the first few years of life.[1] However, up to 15 infections per year can still be within the normal range. The high frequency of infections in the first years of life results from the relative immunologic immaturity of young children and their frequent exposure to respiratory pathogens. Factors such as attendance in child care and exposure to secondhand smoke may increase the number of infections.[2-4]

In the healthy host, these infections are self-limited, occur more frequently in the winter than in other seasons, and are associated with periods of wellness in between illnesses. Growth and development are normal. Considering that the average duration of a viral illness is 7 to 10 days, typically, a toddler may be sick for up to 100 days or almost one-third of the year.

## INFECTIONS ASSOCIATED WITH AN UNDERLYING IMMUNE DISORDER

Occasionally, a pediatrician will encounter a child who has a history of infections that number above the normal range. Certain patterns of infections should alert the physician to the possibility of an underlying immunodeficiency. One such pattern is an increased frequency of common infections. Although an immunocompetent child can experience a single serious bacterial infection such as pneumonia, meningitis, or osteomyelitis, repeated serious bacterial infections should alert the pediatrician to the possibility of an underlying disorder. Immunodeficiency may also cause a common infection to manifest uncommonly, with increased severity, prolonged duration, or failure to respond to appropriate treatment. Varicella, a typically benign infection in healthy, immunocompetent children, can cause overwhelming infections in children who have leukemia, and prolonged illness in children who have acquired immunodeficiency syndrome (AIDS). Immunodeficiency may also be suggested by a common infection exhibiting at an uncommon age. Thrush or candidal diaper dermatitis in children older than 1 year suggests a defect in T-cell immunity. Alternatively, immunodeficiency may produce an infection with an opportunistic pathogen (ie, *Pneumocystis jiroveci*, *Cryptococcus neoformans*). Rarely, immunodeficiency may become apparent as an infection after the administration of a live virus vaccine.

## ▶ NONIMMUNOLOGIC DISORDERS ASSOCIATED WITH ENHANCED SUSCEPTIBILITY TO INFECTIONS

Host defense against microbial pathogens involves anatomic, physiologic, and inflammatory barriers. Defects in any of these systems can lead to recurrent infections. In general, recurrent bacterial infections at the same anatomic site that are not associated with other infections or other signs of an underlying syndrome should suggest the possibility of an anatomic defect that may be either congenital or acquired. This circumstance is true especially of children who have urinary tract infections and otitis media. About 62% of children younger than 1 year have more than 1 episode of otitis media, and 17% have 3 or more episodes.[5] The increased susceptibility of young children to otitis media results from an age-related dysfunction of the eustachian tubes and is rarely associated with underlying immunodeficiency. Anatomic defects leading to recurrent infections may also occur in other organ systems. Recurrent meningitis may occur as the result of an occult cerebral spinal fluid leak. Recurrent pneumonia may result from various nonimmunologic causes such as alteration of the normal barrier as a result of foreign body aspiration, tracheoesophageal fistula, or gastroesophageal reflux. Impaired function of mucociliary transport, as seen in cystic fibrosis and immotile cilia syndromes, also leads to recurrent pneumonia. Besides anatomic defects, recurrent or unusual infections can also occur as a result of alteration in the normal microbial flora associated with antibiotic use (eg, *Clostridium difficile* colitis) and circulatory disorders such as venostasis.

Certain types of infection may be associated with recurrent disease in the absence of recognized immunodeficiency. Recurrent soft tissue and skin infections with *Staphylococcus aureus* and colitis with *C difficile* fit this pattern, in which recurrence is thought to result primarily from bacterial characteristics that lead to persistence despite antimicrobial therapy. Treatment is therefore directed at eliminating underlying infection.

Allergic conditions may be confused with recurrent infections. Allergic rhinitis may be misdiagnosed as recurrent upper respiratory tract infection, and asthma may be misdiagnosed as recurrent pneumonia. When repeated episodes of pneumonia are the sole presentation of recurrent infection, the physician should consider the possibility of reactive airway disease, which can produce recurrent respiratory symptoms in association with pulmonary infiltrates.

## ▶ SECONDARY IMMUNODEFICIENCIES

Abnormalities of the immune system may be categorized as either primary or secondary. Secondary immunodeficiencies, more common than primary, are either acquired or a consequence of a nonimmunologic process, including infection, malignancy, medication (ie, cytotoxic, immunosuppressive), malnutrition, splenic dysfunction, and metabolic disorders (Table 64-1). Improvements in medical care have led to an increase in the number of children with secondary immunodeficiencies, including those with organ transplants, rheumatologic diseases, and malignancies. New therapies have also led to new risk factors for unusual infections. For example, anticytokine therapies such as antitumor necrosis factor-a for rheumatoid diseases and Crohn disease have been associated with an increased susceptibility to tuberculosis and histoplasmosis.[6,7] Similarly, the implantation of foreign materials (ie, heart valves, catheters) is associated with an increased risk for infection. Improved postnatal

**Table 64-1**
**Secondary Immunodeficiencies**

| CAUSE | DISEASE |
|---|---|
| Infection | HIV; congenital rubella |
| Malignancy | Leukemia; lymphoma |
| Metabolic | Uremia; malnutrition; protein-losing enteropathy; diabetes; galactosemia |
| Chromosomal | Down syndrome; Bloom syndrome |
| Medications | Corticosteroids; chemotherapy; antirejection medication |
| Splenic dysfunction | Splenectomy; sickle cell disease; congenital asplenia |

*HIV*, human immunodeficiency virus.

care has led to improved survival of premature neonates, who exhibit a variety of immune deficits that put them at increased risk for infection.

The spleen serves as a filter to remove infectious agents from the circulation and as a site for maturation of the immune response. Splenic dysfunction and its associated immunodeficiency can result from a variety of disorders, including congenital absence, surgical removal, hemoglobinopathies, and infiltrative diseases. Affected patients typically experience increased susceptibility to bacterial pathogens, especially encapsulated organisms.

Human immunodeficiency virus (HIV) infection, which produces a combined deficiency in both humoral and cellular immunity (AIDS) and is an important cause of secondary immunodeficiency, may be acquired congenitally or horizontally. Children infected with HIV can develop symptoms related to a variety of infection types (ie, opportunistic, recurrent, atypical), depending on the immune status of the child. Older children, who acquire HIV infection horizontally, may develop a primary syndrome in association with the HIV infection itself, which is clinically similar to other viral illnesses (ie, influenza, infectious mononucleosis). Recent advances in HIV therapy have helped decrease the morbidity and mortality associated with this disease, making early recognition and prompt intervention essential for optimal management. Other viral infections may impair the immune response in more subtle ways. For example, preceding influenza infection is readily recognized as a risk factor for superinfection with bacterial pneumonia.

Malnutrition, resulting from protein, mineral, or vitamin deficiency, is an extremely important cause of secondary immunodeficiency in many areas of the world and has been linked to increased susceptibility to a variety of infections, including measles, pneumocystis, and tuberculosis.

## ▶ PRIMARY IMMUNODEFICIENCY

Primary immunodeficiencies, far less common than secondary, are caused by intrinsic defects in the immune system that are genetically determined. Excluding selective immunoglobulin A (IgA) deficiency, primary immunodeficiencies occur at an incidence of 1 in 10,000 births.[8,9] Because many of these syndromes are X-linked, boys are affected more commonly than girls. Most children who have primary immunodeficiencies are symptomatic within the first few years of life, with several exceptions, including common variable immunodeficiency and deficiencies of the terminal complement components. Primary immunodeficiencies may involve the innate or adaptive immune system and are classified by the specific component of the immune system that is affected (eg, humoral, cellular, complement, and phagocytic). As our understanding of immunity and genetics has grown, there has been increased recognition of primary immune deficiency states, including defects in the innate (eg, toll-like and dectin receptors) and cellular (eg, helper T cells subtype 17 [Th17]) immune responses. There has also been improved understanding of the basis of immunodeficiency for certain syndromes. For example, defects in the Th17 immune response are now recognized to contribute to the immunodeficiecny associated with hyper-IgE syndrome. Defects in various arms of the immune system are associated with enhanced susceptibility to infections by particular types of pathogens (see later). Hence, the type of infecting pathogen may be useful in guiding the evaluation of a child with a suspected immunodeficiency. Associated clinical findings, which can be nonspecific or syndrome specific, may also suggest a primary immunodeficiency. A child who has serious recurrent infections will often experience growth failure. However, other physical, historical, and laboratory findings associated with primary immunodeficiency syndromes can be found (Table 64-2). The specific timing of infections may also serve as an important clue to the nature of immunodeficiency. For example, antibody deficiency states are not generally recognized within the first few months of life because of the presence of maternal antibody. In contrast, severe combined immunodeficiency, complete DiGeorge syndrome, congenital neutropenia, and leukocyte adhesion defect typically present with infections early in life.

### *Defects in Humoral Immunity*

Defects in humoral immunity, the antibody-mediated arm of the immune system, represent 50% to 70% of symptomatic primary immunodeficiencies. The defects occur at various stages of B-cell development and result in a wide variety of clinical presentations. Syndromes range in severity from a total absence of mature B cells to an isotype deficiency to a defective antibody response against polysaccharide antigens (Table 64-3). Given the protective effects of maternally acquired antibody, even the most severely affected children (eg, those who have a total absence of antibody production) do not become symptomatic until after

**Table 64-2**
**Signs Associated With Primary Immunodeficiencies**

| SIGN | ASSOCIATED SYNDROME |
|---|---|
| Intractable diarrhea and malabsorption | SCID; XLA; CVID |
| Rheumatologic conditions | CVID; IgA deficiency; XLA |
| Hepatosplenomegaly, lymphadenopathy | Hyper-IgM syndrome |
| Absence of lymph tissue | XLA |
| Thrombocytopenia | Wiskott-Aldrich syndrome |
| Eczema | Wiskott-Aldrich syndrome; chronic granulomatous disease; Job syndrome |
| Oculocutaneous albinism | Chédiak-Higashi syndrome |

*CVID,* common variable immunodeficiency; *SCID,* severe combined immunodeficiency; *XLA,* X-linked agammaglobulinemia.

**Table 64-3**
**Humoral Immunodeficiencies**

| SYNDROME | CLINICAL FEATURES | ASSOCIATED FEATURES |
|---|---|---|
| X-linked agammaglobulinemia | Susceptibility to encapsulated bacterial pathogens<br>Sinopulmonary and gastrointestinal infections, sepsis, meningitis<br>Enhanced susceptibility to enterovirus and rotavirus<br>Symptomatic polio infection following live polio vaccination | Asymmetrical arthritis; dermatomyositis; malabsorption; absence of tonsils, adenoids, and lymph nodes |
| Transient hypogammaglobulinemia of infancy | Recurrent sinopulmonary infections; generally improves by 3–4 yr | May develop IgA deficiency |
| Hyper-IgM syndrome | X-linked<br>Recurrent bacterial infections including encapsulated pathogens<br>Infections associated with T-cell defects (eg, *Pneumocystis carinii*) also seen | Low levels of IgG, IgA, and IgE<br>Neutropenia, thrombocytopenia; T-cell defects |
| Common variable immunodeficiency | Sinopulmonary infections<br>Bronchiectasis<br>Giardiasis | Most common in second and third decade<br>Noncaseating granulomas; malabsorption; autoimmune disease |
| IgA deficiency | Very common (1 in 400 individuals) but usually asymptomatic<br>Recurrent pulmonary infections leading to bronchiectasis | Systemic lupus erythematosus; rheumatoid arthritis; chronic diarrhea<br>Allergic reactions to gammaglobulin preparations<br>IgG subclass deficiency in some |
| Specific antibody deficiency with normal immunoglobulins | Recurrent bacterial infections of the respiratory tract | |
| IgG subclass deficiency | Normal immunoglobulin levels but with impaired antibody responses to polysaccharide antigens<br>Clinical significance not well delineated | |

the first few months of life. Children who have defects in the humoral immune system are characteristically susceptible to recurrent sinopulmonary infections with encapsulated bacteria, including *Streptococcus pneumonia* and *Haemophilus influenzae*. X-linked agammaglobulinemia (Bruton agammaglobulinemia), one of the first primary immunodeficiencies to be described, is associated with a complete absence of mature B cells. Affected children have poor lymph tissue development, and a physical examination may reveal the absence of lymph nodes and tonsils. Although these children are generally not more susceptible to viral illnesses, they may experience severe or persistent enterovirus and rotavirus infections. Oral vaccination with live attenuated polio (no longer available in the United States) should be avoided because of the risk for vaccine-associated disease. Persistent *Campylobacter* species infections also may occur. Children who have defects in humoral immunity are also predisposed to autoimmune disorders, such as dermatomyositis and asymmetrical arthritis. Chronic lung disease may also occur. Treatment for antibody deficiency disorders depends on the type of disorder. Lifelong replacement therapy with intravenous immunoglobulin (IVIG) is indicated for X-linked agammaglobulinemia.

### Combined Defects in Cellular and Humoral Immunity

Combined defects in cellular immunity and humoral immunity make up the second largest group of primary immunodeficiencies. Isolated defects in cellular immunity, which is mediated primarily by T lymphocytes, with preserved antibody function are very uncommon because T cells play a critical role in B-cell function and development. A deficiency in the production and response to T-cell cytokines such as interferon-g is a rare exception. Most children with defects in T-cell immunity have associated defects in antibody immunity. In addition to bacterial infections, affected children are characteristically more susceptible to fungal, mycobacterial, and viral infections. These children may experience recurrent or persistent candidiasis (or both) in the form of thrush and diaper candidiasis. Common viral infections of childhood (eg, varicella) may cause severe or recurrent disease in affected children. Table 64-4 lists some of the more common combined immunodeficiency syndromes.

Severe combined immunodeficiency (SCID) is the prototypical combined immunodeficiency syndrome and actually represents a collection of diseases. A variety of defects may result in SCID, including those affecting the following systems: cytokine receptors, signaling pathways, enzymes of the nucleotide salvage pathway, and major histocompatibility complex. In the first few months of life, children with SCID typically experience intractable diarrhea, failure to thrive, recurrent candidiasis, and *P jiroveci* pneumonia. Definitive therapy depends on the type of SCID and may involve bone marrow transplantation or enzyme or gene therapy.

**Table 64-4**
**Combined Immunodeficiencies**

| SYNDROME | CLINICAL FEATURES | ASSOCIATED FEATURES |
|---|---|---|
| DiGeorge syndrome | Clinically variable<br>Increased viral and fungal infections | Hypocalcemia; hypoparathyroidism; congenital heart disease; abnormal facies |
| Severe combined immunodeficiency (SCID) | Both B-cell and T-cell deficiencies present<br>Includes a variety of disorders that have multiple modes of inheritance<br>Presents early in life (within first 3 mo of age) with recurrent or severe infections with all types of pathogens | Failure to thrive; diarrhea<br>Most common (50%) form is X-linked<br>Thymic hypoplasia<br>Cartilage-hair hypoplasia with certain forms of SCID<br>At increased risk for graft-versus-host disease with red blood cell transfusions |
| Ataxia telangiectasia | Recurrent sinopulmonary infections | Truncal ataxia; mental retardation; thymic hypoplasia; telangiectasia of skin and conjunctiva; glucose intolerance; increased risk for malignancy |
| Wiskott-Aldrich syndrome | Recurrent sinopulmonary infections | Eczema; thrombocytopenia; increased risk for malignancy |

Wiskott-Aldrich syndrome is an X-linked disorder associated with the triad of thrombocytopenia, eczema, and recurrent infections. This disorder is thought to be related to a deficiency in T-cell activation. Affected infants often experience bleeding in the first few years of life. These children may have low IgM levels but normal IgG levels.

Ataxia-telangiectasia is an autosomal recessive disorder that produces progressive ataxia, conjunctival telangiectasias, decreased IgA levels, and altered T-cell function. Children with ataxia-telangiectasia may have thymic hypoplasia, insulin resistance, or gonadal atrophy and are at increased risk for hematologic malignancies.

### Defects in Phagocytic Immunity

The phagocytic arm of the immune response includes neutrophils and monocytes. Phagocytes form the first line of defense against many pathogens and are considered part of the nonspecific immune response. Defects in phagocytic immunity range from the absence of a particular cell type (ie, congenital neutropenia, cyclical neutropenia) to defects in chemotaxis (leukocyte adhesion disorder) to defects in effector function (chronic granulomatous disease) (Table 64-5). Affected children typically experience recurrent skin infections and abscesses in addition to sinopulmonary infections. Children with defects in phagocytic oxidative burst (ie, chronic granulomatous disease) are particularly susceptible to infections caused by organisms (*Staphylococcus*, *Nocardia*, and *Aspergillus* species) that are catalase positive and thus able to degrade hydrogen peroxide. Other clinical features associated with defects in phagocytic immunity include poor wound healing, delayed umbilical cord separation, gingivitis, and eczema.

### Defects in the Complement System

Complement acts to lyse target cells and, as an opsonin, promotes the phagocytosis of microbial pathogens. Defects in the complement system are the least common among the

**Table 64-5**
**Phagocytic Immunodeficiencies**

| SYNDROME | CLINICAL FEATURES | ASSOCIATED FEATURES |
|---|---|---|
| Chronic granulomatous disease (CGD) | Often X-linked<br>Recurrent infection of skin, lungs, liver, lymph nodes, and bone<br>Infections with catalase-positive organisms (*Staphylococci* spp, *Escherichia coli*, *Aspergillus fumigatus*, and *Candida albicans*) | Eczema; lymphadenopathy; hepatosplenomegaly |
| Chédiak-Higashi syndrome | Autosomal recessive<br>Recurrent pyogenic infections with organisms similar to those seen in CGD | Ocular albinism; lymphoreticular malignancies<br>Neutrophils have abnormally large granules |
| Job syndrome | Recurrent sinopulmonary infections and skin abscesses | Eczema; red hair; coarse facies; high IgE levels |
| Leukocyte adhesion defect | Autosomal recessive<br>Recurrent bacterial infections and necrotic skin lesions | Leukocytosis with absence of neutrophils at infection site<br>Severe gingivitis with early loss of teeth<br>Delayed separation of umbilical cord |

primary immunodeficiencies. Congenital deficiencies in the late or terminal components of the complement system (C5, C6, C7, C8, and C9) are inherited as autosomal recessive traits and result in recurrent neisserial infections. In contrast to many of the primary immunodeficiencies, terminal complement deficiencies tend to manifest in older children and in adolescents, typically with recurrent meningococcal infection (meningitis or meningococcemia) or gonococcal arthritis. Deficiency in the C3 component results in an increased susceptibility to encapsulated bacterial pathogens and may be difficult to distinguish from antibody deficiencies except that it tends to occur at an earlier age, within the first few months of life.

## ▶ EVALUATION OF THE CHILD WITH POSSIBLE PRIMARY IMMUNODEFICIENCY

### *History*

An evaluation for a primary immunodeficiency should be performed after nonimmunologic and secondary immunodeficiency syndromes have been considered. A complete history should be obtained for all children being evaluated for recurrent infections, including a history of risk factors for HIV infection (either personal for adolescents or parental when congenital transmission is a possibility): drug use, prostitution, blood-product transfusion, multiple sexual partners, or history of sexually transmitted infection and homosexual behavior. Particular attention should be paid to documenting the characteristics of previous infections, including the types of pathogens and infections, duration of illnesses, and need for hospitalizations. Because many of the primary immunodeficiencies are hereditary, a detailed family history is important. A complete review of systems should be obtained, with attention paid to known associated features of immunodeficiency syndromes, including failure to thrive. The immunization history is important because failure to make protective antibodies in response to immunizations can be indicative of immunodeficiency.

### *Physical Examination*

A complete physical examination should be performed. Many children who have immunodeficiency appear chronically ill. Growth parameters (height, weight, and head circumference percentiles) should be obtained to determine the presence of failure to thrive. Physical signs that may indicate underlying immunodeficiency include absence of tonsils and the presence of generalized lymphadenopathy and hepatosplenomegaly. Skin lesions (eczema, abscesses, and seborrhea) and mucous membrane involvement (telangiectasia, mucositis) are observed with some immunologic disorders. Signs of recurrent infection (eg, dull, retracted tympanic membranes) and evidence of ongoing infection (eg, thrush) may be present. Specific signs associated with a particular immunodeficiency syndrome, such as oculocutaneous albinism in Chédiak-Higashi syndrome, may be present.

### *Laboratory Evaluation and Referral*

Laboratory evaluation for a child who is thought to have an immunodeficiency should be guided by the type of infections the child is experiencing. Initial screening tests usually include complete blood count and differential, serum immunoglobulin levels (IgG, IgA, and IgM), and lymphocyte count. Most primary immunodeficiency syndromes will be associated with abnormal serum immunoglobulin levels. HIV testing should be strongly considered, as indicated by the history and physical findings. In an area that has a high prevalence of HIV infection, testing should be considered even if no obvious risk factor can be identified. Other tests of humoral immunity include B-cell number, antibody levels to various antigens, and IgG subclass determinations. Tests of cellular immunity include delayed-type hypersensitivity (ie, mumps, *Trichophyton* species infection, tetanus toxoid), T-cell enumeration, and lymphoproliferative responses. Table 64-6 lists the initial screening tests to be considered for each component of the immune system. Antibody and T-cell studies must be analyzed in the context of age-adjusted normal values and may be affected by acute illnesses. Likewise, delayed-type hypersensitivity responses are unreliable in children younger than 1 year. Radiologic studies are used primarily in the diagnosis or management of associated infections, although the absence of a thymic shadow can be indicative of DiGeorge syndrome or SCID. Regardless of the results of initial screening tests, referral to a specialist, either immunologist or infectious diseases expert, should be considered for children who have signs and symptoms suggestive of immunodeficiency (Box 64-1).

### Treatment

Treatment of primary immunodeficiency is condition specific. Patients with humoral and combined immunodeficiencies may benefit from the administration of IVIG as replacement therapy. The initial regimen is 300 to 400 mg/kg every 3 to 4 weeks and should be adjusted based on the patient's response. The trough concentration of antibody should be at least

**Table 64-6**
**Laboratory Examination**

| IMMUNODEFICIENCY | SCREENING TESTS | GENERAL COMMENTS |
|---|---|---|
| Humoral (B cell) | Serum immunoglobulin levels (IgG, IgM, IgA)<br>Antibody titers against protein (diphtheria, tetanus toxoid) and polysaccharide *(Haemophilus, Pneumococcus* spp*)* antigens | Antibody levels must be interpreted with respect to age-appropriate values. High or low levels can be significant. Specific antibody responses must be interpreted in the context of vaccine history. |
| Cellular (T cell) | Lymphocyte count, anergy testing, lymphoproliferative assays | Total lymphocyte count is obtained by multiplying total white blood cell count by the percentage of lymphocytes.<br>Value <1,500 mcL is considered lymphopenia.<br>Anergy testing not reliable for children <1 yr. |
| Phagocytic (macrophage or neutrophil) | Complete blood count<br>IgE level<br>Nitroblue tetrazolium (NBT) test, flow cytometric respiratory burst assay | Abnormal neutrophil structure may be present.<br>IgE level elevated in Job syndrome. |
| Complement | $CH_{50}$ assay | Screening assay for components of classic complement pathway.<br>May not be sensitive for limited deficiencies in individual complement components. |

BOX 64-1

### *Reasons for Referral for Suspected Immunodeficiency*

- Recurrent serious (ie, sepsis, pneumonia, meningitis) bacterial infection
- Serious bacterial infection in the context of failure to thrive
- Infection with an opportunistic pathogen (ie, *Pneumocystis, Cryptococcus* spp infection)
- Vaccine-associated infection
- Unusual age for infection (ie, early zoster, late thrush)
- Unusual severity or chronicity for a given infection
- Family history of immunodeficiency

500 mg/dL.[10] Replacement IVIG is not indicated for all types of humoral deficiency. Furthermore, patients with IgA deficiency may develop anaphylaxis to certain brands of IVIG that contain small amounts of IgA. Other therapies include bone marrow transplantation (SCID, Wiskott-Aldrich, DiGeorge syndrome), enzyme replacement (certain forms of SCID), and cytokine therapy (interleukin-2 deficiency). Recently, interferon-g treatment has been demonstrated to decrease the number of infections in patients with chronic granulomatous disease.[11] The genetic basis for many of the primary immunodeficiencies is now known, and prenatal screening is increasingly available.

Pending a complete immunologic evaluation, children who are thought to have immunodeficiency syndromes should not receive live attenuated vaccines, such as varicella and measles, to avoid the possibility of vaccine-associated infection. Vaccine recommendations for specific immunodeficiencies can be found in the American Academy of Pediatrics *Red Book: Report of the Committee on Infectious Diseases*.[12] Blood transfusion, when needed, should be with cytomegalovirus-negative, irradiated cells to prevent the possibility of cytomegalovirus infection and graft-versus-host disease.

## TOOLS FOR PRACTICE

### Engaging Patient and Family

- *Recurrent Infections* (fact sheet), Riley Hospital for Children at Indiana University Health (iuhealth.org/riley/pediatric-allergy-and-asthma/recurrent-infections)
- *Primary Immunodeficiency Disease* (Web page), American Academy of Allergy, Asthma, and Immunology (www.aaaai.org/conditions-and-treatments/primary-immunodeficiency-disease.aspx)

### Medical Decision Support

- *About Primary Immunodeficiencies* (Web page), The Immune Deficiency Foundation (primaryimmune.org/about-primary-immunodeficiencies)

## REFERENCES

1. Wald ER, Guerra N, Byers C. Upper respiratory tract infections in young children: duration of and frequency of complications. *Pediatrics*. 1991;87:129–133
2. Klein JO. Infectious diseases and day care. *Rev Infect Dis*. 1986;8:521–526
3. Hurwitz ES, Gunn WJ, Pinsky PF, Schonberger LB. Risk of respiratory illness associated with day-care attendance: a nationwide study. *Pediatrics*. 1991;87:62–69

4. Peat JK, Keena V, Harakeh Z, Marks G. Parental smoking and respiratory tract infections in children. *Paediatr Respir Rev.* 2001;2(3):207–213
5. Teele DW, Klein JO, Rosner B. Epidemiology of otitis media during the first seven years of life in children in greater Boston: a prospective, cohort study. *J Infect Dis.* 1989;160:83–94
6. Nunez MO, Ripoll NC, Carneros Martin JA, et al. Reactivation tuberculosis in a patient with anti-TNF-alpha treatment. *Am J Gastroenterol.* 2001;96(5):1665–1666
7. Wood KL, Hage CA, Knox KS, et al. Histoplasmosis after treatment with anti-tumor necrosis factor-alpha therapy. *Am J Respir Crit Care Med.* 2003;167:1279–1282
8. Affentranger P, Morell A, Spath P, Seger R. Registry of primary immunodeficiencies in Switzerland. *Immunodeficiency.* 1993;4(1–4):193–195
9. Stray-Pedersen A, Abrahamsen TG, Frøland SS. Primary immunodeficiency diseases in Norway. *J Clin Immunol.* 2000;20(6):477–485
10. American Academy of Pediatrics. Passive immunization. In: Pickering LK, Baker CJ, Kimberlin DW, Long SS, eds. *Red Book: 2012 Report of the Committee on Infectious Diseases.* 29th ed. Elk Grove Village, IL: American Academy of Pediatrics; 2012:56–57
11. Marciano BE, Wesley R, De Carlo ES, et al. Long-term interferon-gamma therapy for patients with chronic granulomatous disease. *Clin Infect Dis.* 2004;39:692–699
12. American Academy of Pediatrics. Immunization in special clinical circumstances. In: Pickering LK, Baker CJ, Kimberlin DW, Long SS, eds. *Red Book: 2012 Report of the Committee on Infectious Diseases.* 29th ed. Elk Grove Village, IL: American Academy of Pediatrics; 2012:69–109

# Chapter 65

# Red Eye/Pink Eye

*Judith B. Lavrich, MD; Sebastian Heersink, MD*

Red eye in children can be difficult to diagnose and manage because, as a physical finding, it has many possible causes, variable presentations, and severity ranging from asymptomatic to vision threatening. The most common causes of a red eye in a child are infectious (bacterial, viral, or parasitic); inflammatory; allergic; traumatic, from a foreign body and corneal abrasion; or related to an underlying systemic cause. In general, red eye associated with pain, photophobia, or blurry vision indicates a serious ocular disease and should be considered for referral.[1,2]

The first step in determining the cause of a child's red eye is identifying the location of the redness and swelling: is it isolated to the eyelid itself, or does it involve the conjunctiva, either diffusely, or focally around the cornea (ciliary flush, Figure 65-1)? The location provides clues to the underlying problem, which helps direct the history taking and organize the differential diagnosis. (See Table 65-1.)

## ▶ HISTORY

A detailed history should be obtained, with specific attention paid to the onset and progression of the redness, prior episodes of redness, possible trauma or injury, prior ocular surgery, use of contact lenses, and personal contact with similarly affected individuals. In young children, the history of trauma or chemical injury can be difficult to obtain, so this possibility

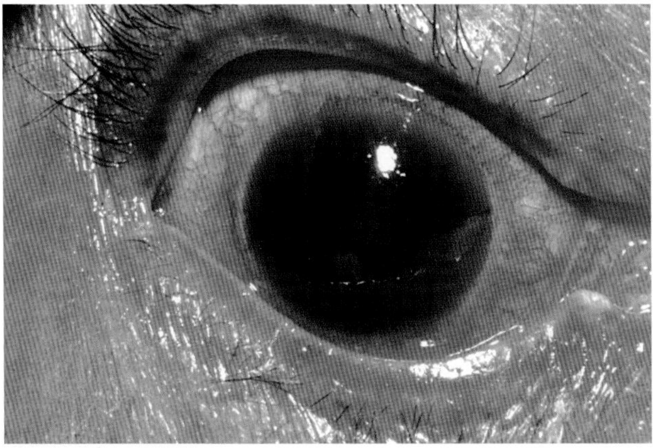

**Figure 65-1**
Ciliary flush.

**Table 65-1**
**Causes of Red Eye by Location of Redness**

| | |
|---|---|
| Eyelid | Preseptal cellulitis |
| | Orbital cellulitis |
| | Eyelid tumors |
| | Allergic dermatitis |
| | Chalazia and hordeola |
| | Blepharitis |
| | Trauma |
| Conjunctiva | Viral |
| | Bacterial |
| | Chemical |
| | Allergic |
| | Vernal |
| | Phlyctenulosis |
| | Subconjunctival hemorrhage |
| | Papilloma |
| Cornea | Abrasion |
| | Corneal infection: bacterial, viral, fungal, or parasitic |
| | Foreign body |
| Intraocular | Iritis, uveitis |
| | Hyphema |
| Focal inflammation over involved area | Scleritis |
| | Episcleritis |
| | Ocular myositis |

needs to be considered on examination. Symptoms including itching, pain, photophobia, visual disturbance, tearing, mucous discharge, nasal discharge, and fevers should be elicited. In cases in which both eyes are affected, the sequence and timing of symptom onset are important to know: did both eyes become red initially, or was one affected before the other?

## ▶ PHYSICAL EXAMINATION

If possible, assessing visual acuity should be the first step of any eye examination. In small children, the ability to fixate on and follow a toy is often all that can be gathered about their vision. Careful examination of ocular structures with a penlight should be next. Starting with the lids, look for redness, crusting, clogged meibomian glands, redness at the lid margin, and thickening of the lid margin. Next, moving inward toward the eye, examine the conjunctiva, including everting the lids and looking for a foreign body (Figure 65-2). To look under the upper lid, place a cotton-tipped swab on the outside of the upper lid 1 cm above the lash line and gently evert the lid over the cotton swab. (This technique is demonstrated at www.nlm.nih.gov/medlineplus/ency/imagepages/19662.htm.) Then, determine whether the

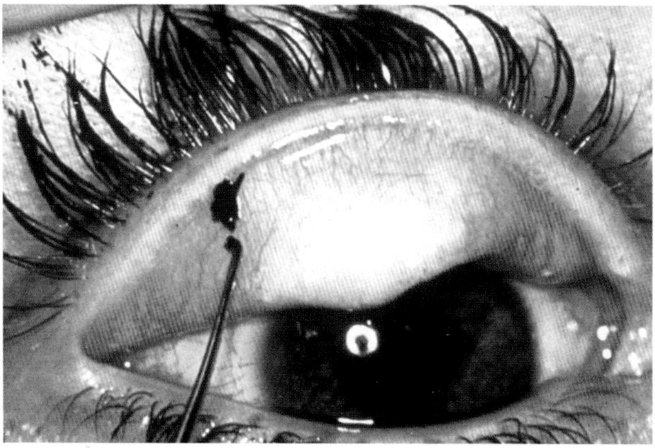

**Figure 65-2**
Foreign body in the conjunctiva.

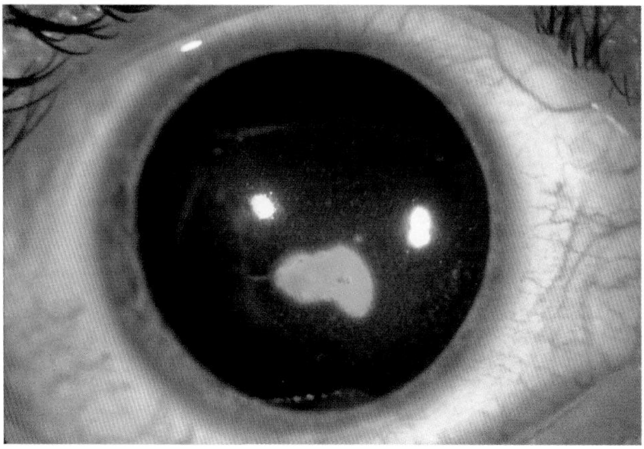

**Figure 65-3**
Corneal abrasion.

conjunctival redness is diffuse or sectoral. Fine follicles in the conjunctiva overlying the lid indicate a viral infection, whereas edema suggests allergic conjunctivitis. The cornea should then be evaluated for opacities, foreign bodies, and disruption of the light reflex. The use of fluorescein and a cobalt blue light can highlight any corneal abrasions (Figure 65-3). Next, examine the pupils: check for size, shape, and reactivity. A mid-dilated pupil would suggest iritis. An irregular pupil may suggest trauma and possible intraocular foreign body. Beyond the eye, attention should be paid to preauricular lymph nodes (viral conjunctivitis), stiff or tender joints (juvenile idiopathic arthritis, or JIA).

## ▶ DIFFERENTIAL DIAGNOSIS AND MANAGEMENT

### *Eyelid Abnormalities*

#### Preseptal and Orbital Cellulitis

Signs of preseptal cellulitis include tenderness, conjunctival swelling, and redness. As the name suggests, preseptal cellulitis (Figure 65-4) occurs anterior to the orbital septum,

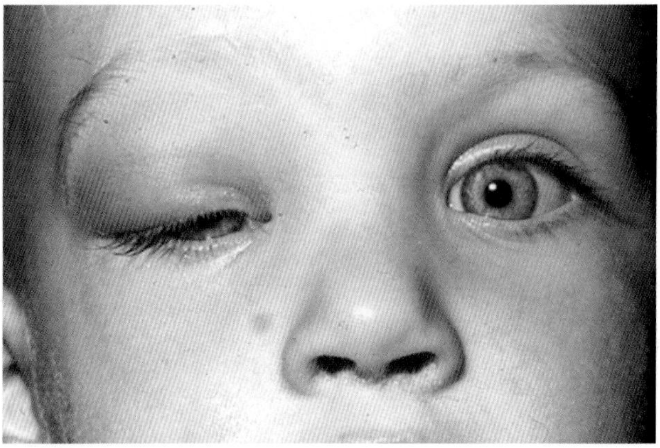

**Figure 65-4**
Preseptal cellulitis.

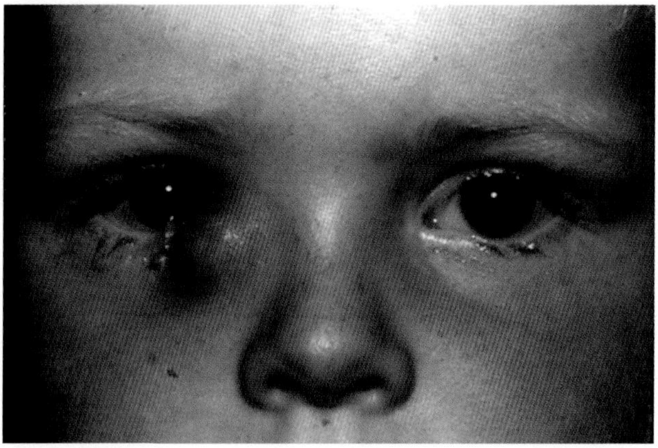

**Figure 65-5**
Dacryocystitis.

and therefore has *no* associated double vision, decreased vision, proptosis (eyeball pushed forward), limited motility, or pain with eye movement. These signs would indicate a more severe condition with orbital involvement. Common causes of preseptal cellulitis in children are trauma (laceration, insect bite, or puncture wound) or adjacent infections (sinusitis, herpetic dermatitis, infected chalazion, or dacryocystitis—an infected tear drainage duct) (Figure 65-5). For patients with mild to moderate preseptal cellulitis, laboratory evaluation is not usually needed. For highly febrile patients or severe preseptal cellulitis, a complete blood cell count (CBC) and blood culture should be considered. A computed tomography (CT) scan with contrast of the orbits and sinuses provides details related to bony structures or radiopaque foreign bodies and should be performed in cases of significant trauma or suspected foreign body, sinus disease, suspected orbital involvement, or abscess formation.

Signs of orbital cellulitis may include tenderness, conjunctival swelling and redness, double vision, decreased vision, proptosis, limited motility (Figure 65-6), pain with eye movement, fever, and in severe cases, pupillary involvement. The most common cause of orbital cellulitis in children is concomitant sinus disease with penetration through the thin

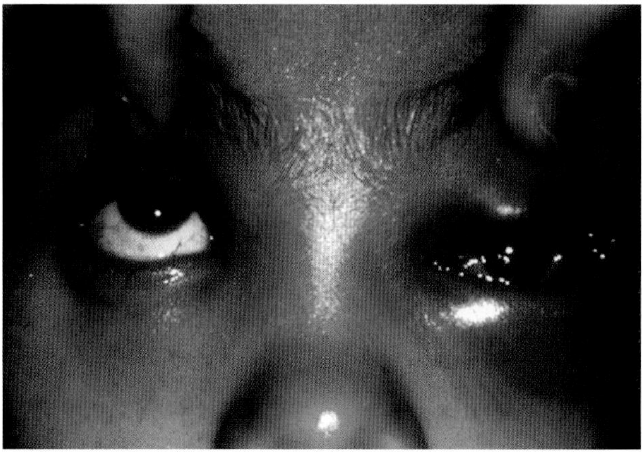

**Figure 65-6**
Orbital cellulitis.

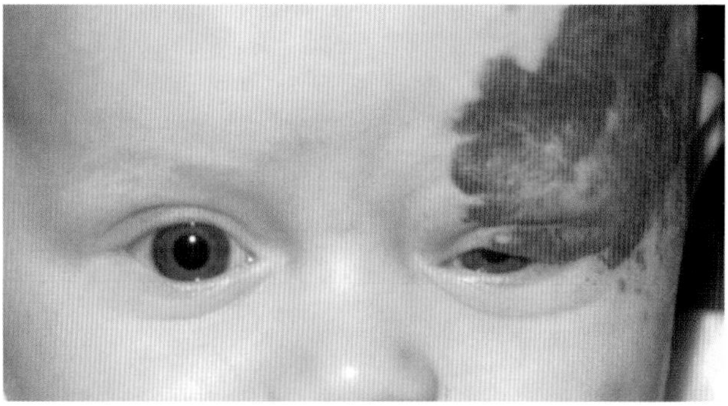

**Figure 65-7**
Capillary hemangioma.

bones of the orbital walls; but it can also result from dental infection, hematogenous spread, or orbital trauma. In cases of suspected orbital cellulitis, vital signs, mental status, neck flexibility, and facial sensation should be evaluated. Laboratory evaluation should include a CBC and blood culture. Computed tomography scanning of the orbits and sinuses with and without contrast should be performed to evaluate for foreign bodies, sinus disease, and abscess formation. Orbital tumors such as neuroblastoma, rhabdomyosarcoma, and lymphangioma can masquerade as orbital cellulitis. For better delineation of soft tissue details, and particularly if the physician also suspects an intracranial complication, magnetic resonance imaging may be needed. Admission for broad-spectrum intravenous antibiotics and possible surgical drainage is mandatory.

## Eyelid Tumors

Capillary hemangiomas (Figure 65-7) and the port wine stain of Sturge-Weber syndrome can cause redness and swelling of the lid. In these conditions, which progress slowly over months, the visual axis can become obstructed leading to amblyopia—affected patients should be referred to an ophthalmologist for evaluation.

## Allergic Reactions

Contact dermatitis (Figure 65-8), insect bites, or bee stings can mimic preseptal cellulitis but can be differentiated by the significant itching, limited pain, and boggy rather than tense edema. Treatment options include oral antihistamines, topical or oral steroids, and cool compresses.

## Hordeola and Chalazia

Hordeola, commonly known as styes, and chalazia are localized inflammatory reactions to blocked oil glands (meibomian glands) in the eyelid margin. These lesions have focal areas of tense, firm, and often painful swelling with visible concretions in the oil glands near the areas of swelling (Figure 65-9). Treatment includes hot compresses with light massage and an antibiotic ointment (erythromycin, bacitracin) applied to the eyelash margin twice daily. If there is no resolution in 4 to 6 weeks, or if there is significant worsening, patients should be referred for evaluation of possible surgical drainage.

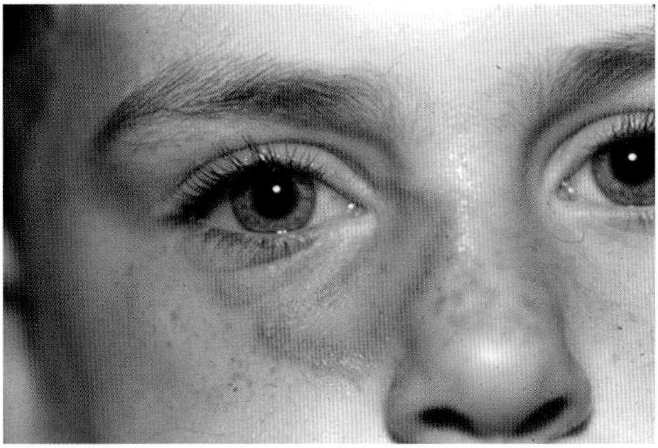

**Figure 65-8**
Contact dermatitis.

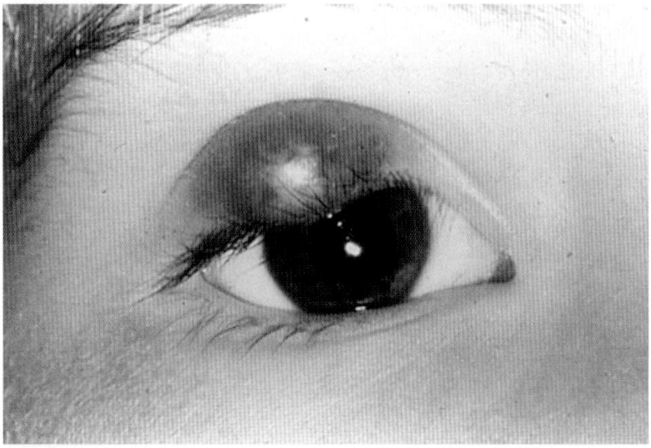

**Figure 65-9**
Chalazion.

## Blepharitis

Blepharitis is a common, chronic inflammation and redness of the eyelid margin with blockage of the meibomian glands and associated crusting of the lashes. It is treated with lid scrubs using nonirritating products such as baby wash or baby shampoo to remove crusting, warm soaks to help drain the meibomian glands, and antibiotic ointment to the lids to reduce the bacterial load on the skin.

## Trauma

Trauma to the eye often leads to edema and ecchymosis of the eyelids, making examination difficult. The lids may be so tense that a lid speculum may be needed to open them, if the physician is comfortable using this instrument. If the eyelids cannot be opened with effort, a retrobulbar hemorrhage should be suspected, and emergent ophthalmologic consult should be obtained. Avoid putting any pressure on the eye until it is confirmed that the globe is intact.

### *Conjunctival Abnormalities*

Conjunctival redness can be either focal or diffuse, and the differential diagnosis includes viral or bacterial infection, chemical exposure, an allergic reaction, subconjunctival hemorrhage, a viral papilloma, or Kawasaki disease. For an overview of distinguishing characteristics among causes of conjunctivitis, see Table 65-2. Rarely, nondraining conjunctivitis can be caused by leptospirosis, tularemia, or toxin-mediated staphylococcal or streptococcal disease.

**Table 65-2**
**Differentiating Types of Conjunctivitis**

| | BACTERIAL | VIRAL | ALLERGIC | PROBABLE REFERRAL |
|---|---|---|---|---|
| **Presentation** | Unilateral or bilateral | Usually unilateral, then spreads to other eye | Usually bilateral; can be unilateral | |
| **Season** | Common in winter | Spring or fall | Spring or fall | |
| **Onset** | Concurrent with otitis media | Concurrent systemic viral infection | Acute or chronic | |
| **Symptoms** | Crusting on eyelashes<br>Gluey or sticky eyelids ± fever | Tearing<br>Eye irritation ± fever | Itching<br>Swelling of lids<br>Conjunctival edema | Light sensitivity<br>Pain<br>Blurred vision |
| **Discharge type** | Purulent, thick, yellow/green | Serous or mucoid | Stringy, whitish, ropey, if any | |
| **Patient type** | Younger children<br>Contact lens wearer | Any age | >2 yr | Red eye for ≥2 wk |
| **Examination findings** | Papules on conjunctiva | Follicles on palpebral conjunctiva<br>Frequent preauricular nodes | Conjunctival edema and injection | |

## Viral Conjunctivitis

The most common cause of conjunctivitis is a viral infection. Viral conjunctivitis is often highly contagious. Adenovirus is the most common viral pathogen. Rarely, herpes simplex virus (HSV) can cause conjunctivitis, but there are often typical HSV satellite lesions on the skin near the eye. Corneal involvement may also occur with HSV and is often accompanied by photophobia and more intense pain. (See Herpetic Keratitis.) Spreading through the copious watery discharge of an infected individual from eye to hand to eye, viral conjunctivitis quite commonly affects entire households or sports teams. In addition to itching, burning, or gritty sensation that typically starts in 1 eye and involves the fellow eye 2 to 5 days later, patients often complain of watery discharge, rhinorrhea, and sore throat. Patients can sometimes recall a recent exposure to a sick contact or someone with a red eye. There is often preauricular lymphadenopathy, and the conjunctiva will often have follicles, or bumps of lymphoid aggregates best seen with fluorescein (Figure 65-10). Severe cases sometimes have pseudomembranes of fibrin that cause scant bleeding when removed with cotton tips, as well as corneal subepithelial infiltrates, aggregates of immune cells. These signs occur 1 to 2 weeks after onset of symptoms and warrant referral to an ophthalmologist. Treatment is supportive, with a focus on minimizing contagion. Patients and parents should be instructed to wash their hands often and not share towels or bed linens. In the absence of systemic signs of illness such as fever, children with conjunctivitis should not be removed from school unless they are unable to participate in activities, the care of their classmates would be compromised by their need for special attention, or their exclusion has been recommended by a physician or department of health. In group care settings, if 2 or more children are infected with conjunctivitis at the same time, it is appropriate to seek the advice of a health care provider or department of health.[3,4]

For nonspecific viral conjunctivitis or adenovirus, chilled preservative-free artificial tears 4 to 8 times a day and cool compresses several times a day are recommended for symptomatic relief. Currently, topical ganciclovir ophthalmic gel is being used off-label to treat adenoviral infections, as recent small case studies have shown its effectiveness. HSV conjunctivitis should be referred to an ophthalmologist for a more complete examination and antiviral therapy because it can be a vision-threatening infection.

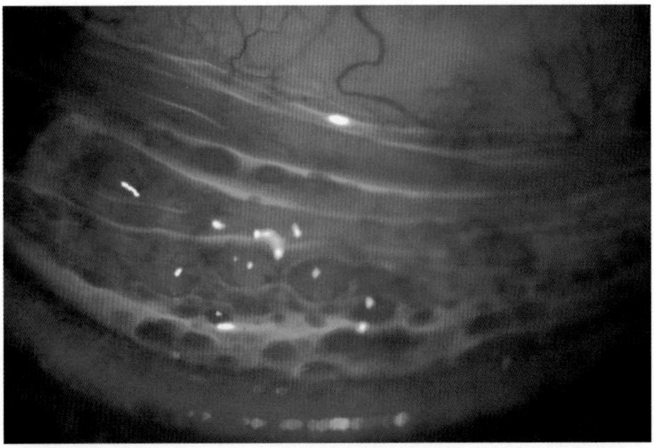

**Figure 65-10**
Viral conjunctivitis.

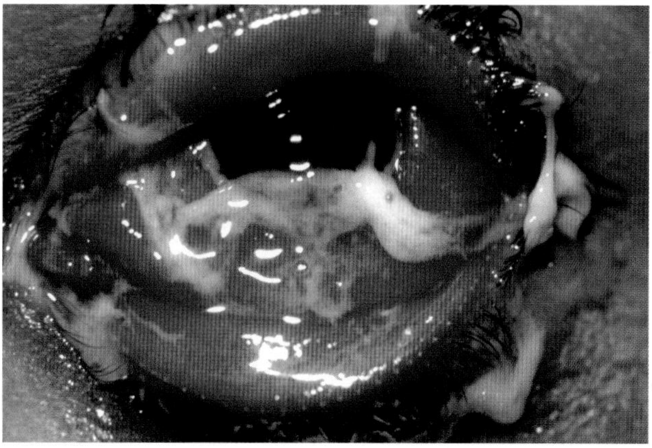

**Figure 65-11**
Bacterial conjunctivitis.

## Bacterial Conjunctivitis

Compared with viral conjunctivitis, bacterial conjunctivitis is less common and often has a purulent rather than a watery discharge (Figure 65-11) and less of a follicular reaction. Cultures are not routinely performed. Common bacteria include *Staphylococcus aureus, Staphylococcus epidermidis*, *Streptococcus pneumoniae*, and *Haemophilus influenzae.* Topical antibiotic treatment is often successful, either with drops (trimethoprim-polymyxin B, moxifloxacin, or gentamicin 4 times a day for 7 to 10 days), or with an ointment (bacitracin-polymyxin B or erythromycin 4 times a day for 5 to 7 days). A fluoroquinolone gel (besifloxacin) is also approved for use, twice daily for 7 days.

In neonates with conjunctivitis, bacterial infection must be ruled out. With a hyperacute onset and copious discharge, gonococcus should be the first consideration because it can perforate a healthy cornea within 24 hours. Gonorrheal infection usually manifests 3 to 4 days after birth. Chlamydial infection can cause pneumonia as well as conjunctivitis and usually occurs within the first month of life. Cultures should be taken with special media. Presumptive treatment pending culture results involves intravenous ceftriaxone for *Neisseria gonorrhoeae* and oral erythromycin for chlamydia. Erythromycin has been associated with infantile hypertrophic pyloric stenosis (IHPS) when administered to infants younger than 6 weeks. Because the risk for IHPS after azithromycin has not been established and at least some evidence suggests it may be lower, some physicians prefer it in place of erythromycin, which the American Academy of Pediatrics continues to recommend. An ophthalmology consultation should be considered.

Of note, nasolacrimal duct obstruction, like bacterial conjunctivitis, can produce mucopurulent drainage, but the conjunctiva typically remains white and noninflamed. Pressure over the nasolacrimal sac, inferior to the medial canthus, will cause reflux of watery mucoid discharge.

In teenagers, bacterial conjunctivitis can represent a sexually transmitted disease, either gonorrhea or chlamydia. Gonorrhea typically produces hyperacute conjunctivitis with copious purulent discharge. Cultures should be taken, and the patient and sexual partners should be treated systemically for gonorrhea, usually with ceftriaxone. Chlamydia usually causes a chronic conjunctivitis with scant discharge and beefy inflamed conjunctiva. It should be suspected when topical antibiotics fail to improve a bacterial conjunctivitis. Treatment of patient and contacts is with oral azithromycin or doxycycline; however, the latter should be avoided in children younger than 8 years because of potential permanent staining of teeth.

## Chemical Conjunctivitis

Exposure to a chemical irritant can produce rapid conjunctival inflammation. For children who have gotten a household chemical into an eye, the most important treatment is immediate and copious irrigation with the nearest source of water. When the child is brought to medical attention, the pH of the conjunctival surface should be checked (basic solutions penetrate deeper and cause more damage than acids), and irrigation should not be discontinued until the pH remains 7.0 for several minutes after an interruption. If there are areas of white clear conjunctiva or corneal clouding, which suggest necrosis, the child should be urgently referred to an ophthalmologist for aggressive treatment. In most cases, however, artificial tears and topical antibiotic eyedrops are sufficient.

## Allergic Conjunctivitis

Allergic conjunctivitis may be acute or chronic, but it is almost always associated with itching. Discharge may be clear, with some mucus, or stringy and white. Conjunctival edema with associated redness may appear as an intensely swollen eye (Figure 65-12). Treatment of allergic conjunctivitis includes cool compresses, topical antihistamines and mast cell stabilizers, oral antihistamines, topical steroids, and rarely oral steroids.

Vernal conjunctivitis is a subset of allergic conjunctivitis that occurs most often in the springtime every year in young boys with a family history of allergies. On examination, there is often a ring of swollen, gelatinous conjunctiva with or without whitish-yellow deposits, and papillae are common on the tarsal conjunctiva (Figure 65-13).

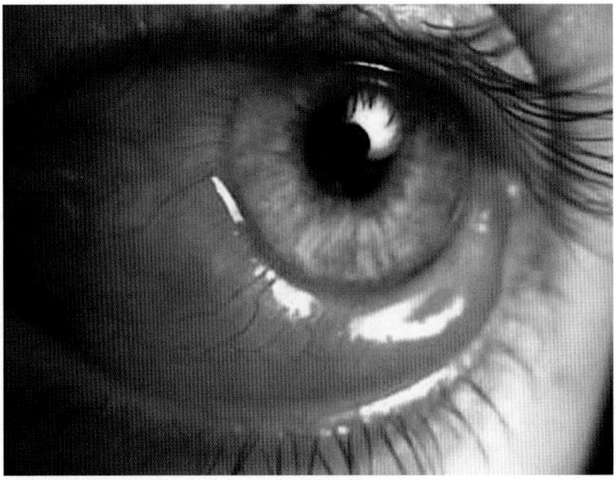

**Figure 65-12**
Allergic conjunctivitis.

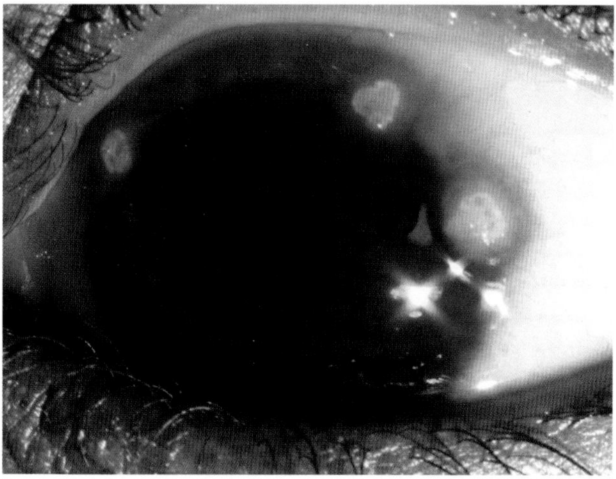

**Figure 65-13**
Vernal conjunctivitis.

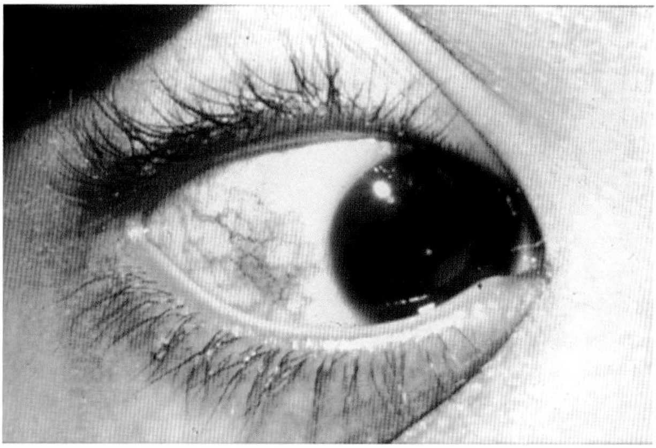

**Figure 65-14**
Phlyctenule.

Phlyctenulosis, another subset of allergic conjunctivitis, is a delayed hypersensitivity reaction that is often bilateral and results in a white, raised lesion on either the conjunctiva or peripheral cornea, with dilated blood vessels at its borders (Figure 65-14). The most common precipitant is exposure to staphylococci, but it can also be associated with tuberculosis or histoplasmosis, so in cases without signs of blepharitis, a test for tuberculosis and a chest radiograph are warranted. Treatment is the same as for blepharitis, with the addition of interventions to treat the allergic component. Patients with significant irritation may require topical steroids and should be referred.

## Subconjunctival Hemorrhage

Subconjunctival hemorrhage is easily diagnosed by its often strikingly large patch of bright red on an otherwise white conjunctiva, usually in an asymptomatic patient (Figure 65-15).

It can occur after a vaginal delivery, with Valsalva maneuver, with use of antiplatelet medications, from a severe cough as with pertussis, or from trauma. Nonaccidental trauma should be considered in atypical cases. When there are recurrent subconjunctival hemorrhages, a bleeding disorder or blood dyscrasia should be considered. No treatment is needed for a subconjunctival hemorrhage, which will resolve over 2 to 3 weeks. It is worth counseling patients and parents that, as with most ecchymoses, the lesion may expand slightly and change colors as it resolves.

## Conjunctival Papilloma

Commonly a benign, self-limited lesion caused by human papillomavirus 6 or 11, a conjunctival papilloma is a fleshy nodule with a sunburst vascular pattern (Figure 65-16). For large, multiple, recurrent, or cosmetically disturbing lesions, treatment options include cryotherapy, surgical excision, and oral cimetidine.[5]

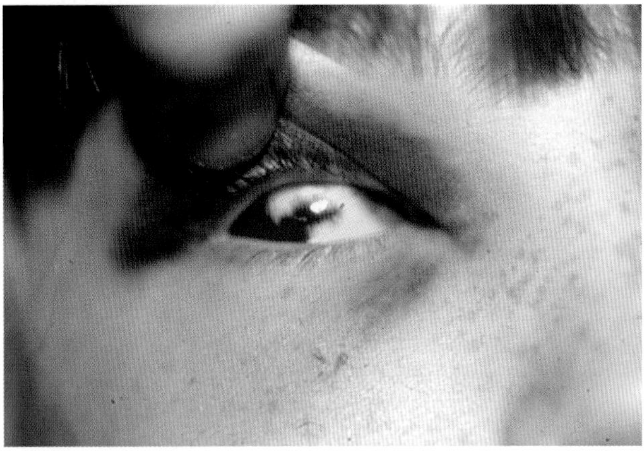

**Figure 65-15**
Subconjunctival hemorrhage.

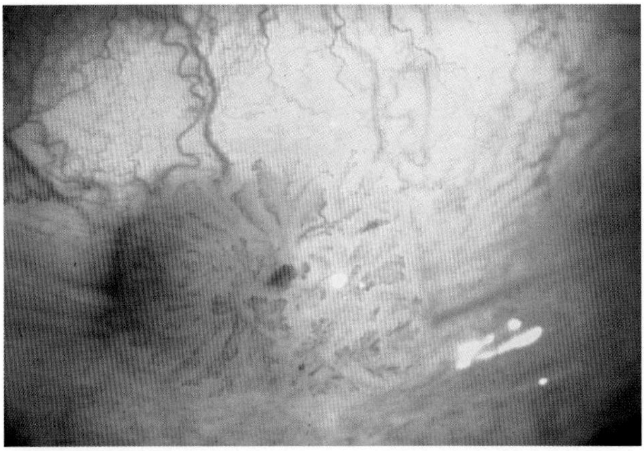

**Figure 65-16**
Conjunctival papilloma.

## Kawasaki Disease

The bilateral nonexudative conjunctivitis of Kawasaki disease, an acute vasculitis, is associated with fever, mucosal erythema, rash, cervical lymphadenopathy, and the potential for coronary artery aneurysms. The conjunctivitis is usually self-limited and can be treated with artificial tears.[6]

### *Corneal Abnormalities*

## Corneal Abrasion/Foreign Body

Corneal abrasions classically have a very painful presentation, and the patient will complain of a foreign body sensation, tearing, and often photophobia. Patients often recall a sudden onset after being hit or scratched in the eye. Examination is often difficult, but instillation of anesthetic drops, such as proparacaine 0.5%, facilitates examination. The corneal abrasion is easily identified with a Wood lamp and fluorescein. In patients with a corneal abrasion, a foreign body should be suspected, and the undersurface of the eyelids should be examined. A corneal foreign body (Figure 65-17) can be removed with a moist cotton-tipped applicator if superficial, but deeper ones should be referred to an ophthalmologist.

## Corneal Ulcer

Bacterial, fungal, viral, or parasitic organisms can cause ulceration, a sight-threatening condition that requires urgent ophthalmologic evaluation if there is corneal opacity, decreased vision, or ocular pain (Figure 65-18). Because contact lenses are a significant cause of corneal infections, an ophthalmologist should evaluate patients who develop a red eye and wear contact lenses.

## Herpetic Keratitis

Both HSV and varicella-zoster virus (VZV) can infect the eye. Whereas VZV typically spreads to the eye from the face or eyelid, HSV can infect the cornea directly. Examination of the cornea with fluorescein reveals a dendritic branching epithelial defect (Figure 65-19).

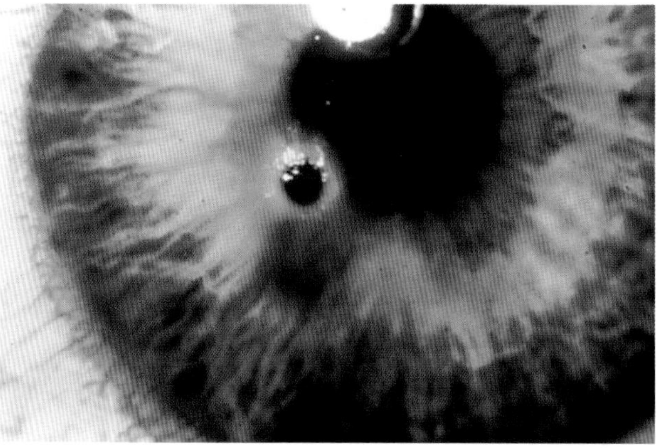

**Figure 65-17**
Corneal foreign body.

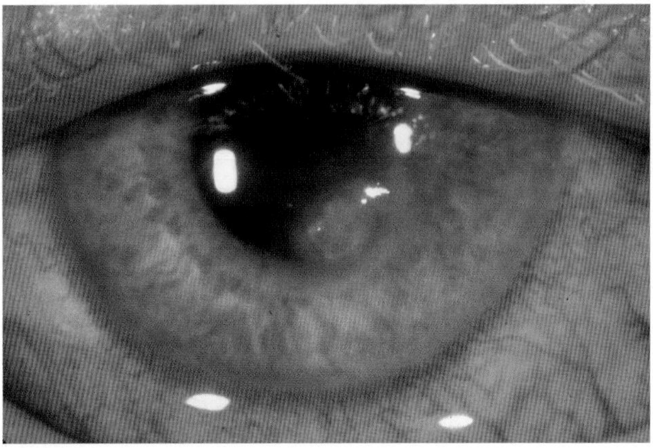

**Figure 65-18**
Corneal ulcer.

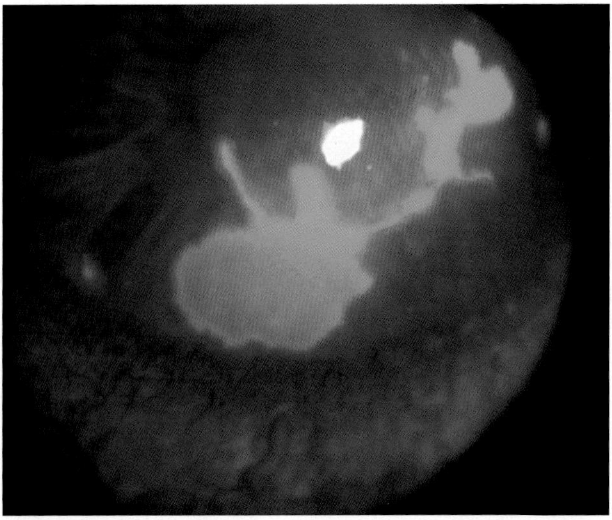

**Figure 65-19**
Herpetic keratitis.

If herpes is suspected, an ophthalmologic evaluation is urgently warranted to evaluate for intraocular involvement and intraocular pressure elevation. Treatment of both HSV and VZV involves either oral antivirals (acyclovir, valacyclovir) or topical antiviral eyedrops (trifluridine) or gel (gancyclovir).[7] If patients with a history of herpetic keratitis develop red eye, they should be seen by an ophthalmologist because recurrence is common. Corneal HSV disease often causes corneal scarring, which can be sight threatening.

### *Intraocular Abnormalities*

Corneal and ciliary flush (Figure 65-1) is a violaceous, extreme engorgement of vessels at the corneal limbus that indicates involvement of deeper ocular structures. A patient with this finding should always be referred to an ophthalmologist. The differential diagnosis includes corneal infection, iritis, uveitis, and hyphema.

## Iritis/Uveitis

Iritis and uveitis are inflammatory disorders within the eye often associated with sarcoidosis, HSV, syphilis, tuberculosis, lupus, or autoimmune arthritides—including JIA and the HLA-B27–positive spondyloarthropathies. Affected patients complain of photophobia, pain, and blurred vision and usually have ciliary flush and a mid-dilated pupil. In patients with a first episode of unilateral iritis, no workup is indicated because it will have an unidentified cause. However, in the case of recurrent or bilateral disease, or if the medical history suggests a systemic disorder, an underlying cause should be sought and treated. The laboratory workup includes antinuclear antibody, erythrocyte sedimentation rate, serum uric acid level, antineutrophil cytoplasmic antibody, rapid plasma reagin, and fluorescent trepenmal antibody absorption. In children with JIA, frequent screening for uveitis is critical because the inflammation is commonly asymptomatic with few external findings and if left untreated can lead to blindness.[8] Young patients with pauciarticular JIA should be evaluated every 3 months for 7 years. Treatment includes topical and/or oral steroids to control the disease and cycloplegia to prevent iris adhesions and reduce photophobia. In the event of long-term steroid use, intraocular pressure should be monitored.

## Hyphema

A hyphema is blood collected in the anterior chamber of the eye, which is located behind the cornea and in front of the lens (Figure 65-20). In children it is almost exclusively a result of trauma, but in the absence of trauma, tumors and coagulopathies should be suspected. Affected patients should be referred to an ophthalmologist because treatment includes monitoring of intraocular pressure, cycloplegia to prevent iris movement and adhesions, topical steroids to decrease inflammation, and reduced patient activity to prevent a rebleed.

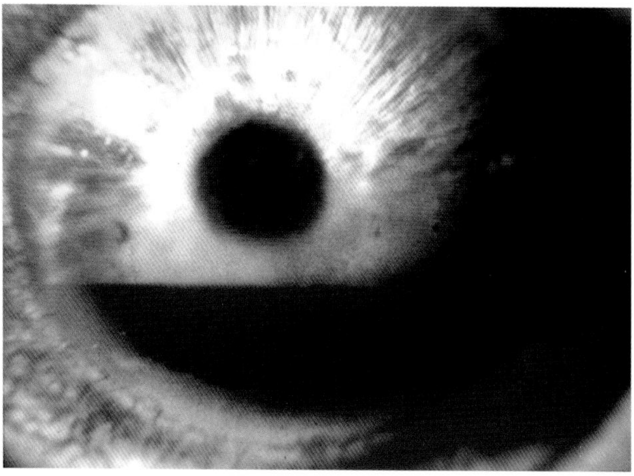

**Figure 65-20**
Hyphema.

## Other Inflammatory Conditions

Scleritis, episcleritis, and ocular myositis are rare inflammatory conditions that cause a focal conjunctival redness. Episcleritis and scleritis can be distinguished because episcleritis has minimal discomfort, in sharp contrast to the severe pain of scleritis. The inflammation of myositis is seen overlying the affected extraocular muscle, and often patients develop a head tilt to avoid using the sore muscle. The workup for these conditions is the same as for recurrent iritis. Treatment of episcleritis includes oral nonsteroidal anti-inflammatory drugs (NSAIDs, eg, ibuprofen) alone or accompanied by topical steroids. For scleritis and ocular myositis, ophthalmologic consultation should be obtained: treatment typically begins with NSAIDs; but if there is no improvement, systemic steroids with possible steroid-sparing immunosuppressive agents should be used.

In conclusion, the pediatrician can successfully perform the diagnosis and management of the red eye in children when attention is paid to the history, location of redness, and ocular structures involved. Accurate diagnosis allows for appropriate treatment and the proper timing of referrals.

### REFERENCES

1. Greenberg MF, Pollard ZF. The red eye in childhood. *Pediatr Clin North Am.* 2003;50:105–124
2. Elkington AR, Khaw PT. ABC of eyes. The red eye. *Br Med J (Clin Res Ed).* 1988;296:1720–1724
3. American Academy of Pediatrics. Children in out-of-home child care. In: Pickering LK, Baker CJ, Kimberlin DW, Long SS, eds. *Red Book: 2012 Report of the Committee on Infectious Diseases.* Elk Grove Village, IL: American Academy of Pediatrics; 2012:144
4. American Academy of Pediatrics. Adenovirus infections. In: Pickering LK, Baker CJ, Kimberlin DW, Long SS, eds. *Red Book: 2012 Report of the Committee on Infectious Diseases.* Elk Grove Village, IL: American Academy of Pediatrics; 2012:222
5. Shields CL, Lally MR, Singh AD, Shields JA, Nowinski T. Oral cimetidine (Tagamet) for recalcitrant, diffuse conjunctival papillomatosis. *Am J Ophthalmol.* 1999;128:362–364
6. Newburger JW, Takahashi M, Gerber MA, et al. Diagnosis, treatment, and long-term management of Kawasaki disease: a statement for health professionals from the Committee on Rheumatic Fever, Endocarditis, and Kawasaki Disease, Council on Cardiovascular Disease in the Young, American Heart Association. *Pediatrics.* 2004;114:1708–1733
7. A controlled trial of oral acyclovir for iridocyclitis caused by herpes simplex virus. The Herpetic Eye Disease Study Group. *Arch Ophthalmol.* 1996;114:1065–1072
8. Durkin SR, Casey TM. Beware of the unilateral red eye: don't miss blinding uveitis. *Med J Aust.* 2005;182:296–297

# Chapter 66

# School Absenteeism and School Refusal

*Ronald V. Marino, DO, MPH*

A major developmental task of childhood is separating from the family and accepting the functional demands of society. One of the most obvious indicators that this process may not be proceeding normally is lack of attendance at school. Assessing a child's school attendance and functioning in the context of biopsychosocial health supervision is the responsibility of child health professionals.

Nonattendance may be the consequence of a variety of underlying causes. *Absenteeism* is generally considered to be parentally sanctioned nonattendance, most commonly attributed to medical illness. *Truancy* is nonattendance without parental consent, in which the time allegedly spent at school is often spent engaging in antisocial behaviors or rebelling against authority. *School refusal* is characterized by inappropriate fear about leaving home, inappropriate fear of school, or both.

## ▶ ABSENTEEISM

Excessive absenteeism is important to health care professionals because it is an excellent marker for both physical and mental health problems (Box 66-1). It also is negatively correlated with social adjustment and academic performance. In fact, excessive absenteeism and failure to read at the appropriate level in the third grade are the 2 strongest predictors of subsequent dropping out of school. According to the National Center for Education Statistics for 2005, 19% of fourth-graders and 20% of eighth-graders missed at least 3 days of school in the past month. More specifically, 7% of fourth-graders and 7% of eighth-graders missed at least 5 days of school in the past month. National surveys indicate that healthy children average 4 or 5 absences a school year, whereas children who have a chronic disease typically are absent at least twice as often.[1,2] Educators think that missing more than 10 days in a 90-day semester results in difficulty staying at grade level.[3]

Acute physical health problems are given as the reason for nonattendance 75% of the time. However, the variability in absenteeism among children who have the same medical condition suggests that individual and family responses to the physical condition are more important than the actual condition in determining attendance.[3] The decision not to attend school reflects subtle and complex relationships among the physical, social, and psychological states of the student, family, and community. Individual rates of absenteeism tend to be stable for a given child and also for a given school district.

Box 66-1

## *Chronic School Absence: Differential Diagnosis*

- School refusal
- Parental overresponse to minor illnesses
- Chronic physical disease with poor adaptation
- Learning disability with poor adaptation
- Untreated mental health issues (eg, anxiety, depression)
- Bullying
- Truancy
- Substance abuse
- Psychosis
- Teenage pregnancy
- Family dysfunction (including violence and abuse)

The health conditions most commonly associated with nonattendance include upper respiratory tract infections, headaches, abdominal distress, menstrual cramps, and sleep disorders.[3,4] Parental characteristics associated with excessive absenteeism include lower socioeconomic class, cigarette smoking, chronic parental illness (including mental illness), lower educational expectations, and vulnerable child syndrome.[5–7] A plethora of nonmedical conditions, including transportation difficulties, illness of other family members, religious holidays, family vacations, inclement weather, and professional appointments, are also reasons children miss school. Chronically ill children typically miss more school than their healthy peers. This tendency may result from a wide variety of causes, including acute exacerbations of the underlying condition, health care visits, side effects of medications, and parental misconceptions about the child's ability to attend school. Healthy adjustment by the child and family to the chronic condition minimizes the potential effect of the increase in school days missed. A significant increase in absenteeism over baseline is always a warning sign. Exploring the reasons why a particular child seeks to avoid school is the physician's responsibility. Sudden changes in school attendance may be the first concrete symptom of family dysfunction, mental illness, physical deterioration of the student or a family member, alcohol or drug abuse, or school refusal.

## ▶ SCHOOL REFUSAL

Difficulties attending school despite caretakers' support have been a problem for children, families, schools, and physicians since the early 20th century. Initial views of school refusal focused on truancy and its link to delinquency. In 1932, Broadwin focused attention on the frequent role of anxiety in attendance difficulties, and, in 1939, Patridge[8] labeled this clinical condition *psychoneurotic truancy*. Johnson et al[9] introduced the term *school phobia* in 1941, stressing that the child's anxiety about separating from mother was displaced to fear of attending school. This view was strengthened further in the 1950s, when Estes et al[10] concluded that school phobia was a variant of separation anxiety.

This view and nomenclature persisted until the late 1970s, when the term *school refusal* was introduced. The term has descriptive merits that recognize the heterogeneity of the underlying disorders. These disorders include, but are not limited to, major depression, simple and social phobia, or separation anxiety disorder. Criteria for making this diagnosis include severe difficulty in attending school or refusal to attend school, severe emotional upset when attempting to go to school, absence of significant antisocial disorders, and staying at home with the parent's knowledge.

A variety of physical symptoms often accompany the child's request to not attend school. Symptoms can be quite impressive to parents and may emulate organic medical problems.

## Prevalence

The prevalence of school refusal varies widely and has been estimated to be between 0.4% and 18%.[11–13] The incidence of school refusal has 2 peaks—the first is associated with entering primary school (4–6 years), and the second is at the age of 11 to 12 years, a time of change from elementary to intermediate school, as well as the onset of early adolescence. The American Academy of Pediatrics estimates that 5% of elementary school children and 2% of junior high students experience this disorder. The symptoms of school refusal are associated with several psychiatric disorders. In an outpatient sample of referred children, 22% had separation anxiety disorder, 11% had generalized anxiety disorder, 8% had oppositional defiant disorder, and 5% had major depressive disorder. Of note is that 20% to 30% of school-refusing children do not qualify for any specific psychiatric diagnosis.[11,14]

## Child-Related Factors

Children who have school refusal usually have at least average intelligence and academic achievement. Cultural norms encourage girls to admit fear and discourage boys from doing the same. The actual incidence of school refusal is nearly identical between the sexes.[12] Younger children report more fear of being scolded or of performing before a group, whereas older children seem to be more intimidated by tests and the possibility of failure. Vague somatic symptoms, typically offered as a rationale for nonattendance, may belie the underlying anxiety that is frequently present. Symptoms may amplify in response to parental pressure to attend and/or excel in school. Overdependency or concern about the well-being of a parent is also a common underlying dynamic. Serious or chronic illness in the parent may lead to school refusal. Depression has often been noted, as have panic disorder and agoraphobia. Because there are reports of suicide among school refusers, any reference to this possibility must be addressed seriously.

## Family Factors

The family context is always a major factor because marital conflict or constricted communication patterns are often found in families with school refusers. The child's presence at home as a result of physical illness may provide a cohesive force to an otherwise unstable marital relationship. Families of youths with school refusal behavior are often marked by poverty, poor cohesion and considerable conflict, enmeshment, isolation and detachment.[15,16]

Common patterns of communication in families in which school refusal occurs have been described:[18] Both parents are overly concerned and solicitous of the child's medical problem; 1 parent, typically the mother, is overprotective and concerned, whereas the other overtly disagrees; and 1 parent, typically the mother, is overinvolved in caring for the child's every need, whereas the other parent is emotionally absent. Because children are reared in many diverse family situations, physicians must remain open and attentive to family structure and dynamics in order to develop an effective treatment plan.[19]

### School Environment Factors

The role of the school environment in school refusal has received little attention. Institutional factors such as changing classrooms or lack of privacy in the school bathroom have been associated with fear of school. The physical environment may include uncomfortable temperatures, mold, or allergens, which predispose to illness or student discomfort. Humiliation caused by an insensitive teacher may also be a precipitating stressor in the onset of clinical symptoms. Temperamental mismatch among teacher, student, and parents may serve a maintaining role.

Bullying and social humiliation are increasing in frequency and victims often develop somatic symptoms as a coping mechanism.[20] The increased use of social media has created a new and potentially dangerous phenomenon in cyber bullying. Cyber bullying is defined as willful and repeated harm inflicted through the use of computers, cell phones, and other electronic devices. More than 20% of 4,400 randomly selected 11- to 18-year-olds indicated they had been subjected to cyber bullying at some point in their lives.[21] In 2005, 24% of students aged 12 to 18 years reported gangs at their schools; this was more common among urban (36%) than suburban (21%) or rural (16%) schools. In addition, 28% of students aged 12 to 18 years were reportedly bullied at school in the past 6 months. Most said bullying occurred 1 to 2 times in 6 months, but 25% were bullied 1 to 2 times per month, 11% were bullied 1 to 2 times per week, and 8% were reportedly bullied almost daily.[22] Both traditional and cyber bullying have been implicated as sources of severe emotional distress among victims, even leading to suicide. Violence in secondary schools provides children a seemingly appropriate reason for refusing to attend school. Twenty-six percent of junior and senior high school students have been assaulted on school grounds, 20% of students admitted bringing a knife or gun to school, and 10% admitted not going to school because of fear of violence.[13,23] Media attention to school violence may further accelerates a child's anxiety and school refusal. Clearly, school-associated stressors are emerging as a concern in understanding and treating school refusal.

### Associated Stressors

While exploring factors related to the child, parent, family, and school environment, the physician must also search for a precipitating event or stress that may have tipped the balance in causing a child to refuse to attend school. Illness or injury of a family member or of the child may be the initial reason for nonattendance. Similarly, the death of a relative or close friend may precipitate the refusal. Moving to a new home, community, or school also may contribute to refusal. The longer a child has been out of school, the more difficult and stressful returning can become.

### Clinical Management

In 1958, Eisenberg[24] stated, "[I]t is essential that the paralyzing force of the school phobia on the child's whole life be recognized. The symptom itself serves to isolate him from normal experience and makes further psychological growth almost impossible. If we do no more than check this central symptom, we have nonetheless done a great deal." The foundations of any clinical treatment plan are rapport, trust, and respect. The initial interview should serve not only as a means of gathering data, but also as the start of a therapeutic alliance. Physicians should use a sensitive, holistic approach to data gathering, because the history-taking technique provides the first opportunity for creating a healing rapport. Factors related to the child, parents, family, and school environment must be investigated when exploring school maladaptation. An open mind that recognizes the unique and complex interactions of temperament, stressful life events, family systems function, learning style, parental medical or psychiatric conditions, and school system variables will be helpful in solving this problem. The child must understand that involving a physician in treatment reflects the seriousness of the symptoms and marks a turning point in changing the avoidant behavior.

Organic disease should be ruled out through a thorough history and physical examination, coupled with judicious laboratory evaluation. Time spent in conducting a thorough medical examination communicates the physician's sincere acceptance of the child's symptoms as being real. Parents are better able to confront the lack of organic disease when a physician who is completely familiar with the child's history and physical examination discusses the subject with them. A biopsychosocial approach from the outset also aids family acceptance of psychiatric concerns. The laboratory should be used in a symptom-specific, noninvasive, cost-effective manner consistent with ruling out possible organic disease. Additionally, addressing the potential contributions of parental disorders or specific environmental problems will be helpful in formulating a treatment plan.

The parents, physician, and school personnel must all agree that returning to school as quickly as possible is the immediate goal of treatment. Allowing the child to stay home while awaiting laboratory data results or using home tutors only delays the inevitable and makes the return to school more difficult. A specific plan must be developed to respond to clinical symptoms. Objective criteria for school absence, such as a measured fever, should be consistently used in modifying performance expectations, both at home and in school. Parents in doubt should seek the guidance of the child's physician regarding the significance of acute symptoms before keeping the child home. In addition, the significant attachment figures in the child's life must make it clear they will adhere to the therapeutic program consistently and persistently. In most cases of school refusal, especially in the elementary years, the aforementioned program, carried out by the primary care pediatrician, is curative. Other treatment modalities, typically used by a mental health professional, include desensitization, psychotherapy, hypnotherapy, cognitive restructuring, and behavior modification. A variety of psychopharmacologic agents have been used to manage anxiety- or depression-based school refusal. selective serotonin reuptake inhibitors (SSRIs) predominate the scant literature and have been found to be useful in some individuals.[13] Concerns about a possible relationship between SSRIs and risk of suicide in children and adolescents have reduced the number of primary care physicians willing to prescribe these medications. Children who are recalcitrant to behavioral interventions may require referral to a mental health specialist. Suggested criteria for mental health referral are listed in Box 66-2.

Mental health professionals typically employ cognitive behavioral therapy with or without SSRIs.[25–27] Severe cases may require inpatient treatment.[28]

## Prognosis

Most children who refuse to attend school quickly overcome the difficulty with appropriate clinical management. Intermittent relapses associated with stress or new separation

Box 66-2

## *Criteria for Mental Health Referral*

- Unresponsive to management
- Out of school for 2 months
- Onset in adolescence
- Psychosis
- Depression
- Panic reactions
- Parental inability to cooperate with treatment plan

**Table 66-1**

**Long-term Sequelae in Children With School Refusal**

| OUTCOME | PREVALENCE |
|---|---|
| Interrupted compulsory school | 18% |
| Did not complete high school | 45% |
| Adult psychiatric outpatient care | 43% |
| Adult psychiatric inpatient care | 6% |
| Criminal offense | 6% |
| Still living with parents after 20-year follow-up | 14% |
| Married at 20-year follow-up | 41% |

From Fremont WD. School refusal in children and adolescents. *Am Fam Physician*. 2003;68(8): 1555–1560. Data from Bernstein GA, Hektner JM, Borchardt CM, McMillan MH. Treatment of school refusal: one-year follow-up. *J Am Acad Child Adolesc Psychiatry*. 2001;40(2):206–213; Flakierska-Praquin N, Lindström M, Gillberg C. School phobia with separation anxiety disorder: a comparative 20- to 29-year follow-up study of 35 school refusers. *Compr Psychiatry*. 1997;38(1):17–22.

experiences, such as camp or sleepovers, occur in approximately 5% of children. Children who require psychiatric management do not fare as well.[23] Most published series in the psychiatric literature reveal significant cohorts of patients requiring ongoing therapy and having persistent difficulties in emancipating themselves from their family.[24,29] Phobias, depression, and anxiety are more common in adults who have a history of childhood school refusal.[30] Table 66-1 lists long-term sequelae in children with school refusal.[31]

## *Prevention*

Anticipatory guidance is an excellent means of primary prevention, and allows the primary care physician to advise parents on developmentally appropriate separation guidelines. For example, by the time an infant is 6 months of age, the parents should be able to spend some evenings out alone. By 1 year of age, peer contact should be encouraged. Toddlers should experience babysitters while awake. By age 3 years, the child should experience being away from home without a parent, such as in a playgroup or at a neighbor's home. Age 4 years is a good time to consider preschool for the child. Such guidance can be shared in the context of routine health supervision. Parents should also be discouraged from keeping children home because of minor illness, and physicians must avoid unnecessary medical restrictions.

Preventing vulnerable child syndrome is also important when caring for ill children. This disorder arises when parents think that their child's life has been threatened significantly, and it results in separation difficulties, overprotection, bodily concerns, and underachievement in school.[7] Parents need to be informed about the true significance and prognosis of any medical difficulty the child has experienced. Physicians have a responsibility to avoid creating iatrogenic misconceptions about a child's health. They can accomplish this task by using everyday language as much as possible, rather than medical jargon, and by demystifying anxiety associated with insignificant findings, such as a functional murmur. Parents need to be reassured that children who have recovered fully from an acute illness are at no increased risk for future illness. By inquiring about children's school attendance and promoting healthy parenting styles, primary care physicians can help prevent school refusal.

## ▶ TRUANCY AND DROPPING OUT

Truancy is a good predictor of dropping out at a later date. Many schools in inner cities report daily absence rates above 20%, with most of this thought to be the result of truancy; an equal or greater percentage of inner-city school children never finish high school. Truancy is a serious social problem that can have lifelong consequences. Unemployment or underemployment, criminal behavior, marital problems, and chronic social maladjustment are often seen in children with truancy or children who drop out. These same long-term outcomes have been identified in groups of children who have learning disabilities. One risk factor for truancy is learning disability and its associated school failure.

Truancy also has been noted among children who have a history of having been sexually abused. Other risk factors are low socioeconomic status, conduct disorder, gang membership, substance abuse, cigarette smoking, and family discord. Early recognition of children at risk should prompt immediate intervention to promote optimal adjustment. Mobilization of resources in the school, community, and family is critical to help prevent progression from truancy to dropping out. Creative programs to foster school attendance and success have been conducted with variable results. An emerging new truancy variant is the child who goes to school or its immediate environment but does not attend class. This child is participating in the social aspects of the school community but is shunning the academics. Medical physicians can assume an advocacy role in guiding and supporting therapeutic interventions in the educational and social welfare arenas.

## ▶ CONCLUSION

Absenteeism is a symptom that has multiple causes. Because success in school is often the foundation for continuing success in life, health care professionals must devote thoughtful attention to understanding and treating absentees. Using a biopsychosocial model and mobilizing multidisciplinary resources are the keys to clinical success.

### *TOOLS FOR PRACTICE*

#### Medical Decision Support

- *AAP Council on School Health* (Web page), American Academy of Pediatrics (www.schoolhealth.org)
- *Adolescent and School Health* (Web page), Centers for Disease Control and Prevention (www.cdc.gov/HealthyYouth)

- *Managing Infectious Diseases in Child Care and Schools* (book), American Academy of Pediatrics (shop.aap.org)
- *School Health: Policy & Practice,* 6th ed (book), American Academy of Pediatrics (shop.aap.org)

## AAP POLICY STATEMENTS

American Academy of Pediatrics Committee on Child Abuse and Neglect and Section on Adoption and Foster Care; American Academy of Child and Adolescent Psychiatry; National Center for Child Traumatic Stress. Understanding the behavioral and emotional consequences of child abuse. *Pediatrics.* 2008;122(3):667–673. Reaffirmed August 2012 (pediatrics.aappublications.org/content/122/3/667)

Thackeray JD, Hibbard R, Dowd MD; American Academy of Pediatrics Committee on Child Abuse and Neglect, Committee on Injury, Violence, and Poison Prevention. Intimate partner violence: the role of the pediatrician. *Pediatrics.* 2010;125(5):1094–1100. Reaffirmed January 2014 (pediatrics.aappublications.org/content/125/5/1094)

Jenny C, Crawford-Jakubiak JE; American Academy of Pediatrics Committee on Child Abuse and Neglect. The evaluation of children in the primary care setting when sexual abuse is suspected. *Pediatrics.* 2013;132(2):e558–e567 (pediatrics.aappublications.org/content/132/2/e558)

Kellogg ND; American Academy of Pediatrics Committee on Child Abuse and Neglect. Evaluation of suspected child physical abuse. *Pediatrics.* 2007;119(6):1232–1241. Reaffirmed May 2012 (pediatrics.aappublications.org/content/119/6/1232)

American Academy of Pediatrics Committee on School Health. Home, hospital, and other non–school-based instruction for children and adolescents who are medically unable to attend school. *Pediatrics.* 2000;106:1154–1155 (pediatrics.aappublications.org/content/106/5/1154)

American Academy of Pediatrics Committee on School Health. Out-of-school suspension and expulsion. *Pediatrics.* 2003;112:1206–1208. Reaffirmed May 2008 (pediatrics.aappublications.org/content/112/5/1206)

Taras H, Duncan P, Luckenbill D, et al, eds. *Health, Mental Health, and Safety Guidelines for Schools.* Elk Grove Village, IL: American Academy of Pediatrics; 2004. AAP endorsed

## REFERENCES

1. Fowler MG, Johnson MP, Atkinson SS. School achievement and absence in children with chronic health conditions. *J Pediatr.* 1985;106:683–687
2. Klerman LV. School absence—a health perspective. *Pediatr Clin North Am.* 1988;35:1253–1269
3. Weitzman M, Klerman LV, Alpert JJ, et al. Factors associated with excessive school absence. *Pediatrician.* 1986;13:74–80
4. Bernstein GA, Massie ED, Thuras PD, et al. Somatic symptoms in anxious-depressed school refusers. *J Am Acad Child Adolesc Psychiatry.* 1997;36:661–668
5. Charlton A, Blair V. Absence from school related to children's and parental smoking habits. *BMJ.* 1989;298:90–92
6. Cassino C, Auerbach M, Kammerman S, et al. Effect of maternal asthma on performance of parenting tasks and children's school attendance. *J Asthma.* 1997;34:499–507
7. Green M, Solnit AJ. Reactions to the threatened loss of a child: a vulnerable child syndrome. Pediatric management of the dying child, Part III. *Pediatrics.* 1964;34:58–66
8. Patridge JM. Truancy. *J Mental Sci.* 1939;85:45–81
9. Johnson AM, Falstein EI, Szurek SA, et al. School phobia. *Am J Orthopsychiatry.* 1941;11:702–711
10. Estes HR, Haylett CH, Johnson M. Separation anxiety. *Am J Psycother.* 1956;10(4):682–695
11. Granell de Aldaz E, Vivas E, Gelfand DM, Feldman L. Estimating the prevalence of school refusal and school related fears. a Venezuelan sample. *J Nerv Mental Dis.* 1984;172(12):722–729
12. American Academy of Pediatrics. *School Health: Policy & Practice.* 5th ed. Nader PR, ed. Elk Grove Village, IL: American Academy of Pediatrics; 1993

13. Kearney CA. School absenteeism and school refusal behavior in youth: a contemporary review. *Clin Psychol Rev*. 2008;28:451–471
14. Hella B, Bernstein GA. Panic disorder and school refusal. *Child Adolesc Psychiatr Clin N Am*. 2012;21:593–606
15. Berg I. Absence from school and mental health. *Br J Psychiatry*. 1992;161:154–166
16. Hansen C, Sanders SL, Massaro S, Last CG. Predictors of severity of absenteeism in children with anxiety-based school refusal. *J Clin Child Psychol*. 1998;27:246–254
17. Chapan G. 2007. *Family environment and school refusal behavior in youth*. Paper presented at the meeting of the Anxiety Disorder Association of America, St. Louis, MO
18. Nader PR, Bullock D, Caldwell B. School phobia. *Pediatr Clin North Am*. 1975;22:605–617
19. Hersov L. School refusal. *Br Med J*. 1972;3:102–104
20. Torrens Armstrong AM, McCormack Brown KR, Brindley R, Coreil J, McDermott RJ. Frequent fliers, school phobias, and the sick student: school health personnel's perceptions of students who refuse school. *J Sch Health*. 2011;81:552–559
21. Patchin JW; Cyberbullying Research Center. 2010 data. www.cyberbullying.us/2010-data
22. National Center for Education Statistics. Student reports of bullying and cyber-bullying: results from the 2011 School Crime Supplement to the National Crime Victimization Survey. http://nces.ed.gov/pubs2013/2013329.pdf (Accessed February 10, 2015)
23. New York State Education Department, Division of Criminal Justice Services. Study: 1 in 5 students were armed. *Newsday*. February 14, 1994:19
24. Eisenberg L. School phobia: a study in the communication of anxiety. *Am J Psychiatry*. 1958;114:712–718
25. Last CG, Hansen C, Franco N. Cognitive-behavioral treatment of school phobia. *J Am Acad Child Adolesc Psychiatry*. 1998;37:404–411
26. Bernstein GA, Borchardt CM, Perwien AR, et al. Imipramine plus cognitive-behavioral therapy in the treatment of school refusal. *J Am Acad Child Adolesc Psychiatry*. 2000;39:276–283
27. Walkup JT, Albano AM, Piacentini J, et al. Cognitive behavioral therapy, sertraline, or a combination in childhood anxiety. *N Engl J Med*. 2008;359:2753–2766
28. Walter D, Hautmann C, Rizk S, et al. Short term effects of inpatient cognitive behavioral treatment of adolescents with anxious-depressed school absenteeism: an observational study. *Eur Child Adolesc Psychiatry*. 2010;19:835–844
29. Flaierska-Praquin N, Lindström M, Gillberg C. School phobia with separation anxiety disorder: a comparative 20- to 29-year follow-up study of 35 school refusers. *Compr Psychiatry*. 1997;38(1):17–22
30. Bernstein GA, Hektner JM, Borchardt CM, McMillan MH. Treatment of school refusal: one-year follow-up. *J Am Acad Child Adolesc Psychiatry*. 2001;40:206–213
31. Fremont WP. School refusal in children and adolescents. *Am Fam Physician*. 2003;68(8):1555–1560

# Chapter 67

# Scrotal Swelling and Pain

*Lane S. Palmer, MD*

Scrotal swelling can be particularly frightening for boys and their families, and because the differential diagnosis includes conditions that demand emergent treatment, it poses a challenge to pediatricians. A helpful organizing strategy during evaluation is to classify the scrotal swelling as either painful or painless and as acute or chronic (Box 67-1). Rapid and accurate evaluation of a boy with scrotal swelling depends on a thorough history and a physical examination of the genital area and abdomen that includes both inspection and palpation. Laboratory tests may be helpful but are not usually decisive, whereas imaging studies can be helpful in confirming a diagnosis and guiding management.

## ▶ EVALUATION OF THE CHILD WITH SCROTAL SWELLING

The history should be taken from both the child (when possible) and the parent. The physician must determine whether the swelling or pain is a single event or recurrent and whether it is acute or chronic. The exact timing of the onset of symptoms is vital, particularly in the presence of acute pain and swelling. The nature of the pain must be determined: sharp, dull, constant, intermittent, constant with intermittent increases in intensity, or associated with nausea or vomiting. The location of the pain needs to be ascertained (ie, in the scrotum, specifically the testis; radiation into the abdomen or from the abdomen into the scrotum; laterality of the swelling and pain). Associated factors such as activity or positions that alleviate or aggravate the pain and swelling should be elicited. The nature of the swelling is important: specifically, whether the swelling changes in size during the course of a single day or whether it is constant or, in general, increasing or decreasing with time. Other important considerations include recent trauma, sexual activity, use of medications, the presence of rashes, weight loss, and nausea and vomiting.

The physical examination should include the abdomen, groin, and scrotum. Palpation of the abdomen and groin is important in determining whether an intraabdominal process is extending into the scrotum. Inspection of the scrotum should look for laterality of the process, scrotal erythema, and orientation of the testis, whereas palpation will determine the presence and symmetry of cremasteric reflexes, testicular position, tenderness, localization of the swelling to the intrascrotal contents, or the presence of proximal extension into the cord.

In general, laboratory tests are of limited value. The white blood cell count may be elevated in the setting of infection. Urinalysis may be helpful in distinguishing orchitis from torsion of the spermatic cord or testicular appendage when white blood cells or nitrites are present.

Box 67-1

## *Causes of Scrotal Swelling*

**ACUTE, PAINFUL SCROTAL SWELLING**

- Torsion of spermatic cord
- Torsion of appendix, testis, epididymis
- Acute epididymitis, orchitis
- Mumps orchitis
- Henoch-Schönlein purpura
- Trauma
- Insect bite
- Thrombosis of spermatic vein
- Fat necrosis
- Hernia
- Folliculitis
- Dermatitis, acute

**PAINLESS SCROTAL SWELLING**

- Tumor
- Idiopathic scrotal edema
- Hydrocele
- Henoch-Schönlein purpura
- Hernia

**CHRONIC SCROTAL SWELLING**

- Hydrocele
- Hernia
- Varicocele
- Spermatocele
- Sebaceous cyst
- Tumor

Imaging studies can be useful in differentiating among possible diagnoses. Ultrasound of the scrotum can be used to determine whether the scrotal swelling is fluid filled or solid, arising from the abdomen extending into the groin, limited to the scrotum, or arising from the testis or spermatic cord structures. Ultrasound with Doppler can assess the flow of blood into the testis, helping to differentiate torsion of the testis from an inflammatory process. Nuclear scintigraphy using technetium-99m pertechnetate is another way to evaluate blood flow to the testis; absence of flow results in a cold spot and suggests torsion, whereas inflammation results in increased flow to the same area. Nuclear scanning is less limited by the user variability associated with ultrasound and does not require placing a probe over a tender area. However, the study uses ionizing radiation and takes longer to perform than ultrasound, thus limiting its utility when time is of the essence. The sensitivity and specificity of the 2 modalities are similar.

## ▶ ACUTE SCROTAL SWELLING WITH PAIN

The sudden onset of scrotal swelling and pain can be a surgical emergency and therefore warrants urgent evaluation and management. The primary clinical entities that constitute this constellation of signs and symptoms include torsion of the testicle, torsion of the testicular appendages, and epididymitis-orchitis (Figure 67-1).

### *Torsion of the Testicle*

Testicular torsion is the twisting of the spermatic cord, with resulting compromise of the blood supply to the testis. This compromise and the risk it poses for testicular loss makes torsion a surgical emergency. In the neonate, the torsion occurs on the cord above the insertion of the tunica vaginalis (ie, extravaginal torsion). In the adolescent, the *bell clapper deformity* leads to torsion on the cord within the confines of the tunica vaginalis (ie, intravaginal torsion). Torsion of the spermatic cord first causes venous congestion, which

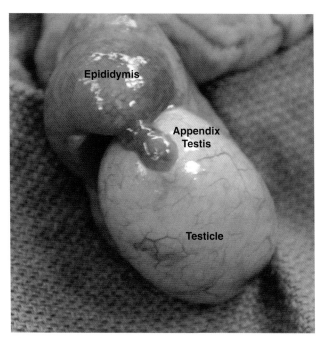


**Figure 67-1**
Structures of the scrotum.

is followed by compromise of arterial blood flow. Spermatogenesis may be compromised after 4 to 6 hours of ischemia.[1] Similarly, testicular salvage is time dependent, with universal loss of the testis after 24 hours of torsion. A familial tendency has been described, and although the mode of inheritance remains ill-defined, 1 family with 3 generations has been identified.[2] In addition, there may be some seasonal variation in the presentation of acute testicular torsion with a predilection for the colder months,[3,4] although this has not been true in all series.[4]

## Incidence

Testicular torsion occurs in 1 in 4,000 boys. Although a peak in incidence occurs in the neonatal period, testicular torsion more commonly occurs between the ages of 12 and 18 years. Nevertheless, testicular torsion should not be excluded from the differential diagnosis of acute scrotal swelling and pain based on age.

## Evaluation

The history typically describes acute onset of constant, severe scrotal pain aggravated by physical activity and sometimes alleviated by being still. If periods of acute respite from the pain occur, then intermittent torsion and detorsion should be considered. Nausea and vomiting may occur. The patient may have a history of incidental antecedent scrotal trauma, but the onset of pain usually occurs during periods of rest or sleep. Characteristic findings on physical examination include scrotal erythema and swelling of the involved hemiscrotum. Further inspection may reveal a higher-than-normal position of the testis within the scrotum and may also demonstrate a horizontal rather than the normal vertical orientation of the testicle. Evaluation of the cremasteric reflex should begin on the contralateral side, along with palpation of the apparently unaffected testis to confirm normal size and position. Unilateral loss of the cremasteric reflex on the side of the swelling and pain highly correlates with the presence of torsion.[5] The testis should then be palpated despite the pain the maneuver may cause to help differentiate torsion from epididymitis. With torsion, exquisite pain is elicited on palpation from the testis, as well as from the epididymis and distal spermatic cord. In some instances, the actual point of torsion of the spermatic cord can be palpated. An associated hydrocele may be palpated and confirmed by transillumination. A tense or large hydrocele often makes the examination difficult. Urinalysis is unremarkable, and although the white blood cell count may be mildly elevated, it is not discriminating. Imaging by nuclear scintigraphy[6,7] or Doppler ultrasound[8,9] should be performed if the diagnosis of testicular torsion is in question, but only when it will not unduly delay surgical exploration if a torsion exists, adding to the risk for testicular loss. The absence of blood flow on Doppler and the presence of heterogeneous parenchyma are indicative of a "missed torsion" and a nonsalvageable testis.[10]

## Treatment

Surgical intervention is not only indicated when testicular torsion is strongly suspected, but also should be considered in equivocal cases when torsion cannot be convincingly excluded. The likelihood of salvaging the testis, the goal of surgical exploration, is highest when surgery occurs shortly after the onset of pain; the chance for a successful outcome dissipates rapidly with time (Figure 67-2). With surgery, the affected testis is explored first, and when torsion

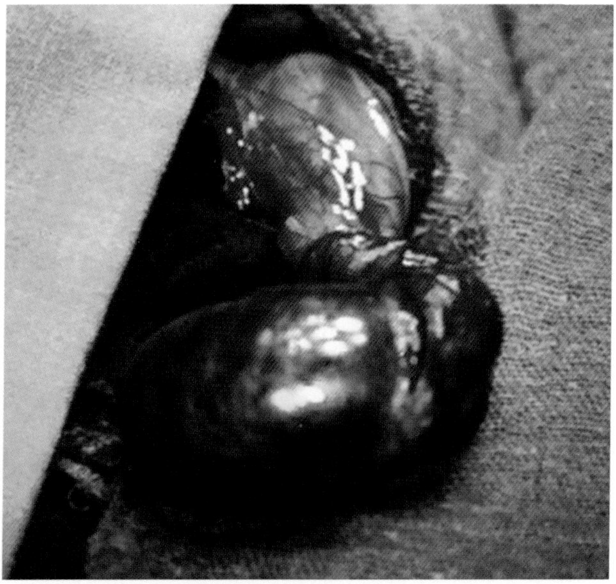

**Figure 67-2**
Intraoperative photograph of nonsalvageable testis after prolonged period of pain.

is present, the cord is detorsed. The contralateral testis, which may have the same anatomic defect, is explored and fixed in place to avert a future metachronous torsion. The affected gonad is then reinspected and the possibility of salvage determined. If the testis can be saved, then it is fixed in the scrotum. Subsequent atrophy may still result because of the vascular insult,[11] and fertility may be compromised as well.[12]

When testicular torsion is diagnosed, manual detorsion can be attempted while surgery is being arranged. The testis is twisted either clockwise or counterclockwise. When twisting in 1 direction has not succeeded, an attempt in the opposite direction can be made. When the procedure is successful, the return of blood flow to the testis provides rapid relief from pain. If manual detorsion can be accomplished preoperatively, then the surgical intervention to tack down the testes can be performed electively.[13]

### Neonatal Testicular Torsion

Neonatal testicular torsion can exhibit at delivery as a nontender hard scrotal mass. Salvage in these cases is rare, and emergent exploration is futile.[14] At exploration, the contralateral testis should be anchored and the nonviable testis removed. Although neonatal torsion can occur after delivery, this is very uncommon and then is more typical of torsion in the older patient, with a greater potential for salvage if intervention is rapid.

### Torsion of the Appendix Testis

#### Evaluation

Torsion of the appendix testis or appendix epididymis may lead to a clinical picture similar to that of the more consequential and urgent torsion of the spermatic cord. The appendix testis is a vestige of the Müllerian duct system and hangs from the anterior surface of the testis where it meets the head of the epididymis. When it torses, inflammation and swelling of the testis and epididymis ensues, causing testicular pain and scrotal erythema. The onset of pain and swelling is commonly acute but can be progressive, usually occurring during periods of rest. The pain can be severe, but nausea and vomiting are less common than with testicular torsion. The physical examination may demonstrate hemiscrotal erythema and swelling. The *blue dot sign*, with the necrotic appendage visible through the scrotal skin, can help make the diagnosis.[15] A normal cremasteric reflex is present bilaterally, and the testis is normally positioned within the scrotum. Testicular discomfort, if present, is typically mild, but point tenderness may be elicited from the uppermost pole of the testis near the head of the epididymis—the location of the appendages. On palpation, the examiner may feel a 3- to 5-mm tender indurated mass on the upper pole. In some cases, the inflammatory process resulting from torsion of the appendage can lead to physical findings that make differentiating from true spermatic cord torsion impossible. In these cases, imaging may be helpful because either scrotal Doppler ultrasound or nuclear scintigraphy will demonstrate normal or increased flow to the ipsilateral testis.

#### Treatment

The management of the torsed appendage is nonsurgical. The patient should rest and use nonsteroidal pain relievers and cold compresses for several days to reduce the inflammation, swelling, and pain. Surgical intervention is indicated only when the diagnosis of acute testicular torsion cannot be excluded. In these cases, the infarcted appendage is removed at surgical exploration.

## Acute Epididymitis-Orchitis

### Evaluation

Acute inflammation of the epididymis or testis occurs in both young and older boys. Uncommon in the younger child, it usually results from an anomaly of the urinary tract, either congenital or acquired, which can often be identified by renal and bladder sonography.[16] Renal duplications and posterior urethral valves are among the more common anomalies. Traditionally, a voiding cystourethrogram has been a routine part of the evaluation, but its yield is low with a normal ultrasound and a sterile urine. In children who perform intermittent catheterization, epididymo-orchitis can occur from the retrograde passage of bacteria back from the ejaculatory ducts at the level of the prostate to the testis and epididymis.[17]

In the older child and adolescent, the history and physical examination may help distinguish epididymitis or orchitis from testicular torsion or appendix torsion, but this is not always the case. The history can reveal an acute or more protracted onset of pain. The patient may have fever or dysuria. Epididymal inflammation may arise after scrotal trauma. In the adolescent patient, a history of sexual activity or a urethral discharge helps guide antibiotic treatment. The physical examination reveals scrotal erythema and swelling and an intact cremasteric reflex. Palpation during the early phase of the inflammatory process demonstrates tenderness limited to the epididymis, whereas in the later phase, the tenderness and inflammation include both the epididymis and testis, and the distinction between the 2 structures may be difficult to appreciate. The Prehn sign (relief of pain with testicular elevation) may be positive.

Laboratory and radiologic imaging are useful in these cases. Urinalysis may prove positive for white blood cells and nitrite but is often unremarkable among adolescents. The white blood cell count is usually elevated. Ultrasound and nuclear scintigraphy studies demonstrate either normal symmetrical blood flow or increased blood flow to an enlarged epididymis or testis.

### Treatment

Management of epididymo-orchitis requires antibiotic therapy that is based on the results of the urine culture and sensitivities. In the sexually active adolescent, the choice of antibiotic coverage must also include coverage of gonococcal and nongonococcal sexually transmitted infections. Additionally, anti-inflammatory agents, scrotal elevation, and rest should be prescribed.

## Other Causes of Acute Swelling and Pain of the Scrotum

### Henoch-Schönlein Purpura

Henoch-Schönlein purpura is a systemic vasculitis that can cause abdominal pain, joint pain, renal disease, and bleeding from the gastrointestinal tract and may involve the scrotal wall in a minority of cases. The onset may be insidious or acute, producing a variable degree of erythema and edema. In more severe cases, the process may involve the testis and epididymis, mimicking testicular torsion.[18] The presence of concurrent Henoch-Schönlein purpura and testicular torsion has been reported; therefore, if torsion is a consideration, then imaging with either Doppler ultrasound or nuclear scintigraphy is indicated to evaluate testicular blood flow. Surgical exploration may be needed in equivocal cases.

### Focal Fat Necrosis

Focal fat necrosis can result in scrotal pain and swelling,[19] usually after trauma, in an obese boy. The examination demonstrates pain and swelling limited to the scrotum and not the testis; however, the examination can be limited by the discomfort and the degree of obesity. If properly diagnosed, then management consists of rest and anti-inflammatory agents. When spermatic cord torsion cannot be excluded clinically, either an imaging study or immediate surgical exploration is indicated.

### Trauma

Injuries can vary from zipper entrapment of scrotal skin to more severe blunt or straddle trauma affecting the scrotal contents. The history can be definitive. The physical examination must include both hemiscrotums and the surrounding structures (penis, perineum), assessing for swelling, ecchymosis, and bleeding. Palpation may be limited by the degree of swelling or blood within the scrotum. The tenderness may be limited to the testis or the epididymis, depending on the extent of the trauma. Scrotal ultrasound can document the integrity of the testis and of the tunica albuginea and the adequacy of blood flow.[20] Testicular or spermatic cord contusions are managed symptomatically, whereas testicular rupture may require surgical exploration, evacuation of the hematoma, debridement, and repair (when possible); however, a nonsurgical approach has been reported.[21]

### Mumps Orchitis

Mumps orchitis can occur at any age but is more common among adolescents. Rarely occurring in isolation, the pain and swelling usually occur within 1 week after parotitis. The physical examination demonstrates a tender testis. Treatment is symptomatic. Infertility may occur when mumps orchitis results in atrophy of both testicles.[22]

### Scrotal Skin Disease

Insect bites, folliculitis, and allergic dermatitis may cause erythema and edema of the scrotal wall. The history may be of limited utility. The examination reveals redness and edema limited to the scrotum, with a normal testicle and spermatic cord. Idiopathic scrotal edema affects children younger than 14 years, with acute erythema, edema, and mild scrotal wall tenderness, sparing the testis and cord.[23] The process resolves spontaneously. The management includes rest and scrotal elevation.

## ▶ SCROTAL SWELLING WITHOUT PAIN

### *Inguinal Hernias and Hydroceles*

Hernias and hydroceles, the most common causes of scrotal swelling, fall along a continuum (Figure 67-3). They are more common in premature infants and are predominately

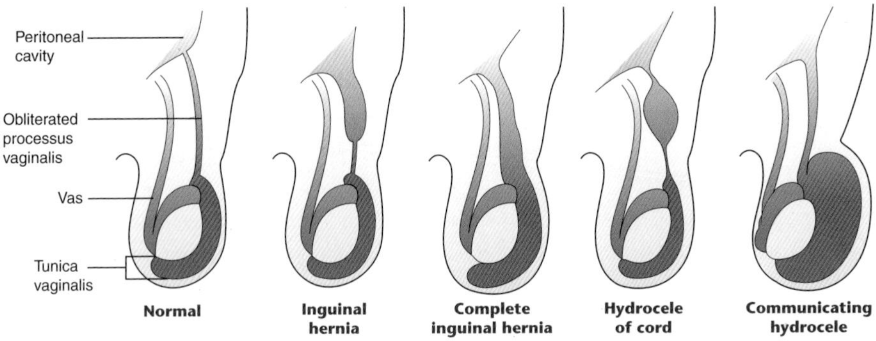


**Figure 67-3**
Diagram of the continuum of hernia and hydrocele.

right sided. Most inguinal hernias and hydroceles are caused by persistent patency of the processus vaginalis (PPV), a peritoneal evagination that accompanies the testis during its abdominal-scrotal descent. The layers of the processus vaginalis condense late in gestation or early postnatally. Obliteration of the processus vaginalis only around the testis leads to an indirect inguinal hernia with the protrusion of fluid (or other contents) through the internal ring to the end of the pouch and potentially to the scrotum. A communicating hydrocele occurs when fluid travels through a PPV into the tunica vaginalis around the testis. A scrotal hydrocele occurs after complete obliteration proximally with patency distally. Hydroceles of the cord occur when the processus vaginalis obliterates proximally and distally, leaving a patent area in the midportion with retained fluid.

Inguinal hernias and hydroceles may be asymptomatic or may have a spectrum of symptoms. A hernia can occur at any age as an inguinal swelling extending toward and potentially reaching the scrotum. The swelling expands with increases in intraabdominal pressure (eg, crying, bowel movements, coughing, exercise). The parent or child will often report the swelling to be smallest in the morning and greatest later in the day. When omentum is in the hernia sac, the likelihood of spontaneous reduction is low, and periods of discomfort can occur. An incarcerated hernia can produce pain, fever, nausea, vomiting, and irritability. A hydrocele is usually an asymptomatic bulge in the scrotum. In many instances, whether the hydrocele is acute or whether the scrotum has been chronically enlarged is unclear. The patient may have a history of trauma to the scrotum that stimulates the production of serous fluid. When the scrotum changes sizes during the day, the physician should suspect a communicating hydrocele.

## Evaluation

The physical examination is often sufficient to distinguish among these entities. The examiner should feel for the testis first and keep it in mind during the rest of the examination so as to avoid confusing it with the contents of an incarcerated hernia. A bulge in the inguinal region with fluid that can be gently reduced back into the abdomen is diagnostic of an inguinal hernia. In the cooperative child who can increase his intraabdominal pressure, this procedure may be repeatedly demonstrated particularly with the child standing. When the fluid is limited to the testis and the spermatic cord can be palpated above the fluid, a hydrocele is present. The presence of a thickened spermatic cord or a *silk stocking sign* (the feel of the layers of the processus vaginalis being rubbed against each other) is suggestive of a PPV or a hernia, which is helpful in distinguishing a scrotal hydrocele from a communicating hydrocele. Hydroceles transilluminate, but so can the incarcerated bowel of an infant. A hydrocele of the spermatic cord feels distinct from the testis and is round or ovoid, possibly mimicking the presence of an additional testis. Hydroceles, whether communicating, scrotal, or of the cord, are rarely associated with tenderness on palpation.

Ultrasound can be useful to delineate the scrotal contents, especially when a large or tense hydrocele limits the physical examination, and to determine the cystic or solid nature of a tense scrotal mass (eg, hydrocele, tumor) or spermatic cord mass (eg, hydrocele of the cord, paratesticular tumor). Laboratory tests are useful only in cases of incarcerated inguinal hernias, with an elevated white blood cell count and possible acidosis.

### Treatment

Inguinal hernias and communicating hydroceles should be repaired on diagnosis to prevent incarceration. The risk for incarceration increases with time and is more likely in the young child or infant. Communicating hydroceles should also be repaired on diagnosis to avert progression. Surgery is performed inguinally, during which the sac is isolated from the cord structures and ligated at the level of the internal ring. The likelihood of a PPV on the contralateral side is highest in younger children, and the need for contralateral exploration remains controversial. However, diagnostic laparoscopy through the isolated ipsilateral sac allows visualization of the contralateral ring[24] (Figure 67-4). If the internal ring is open, then contralateral surgical correction proceeds. Most hydroceles resolve spontaneously by 1 year and should be repaired if they persist beyond this age. However, if the hydrocele is painful, tense, and large, then surgery should proceed sooner. In younger children, the surgical approach is inguinal; in older boys and adolescents, a scrotal approach is appropriate.

## Tumors

Testicular tumors are uncommon in children, accounting for 1% to 2% of all solid tumors, but occur in all age groups. Fortunately, about 74% of prepubertal testis tumors are benign.[25] Tumors are usually displayed as a hard, painless (or a vague, heavy-feeling) mass in the testicle detected by the child, parent, or examining physician. On palpation, the mass is harder than the substance of the testis, but this distinction may be difficult to discern. The mass may bulge from the surface of the testis. Tumors do not transilluminate. Scrotal ultrasound is used to delineate the mass and in some cases help to assess whether the mass is likely to be benign (anechoic). Preoperative tumor markers ($\alpha$-fetoprotein [AFP], $\beta$-human chorionic gonadotropin) should be drawn and used for postoperative monitoring. AFP cannot be used effectively as a tumor marker until it is no longer produced at about 8 months of age. Staging depends on serum markers, computed tomography (CT) imaging of the retroperitoneum and chest, and pathology. The surgical approach depends on the nature of the mass. All cases are approached through an inguinal incision in case the mass is malignant. Mature teratoma, the most common testis tumor among prepubertal males, is benign and is managed by testis-sparing surgery. Immature teratoma has also been successfully managed without removing the testis.[25,26] Yolk sac tumor is the second most common tumor and presents with elevated AFP levels (recall caveat above). Radical orchiectomy is curative in more than 90% of cases

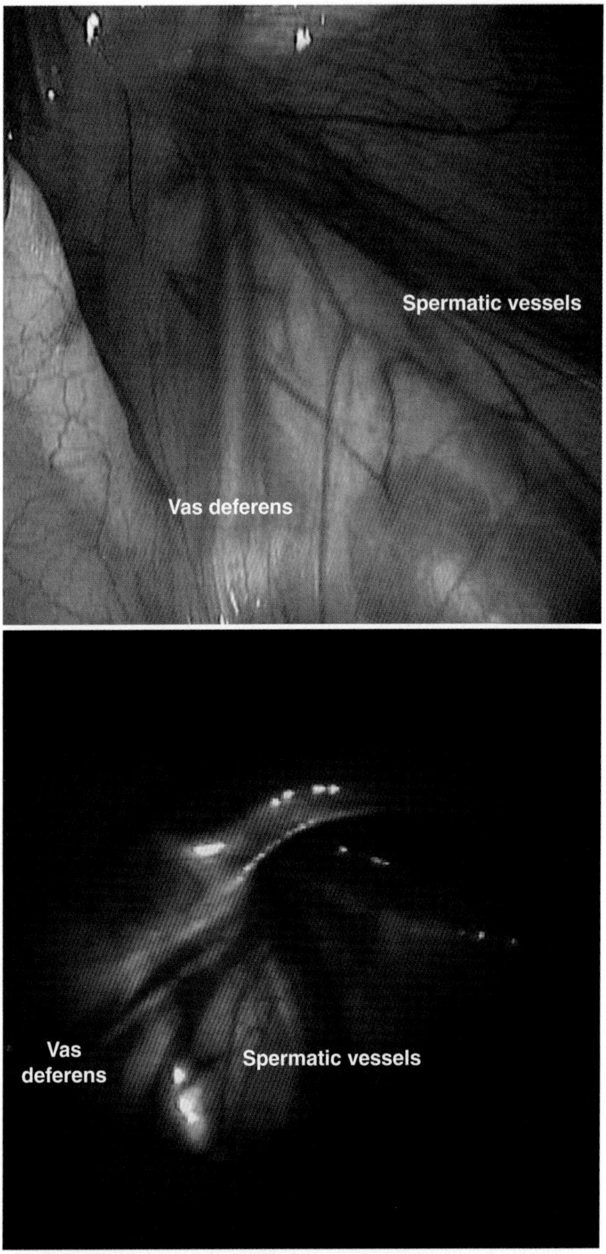


**Figure 67-4**
Laparoscopic appearance of a closed *(top)* and an open *(bottom)* internal inguinal ring. The ring appears at junction of the vas deferens and the internal spermatic vessels.

(stage 1); platinum-based chemotherapy and possible retroperitoneal lymph node dissection may be needed for higher stage disease. Boys with Leydig cell tumors present with a solid testis mass and precocious puberty and can be treated with tumor enucleation. Gonadoblastoma occurs in dysgenetic gonads of children with disorders of sexual differentiation carrying a Y chromosome.

### Varicoceles

Varicoceles, which are dilations of the spermatic veins or pampiniform plexus, are present in 15% of male adolescents and adults and may have a negative impact on fertility. The dilated veins are usually asymptomatic and are detected either by the patient or by the physician during routine physical examination, usually between 10 and 15 years of age. On occasion, the patient may report some heaviness or a *dragging* feeling in the scrotum. A predilection for the left side exists, reflecting the anatomy of the left gonadal vein entering the left renal vein at a right angle. The right gonadal vein enters the vena cava directly at an angle, precluding reflux of venous blood. The presence of bilateral or right-sided varicoceles warrants an abdominal and pelvic ultrasound or CT scan to evaluate for a possible mass occluding venous return. Physical examination should be performed with the patient in the supine and standing positions; the varicocele is usually decompressed in the supine position and present in the standing position. Inspection may reveal the classic *bag of worms* of dilated veins (grade 3 of 3). In other cases, increased blood pooling in the veins can be prompted by a Valsalva maneuver (grade 2 of 3). Less commonly, a varicocele is detected only by ultrasound (grade 1 of 3). Testicular size, most accurately assessed by ultrasound, should be measured[27]; a significant loss of testicular volume is one indication for surgery. Other indications for repair include abnormal semen analysis (older adolescent patients), very large varicoceles, and pain. Corrective measures include open surgery, laparoscopic surgery, or radiologic ablative techniques—all aimed at occluding direct venous return through the internal spermatic vein to improve the likelihood of normal fertility. In most cases, the testis will subsequently increase in size to equal that of the contralateral testis.[28]

### Spermatoceles and Epididymal Cysts

Spermatoceles and epididymal cysts represent sperm-filled cystic lesions attached to the upper pole of the testis. They are separate from the testis and can be transilluminated. Painless and round, they usually remain stable in size but can sometimes enlarge. Management consists typically of observation, but surgery may be indicated when pain or significant enlargement is present. Postoperative scarring can obstruct the epididymal ductal system and lead to infertility.[29]

## When to Refer

- Acute painful scrotal swelling
- Acute hydrocele
- Hernia
- Scrotal trauma
- Cellulitis of scrotum
- Varicocele
- Testicular mass
- Paratesticular mass

### TOOLS FOR PRACTICE

#### Engaging Patient and Family

- *Hydroceles and Inguinal Hernias* (fact sheet), American Urological Association (www.urologyhealth.org/urology/index.cfm?article=129)

- *Neonatal Testicular Torsion* (fact sheet), American Urological Association (www.urologyhealth.org/urology/index.cfm?article=7)
- *Testicular Trauma* (fact sheet), American Urological Association (www.urologyhealth.org/urology/index.cfm?article=35)

## REFERENCES


1. Bartsch G, Frank S, Marberger H, Mikuz G. Testicular torsion: late results with special regard to fertility and endocrine function. *J Urol.* 1980;124:375–378
2. Cubillos J, Palmer JS, Friedman SC, et al. Familial testicular torsion. *J Urol.* 2011;185(6 Suppl): 2469–2472
3. Lyronis ID, Ploumis N, Vlahakis I, Charissis G. Acute scrotum -etiology, clinical presentation and seasonal variation. *Indian J Pediatr.* 2009;76:407–410
4. Srinivasan AK, Freyle J, Gitlin JS, Palmer LS. Climatic conditions and the risk of testicular torsion in adolescent males. *J Urol.* 2007;178:2585–2588
5. Rabinowitz R. The importance of the cremasteric reflex in acute scrotal swelling in children. *J Urol.* 1984;132:89–90
6. Falkowski WS, Firlit CF. Testicular torsion: the role of radioisotopic scanning. *J Urol.* 1980;124: 886–888
7. Mendel JB, Taylor GA, Treves S, et al. Testicular torsion in children: scintigraphic assessment. *Pediatr Radiol.* 1985;15:110–115
8. Baker LA, Sigman D, Mathews RI, Benson J, Docimo SG. An analysis of clinical outcomes using color doppler testicular ultrasound for testicular torsion. *Pediatrics.* 2000;105:604–607
9. Nussbaum Blask AR, Bulas D, Shalaby-Rana E, et al. Color Doppler sonography and scintigraphy of the testis: a prospective, comparative analysis in children with acute scrotal pain. *Pediatr Emerg Care.* 2002;18:67–71
10. Kaye JD, Shapiro EY, Levitt SB, et al. Parenchymal echo texture predicts testicular salvage after torsion: potential impact on the need for emergent exploration. *J Urol.* 2008;180:1733–1736
11. Sessions AE, Rabinowitz R, Hulbert WC, Goldstein MM, Mevorach RA. Testicular torsion: direction, degree, duration and disinformation. *J Urol.* 2003;169:663–665
12. Nagler HM, White RD. The effect of testicular torsion on the contralateral testis. *J Urol.* 1982;128:1343–1348
13. Cornel EB, Karthaus HF. Manual derotation of the twisted spermatic cord. *BJU Int.* 1999;83: 672–674
14. Kaye JD, Levitt SB, Friedman SC, et al. Neonatal torsion: a 14-year experience and proposed algorithm for management. *J Urol.* 2008;179:2377–2383
15. Dresner ML. Torsed appendage. Diagnosis and management: blue dot sign. *Urology.* 1973;1:63–66
16. Siegel A, Snyder H, Duckett JW. Epididymitis in infants and boys: underlying urogenital anomalies and efficacy of imaging modalities. *J Urol.* 1987;138:1100–1103
17. Lindehall B, Abrahamsson K, Hjälmās K, et al. Complications of clean intermittent catheterization in boys and young males with neurogenic bladder dysfunction. *J Urol.* 2004;172:1686–1688
18. Khan AU, Williams TH, Malek RS. Acute scrotal swelling in Henoch-Schönlein syndrome. *Urology.* 1977;10:139–141
19. Hollander JB, Begun FP, Lee RD. Scrotal fat necrosis. *J Urol.* 1985;134:150–151
20. Buckley JC, McAninch JW. Use of ultrasonography for the diagnosis of testicular injuries in blunt scrotal trauma. *J Urol.* 2006;175:175–178
21. Cubillos J, Reda EF, Gitlin J, Zelkovic P, Palmer LS. A conservative approach to testicular rupture in adolescent boys. *J Urol.* 2010;184:1733–1738
22. Philip J, Selvan D, Desmond AD. Mumps orchitis in the non-immune postpubertal male: a resurgent threat to male fertility? *BJU Int.* 2006;97:138–141
23. Kaplan GW. Acute idiopathic scrotal edema. *J Pediatr Surg.* 1977;12:647–649

24. Miltenburg DM, Nuchtern JG, Jaksic T, Kozinetiz C, Brandt ML. Laparoscopic evaluation of the pediatric inguinal hernia—a meta-analysis. *J Pediatr Surg.* 1998;33:874–879
25. Pohl HG, Shukla AR, Metcalf PD, et al. Prepubertal testis tumors: actual prevalence rate of histological types. *J Urol.* 2004;172:2370–2372
26. Shukla AR, Woodward C, Carr MC, et al. Experience with testis sparing surgery for testicular teratoma. *J Urol.* 2004;171:161–163
27. Diamond DA, Paltiel HJ, DiCanzio J, et al. Comparative assessment of pediatric testicular volume: orchidometer versus ultrasound. *J Urol.* 2000;164:1111–1114
28. Atassi O, Kass EJ, Steinert BW. Testicular growth after successful varicocele correction in adolescents: comparison of artery sparing techniques with the Palomo procedure. *J Urol.* 1995;153:482–483
29. Zahalsky MP, Berman AJ, Nagler HM. Evaluating the risk of epididymal injury during hydrocelectomy and spermatocelectomy. *J Urol.* 2004;171:2291–2292
30. Shukla RB, Kelly DG, Daly L, Guiney EJ. Association of cold weather with testicular torsion. *Br Med J (Clin Res Ed).* 1982;285(6353):1459–1460

# Chapter 68

# Self-harm

*Nancy Heath, PhD; Jessica R. Toste, PhD; Timothy R. Moore, PhD; Frank Symons, PhD*

## ▶ FOUNDATIONS OF SELF-INJURY

Self-injury in children and youth may be grouped into 2 classifications: self-injury with intent to die (suicidal behaviors) and self-injury without intent to die (nonsuicidal self-injurious behaviors). Two of the best-known behaviors within the nonsuicidal classification are *nonsuicidal self-injury* (NSSI), occurring in typically developing children and youth, and *self-injurious behavior* (SIB), most common among children and youth with intellectual and developmental disabilities. Although cases of NSSI are seen more commonly than SIB in clinical practice, SIB is generally the more severe behavior. However, both forms of self-injury pose significant challenges to pediatricians. The chapter describes the independent and converging characteristics and features of each of these presentations of self-injury.

### *Definition and Types of Self-injury*

Nonsuicidal self-injury refers to the deliberate destruction of one's own body tissue, occurring without suicidal intent and for purposes not socially sanctioned. Thus, NSSI excludes piercings and tattoos. Most commonly, NSSI includes superficial to moderate self-cutting, burning, scratching, and bruising. NSSI occurs among typically developing children and adolescents. This behavior is often engaged in repetitively over long periods of time, with increasing severity, and has been found to be a significant risk factor for future suicidal behaviors.[1] Furthermore, these self-inflicted injuries can result in medical complications, infection, or permanent scarring. Historically, this behavior has also been referred to as *self-mutilation*, *self-harm*, and *parasuicide*. The definition of NSSI excludes extreme forms of body mutilation (eg, amputation, enucleation) seen in patients with psychosis, as well as stereotypical self-injury seen among individuals with intellectual and developmental disabilities (IDD).

SIB among children and youth with IDD shares a similar definition with NSSI. SIB is defined as physical acts directed to one's own body that result in or produce tissue damage, or have the possibility of producing tissue damage if left unchecked. However, the most common forms of SIB are different from those of NSSI, and may include head banging, biting, scratching, pinching, and rubbing. Chronic SIB poses tremendous challenges for affected individuals and their families. Indeed, SIB is among the most disturbing and serious of all behaviors exhibited by children with IDD, because it has profound implications for a child's health and quality of life. SIB often leads to increased risk for institutionalization and social stigmatization, and decreased opportunities to learn.

## Epidemiology

The onset of NSSI most commonly occurs in early adolescence (12–14 years), although it is increasingly common for this behavior to occur among prepubertal children.[2] Research has found that between 14% and 20% of adolescents in community samples report having engaged in NSSI at least once during their lifetime. Studies of mental health issues in college students have reported comparable lifetime prevalence estimates, suggesting that rates of NSSI are similar from adolescence to young adulthood. Currently, there has been no research investigating the prevalence of NSSI among prepubertal children in the general population; however, there is a clear indication from retrospective reports of self-injurers, as well as anecdotal reports (eg, physicians, school professionals) that NSSI does occur among children. In contrast to studies conducted with community samples, lifetime prevalence estimates of NSSI among clinical adolescent samples are substantially higher, with rates ranging from 60% to 80%.[3]

Interestingly, while research has found NSSI rates to be much higher among females in clinical settings,[4] the same pattern is not consistently found in community samples. Some studies have found a female predominance in the behavior,[5,6] while others conclude that there may be little or no gender difference in occurrence of NSSI.[7–10] In a review of the literature of NSSI among adolescents, Heath and colleagues[11] found that studies reporting gender differences have included overdose and medication abuse, which have been found to be largely female behaviors. Investigations that are limited to cutting, burning, self-hitting to bruise, and other forms of tissue damage have failed to find a gender difference. Thus, it is important to avoid the assumption that NSSI is a predominantly female behavior in community practice, even though girls are more likely to be seen in clinical settings.

Findings regarding age of onset and gender patterns for SIB are notably different from those for NSSI. SIB occurs at all levels of IDD across the lifespan, with greater frequency typically reported among children with more severe intellectual impairments. The specific age of onset is typically unknown, but reports documenting SIB have included children as young as 18 months.[12] Epidemiologic estimates vary depending on study design and participant characteristics, but it is estimated that approximately 20% of individuals with IDD living in large aggregate care facilities exhibit some form of self-injury.[13] Unlike NSSI, there are clear gender differences in occurrence of SIB, with males overrepresented by a ratio of approximately 4 to 1. There have been no studies directly addressing ethnic differences in the prevalence of NSSI or SIB among children with IDD.

## Etiology and Function

For many years, self-injury occurring outside of the IDD population was believed to be indicative of severe psychiatric disorders, particularly borderline personality disorder (BPD).[14,15] However, emerging research has shown that NSSI is not limited to individuals with BPD. Research has revealed that this behavior serves a number of different functions.[16–18] These may be understood as falling into 2 broad categories: functions that serve an internal or automatic purpose (eg, to elicit a calm feeling or eliminate tension) or functions that serve an external or social purpose (eg, as a form of communication or to elicit a response). For most individuals who engage in NSSI, emotion regulation difficulties are at the root of this behavior.[16,19–22] These youth experience their intense negative emotions as intolerable and use NSSI to gain relief.

Although use of NSSI to regulate internal states or emotions has received the most support in the literature, for a minority of youth it seems that social factors may also play a role in this behavior.[11,23] It has been suggested that in these cases NSSI serves as a form of communication to parents and peers when alternative forms of communication are perceived as being ineffective.[17] Thus, for typically developing youth, the primary function of the behavior is to obtain relief from an internal state or experience. In contrast, as discussed below, SIB among children and youth with IDD is most often found to serve an environmental or social function (eg, to gain attention from others or to escape from task demands); however, it is recognized that an automatic function may also be involved in many cases (eg, to attain relief from pain caused by an underlying medical condition).

Advances in behavioral assessment technology have led to remarkable progress in identifying environmental[24–26] and biologic[27,28] variables underlying SIB. While the etiology of SIB may be related to an undiagnosed painful medical condition in some cases,[29] the specific etiology of SIB is unknown in most cases. Little is known about the behavioral or biologic mechanisms influencing the early development of SIB in young children with IDD.[30] Communication impairment associated with IDD is a primary risk factor, as is the overall severity of the intellectual impairment.

### Co-occurring Disorders

Research on co-occurrence is crucial for knowing how to assess and treat youth who engage in different forms of self-injury. For example, because the underlying functions of NSSI are similar to those of other mental health issues, it is necessary to be aware of which conditions tend to occur with NSSI and how to effectively assess and monitor them. Some of the most commonly co-occurring disorders include mood disorder, anxiety disorder, impulse control/conduct problems, uncontrolled anger, BPD, alcohol or substance abuse, eating disorders, and suicidality.[31]

Similarly, a number of IDD-related syndromes tend to occur with SIB. The most common of these include Lesch-Nyhan syndrome, fragile X syndrome, Cornelia deLange syndrome, Prader-Willi syndrome, and Rett syndrome.[32,33] Whether there are mechanisms specific to any single genetic disorder and the expression of SIB is unclear but unlikely.

## ▶ EVALUATION

Diagnostic and treatment approaches to NSSI and SIB differ substantially. NSSI is largely hidden and may range in severity or treatment needs; therefore, much of the focus for the physician is on early risk assessment and referral to appropriate treatment. In contrast, SIB necessitates an initial ruling out of a possible underlying medical condition followed by the need for a full behavioral evaluation by a behavior analyst certified by the Behavior Analyst Certification Board (BACB.com). Interestingly, despite the obvious differences between the diagnostic approaches to NSSI and SIB, both share the difficulty of preconceived notions regarding the behavior (based on common misconceptions) and the lack of consideration of both internal and external functions. For clarity, the following section is divided into separate, brief reviews of NSSI and SIB.

## *Nonsuicidal Self-injury*

### Signs and Symptoms

A particularly challenging aspect of NSSI among children and youth is that it is a largely hidden behavior. Most youth engaging in the behavior make great efforts to keep the behavior secret, perhaps revealing only to friends or peers in online communities.[34] Despite the child's reluctance to reveal the behavior, physical examination of the child will reveal fresh injuries, scars, burns, or unexplained bruises that are clearly indicative of NSSI. Some individuals will limit themselves to pin or razor blade scratching that they may explain as "cat scratches." Awareness of NSSI in typically developing youth ensures that physicians are cautious in their interpretation of signs of injury (eg, bruising, burning, or cutting) as signs of physical abuse (intentional harm by another).

One of the most significant obstacles to identification of NSSI by physicians is a lack of awareness of this behavior. It is widely thought that self-injury is largely a female behavior and limited to self-cutting; thus, NSSI is often overlooked in males or when other methods of injury are involved. Rather than understanding the underlying emotion regulation or "coping" function, physicians who encounter cases of NSSI often misidentify it as a suicide attempt or physical abuse, or assume that there are underlying disorders (eg, BPD, eating disorders). Additionally, physicians must recognize the high rate of occurrence for NSSI in youth and that the behavior is not limited to specific social cliques (eg, "emos" or "goths").

### Diagnostic Approach

Of particular importance is the need to distinguish between NSSI and suicidal behaviors. In the past, researchers have often failed to distinguish between self-injury with and without suicidal intent.[11] However, suicide attempts and NSSI are distinct behaviors and should be understood, managed, and treated differently. Suicide attempts are behaviors that may or may not result in injury, for which there is intent to die. In contrast, NSSI is a behavior in which immediate tissue damage is present, but for which there is no intent to die. In essence, suicidal behaviors express a wish to stop living, whereas NSSI is reported by the youth as an attempt to feel better without any conscious desire to die. Nevertheless, these behaviors are not mutually exclusive, and some youth engage in both, albeit at different times and with different intents. Therefore, it is important to evaluate for both suicidal and nonsuicidal self-injury.

### Risk Assessment and Effective Referral

A key role of the pediatrician is to complete a risk assessment to determine the current risk level and make appropriate referrals. Assessment includes evaluation of risk for suicide, physical injury, and the presence of other co-occurring risk factors. In determining risk-level status, the physician must recognize that there is no simple formula for determining whether a youth is at high or low risk. Nevertheless, if there is increased risk for suicide or physical injury, or if there are significant mental health concerns, then the risk-level status of the patient increases. Despite the extensive list of factors contributing to risk stratification, many patients who self-injure remain in the low-risk category. These patients may have mild, nonclinical levels of depression, anxiety, negative body image, or self-derogation and may seem to be functioning extremely well academically, socially, and within their home environment. Despite this apparent positive presentation, research has found that engaging in NSSI (even if only a few times) indicates problematic emotional regulation and a need for intervention to develop more adaptive coping strategies.[35] Furthermore, it is known that risk level for suicide by individuals who engage in NSSI is substantial and subject to change over time; thus, regular reassessment is essential.

### *Self-injurious Behavior*

#### Signs and Symptoms

The physician should be aware that SIB injuries can have pattern-mark appearances and can be mistaken for physical abuse. Children with developmental disabilities, however, may be at higher risk for abuse or neglect. Careful history, risk assessment, and physical examination are warranted.

Presence of SIB often includes biting of the hands, arms, or lips; banging the head on solid surfaces; hitting the head or face with a closed fist or open palm; eye-poking; or scratching, picking, pinching, or rubbing skin.[36] Mild, moderate, or permanent tissue damage and disfigurement, possibly life threatening, can occur if SIB is left untreated.[37]

#### Diagnostic Approach

Behavioral evaluation of SIB is predicated on 3 empirically based assumptions: (1) SIB is functional, learned behavior (ie, a function, in part, of its circumstances and consequences); (2) the momentary likelihood of SIB is influenced by antecedent stimulus conditions (ie, it occurs more often in the presence of certain people, places, materials, demand contexts, and biological states than in others); (3) intervention linked to function (ie, related to antecedents and consequences) rather than form alone will result in superior, clinically significant outcomes.[38–40] Behavioral evaluations require effort, time, and trained staff to administer and interpret, but lead to effective interventions more quickly than alternatives not based on behavioral function.

#### Functional Assessment and Analysis of Behavior

Physicians who eliminate the possibility of underlying medical conditions and determine that SIB warrants evaluation should refer the patient to a board-certified behavior analyst (BCBA). State-by-state and provincial listings of BCBAs are available. Two broad categories of clinical evaluation procedures are available: functional assessment[41–44] and functional analysis.[24,45] Both types of evaluations are designed to generate information about environmental antecedents to, and contingent consequences of, behavior that can be directly linked to interventions. Functional assessments generate descriptive accounts of contextual and antecedent precursors to behavior as well as outcomes produced by behavior. The functional assessment interview[42] is typically administered face to face, and it can be completed in approximately 1 hour (shorter or longer depending on the complexity of the behavior and level of information desired). The Questions About Behavioral Function,[43] Functional Analysis Screening Tool,[41] and Motivation Assessment Scale[44] are more time-efficient survey forms that can be completed by caregivers at home or school. It is best practice to corroborate any interview and survey information with observations of the behavior, because these instruments have been found to generate different hypotheses about the function of SIB than observational accounts such as experimental functional analysis.[46,47] Nevertheless, strong hypotheses of the function of SIB can be generated by these types of descriptive functional assessments and effective interventions can be developed based on those hypotheses.

Experimental functional analysis involves systematic manipulation of the antecedents to, and consequences for, SIB, and direct observation of the effects of these consequences.[24] Typically, children are evaluated in clinical settings and the occurrence of SIB is compared across test and control conditions to determine whether SIB is sensitive to social consequences. The usual consequences evaluated are possible positive and negative reinforcers in the form of attention from others, escape from task demands, access to tangible items, or other preferred situations. When the presentations of antecedent and consequence stimuli are arranged systematically in a single-subject experimental design, causal claims between SIB and its consequences can be made. Experimental functional analysis requires highly trained professionals to administer and interpret (and is therefore more costly), but the tradeoff is confirmation of the environment–behavior relationship responsible for the maintenance of SIB, resulting in more prompt implemenation of the proper intervention.

## ▶ MANAGEMENT AND TREATMENT

Effective treatment of NSSI begins with appropriate assessment. This includes a full history of the behavior, including age of onset; incidence over time; and specific aspects of the behavior over time, including the history of method(s), frequency, location(s), number of injuries per episode, and medical severity of injuries. These variables may change with time, indicating an overall profile of increasing severity or a pattern of waxing and waning reflective of periods of stress.[35] Currently, the only treatment approach for NSSI that has some empirical support (including randomized controlled trials) is dialectal behavior therapy (DBT)[48] which has been found to be effective both with adults and adolescents.[49] However, none of these studies used community samples of youth engaging only in NSSI; rather, this approach has been found to be effective with individuals with severe NSSI and co-occuring suicidal behaviors. DBT focuses on specific treatment goals arranged in a hierarchy of importance as follows: (a) decreasing life-threatening and NSSI behaviors; (b) eliminating behaviors that interfere with therapy; (c) decreasing behaviors that interfere with quality of life (eg, substance abuse, high-risk sex); and (d) skills training in mindfulness, distress tolerance, emotion regulation, and interpersonal effectiveness to help manage psychological distress.[50,51] This approach is intensive and demanding of resources, requiring a therapist trained in DBT. Although DBT has been referred to as the "gold standard" of treatment, less intensive treatment approaches that incorporate the key elements of mindfulness, distress tolerance, emotion regulation, and interpersonal skills to some degree may be effective with community samples of youth who engage in NSSI.[52,53] Regardless, at a minimum the physician working with the youth must be aware of the elements of DBT.

A child with IDD presenting with SIB should be evaluated for any possible illness or the likelihood of an acute or chronic condition that may be painful. Treating the underlying medical condition may lead to reduced SIB. For behavioral assessment, referral to a qualified specialist (eg, BCBA) is recommended. The evidence for SIB treatment based on behavioral evaluation is large and growing.[54,55] Best practice calls for linking behavioral evaluation results directly to intervention strategies that include modifications to the antecedent environment in order to limit the presence of variables known to be associated with the onset of self-injury,[56] and approaches to decreasing self-injury that emphasize reinforcement of desired behavior[57–59] and de-emphasize the use of punishment.[54] Specifics of any treatment regimen should be individualized with respect to the patient's preferences, strengths, needs, and scope of SIB, as well as consideration of the caregivers' preferences, strengths, capacities, and available family and community supports.[60,61] Studies of neurobiologic factors associated with SIB have identified a role for opioidergic, dopaminergic, and serotonergic systems in the pathophysiology of SIB. These findings are in line with the results of a growing body of controlled psychopharmacologic studies demonstrating that SIB can be reduced to different degrees by agents that have actions in these neurochemical systems. One main difficulty to date is that it is not clear who will respond to what medication under what circumstances.[33]

### *Ongoing Care*

The main consideration in the ongoing care of patients who have engaged in NSSI is the need for regular follow-up and suicide risk assessment. Although many individuals will stop and not resume the behavior (exact numbers are unclear at this time), some youth will relapse and show a sharp escalation in severity following a stressor. While the prognosis is excellent for most youth who engage in NSSI at a low or moderate severity level, as a group they remain at significantly greater risk for suicide. Similarly, while tremendous advances have been made in the past 3 decades in our understanding and treatment of SIB, there is little evidence that the scientific community has effectively reduced the long-term burden of SIB on families and society. Prevalence estimates continue to suggest approximately 20% of people with IDD exhibit SIB,[62] suggesting an ongoing need for intensive intervention with an emphasis on sustainability by incumbent supports.

### *Self-injury Similarities and Differences*

In summary, self-injury is generally understood to be a completely different phenomeon in typically vs atypically developing children and youth. While there are many differences in presentation and treatment approaches, these behaviors can be understood as possibly serving either an automatic or social function in both populations. Furthermore, it is essential in both instances to evaluate for the underlying functions in order to understand the reinforcers of these behaviors. Treatment for NSSI and SIB requires a detailed analysis and understanding of what is reinforcing the behavior and ultimately trying to interrupt this reinforcement chain. Effectively disrupting the response-reinforcer contingency depends, in part, on recognizing that self-injury elicits reactions from individuals in the patient's or individual's environment, which can create a complex situation (ie, it is a natural response on the part of a physician to want to react and stop an individual from harming himself). Documentation and clear communication to share information about any planned intervention is essential to effective outcomes.

## When to Refer

**NSSI**

- Following initial risk assessment
- Emotional regulation difficulties or poor coping strategies

## When to Admit

**NSSI**

- Threat of suicide
- Serious physical injury
- Underlying psychiatric conditions

### *TOOLS FOR PRACTICE*

**Engaging Patient and Family**

- *S.A.F.E. Alternatives* (Web site), (www.selfinjury.com)
- *Self-injury Outreach and Support* (Web site), (sioutreach.org)

**Medical Decision Support**

- *Certificant Registry* (Web page), Behavior Analyst Certification Board (www.bacb.com/index.php?page=100155)
- *Five Things to Know About Non-Suicidal Self-Injury* (article), *Canadian Medical Association Journal*, Vol 185, Issue 6, 2013
- *Self-Injury Trauma (SIT) Scale: A Method for Quantifying Surface Tissue Damage Caused by Self-Injurious Behavior* (article), *Journal of Applied Behavior Analysis*, Vol 23, Issue 1, 1990
- *Pediatric Symptom Checklist* (screen), Massachusetts General Hospital (www.massgeneral.org/psychiatry/services/psc_forms.aspx)
- *Strengths & Difficulties Questionnaire* (screen), Youth in Mind, Ltd. (www.sdqinfo.com)
- *Adapted SAD PERSONS* (screen), American Academy of Pediatrics (pediatrics.aappublications.org/content/125/Supplement_3/S195.full.pdf)

### *REFERENCES*


1. Joiner T. *Why People Die by Suicide.* Cambridge, MA: Harvard University Press; 2005
2. Rodham K, Hawton K. Epidemiology and phenomenology of nonsuicidal self-injury. In: Nock MK, ed. *Understanding Nonsuicidal Self-Injury: Origins, Assessment, and Treatment.* Washington, DC: American Psychological Association; 2009
3. Heath NL, Schaub K, Holly S, Nixon MK. Self-injury today: review of population and clinical studies in adolescents. In: Nixon MK, Heath NL, eds. *Self-Injury in Youth: The Essential Guide to Assessment and Intervention.* New York, NY: Routledge/Taylor & Francis Group; 2009
4. Claes L, Vanderycken W, Vertommen H. Eating-disordered patients with and without self-injurious behaviors: a comparison of psychopathological features. *Eur Eat Disords Rev.* 2003;11(5):379–396
5. Laye-Gindhu A, Shonert-Reichl K. Nonsuicidal self-harm among community adolescents: understanding the "whats" and "whys" of self-harm. *J Youth Adolesc.* 2005;34(5):445–457
6. Nixon MK, Cloutier P, Jansson SM. Nonsuicidal self-harm in youth: a population-based survey. *CMAJ.* 2008;178:306–312
7. Lloyd-Richardson EE, Perrine N, Dierker L, Kelley ML. Characteristics and functions of non-suicidal self-injury in a community sample of adolescents. *Psychol Med.* 2007;37:1183–1192
8. Muehlenkamp JJ, Gutierrez PM. Risk for suicide attempts among adolescents who engage in nonsuicidal self-injury. *Arch Suicide Res.* 2007;11:69–82
9. Muehlenkamp JJ, Gutierrez PM. An investigation of differences between self-injurious behavior and suicide attempts in a sample of adolescents. *Suicide Life Threat Behav.* 2004;34:12–23
10. Izutsu T, Shimotsu S, Matsumoto T, et al. Deliberate self-harm and childhood hyperactivity in junior high school students. *Eur Child Adolesc Psychiatry.* 2006;15:172–176
11. Heath NL, Ross S, Toste JR, Charlebois A, Nedecheva T. Retrospective analysis of social factors and nonsuicidal self-injury among young adults. *Can J Behav Sci.* 2009;41(3):180–186

12. Moore TR, Gilles E, McComas JJ, Symons FJ. Functional analysis and treatment of self-injurious behaviour in a young child with traumatic brain injury. *Brain Inj.* 2010;24:1511–1518
13. Rojahn J. Epidemiology and topographic taxonomy of self-injurious behavior. In: Thompson T, Gray BB, eds. *Destructive Behavior in Developmental Disabilities: Diagnosis and Treatment.* Thousand Oaks, CA: Sage; 1994
14. Gerson J, Stanley B. Suicidal and self-injurious behavior in personality disorder: controversies and treatment directions. *Curr Psychiatry Rep.* 2002;4:30–38
15. Paris J. Understanding self-mutilation in borderline personality disorder. *Harv Rev Psychiatry.* 2005;13:179–185
16. Klonsky ED. The functions of deliberate self-injury: a review of the evidence. *Clin Psychol Rev.* 2007;27(2):226–239
17. Nock MK. Actions speak louder than words: an elaborated theoretical model of the social functions of self-injury and other harmful behaviors. *Appl Prev Psychol.* 2008;12:159–168
18. Nock MK, Prinstein MJ. A functional approach to the assessment of self-mutilative behavior. *J Consult Clin Psychol.* 2004;72:885–890
19. Chapman AL, Gratz KL, Brown MZ. Solving the puzzle of deliberate self-harm: the experiential avoidance model. *Behav Res Ther.* 2006;44:371–394
20. Heath NL, Toste JR, Nedecheva T, Charlebois A. An examination of non-suicidal self-injury in college students. *J Ment Health Couns.* 2008;30(2):137–156
21. Klonsky ED. The functions of self-injury in young adults who cut themselves: clarifying the evidence for affect-regulation. *Psychiatry Res.* 2009;166(2–3):260–268
22. Nock MK, Prinstein MJ. Contextual features and behavioral functions of self-mutilation among adolescents. *J Abnorm Psychol.* 2005;114:140–146
23. Hilt LM, Nock MK, Lloyd-Richardson EE, Prinstein MJ. Longitudinal study of nonsuicidal self-injury among young adolescents. *J Early Adolesc.* 2008;28(3):455–469
24. Iwata BA, Dorsey MF, Slifer KJ, Bauman KE, Richman GS. Toward a functional analysis of self-injury. *J Appl Behav Anal.* 1994;27:197–209
25. Sprague JR, Horner RH. Functional assessment and intervention in community settings. *Ment Retard Dev Disabil Res Rev.* 1995;1:89–93
26. Wacker DP, Berg WK, Harding JW, et al. Evaluation and long-term treatment of aberrant behavior displayed by young children with disabilities. *J Dev Behav Pediatr.* 1998;19:260–266
27. Carr EG, Smith CE. Biological setting events for self-injury. *Ment Retard Dev Disabil Res Rev.* 1995;1:94–98
28. Sandman CA, Hetrick W, Taylor DV, Chicz-DeMet A. Dissociation of POMC peptides after self-injury predicts responses to centrally acting opiate blockers. *Am J Ment Retard.* 1997;102:182–199
29. Bosch J, Van Dyke C, Smith SM, Poulton S. Role of medical conditions in the exacerbation of self-injurious behavior: an exploratory study. *Ment Retard.* 1997;35:124–130
30. Richman DM. Annotation: early intervention and prevention of self-injurious behaviour exhibited by young children with developmental disabilities. *J Intellect Disabil Res.* 2008;52:3–17
31. Lofthouse N, Muehlenkamp JJ, Adler R. Nonsuicidal self-injury and co-occurrence. In: Nixon MK, Heath NL, eds. *Self-Injury in Youth: The Essential Guide to Assessment and Intervention.* New York, NY: Routledge Press/Taylor & Francis Group; 2009
32. MacLean WE, Symons F. Self-injurious behavior in infancy and young childhood. *Infants Young Child.* 2002;14(4):31–41
33. Schroeder S, Thompson T, Oster-Granite ML. *Self-Injurious Behavior: Genes, Brain, and Behavior.* Washington, DC: American Psychological Association; 2002
34. Adler PA, Adler P. The demedicalization of self-injury: from psychopathology to sociological deviance. *J Contemp Ethnog.* 2007:36(5):537–550
35. Heath NL, Nixon MK. Assessment of nonsuicidal self-injury in youth. In: Nixon MK, Heath NL, eds. *Self-Injury in Youth: The Essential Guide to Assessment and Intervention.* New York, NY: Routledge Press/Taylor & Francis Group; 2009

36. Symons FJ, Thompson T. Self-injurious behaviour and body site preference. *J Intellect Disabil Res.* 1997;41(Pt 6):456–468
37. Luiselli JK, Matson JL, Singh NN, eds. *Self-injurious Behavior: Analysis, Assessment, and Treatment.* New York, NY: Springer; 1992
38. Carr EG, Durand VM. Reducing behavior problems through functional communication training. *J Appl Behav Anal.* 1985;18:111–126
39. Day HM, Horner RH, O'Neill RE. Multiple functions of problem behaviors: assessment and intervention. *J Appl Behav Anal.* 1994;27:279–289
40. Repp AC, Felce D, Barton LE. Basing the treatment of stereotypic and self-injurious behaviors on hypotheses of their causes. *J Appl Behav Anal.* 1988;21(3):281–289
41. Florida Center on Self-Injury. Functional Analysis Screening Tool. http://adapt-fl.com/files/FAST.pdf (Accessed February 10, 2015)
42. O'Neill RE, Albin RW, Storey K, Horner RH, Sprague JR. *Functional Assessment and Program Development for Problem Behavior: A Practical Handbook.* Stamford, CT: Cengage Learning; 2014
43. Paclawskyj TR, Matson JL, Rush KS, Smalls Y, Vollmer TR. Questions about behavioral function (QABF): a behavioral checklist for functional assessment of aberrant behavior. *Res Dev Disabil.* 2000;21:223–239
44. Durand VM, Durand DB. Identifying the variables maintaining self-injurious behavior. *J Autism Dev Dis.* 1988;18(1):99–117
45. Northup J, Wacker D, Sasso G, et al. A brief functional analysis of aggressive and alternative behavior in an outclinic setting. *J Appl Behav Anal.* 1991;24:509–522
46. Hall SS. Comparing descriptive, experimental and informant-based assessments of problem behaviors. *Res Dev Disabil.* 2005;26:514–526
47. Paclawskyj TR, Matson JL, Rush KS, Smalls Y, Vollmer TR. Assessment of the convergent validity of the Questions About Behavioral Function scale with analogue functional analysis and the Motivation Assessment Scale. *J Intellect Disabil Res.* 2001;45:484–494
48. Lynch TR, Cozza C. Behavior therapy for nonsuicidal self-injury. In: Nock MK, ed. *Understanding Nonsuicidal Self-Injury: Origins, Assessment, and Treatment.* Washington, DC: American Psychological Association; 2009
49. Miller AL, Muehlenkamp JJ, Jacobson CM. Special issues in treating adolescent nonsuicidal self-injury. In: Nock MK, ed. *Understanding Nonsuicidal Self-Injury: Origins, Assessment, and Treatment.* Washington, DC: American Psychological Association; 2009
50. Miller AL, Rathus JH. Dialetical behavior therapy: adaptations and new applications. *Cog Behav Pract.* 2000;7:420–425
51. Miller AL, Rathus JH, Linehan MM. *Dialectical Behavior Therapy With Suicidal Adolescents.* New York, NY: The Guilford Press; 2006
52. Gratz KL, Chapman AL. *Freedom From Self-Harm: Overcoming Self-Injury With Skills From DBT and Other Treatments.* Oakland, CA: New Harbinger Publications, Inc; 2009
53. Hollander M. *Helping Teens Who Cut: Understanding and Ending Self-injury.* New York, NY: The Guilford Press; 2008
54. Kahng S, Iwata BA, Lewin AB. Behavioral treatment of self-injury, 1964 to 2000. *Am J Ment Retard.* 2002;107:212–221
55. Tiger JH, Hanley GP, Bruzek J. Functional communication training: a review and practical guide. *Behav Anal Pract.* 2008;1:16–23
56. Kern L, Clarke S. Antecedent and setting event interventions. In: Bambara LM, Kern L, eds. *Individualized Supports for Students With Problem Behaviors: Designing Positive Behavior Support Plans.* New York, NY: Guilford; 2005
57. Durand VM, Carr EG. Functional communication training to reduce challenging behavior: maintenance and application in new settings. *J Appl Behav Anal.* 1991;24:251–264
58. Petscher ES, Rey C, Bailey JS. A review of empirical support for differential reinforcement of alternative behavior. *Res Dev Disabil.* 2009;30(3):49–425

59. Wacker DP, Berg WK, Harding JW, et al. Treatment effectiveness, stimulus generalization, and acceptability to parents of functional communication training. *Educ Psychol.* 2005;25:233–256
60. Lucyshyn JM, Albin RW, Nixon CD. Embedding comprehensive behavioral support in family ecology: an experimental, single-case analysis. *J Consult Clin Psychol.* 1997;65:241–251
61. Moes DR, Frea WD. Using family context to inform intervention planning for the treatment of a child with autism. *J Pos Behav Interv.* 2002;2(1):40–46
62. Lowe K, Allen D, Jones E, et al. Challenging behaviours: prevalence and topographies. *J Intellect Disabil Res.* 2007;51:625–636

# Chapter 69

# Self-stimulating Behaviors

*Richard M. Sarles, MD; Sarah Edwards, DO*

Repetitive and self-stimulating behaviors, such as head banging, head rolling, rocking, thumb sucking, and masturbation, as well as habits such as hair pulling and nail biting, are of concern to both parents and pediatricians. Research has suggested that commonalities exist among repetitive behaviors, sometimes classified as *stereotypies,* and that they represent an interaction of the stage of neuromotor development with environmental influences (eg, restrictive car seats and cribs) and are a homeostatic mechanism that serves to regulate stimulation from the environment. Many of these behaviors, such as head banging, head rolling, and rocking, typically appear before 12 months of age, peak soon thereafter, and subsequently decline rapidly. Thumb sucking (25%) and nail biting (23%) are the most common behaviors described in preschool children, with only 4% developing motor stereotypies.[1] Young children practice self-stimulation through thumb sucking and genital play, with a peak at age 2½ years.[2] In general, most of these behaviors are self-limited to the preschool period and are usually viewed as normal, common, and expected behaviors. These habits generally do not signify psychological maladjustment. They often require little intervention other than reassuring the parents and suggesting adequate interaction with their child.[3]

## ▶ HEAD BANGING AND ROCKING

*Head banging* consists of rhythmic movements of the head against a solid object, such as the crib mattress or headboard, and is often associated with rocking the head and the entire body.[4,5] It is observed most commonly at bedtime or at times of fatigue or stress and may vary in duration from several minutes to hours. Head banging often continues even when the child is asleep. The age of onset shows wide variability, but the behavior is witnessed most commonly during the preschool years. The reported incidence of head-banging or rocking behavior varies between 3% and 20%, with a male-to-female ratio of approximately 3:1. Occasionally a family history of such behavior can be found, but only 20% of siblings of children who rock exhibit similar or other rhythmic pattern disturbances.[6]

Various theories have been developed to understand these self-limited but often disturbing behaviors.[3] Rocking is thought to be a soothing, pleasurable experience that every infant encounters in utero and that most infants encounter from the neonatal period onward. The pleasure from movement is repeated throughout life, from being rocked in the mother's arms during early childhood, for example, to jumping rope and playing on swings in childhood, to dancing in adulthood. Individual constitutional patterns in childhood account for a wide variability in the amount of stimulation any particular child may require. However, in certain children, such as those who are hearing or sight impaired, emotionally disturbed, or severely intellectually disabled, marked rhythmic movements are commonly found. In these cases the movements may represent a compensatory reaction for a lack of stimuli or the inability to integrate stimuli. Head banging in children with severe disabilities can be a form of functional communication. For example, a child may increase head banging to receive parental attention or to avoid task demands. In addition, the child who has no disability but who is inactive because of physical illness generally shows a need for motor release that is often characterized by bed rocking or other rhythmic body movements, which generally disappear once normal mobility is restored.

Physical and neurologic examinations show these children to be predominantly within normal limits, and electroencephalogram studies are not indicated because the findings are generally not helpful. These behaviors seem to be linked to maturational patterns and correlate closely with teething and other transitions of growth and development, perhaps as a mechanism for increasing or reducing arousal and maintaining homeostasis. Even though psychosocial growth and development are apparently not disturbed in these children and studies indicate no connection between rocking behavior and parental divorce or separation, the question of inadequate stimulation for the child should be raised, and the presence of family turmoil and stress should be investigated.

Treatment is generally directed toward assuring the parents that head banging cannot cause brain injury and that the child will show no adverse neurologic effects in later life; children who engage in head-banging behavior usually grow up as typical, coordinated children. Securing the crib to prevent rolling may help during the limited rocking behavior, but crib bumpers are not recommended because of concerns of suffocation, strangulation, or entrapment. Sedation in the form of diphenhydramine may prove effective, but psychotropic medication is generally unnecessary and is thus discouraged. Parents should not visit the child frequently at night, because doing so could reinforce what may become an attention-seeking behavior. Rarely, if ever, do fractures of the skull or cerebral hemorrhages result from head banging in typically developing children, but soft-tissue swelling and scalp contusions have been reported. Intracranial injuries and retinal detachment have been reported in children with autism and severe intellectual disabilities, and a protective helmet may be advised in severe cases. Consultation with a child psychiatrist or psychologist is indicated if the head-banging or rocking behavior persists beyond 3 years of age. For children who show a lack of social interaction or a preoccupation with themselves or with self-stimulatory behavior, consultation is indicated.

## ▶ THUMB SUCKING AND NAIL BITING

Thumb sucking occurs almost universally in infancy but varies among cultures. Infants may place virtually every object they encounter in their mouth unless parents, for safety reasons, restrict the object choice.

The pleasurable sensations associated with the double tactile experience of sucking and being sucked and the feelings of security and comfort that these experiences evoke tend to reinforce this behavior. Many families substitute artificial pacifiers as a more socially acceptable means of oral pleasure, and children themselves often spontaneously suck a security blanket, a doll, or a stuffed animal. Thumb sucking usually occurs during times of stress or boredom and at bedtime. Young children may suck their thumb to help themselves fall asleep. Social and family pressures generally limit thumb sucking to the preschool years. However, the habit may persist into adolescence. Approximately 25% to 40% of American children engage in finger sucking during the preschool years and 10% to 20% continue beyond 6 years of age.[7]

Nail biting is an extension or permutation of the habit of thumb sucking. Some experts consider this behavior a form of more overt self-aggression; others would define nail biting simply as a variation of thumb sucking because this behavior is also seen typically during times of stress. An estimated 25% of preschoolers and 33% of children ages 7 to 10 years bite their nails. Adolescent rates of nail biting are as high as 45%. Thus nail biting, in contrast to thumb sucking, often continues throughout development, but decreases to adult rates of 10%. Gender differences do not appear until adolescence when the incidence of nail biting is greater for males.[8] A family history exists in most cases, but this habit is so common that such an apparent association may be of no significance. Children from higher socioeconomic groups and higher levels of parental education seem to demonstrate oral habits more often, but no clear correlation has been found with the number of children in the family, birth order, type of feeding, or feeding schedule.[9]

Thumb sucking, nail biting, and cuticle biting or picking may be harmful to dentition and increase the risk of dental malocclusion and the incidence of digital cutaneous infections. There is a higher probability of malocclusion if thumb sucking continues after the eruption of permanent teeth.[7,9] In addition, thumb sucking that persists into school age can bring on teasing from peers and criticism from teachers and family, leaving the child with decreased self-esteem and increased psychological distress.

Clarifying with parents the nature of these habits is important, as is encouraging them to avoid punishing or shaming the child for them. An underlying cause of tension should always be investigated, but simple behavioral therapy (based on positive reinforcement) is often sufficient to alleviate the habit. The parents should be advised to avoid punishment, threats, or anger. Encouragement in the place of restrictions is helpful in engaging children in their own program to decrease or eliminate the behavior.

Bitter-tasting commercial preparations applied to the fingers may be used as a reminder for the child, but these preparations are generally inadequate unless supplemented by consistent positive reinforcement. The choice of reinforcement reward should be the child's and might take the form of extra television privileges, dessert, or other special treats. A combination of aversive taste treatment and a reward system seems to be effective in treating chronic thumb sucking.[10] Weekly visits to the physician for the first month of treatment are important to reinforce the change in behavior. Hypnosis is another treatment that is often successful and poses no danger; psychotropic medications, on the other hand, are of little value. If these habits are linked to other signs of emotional distress or if there is excessive nail biting and cuticle picking, referral to a specialist in behavioral disorders is warranted to investigate other mental health issues such as anxiety or a body-focused repetitive behavior disorder.[11]

## ▶ MASTURBATION

Childhood masturbation is almost universal and often causes great parental concern. Genital exploration and touch typically begin around 2 months of age and evolve into masturbatory activities that peak at 4 to 5 years of age and again in adolescence.[2,12] Such activity may vary from direct manual genital stimulation to movements of the thighs against each other. Rhythmic swaying or thrusting motions of the child while straddling a hobby horse, pillow, stuffed animal, or other objects also are common methods of masturbation. Infants and children are capable of a physiologic orgasmic response similar to that experienced by the adult, except for the absence of ejaculation in the male child, as demonstrated by the common practice in Europe in the late 1800s of masturbating an irritable child to induce relaxation and sleep. Occasionally, this orgasmic response has been incorrectly thought to represent a convulsive or movement disorder in infants and children leading to unnecessary and expensive neurological workup.[12] Masturbatory activity is generally initiated as a response to the learned pleasure associated with touching of the genitalia that is first experienced in infancy during normal body exploration. Masturbation will continue as a lifelong pleasurable experience unless suppressed by parents or other adults.

The physician needs to educate parents about healthy childhood sexual development. Physicians should counsel parents on masturbatory practices and emphasize that masturbation is a normal, harmless, and healthy practice that helps the child to derive pleasure from the child's own body. Many parents may have received negative messages as children about their sexual development, and this has led them to view typical sexual behaviors as problematic. Myths must be dispelled concerning the belief that masturbation is a definitive sign of sexual abuse, that it may cause intellectual disability, physical deformity, blindness, poor physical and mental health, facial pimples, hair on the palms of the hand, homosexuality, and sexual perversions. Parents should be aware that masturbation occurs almost universally in children and should be encouraged to avoid punishing or shaming their child for a normal behavior. Negative parental reactions will not reduce the frequency of masturbation, but can lead to feelings of guilt and shame in children. If parents observe masturbatory activity in their child, they may want to suggest to the child the inappropriateness of manipulating their genitalia in public places or in front of others and inform the child that certain practices, such as using the toilet and masturbating, are best carried out in private.[13,14]

Because local genital irritation, *Candida* infection, or pinworms in rare cases may cause a child to repeatedly touch their genitals, a physical examination helps to exclude such possibilities. Compulsive, overt masturbation among children and adolescents may lead to social ridicule and condemnation, or it may signify a deeper emotional problem. Consultation with a specialist in behavioral disorders of children and adolescents is indicated if the physician suspects that the masturbatory activity is excessive, compulsive, or not easily redirectable or may indicate the presence of a more complicated, troublesome emotional problem. Any masturbatory actions that involve self-harm or are coercive of other children are concerning and warrant additional evaluation and consultation.

The pediatrician should be aware that even with the current societal trends toward sexual openness and enlightenment, myths and feelings concerning masturbation often are deep seated and persistent. Thus, counseling and advice given by the pediatrician may be met with covert or overt resistance by parents or school authorities. The pediatrician should be well prepared to educate persons responsible for the growth and development of children.

## ▶ HAIR PULLING AND TWISTING

Recurrent hair pulling and twisting *(trichotillomania)* is a form of self-stimulating behavior that often indicates the presence of psychological stress. The scalp is the most common area affected; eyebrows and eyelashes are the next most likely sites. The obvious cosmetic damage often results in ridicule by peers and shame for the child. The formation of a hairball, or *trichobezoar,* in the stomach if the child ingests the hair is a serious problem that often results in hospitalization for surgical removal of the accumulated matted hair. This behavior has been reported across all age groups and has a bimodal onset with peaks in the preschool years and in early adolescence (ages 11–13 years).[15] Onset in very early childhood shows no gender bias; however, this behavior becomes more common in females with increasing age.[16] The *Diagnostic and Statistical Manual of Mental Disorders,* Fifth Edition, groups trichotillomania with the obsessive-compulsive and related disorders because it is a recurrent, body-focused, repetitive behavior.[11] Two types of trichotillomania have been described in clinical practice, both of which can coexist in the same individual. In the *focused* type, which is associated with tension before and relief after the hair is pulled, time is set aside to pull the hair. In the second, *automatic* type, the patient is generally unaware of the behavior during the hair pulling or twisting itself and often recognizes the action as senseless and undesirable.[17]

Treatment is usually indicated and behavioral and cognitive behavioral therapy should be used as first-line treatment.[18] Local irritation from a dermatologic condition is rarely the cause of this disorder, but the possibility should be investigated. Referral to a mental health professional is often warranted to investigate possible underlying causes of tension, anxiety, depression, or obsessive-compulsive disorder. Psychotherapy may be required in many of these cases. Research does not support the use of selective serotonin reuptake inhibitors (SSRIs) to treat trichotillomania, but SSRIs can treat comorbid anxiety in children and adolescents.[19,20] Although studies of the treatment of adult trichotillomania showed significant benefit using N-acetylcysteine (NAC), research had not supported the benefit of NAC for the treatment of children.[21]

## ▶ SPECIAL PROBLEMS IN CHILDREN WITH SEVERE MENTAL HEALTH DISORDERS

A broad spectrum of self-stimulating behaviors may be seen in children with developmental disabilities and severe mental health disorders. The behaviors, including body twirling or spinning and hand or arm flapping, are often seen in cases of infantile autism or childhood schizophrenia. Excessive rocking behavior is common in severely intellectually disabled and emotionally disturbed children. In addition, severe self-mutilating behaviors, such as compulsive self-biting, severe head banging, and skin gouging, may be seen in these disorders and are characteristic of certain metabolic or genetic disorders, such as Lesch-Nyhan syndrome and Cornelia de Lange syndrome.[22] Patients who have Prader-Willi syndrome often demonstrate severe skin picking.[23]

These behaviors are part of a symptom complex in a severe disorder, in contrast to the generally isolated behaviors in typically developing children. The cause is generally linked to the basic disorder and may also reflect the lack, or disordered integration, of sensory stimuli. As previously mentioned, these behaviors can be reinforced by parental/adult reactions and often serve a communication function, eg, the child increases the self-stimulating behavior to receive attention and avoid unpleasant tasks.

All of these cases require treatment for the basic disorder and generally demand special behavioral treatment beyond the scope and expertise of the primary care physician. When the behavior is severe, institutionalization is often required, and methods of treatment include the application of aversive behavior modification techniques; the use of arm and neck restraints, head helmets, and psychotropic medications; and the institution of psychotherapeutic behavioral programs.

## When to Refer

- Persistence of head banging or rocking beyond the age of 3 years
- Preoccupation with self-stimulating behavior to the point that it interferes with healthy social and emotional interaction
- Presence of accompanying symptoms such as decreased socialization or other behavioral problems
- Causing tissue damage

### TOOLS FOR PRACTICE

#### Engaging Patient and Family

- *Common Childhood Habits* (fact sheet), American Academy of Pediatrics (www.healthychildren.org/English/family-life/family-dynamics/communication-discipline/Pages/Common-Childhood-Habits.aspx)
- *Thumbsucking* (audio) American Academy of Pediatrics (www.healthychildren.org/English/ages-stages/baby/crying-colic/Pages/Thumbsucking.aspx)
- *Pacifiers and Thumb Sucking* (fact sheet), American Academy of Pediatrics (www.healthychildren.org/English/ages-stages/baby/crying-colic/Pages/Pacifiers-and-Thumb-Sucking.aspx)

### REFERENCES

1. Foster LG. Nervous habits and stereotyped behaviors in preschool children. *J Am Acad Child Adolesc Psychiatry*. 1998;37:711–717
2. Jellinek M, Patel BP, Froehle MC. *Bright Futures in Practice: Mental Health. Volume 1. Practice Guide.* Arlington, VA: National Center for Education in Maternal and Child Health; 2002
3. Lourie RS. The role of rhythmic patterns in childhood. *Am J Psychiatry*. 1949;105:653–660
4. Werry JS, Carlielle J, Fitzpatrick J. Rhythmic motor activities (stereotypies) in children under five: etiology and prevalence. *J Am Acad Child Adolesc Psychiatry.* 1983;22:329–336
5. Leekam S, Tandos J, McConachie H, et al. Repetitive behaviours in typically developing 2-year-olds. *J Child Psychol Psychiatry*. 2007;48:1131–1138
6. Kravitz H, Rosenthal V, Teplitz Z, et al. A study of head-banging in infants and children. *Dis Nerv Sys.* 1960;21:203–208
7. Leung AK, Robson WL. Thumb sucking. *Am Fam Physician*. 1991;44:1724–1728
8. Leung AK, Robson WL. Nailbiting. *Clin Pediatr (Phila)*. 1990;29:690–692
9. Johnson ED, Larson BE. Thumb-sucking: literature review. *ASDC J Dent Child.* 1993;60:385–391
10. Friman PC, Leibowitz JM. An effective and acceptable treatment alternative for chronic thumb- and finger-sucking. *J Pediatr Psychol.* 1990;15:57–65

11. American Psychiatric Association. *Diagnostic and Statistical Manual of Mental Disorders.* 5th ed. Arlington, VA: American Psychiatric Association; 2013
12. Yang ML, Fullwood E, Goldstein J, Mink JW. Masturbation in infancy and early childhood presenting as a movement disorder: 12 cases and a review of the literature. *Pediatrics.* 2005;116:1427–1432
13. Strachan E, Staples B. Masturbation. *Pediatr Rev.* 2012;33:190–191
14. Kellogg ND; American Academy of Pediatrics Committee on Child Abuse and Neglect. Clinical report—the evaluation of sexual behaviors in children. *Pediatrics.* 2009;124:992–998
15. Bruce TO, Barwick LW, Wright HH. Diagnosis and management of trichotillomania in children and adolescents. *Paediatr Drugs.* 2005;7:365–376
16. Duke DC, Keeley ML, Geffken GR, Storch EA. Trichotillomania: a current review. *Clin Psychol Rev.* 2010;30:181–193
17. Harrison JP, Franklin ME. Pediatric trichotillomania. *Curr Psychiatry Rep.* 2012;14:188–196
18. Tolin DF, Franklin ME, Diefenbach GJ, Anderson E, Meunier SA. Pediatric trichotillomania: descriptive psychopathology and an open trial of cognitive behavioral therapy. *Cogn Behav Ther.* 2007;36:129–144
19. Bloch MH, Landeros-Weisenberger A, Dombrowski P, et al. Systematic review: pharmacological and behavioral treatment for trichotillomania. *Biol Psychiatry.* 2007;62:839–846
20. Ginsburg GS, Becker EM, Keeton CP, et al. Naturalistic follow-up of youths treated for pediatric anxiety disorders. *JAMA Psychiatry.* 2014;71:310–318
21. Bloch MH, Panza KE, Grant JE, Pittenger C, Leckman JF. N-Acetylcysteine in the treatment of pediatric trichotillomania: a randomized, double-blind, placebo-controlled add-on trial. *J Am Acad Child Adolesc Psychiatry.* 2013;52:231–240
22. Harris JC. Destructive behavior: aggression and self injury. In: Harris JC, ed. *Developmental Neuropsychiatry: The Fundamentals,* New York, NY: Oxford University Press; 1995
23. Donaldson MD, Chu CE, Cooke A, et al. The Prader-Willi syndrome. *Arch Dis Child.* 1994; 70:58–63

### Short Stature Associated With Syndromes and With Being Born Small for Gestational Age

Short stature associated with a syndrome should be considered when a very short child has a dysmorphic appearance, particularly if born small for gestational age (SGA) (eg, birth weight of ≤2,500 g at term).

Turner syndrome should be a consideration in any girl whose height is well below the third percentile, but certain features make the diagnosis more likely. Lymphedema in the newborn period or frequent ear infections well past 2 years of age are common. The most common physical findings include a narrow, high-arched palate, cubitus valgus (a large angle at the elbow when the arms are stretched out), and upturned fingernails.[3] The classic webbed neck is seen in only 40%. Approximately 15% have congenital heart disease, usually coarctation of the aorta. Mean birth weight is 2,785 g; thus, many patients are not born SGA.

Many less common syndromes exist in which dysmorphic features are associated with short stature. In Russell-Silver syndrome, the most characteristic features are a history of being born SGA and having a triangular face with a down-turned mouth. Noonan syndrome may be suggested by the finding of pulmonic stenosis and facial features that include a flat nasal bridge, hypertelorism, and ptosis.

Short stature associated with SGA is diagnosed when a child born SGA fails to catch up to the normal range in height by 2 years of age. Many of these children have no dysmorphic features, and no defined cause can be found for their intrauterine growth restriction.

### Chronic Illness and Nutritional Disorders

A chronic illness or nutritional disorder should be considered in short children whose weight is further below the curve than their height (or whose body mass index is below the 10th percentile for age).

Inadequate calories, rarely a result of poverty in the United States because high-calorie foods are inexpensive, is sometimes seen in the setting of a child who is on a self-imposed or parent-imposed restrictive diet to avoid gaining weight or to lower cholesterol levels. The extreme example of this situation is anorexia nervosa.

Inflammatory bowel disease, though rarely the cause of undiagnosed short stature, may be suspected in a child whose growth has been normal but then shows a marked falloff in both height and weight, particularly in the presence of gastrointestinal (GI) symptoms such as abdominal pain, early satiety, and blood in the stool.[4] Growth attenuation may start when GI symptoms are relatively mild or even before they become apparent.

Celiac disease, or gluten enteropathy, is a common cause of short stature in Europe (up to 8% in some studies), although its frequency in the United States seems to be much lower.[5] Abdominal pain, distension, and loose stools may suggest the diagnosis, but most short children with celiac disease have few if any GI symptoms.

Renal disease can cause short stature, but only rarely is it diagnosed solely because of an abnormal growth curve. Renal tubular acidosis and chronic renal failure are the 2 renal conditions that can cause growth failure and that can be ruled out by appropriate screening tests.

### Poor Growth Associated With Medications

Children treated with stimulant medications for attention-deficit disorder may have growth attenuation starting either at the time the medications are begun or between 9 and 12 years of age. One recent study, which included younger patients with a mean age of 4.4 years, found a 20% reduction in height velocity and a 50% reduction in weight gain in treated children.[6] Although the common belief asserts that decreased appetite is responsible for the slow growth, many of these children are not underweight, and the explanation for their slow linear growth is still unknown.

Chronic glucocorticoid therapy is another cause of short stature, mostly seen in children with such conditions as rheumatoid arthritis and inflammatory bowel disease treated with daily oral prednisone. The effect on the growth of children treated long-term with inhaled corticosteroids for asthma is clearly much less than for systemic glucocorticoids, although monitoring of linear growth may occasionally detect evidence of growth suppression.

### Endocrine Disorders

The Utah Growth Study reported that less than 5% of short, slowly growing children had a defined endocrine disorder.[2] A major clue that an endocrine cause may exist is that height is often more affected than weight.

Growth hormone (GH) deficiency is not a common cause of short stature. In the Utah Growth Study the incidence in school aged children was estimated at 1:3,480.[2] A 2004 study from Belgium, which considered all children diagnosed with GH deficiency between 1985 and 2001, estimated the incidence at 1:5,600.[7] The diagnosis should be suspected in children who are well below the third percentile in height and falling further below over time. One suggestive physical finding is an increase in subcutaneous fat that is greater in the trunk area than elsewhere. Most cases are congenital; birth weight is usually normal but a falloff in growth occurs starting late in the first or in the second year of life. In the much less common acquired cases, a period of normal growth is followed by deceleration; central nervous system symptoms such as severe recurrent headaches may be part of the clinical picture. Once a diagnosis of acquired GH deficiency is established, the endocrinologist will order brain imaging to look for a tumor in the area of the pituitary gland. Milder or partial forms of GH deficiency are difficult to distinguish from CGD and FSS based on growth pattern, physical findings, and laboratory tests. The apparently higher frequency of GH deficiency in recent years is, in large part, because GH testing done in the United States has many false-positive results, and many normally growing children fail the test using the accepted cutoff of 10 ng/mL.[8]

Acquired hypothyroidism, when severe, can cause slowing of growth or even complete growth arrest. Other symptoms, including fatigue and cold intolerance, are often present, and most children will have a goiter. Acquired hypothyroidism needs to be excluded as a possibility in any child with documented growth deceleration, even if height is still above the third percentile.

Although iatrogenic Cushing syndrome is not uncommon, true endogenous Cushing syndrome is extremely rare. Rapid weight gain in the trunk, rather than generalized in distribution, accompanied by a slowing of linear growth are the key findings. Moon facies and purple abdominal striae are often seen, as well as increased skin pigmentation.

### Idiopathic Short Stature

*Idiopathic short stature* (ISS) is a term used to describe moderately to severely short children who do not meet the criteria for CGD and FSS (eg, they often have a subnormal rate of growth); and in whom no cause for their poor growth is found after extensive testing. Studies have shown that most children with ISS respond to a variable degree to GH and see a modest average improvement in adult height.[9,10] The US Food and Drug Administration (FDA) in 2003 approved GH for children at or below the first percentile with an anticipated adult height (based on bone age) below the normal range.[9] However, some insurance companies refuse to cover GH to treat ISS, arguing that no medical condition causing the growth problem exists and that treatment is cosmetic.

## ▶ EVALUATION

### History

The most helpful information in evaluating the short child is the growth curve. If the growth rate has been normal for the previous 2 or more years, then the child most likely has CGD or FSS and is unlikely to have a defined, treatable cause. A single height point that falls off the established curve is often a measurement error and should be rechecked. A history of stimulant medications or glucocorticoid use might be a key piece of information. Many children with chronic growth-limiting illnesses have a decreased energy level and may have a poor appetite, although many short, healthy children are also described as picky eaters. An abnormal stool history should make the PCP think of malabsorption, celiac disease, or inflammatory bowel disease.

Heights of parents and grandparents and growth percentiles of siblings should be reviewed because they may suggest FSS in a healthy child who is short but growing at a normal rate. Approximately two-thirds of children with CGD have a family history of a parent who was a late maturer (eg, mother's menarche after age 14 or a father who continued to grow after high school).

### Physical Examination

Most short children do not have any physical findings that point to a specific diagnosis. A child with decreased subcutaneous fat stores and weight more affected than height may simply not be getting enough calories or may have bowel disease or another chronic illness. Conversely, a short child who is relatively pudgy (particularly if excess rippled fat is present over the trunk) may have GH deficiency. Dysmorphic features may provide a clue to a syndrome associated with short stature. In girls, the PCP should look for, among other things, a high-arched palate, cubitus valgus, and fingernails that bend upward, which may point to a diagnosis of Turner syndrome. An enlarged thyroid may be the only clue that a short child has hypothyroidism. Pubertal staging should be done on any short child who is 10 years or older. A short, healthy 14-year-old boy (or, less often, a short, healthy 13-year-old girl) who is still prepubertal is most likely to have a diagnosis of CGD. A child who has a flattened growth curve at 13 to 16 years of age and who, by examination, is found to be in the late stages of puberty has completed or has nearly completed growing, and nothing can be done to increase the individual's adult height.

### Laboratory Evaluation

Primary care physicians should resist the temptation to order multiple laboratory tests for a child who is only mildly short (at or above the third percentile) and whose growth rate seems to be normal. In this situation, a clinically significant abnormal test result that will explain why the child is short is rarely found. Most growth specialists prefer either to order a very few tests on such children or to perform no tests at all, particularly if everything points to a diagnosis of CGD or FSS.

Ordering screening tests in advance of a visit with a specialist might be appropriate if the child's height is well below the third percentile or if growth deceleration that cannot be explained by medication is well-documented. However, the specialist can order any needed test at the first consultation.

Insulin-like growth factor 1 (IGF-1) is still the best screening test if GH deficiency is suspected, although many children with CGD have IGF-1 levels that are borderline low for age. IGF-binding protein 3 has not lived up to its initial promise as a better screening test for GH deficiency than IGF-1, and it is not worth ordering routinely. A random GH level is of no value because of the pulsatile nature of GH secretion.

Thyroid testing should be limited to free thyroxine (T4) and thyroid-stimulating hormone (TSH) assessment, which will identify both primary and secondary hypothyroidism. Triiodothyronine (T3), T3 uptake, and thyroid antibodies are not helpful as screening tests for short children. A borderline increased TSH (in the 5.5- to 10-mcU/mL range) with a normal free T4 is usually a normal variation and will not explain poor growth.

Complete blood count and erythrocyte sedimentation rate are mainly useful in the occasional child in whom inflammatory bowel disease is suspected. A microcytic anemia may be a clue to occult GI blood loss. Either tissue transglutaminase immunoglobulin A (IgA) antibody or antiendomyseal antibody are good tests to screen for celiac disease. Antigliadin IgG and IgA are much less specific and are not worth the extra cost.

A comprehensive metabolic profile will rule out electrolyte disturbances, kidney disease, and liver disease, all of which are rare causes of short stature.

### *Imaging Studies*

The only radiographic examination that should be considered is the bone age film, which is not a very useful diagnostic test because most children who are short for any reason (aside from genetic short stature) will have a bone age delay of a year or more. The clinician may order a bone age film in a child over 7 to make a height prediction when either CGD or FSS is suspected.

## ▶ MANAGEMENT

Healthy children who are at or above the third percentile and growing at a normal rate need not be referred to a specialist because the chances of finding a treatable cause for their short stature are small. If the parents insist on seeing a specialist, then they should be told that the child will not likely need or be eligible for coverage of GH therapy.[11] Such children should have their growth carefully measured and plotted at each visit to make sure they are not dropping below the third percentile in height. A few children report having poor self-esteem because they are shorter than most of their peers, and they may be subjected to teasing or bullying; referral to a psychologist may be more helpful than to an endocrinologist.

Infants or children who are maintaining linear growth at or above the third percentile but whose weight is consistently below or has recently fallen below the third percentile almost never have an endocrine problem. If weight gain is slow but fairly consistent in a thin child, this may be a norrmal variation; parents may say that they were thin at the same age. If weight gain is persistently poor or there is weight loss, then referral to a GI or nutrition specialist should be considered.

The child who is still in the normal range but who is crossing percentiles may present a dilemma. Between 6 and 24 months, such percentile shifts in height and weight are common, especially in patients with CGD, and a stable growth curve is usually established between 2 and 3 years of age[12]; therefore referral may be deferred if the child is healthy.[10] If the child crosses 1 percentile channel (eg, from the 25th to the 10th percentile) over 3 or more years, and if the history and examination reveal nothing abnormal, then a cause will not likely be found. Children who cross more than 1 percentile channel in a period of less than 3 years have a greater chance of having a definable cause for their short stature. The most common cause of this growth pattern is the use of stimulant medication in children with attention-deficit disorder.

Parents of children who are short enough to be referred can be told that screening tests and a period of observation are needed before any decision can be made regarding the possible need for GH therapy. Such children are best referred between the ages of 3 and 6; children who are pubertal or on the verge of puberty are usually too old to derive much benefit from GH therapy.

## When to Refer

- Any child whose height is below the third percentile, particularly if the height is falling further below the normal range over time. Children who are below the first percentile have an even better chance of qualifying for GH therapy because they are more likely to have true GH deficiency; and if they do not have GH deficiency, then they may still meet the FDA criteria for GH treatment for ISS.
- A child with a history of intrauterine growth retardation who was born SGA and who has not caught up to the normal range by age 2 years or older. The FDA has approved the use of GH in such children without the need for GH testing. A dysmorphic child with a history of intrauterine growth retardation should also be referred to a geneticist to try to make a specific diagnosis.
- A child who is within the normal range in height but has experienced a drop-off in linear growth of more than 1 percentile channel over a period of less than 3 years, or who has shown documented growth arrest for a year.
- A child with short stature who has not started puberty by age 14. This situation occurs mostly in boys with CGD; and in many cases, when the boy is anxious to start his growth spurt sooner rather than later, treating such boys with a brief course of testosterone injections is appropriate.

### *TOOLS FOR PRACTICE*

#### Engaging Patient and Family

- *The Short Child: A Parents' Guide to the Causes, Consequences, and Treatment of Growth Problems* (book), Warner Wellness Books

#### Medical Decision Support

- *Clinical Longitudinal Standards for Height and Height Velocity for North American Children* (article), *The Journal of Pediatrics*, Volume 107, Issue 3, 1985
- *Utah Growth Study: Growth Standards and the Prevalence of Growth Hormone Deficiency* (article), *The Journal of Pediatrics*, Volume 125, Issue 1, 1994

## REFERENCES


1. Tanner JM, Davies PS. Clinical longitudinal standards for height and height velocity for North American children. *J Pediatr.* 1985;107:317–329
2. Lindsay R, Feldkamp M, Harris D, Robertson J, Rallison M. Utah Growth Study: growth standards and the prevalence of growth hormone deficiency. *J Pediatr.* 1994;125:29–35
3. Frias JL, Davenport ML; American Academy of Pediatrics Committee on Genetics and Section on Endocrinology. Health supervision for children with Turner syndrome. *Pediatrics.* 2003;11:692–702
4. Savage MO, Beattie RM, Camacho-Hubner C, et al. Growth in Crohn's disease. *Acta Paediatra.* 1999;88(suppl):89–92
5. Rossi TM, Albini CH, Kumar V. Incidence of celiac disease identified by the presence of serum endomysial antibodies in children with chronic diarrhea, short stature, or insulin-dependent diabetes mellitus. *J Pediatr.* 1993;123:262–264
6. Swanson J, Greenhill L, Wigal T, et al. Stimulant-related reductions of growth rates in the PATS. *J Am Acad Child Adolesc Psychiatry.* 2006;45:1304–1313
7. Thomas M, Massa G, Craen M, et al. Prevalence and demographic features of childhood growth hormone deficiency in Belgium during the period 1986-2001. *Eur J Endocrinol.* 2004;151:67–72
8. Mauras N, Walton P, Nicar M, Welch S, Rogol AD. Growth hormone stimulation testing in both short and normal statured children: use of an immunofunctional assay. *Pediatr Res.* 2000;48:614–618
9. Lescheck EW, Rose SR, Yanovski JA, et al. Effect of growth hormone treatment on adult height in peripubertal children with idiopathic short stature: a randomized, double-blind, placebo-controlled trial. *J Clin Endocrinol Metab.* 2004;89:3140–3148
10. Wit JM, Rekers-Monbarg LT, Cutler GB, et al. Growth hormone (GH) treatment to final height in children with idiopathic short stature: evidence for a dose effect. *J Pediatr.* 2005;146:48–53
11. Allen DB. rhGH treatment for short stature: panacea or Pandora's box? *AAP News.* 2010;31(3):16
12. Horner JM, Thorsson AV, Hintz RL. Growth deceleration patterns in children with constitutional short stature: an aid to diagnosis. *Pediatrics.* 1978;62:529–534

# Chapter 71

# Sleep Disturbances (Nonspecific)

*Mark L. Splaingard, MD; Anne May, MD*

Sleep is necessary for human development and well-being, yet it has unique vulnerabilities in childhood that can manifest, for example, as central congenital hypoventilation syndrome or the inability of most primary school–aged children to awaken to very loud noises such as fire alarms during slow-wave sleep.[1] Estimates of prevalence in children vary most widely for behavioral sleep problems like insomnia, as opposed to organic sleep problems like obstructive sleep apnea (OSA), with interesting cultural and ethnic variations. Underreporting by parents and underdiagnosis by primary care physicians have been issues,[2] with sleep problems conservatively estimated to occur in approximately 25% of healthy children younger than 5 years and in up to 80% of children with special needs. Because many sleep difficulties can be managed successfully in the primary care setting, pediatricians are ideally positioned to anticipate, recognize, and treat most sleep problems and to refer children to a specialist when appropriate. Successful management of pediatric sleep problems often results in improved sleep and daytime function for all members of the household.[3]

A strong subjective component can be found for many pediatric sleep problems, as in the typical case of the toddler with night awakenings who wants to get in the parental bed:

- The parents in family A do not consider this desire as a problem. Both parents are good sleepers and do not care if their child sleeps in their bed.
- The parents in family B believe strongly that the child does not belong in their bed and that their bedroom is the only place they have to themselves.
- The mother in family C lives with her own mother and is raising two children. They live in a small apartment in which the two children share a bed.
- The parents in family D own a bed-and-breakfast business and live on the premises. They do not want their child in their bed but cannot afford to have a crying child wake the guests.
- The parents in family E have let their child into their bed in the past, but another infant is due in 3 months, and they would like their child to transition to spending the night in her own bed.

These examples illustrate the variety of responses to a common sleep issue in the young child. All of these families have caring parents and normally developing toddlers. Some of the parents regard the behavior as a sleep problem, whereas others do not. The parents in family B are more likely to consult a pediatrician about the child's sleep than the parents in family A.

Some sleep problems such as OSA are more likely to be acknowledged as problems by most families, although perceptions may vary. A hearing-impaired parent may not complain of a child's snoring. A parent who is a light sleeper is more likely to take note of a child's sleep disruptions than a parent who is a sound sleeper. Parents frequently consult pediatricians about sleep issues, and the pediatrician should recognize the range of sleep problems and the variability in parental perception of these problems.[4]

## ▶ DEVELOPMENT OF SLEEP

The development of physiologic sleep patterns is predictable (Table 71-1). It begins in utero; by 28 weeks gestational age, rapid eye movement (REM), or active sleep, can be discerned via fetal ultrasound. Non–rapid eye movement (NREM), or quiet sleep, appears at 32 weeks gestational age. At term, newborns have discrete sleep cycles, lasting 50 to 60 minutes, with

**Table 71-1**
**Sleep Developmental Milestones**

| GESTATIONAL AGE (WK) | SLEEP PATTERNS |
|---|---|
| 10 | Spontaneous fetal movements are identified. |
| 24 | Neither quiet nor active sleep can be identified between 24 and 26 weeks. Early premature (24–27 weeks) neonates have atypical sleep state characteristic of active and quiet sleep. |
| 28 | Active sleep is identified by 28 to 30 weeks by eye, body, and irregular respiratory movements. Chin tone does not become tonic before 36 weeks. Rhythmic cycling period of activity and quiescence is identified between 28 and 32 weeks. |
| 30 | Typical sleep states begin to emerge at 30 weeks. |
| 32 | Tracé alternant pattern associated with quiet sleep appears at 32 to 34 weeks. Occipital predominance of delta activity is striking at 31 to 32 weeks. At 32 weeks, EEG differences among wakefulness, active sleep, and quiet sleep develop. |
| 34 | Active sleep is 60% of TST. |
| 37 | Sleep organization at 37 weeks similar to term newborn. |
| 40 | Sleep onset through active/REM (REM within 15 minutes of sleep onset). Three distinct sleep states in term newborn: (1) REM (active), (2) NREM (quiet), and (3) indeterminate. Newborn sleeps 16 to 17 of 24 hours. Active sleep 50% of TST in term infant. Newborn sleep cycle is 50 to 60 minutes (range, 30–70 minutes), 58% active, and 39% quiet. Periodic breathing is noted, particularly in active sleep. |
| 46 | Tracé alternant present in quiet sleep in normal infants is not seen after 46 weeks. |
| 48 | Sleep spindles appear. Premature infants show spindle development approximately 4 weeks in advance of full term. Periodic breathing becomes rare after 48 weeks. |
| 3 months | NREM sleep stages begin to appear. By 3 months, sleep-onset REM is no longer present. By 3 months, 60% of sleep is quiet sleep, and 40% is active sleep. Lack of sleep spindles after 3 months is associated with hypothyroidism. |
| 4 months | Sleep shifts to nighttime *settling* by 12 to 16 weeks. Slow-wave sleep recognized at 3 to 4 months. Adult sleep stages at 4 to 5 months. Infant asleep 14 to 15 hours a day by 4 months. By 16 weeks, sustained wake periods are as long as 3 to 4 hours. |
| 6 months | By 6 months, 90% of infants have more NREM sleep than REM sleep. |
| 8 months | REM sleep occupies 30% of TST. Total sleep duration is 13 to 14 hours a day by 6 to 8 months of age. |

*EEG,* electroencephalogram; *NREM,* non–rapid eye movement; *REM,* rapid eye movement; *TST,* total sleep time.

awakenings every 2 to 6 hours. These sleep cycles are composed of alternating periods of equal amounts of quiet and active sleep. Quiet sleep is characterized by body stillness, regular respirations, and normal muscle tone. During active sleep, the infant has decreased muscle tone with frequent body movements, including eye movements and irregular respirations. The total daily amount of reported sleep at 1 month of age ranges widely from 9 to 19 hours, with an average of 14 hours (Table 71-2).

By 4 months of age, mature sleep stages begin to emerge, and day–night sleep patterns are well consolidated. Infants have their longest sleep periods at night and 3- to 4-hour periods of wakefulness during the day. By 6 months, circadian rhythms begin to display activity similar to rhythms in adults and are well established by 1 year of age. By 3 years of age, the child reaches an adult pattern of sleep, with each discrete cycle of NREM and REM sleep lasting 70 to 100 minutes.[6]

At the beginning of the night, a child progresses rapidly through stage N1 and stage N2 sleep and enters slow-wave sleep (stage N3) for much of the first third of the night. During

**Table 71-2**
**Average Sleep by Age**

| AGE | TOTAL SLEEP DURATION (hr) | 2%–98% | MEAN DAYTIME SLEEP DURATION (hr) | DAYTIME NAPPING CHILDREN (%) |
|---|---|---|---|---|
| 1 mo | 14 | 9–19 | 5.5 | 100 |
| 3 mo | 14 | 10–18.5 | 5.0 | 100 |
| 6 mo | 14.2 | 10.4–18.1 | 3.4 | 100 |
| 9 mo | 13.9 | 10.5–17.4 | 2.8 | 100 |
| 12 mo | 13.9 | 11.4–16.5 | 2.4 | 100 |
| 18 mo | 13.6 | 11.1–16 | 2.0 | 96 |
| 2 yr | 13.2 | 10.8–15.6 | 1.8 | 87 |
| 3 yr | 12.5 | 10.3–14.8 | 1.7 | 50 |
| 4 yr | 11.8 | 9.7–14.0 | 1.5 | 35 |
| 5 yr | 11.4 | 9.5–13.3 | 0 | 8 |
| 6 yr | 11.0 | 9.3–12.6 | 0 | 5 |
| 7 yr | 10.6 | 9.2–12.1 | 0 | 1 |
| 8 yr | 10.4 | 9.0–11.7 | 0 | 0 |
| 9 yr | 10.1 | 8.8–11.4 | 0 | 0 |
| 10 yr | 9.9 | 8.6–11.1 | 0 | 0 |
| 11 yr | 9.6 | 8.3–10.9 | 0 | 0 |
| 12 yr | 9.3 | 8.0–10.7 | 0 | 0 |
| 13 yr | 9.0 | 7.7–10.4 | 0 | 0 |
| 14 yr | 8.7 | 7.3–10.1 | 0 | 0 |
| 15 yr | 8.4 | 7.0–9.9 | 0 | 0 |
| 16 yr | 8.1 | 6.6–9.6 | 0 | 0 |

Adapted from Iglowstein I, Jenni OG, Molinari L, Largo RH. Sleep duration from infancy to adolescence: reference values and generational trends. *Pediatrics*. 2003;111(2):302–307.

slow-wave sleep, the child is difficult to awaken. (Many parents will recognize this period as the time of night that they can vacuum or listen to loud music without waking the child.) Subsequent sleep cycles have decreased amounts of slow-wave sleep and increased amounts of stage N2 sleep and REM sleep. Dreaming takes place mainly during REM sleep. REM episodes become longer and more intense later in the sleep period; thus, children are more likely to complain of bad dreams during the last portion of the night. In addition, sleep-disordered breathing (SDB) is likely to be most prominent during REM sleep. This tendency is important to recognize, given that this time of night is when parents are least likely to be awake and watching the sleep patterns of their children.

The amount of sleep that children need varies by age, but most children in the early school years need at least 10 hours of sleep (see Table 71-1). Children who are sleep deprived are sometimes sleepy but are more often irritable, inattentive, or hyperactive. Adolescents need sleep as much as younger children do, but they are less likely to get as much sleep as they need.

Humans have internal clocks that operate on a cycle of approximately 24 hours. These 24-hour cycles, known as *circadian rhythms,* are controlled by the hypothalamic suprachiasmatic nucleus. Most people have cycles that are not exactly 24 hours in length, and external time cues help reinforce the 24-hour schedule. The time cues are known as *zeitgebers* (German for *time givers*). The most powerful cue is exposure to bright light; other cues include social interaction, food, and exercise. Circadian rhythms are usually synchronized or *entrained* with light–dark cycles. Infants develop these circadian rhythms over the first few months of life, with rhythmic secretion of melatonin by 12 weeks in term infants. Circadian rhythm sleep disorders occur when a person's sleep is of normal duration but occurs at a time that does not allow adequate sleep in the context of the person's life. For example, an adolescent who is unable to fall asleep until 4:00 am and cannot wake before noon is said to have a circadian rhythm disorder (sleep-phase delay) and is likely to have problems functioning in a usual school environment. If, however, a person with the same sleep-phase delay works at night, then the sleep-phase delay is not considered a disorder.

## ▶ SLEEP EVALUATION

Children rarely complain of sleeping problems. A parent or other caregiver usually initiates the diagnostic evaluation. The most common complaints are the child's inability to fall asleep or remain asleep, daytime sleepiness, and abnormal behaviors during sleep (snoring, gasping, or yelling). In sorting out a concern about sleep, history is the major initial diagnostic tool.

Questionnaires for general screening or for evaluating sleep complaints may be helpful in gathering data in busy practices. One simple, 5-item pediatric sleep screening instrument is BEARS (**B**edtime problems, **E**xcessive daytime sleepiness, **A**wakenings at night, **R**egularity and duration of sleep, and **S**noring).[7] The key areas explored on the BEARS parent questionnaire can lead to further open-ended questions by the practitioner to determine the level of parental concern (or to elicit maladaptive patterns if no concern is expressed) and to help formulate a differential diagnosis (Table 71-3). Having the parents keep a sleep chart is helpful (Figure 71-1); it may demonstrate a consistent pattern, which may improve with the use of sleep hygiene principles (Box 71-1). A general medical, developmental, and mental health history assessment should include any medications, herbal products, drugs, alcohol,

**Table 71-3**
**Questions to Clarify Sleep Problems**

| QUESTIONS | TO CLARIFY |
|---|---|
| **TO THE PARENTS** | |
| Do you have any concerns about the child's sleeping? | Problem versus disorder |
| How do you think the child is sleeping compared with other children of similar age? | Traumas or stress |
| When and how did the child's sleep problems start? | Secondary gain |
| Did other changes in the child's life occur around this time? | Traumas or stress |
| • What methods have you tried to solve this problem?<br>• What ideas have you had about solving this problem?<br>• What have others told you about this problem? | |
| What is the atmosphere in the room where the child sleeps with regard to temperature, darkness, noise, presence of siblings, and type of bed? | Environmental sleep disorder |
| When is the last time the child eats before falling asleep? | Inadequate sleep hygiene<br>Sleep-onset association disorder |
| Does the child consume any caffeine or nicotine in the evening? | Insomnia caused by substance or drug effects |
| What is the child doing just before bedtime? | Inadequate sleep hygiene<br>Limit-setting disorder<br>Bedtime resistance |
| What routines do you use to put the child to bed? | Inadequate sleep hygiene<br>Limit-setting disorder<br>Bedtime resistance |
| What exactly do you do at bedtime? | Sleep-association disorder |
| How does the child act at bedtime? | Bedtime resistance |
| Where and with whom does the child sleep? | Sleep-association disorder |
| What does your spouse or partner think about this arrangement? | Family conflict |
| Who else has something to say about the child's sleeping? | Family conflict |
| Is the child already asleep when you put him or her in the crib or bed? | Sleep-association disorder |
| What time is the child put in bed? | Limit-setting disorder<br>Inadequate sleep hygiene<br>Circadian disorders |
| What time is the child asleep? | Limit-setting disorder<br>Inadequate sleep hygiene<br>Circadian disorders |
| Does the child do anything unusual during sleep?<br>Snoring, gasping, apnea? | Sleep-disordered breathing |
| Leg kicking, thrashing? | Periodic limb movements, restless leg syndrome |
| Bed wetting? | Nocturnal enuresis |
| Shaking, screaming? | Nocturnal seizures<br>Parasomnias |

*Continued*

**Table 71-3**
**Questions to Clarify Sleep Problems—cont'd**

| QUESTIONS | TO CLARIFY |
|---|---|
| **TO THE PARENTS** | |
| What times does the child wake up? | Night feeders<br>Sleep-association disorder |
| How does the child appear, or what does he or she do after waking? | Parasomnias<br>Developmental night waking<br>Trained night feeders<br>Seizures |
| What works to resettle the child? | Sleep-association disorder<br>Trained night waking<br>Trained night feeding<br>Gastroesophageal reflux |
| How is that process for you? | Secondary gain |
| Does the child snore or seem to stop breathing during the night? | Sleep-related breathing disorder |
| What time is the child up for the day? | Circadian disorders<br>Mood disorders |
| Is the schedule the same on weekends, or does the child sleep in? | Limit-setting disorder or sleep-phase delay |
| How does the child wake up in the morning? | Circadian disorder or sleep-phase delay |
| When you wake the child, does he or she seem rested and cheerful? | Circadian disorder or sleep-phase delay<br>Inadequate sleep |
| What time does the child eat in the morning? | Circadian disorder or sleep-phase advance<br>Limit-setting disorder |
| If older than 3 years, does the child remember what happened during the night? | Parasomnia (not remembered)<br>Nightmares (remembered)<br>Panic attacks (remembered) |
| Does the child fall asleep during the day? If so, then when, where, and for how long? | Circadian disorders<br>Idiopathic hypersomnia or narcolepsy |
| How is the child settled for naps? | Sleep-association disorder<br>Limit-setting disorder |
| Does the child sleep differently at other people's houses? If so, then how? | Sleep-association disorder<br>Limit-setting disorder |
| Has the child ever been given any medications for sleep? | Insomnia caused by a psychiatric or behavioral condition |
| What was the medication? How did it work? | |
| Has anyone in the family ever had sleep problems? Did either of you have sleep problems as kids? | Genetic factors (short or long sleeper) |
| **TO THE CHILD** | |
| What do you think about before you go to sleep? | Anxiety or mood disorder<br>Limit-setting disorder |

**Table 71-3**
**Questions to Clarify Sleep Problems—cont'd**

| QUESTIONS | TO CLARIFY |
|---|---|
| **TO THE CHILD** | |
| How do you feel when you wake up in the night? | Nightmares<br>Disorders of arousal<br>Anxiety or mood disorders |
| Do you still feel sleepy in the morning? | Inadequate sleep<br>Circadian disorder or sleep-phase delay |
| How do you feel about this sleeping problem? | Anxiety<br>Secondary gain |
| What do you think your parents should do about this? | Secondary gain |
| How are your concentration and grades at school? | Sleep-related breathing disorder<br>Sleep-phase delay<br>Periodic limb movements disorder<br>Narcolepsy<br>Idiopathic hypersomnia |

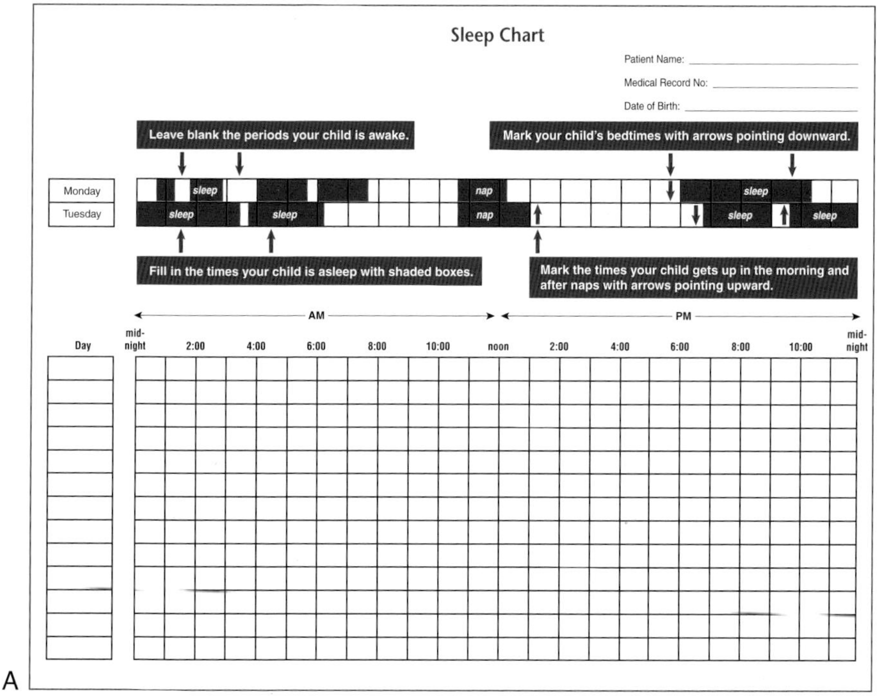


**Figure 71-1**
**A**, Sleep log.

*Continued*

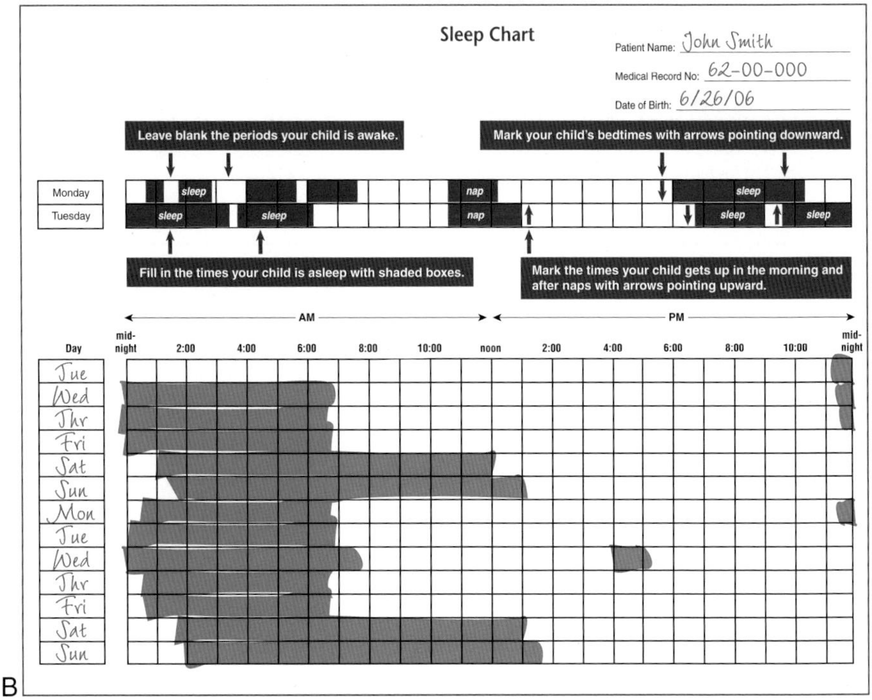


**Figure 71-1, cont'd**
**B**, Sleep log showing sleep-phase delay.

or tobacco use. Given that many sleep disorders have a strong familial component, a history of parental sleep issues may be helpful.

Parental perceptions and differences of opinion about sleep often are critical in problem-solving efforts. Co-sleeping (one or both parents sharing a bed with one or more children) serves as a good example of this point. Co-sleeping is a common practice in many cultures and households. When it is agreeable to both parents, co-sleeping is not associated with greater-than-average behavioral or emotional problems in the child. If, however, co-sleeping is a source of discord between parents or reflects a parent's inability to manage the child's behavioral bedtime problems, then it should be addressed as a sleep problem. When co-sleeping is planned, parents should agree on the desired duration. The pediatrician may help the parents by telling them that this arrangement is easier to change before 6 months of age (if an end is intended during infancy). Bed sharing with infants remains controversial particularly with mothers who smoke and when the infant is younger than 11 weeks.

Parental mental health needs to be screened in assessing sleep difficulties because the emotional stability of parents may affect both the perception of problems in children and the ability to carry out a treatment plan. Histories from babysitters or relatives who observe the child's sleep may be diagnostic, especially when problems seen at home are not seen in these settings. The family may provide audiotapes or videotapes that may be helpful.

**BOX 71-1**

## *Sleep Hygiene Principles*

General principles of sleep hygiene apply at any age, but specifics may vary with the child's age.

1. Establish a good sleep environment that is dark, quiet, and comfortable and has a steady, slightly cool temperature. Sleep should be in the same place for night and naps as much as possible. The bed or crib should be used as a place for sleep and not as play area or playpen while awake.
2. Establish a soothing bedtime routine that involves friendly interaction between the parent and the child. This routine may include a snack and then tooth brushing, use of the toilet, and then story, prayer, or talking time with children in their own bed. The parent should leave the room while the child is still awake.
3. Infants should be fed in a parent's arms and placed in the crib without a breast or a bottle in their mouth. Avoid excessive feeding close to bedtime to reduce the need to void during the night.
4. The child should be put to bed when moderately tired to reduce bedtime resistance.
5. For children whom the parents would like to have sleep in their own crib, teach them the skill of falling asleep on their own by avoiding pacifiers or body contact with the parent as they drift to sleep (self-soothing). This method enables children to go back to sleep on their own after waking during the night.
6. Avoid changing the routine because of demands or tantrums at bedtime, which can quickly develop into a pattern.
7. No television, computer, or any electronic screens should be in the child's room because research shows that video screens will prolong sleep onset and delay bedtime. It is advisable to enforce an electronic curfew for older children and adolescents to fascilitate preparation for sleep without distraction and also prevent further use during the night without parental supervision.
8. Try to keep a consistent schedule for bedtime, naps, and morning wake up, which will help the child maintain regular circadian rhythms. Naps should not be taken too close to bedtime.
9. Remember that television programs and movies may be frightening or stimulating. Arguments between parents or other family members may also be distressing. Try to keep the household atmosphere calm in the evening.
10. Keep track of activities that seem to lead to sleeping problems. If active play or video games lead to problems, then stop them 1 or 2 hours before bedtime. Caffeine and nicotine can disrupt sleep. Avoid caffeine at least 6 hours before bedtime.

The history is often diagnostic, but some patients need an overnight sleep study for further assessment. An overnight sleep study or polysomnogram consists of the following:

- Electroencephalogram (EEG) to identify sleep stages
- Electromyelogram of chin activity to help identify decreased tone during REM sleep
- Leg electromyelogram to measure leg movements
- Electrooculogram to identify eye movements seen in REM sleep
- Electrocardiogram to monitor cardiac rate and rhythm
- Nasal and oral thermistors to measure airflow
- Thoracic and abdominal belts to measure chest and abdominal movements during breathing (helpful in demonstrating increased or decreased respiratory effort)
- Pulse oximetry to measure oxygen saturation
- End-tidal carbon dioxide monitoring to indirectly measure hypoventilation

All of these measurements provide clinically useful information about sleep stages, sleep disruption, respiratory status during all sleep stages, leg movements, and changes in cardiac rate and rhythm during sleep. The sleep study also provides a picture of the relationship of sleep-related measurements. For instance, OSA may cause arousals, cardiac deceleration, and oxygen desaturation; these findings may be mild during NREM sleep but profound during REM sleep.

Overnight sleep studies are attended by a sleep technologist who attaches monitoring sensors and adjusts them during the night. The technologist also provides observations about the child's sleep that may be invaluable in making an accurate diagnosis.

Extended-montage video electromyelograms may be incorporated into the polysomnogram to diagnose nocturnal seizures. Haplotyping, karyotyping, or fluorescent in situ hybridization studies can be helpful for diagnosing some of the genetic conditions associated with sleep disorders such as congenital central hypoventilation syndrome, Rett syndrome, Smith-Magenis syndrome, and Prader-Willi syndrome.

## ▶ CLASSIFICATION OF SLEEP DISTURBANCES

Sleep disturbances in children can be categorized according to the *International Classification of Sleep Disorders*, second edition.[8]

- Behavioral insomnia of children
- Sleep-related breathing disorders
- Circadian rhythm disorders
- Parasomnias
- Sleep-related movement disorders
- Hypersomnias

## ▶ MATURATIONAL OR BEHAVIORAL ISSUES

### *Day–Night Reversals*

The earliest parental complaint about sleep is often day–night reversal, occurring around 2 weeks of age. This problem is predictable because consolidated nocturnal sleep has not yet developed. Parental concerns provide the pediatrician a valuable opportunity to assess parental coping skills and help parents understand the normal unfolding of the child's physiologic regulation. Day–night reversals can be shifted by establishing a general bedtime, keeping the lights off or low, and keeping handling and interaction to a minimum during nighttime feedings. In the morning, lights should be bright and social interaction encouraged. Lack of sleep at this age is unusual and should alert the clinician to medical problems, especially if associated with irritability.

### *Delayed Settling*

Another common problem is a delay in the much desired milestone of sleeping through the night. One definition of settling or sleeping through the night is 5 hours of continuous sleep after midnight for 4 consecutive weeks. Unrealistic parental expectations for sleeping through the night are common, and pediatricians need to carefully address misperceptions about how well a child should sleep. Anders observed that 44% of parents of 2-month-olds reported that their child slept throughout the night when, in fact, actual recording on time-lapse videotape showed that only 15% actually slept throughout the night without awakening.[9]

The issue of sleeping through the night may have important ramifications for the breastfeeding infant. Despite the widely recognized and undisputed advantages of human milk for infants, the duration of lactation in the United States is still well below the recommended goal of 50% at 6 months in all ethnic groups.[10] The perceptions of normal maternal and infant sleep patterns may be an important factor in failure to sustain lactation. Although breastfed infants are typically assumed to feed more frequently and have shorter meal intervals than bottle-fed infants, widely disparate differences in sleep patterns, crying, fussiness, and colic behavior between breastfed and bottle-fed infants have been reported. The perception that breastfed infants typically *settle* at an older age than bottle-fed infants and awaken more frequently at night is quoted in the popular press as an *advantage* of formula feeding. As a corollary, a mother's need for an uninterrupted night's sleep may inadvertently promote the early cessation of breastfeeding.

In fact, breastfeeding need not be associated with increased night wakening by 12 weeks of age; both breastfed and bottle-fed infants can respond to behavioral interventions aimed at increasing sleep time during the night.[11-13] Additional evidence is emerging that continuing lactation can actually increase maternal slow-wave (restorative) sleep because of increased circulating prolactin levels.[14] The circadian rhythm of tryptophan secretion in mother's milk may help promote nocturnal infant sleep and is being mimicked by investigation of varying amounts of tryptophan in day–night formulas.[15]

Infants who appear to have a low threshold of sensitivity by temperamental disposition also tend to settle later. Premature infants tend to settle around the time expected for their gestational age, although variability is greater than among full-term infants. Delays in central nervous system (CNS) maturation often are associated with delays in settling. Infants with frank neurologic impairments may not only be delayed in settling but also have other medical issues that need to be addressed to allow settling to occur.

## Sleep-Onset Associations

Infants and children develop habits of falling asleep in accustomed circumstances, such as in a bed, in a parent's arms, or while being fed. These sleep-onset associations may begin in the first 2 months of life and are one of several behavioral causes for insufficient sleep outlined in Table 71-4. Sleep-onset association may be viewed as a problem by the family when a child older than 6 months needs prolonged parental assistance to fall asleep at the beginning of the night and after each nocturnal arousal. This pattern is a conditioned response, and the child is unable to fall asleep unless the conditions allowing sleep onset are recreated. Parents may complain that their own sleep is severely disrupted because they need to help the infant resettle several times each night. Treatment is straightforward—the child learns to make the transition from wake to sleep without expecting a parent's participation. Parents should be advised to place the infant while still awake into the crib for both night and naps starting by 48 weeks postgestational age. A helpful tactic is for the infant's bedding to have the mother's scent for comfort. If a problematic sleep-onset association has already developed, then parents may need to institute a graduated extinction program (see below) to help infants older than 6 months learn to fall asleep on their own over several weeks.[16]

Although graduated extinction is a very effective treatment, parental distress is a common issue during the initial portions of employing an extinction strategy. Warning parents what to expect and addressing fears about harming or creating a sense of abandonment in the child

**Table 71-4**
**Causes of Insufficient Sleep in Children**

| | PREVALENCE | TREATMENT |
|---|---|---|
| **BEHAVIORAL** | | |
| Sleep-onset association disorder | 30%–40% | Education, extinction strategy |
| Limit-setting disorder | | Education, family counseling |
| Adjustment disorder | | Education, family counseling |
| Chronic sleep deprivation | Common | Education in sleep hygiene |
| Early school starting times | | Education; advocacy (petition school boards and legislature for later school start times) |
| Parent work schedule | | Education |
| Social activities | | Education |
| Idiopathic insomnia (diagnosis of exclusion; often made retrospectively) | Unknown | Good sleep hygiene; hypnotics under investigation |
| Circadian rhythm disorder | | Education, morning light therapy |
| Delayed sleep phase | | Advance sleep phase |
| Sleep entrainment | | Intense sensory clues; regular or strict daily schedule; melatonin |
| Hypothalamic tumor | | Intense sensory clues; regular or strict daily schedule; melatonin |
| Blindness | | Intense sensory clues; regular or strict daily schedule; melatonin |
| Mental retardation | | Intense sensory clues; regular or strict daily schedule; melatonin |

Reprinted from Givan DC. The sleepy child. *Pediatr Clin North Am.* 2004;51:15–31. Copyright 2004, with permission from Elsevier.

may alleviate some parental concern. Successful treatment will require consistency, and it is important that all nighttime caregivers are able to implement the extinction technique. If the parents are uncertain that they will be able to consistently implement extinction strategy, it may be advisable to delay treatment until that is possible. Parents should be educated that the extinction process may take longer if the disruptive sleep pattern becomes more well-established as the child becomes older.[17]

### Limit-Setting Disorder

Bedtime routines should take 30 minutes or less. Consistently longer bedtime routines may reflect parental difficulty in setting limits. Prolonged bedtime routines are often associated with multiple curtain calls for stories, hugs, water, and trips to the toilet. Toddlers and preschool children no longer sleeping in a crib may reappear after being put to bed, thus prolonging the routine. These curtain calls are unintentionally reinforced by the parental attention needed to return the child to bed, even if done with obvious displeasure.

The best management of prolonged bedtime routines is prevention through reasonable daily schedules, assurance of adequate special individual time with each parent every day, and careful limit setting. This approach reduces the child's separation anxiety as well as parental guilt. The bedtime routine should be limited to a defined set of activities or length of time. Parents may then either notify the child that they will not respond to further requests, or say "only one more" and adhere to this declaration. Parents should be warned to avoid responding to the excuses that will likely ensue. Having the parent promise to check the child frequently can also be reassuring. Bedtime should occur when the child is tired to enhance his or her tendency to fall asleep. Naps should not occur close to bedtime.

Positive reinforcement may enhance limit setting. Children who stay in bed without calling out may be motivated by simple rewards with stickers in the morning or an extra story the following night. Parents may need coaching on limit setting or referral to a psychologist if discipline is a major problem, or they may benefit from marital counseling if significant discord exists regarding family life.

### Bedtime Fears

Preschool and early school-aged children often have bedtime fears, which are often generated by stresses such as separation from parents, aggressive peers, sibling birth, or the death of a grandparent. Exposure to frightening movies or video games can also contribute. The child's fears should be acknowledged, and he or she should be reassured that the parents will keep him or her safe. A ritual of the adult *spraying for monsters* may be helpful. Having the child help the parent buy a special flashlight to check out the room at night provides a sense of mastery. Older children benefit from relaxation exercises accompanied by empowerment stories. A nightlight may be helpful.

### Primary Insomnia

Primary insomnia can be seen in normal children but is generally transient and is a diagnosis of exclusion. It must last at least 1 month, interfere significantly with functioning or cause significant distress, and not be part of another medical, sleep, or mental disorder. The symptoms and signs of inadequate sleep are listed in Box 71-2.

Medication for primary insomnia in healthy children is controversial, but medications such as diphenhydramine, clonidine, and melatonin have been used in pediatric insomnia. Indiscriminate medication use can mislead physicians and families about the causes of insomnia and ignore the behavioral management needed.[18]

A disruptive sleeping environment may cause either sleep onset or sleep maintenance insomnia. Excessive noise or light, uncomfortable bedding, excessive room temperature,

**Box 71-2**

#### *Symptoms and Signs of Inadequate Amount of Sleep*

1. Excessive daytime sleepiness (rare in young children)
2. Hyperactivity–impaired attention
3. Poor school performance–impaired concentration, vigilance
4. Behavior problems–bad mood, irritability
5. Obesity–possible link to inadequate sleep
6. Failure to thrive

interference of pets, or outside noises are commonly found. Treatment is simply to eliminate or correct the environmental condition or distraction.

### Other Difficulties Falling Asleep

Dyssomnia, the term for insomnia that does not meet disorder criteria, occurs mainly in preschool-aged and older children. This problem includes environmental sleep disorder caused commonly by noise, pets, and temperature extremes. Revising the household routine to allow quiet for adequate sleep is necessary to resolve this dilemma (Table 71-5).

## Awakenings From Sleep

Waking at night occurs in more than 80% of children and, of course, in infants who still need to feed. Night waking is only problematic when the child cannot return to sleep on

**Table 71-5**
**Causes of Sleep Fragmentation in Children**

| | PREVALENCE | TREATMENT |
|---|---|---|
| Behavioral | 30%–40% of persons with sleep fragmentation | |
| Sleep-onset association | | Education |
| **PARASOMNIAS** | | |
| Sleep terrors | | Education, good sleep hygiene, medication (rarely) |
| Sleep talking | | Education, good sleep hygiene |
| Somnambulism | | Education, good sleep hygiene, review safety issues |
| Confusional arousals | | Education, good sleep hygiene |
| **SLEEP-RELATED BREATHING DISORDER** | | |
| Sleep apnea | 2% | Adenotonsillectomy, nasal CPAP |
| Upper airway resistance syndrome | Unknown | Adenotonsillectomy, nasal CPAP |
| **OTHER MEDICAL** | | |
| Asthma<br>Cystic fibrosis<br>Gastroesophageal reflux<br>Nocturnal seizure | | Medical management<br>Medical management<br>Medical management<br>Anticonvulsants |
| Periodic leg movements of sleep | 3.9%–10% of adults; 2% of children; 20% of children with attention-deficit/hyperactivity disorder | Iron replacement therapy; dopamine agonists; gabapentin |
| **ENVIRONMENT** | | |
| Co-sleeping, noise, pets | | Education, safety issues |

*CPAP,* continuous positive airway pressure.
Reprinted from Givan DC. The sleepy child. *Pediatr Clin North Am.* 2004;51:15–31. Copyright 2004, with permission from Elsevier.

his or her own. As many as 20% of 2-year-olds, 14% of 3-year-olds, and 6.5% of 5- to 12-year-olds have problematic night awakenings.[19] Common causes and treatment of sleep fragmentation and disrupted sleep continuity are outlined in Table 71-5.

## Sleep-Onset Association Disorder

**TRAINED NIGHT FEEDING.** In Western industrialized societies, between 60% and 70% of either breastfed or bottle-fed infants are reported to be settling or sleeping through the night by 12 weeks of age without any specific behavioral interventions.[12,20] Nonetheless, some infants older than 6 months who wake up during the night are immediately fed to encourage their return to sleep. Their sleep cycle may be changed by the introduction of food to produce an arousal—basically, learned hunger—and they will consume a full feeding during the night. Trained night feeding should generally not be diagnosed before 6 months postterm because of the frequent need for a feeding during the night in younger or premature infants. Infants who learned to sleep through the night and subsequently begin waking during the night and seem genuinely hungry are probably ready for solids (if they are older than 4 to 6 months) or need increased volumes or number of feeds during the day and evening if they are formula fed. Breastfed infants may respond better to more frequent evening feedings (cluster feeding) of smaller but richer (higher lipid content) human milk.

Trained night feeding can be prevented by teaching parents ways to recognize when an infant is fussy because of hunger and when fussiness arises from other causes, such as boredom. Parents should not automatically feed a fussy infant unless the infant appears hungry. Parents who go to their infants older than 4 months at the first sound of stirring should also be encouraged to allow their infants the opportunity to return to sleep without intervention. Expectations of the appropriate need for a late (eg, 10:00 pm) feeding should be clarified. Daytime feeding intervals can be adjusted gradually and any sleep associations retrained simultaneously. If night feedings are an established pattern, then the formula-fed infant can be fed 1 oz less each night. This tactic will usually help resolve trained night feeding in approximately 1 week.

**TRAINED NIGHT WAKING.** Waking at night without requiring a feeding in the infant between 4 and 8 months of age is called *trained night waking*. This pattern often begins when the infant is ill or subjected to travel or some other change in routine, but the pattern may persist because the child gets a secondary reward from the parent's attention. One parent may believe that quieting the infant quickly is necessary to avoid disturbing other family members or neighbors. In some instances, parents who have little time to spend with the child during the day enjoy this time with the child and reinforce the night waking by playing with him or her. Trained night waking is also increasingly common in infants who have difficult temperaments.

Management of trained night waking that causes persistent family disruption requires management of the precipitant stress and, ideally, collaboration with the spouse or neighbors to tolerate some crying during the treatment. Bedtime routines need to be established, perhaps with bedding or infant clothing with a maternal scent, and the infant should be put into bed awake. Daytime naps should be limited to 2 hours to consolidate the longest sleep period at night. When awakening during the night, the infant should be allowed 1 to 2 minutes of crying before being checked, but not fed, and then checked every 2 to 5 minutes in most circumstances. The infant may be touched but not picked up, rocked, or cuddled. For success, this approach may require the more involved parent to take a shower, turn up music, or find some other distraction. Brief sedation with diphenhydramine for the infant should rarely be needed to help modify this habit if the graded extinction techniques described previously are strictly applied.

**DEVELOPMENTAL NIGHT WAKING.** Although most infants are sleeping through the night by 6 months of age, many begin awakening again around 8 to 10 months of age. This new behavior, called *developmental night waking*, corresponds to several coincident developmental processes, including increased mobility, fear reactions to strangers, and object permanence (ability to remember and seek something or someone, like a parent, that is out of sight).

The best management is advising parents at the 6-month well visit to expect a recurrence of night waking. Because of differences in cultures, not all parents will see this circumstance as a problem. For parents who do, they should be advised to wait a few minutes before going to the infant but to avoid feeding or other reinforcement. If waking is already established, then the parents should have the contributing developmental forces explained and be advised to create a bedtime routine, including a transitional object and a dim nightlight. When the infant awakens, he or she should be given at least 2 minutes to self-soothe, with some fussing tolerated as part of the process. If fussing continues, then one parent can go to reassure the child briefly, without touching or feeding, and settle down within sight to sleep the rest of the night without talking to the child. The child often becomes enraged instead of fearful, which is more tolerable to the parent, who can see that the child is safe. Some parents are more comfortable than others with this plan. For children who are no longer constrained to a crib, the parent must prevent body contact with the child by giving him or her the alternative that the parent will leave the room to avoid establishing a sleep association. Further interactions should be brief and minimally interactive. Eventually, the child will no longer require the parent's presence to return to sleep after nocturnal awakenings.[17]

## Sleep-Related Breathing Disorder

The pediatrician is often confronted with the problem of what to do with the child who snores. Snoring is common; OSA is less common.

Young children with SDB are usually not obese, unlike typical adult patients. Some groups of children are at particularly high risk for SDB, including those with craniofacial anomalies, chromosomal syndromes, and neuromuscular disorders. Children with Down syndrome, Prader-Willi syndrome, cleft palate, achondroplasia, muscular dystrophy, cerebral palsy, and other underlying disorders should be routinely screened for sleep problems.[21] Although children with Down syndrome, for instance, typically have learning difficulties, treatment of SDB may result in improved daytime performance.

While many children with obstructive SDB improve after adenotonsillectomy, those with either obesity or asthma are more likely not to have complete resolution of symptoms.[22] On occasion, nasal continuous positive airway pressure (CPAP) or even tracheostomy may be required.

The question of whether all children should have sleep studies before undergoing adenotonsillectomy is controversial. However, certain groups of children are clearly at higher risk for perioperative complications and may warrant polysomnograms as part of a preoperative evaluation, especially if outpatient surgery is being contemplated. Children younger than

3 years, children with morbid obesity or chromosomal or craniofacial anomalies, children with underlying neuromuscular disorders, and those with other underlying medical conditions that make them higher-risk surgical patients should be considered for preoperative polysomnograms.[22-24]

## Circadian Rhythm Sleep Disorder

The most common circadian rhythm disorder causing insomnia is a sleep-phase delay that is commonly seen in adolescents. Because the natural circadian cycle is approximately 24.5 hours, some individuals are vulnerable to shifting sleep cycles by approximately 30 minutes a day. This shift often results in difficulty waking in time for school in the morning. Morning battles with parents about waking for school are common. Phase-delayed adolescents often sleep very late on weekends and vacations and then find falling asleep at a reasonable bedtime even more difficult. Changing adolescent sleep-phase delay is very difficult and requires intense commitment and active participation of the adolescent and parents with the use of bright light exposure in the morning and consistent wake times all 7 days of the week.

Some children who are deprived of normal circadian stimuli develop circadian rhythm disorders. Because zeitgebers that entrain normal circadian rhythm include light (especially sunlight that may be 100,000 lux), exercise, social activities, and eating, the fact that a child with cerebral palsy who is blind, wheelchair dependent, and fed by gastrostomy tube has difficulty with a varying sleep time is not surprising.

Other children have circadian rhythm problems that reflect a chaotic home life. Some families do not adhere to predictable routines, allowing children to set their own schedules, resulting in seemingly bizarre sleep patterns. A circadian rhythm disorder may be differentiated from an oppositional disorder by the child's behavior pattern. A child with a circadian rhythm disorder may not resist going to bed but is unable to fall asleep. In the morning, the child is difficult to arouse and does not feel rested.

A sleep-phase advance usually occurs in infants or toddlers who fall asleep early (7:00 pm) but then awaken early in the morning (3:00 am). Different types of circadian shift can be adjusted by simultaneously shifting naps, bedtime, waking time, and meals to a desired schedule that matches the child's total daily sleep needs.

In difficult cases, the child can wear an actigraph, a small portable device similar to a large wristwatch, for several weeks. The device senses physical motion by means of an accelerometer and stores the information. Actigraphy provides a graphic illustration of a child's sleep–wake schedule and can be a useful, noninvasive method for assessing specific sleep disorders such as insomnia, excessive daytime sleepiness, and circadian rhythm disorders (Figure 71-2).

## Parasomnias (Partial Arousal Disorders)

Parasomnias are unusual behaviors or experiences that occur during sleep or the transition between sleep and wake. Parasomnias associated with partial arousal from slow-wave sleep are common in children. They include confusional arousals, sleep terrors, and sleepwalking disorder (somnambulism). All of these episodes occur during arousal from slow-wave sleep, usually in the first third of the night. The child appears confused or frightened and is unresponsive to parental intervention. The child is not fully awake and does not remember the event in the morning.

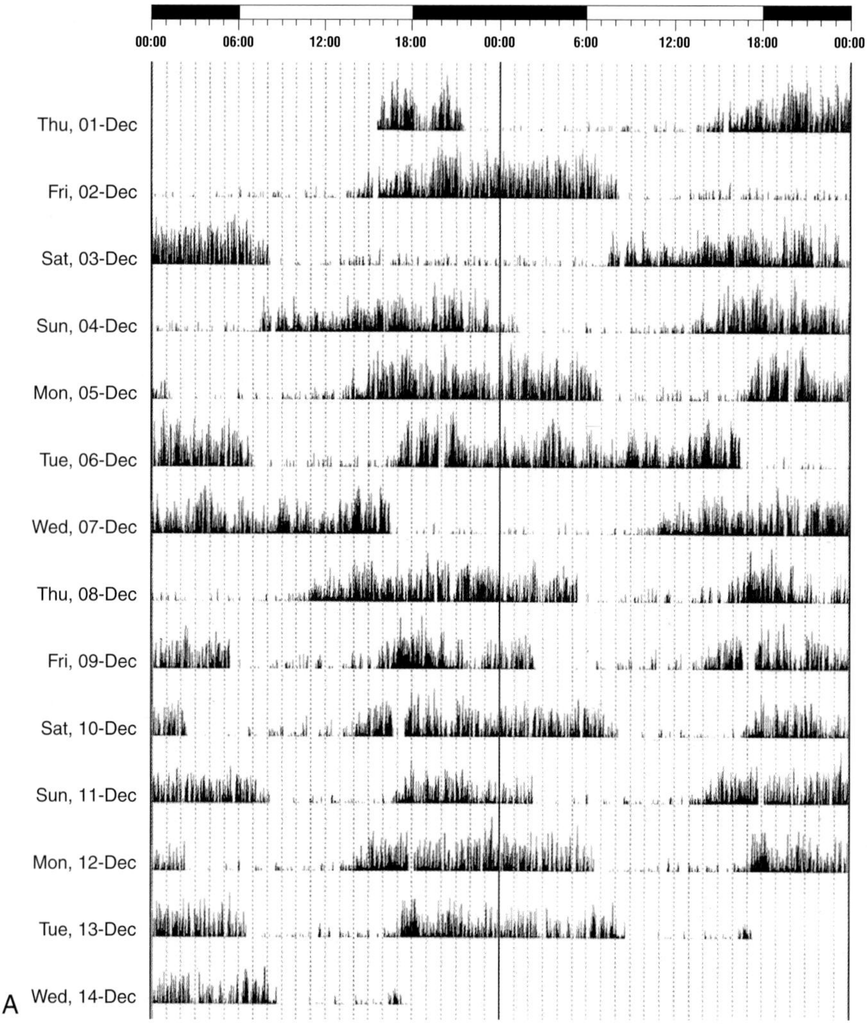


**Figure 71-2**
Ten-year-old child with Down syndrome and nighttime G-tube feeding after brain injury. **A**, Random sleeping pattern with the child frequently awake at night.

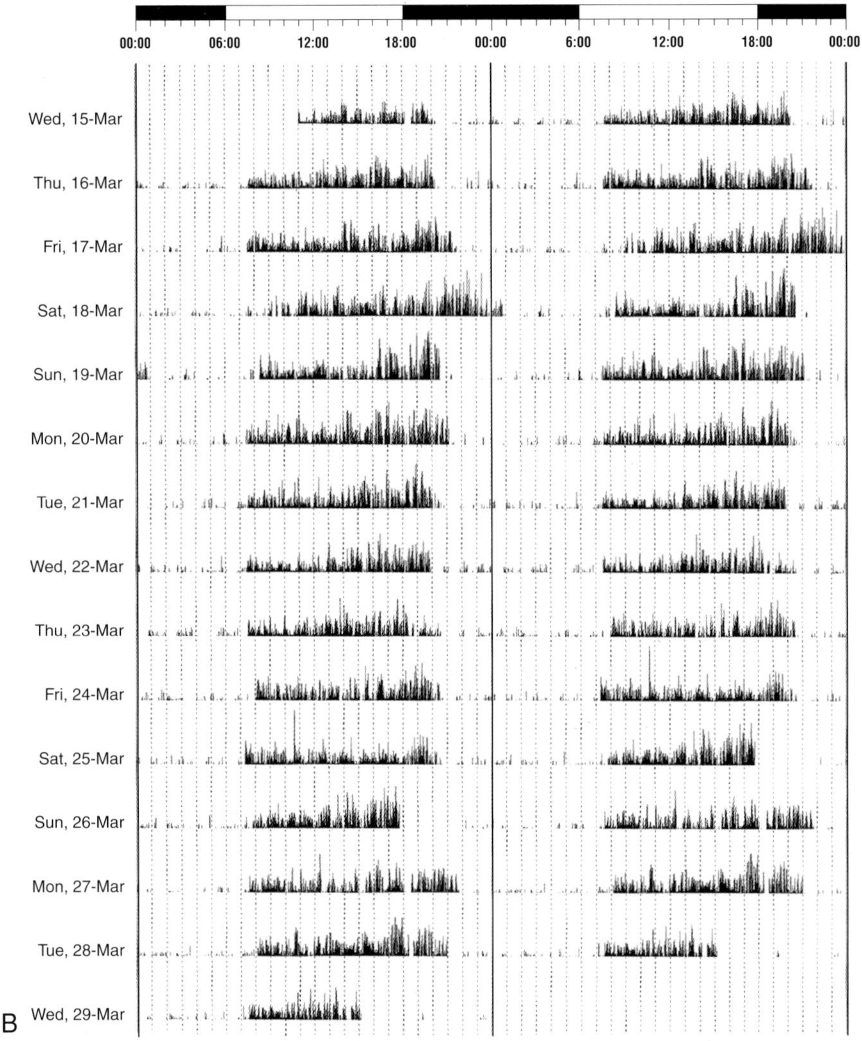


**Figure 71-2, cont'd**

**B,** Stabilized sleeping pattern using nighttime melatonin and morning phototherapy, and stopping G-tube feedings at night.

Symptoms most often begin in childhood and resolve spontaneously, occasionally persisting into adulthood (0.5%). Diagnosis is based on the timing of these symptoms (generally during the first third of the night), the typical presentation, and the child's lack of recall of the events when awake the next morning (morning amnesia). A strong familial component exists, and history often reveals that one or both parents had similar behaviors as children.

**CONFUSIONAL AROUSALS.** Young children may experience partial arousals from slow-wave sleep, during which they sit up, mumble, and may appear awake; they seem confused and nonresponsive to parental questions. The prevalence of confusional arousals was 17% between ages 3 and 13 years in one study.[25] Children may sometimes thrash about and respond combatively to parental attempts to intervene. Confusional arousals usually occur in the first third of the night, but a child may occasionally have multiple arousals, extending into the second half of the night, generally decreasing in intensity. Confusional arousals are most common when children are overtired or ill. Management includes reassurance that the episodes are generally benign, minimal intervention during episodes, and removal of potential safety hazards from the child's bedroom. Treating disorders that may fragment sleep such as OSA and restless leg syndrome can be helpful. In severe cases, a few weeks of a benzodiazepine, such as lorazepam, at bedtime may interrupt the sequence by reducing slow-wave sleep. However, rebound occurs with discontinuation of the medication, often with an increasing number of events. A sleep study may help to confirm the diagnosis and detect precipitating events such as OSA or nocturnal seizures in severe or atypical cases.

**SLEEP TERRORS.** Sleep terrors are partial awakenings from slow-wave sleep characterized by physiologic arousal including pallor, sweating, pupillary dilation, piloerection, and tachycardia. The child may sit up and scream and may appear terrified. The child may thrash or run and is not responsive to attempted parental comforting. The child does not remember the event in the morning. Sleep terrors occur in 3% of children, usually starting between 18 months and 5 years. These episodes do not reflect emotional disturbance, although, as with all NREM parasomnias, occurrence is increased with illness, stress, or sleep deprivation. A family history of sleep terrors, enuresis, somnambulism, or sleep talking is often present. Sleep terrors may be precipitated by fatigue, stress, a full bladder, or loud noises. They tend to occur in bouts for several weeks and then disappear only to recur several weeks later. Parents need reassurance about the benign nature of sleep terrors and their tendency to resolve in approximately 95% of children by 8 years of age. The bladder should be emptied routinely before bedtime, and the environment should be kept dark and quiet. The bouts may occasionally be interrupted by waking the child 15 minutes before the expected episode, generally occurring approximately 1 hour into sleep each night for approximately a week. A 30- to 60-minute afternoon nap can also reduce the depth and amount of stage IV sleep and may decrease the number of episodes. Treatment with benzodiazepines can reduce the frequency of these events by altering slow-wave sleep, but episodes may recur when the child is weaned or when tolerance occurs. An investigation for nocturnal seizures with full EEG as part of a sleep study is indicated in intractable cases or those that have their onset in adolescence.

**SLEEPWALKING DISORDER (SOMNAMBULISM).** Approximately 15% of children sleepwalk at some time. Between 1% and 6% have 1 to 4 episodes per week, mostly between ages 4 and 12 years.[26] Sleepwalking, as with other disorders of arousal, occurs mainly during slow-wave stage N3 sleep, generally in the initial 120 minutes of sleep. During sleepwalking, children are difficult to arouse, are uncoordinated, and tend to wander in illogical places, often urinating outside the toilet. Chronic sleepwalkers need to be carefully safeguarded so that they do not injure themselves. Door and window alarms and locks may be necessary. Amnesia of the event in the morning is common. Sleepwalking can usually be differentiated by history (regular timing, same movements) or videotapes from dissociative states or seizures; however, occasionally, extended EEG as part of a sleep study may be necessary.

## Nightmare Disorder

Nightmares are an extremely common parasomnia occurring during REM sleep and are most common in the last third of the sleep period. The dream content often is recalled as frightening and reflects daytime stresses. Although children clearly dream by 14 months of age, nightmares are most common between 3 and 6 years, occurring in 10% to 50% of children. At these ages, children have the verbal skills to describe dreams. They also have vivid imaginations and fears.

Nightmares are uniformly part of posttraumatic stress disorder; they may increase after withdrawal of REM-suppressing substances such as alcohol and antidepressants.

A child who wakes from a frightening dream should be comforted, keeping the intervention brief to avoid secondary gain. The same concerns listed for bedtime fears should be addressed when nightmares are frequent. Children who have chronic nightmares have been shown to improve with targeted relaxation exercises and stories in which the child masters a situation. Children can prepare to have good dreams through rehearsal and imaging at bedtime. Severe nightmares may respond to bedtime medications, although counseling is mandatory if the condition is of a severity to warrant medication.

### Violent Behavior During Sleep

An REM behavior disorder (RBD) has been described in which normal REM atonia does not occur. Dream content can be physically acted out, sometimes in violent ways. RBD is very rare in healthy children but has been seen in autistic children or in association with neurologic disorders. A clue to diagnosis is that abnormal behaviors occur during the last third of the night, unlike NREM motor parasomnias, which typically occur during slow-wave sleep during the first third of the sleep period. Diagnosis requires a sleep study and neuroimaging studies. Treatment with clonazepam has been beneficial in autistic children and is the most common treatment in adults.

### Other Parasomnias

Bruxism is grinding the teeth during sleep and has been reported in more than 50% of children, with a mean age of onset of 10.5 years. No longitudinal studies demonstrating the natural history of bruxism have been conducted, but dental evidence of bruxism can be identified in 10% to 20% of the general population. Bruxism can also be caused by dental malocclusion or neurologic or psychiatric conditions. Tooth guards can protect the teeth and reduce potential damage to the temporomandibular joint. If stress or anxiety is a trigger, then relaxation exercises at bedtime may be helpful.

## ▶ SLEEP-RELATED MOVEMENT DISORDERS

### Restless Legs Syndrome and Periodic Limb Movements of Sleep

Restless legs syndrome occurs in about 2% of children between 8 and 17 years of age.[27] It is characterized by uncomfortable sensations in the legs, which are worse at rest ("like worms crawling under my skin"). These sensations are present in the evening, are associated with the need to move, and are temporarily relieved by movement. They are sometimes confused with growing pains. They may interfere with the child's ability to fall asleep. A strong familial component exists. Periodic limb movements of sleep are repetitive, brief leg twitches, occurring more than 5 times per hour in children. Leg movements or jerks may occur with resumption of a breath after a central apnea or with a loud snort or snore at the termination of an obstructive apnea. They may cause arousals, fragmenting the continuity of sleep and leading to a complaint of sleep maintenance insomnia. Although the two syndromes are not identical, many patients experience both. In children, limb movements may be exacerbated by iron deficiency or the use of antidepressant medication. They are more common in children with attention-deficit/hyperactivity disorder (ADHD). Treatment may include iron supplements, clonidine, gabapentin, or dopaminergic agents, depending on the age of the child.

### Sleep–Wake Transition Disorder

Rhythmic movements while falling asleep are common in infants and toddlers. Rhythmic movement disorders include head banging and body rocking. Some rhythmic activity at bedtime occurs in more than half of 9-month-olds, decreasing to one-third at 18 months, and to less than one-fourth at 2 years of age. Head banging is typically monotonous, occurring 60 to 80 times per minute, usually for less than 15 minutes. Usually benign, head banging may occasionally be caused by CNS injury, headache, inner ear abnormality, sensory deprivation (including visual or hearing impairment), neglect, or abuse. Children of intense temperament are especially likely to bang. Although head banging usually does not cause brain injury, it can be traumatic if the bed is unstable or if safety precautions are not taken in the environment. The condition may be reduced by kinesthetic stimulation during the evening and holding the child as part of the bedtime routine. Sleep restriction (ie, limiting the time the child lies in bed before falling asleep) and mild sedation have been shown to be helpful in difficult cases. Parents often need reassurance of the generally benign nature of these behaviors.

## ▶ HYPERSOMNIA

Excessive daytime sleepiness (EDS) can be caused by insufficient sleep (see Table 71-4), fragmented sleep (see Table 71-5), or increased sleep drive (Table 71-6). Although some sleepy children appear to have difficulty remaining awake, many sleepy children may exhibit hyperactivity, restlessness, poor concentration, impulsivity, aggressiveness, or irritability. Sleepiness needs to be differentiated from weakness or fatigue. The major sleep disorders causing primary hypersomnia in children are narcolepsy and idiopathic hypersomnia.

**Table 71-6**
**Excessive Sleepiness in Children—Causes of Increased Sleep Drive**

| DIAGNOSIS | PREVALENCE | TREATMENT |
|---|---|---|
| Narcolepsy | 0.2% | Stimulant medication, attention to sleep hygiene, treatment of coexisting sleep problems (periodic limb movement disorder, obstructive apnea) |
| **TEMPORARY HYPERSOMNOLENCE** | | |
| | | None specifically |
| Acute medical illness<br>Illicit drug use<br>Medications | | |
| **RECURRENT HYPERSOMNOLENCE** | | |
| Depression | Common | Antidepressants |
| Kleine-Levin syndrome | Rare | Lithium; carbamazepine; monitor serum levels for both drugs |
| Menstruation related | Rare | Oral contraceptives |
| **IDIOPATHIC HYPERSOMNOLENCE** | | |
| | | Stimulant medication |

Reprinted from Givan DC. The sleepy child. *Pediatr Clin North Am.* 2004;51:15–31. Copyright 2004, with permission from Elsevier.

## Narcolepsy

Narcolepsy is a potentially disabling syndrome of irresistible daytime sleep attacks, abnormally fast transitions to REM sleep from awake, and disrupted nighttime sleep. It occurs in 0.04% of whites and 0.07% of blacks. As many as one-third of adults with narcolepsy report onset of symptoms before 15 years of age, but diagnosis is frequently delayed at least a decade. Loss of muscle tone with emotions while awake (cataplexy), inability to move for a few seconds to minutes on awakening (sleep paralysis), and visual aura or dream states while falling asleep (hypnagogic hallucinations), along with EDS, make up the complete narcolepsy tetrad seen in 30% of affected persons. Approximately 90% of patients with narcolepsy with cataplexy are positive for HLA DQB1*0602. Narcolepsy is seen in children, but peak age of onset of symptoms is 15 to 25 years. Cataplexy—brief episodes of bilateral muscle weakness, usually associated with laughter or strong emotion, that may result in falling, head bobbing, or jaw sagging—is highly specific to narcolepsy but may not be seen in more than 50% of cases. Diagnosis of narcolepsy without documented cataplexy can be made by overnight polysomnography showing absence of other sleep diagnoses and a multiple sleep latency test (5 nap opportunities, separated by 2 hours, immediately following the overnight sleep study) showing rapid sleep onset periods (mean, <8 minutes) with at least 2 naps containing REM sleep. Differential diagnosis includes hydrocephalus, postviral infection (mononucleosis), previous CNS trauma, or idiopathic hypersomnia. Absence of HLA DQB1*0602 does not exclude the diagnosis of narcolepsy, especially without cataplexy. Given that 20% of the general population is positive for HLA DQB1*0602, this test is not specific for possible narcolepsy patients with EDS. Recent research shows that narcolepsy with cataplexy results from the loss of approximately 70,000 hypothalamic neurons producing the neuropeptide hypocretin.

Narcolepsy treatment may include the use of stimulants such as modafinil or methylphenidate to address excessive daytime sleepiness, antidepressants such as venlafaxine to control cataplexy, regular adequate sleep, 2 to 3 planned 30-minute daytime naps, and timing of activities at optimal hours of alertness.[28] Education of the patient, family members, and school personnel is important. Support for handling the difficulties of this lifelong chronic condition is such that referral to a pediatric sleep disorders center is indicated, but often primary care physicians may be required to monitor compliance with medications for participation in activities such as sports, school testing, and driving.

## Idiopathic Hypersomnia

Idiopathic hypersomnia is a disorder of constant and severe EDS, despite adequate nocturnal sleep. Idiopathic hypersomnia is, by definition, a diagnosis of exclusion. A complete evaluation for other causes of hypersomnia must be undertaken, including neurologic disorders (hydrocephalus or CNS tumors), primary sleep disorders (OSA), mood disorders, chronic fatigue syndrome, and medical disorders (acute and chronic infections including mononucleosis, metabolic disorders, or muscle diseases). Although the mean sleep latency is short in idiopathic hypersomnia, similar to narcolepsy, affected patients do not have the 2 sleep-onset REM periods that characterize narcolepsy. Treatment of idiopathic hypersomnia includes attention to sleep hygiene issues, use of stimulant medications, and thorough review of safety issues such as driving or operating machinery.[29]

## ▶ SLEEP DISORDERS ASSOCIATED WITH PSYCHIATRIC OR BEHAVIORAL DISORDERS

Although sleep problems may occur in association with almost any mental health disorder (Table 71-7), mood disorders are among the most common. Depression may cause sleep-onset insomnia, although this condition is less common in young children than in other age groups. The early-morning waking of depressed adults is not usually seen before puberty and only rarely among adolescents, for whom hypersomnia is a more common complaint than insomnia.[30] The sleep problems that are intrinsic to depression are complicated by intrusive thoughts or worries that may interfere with sleep maintenance. Treatments of sleeping problems in depressed children may include cognitive behavioral therapy and antidepressants.[31]

Children with bipolar disorder may have a dramatically reduced need for sleep (<4 hours a day) during the manic phase. Anxiety and panic disorders may result in difficulties falling asleep because of specific or nonspecific fears, as well as difficulties returning to sleep if aroused during the night. Children who have been abused have frequent sleep problems, including nightmares, increased activity during sleep, and sleep-onset and sleep-maintenance insomnia.[32]

Personality disorders in adolescence have been associated with sleep-onset insomnia. Psychoses may include troubling intrusive thoughts, especially at night.

**Table 71-7**
**Behavioral and Psychiatric Disorders Associated With Sleep Problems in Children**

| DIAGNOSIS | SLEEP PROBLEMS |
|---|---|
| Depression | Sleep-onset or maintenance insomnia seen in 50%<br>Early morning awakenings<br>EDS seen in 25%<br>Sleep complaints are the most prevalent symptoms of major depression in adolescents |
| Bipolar disorder | Decreased need for sleep without fatigue<br>Insomnia |
| Seasonal affective disorder | Prevalence 3%–4% in children with EDS, fatigue in winter |
| Anxiety disorder | Increased night awakenings, nighttime fears<br>Increased sleep-onset insomnia, bedtime problems<br>Increased EDS |
| Obsessive compulsive disorder | Decreased total sleep time |
| Autism, pervasive developmental disorder | Sleep-onset insomnia, difficulty settling at night, prolonged and frequent nocturnal awakenings<br>Shortened duration of sleep<br>Irregular sleep–wake pattern<br>Parasomnia (including rapid eye movement behavioral disorder) |
| Attention-deficit/hyperactivity disorder | Sleep-onset or maintenance insomnia<br>Nocturnal wakening, obstructive sleep apnea, excessive periodic limb movements |

*EDS,* excessive daytime sleepiness.
Derived from Ivananko A, Crabtree VM, Gozal D. Sleep in children with psychiatric disorders. *Pediatr Clin North Am.* 2004;51:51–68.

Insomnia or hypersomnia caused by substance abuse should be considered in sleep disorders in older children and adolescents. Alcohol can induce sleep, but it causes sleep fragmentation in the latter portion of the night. When alcohol is metabolized (1 beer, 5 oz of wine, or 1 oz of liquor per hour), sympathetic tone increases, leading to abrupt arousals and sleep maintenance insomnia. Withdrawal from chronic alcohol abuse may cause severe insomnia. Stimulants such as cocaine and amphetamines can cause severe insomnia. Some antidepressants such as fluoxetine may cause insomnia, whereas others such as tricyclics, trazodone, or mirtazapine may cause EDS. Antidepressants may eliminate REM atonia, thus precipitating RBD. Atypical antipsychotics such as aripiprazole may cause stimulation, whereas others such as olanzapine cause sedation.

## ▶ DEVELOPMENTAL DISORDERS

Learning disabilities are associated with increased rates of sleep disturbance, including night waking and trouble falling asleep. Half of these sleep difficulties persist for more than 3 years.[33] Systematic review of the literature suggests that children with ADHD have higher daytime sleepiness, more movements during sleep, and higher apnea-hypopnea indexes compared with controls. Reported sleep problems also include trouble settling to sleep and multiple awakenings from sleep.[34] Medications used to treat ADHD may prolong sleep-onset latency. Clonidine at bedtime has been found to be effective in improving the sleep of 85% of these children when behavioral measures failed.[35]

Many children with autism have serious sleep problems, with difficulties falling asleep, waking in the night, and early-morning waking. Children with autism frequently have insomnia that may benefit from behavioral interventions, melatonin, or medications.[36] Asperger syndrome has been associated with insomnia and RBD. Children who have Tourette syndrome have increased parasomnias.

## ▶ SLEEP DISORDERS ASSOCIATED WITH MEDICAL PROBLEMS

Sleep problems are seen in a variety of medical conditions (Table 71-8).

### *Neurologic Disorders*

Any CNS impairment can result in dysregulation of the sleep cycle. As many as 85% of children who have major developmental disabilities may experience chronic sleep problems.[37] Behavioral sleep problems in these children can be improved by establishing a bedtime routine and putting the child to bed when sleep onset is likely to occur quickly. If the child has persistent difficulty falling asleep, then establishing a new pattern may be helpful by delaying the usual bedtime for 30 minutes and then removing the child from bed if sleep does not occur in 15 to 20 minutes. After removing the child from bed, the parent should keep him or her awake for 30 minutes. This procedure is repeated until the child falls asleep within 15 minutes of being put in bed. Wake-up time is kept constant. Daytime naps are not allowed for children older than 4 years.

Other factors such as timing of medications, need for repositioning during the night, pain, nighttime feedings, and caregiver anxiety can contribute to sleep problems in the neurologically impaired child. Melatonin at bedtime has been shown to be helpful in some children who have CNS problems or blindness as the cause of their sleep disturbance. Melatonin should be used cautiously in children with seizure disorders.

### Table 71-8
### Medical Disorders Associated With Sleep Problems in Childhood

| DIAGNOSIS | SLEEP PROBLEMS |
|---|---|
| Asthma | Circadian variation in |
| | • Peak expiratory flow (nadir at 4:00 am)<br>• Cutaneous immediate hypersensitivity to house dust allergen<br>• Airway inflammation<br>Sleep-related changes<br>• Decrease in lung volumes and increase airway resistance<br>• Increase airway resistance and decrease intrapulmonary blood volume<br>• Decrease mucociliary clearance<br>• Nocturnal gastroesophageal reflux |
| | Frequent nocturnal awakenings and decrease stage 4 sleep |
| Cystic fibrosis | OSA can be common in children <7 years.<br>Nocturnal oxygen desaturation in children >7 years<br>• Hypoventilation, especially in REM sleep caused by de-recruitment of ventilatory muscles<br>• Ventilation–perfusion mismatch caused by decreased functional residual capacity<br>• Occurs more frequently with forced expiratory volume <65% or resting oxygen saturation while sitting <94% |
| Craniofacial abnormalities (Pierre Robin sequence, Goldenhar syndrome, Down syndrome, Treacher Collins syndrome, velocardiofacial syndrome, cleft lip and palate) | Upper airway obstruction<br>Nocturnal hypoventilation |
| Gastroesophageal reflux | Increased night awakening and pain<br>Delayed sleep onset<br>May result in nocturnal stridor, cough, and wheezing |
| Down syndrome | Upper airway obstruction with OSA in 30%–60%<br>Decreased REM sleep associated with low IQ |
| Sickle cell disease | Episodic and continuous nocturnal hypoxemia in 40% of children caused by either OSA or primary lung disease |
| Obesity | OSA<br>• Obesity hypoventilation syndrome: Hypercapnia, hypoxemia, and daytime somnolence.<br>• 95% of children with Prader-Willi syndrome have excessive daytime sleepiness. |
| Scoliosis or congenital neuromuscular disorder (Duchenne muscular dystrophy, spinal muscular atrophy) | Nocturnal hypoventilation<br>Nocturnal hypoxemia—excessive daytime sleepiness, morning headaches<br>OSA<br>Restless sleep<br>Frequent awakenings |

**Table 71-8**
**Medical Disorders Associated With Sleep Problems in Childhood—cont'd**

| DIAGNOSIS | SLEEP PROBLEMS |
|---|---|
| Traumatic brain injuries | Sleep-onset and maintenance insomnia<br>Excessive daytime sleepiness<br>Dreaming disturbances<br>Nocturnal hypoventilation |
| Spina bifida | Obstructive, central, or mixed apnea<br>Nocturnal hypoventilation may cause severe excessive daytime sleepiness |

*OSA,* obstructive sleep apnea; *REM,* rapid eye movement.
Derived from Bandla H, Splaingard M. Sleep problems in children with common medical disorders. *Pediatr Clin North Am.* 2004;51:203–227.

Kleine-Levin syndrome, a rare disorder with episodes of severe daytime sleepiness, hyperphagia, and hypersexuality lasting hours to weeks, may be seen in adolescence. Tumors of the third ventricle or posterior hypothalamus may also cause daytime sleepiness. Brainstem lesions or Chiari malformation type II, which are common in children with myelomeningoceles, can cause severe central apnea or vocal cord paralysis causing obstructive apnea.

## Sleep-Related Epilepsy

Approximately 20% of epileptic patients have seizures only during sleep, most often at the time of sleep–wake transitions. Seizures occurring during the night may disrupt sleep by causing multiple awakenings. The possibility of a seizure disorder should be considered in adolescents with new-onset parasomnias. Atypical seizures may produce EDS.

## Sleep-Related Headaches

Most headaches occurring during sleep occur during REM sleep. Cluster headaches are more frequent at night than in the daytime and often disrupt sleep. Headaches on awakening are unusual; the child should be evaluated carefully for the presence of increased intracranial pressure or hypercapnia caused by hypoventilation (eg, Duchenne muscular dystrophy).

## Degenerative Disorders

Degenerative brain disorders result in frequent awakenings, difficulty falling asleep, early-morning waking, sleep deprivation, and daytime sleepiness.

## Other Medical Disorders

Any condition causing pain at night, such as juvenile idiopathic arthritis, can result in disrupted sleep.[38] Eczema that causes associated scratching results in frequent awakenings. Painful menstrual cramps may also disrupt sleep.

## Sleep-Related Asthma

Asthma episodes are increased during sleep, presumably because the neuroendocrine regulators of respiration are sensitive to diurnal regulation. Children who have sleep-related asthma have fragmented sleep and may develop anxiety associated with breathing discomfort. This disruption may lead to bedtime resistance and insufficient nocturnal sleep, leading to problems outlined in Box 71-2. In one study of children with asthma, 34% awakened at least once a week, and 5% awakened every night from asthma symptoms. Daytime sequelae were common, with 59% reporting daytime sleepiness and 51% reporting difficulty with concentration. These complaints all improved with successful asthma management.[39,40]

### Gastroesophageal Reflux Disease

Gastroesophageal reflux disease (GERD) may produce sleep problems in a variety of ways. The reflux can be painful, resulting in night waking and crying. Reflux has also been associated with both central and obstructive apnea and with apparent life-threatening events in infants and young children. The diagnosis of GERD may not always be obvious, owing to lack of usual signs, including excessive spitting up, reswallowing motions, increased fussiness, refusal of feedings, and failure to thrive. Esophagoscopy, assessing for esophageal erosions, may be needed to determine the cause of nighttime pain. Failure to be consoled while being held can be a clue that the child is suffering pain. Holding the child upright reduces the amount of acid in the esophagus and may comfort a child with reflux. See Chapter 83, Vomiting, for further discussion of gastroesophageal reflux.

## When to Refer

- If the physician is unable to relieve a sleep disturbance after working with the family over the course of 6 weeks, then assistance may be needed either from a sleep specialist or from a family therapist or psychologist. The physician should always consider, and generally respect, a family that really does not care to change a sleeping situation that would seem to be a sleep disturbance to others. Children with chronic, physically based sleep disorders, such as narcolepsy and SDB requiring CPAP, benefit from referral to a sleep disorders center for treatment and group support.
- Alternative therapies have been devised by many cultures to restore the essential health-giving function of sleep. Herbal remedies such as chamomile and other soothing teas are common. Any treatment that involves scheduled rest and mental preparation for sleep would be expected to result in improvement.

## When to Admit

- Primary sleep disturbances rarely require hospitalization, other than the overnight stay needed for a sleep study. Exceptions may include severe SDB with life-threatening oxygen desaturations, arrhythmias, or cor pulmonale. Hospitalization may be needed for some of the underlying disorders, such as CNS tumors or serious depression that may initially present symptoms of a sleep disorder. Admission for video EEG monitoring of movements during sleep that suggest seizures may be required.

## TOOLS FOR PRACTICE

### Engaging Patient and Family

- *Fostering Comfortable Sleep Patterns in Infancy* (fact sheet), Bright Futures (www.brightfutures.org/mentalhealth/pdf/families/in/sleep_patterns.pdf)
- *Sleep: What Every Parent Needs to Know,* 2nd ed (book), American Academy of Pediatrics (shop.aap.org)

- *Sleep (Baby 0–12 mos.)* (Web page), American Academy of Pediatrics (www.healthychildren.org/English/ages-stages/baby/sleep/Pages/default.aspx)
- *Sleep Apnea and Your Child* (handout), American Academy of Pediatrics (patiented.solutions.aap.org)
- *Sleep Problems in Children* (handout), American Academy of Pediatrics (patiented.solutions.aap.org)
- *Parenting Tips for Better Sleep* (fact sheet), American Academy of Pediatrics (www2.aap.org/sections/dbpeds/pdf/sleeptips.pdf)

## AAP POLICY STATEMENTS

Millman RP, Working Group on Sleepiness in Adolescents/Young Adults; American Academy of Pediatrics Committee on Adolescence. Excessive sleepiness in adolescents and young adults: causes, consequences, and treatment strategies. *Pediatrics.* 2005;115(6):1774–1786 (pediatrics.aappublications.org/content/115/6/1774.full)

Marcus CL, Brooks LJ, Draper KA, et al. Clinical practice guideline: diagnosis and management of childhood obstructive sleep apnea syndrome. *Pediatrics.* 2012;130(3):576–584 (pediatrics.aappublications.org/content/130/3/576.full)

Marcus CL, Brooks LJ, Draper KA, et al. Technical report: diagnosis and management of childhood obstructive sleep apnea syndrome. *Pediatrics.* 2012;130(3):e714–e755 (pediatrics.aappublications.org/content/130/3/e714.full)

American Academy of Pediatrics Task Force on Sudden Infant Death Syndrome. SIDS and other sleep-related infant deaths: expansion of recommendations for a safe infant sleeping environment. *Pediatrics.* 2011;128(5):1030–1039 (pediatrics.aappublications.org/content/128/5/1030.full)

## REFERENCES


1. Smith GA, Splaingard M, Hayes JR, Xiang H. Comparison of a personalized parent voice smoke alarm with a conventional residential tone smoke alarm for awakening children. *Pediatrics.* 2006;118:1623–1632
2. Meltzer LJ, Johnson C, Crosette J, Ramos M, Mindell JA. Prevalence of diagnosed sleep disorders in pediatric primary care practices. *Pediatrics.* 2010;125(6):e1410–e1418
3. Minde K, Faucon A, Falkner S. Sleep problems in toddlers: effects of treatment on their daytime behavior. *J Am Acad Child Adolesc Psychiatry.* 1994;33:1114–1121
4. Riter S, Wills L. Sleep wars: research and opinion. *Pediatr Clin North Am.* 2004;51:1–13
5. Iglowstein I, Jenni OG, Molinari L, Largo RH. Sleep duration from infancy to adolescence: reference values and generational trends. *Pediatrics.* 2003;111(2):302–307
6. Sheldon SH. *Evaluating Sleep in Infants and Children.* Philadelphia, PA: Lippincott-Raven Publishers; 1996
7. Owens JA, Dalzell V. Use of the 'BEARS' sleep screening tool in a pediatric residents' continuity clinic: a pilot study. *Sleep Med.* 2005;6:63–69
8. Sateia MJ. *The International Classification of Sleep Disorders: Diagnostic and Coding Manual.* 2nd ed. Westchester, IL: American Academy of Sleep Medicine; 2005
9. Anders TF. Night-waking in infants during the first year of life. *Pediatrics.* 1979;63:860–864
10. Gartner LM, Morton J, Lawrence RA, et al. Breastfeeding and the use of human milk. *Pediatrics.* 2005;115:496–506
11. Pinilla T, Birch LL. Help me make it through the night: behavioral entrainment of breast-fed infants' sleep patterns. *Pediatrics.* 1993;91:436–444
12. St James-Roberts I, Sleep J, Morris S, Owen C, Gillham P. Use of a behavioural programme in the first 3 months to prevent infant crying and sleeping problems. *J Paediatr Child Health.* 2001;37:289–297
13. Nikolopoulou M, St James-Roberts I. Preventing sleeping problems in infants who are at risk of developing them. *Arch Dis Child.* 2003;88:108–111

14. Blyton DM, Sullivan CE, Edwards N. Lactation is associated with an increase in slow-wave sleep in women. *J Sleep Res.* 2002;11:297–303
15. Cubero J, Narciso D, Terrón P. Chrononutrition applied to formula milks to consolidate infants' sleep/wake cycle. *Neuro Endocrinol Lett.* 2007;28:360–366
16. Kuhn BR, Elliott AJ. Treatment efficacy in behavioral pediatric sleep medicine. *J Psychosom Res.* 2003;54:587–597
17. Owens JA, Mindell JA. Pediatric insomnia. *Pediatr Clin North Am.* 2011;58(3):555–569
18. Pelayo R, Chen W, Monzon S, Guilleminault C. Pediatric sleep pharmacology: you want to give my kid sleeping pills? *Pediatr Clin North Am.* 2004;51:117–134
19. Blader JC, Koplewicz HS, Abikoff H, Foley C. Sleep problems of elementary school children. A community survey. *Arch Pediatr Adolesc Med.* 1997;151:473–480
20. Parmelee AH, Wenner WH, Schulz HR. Infant sleep patterns: from birth to 16 weeks of age. *J Pediatr.* 1964;65:576–582
21. Marcus CL. Sleep-disordered breathing in children. *Am J Respir Crit Care Med.* 2011;164(1):16–30
22. Bhattacharjee R, Kheirandish-Gozal L, Spruyt K, et al. Adenotonsillectomy outcomes in treatment of obstructive sleep apnea in children: a multicenter retrospective study. *Am J Respir Crit Care Med.* 2010;182:676–683
23. McColley SA, April MM, Carroll JL, Naclerio RM, Loughlin GM. Respiratory compromise after adenotonsillectomy in children with obstructive sleep apnea. *Arch Otolaryngol Head Neck Surg.* 1992;118:940–943
24. Rosen GM, Muckle RP, Mahowald MW, Goding GS, Ullevig C. Postoperative respiratory compromise in children with obstructive sleep apnea syndrome: can it be anticipated? *Pediatrics.* 1994;93:784–788
25. Laberge L, Tremblay RE, Vitaro F, Montplaisir J. Development of parasomnias from childhood to early adolescence. *Pediatrics.* 2000;106:67–74
26. Anders TF, Eiben LA. Pediatric sleep disorders: a review of the past 10 years. *J Am Acad Child Adolesc Psychiatry.* 1997;36:9–20
27. Picchietti D, Allen RP, Walters AS, et al. Restless legs syndrome: prevalence and impact in children and adolescents—the Peds REST study. *Pediatrics.* 2007;120:253–266
28. Aran A, Einen M, Lin L, et al. Clinical and therapeutic aspects of childhood narcolepsy-cataplexy: a retrospective study of 51 children. *Sleep.* 2010;33:1457–1464
29. Sheldon SH, Ferber R, Kryger MH. *Principles and Practice of Pediatric Sleep Medicine.* Philadelphia, PA: Elsevier Saunders; 2005
30. Dahl RE, Ryan ND, Matty MK, et al. Sleep onset abnormalities in depressed adolescents. *Biol Psychiatry.* 1996;39:400–410
31. Lofthouse N, Gilchrist R, Splaingard M. Mood-related sleep problems in children and adolescents. *Child Adolesc Psychiatr Clin N Am.* 2009;18(4):893–916
32. Glod CA, Teicher MH, Hartman CR, Harakal T. Increased nocturnal activity and impaired sleep maintenance in abused children. *J Am Acad Child Adolesc Psychiatry.* 1997;36:1236–1243
33. Wiggs L, Stores G. Severe sleep disturbance and daytime challenging behaviour in children with severe learning disabilities. *J Intellect Disabil Res.* 1996;40(Pt 6):518–528
34. Cortese S, Konofal E, Yateman N, Mouren MC, Lecendreux M. Sleep and alertness in children with attention-deficit/hyperactivity disorder: a systematic review of the literature. *Sleep.* 2006;29(4):504–511
35. Prince JB, Wilens TE, Biederman J, Spencer TJ, Wozniak JR. Clonidine for sleep disturbances associated with attention-deficit hyperactivity disorder: a systematic chart review of 62 cases. *J Am Acad Child Adolesc Psychiatry.* 1996;35:599–605
36. Johnson KP, Giannotti F, Cortesi F. Sleep patterns in autism spectrum disorders. *Child Adolesc Psychiatr Clin N Am.* 2009;18(4):917–928
37. Piazza CC, Fisher WW, Sherer M. Treatment of multiple sleep problems in children with developmental disabilities: faded bedtime with response cost versus bedtime scheduling. *Dev Med Child Neurol.* 1997;39:414–418

38. Zamir G, Press J, Tal A, Tarasiuk A. Sleep fragmentation in children with juvenile rheumatoid arthritis. *J Rheumatol.* 1998;25:1191–1197
39. Stores G, Ellis AJ, Wiggs L, Crawford C, Thomson A. Sleep and psychological disturbance in nocturnal asthma. *Arch Dis Child.* 1998;78:413–419
40. Splaingard M. Sleep problems in children with respiratory disorders. *Sleep Med Clin.* 2008;3(4):589–600

# Chapter 72

# Speech and Language Concerns

*Maris Rosenberg, MD; Nancy Tarshis, MA, MS*

## ▶ INTRODUCTION

Speech and language delay, arguably the most common developmental concern parents have about their young children, occurs with an estimated prevalence of 2% to 19%.[1–5] The delay can occur alone, or signal the presence of other developmental disorders such as intellectual disability, autistic spectrum disorders, or hearing impairment. In keeping with the recommendations of the American Academy of Pediatrics (AAP),[6] the pediatrician should perform developmental surveillance and screening to identify children at risk, refer for appropriate evaluation, and implement intervention as early as possible. Speech and language impairments have academic, social, and behavioral implications, and appropriate intervention can maximize a child's outcome.

Parents commonly focus on their child's verbal communication and consult the pediatrician when there are concerns. A working knowledge of risk factors for communication delays, normal speech and language milestones, and red flags for language delays and associated developmental problems is essential in providing appropriate pediatric primary care.[7]

## ▶ LANGUAGE DEVELOPMENT

Language, as the primary vehicle for communication, is a socially shared code or conventional system for representing concepts through an arbitrary set of rule-governed symbols (speech sounds/phonemes) and symbol combinations. A social tool through which we share ideas and rules of behavior and develop our attachments to people and places, language is a rule-governed yet generative system that permits speakers to create an endless number of meaningful utterances to communicate thoughts, feelings, information, and ideas.

A summary of typically acquired speech and language milestones is presented in Table 72 1.

## ▶ RISK FACTORS FOR LANGUAGE DELAYS

Risk factors for language delays are similar to those for developmental disorders in general. In a review for the US Preventive Services Task Force, the most common risk factors reported were a family history of speech and language delay, male gender, and perinatal factors. Other, less commonly reported risk factors included educational level of the parents,

**Table 72-1**
**Developmental Milestones**

| AGE | DEVELOPMENTAL MILESTONES |
|---|---|
| 0–6 mo | Cooing<br>Babbling<br>Differentiated cries |
| 6–9 mo | Canonical babbling (reduplicated babbling, eg, "bababa")<br>Response to name<br>Comprehension of familiar words in context |
| 9–15 mo | First words<br>Directed point (initially with hand, then with 1 finger) |
| 18–24 mo | Uses own name<br>2-word sentences (by 24 mo)<br>Knows 5 body parts |
| 24–30 mo | Pretend play with familiar objects<br>3-word sentences<br>Points to action words in pictures<br>Answers simple, concrete "wh-" questions (eg, who, what)<br>Uses 50+ words |
| 30–36 mo | Names most familiar things and pictures<br>Begins to recognize same and different<br>Helps tell a familiar story<br>Uses descriptive words (adjectives)<br>Uses 200–1,000 words<br>Speech is nearly all intelligible to any listener. |
| 3–4 yr | Comprehends 1,000 words<br>Points to common objects by function<br>Responds to commands involving 2 actions<br>Uses at least 800 words<br>Responds to simple "how" questions<br>Asks "what" and "who" questions<br>Uses plurals and verb tense markers<br>Talks about events out of the here and now |
| 4–5 yr | Understands most of what is said to him or her<br>Tells a personal story with a beginning, middle, and end<br>Can listen and answer questions about a story<br>Speech is fully intelligible.<br>Can recognize and produce rhymes |

childhood illness, and family size.[5] A careful history eliciting any prenatal, perinatal, or postnatal adverse events and a detailed family history focusing on developmental disorders, academic achievement, and social functioning are essential in determining which children are at greater risk. Environmental factors clearly play a role in determining language development. Children who live in disadvantaged environments with less language stimulation and greater psychosocial stress are at greater risk for language delay than children from more advantaged backgrounds.

Table 72-2 states the red flags in language and play that may signal the existence of a language or other developmental disorder.

**Table 72-2**
**Red Flags in Language and Play**

| AGE | WARNING SIGNS AND RED FLAGS |
|---|---|
| 0–12 mo: play | Restricted repertoire of skills |
| | Does not follow objects that fall |
| | Little purposeful play |
| | Reduced or absent imitation |
| | Reduced object permanence |
| | No interactive games |
| 0–12 mo: sensory motor | Does not reach or swat at objects |
| | Overly reactive to stimuli |
| | Extreme irritability |
| 0–12 mo: socioemotional | Overly clingy |
| | No apparent attachments |
| | No awareness of danger |
| | Difficulty modulating emotions |
| | Reduced range of affect |
| 0–12 mo: speech and language | Difficulty sucking and feeding |
| | Averts gaze |
| | Fails to make a variety of sounds |
| | Fails to respond to name |
| | Undifferentiated crying |
| 12–24 mo: play | No container play |
| | No early problem solving |
| | Does not go to adults for help |
| | Very rigid play |
| | Focuses on irrelevant parts of toys such as wheels of car |
| | Does not include adults in play; prefers to play alone |
| | No interest in playing symbolically |
| | No spontaneous pretend play |
| | Restricted range of interests |
| | No early problem solving |
| 12–24 mo: socioemotional | Short attention span |
| | Does not seek to engage with others |
| | Tunes out |
| | Avoids eye contact |
| 12–24 mo: speech and language | No specific *mama* or *dada* |
| | Does not point |
| | Cannot follow simple directives without gesture |
| | Reduced vocabulary |
| | No word combinations |

*Continued*

**Table 72-2**
**Red Flags in Language and Play—cont'd**

| AGE | WARNING SIGNS AND RED FLAGS |
|---|---|
| 24–36 mo: play | Little or no symbolic play |
| | Not able to sequence events in play |
| | Not interested in playing with peers |
| | Restricted range of skills and interests |
| | Lines up toys rather than playing with them |
| 24–36 mo: speech and language | Avoids eye contact |
| | Reduced communicative intent |
| | Difficulty following directions |
| | Lack of verbal expression |
| | Reduced reciprocity and turn taking |
| | Talking better than listening |
| | Poor conversation skills |
| 3–4 yr: play | Cannot take turns or play cooperatively with peers (prefers solitary play) |
| | Little interest in toys |
| | Insists on sameness in routine |
| | No idea how to approach new skills or toys |
| | Cannot use blocks to build simple structures |
| 3–4 yr: language | Does not engage in back-and-forth communication for purely social reasons |
| | Does not talk about what communicative partners are talking about |
| | Uses language that is repetitive or recycled from other contexts |
| 4–5 yr: play | Cannot follow simple rules in play |
| | Prefers solitary play |
| | Insists on sameness in play |
| | Reacts strongly to change |
| | Does not engage in symbolic or imaginative play |
| | Does not integrate other children in play |
| 4–5 yr: language | Weak ability to hold a conversation |
| | Cannot tell a personal narrative |
| | Difficulty with sequencing information |
| | Uses language that is repetitive or recycled from other contexts |

## ▶ ROLE OF THE PRIMARY CARE PHYSICIAN: SURVEILLANCE AND SCREENING

Performing developmental surveillance at all health maintenance visits implies eliciting parental concerns, acknowledging risk and protective factors, performing longitudinal observations, and keeping an accurate, ongoing record.

The use of standardized general developmental screening instruments is recommended at ages 9, 18, and 30 months or whenever concerns arise in the course of surveillance.[6] In addition, the recommendation for screening for autistic spectrum disorders at 18 and 24 months allows additional insight into the development of communication and social skills. After a systematic review in 2006,[5,8,9] the US Preventive Services Task Force concluded that there is no single screening instrument that serves as a gold standard for screening specifically for language disorders, and there were no universally agreed-on recommendations for age or interval for speech and language screening. However, it is generally agreed that use of standardized screening instruments can assist the pediatrician in assessing a young child's general development and making decisions as to whether referral for further evaluation by developmental specialists would be appropriate. Screening instruments vary in format and applicability to particular populations.[9] Table 72-3 provides a partial list of both general and language-specific screening instruments that can be used in the primary care setting. The resource provided by the AAP Developmental Screening task force lists additional tools.[6]

## ▶ LANGUAGE DISORDERS

A language disorder as defined by the American Speech and Hearing Association can be classified as any disturbance to an individual's ability to develop and produce spoken or written language. This encompasses both the ability to comprehend and the ability to express language at an age-appropriate level. Language disorders, both developmental and acquired, represent a heterogeneous set of difficulties that range from mild to severe. Children with receptive language deficits have difficulty comprehending language. Of note, a receptive deficit is rarely seen in isolation, and in typical development, comprehension precedes expression of new and more mature language forms. Difficulty with comprehension manifests as reduced understanding of conversation and problems both with following directions and interpreting the intentions of others. Receptive language generally develops in advance of expressive language, except in very rare circumstances (eg, hydrocephalus, severe language processing disorder, and in autism spectrum disorders). Children with expressive language deficits have problems using language to express their most basic wants and needs as well as more sophisticated thoughts, feelings, and intentions. They may have a hard time putting words into sentences; sentences may be simple and short with confused syntax or verb tense errors, or there may be difficulty finding the right words. A child's vocabulary might be below the level of other children the same age; or the child might use words and phrases repetitively or pick up scripts from videos, commercials, and television. Language impairment might also become apparent as a deficit in stringing sentences together to tell a cohesive story or personal narrative.

A language disorder can be characterized by deficits in the form (comprehension and expression of linguistic rules and syntax), the content (vocabulary and semantics), or the use (discourse pragmatics) of language. Difficulty acquiring and using the rules applicable to the sounds, words, phrases, and sentences or the surface features of what is being said constitutes

**Table 72-3**
**General and Language-Specific Screening Instruments**

| TOOL | TIME FOR ADMINIS-TRATION | AGE RANGE | TYPE OF TOOL | LANGUAGES AVAILABLE | FOR FURTHER INFORMATION |
|---|---|---|---|---|---|
| **Ages & Stages Questionnaires** | 10–15 min | 4–60 mo | Parent-completed General developmental screen | English, Spanish, French, Korean | Paul H. Brookes Publishing: www.brookespublishing.com |
| **Batelle Development Inventory Screen** | 10–30 min | 0–95 mo | Direct-administration General developmental screen | English, Spanish | Riverside Publishing Co. www.riverpub.com |
| **Brigance Screens II** | 10–15 min | 0–90 mo | Direct-administration General developmental screen | English, Spanish | Curriculum Associates, Inc. www.curriculumassociates.com |
| **Denver Developmental II** | 10–20 min | 0–72 mo | Direct-administration General developmental screen | English, Spanish | Denver Developmental Materials www.denverii.com |
| **Parents' Evaluation of Developmental Status (PEDS, PEDS-DM)** | 2–10 min | 0–96 mo | Parent-completed General developmental screen | English, Spanish, and multiple other languages | Ellsworth & Vandermeer Press, LLC www.pedstest.com |
| **Capute Scales (CAT/Clams)** | 15–20 min | 3–36 mo | Direct-administration CLAMS specific for language | English, Spanish, Russian | Paul H. Brookes Publishing: www.brookespublishing.com |
| **Early Language Milestone Scales** | 1–10 min | 0–36 mo | Direct-administration Language screen | English | Pro-ed Inc: www.proedinc.com |
| **Language Development Survey** | 10 min | 18–35 mo | Parent-completed Language screen | English, Spanish | ASEBA www.aseba.org |
| **Communication and Symbolic Behavior Scales Developmental Profile (CSBS-DP) Infant-Toddler Checklist** | 5–10 min | 6–24 mo | Parent-completed Language screen | English | Paul H. Brookes Publishing: www.brookespublishing.com |
| **Modified Checklist for Autism in Toddlers (M-CHAT)** | 2–3 min | 16–30 mo | Parent-completed Autism screen followed by questionnaire for positive items | Multiple languages | Available free from First Signs: https://www.firstsigns.org/downloads/m-chat.PDF |

a deficit in the *form* of language. For children with disorders of *content*, speaking may come easily, but often what they have to say lacks substance. Their discourse is missing the essential ingredients such as objects, events, relations between people, and cultural references that give meaning to the utterance. Pragmatic deficits result in weakness in language *use*, in managing and understanding the why, when, and where aspects of discourse. Children with this difficulty have a hard time selecting and maintaining topics, taking turns in conversation, choosing their style of speech to match the listener or context, using intonation to signal intention, and understanding the nonverbal aspects of language such as proximity, body posture, facial expression, and flexible gaze shifting.

Language-based learning disabilities present as problems with reading, spelling, or writing in addition to the aforementioned oral language deficits. Typically, children with such disabilities have trouble expressing ideas, finding words, learning new vocabulary, comprehending questions, following directions, and retaining written material. They struggle learning the alphabet, spelling rules, multiplication tables, and other rote-memorized information, all of which make it difficult to achieve academically.

## ▶ SPEECH DISORDERS

Speech disorders manifest as articulation errors past the age of expectation. *Articulation* is the movement of the speech mechanism (palate, lips, tongue, jaw, larynx) to create sound. *Phonology* is the rule system that governs how speech sounds interact with one another. A child with a lisp has a problem with articulation; a child who substitutes all K sounds with T ("otay" for okay) has a phonological problem. For pediatricians, knowing when to refer for evaluation is key. As a guideline, a 2-year-old should be 50% intelligible, a 3-year-old 75%, and a 4-year-old fully intelligible to a stranger, not just family and familiar adults.

A child might present with speech problems for several reasons. Some errors are developmental and will resolve in time, and others will need intervention. Some errors are related to the architecture of the mouth, and others are rule-based errors (phonologic). If the errors persist, or the child expresses frustration, an evaluation is in order. When a child makes errors that are inconsistent, a motor speech disorder should be suspected. Apraxia is a motor speech disorder caused by a difficulty planning and executing speech sounds that cannot be attributed to muscle weakness or paralysis. Key characteristics include limited repertoire of vowels and vowel errors. The error patterns are typically highly variable, with unusual and idiosyncratic error patterns. Errors increase with the length and complexity of utterances, such as in multisyllabic or phonetically challenging words. If apraxia is suspected, a child should be evaluated as soon as possible because the earlier intervention begins, the better the outcome. *Stuttering* or *dysfluency* is a speech disorder characterized by breaks in fluency that can affect sounds, syllables, or words. In young children there can be a period of normal dysfluency between 2 and 4 years of age. The decision to refer for evaluation should be based on how long dysfluency has persisted, whether there is a family history, the type of repetitions, and secondary behaviors. Indications for evaluation include dysfluency that persists for more than 6 months, family history of stuttering, awareness of difficulty, or anxiety or frustration related to speaking. In addition, if breaks in fluency are partial words, single sounds, silent or accompanied by any secondary or atypical behaviors, or if the balance of dysfluent speech to fluent speech is more than 10% of the overall communication, evaluation should be initiated.

## ▶ DIFFERENTIAL DIAGNOSIS

Delays in speech and language milestones are often the first indication of the presence of a developmental disorder. Hearing loss is an important consideration in any child who exhibits delayed acquisition of language milestones or unclear or atypical patterns of speech. Careful history and observation may suggest accompanying delays in other domains indicating more global involvement, as in intellectual disability. Subtle delays in communication can be apparent even before verbal communication is questioned. The phenomenon of joint attention, as evidenced by gaze sharing or pointing, can be documented as early as 8 to 10 months of age. The absence of joint attention should alert the physician to the possibility of an autism spectrum disorder. In the absence of the above conditions, *specific language impairment* (SLI), refers to the developmental disorders affecting primarily receptive, expressive, or mixed receptive-expressive language impairments, whereas *phonologic disorders* refer to conditions affecting the clarity of speech.

## ▶ THERAPEUTIC CONSIDERATIONS: WHAT THE PEDIATRICIAN NEEDS TO KNOW

Once a speech and language delay is suspected, referral for diagnostic evaluation is critical to determine the extent of impairment, characterize the nature of the disability, and suggest strategies for intervention. Referral for early intervention evaluation for children from birth to age 3 years, or to the Department of Education for children 3 years and older, offers a means of evaluation within a mandated time frame and services based on the evaluation results. Ideally, this evaluation is conducted by a multidisciplinary team, on which the speech and language pathologist (SLP) plays a key role. The SLP will gather information regarding communication across a variety of contexts. He or she will evaluate the child's ability to comprehend directions, stories, and other communication as well as vocabulary, grammar, and syntax and use of language for a variety of purposes. In certain circumstances, based on the presenting problems, speech sound development, literacy skills, writing, reading comprehension, and fluency will also be evaluated. This assessment should contain informal components such as pretend play in young children and conversation and storytelling in older children. Formal testing with standardized instruments can corroborate and elucidate informal findings and should always be considered.

The pediatrician should order a formal hearing test to be done by an audiologist. Speech and language therapy should not be delayed pending definitive audiologic evaluation, however, because it may take months for an uncooperative child to have a hearing test completed. A formal hearing test should be ordered as part of the multidisciplinary evaluation, and hearing status should be followed according to recommendations of the audiologist as therapy progresses.

Any child with significant exposure to a second language or dialect is considered bilingually-exposed. Regardless of the type of exposure, simultaneous or sequential, such a child must be evaluated in both languages to determine the presence or absence of language impairment. Many children who are bilingually exposed may go through a short period of language loss, especially if recently exposed to a new language. There may be a delay in mastering some grammatical aspects of both languages, and vocabulary may be judged to be insufficient if words in both languages are not considered. Such children should be assessed by a qualified *bilingual* SLP. If a language impairment is documented in a bilingually exposed child, it is important to determine the dominant language when initiating therapy.

## ▶ PROGNOSIS

Based on their presentation and degree of severity, language disorders may resolve with intervention by the time a child enters the early school years. More often, they persist to some degree for the lifetime of the individual. Children identified with speech and language delays in toddler and preschool years are known to be at special risk for behavioral difficulties and for problems with socializing. The association between communication difficulties and externalizing disorders (attention deficit/hyperactivity disorder, oppositional defiant disorder) and internalizing disorders (anxiety disorders, depression) has also been described.[3] The link between early language and later learning problems is also well documented. Children identified with communication impairments at age 4 to 5 years are likely to have significantly more difficulty in reading, writing, and overall academic achievement at ages 7 to 9 years. In addition, these children have more difficulty with peer relationships and less satisfaction with school than their peers.[10]

A multitude of factors determine the outcome of children with speech and language impairments. Important considerations include nonverbal intelligence, type and degree of language disability, and response to intervention. Preschool-aged children with primarily expressive phonologic impairments tend to have a lower risk for later reading problems than those who demonstrate difficulty with phonologic awareness (eg, rhyming, letter–sound association). It is generally agreed that children with language problems that persist until kindergarten entry have a high risk for continuing problems throughout the school years.[3] Parents should be counseled that providing a language-rich environment, stressing verbal interaction and literacy, is recommended, in addition to specific therapy, to mediate the effects of a language delay (eg, the Reach Out and Read program, www.reachoutandread.org).

## ▶ CONCLUSION

Speech and language delays are common and are readily detected in the context of the developmental surveillance and screening that are part of primary pediatric care. These delays may be associated with impairments limited to the domains of speech and language or may signal the presence of conditions such as hearing impairment, intellectual disability, or autistic spectrum disorders. Using the knowledge of risk factors and attention to "red flags" suggesting these disorders is the first step to referral for appropriate evaluation and interventions to minimize associated difficulties with learning, behavior, and socialization.

### *TOOLS FOR PRACTICE*

#### Engaging Patient and Family

- *American Speech-Language Hearing Association* (Web site), American Speech-Language Association (www.asha.org)
- *Is Your Toddler Communicating With You?* (handout), American Academy of Pediatrics (patiented.solutions.aap.org)
- *Language Delay* (fact sheet), American Academy of Pediatrics (www.healthychildren.org/English/ages-stages/toddler/Pages/Language-Delay.aspx)

- *Language Development: 1 Year Olds* (fact sheet), American Academy of Pediatrics (www.healthychildren.org/English/ages-stages/toddler/Pages/Language-Development-1-Year-Olds.aspx)
- *Language Development: 2 Year Olds* (fact sheet), American Academy of Pediatrics (www.healthychildren.org/English/ages-stages/toddler/Pages/Language-Development-2-Year-Olds.aspx)
- *Learn the Signs. Act Early.* (Web page), Centers for Disease Control and Prevention (www.cdc.gov/ncbddd/actearly/index.html)

## AAP POLICY STATEMENT

American Academy of Pediatrics Council on Children with Disabilities, Section on Developmental and Behavioral Pediatrics, Bright Futures Steering Committee, Medical Home Initiatives for Children With Special Needs Project Advisory Committee. Identifying infants and young children with developmental disorders in the medical home: an algorithm for developmental surveillance and screening. *Pediatrics.* 2006;118(1):405–420. Reaffirmed December 2009 (pediatrics.aappublications.org/content/118/1/405.full)

## REFERENCES

1. Pinborough-Zimmerman J, Satterfield R, Miller J, et al. Communication disorders: prevalence and comorbid intellectual disability, autism, and emotional/behavioral disorders. *Am J Speech Lang Pathol.* 2007;16:359–367
2. McLeod S, Harrison LJ. Epidemiology of speech and language impairment in a nationally representative sample of 4- to 5-year-old children. *J Speech Lang Hear Res.* 2009;52:1213–1229
3. Simms MD. Language disorders in children: classification and clinical syndromes. *Pediatr Clin North Am.* 2007;54:437–467
4. McQuiston S, Kloczko N. Speech and language development: monitoring process and problems. *Pediatr Rev.* 2011;32:230–238; quiz 239
5. Nelson HD, Nygren P, Walker M, Panoscha R. Screening for speech and language delay in preschool children: systematic evidence review for the US Preventive Services Task Force. *Pediatrics.* 2006;117:e298–e319
6. American Academy of Pediatrics Council on Children With Disabilities, Section on Developmental and Behavioral Pediatrics, Bright Futures Steering Committee, Medical Home Initiatives for Children With Special Needs Project Advisory Committee. Identifying infants and young children with developmental disorders in the medical home: an algorithm for developmental surveillance and screening. *Pediatrics.* 2006;118(1):405–420
7. Schum RL. Language screening in the pediatric office setting. *Pediatr Clin North Am.* 2007;54:425–436, v
8. US Preventive Services Task Force. Screening for speech and language delay in preschool children: recommendation statement. *Pediatrics.* 2006;117:497–501
9. Drotar D, Stancin T, Dworkin PH, Sices L, Wood S. Selecting developmental surveillance and screening tools. *Pediatr Rev.* 2008;29:e52–e58
10. McCormack J, Harrison LJ, McLeod S, McAllister L. A nationally representative study of the association between communication impairment at 4-5 years and children's life activities at 7-9 years. *J Speech Lang Hear Res.* 2011;54:1328–1348

# Chapter 73

# Splenomegaly

*Marina Reznik, MD, MS; Philip O. Ozuah, MD, PhD*

*Splenomegaly* is an enlargement of the spleen resulting from abnormalities of its lymphoid, reticuloendothelial, or vascular components. Although splenomegaly is often considered to be an ominous clinical finding, certain normal variants have been found. In children, as a result of the thinness of the abdominal musculature, a palpable spleen is commonly encountered.[1] Thus a soft spleen is normally palpable in 15% to 30% of neonates. By 1 year of age, 10% of healthy children have a palpable spleen. Even after 10 years of age, 1% of children have a palpable spleen.

Wide interobserver variability exists in the ability to appreciate an enlarged spleen on examination; this variability is not generally associated with clinical experience.[2] The spleen moves downward with inspiration and enlarges diagonally across the midline toward the right iliac fossa.

An enlarged spleen may extend into the pelvis; thus, when examining a child with suspected splenomegaly, the physician should start palpating in the right lower quadrant and move across the abdomen toward the left upper quadrant. As the spleen enlarges, it replaces the tympany of the stomach and colon with the dullness of a solid organ. Percussion cannot confirm splenic enlargement, but it can raise suspicion of it.[3] If tympany is prominent, especially laterally, then splenomegaly is not likely. In addition, a change from tympany to dullness on inspiration when percussing at the lower interspace in the left anterior axillary line suggests splenic enlargement.[3]

Spleen size is conventionally recorded as "centimeters below the costal margin" in the midclavicular and anterior axillary lines. Measuring this span with a rigid ruler gives the most reproducible measurement.[4]

Spleen length is correlated with age, height, weight, and body surface area in a nonlinear fashion, similar to the liver.[5–7] No sex-based differences in spleen size have been found. Imaging of the spleen with ultrasonography, high-frequency ultrasonography, radioactive (technetium-99m) sulfur colloid scintigraphy, computed tomography (CT), or magnetic resonance imaging (MRI) can be an important adjunct to the physical examination in defining pathologic changes in this organ.[8–10] Contrast-enhanced sonography is a novel technique that allows real-time assessment of the spleen.[11–13]

## ▶ DIFFERENTIAL DIAGNOSIS

When assessing a child with splenomegaly, the major splenic functions should be kept in mind: its hematopoietic, phagocytic, and immunologic roles and its role as a reservoir for blood-borne elements. The spleen is a major hematopoietic organ during fetal life. However, it is capable of resuming extramedullary hematopoiesis in children and adults with bone marrow failure. The spleen removes the senescent and abnormal red blood cells, as well as particulate material, from the blood. A major lymphoreticular organ that acts as a filter for infectious organisms in the blood, the spleen also acts as a site of immunoglobulin M and properdin production. Finally, the spleen acts as a reservoir for platelets, reticulocytes, and plasma proteins, especially factor VIII. Because the spleen has so many functions, splenomegaly may be caused by systemic infections, by an increase in normal splenic process (as seen in hemolytic anemia), by infiltration of storage diseases or malignancies, by congestion from splenic or portal vein obstruction, or by inflammatory diseases. The spleen is the organ most commonly injured following blunt abdominal trauma.[14] Engorgement caused by splenic trauma with subcapsular hemorrhage may manifest as an enlarged, tender spleen. The differential diagnosis of splenomegaly is provided in Box 73-1.

## Infections

In infectious processes, splenomegaly results from hypertrophy of lymphatic and reticuloendothelial elements. Viral infections are the most common causes of splenomegaly in children. The splenic enlargement is usually transient and mild to moderate in severity.

BOX 73-1

### *Differential Diagnosis of Splenomegaly*

**INFECTIONS**

- Viral: Epstein-Barr virus, cytomegalovirus, human immunodeficiency virus (HIV)
- Bacterial: acute bacterial infections, subacute bacterial endocarditis, congenital syphilis, tuberculosis
- Parasitic: malaria, toxoplasmosis, leishmaniasis
- Fungal: candidiasis, histoplasmosis, coccidioidomycosis

**HEMATOLOGIC DISORDERS**

***Hemolytic Anemias–Congenital and Acquired***

- Red cell membrane defects: hereditary spherocytosis, hereditary elliptocytosis
- Red cell hemoglobin defects: sickle cell disease and related syndromes, thalassemia
- Red cell enzyme defects: glucose-6-phosphate dehydrogenase deficiency, pyruvate kinase deficiency, etc
- Autoimmune hemolytic anemia

***Extramedullary Hematopoiesis***

- Thalassemia major, osteopetrosis, myelofibrosis

**INFILTRATIVE DISORDERS**

- Leukemias
- Lymphomas
- Lipidoses
- Mucopolysaccharidosis
- Langerhans cell histiocytosis

**CONGESTIVE SPLENOMEGALY**

- Portal vein thrombosis
- Hepatic cirrhosis
- Congestive heart failure
- Hepatic portal or splenic vein obstruction

**INFLAMMATORY DISEASES**

- Systemic lupus erythematosus (SLE)
- Juvenile idiopathic arthritis (JIA)
- Serum sickness
- Sarcoidosis
- Immune thrombocytopenias and neutropenias

**PRIMARY SPLENIC DISORDERS**

- Splenoptosis (wandering spleen)
- Cysts
- Hemangiomas and lymphangiomas
- Subcapsular hemorrhage
- Accessory spleen

Infectious mononucleosis from Epstein-Barr virus, cytomegalovirus, and HIV infections leads to a greater degree of splenic enlargement. Specifically, splenomegaly occurs in 50% to 75% of cases of infectious mononucleosis. Subacute bacterial endocarditis, tuberculosis, and other chronic bacterial infections may cause splenic enlargement. Septicemia from meningococcus or pneumococcus may also be associated with splenomegaly. Malaria and visceral leishmaniasis are common causes of splenomegaly in areas endemic for these diseases.[15,16] Progressive disseminated histoplasmosis can occur in healthy children younger than 2 years who have been exposed to fungus in endemic areas of the eastern and central United States (Mississippi, Ohio, and Missouri River valleys). Early manifestations of this disease include fever, failure to thrive, and hepatosplenomegaly.

### Hematologic Disorders

Splenomegaly associated with hemolytic states, such as membranopathies, hemoglobinopathies, and autoimmune hemolytic anemia, results from engorgement of the splenic sinusoids by abnormal red blood cells, as well as by increased phagocytic activity (work hypertrophy) of the reticuloendothelial elements. Splenic enlargement as a result of extramedullary hematopoiesis occurs in diseases associated with increased demand on the bone marrow for cell production (thalassemia major). Measurement of the spleen's size and recording the result are an essential part of every physical examination in children with sickle cell disease. It is important to have this baseline information because a rapidly enlarging spleen with a falling hematocrit, pallor, dyspnea, weakness, and left-sided abdominal pain suggests the diagnosis of acute splenic sequestration crisis—a leading cause of death in children with sickle cell anemia and a medical emergency that requires prompt recognition and treatment.

### Infiltrative Disorders

The spleen is commonly enlarged in untreated leukemias and lymphomas, including Hodgkin disease. Malignant infiltration of the spleen often produces a massively enlarged, firm spleen that crosses the midline of the body. In the lipidoses and mucopolysaccharidoses, the phagocytic reticuloendothelial elements of the spleen accumulate large amounts of lipid and mucopolysaccharide, respectively. In Langerhans cell histiocytosis, the spleen is infiltrated by histiocytes.

### Congestive Splenomegaly (Banti Syndrome)

Splenomegaly may occur from obstruction of the hepatic, portal, or splenic veins. The most common causes include portal vein thrombosis, hepatic cirrhosis, and congestive heart failure. Umbilical vein catheterization or septic omphalitis in neonates may also result in obliteration of these vessels. Congestive splenomegaly is the most common cause of hypersplenism (the term used to describe patients with splenomegaly, peripheral blood cytopenias from excessive splenic function, and increased bone marrow production of the affected blood cells).

### Inflammatory Diseases

Splenomegaly seen in inflammatory diseases such as systemic lupus erythematosus (SLE), juvenile idiopathic arthritis (JIA), sarcoidosis, and serum sickness is the result of increased numbers of reticuloendothelial cells that remove antibody-coated cells and proteins. Lymphoid hyperplasia may occur as a result of accelerated antibody production in the spleen.

### Primary Splenic Disorders

Splenoptosis, or wandering spleen, is a congenital fusion anomaly of dorsal mesogastrium that results in a spleen of normal size that moves freely within the peritoneal cavity.[17] A patient with splenoptosis usually has an asymptomatic abdominal mass.[18] Splenic cysts may mimic splenomegaly. Two types of splenic cysts have been identified: those that are congenital (epidermoid) and those that are acquired (pseudocyst) from trauma or infarction. Cysts are generally asymptomatic and are confirmed by radiologic studies. Abdominal trauma may cause subcapsular hemorrhage of the spleen that results in abdominal pain and splenomegaly. Accessory spleens, which are found in 15% of individuals, may also mimic splenomegaly.[4]

## ▶ EVALUATION

### History

The cause of splenomegaly can be determined by history and physical examination in addition to laboratory tests and, if necessary, radiographic studies. A thorough history, including travel and family history, may provide valuable clues to the possible cause of splenomegaly. In a child with a history of a fever, pharyngitis, malaise, and splenomegaly, a viral cause (Epstein-Barr virus, cytomegalovirus) should be considered. Malaria or histoplasmosis may be the cause if the patient has recently traveled to areas endemic for these diseases. In the patient with fever, night sweats, malaise, weight loss, rash, arthralgia, and bone pain, an underlying inflammatory, infectious, or malignant process should be suspected. A newborn with unexplained jaundice and a family history of anemia, jaundice, splenomegaly, or splenectomy most likely has a congenital hemolytic anemia. A history of umbilical vein catheterization or omphalitis in the neonatal period may suggest a diagnosis of portal vein thrombosis.

### Physical Examination

The normal palpable spleen is soft, smooth, and nontender and is less than 1 to 2 cm below the left costal margin. A pathologically enlarged spleen is usually firm, has an abnormal surface, and is often associated with signs and symptoms of an underlying disease. An enlarged spleen may be tender if it has enlarged quickly (splenic sequestration, splenic trauma with subcapsular hemorrhage). When portal hypertension causes splenomegaly, dilation of the superficial abdominal veins can be noted at physical examination. Findings of a rash, arthritis, mucosal ulcerations, and splenomegaly may suggest an autoimmune disorder. Although a palpable spleen may be a normal variant, the concomitant finding of hepatomegaly is usually pathologic and should prompt further investigation.

### Laboratory Evaluation

The initial laboratory testing of a child with splenomegaly should include a complete blood count with a white blood cell differential, reticulocyte count, and examination of the peripheral blood smear. Further laboratory investigations should be directed at the suspected diagnosis, as indicated by the history, physical examination, and the results of the initial laboratory tests.

### Imaging Studies

Radiologic confirmation of a mass in the left upper quadrant should be performed if any question exists about the nature of the mass. Retroperitoneal tumors such as neuroblastoma and Wilms tumor may be mistaken for an enlarged spleen. Ultrasonography is used to quantify splenic enlargement and to differentiate the spleen from other left-upper-quadrant abdominal masses. CT scanning has been used to evaluate splenic trauma and focal splenic pathology. Contrast-enhanced ultrasonography is a novel technique used to detect bleeding sites and hematomas in splenic trauma.[13] MRI of the spleen can further clarify abnormalities in size and shape and can define parenchymal disease. Technetium-99m sulfur colloid scan is used to assess splenic function.

## ▶ TREATMENT

Treatment of splenomegaly should be aimed at the underlying disease entity. Patients who have bacterial infections should receive appropriate antimicrobial therapy. Viral causes of splenomegaly generally respond to supportive care. With splenomegaly from infectious mononucleosis, patients should refrain from contact or collision sports until the illness has completely resolved clinically and the spleen has returned to a normal size, generally at least 4 weeks from the onset of illness. Some experts suggest a sonographic evaluation of spleen size to help decide when the patient can resume full athletic activity.[19,20]

Splenectomy may be indicated to help control or stage some diseases that cause splenomegaly. Such diseases include hereditary spherocytosis, autoimmune thrombocytopenia or hemolysis, and lymphoma (Hodgkin lymphoma). Splenectomy may also be indicated for the treatment of chronic, severe hypersplenism. Laparoscopic splenectomy is being performed more commonly in children and has been found to be a safe procedure, with a shorter hospital stay, compared with open splenectomy.[21–25] During the past decade, partial splenectomy has become a viable therapeutic alternative to total splenectomy. Removal of up to 90% of the enlarged spleen usually provides relief from splenomegaly while retaining sufficient splenic tissue for immune competence.[4] Partial splenectomy has been used successfully in children with hereditary spherocytosis,[26,27] nonparasitic splenic cysts, sickle cell disease, and thalassemia. All children without spleens are at risk for fulminant bacteremia, sometimes referred to as overwhelming postsplenectomy infection (OPSI),[4] particularly from *Streptococcus pneumoniae, Haemophilus influenzae* type b, and *Neisseria meningitidis,* and should receive needed immunizations at least 2 weeks before surgery if possible. Twice-daily penicillin prophylaxis against pneumococcal infections (in addition to immunization) is recommended for these children if they are younger than 5 years and for at least 1 year after splenectomy. Some experts continue prophylaxis throughout childhood and into adulthood for particularly high-risk patients with asplenia.[31]

### When to Refer

- Splenomegaly with concomitant adenopathy or hepatomegaly
- Palpation of a hard spleen
- Suspicion of malignancy or other infiltrative disorders
- Evidence of hemolytic anemias

### When to Admit

- Splenic sequestration in sickle cell disease
- Injury to the spleen from abdominal trauma

## REFERENCES


1. Pearson HA. The spleen and disturbances of splenic function. In: Nathan DG, Orkin SH, Lampert R, eds. *Nathan and Oski's Hematology of Infancy and Childhood.* 5th ed. Philadelphia, PA: WB Saunders; 1997
2. Tamayo SG, Rickman LS, Mathews WC, et al. Examiner dependence on physical diagnostic tests for the detection of splenomegaly: a prospective study with multiple observers. *J Gen Intern Med.* 1993;8:69–75
3. Barkun AN, Camus M, Green L, et al. The bedside assessment of splenic enlargement. *Am J Med.* 1991;91:512–518
4. Ware RE. Autoimmune hemolytic anemia. In: Orkin SH, Nathan DG, Ginsburg D, Look AT, Fisher DE, Lux SE, eds. *Nathan and Oski's Hematology of Infancy and Childhood.* 7th ed. Philadelphia, PA: Saunders; 2009
5. Rosenberg HK, Markowitz RI, Kolberg H, et al. Normal splenic size in infants and children: sonographic measurements. *Am J Roentgenol.* 1991;157:119–121
6. Megremis SD, Vlachonikolis IG, Tsilimigaki AM. Spleen length in childhood with US: normal values based on age, sex, and somatometric parameters. *Radiology.* 2004;231:129–134
7. Safak AA, Simsek E, Bahcebasi T. Sonographic assessment of the normal limits and percentile curves of liver, spleen, and kidney dimensions in healthy school-aged children. *J Ultrasound Med.* 2005;24:1359–1364
8. Paterson A, Frush DP, Donnelly LF, et al. A pattern-oriented approach to splenic imaging in infants and children. *Radiographics.* 1999;19:1465–1485
9. Doria AS, Daneman A, Moineddin R, et al. High-frequency sonographic patterns of the spleen in children. *Radiology.* 2006;240:821–827
10. Tu DG, Tu CW, Tsai YC. Detection of viable autotransplanted splenic tissue by Tc-99m sulfur colloid. *J Trauma.* 2007;62:1313
11. Catalano O, Sandomenico F, Matarazzo I, Siani A. Contrast-enhanced sonography of the spleen. *AJR Am J Roentgenol.* 2005;184:1150–1156
12. Thorelius L. Emergency real-time contrast-enhanced ultrasonography for detection of solid organ injuries. *Eur Radiol.* 2007;17(Suppl 6):F107–F111
13. Xu HX. Contrast-enhanced ultrasound: the evolving applications. *World J Radiol.* 2009;1:15–24
14. Lynn KN, Werder GM, Callaghan RM, et al. Pediatric blunt splenic trauma: a comprehensive review. *Pediatr Radiol.* 2009;39:904–916
15. Maroushek SR, Aguilar EF, Stauffer W, Abd-Alla MD. Malaria among refugee children at arrival in the United States. *Pediatr Infect Dis J.* 2005;24:450–452
16. Tanoli ZM, Rai ME, Gandapur AS. Clinical presentation and management of visceral leishmaniasis. *J Ayub Med Coll Abbottabad.* 2005;17:51–53
17. Balik E, Yazici M, Taneli C, Ulman I, Genç K. Splenoptosis (wandering spleen). *Eur J Pediatr Surg.* 1993;3:174–175
18. Maschio M, Cozzi G, Sanabor D, et al. Splenomegaly as presentation of a wandering spleen. *J Pediatr.* 2010;157:859.E1
19. Buescher ES. Infections associated with pediatric sport participation. *Pediatr Clin North Am.* 2002;49:743–751
20. Hosey RG, Kriss V, Uhl TL, et al. Ultrasonographic evaluation of splenic enlargement in athletes with acute infectious mononucleosis. *Br J Sports Med.* 2008;42:974–977
21. Rescorla FJ, Engum SA, West KW, et al. Laparoscopic splenectomy has become the gold standard in children. *Am Surg.* 2002;68:297–301
22. Qureshi FG, Ergun O, Sandulache VC, et al. Laparoscopic splenectomy in children. *JSLS.* 2005;9:389–392
23. Carmona J, Lugo Vicente H. Laparoscopic splenectomy for infarcted splenoptosis in a child: a case report. *Bol Asoc Med P R.* 2010;102:47–49
24. Hansen EN, Muensterer OJ. Single incision laparoscopic splenectomy in a 5-year-old with hereditary spherocytosis. *JSLS.* 2010;14:286–288
25. Rescorla FJ, West KW, Engum SA, Grosfeld JL. Laparoscopic splenic procedures in children: experience in 231 children. *Ann Surg.* 2007;246:683–688

26. Slater BJ, Chan FP, Davis K, Dutta S. Institutional experience with laparoscopic partial splenectomy for hereditary spherocytosis. *J Pediatr Surg*. 2010;45:1682–1686
27. Hollingsworth CL, Rice HE. Hereditary spherocytosis and partial splenectomy in children: review of surgical technique and the role of imaging. *Pediatr Radiol*. 2010;40:1177–1183
28. Kaiwa Y, Kurokawa Y, Namiki K, Matsumoto H, Satomi S. Laparoscopic partial splenectomies for true splenic cysts. A report of two cases. *Surg Endosc*. 2000;14:865
29. Vick LR, Gosche JR, Islam S. Partial splenectomy prevents splenic sequestration crises in sickle cell disease. *J Pediatr Surg*. 2009;44:2088–2091
30. al-Salem AH, al-Dabbous I, Bhamidibati P. The role of partial splenectomy in children with thalassemia. *Eur J Pediatr Surg*. 1998;8:334–338
31. American Academy of Pediatrics. Immunocompromised children. In: Pickering LK, Baker CJ, Kimberlin DW, Long SS, eds. *Red Book: 2012 Report of the Committee on Infectious Diseases*. 29th ed. Elk Grove Village, IL: American Academy of Pediatrics; 2012:72–90
32. Bickley LS, Szilagi PG, Bates B. *Bates' Guide to Physical Examination and History Taking*. 10th ed. Philadelphia, PA: Wolters Kluwer/Lippincott Williams & Wilkins; 2009

# Chapter 74

# Stridor

*Alfin G. Vicencio, MD; John P. Bent, MD*

## ▶ DEFINITION

Stridor is typically a high-pitched, monophonic noise caused by turbulent airflow through a partially obstructed extrathoracic airway, heard predominantly on inspiration. Although obstruction of large intrathoracic airways (ie, main-stem bronchi, mid and distal trachea) can produce a similar noise on expiration, these lesions are more thoroughly covered in Chapter 85, Wheezing, and will not be discussed here.

During the normal respiratory cycle, rhythmic expansion and contraction of the thorax leads to dynamic changes in thoracic pressures, allowing air to flow into and out of the lungs. (For a schematic representation, see Figure 85-1, Chapter 85, Wheezing.) During expiration the volume of the thoracic cavity decreases, creating positive pressures within the thorax. Airways located within the thorax are directly subjected to these positive pressures and thus are more prone to obstruction during expiration, leading to turbulent airflow and wheezing. On inspiration the thoracic cavity expands, resulting in negative intrathoracic pressures and improved patency of intrathoracic airways. However, because the intraluminal airway pressure drops to allow inflow of air, and because the extrathoracic airways (nose, nasopharynx, oropharynx, and larynx) may collapse from transmitted negative intrathoracic pressures, this portion of the airway is susceptible to obstruction, and thus stridor, during inspiration.

Because the extrathoracic airways extend from the nose to the proximal trachea, high-pitched laryngeal stridor must be differentiated from other abnormal inspiratory noises, such as stertor, a noisy, rumbling-type noise similar to snoring, which can be heard with partial airway obstruction in the oropharynx or nasopharynx. Accurately recognizing stridor will facilitate the ensuing diagnostic tests, given that the offending lesion is likely to be in or around the glottic region, a relatively focused anatomic area.

## ▶ DIFFERENTIAL DIAGNOSIS

Because stridor reflects obstruction of a large centralized airway and can range in severity from mild to life-threatening, ensuring airway patency should precede the generation of a differential diagnosis. For the child who has signs of severe respiratory compromise—distressed appearance, severe retractions, nasal flaring, pallor or cyanosis, altered mental status—initial measures should focus on maintaining the airway and, if possible, relieving the obstruction. Only personnel skilled at airway management should attempt intubation, if required, and such a procedure should be performed in as controlled a setting as possible. In select situations for which medical intubation might prove difficult (ie, suspected epiglottitis in a patient with high fever, drooling, and severe respiratory distress), surgical support should be present before airway manipulation in the event that tracheostomy is required. Luckily, most cases of stridor that the general pediatrician encounters can be approached with a succinct, focused history and physical examination followed by directed diagnostic tests.

The most common causes of stridor in the pediatric age group, laryngomalacia and viral croup, can be easily recognized by the experienced physician after obtaining a focused history and physical examination (see Evaluation). However, because the differential diagnosis of stridor is extensive and includes anything that obstructs the extrathoracic airway, a major challenge for the pediatrician is identifying select patients who have less common causes of obstruction and thus require specific diagnostic tests and different management (Table 74-1). For example, laryngomalacia, vocal cord dysfunction, subglottic stenosis, laryngeal papillomatosis, glottic cysts, laryngeal webs, subglottic hemangiomas, foreign bodies, retropharyngeal abscesses, and laryngeal fractures can all compromise the extrathoracic airway and cause stridor.[1] In most cases a careful stepwise evaluation by the astute pediatrician will lead to the correct diagnosis.

## ▶ EVALUATION

### *History*

Once airway patency has been ensured, a focused history should be elicited. Age of initial presentation and a description of the events surrounding the onset of symptoms can provide important clues to the underlying diagnosis. A commonly encountered patient is one whose stridor is preceded by fever, upper respiratory symptoms, and a *barky* or *seal-like* cough. This history, which may include repeated and similar episodes in the past, is consistent with viral croup and is easily recognized by an experienced pediatrician. Stridor beginning in the first few weeks of life that is present only during specific phases of alertness such as eating, sleeping, or excitement suggests congenital laryngomalacia as the underlying cause. Indeed, laryngomalacia is the most common cause of congenital stridor in infancy. In comparison, continuous stridor that begins soon after birth might suggest a congenital and fixed lesion such as a laryngeal web or, particularly in an infant with cutaneous hemangioma, subglottic hemangioma (obstruction associated with subglottic hemangiomas typically is mild at birth and worsens over the first 6 months of life).

Stridor that develops shortly after a prolonged intubation likely results from subglottic stenosis or granulation tissue and is often seen in premature infants who required mechanical ventilation during the neonatal period. A less common but important patient to recognize is one with a history of Arnold-Chiari malformation or hydrocephalus. Because increasing intracranial pressure can result in bilateral vocal cord paralysis, such patients should receive appropriate and emergent care to prevent brainstem herniation. Similarly, a stridulous toddler with a history of choking or placing small objects in the mouth should be evaluated for the presence of a foreign body. Recurrent respiratory papillomatosis is also usually associated with stridor or hoarseness 2 to 3 years after birth, although the infection is acquired through vertical transmission in the birth canal from maternal cervical human papillomavirus infection.

In addition to their onset, the chronicity and progression of symptoms can help identify the underlying cause and can be particularly helpful for patients with presumed

**Table 74-1**
**Causes of Stridor**

| | HISTORY | OBJECTIVE FINDINGS |
|---|---|---|
| Laryngomalacia | • Develops in the first few months of life<br>• Present mostly when agitated or crying | • Predominantly inspiratory<br>• May be positional<br>• Obstruction of glottic space by collapsing supraglottic structures on laryngoscopy |
| Viral croup | • Preceded by upper respiratory tract infection symptoms and fever<br>• No stridor between episodes<br>• May have history of similar episodes in past | • Predominantly inspiratory<br>• No change with position |
| Subglottic stenosis | • Develops after intubation or manipulation of airway<br>• May be continuous | • Predominantly inspiratory but often biphasic<br>• Flat inspiratory and expiratory loop on spirometry<br>• Subglottic narrowing on neck radiograph and direct laryngoscopy |
| Foreign body | • Sudden onset<br>• May have a history of choking | • Predominantly inspiratory if obstruction is extrathoracic<br>• Foreign body may be visualized on radiograph if radiopaque |
| Retropharyngeal abscess | • Fever<br>• Difficulty swallowing | • Often present with stertor<br>• May have drooling<br>• Retropharyngeal mass on lateral neck radiograph |
| Hemangioma | • Worsening stridor<br>• History of cutaneous hemangiomas | • May have cutaneous hemangiomas<br>• Subglottic obstruction on neck radiograph<br>• Hemangioma seen on direct laryngoscopy |
| Bilateral vocal cord paralysis | • History of injury to both recurrent laryngeal nerves<br>• Arnold-Chiari malformation or increased intracranial pressure | • No movement of vocal cords during laryngoscopy |
| Vocal cord cyst | • Hoarse voice<br>• Chronic irritation to vocal cords or airway instrumentation | • Cysts visible on laryngoscopy |
| Laryngeal papillomatosis | • Maternal history of human papillomavirus infection<br>• Hoarse voice<br>• Can develop in the first several years of life | • Papillomas visible on laryngoscopy |
| Laryngeal web | • Develops shortly after birth (congenital)<br>• Develops after airway instrumentation (acquired) | • Web visualized on laryngoscopy |

laryngomalacia or viral croup who do not follow the expected clinical course. Stridor caused by laryngomalacia is typically intermittent and worsens over the first several months of life. As the child becomes older, such episodes become less severe and less frequent. Indeed, for most patients with laryngomalacia, symptoms will completely resolve by the first birthday. Similarly, the likelihood of developing stridor caused by viral croup lessens with age. When the pediatrician is faced with a child whose stridor worsens or persists rather than improves, coexisting or alternate diagnoses should be considered, and appropriate diagnostic testing should be initiated. In addition, persistent symptoms may indicate a different laryngeal abnormality. For example, mild stridor caused by a subglottic hemangioma may initially be attributed to a more common problem such as laryngomalacia. Similar to laryngomalacia, obstruction from a hemangioma tends to worsen after initial presentation as the lesion enlarges. Unlike laryngomalacia, natural resolution of the hemangioma, and thus the stridor, may take several years rather than months. History of a hoarse voice or cry suggests glottic disease and might result from chronic irritation of the vocal cords. Other clues that suggest more ominous conditions include constant stridor, failure to thrive, difficulty swallowing, and severe and sudden onset of symptoms. Last, onset of stridor in an older child or adolescent with no previous history should prompt a more thorough evaluation.

### Physical Examination

Laryngeal stridor represents airway obstruction at the level of the supraglottis, glottis, or subglottis. Although these anatomic regions can be difficult to examine without the use of specific diagnostic tests, several clues from thorough physical examination can help confirm suspicions elicited on history. General inspection of the patient should include an assessment of position—extension of the neck is often described in patients with a serious infection such as epiglottitis or retropharyngeal abscess—as well as any drooling, which might suggest mass effect or edema in the posterior pharynx causing dysphagia in addition to the stridor (of note, these patients often exhibit stertor rather than stridor). Because such entities can be difficult or even dangerous to visualize, attention should focus on keeping the patient calm and maintaining the airway. An oropharyngeal examination might reveal a retropharyngeal bulge, an enlarged epiglottis or a lateral displacement of the uvula, and swelling of a tonsillar pillar from an underlying infection in patients with acute onset of stridor. External examination of the neck might show suprasternal retractions when obstruction is severe and may also reveal displacement of the larynx, a mass obstructing the airway, or signs of trauma. Finally, the quality of the voice should be noted; given that hoarseness, aphonia, or a weak cry suggests vocal cord disease, one should examine the skin for any cutaneous lesions such as hemangiomas. Lastly, improvement of stridor with a jaw thrust could suggest pathology in the region of the epiglottis as opposed to the subglottis.

### Objective Testing

Although a detailed history and physical examination are often sufficient to make a diagnosis of laryngomalacia or viral croup, additional diagnostic tests are warranted for patients whose symptoms and clinical course seem unusual or overly severe. Laboratory testing has limited value in evaluating patients with stridor. Similarly, pulmonary function testing is not often necessary but can confirm suspicions of an extrathoracic obstruction

(Figure 74-1). A simple radiograph of the neck can identify obstructive lesions in the retropharynx, glottis, and subglottic area (Figure 74-2). The classic *steeple sign* on anteroposterior neck radiograph depicts subglottic narrowing but does not distinguish croup from subglottic stenosis. Direct visualization of the airway by flexible laryngoscopy often provides definitive information.

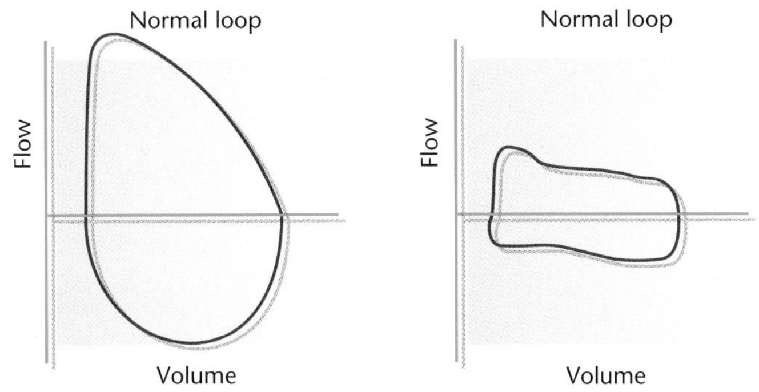


**Figure 74-1**
Findings on spirometry. The normal flow-volume loop has a characteristic shape. In comparison, the flow-volume loop in a patient with severe subglottic stenosis is flat.

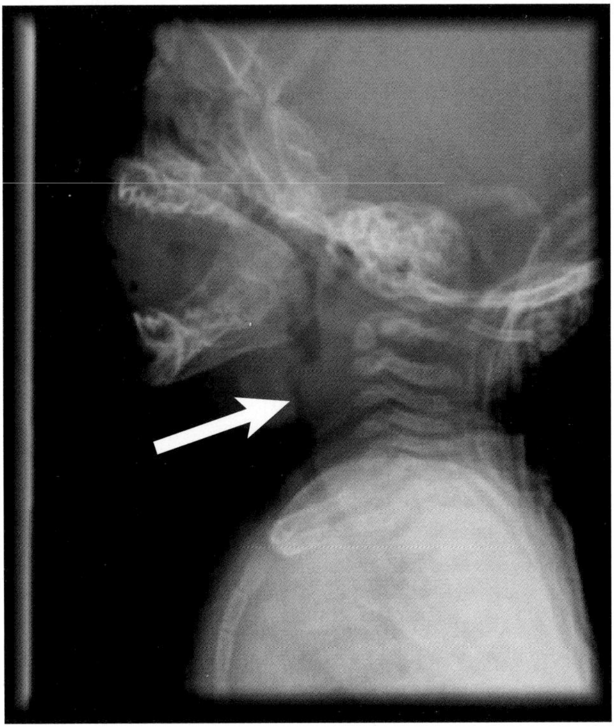

**Figure 74-2**
The neck radiograph demonstrates a mass causing mild obstruction of the subglottic area *(arrow)* in a child with stridor.

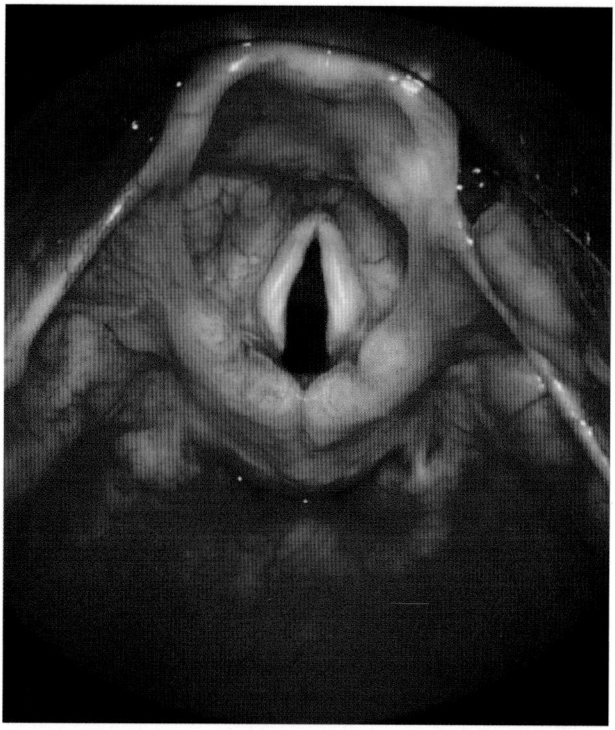

**Figure 74-3**
Normal larynx. Flexible and direct laryngoscopy offers a direct view of the glottis and can identify an abnormality. Shown here is a normal view of the glottis.

Flexible laryngoscopy is a routine procedure for the practicing otolaryngologist. Because the procedure offers direct visualization of the posterior pharynx and glottis (Figure 74-3), numerous other lesions causing laryngeal obstruction can be visualized, leading to a correct diagnosis. In fact, before routine use of office-based flexible laryngoscopy, laryngomalacia was known as *congenital laryngeal stridor,* reflecting physicians' incorrect assumption that all congenital laryngeal stridor might be attributed to a single cause. The procedure is usually well tolerated and can be performed most often with topical anesthesia alone (Figure 74-4). In many instances, laryngoscopy merely confirms the presence of laryngomalacia while excluding other causes of airway obstruction (Figure 74-5, *A* and Figure 74-5, *B*). In cases of severe laryngomalacia, laryngoscopy can also identify specific structures of the larynx that are causing obstruction that might be amenable to surgical correction (Figure 74-5, *C*). Of course, direct visualization of the glottis can also identify other lesions that cause obstruction, as shown in Figure 74-6.

Successful flexible laryngoscopy is often dependent on patient cooperation, particularly with anxious, difficult-to-restrain, and younger school-aged children. Furthermore, although laryngoscopy often provides a clear view of the glottis and supraglottic structures, the subglottic area cannot be well visualized. Indeed, even with a cooperative patient, the presence of severe laryngomalacia might obscure the view of the subglottic area such that a

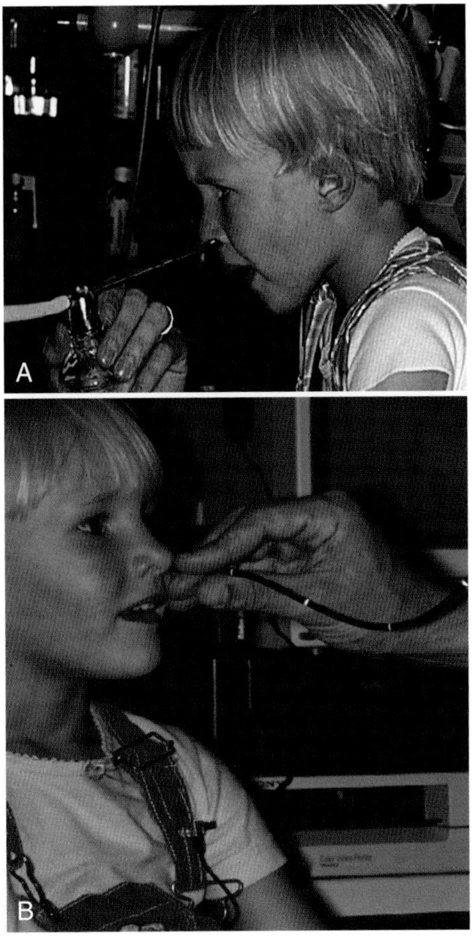

**Figure 74-4**
Flexible laryngoscopy. **A,** Topical anesthetic is applied before performing flexible laryngoscopy. **B,** The procedure is usually well tolerated when performed by an experienced laryngoscopist.

more distal lesion would not be visible. In such cases, direct visualization of the subglottic region and proximal trachea may be indicated to exclude a second lesion. Direct laryngoscopy and bronchoscopy under sedation or general anesthesia can help diagnose and quantify the severity of subglottic stenosis or identify other subglottic lesions that cause obstruction (Figure 74-7).

## ▶ MANAGEMENT

Because patients with laryngomalacia and viral croup are frequently encountered and will include most patients with stridor, the general pediatrician should be comfortable with outpatient management. Most cases of laryngomalacia can be managed with observation alone, with particular attention given to adequate caloric intake and weight gain. For patients with severe episodes of stridor causing hypoxemia or cyanosis, or if symptoms progress over time,

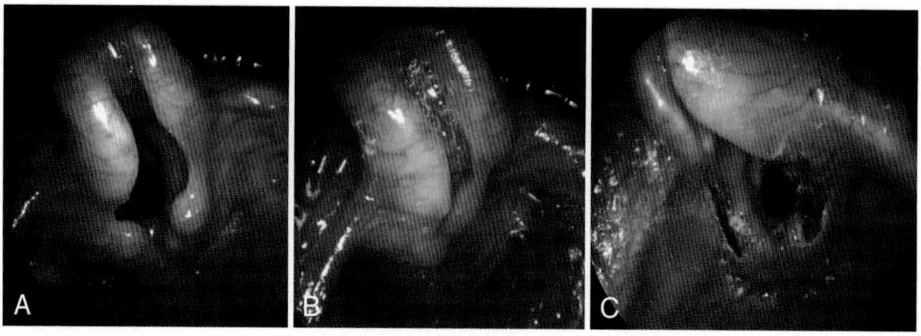

**Figure 74-5**
Laryngomalacia as seen by flexible laryngoscopy. **A,** During expiration the glottis is patent, and no abnormal sound is heard. **B,** During inspiration the epiglottis and arytenoids collapse and compromise the glottic opening, causing inspiratory stridor. **C,** In cases of severe laryngomalacia, surgical resection of redundant tissue can improve the glottic patency even during inspiration.

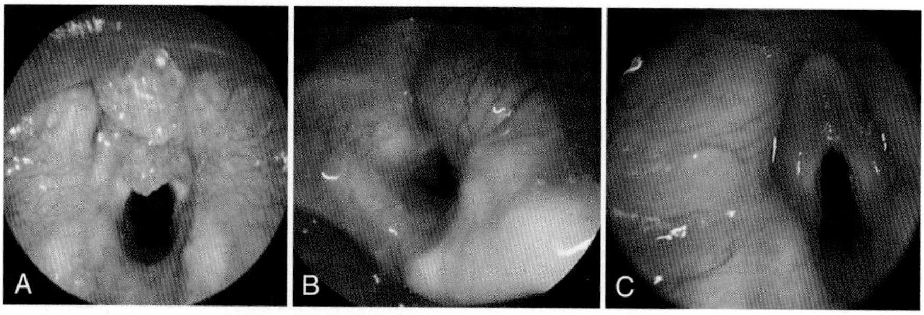

**Figure 74-6**
Obstructive lesions in the glottis. **A,** Laryngeal papilloma. **B,** Anterior saccular cyst. **C,** Glottic web.

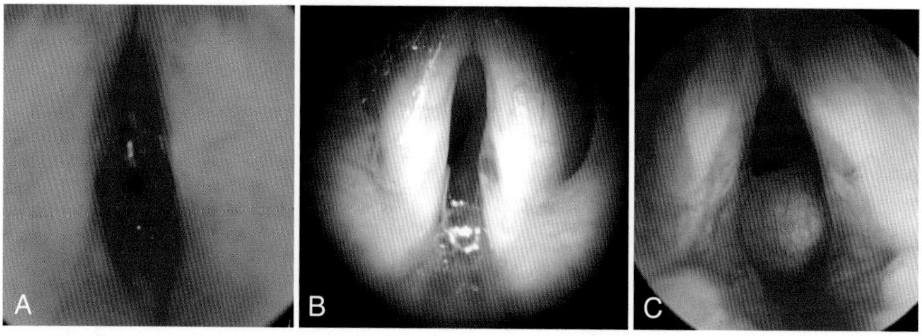

**Figure 74-7**
Obstructive lesions in the subglottic region. **A,** Severe subglottic stenosis. **B,** Right lateral subglottic hemangioma. **C,** Subglottic duct cyst.

additional diagnostic testing is indicated, and referral to a subspecialist may be warranted. In certain instances, laryngomalacia requires surgical management to relieve the obstruction caused by redundant epiglottic folds or arytenoid tissue (see Figure 74-5). Tracheostomy is rarely required. As with laryngomalacia, most patients with viral croup can be managed with close observation alone. For children with more severe obstruction (nasal flaring, retractions), racemic epinephrine and dexamethasone may temporarily relieve symptoms of obstruction and alleviate inflammation, respectively. Hospitalization is indicated for children with hypoxemia, apnea, or poor feeding or dehydration.

As discussed previously, stridor that is continuous, progressive, or severe should prompt the pediatrician to initiate additional diagnostic tests. Referral to a pediatric otolaryngologist for further evaluation by laryngoscopy or bronchoscopy (or both) will facilitate diagnosis of other causes of glottic or subglottic obstruction, which might require surgical management. Laser therapy for a hemangioma or web can provide definitive cure, as can cricoid split and augmentation of the subglottic space for an acquired stenosis.

In summary, the pediatrician evaluating the child with stridor should be aware of the various clinical entities that can present with stridor, be able to recognize by history or physical examination patients who require further evaluation, initiate simple diagnostic tests, and refer to appropriate subspecialty physicians those children with unusual presentations or poor response to conventional therapies.

## When to Refer

- Progressive or continuous stridor
- Poor weight gain or growth associated with persistent stridor
- Repeated hospitalization
- Presence of cutaneous hemangiomas in association with persistent stridor

## When to Admit

- Respiratory distress or hypoxemia
- Inability to eat or drink
- Altered mental status or signs of fatigue
- Stridor associated with signs of increased intracranial pressure

## *TOOLS FOR PRACTICE*

### Engaging Patient and Family

- *What Is a Pediatric Otolaryngologist?* (fact sheet), American Academy of Pediatrics (www.healthychildren.org/English/family-life/health-management/pediatric-specialists/Pages/What-is-a-Pediatric-Otolaryngologist.aspx)

## *REFERENCE*

1. Bent J. Pediatric laryngotracheal obstruction: current perspectives on stridor. *Laryngoscope*. 2006;116:1059–1070

# Substance Use: Initial Approach in Primary Care

*Sharon Levy, MD, MPH; Sarah Bagley, MD*

## ▶ INTRODUCTION

Pediatricians in primary care encounter many youth who have experience with alcohol, marijuana, and other drugs. They may identify a youth because parents or teachers have expressed a concern about use of substances, because the youth has physical signs or symptoms suggesting substance use, because there are nonspecific symptoms that may suggest substance use (eg, declining school performance or attendance, car crash, association with friends who are using substances), or because an asymptomatic youth has a positive substance-use screening test result. Whether the use identified is sporadic or regular, it can have negative health effects related to the direct consequences of the substances or associated risky behaviors. Identifying and addressing substance use to minimize harm is an important task for the primary care physician (PCP). Because substance use is closely associated with morbidity and mortality in this age group, the American Academy of Pediatrics (AAP) recommends that pediatricians achieve competence in identifying and intervening to reduce substance use by youth, as well as supporting the care of youth with substance use disorders (SUDs).[1]

Perceived limitations of time for adequate psychosocial evaluation, discomfort addressing sensitive issues, or lack of familiarity with available therapeutic resources may prevent physicians from thoroughly and appropriately addressing substance use with adolescents. However, as with other disorders, assessment is required in order to determine the appropriate setting and level of care. More often than not, sensitivity to these issues, attention to adolescents' risk behaviors in general, and periodic follow-up in the primary care setting are adequate to help keep adolescents safe and healthy.

## ▶ ADOLESCENT BRAIN DEVELOPMENT

The human brain continues to develop until the middle of the third decade of life. The prefrontal cortex—which controls impulses, attention and organization—matures last, well after the parts of the brain that are involved in pleasure and reward. This developmental "imbalance" is correlated with stimulation seeking and risk-taking behavior that is typical of adolescence. Use of psychoactive substances is one way, albeit dangerous and unhealthy, in which youth may fulfill a natural inclination for stimulation and reward. It is not surprising, therefore, that rates of psychoactive substance use peak in adolescence and early adulthood. Seen in this perspective, substance use can be understood as an (unhealthy) mechanism for fulfilling a normal drive, rather than as purely deviant behavior. Adolescents also may use psychoactive substances for a variety of other reasons: to fit in social situations in which others are using substances; because of expectations that use will be pleasurable; as a form of risk taking or stimulation seeking; or to relax, relieve anxiety, improve mood, or relieve symptoms of a mental health disorder. Identifying the reasons that underlie substance use can help physicians to target counseling, advice, and strategies that are most salient to the adolescent.

Unfortunately substance use, even without symptoms that rise to the level of a "disorder," is associated with significant health problems, including injuries, accidents, unintentional sexual activity, and sexually transmitted infections. Early initiation of substance use is also associated with increased risk of developing a severe SUD (otherwise known as addiction), which is a chronic medical condition that causes neurologic changes. The AAP recommends that physicians routinely screen every adolescent for substance use and deliver an appropriate intervention geared towards preventing or reducing substance use.[1] When a child is referred for specialty care of a substance abuse problem, the AAP recommends that the physician remain involved with the child and family, supporting their positive view of treatment, monitoring progress, and providing complementary primary care services.

## ▶ PREVALENCE OF SUBSTANCE USE

Alcohol, marijuana, and tobacco are the most commonly used substances among youth. By the end of 12th grade, 52% of students report being drunk at least once, as do 12% of eighth-graders. Lifetime rates of use of any illicit drug increased in 2013, driven mainly by increasing rates of marijuana use. Perception of risk related to marijuana use continues to fall, likely foreshadowing continued increases in use over the next few years. Prescription drug misuse continues to be a concern, with 15% of 12th-graders reporting misuse of a prescription drug in the prior year.[2] Rates of tobacco use by youth declined from 1996 to 2010, though over the past few years rates have plateaued. "E-cigarettes," which are electronic devices that vaporize liquid nicotine, are marketed as a tobacco cessation device but are sold in flavors such as bubble gum and cotton candy that are attractive to children who may initiate their "smoking careers" with these devices. Use of tobacco products often precedes use of other substances. Youth who smoke cigarettes are 5 times more likely than nonsmokers to use alcohol, 13 times more likely to use marijuana, and 7 times more likely to use cocaine or heroin.[3]

## ▶ CLASSIFICATION OF SUBSTANCE USE DISORDERS

The *Diagnostic and Statistical Manual, 5th Edition* (*DSM-5*), released in May 2013, included new criteria and replaced the terms "substance abuse" and "substance dependence" with SUD—mild, moderate, or severe. The new diagnostic classification is based on the number of criteria that are met: 2 to 3 constitute a mild disorder, 4 to 5 moderate, and 6 or more severe. Meeting criteria for a mild or moderate SUD indicates particularly hazardous use or that an individual has begun to have problems associated with use. Although there are no clear referral guidelines for adolescents with an SUD unless there is a co-occurring mental illness, those with a mild SUD can likely be managed in primary care. Patients with a moderate SUD may not require a referral to subspecialty care, and the referral decision can be left to the discretion of the PCP and his or her comfort with managing SUDs. Meeting criteria for severe SUD suggests that an individual would likely benefit from specialized treatment for SUDs. However, because many adolescents with a severe SUD will not accept a referral to treatment, PCPs should be prepared to manage these patients in primary care while trying to facilitate completion of the referral. While not an official diagnostic term, "addiction" refers to loss of control or obsessive use of a substance associated with neurologic changes in the brain's reward center. Because there is no cure for addiction, long-term treatment is recommended. Effective, evidence-based treatments, including medication and psychosocial support, are available.

The following sections will describe the physician's role in screening for substance use, assessment of severity, and management of adolescents who are using substances.

## ▶ CONFIDENTIALITY AND SUBSTANCE USE

Given that substance use is one of a number of sensitive topics that may come up in the course of adolescent care, PCPs should have a systematic way to establish "limits" of confidentiality with both youth and parents in the practice. This is particularly important before a pediatrician begins taking the medical history and screening for drug use. Discussions between the pediatrician and patient should remain confidential unless the pediatrician determines that the reported behaviors are putting either the patient or someone else at acute risk of harm. Determining whether a behavior requires breach of confidentiality is a matter of clinical judgment; in most cases reports of occasional tobacco, alcohol, or marijuana use can be kept confidential, though a physician may decide to involve parents if a child is very young or being treated for a medical condition that could be dangerously affected by substance use. Even when there is no reason to breach confidentiality, it is often best to request permission from the youth to engage with parents for their support. In situations where a parent is already aware of use, the youth may be willing to share information, particularly if he or she has agreed to a quit attempt or to engage in further treatment.[4]

## ▶ SCREENING TOOLS

At each health supervision visit with an adolescent or preadolescent patient, pediatricians should include a psychosocial interview to assess family and peer relationships, academic progress, recreational activities, sexual behavior, and drug use. HEADSSS is an acronym that can help physicians to inquire about key domains: home, education, activities, drugs, safety, sexuality, and suicide or depression.[5] Pre-visit questionnaires are also available to capture this information.

This data gathering does not substitute for screening. Standardized, validated tools are recommended when screening for substance use in order to improve sensitivity of report and accuracy of triage based on screen results[6–12] (Table 75-1). Using screening tools minimizes the likelihood that substance use problems or disorders are missed, as commonly occurs when screening on clinical impressions alone.[13]

Screening allows pediatricians to stratify youth into risk categories. Each of the recommended tools does this in a slightly different way, though most include "no use," "lower-risk use," "moderate-risk use," and "high-risk use," with "lower-risk use" corresponding to use without a *DSM-5* SUD and "high-risk" corresponding to a mild, moderate, or severe

**Table 75-1**
**Substance Abuse Screening and Assessment Tools for Use With Adolescents**

| | |
|---|---|
| **BRIEF SCREENS** | |
| S2BI | • 2-question frequency screen<br>• Screens for tobacco, alcohol, marijuana, and other illicit drug use<br>• Discriminates between no use, no SUD, moderate SUD, and severe SUD, based on *DSM-5* diagnoses |
| Brief Screener for Tobacco, Alcohol, and Other Drugs (BSTAD) | • Identifies problematic tobacco, alcohol, and marijuana use in pediatric settings |
| NIAAA Youth Alcohol Screen | • 2-question screen<br>• Screens for friends' use and own use |
| **BRIEF ASSESSMENTS** | |
| Car, Relax, Alone, Friends/Family, Forget, Trouble (CRAFFT) | • A good tool for quickly identifying problems associated with substance use<br>• Not a diagnostic tool |
| Global Appraisal of Individual Needs (GAIN) | • Assesses for both SUDs and mental health disorders |
| Alcohol Use Disorders Identification Test (AUDIT) | • Assesses risky drinking<br>• Not a diagnostic tool |

*DSM-5, Diagnostic and Statistical Management of Mental Disorders, Fifth Edition; SUD,* substance use disorder.

SUD. In this chapter we describe interventions for each of these levels of risk. Some tools do not discriminate between moderate and high risk; in these cases the assessment is used to determine which youth have developed a severe SUD that will benefit most from referral to subspecialty care. Interventions for each stage are described below, in the section on Counseling to Reduce Drug Use and High-Risk Behaviors.

## ▶ ADVICE AND COUNSELING FOR LOW-RISK YOUTH

PCPs should provide youth who are not using substances or are "lower risk" with positive encouragement about their smart and healthy choices. This is an opportunity to provide education about the risks of using substances in addition to anticipatory guidance about how to manage situations when alcohol or other drugs will be available.[1] Importantly, it is recommended that the PCP include a discussion of the risks of impaired driving and help the adolescent plan for times when a driver may have used alcohol or drugs. Students Against Destructive Decisions (SADD) has a helpful framework for physicians to use with patients and parents for driving safety (see Tools for Practice: Engaging Patient and Family at the end of this chapter).[14]

## ▶ PRIMARY CARE OF YOUTH WHO ARE USING SUBSTANCES

### *Assessment*

Assessment is performed with youth whose screen result puts them in the "moderate risk" or "high risk" category in order to determine the problems associated with use and the effect of substance use on their functioning at home, at school, and with peers. Assessment can include questions about age of initiation, frequency, and, for alcohol, quantity of use—information that assists the physician in identifying acute risk (such as very heavy alcohol consumption) as well as personalizing medical advice (such as discussing the effect of daily marijuana use on the adolescent brain). Asking about associated problems, troubles, regrets, and quit attempts may also identify areas of ambivalence that can be incorporated into a discussion of behavior change. These problems can be used as a fulcrum to turn the discussion toward a behavior change plan identified by the youth.

In general, open-ended questions such as "Tell me about your history of alcohol use" encourage more reporting than closed-ended questions. However, physicians may need to prompt adolescents for certain information that is important for formulation. Suggested historical elements are listed in Table 75-2. With a focus on problems associated with substance use, a clinical history can be used as the first step in an intervention. Information about use of tobacco, inhalants, and other psychoactive and illicit substances and misuse of prescription or over-the-counter medications also helps to formulate clinical impressions and treatment recommendations. The National Institute of Alcohol Abuse and Alcoholism's *Alcohol Screening and Brief Intervention for Youth: A Practitioner's Guide* and the AAP Policy Statement on Screening, Brief Intervention, and Referral to Treatment both explain in detail the recommended approach to screening and brief intervention for adolescents.[1,8]

A parent, teacher, or other caregiver may notice nonspecific signs or symptoms that may indicate substance use. If these are reported, the youth should be assessed for a potential SUD through a careful history regardless of screen results. See Table 75-3 for other conditions that may mimic or co-occur with substance use. In addition, certain risk factors such as early initiation of use, family history of SUDs, and co-occurring mental health disorders increase a youth's susceptibility to developing an SUD. When available, this information should be considered in the overall assessment of each patient.

As with screening, an accurate substance use history can be best obtained in an atmosphere of confidentiality, privacy, and trust; it is recommended that parents be excluded from the interview.

**Table 75-2**
**Key Details to Assess in High-Risk Patients**

| SUBSTANCE | KEY HISTORICAL ELEMENTS |
|---|---|
| Alcohol | • Age of first drunkenness<br>• Frequency of drinking episodes<br>• Typical amount of alcohol consumed<br>• Greatest amount of alcohol consumed<br>• History of blackouts, overdose, emergency department visits<br>• Problems associated with alcohol use<br>• Quit attempts |
| Marijuana | • Age at initiation<br>• Frequency of marijuana use<br>• History of paranoia and/or hallucinations<br>• Problems associated with marijuana use<br>• Quit attempts |

**Table 75-3**
**Conditions That May Mimic or Co-occur With Substance Use**

| CONDITION | RATIONALE |
|---|---|
| Learning problems or disabilities | Unidentified learning difficulties can contribute to frustration and stress, school failure, and association with peers who use substances, all of which can increase the chances of developing a substance use disorder (SUD). See Chapter 49, Learning Difficulty, to explore this possibility. |
| Depression or bipolar disorder | Marked sleep disturbance, disturbed appetite, low mood, or tearfulness could indicate that a youth is depressed. Symptoms of depression rapidly alternating with cycles of agitation may suggest bipolar mood disorder. See Chapter 14, Depression. |
| Exposure to adverse childhood experiences (ACE) | Youth who have experienced or witnessed trauma, violence, a natural disaster, separation from a parent, parental divorce or separation, parental substance use, neglect, or physical, emotional, or sexual abuse are at high risk for developing emotional difficulties such as adjustment disorder or posttraumatic stress disorder (PTSD). Consider PTSD if the onset or acceleration of substance use was preceded by an extremely distressing experience. Physicians should speak separately and confidentially with the youth and parents to explore this possibility. Parents are often unaware of exposures that children may have had at school or in the community and may also underestimate the effect on children of major traumas in the family (eg, serious illness in a parent, maltreatment of the child, death or incarceration of a loved one). See also Chapter 6, Anxiety. |
| Other anxiety disorders | Anxiety disorders commonly co-occur with SUDs, and the relationship is bidirectional: anxious youth may be more likely to use substances, and conversely, substance use may cause or precipitate anxiety disorders. |
| Physical illness | Drug or alcohol withdrawal may present as a physical illness and is potentially a medical emergency. Psychiatric symptoms may be associated with medical illness (eg, encephalitis/cerebritis) and may be mistaken for drug intoxication. |
| Psychosis | Though rare, the onset of bipolar disorder or schizophrenia in late adolescence may be subtle and marked only by frightening hallucinations or delusions that the youth does not disclose. These symptoms may result from, precipitate, or accelerate the use of substances. |
| Attention-deficit/hyperactivity disorder (ADHD) | Adolescents with ADHD have higher rates of SUDs than peers. Some studies have suggested that stimulant treatment for adolescents with ADHD may lower the risk of developing an SUD, though findings have been inconclusive. There is no evidence that stimulant treatment increases risk of developing an SUD. See Chapter 45, Inattention and Impulsivity. |

## *Physical Examination*

The medical complications of chronic substance use, although sometimes severe, usually do not appear until after adolescence. Nonetheless, a complete evaluation for an SUD includes a complete physical examination; signs and symptoms of acute intoxication or chronic use should be noted if present. Table 75-4 lists physical signs and symptoms of acute and chronic substance use.

**Table 75-4**
**Physical Findings Potentially Indicating Substance Use and Abuse**

| | ACUTE INTOXICATION | CHRONIC IMPAIRMENT | DRUG(S) TO CONSIDER |
|---|---|---|---|
| **General Appearance** | Altered mood, strange/ inappropriate behavior | Poor dress or hygiene | Any drug |
| **Vital Signs** | | Weight loss | Heroin, cocaine |
| | Hypertension | Hypertension | Cocaine, amphetamine |
| | Hypotension, hypothermia | | Heroin |
| | Hyperthermia | | Cocaine, amphetamine, ecstasy |
| | Tachycardia | | Marijuana, cocaine, amphetamine |
| **Ears, Nose, and Throat** | Conjunctival injection | | Marijuana, inhalants |
| | Dilated pupils | | Cocaine, amphetamines |
| | Constricted pupils | | Opioids |
| | Sluggish pupillary response | | Barbiturates |
| | | Nasal irritation | Cocaine, inhalants, opioids (if sniffing) |
| **Cardiac** | Arrhythmias | Arrhythmias | Methadone, cocaine, amphetamine |
| **Chest** | | Gynecomastia | Marijuana, anabolic steroids |
| **Genitourinary** | | Testicular atrophy, clitoromegaly | Anabolic steroids |
| **Skin** | | Acne, hirsutism | Anabolic steroids |
| | Abscesses, needle track marks | | IV drug use |
| **Neurologic** | Altered sensorium | | Any substance |
| | Ataxia | | Alcohol, barbiturates |
| | Nystagmus | | Barbiturates |
| | Hyporeflexia or hyperreflexia | | Marijuana, cocaine, amphetamine |

## Laboratory Testing

Drug testing may be a useful part of a complete assessment for an SUD, particularly when a parent or other adult is concerned and the adolescent denies use. As with any laboratory test, this procedure yields limited information and should be used only as an adjunct to the history and physical examination. The use of drug testing in general populations (eg, school drug testing programs) has less utility and many associated ethical and legal concerns. Parents may request that the pediatrician perform a urine drug test; however, testing and sharing of the results should only be done with the permission of the adolescent. If an adolescent refuses a test that is indicated, parents can be coached to implement logical consequences as they would in other circumstances, such as refusal to do homework or chores. If there is concern for harm, then the pediatrician should consider breaching confidentiality. Drug testing is a complex laboratory procedure with significant potential for false positive and false negative results; the AAP has produced a clinical report to help guide physicians on how to use this procedure most effectively.

## General Care

PCPs are positioned to provide effective care to youth who are using substances, including youth who also need specialty services.

### Reduce Stress

Consider the child's social environment (eg, family social history, parental depression screening, results of any family assessment tools administered, reports from child care or school). Questions to raise might include the following:

*Is an external problem (adverse experience such as abuse, bullying, or family socioeconomic stress) adding to the youth's stress?* Take steps to explore and reduce stressors, as feasible.

*Are the youth's peers using substances?* Explore options to increase healthy social and recreational activities and reduce contact with peers who are using substances. Youth with severe SUDs can be encouraged to change their phone numbers and eliminate old contacts to avoid being contacted by old friends with whom they previously used drugs. Unfortunately, it is impossible to isolate youth with SUDs from substances. Part of treatment is teaching youths to identify high-risk situations, avoid them when possible, and use strategies to avoid use even when confronted with others who are using. In some communities, youth may be able to attend a recovery high school. Recovery high schools are accredited schools that provide a safe and sober environment for youth with a substance use history to continue their education. Every school has a different approach that includes provision of continued support for students' recovery.

The physician also can acknowledge and reinforce protective factors such as good relationships with at least 1 parent or important adult, prosocial peers, concerned or caring family, help-seeking, and connection to positive organizations.

### Encourage Healthy Habits

Encourage exercise, outdoor time, a healthy and consistent diet, sleep (critically important to mental health), limited screen time, one-on-one time with parents, and time with peers who are not using substances. Offer praise for positive behavior changes, acknowledgment of the youth's strengths, and acknowledgment of the challenges the youth may be facing with transitions including new schools, new friends, new social circles, and new academic demands. Acknowledge that while the patient's friends may be using substances heavily, most of their same-age peers do not binge drink or use drugs.

Encourage involvement in prosocial activities such as youth development, leadership, volunteer, and after-school activities; sports teams, clubs, and mentoring; and faith-based programs. A strengths-based approach that capitalizes on interests, talents, and future goals is most effective.

### Offer Resources

Helpful resources are included in Tools for Practice: Engaging Patient and Family. Provide contact numbers in case of an emergency.

### Monitor Progress

School reports, as well as youth and parent feedback, can be helpful in monitoring progress.

## Counseling to Reduce Drug Use and High-Risk Behaviors

The strategies described below are common elements of evidence-based and evidence-informed psychosocial interventions for the use of substances. They are applicable to the primary care of youth in the early stages of substance use and to the initial management of youth in more advanced stages while readying them for, or awaiting access to, substance abuse specialty care.

*Tailor intervention to stage of use.* Depending on the screening tool used, levels of risk include abstinence, lower risk (ie, use but no SUD), moderate risk (ie, mild or moderate SUD), high risk (ie, youth with a severe SUD), and acute risk, which is determined as part of the assessment of moderate and high risk youth. Interventions for each stage of change are described in Table 75-5.

*Use motivational interviewing techniques* (Table 75-6). The physician can explore ambivalence about use and readiness to enter treatment and negotiate achievable next steps in an empathetic and supportive manner. For high-risk youth, change plans can focus on eliminating highest-risk behaviors (such as driving or riding with an impaired driver) and on engaging in ongoing treatment. The physician should help parents be supportive of behavior change and coach them to avoid inadvertently enabling ongoing use.

*If the youth has a history of either driving or being driven by an individual who has been using alcohol, negotiate a safety plan.* Students Against Destructive Decisions (SADD) has a Contract for Life that can be signed by both a parent and a youth to ensure that the youth has a plan for a safe ride home.[14]

## Referral to Specialty Treatment

The challenge continually posed to pediatricians is to recognize when a patient's substance use becomes significant enough to warrant referral to a treatment program or facility rather than being treated solely in the primary care setting. The AAP statement regarding screening, brief intervention and referral to treatment (SBIRT) provides specific guidance

**Table 75-5**
**Substance Use Spectrum and Goals for Office Intervention**

| STAGE/TRIAGE CATEGORY | DESCRIPTION | OFFICE-BASED INTERVENTION GOALS |
|---|---|---|
| Abstinence | No use of drugs or alcohol | **Positive Reinforcement** Prevent or delay initiation of substance use through positive reinforcement. Include statement about use norms, especially for younger children. |
| No substance use disorder (SUD) | Use of alcohol or marijuana with peers in relatively low-risk situations; without related problems or interference with domains of functioning—such as school, sports, hobbies, or home life. | **Brief Advice** Encourage cessation through brief medically based advice, particularly as it relates to patient's future goals. Promote patient strengths. |
| Mild/moderate SUD | As defined by *DSM-5*. Adolescents with mild/moderate SUDs typically have associated problems or high-risk behaviors associated with use. | **Brief Motivational Intervention** Encourage cessation even for a brief trial period if patient is willing. Reduce potential harm by reducing use and focusing on highest-risk behaviors. Encourage parent involvement to help with follow-through. Follow up with primary physician or allied mental health professional to continue conversation and harm reduction. |
| Severe SUD (addiction) | As defined in *DSM-5*. Loss of control or compulsive drug use, as "dependence" is defined in *DSM-IV-TR*. | **Brief motivational intervention** targeting referral into ongoing treatment. Encourage reducing use and high-risk behaviors and engaging adolescent to accept a referral to treatment. Share diagnosis and referral information with parents, if possible. Follow-up by primary care physician to ensure compliance and encourage long-term treatment. |
| Acute risk | Use associated with acute risk of overdose or in a situation that is physically risky. | **Intervention for safety** may include breaching confidentality to inform parents about use and referral to treatment in a timely fashion. Verbal contracts not to use while awaiting a formal evaluation and advice to parents on how to monitor and what to do in case of escalation may also be helpful. |

From Levy SJ, Kokotailo PK. Substance use screening, brief intervention, and referral to treatment for pediatricians. *Pediatrics*. 2011;128(5):e1330–e1340.

**Table 75-6**
**Sample Framework for Brief Motivational Intervention**

| PROCESS | DESCRIPTION |
|---|---|
| Assessment and summary | Targeted assessment for areas of ambivalence to establish rapport and develop a discrepancy between current status and future goals. Sample questions<br>• *What problems (if any) have you had, related to your use of substances?*<br>• *What regrets (if any) do you have, related to your use of alcohol?*<br>• *What trouble (if any) have you had, related to your use of marijuana?* |
| Brief advice | Offer specific medical advice to quit or cut down substance use as a means for decreasing the types of problems reported during the assessment. Sample statement<br>• *Only you can decide whether or not to drink alcohol. In regard to your health, I recommend you quit.*<br>• *Having a blackout means that you have had enough alcohol to poison your brain cells, at least temporarily.*<br>• *Kids often make bad choices, like the decision to have sex without a condom, when they are drinking.* |
| Planning | Engage patient in setting personal goals and agenda for change and link to follow-up. Sample statement<br>• *It sounds like you really enjoy drinking and also don't want to have another blackout. What could you do to protect yourself?* |

for when to refer patients and to which level of care.[1] Following is a list of indications for specialty referral:

- Child younger than 15 years with a positive screen for moderate- or high-risk substance use.
- Interventions by PCP have not reduced use.
- Drug use is endangering the youth or others.
- Drug use is threatening the achievement of developmentally important goals, such as school attendance and performance, or relationships.
- Co-occurring mental health disorders are present.
- Youth has a history of trauma.
- Youth is using drugs other than alcohol, marijuana, or tobacco.
- Parents are not involved, do not acknowledge concerns, or one or both parents have an active SUD.

If the child is referred to a specialist, the family will probably need assistance in navigating the requirements of their health insurance plan or the public mental health system and selecting an appropriate physician. The PCP and specialist will need to reach agreement on respective roles in the youth's care and establish a mechanism for communicating progress. The PCP can support the youth by encouraging his or her positive view of treatment; monitoring progress in care and observing for co-occurring disorders; coordinating care provided by parents, school, medical home, and specialists; and encouraging parents to seek treatment for tobacco use and other dependencies. Resources available to help physicians in these roles are provided in Tools for Practice at the end of this chapter.

Adolescents (and in some cases their parents) may resist treatment of an SUD. In these cases the following steps may be helpful:

- If a referral is clearly indicated, partner with parents to increase the likelihood of follow-through. Clarify with the youth the relevant laws and protections for minors. In many states, parents can file an order with the police to help enforce house rules. Depending on the situation, it may be necessary to involve the designated child protection agency.
- Provide education and motivational counseling to youth (and family, as appropriate) to reduce harm and improve functioning at home. Even if the youth is unwilling to engage with specific substance use treatment, he or she may be willing to see a licensed clinical social worker or psychologist.

## ▶ SUMMARY

Primary care pediatricians commonly encounter adolescents whose parents or teachers have concerns about their use of substances, who have signs or symptoms of substance use, or who have a positive screening test for substance use. In adolescents who are known to be using substances or who have other concerning signs or history, PCPs can perform a full assessment, including a physical examination and detailed substance use history. Laboratory testing can be used as an adjunct to the history and physical examination.

PCPs are positioned to provide care to youth who are using substances. PCPs can reinforce strengths and healthy behaviors and, by applying evidence-based brief interventions, can often be effective in preventing these youth from escalating their use of substances and in motivating them to decrease their use of substances. PCPs can also recognize those youth who need the care of substance abuse specialists, motivate youth and families to connect with needed services, and offer supportive primary care to youth who are involved in specialty care. If youth and their families resist referral for specialty care, PCPs can monitor the youth's progress and provide primary care interventions aimed at reducing substance use and risky behaviors while increasing their motivation to seek specialty care.

### *TOOLS FOR PRACTICE*

#### Engaging Patient and Family

- *Adolescent Addiction* (Web site), Home Box Office (www.hbo.com/addiction/adolescent_addiction)
- *Become an EX* (Web site), American Legacy Foundation (www.becomeanex.org)
- *Campaign for Tobacco-Free Kids* (Web site), (www.tobaccofreekids.org)
- *Contract for Life* (Web page), Students Against Destructive Decisions (www.sadd.org/contract.htm)
- *Julius B. Richmond Center of Excellence* (Web site), American Academy of Pediatrics (www.aap.org/richmondcenter)
- *National Institute on Drug Abuse* (Web site), (www.drugabuse.gov)
- *National Youth Anti-Drug Media Campaign* (Web Site), Office of National Drug Control Policy (www.abovetheinfluence.com)
- *NIDA for Teens* (Web site), National Institute on Drug Abuse (teens.drugabuse.gov)
- *Talk. They Hear You* (campaign), Substance Abuse and Mental Health Services Administration (teens.drugabuse.gov)
- *Smokefree.gov* (Web site), US Department of Health and Human Services (www.smokefree.gov)
- *The Partnership at Drugfree.org* (Web site), (www.drugfree.org)

### Medical Decision Support

- *Alcohol Screening and Brief Intervention for Youth: A Practitioner's Guide* (book), National Institute of Alcohol Abuse and Alcoholism, American Academy of Pediatrics (www.niaaa.nih.gov/Publications/EducationTrainingMaterials/Pages/YouthGuide.aspx)
- *CRAFFT* (screen), (www.ceasar-boston.org/clinicians/crafft.php)
- *Drug Strategies Treatment Guide* (Web site), DrugStrategies.org (www.drugstrategies.org/youths)
- *Mental Health Initiatives* (Web site), American Academy of Pediatrics (www.aap.org/en-us/advocacy-and-policy/aap-health-initiatives/Mental-Health/Pages/default.aspx)

## AAP POLICY STATEMENTS

American Academy of Pediatrics Committee on Substance Abuse. Substance use screening, brief intervention, and referral to treatment for pediatricians. *Pediatrics.* 2011;128(5):e1330–e1340 (pediatrics.aappublications.org/content/128/5/e1330.full)

Levy S, Siqueira LM; American Academy of Pediatrics Committee on Substance Abuse. Testing for drugs of abuse in children and adolescents. *Pediatrics.* 2014;133(6):1798–1807 (pediatrics.aappublications.org/content/133/6/e1798.full)

American Academy of Pediatrics Committee on Environmental Health, Committee on Substance Abuse, Committee on Adolescence, Committee on Native American Child Health. Tobacco use: a pediatric disease. *Pediatrics.* 2009;124(5):1474–1487. Reaffirmed May 2013 (pediatrics.aappublications.org/content/124/5/1474.full)

American Academy of Pediatrics Committee on Substance Abuse. Alcohol use by youth and adolescents: a pediatric concern. *Pediatrics.* 2010;125(5):1078–1087 (pediatrics.aappublications.org/content/125/5/1078.full)

Best D; American Academy of Pediatrics Committee on Environmental Health, Committee on Native American Child Health, Committee on Adolescence. Secondhand and prenatal tobacco smoke exposure. *Pediatrics.* 2009;124(5):e1017–e1044. Reaffirmed May 2014 (pediatrics.aappublications.org/content/124/5/e1017.full)

Sims TH; American Academy of Pediatrics Committee on Substance Abuse. Tobacco as a substance of abuse. *Pediatrics.* 2009;124(5):e1045–e1053 (pediatrics.aappublications.org/content/124/5/e1045.full)

## REFERENCES

1. American Academy of Pediatrics Committee on Substance Abuse. Substance use screening, brief intervention, and referral to treatment for pediatricians. *Pediatrics.* 2011;128:e1330–40
2. Johnston LD, O'Malley PM, Miech RA, Bachman JG, Schulenberg JE. Monitoring the Future national results on drug use: 1975-2013: overview, key findings on adolescent drug use. Ann Arbor, MI: Institute for Social Research, The University of Michigan; 2014. www.monitoringthefuture.org/pubs/monographs/mtf-overview2013.pdf. Accessed March 20, 2014
3. Abuse NCoAaS. Tobacco: The Smoking Gun. Prepared for the Citizen's Commission to Protect the Truth. Columbia University; 2007
4. Bagley S, Shrier L, Levy S. Talking to adolescents about alcohol, drugs and sexuality. *Minerva Pediatr.* 2014;66:77–87
5. Cohen E, Mackenzie RG, Yates GL. HEADSS, a psychosocial risk assessment instrument: implications for designing effective intervention programs for runaway youth. *J Adolesc Health.* 1991;12:539–44
6. Levy S, Weiss R, Sherritt L, et al. An electronic screen for triaging adolescent substance use by risk levels. *JAMA Pediatr.* 2014;168(9):822–828
7. Kelly S, O'Grady KE, Gryczynski J, Mitchell SG, Kirk A, Schwartz RP. Development and validation of a brief screening tool for adolescent tobacco, alcohol and drug use. In: Association for Medical Education and Research in Substance Abuse (AMERSA) 37th Annual National Conference. Bethesda, MD; 2013. www.amersa.org/Book_of_abstracts_2013.pdf. Accessed March 25, 2014

8. National Institute of Alcohol Abuse and Alcoholism. *NIAAA Alcohol Screening and Brief Intervention for Youth: A Practitioner's Guide.* NIH Publication No. 11-7805; 2011. pubs.niaaa.nih.gov/publications/Practitioner/YouthGuide/YouthGuide.pdf. Accessed March 20, 2014
9. Knight JR, Sherritt L, Shrier LA, Harris SK, Chang G. Validity of the CRAFFT substance abuse screening test among adolescent clinic patients. *Arch Pediatr Adolesc Med.* 2002;156:607–614
10. Dennis ML, Chan YF, Funk RR. Development and validation of the GAIN Short Screener (GSS) for internalizing, externalizing and substance use disorders and crime/violence problems among adolescents and adults. *Am J Addict.* 2006;15(Suppl 1):80–91
11. Babor TF, de la Fuente JR, Saunders J, Grand M. *AUDIT: The Alcohol Use Disorders Identification Test: Guidelines for Use in Primary Care.* Geneva, Switzerland: World Health Organization; 1992
12. Kelly SM, Gryczynski J, Mitchell SG, Kirk A, O'Grady KE. Validity of brief screening instrument for adolescent tobacco, alcohol, and drug use. *Pediatrics.* 2014;133(5):819–826
13. Wilson CR, Sherritt L, Gates E, Knight JR. Are clinical impressions of adolescent substance use accurate? *Pediatrics.* 2004;114:e536–e540
14. Students Against Destructive Decisions. Contract for Life. www.sadd.org/contract.htm. Accessed March 20, 2014

# Chapter 76

# Symptoms of Emotional Disturbance in Young Children

*Mary Margaret Gleason, MD*

Although the child is the patient, the primary care physician (PCP) must remain vigilant that the child's behavior, particularly with respect to social-emotional problems, may reflect difficulty or dysfunction within the child's caregiving context. This chapter outlines the PCP's role in preventing, identifying, and addressing social-emotional problems in young children—a role that is critical because of the numerous associated adverse outcomes, including child and family suffering, school failure, mental and physical illnesses, and fractured social networks throughout the lifespan. This chapter focuses on children in the first 5 years of life, using the term *social-emotional problems* to describe the full range of behavioral difficulties, emotional disturbances, and relationship difficulties that may occur in early childhood, especially in the context of adverse childhood experiences. This chapter will refer to the child's primary caregiver as the parents, who may be biologic parents, grandparents, foster parents, or other.

## ▶ BACKGROUND AND EPIDEMIOLOGY

During early childhood, social-emotional health develops through a complex interaction of a child's genetic makeup, temperament, and social and physical environment, particularly the primary caregiving relationships. Previously, biological risks were not thought to be easily modifiable. However, recent research demonstrates that a child's environment affects social-emotional development directly and can modify gene expression. This in turn influences the structure of the developing brain. Exposure to a wide range of developmental, behavioral, economic, social, educational, biologic, or family stresses (also known as adverse childhood experiences) can overwhelm the child's ability to cope, alter the brain's architecture, and lead to impaired social functioning and impulse control.[1–3] Examples of events that may precipitate toxic stress responses include child neglect; physical, emotional, or sexual abuse; exposure to domestic violence; inconsistent parenting; separation from loved ones; impairment of parents or caregivers (eg, chronic parental depression or substance abuse); natural disasters; poverty; unsafe housing; and chronic illness or delays in the child's development.[3–6] The effect of these stressors on children can vary greatly depending on their developmental stage, their social supports, and the type, intensity, frequency, and duration of the stressors. There is an additive effect of multiple stressors or risk factors, with increased numbers of adverse events related to increased risk of adverse outcomes, likely through the disruption of developmentally normative experiences or the repeated activation of the physiologic trauma responses.[7–9] Therefore, it is important to identify and ameliorate sources of traumatic stress as early as possible. A study by Egger and Angold demonstrated rates of psychopathology in very young children similar to rates in older children.[10] These disorders can persist and interfere with future development and school readiness.[11–14]

A child's relationship with caring and nurturing adults is the most critical factor in developing resilience in the face of the normative stresses of childhood and buffering a child from the adverse effects of toxic stresses. Interventions that support the development of positive parent-child interactions can positively influence a young child's brain development, intelligence, and central nervous system hormonal patterns.[15,16] Specifically, these interventions focus on ensuring that a child experiences sensitive caregiving, in which a caregiver anticipates and responds to a child's unique physical and emotional needs and responds to a child's positive and negative behaviors consistently, persistently, and contingently. Beginning in infancy and continuing through childhood and into adolescence, parents and other caregivers can support their child's pro-social behaviors and emotional regulation by modeling and reinforcing these behaviors and helping a child organize emotions in response to challenging situations. The foremost role of the PCP is in primary prevention—supporting parents and fostering childhood resilience to buffer against the negative effects of toxic stress (topics addressed in the Institute of Medicine *From Neurons to Neighborhoods: The Science of Early Childhood Development*,[3] *Bright Futures*,[4] Substance Abuse & Mental Health Services Administration reports,[5] and the American Academy of Pediatrics (AAP) Policy Statement on Toxic Stress, among others.[6]

## Role of the Primary Care Physician

The PCP can collaborate with local community partners (eg, developmental-behavioral pediatricians, early childhood mental health professionals, early intervention professionals, early childhood educators in child care and schools, child advocates, and public health agencies) to identify and address stressors that put children in their community at high risk for social-emotional problems and to identify and strengthen protective factors. A summary of approaches for screening strategies and interventions can be found on the AAP Early Brain and Child Development Web site (www.aap.org/en-us/advocacy-and-policy/aap-health-initiatives/EBCD/Pages/default.aspx). Each group of PCPs and other early childhood partners will address the issues unique to their community, but some examples may include advocating for the creation of safe outdoor spaces for children's exploration, for domestic violence shelters, for evidence-based nurse visitation programs, for increased access to Head Start or other enriched early childhood caregiving environments, or for appropriate access to prenatal care and postnatal nutrition. Universal prevention approaches also occur within the primary care practice. Physicians can create an environment in which parents feel comfortable raising questions about emotional or behavioral concerns by asking about social-emotional development with open-ended questions, including these topics as part of anticipatory guidance, and including literature promoting social-emotional well-being in the waiting room. For children with overt social-emotional problems, PCPs are often the first professionals who identify the problem as a clinical issue that warrants attention. Therefore, they are responsible for supportive communication about the concern, as well as collaborating with their community partners to enhance access to specialty treatment and monitoring treatment effects.

### *Findings Suggesting Social-Emotional Problems or Risk Factors for Problems*

The symptoms that suggest social-emotional problems for children younger than 5 years can be identified in the child, the caregiver, or the relationship between the child and caregiver. A summary of some the clinical findings that may indicate the need for further assessment can be found in Box 76-1.

### *Tools to Assist With Identification*

Validated, standardized screening instruments may be used to identify children at high risk for having social-emotional problems, either because of parent-reported symptoms or the caregiving environment. Table 76-1 provides examples of general psychosocial screening instrument results that may suggest a child has social-emotional problems. Negative screens indicate that a child is within a lower-risk group, and can be an opportunity for positive feedback or may guide anticipatory guidance. A negative screen should not override clinical judgment if a PCP has concerns because of history or observations. With all parent report measures, but especially in early childhood mental health, it is particularly important to recognize that a parent report reflects that parent's perception of the child's behaviors. Positive screens may indicate that the child has a mental health problem, that the parent is experiencing extreme distress (because of the child or another cause), or that there is a problem within the relationship between the parent and the child. All 3 possibilities have implications for the child's development and warrant clinical attention. Therefore, a positive screen should be followed by further assessment to determine more about the clinical concern.

## ▶ ASSESSMENT

Assessment begins by differentiating the child's symptoms from normal behavior. Children vary in temperament and in their capacity to self-regulate and adapt. Virtually all young children exhibit challenging behaviors at times, especially during periods of adjustment to new environmental circumstances such as birth of a sibling, a move, a new child care arrangement, or a family crisis. Children with social-emotional problems may experience more severe and persistent emotional or behavioral reactions to these normative stresses or even in the absence of an acute stressor. There are also some conditions that may mimic or co-occur with social-emotional problems of young children. Table 76-2 provides a summary of these conditions. Extreme temper tantrums or emotional or behavioral responses to small events such as limit setting can reflect a range of clinical issues. Figure 76-1 provides categories of possible child, parent, or relationship difficulties that should be considered when a parent reports concerns about the child's emotional or behavioral development. Importantly, it should be considered that a maladaptive behavior often represents the only set of tools a child has to cope with an overwhelming emotion, such as anxiety, frustration (with self or other), or distress. Additionally, it is important to address parental concern about social, emotional, or behavioral patterns, even if the PCP does not identify atypical development. Providing parental support around parenting stresses, wondering about alternative attributions for behavior, strategizing around safe, consistent, nurturing responses to difficult behaviors, and close follow-up all may be helpful.

BOX 76-1

## *Symptoms and Clinical Findings Suggesting Social-Emotional Problems in Children Younger Than 5 Years*

### CONCERNS ABOUT THE CHILD'S BEHAVIOR OR EMOTIONS

- Child has regulatory difficulties evidenced by difficulty calming, irregular sleep or feeding patterns, or excessive sensitivity to sensory experiences.
- Child demonstrates difficulty organizing behaviors and demonstrates extreme aggression or severe or persistent tantrums that involve injury or damage to objects.
- Child has experienced significant difficulty adjusting to child care or preschool or has been expelled from child care or preschool.
- Child's activity and impulsivity levels are excessive for developmental age.
- Child's mood is unhappy, irritable, or lacking in true joy more frequently than the average child.
- Child shows more anxiety than others his age, especially related to specific triggers or traumatic reminders, separation from caregiver, or experiencing new situations.
- Child will not talk in public even with reassurance.
- Child has excessively rigid behavioral patterns or "habits" that interfere with typical functioning.

### CONCERNS ABOUT CAREGIVER

- Caregiver is unable to consider the child's strengths, becomes disorganized when talking about the child, or talks about the child using only a negative tone.
- Caregiver does not anticipate a child's need for comfort or does not offer appropriate comfort in new situations or times of distress.
- Caregiver is excessively protective of child and does not allow developmentally appropriate exploration.
- Caregiver is or has been abusive or neglectful (eg, involvement with child protection).

### CONCERNS ABOUT RELATIONSHIP

- Child does not or cannot elicit comfort or reassurance effectively from caregiver in times of distress (eg, immunizations or separations).
- Child (older than 9 months [developmental age]) does not look to caregiver in novel situations or to share joy or excitement.
- Child does not manifest age-appropriate stranger anxiety.
- Child has not met appropriate social milestones related to social reciprocity, peer interactions, adult interactions, or focused attachment (comfort-seeking) behaviors with a primary caregiver.
- Child's relationship with caregiver has been disrupted (eg, foster care, military deployment of parent, death of parent).

### RISK FACTORS FOR INCREASED SUSCEPTIBILITY

- History of maltreatment or significant caregiving disruption (such as is seen in children in foster care, those who have been adopted, or those with other caregiving disruptions)
- Family stressors (eg, poverty, divorce, single parenting, unemployment, limited access to health care, lack of safe and affordable housing or food, social isolation, community violence)
- History of adverse childhood experience in parents
- Parental substance abuse, mental illness, or domestic violence

**Table 76-1**
**General Psychosocial Screening Results Suggesting Social-Emotional Problems**

| SCREENING AREA | SCREENING INSTRUMENT | SCORE |
|---|---|---|
| Child | Baby Pediatric Symptom Checklist (B-PSC) (irritability, inflexibility, difficulties in parenting)<br>Preschool PSC (internalizing, externalizing, attention, and parenting challenges) | A score of 3 or above is considered positive.<br><br>A score of 9 or above is considered positive. |
| | Early Childhood Screening Assessment (assesses emotional and behavioral development in young children 18–60 months old and maternal distress) | A score of 18 or higher on items 1 through 36 indicates a higher than usual risk of disorder. A score above 1 on 37 or 38 may reflect parenting stress. A score of at least 1 on items 39 or 40 suggests risk of caregiver depression. |
| | Ages & Stages Questionnaire: Social-Emotional (ASQ:SE) (useful as early as 4 months to screen for problems in caregiver-infant bond and interaction) | Each measure includes specific instructions about cutoff score for that age. |
| Environment | Edinburgh Postpartum Depression Scale | Score of 12 or above is considered positive. |
| | Parent Health Questionnaire-2 | Any positive response is considered positive. |
| | Abuse Assessment Screen | Positive response to any question indicates high risk of interpersonal violence. |
| | Safe Environments for Every Kid (SEEK) | Positive reponses suggest presence of family stressors. |
| | Caregiver Strain Questionnaire | Score of 7 or more suggests high level of caregiver strain. |
| | Bright Futures Surveillance Questions | Answers suggest social-emotional stressors. |
| | Parenting Stress Index | Results suggest high levels of stress associated with parenting, or within the parent-child relationship. |

The special circumstance of a chronic or significant medical problem should be considered, as it may trigger social-emotional problems in a range of domains. Young children with chronic medical problems are more likely to experience developmental delays and traumatic experiences in the form of medical procedures and separations from parents, and may be seen as particularly vulnerable by their parents because of their medical condition. They may also take medications that may affect mood regulation (eg, steroids) or have primary central nervous system lesions that interfere with emotional, behavioral, or developmental regulation. Similarly, although all children with growth failure should be evaluated for underlying medical problems, psychosocial growth failure can occur in the context of an inadequate caregiving environment, and the role of the caregiving environment as a protective or risk factor should be considered in all cases of growth failure. (See Figure 76-1.)

**Table 76-2**
**Differential Diagnosis of Extreme Emotional or Behavioral Dysregulation**

| DOMAIN | DIFFERENTIAL DIAGNOSIS | RATIONALE |
|---|---|---|
| Normal development | | Extreme responses to normal limits, fatigue, hunger, or new situations are part of typical development in the third and fourth years of life. |
| Developmental delays/frustration | Cognitive and language disabilities | Children with language deficits may experience frustration expressing their needs and desires and therefore may exhibit symptoms of social-emotional problems. Children with intellectual disabilities may function at a level younger than their chronological age and size. This gap between their ability and adult expectations for their behaviors can lead to frustration for the child and caregiver. |
| | Hearing or vision problems | All children who are manifesting atypical development or behavior should be screened for sensory deficits. A complete hearing assessment should be obtained for all young children with delay in language development. |
| | Autism spectrum disorders (ASDs) | Children with ASDs have problems with social relatedness (eg, poor eye contact, preference for solitary activities, lack of joy in sharing with others, lack of empathy), language (delayed expressive language or unusual syntax or prosody), limitations in their range of interest (persistent and intense interest in a particular activity or subject), or atypical mannerisms that can interfere with their ability to function. They may have a need for routine and can become anxious or angry if a routine is disrupted. Accordingly, these children may manifest symptoms of social-emotional problems. In addition, children with ASDs are also at higher than usual risk of comorbid psychiatric disorders that may present in early childhood. |
| Regulatory problem | Sleep problems<br>Feeding disorders | Sleep deprivation as a result of bedtime struggles, night waking, or obstructive sleep apnea can cause irritability and behavioral problems; conversely, social-emotional problems can cause sleep difficulties.<br>Difficulties with feeding—either refusal, sensitivies, or overeating—can cause disruptive or distressed patterns in an infant or toddler, which can occur in a mutually escalating cycle with parental distress around the eating patterns. |

**Table 76-2**
**Differential Diagnosis of Extreme Emotional or Behavioral Dysregulation—cont'd**

| DOMAIN | DIFFERENTIAL DIAGNOSIS | RATIONALE |
|---|---|---|
| Child disruptive behavior problem | Attention-deficit/hyperactivity disorder (ADHD) | High levels of impulsivity, as well as inattentiveness and distractibility, may be seen in very young children with ADHD. It is especially important to assess whether the symptoms occur in multiple settings (as required in ADHD) or whether they are specific to a context or relationship, a pattern that would likely represent an adjustment to that situation. Because of the range of normal activity levels in very young children, ADHD must be distinguished from developmentally inappropriate expectations for young children and from parental symptoms that make normal child behaviors less tolerable, such as depression. In addition, symptoms suggestive of ADHD should be distinguished from lead toxicity and effects of medications such as steroids or sympathomimetics |
| | Disruptive behavior disorders (oppositional defiant disorder, conduct disorder) | Disruptive behaviors in young children may present with extreme oppositional behaviors or conduct disordered symptoms, including aggression. These can occur when a child experiences an inconsistent or coercive caregiving environment. |
| Child mood symptoms | Depression | Very young children can present with all of the symptoms of major depressive disorder, and this diagnosis should be considered in children with extreme sadness or irritability. Associated symptoms include sleep and appetite changes, play or talk centered around death and dying, decreased joy in playing, and concentration difficulties. The validity of the diagnosis of bipolar disorder in preschool has not yet been established. |
| Child anxiety | Anxiety disorders | Preschoolers may present with general anxiety, extreme separation anxiety, school avoidance behaviors, and selective mutism, all often accompanied by extreme distress in the face of the trigger. Similarly, very young children with obsessive-compulsive behaviors may present with behavioral symptoms when asked to interrupt a compulsive behavior. |

*Continued*

**Table 76-2**
**Differential Diagnosis of Extreme Emotional or Behavioral Dysregulation—cont'd**

| DOMAIN | DIFFERENTIAL DIAGNOSIS | RATIONALE |
|---|---|---|
| | Post-traumatic stress disorder and other trauma-related symptoms | In addition, children who have experienced traumatic events may exhibit a set of symptoms similar to the presentation of post-traumatic stress disorder seen in older children (re-experiencing the trauma in thoughts, speech, play, and dreams; emotional and physiologic hyperarousal to reminders of the trauma; avoidance of reminders of the trauma; and numbing symptoms). It is not uncommon for children who have experienced traumatic events to present with disruptive behaviors, perhaps related to their own inability to organize their reactions or because of less consistent parenting after the traumatic event. |
| Parent-child relationship disturbances | Parental mental health problems, substance abuse problems, or severe cognitive limitations | Young children who experience unpredictable or inconsistent parenting, especially if it includes neglectful or dangerous experiences, may present with inconsistent and sometimes dangerous behaviors. Treatment for parents and consideration of child protection involvement is critical in addressing these clinical scenarios. These patterns should be considered in children with a history of foster care or adoption.Depression or other mental illness, bereavement, substance abuse, cognitive disability, or disadvantaged socioeconomic circumstances may prevent a child's caregiver(s) from nurturing the child effectively and may contribute to social-emotional problems in the child. |
| | Disordered attachment or parent-child relationship difficulties | The bond between a child and his caregiver can be affected by characteristics of the child, caregiver, or temperamental "goodness of fit" between child and caregiver. Manifestations of a suboptimal parent-child relationship that increases the risk of attachment problems may include ineffective or inconsistent soothing, nurturing, or disciplinary behaviors of the caregiver, or lack of responsiveness of the child to his caregiver's soothing and nurturing efforts. A parent's own history of unsafe relationships (as a child or in romantic relationships) may shift how a parent thinks about herself in the intimate relationship of parenting and how the parent experiences the child's behaviors and needs. Relationship difficulties may present in the clinic with a parent who experiences the needs of her child as excessive or troublesome, with a child who develops a pattern of maladaptive ways of engaging the parent's attention, or with a child who does not seem to make any attempts to engage the parent even when he might be expected to need comforting. |

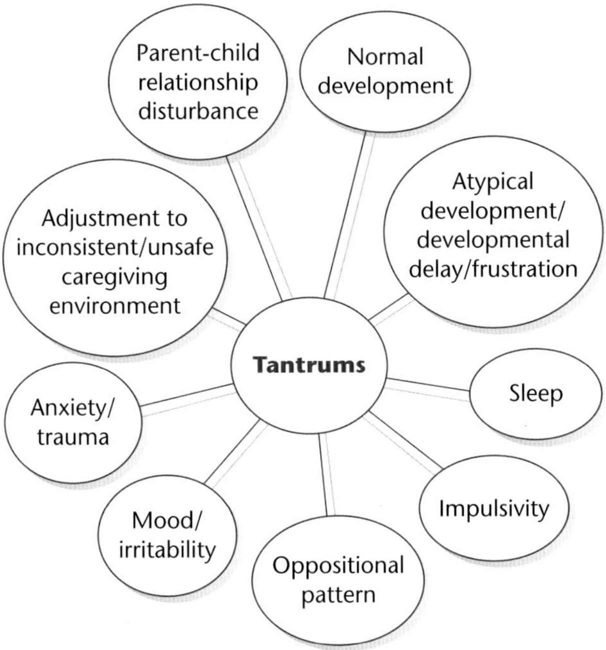


**Figure 76-1**
Differential diagnosis of emotional or behavioral dysregulation.

If a child or caregiver seems to be experiencing symptoms, the PCP can further assess for problems by collecting further information, refer to an appropriate specialist, or review diagnostic criteria for symptoms of disorders in the caregiver-child relationship.

The PCP can information from other caregivers, child care centers, and preschool about eating, sleeping, irritability, and aggression with peers, using behavior or food diaries or validated, structured measures, such as the Baby PSC, Preschool PSC, or Early Childhood Screening Assessment.

Referral may be to a developmental-behavioral pediatrician, mental health professional with expertise in assessment of young children and their families, or early intervention agency.

## ▶ PLAN OF CARE FOR CHILDREN WITH SOCIAL-EMOTIONAL PROBLEMS

The care of a child experiencing social-emotional problems can begin in the primary care setting. Universal screening or active surveillance for social-emotional problems can create an environment in which families feel comfortable discussing social-emotional issues. Following are the elements of providing care to a child with social-emotional problems identified in the primary care setting.

### *Celebrate the Strengths and Engage Child and Family in Care*

Physicians can engage families by recognizing and reinforcing the strengths of child and family and also by acknowledging the distress and emotional costs of the social-emotional concern. The PCP can acknowledge and reinforce protective factors (eg, good relationships with at least 1 parent or important adult, pro-social peers, concerned or caring family, help-seeking, or connection to positive organization[s]). In fostering engagement, it can be useful to use "common factors" techniques[17] to build trust and optimism, including reaching agreement on incremental next steps and, ultimately, therapeutic goals, developing a plan of care (see the following clinical guidance), and determining the role of the PCP. The PCP's role may include providing intervention(s); providing initial intervention while awaiting family's readiness for or access to specialty care; collaborating with a specialist; coordinating with specialist(s), child care, school, or agencies; monitoring progress; and supporting the family's engagement in treatment. Without engagement, most families will not seek or continue in specialty mental health care. This process may require multiple primary care visits.

### Promote Safety

Families whose children experience social-emotional difficulties are at particularly high risk of exposure to unsafe situations. These may include family partner violence, child abuse, or community exposure to violence. In addition, some families may experience safety risks related to housing conditions or a child's access to potentially dangerous medications (diabetes medications, sleeping medications, antihypertensive agents). Assessment for other risks, including weapons in the home, is an important role of the PCP.

### Address Basic Needs

Identifying families' basic needs is perhaps the most important universal intervention for all children with social-emotional problems. Family distress may be reduced by identifying and supporting families with basic needs issues, such as housing, child care, or access to food and a safe place to sleep. Without addressing these needs, it is unlikely that mental health referrals will be successful.

### Support Parental Mental Health

Whether a parent is experiencing a clinical-level problem or distress related to sleep deprivation, it is important for a parent to experience clinical interactions with the PCP as supportive. Even when there are concerns about specific parenting approaches, families will consider changing their behaviors only if they feel that the clinical approach is helpful and that their perspective is respected. Discussion of parental clinical mental health issues like depression or substance abuse, including those identified by screening, may be an important clinical step toward addressing the child's emotional needs.

### Reframe the Child's Behaviors

When a parent seems to perceive a child as overwhelmingly negative or interprets developmentally typical behaviors as intentionally disruptive to the parent, it can be helpful to reframe the behaviors in a way that may allow the parent to experience the same behaviors differently. For example, reframing "clingy and needy" behaviors in toddlers as demonstrating that they are using a parent for emotional support as they begin to venture out to explore their environment may be helpful. Using handouts such as those found on the AAP Early Brain and Child Development resource page or the Circle of Security handout (circleofsecurity.org) or video (www.youtube.com/user/CircleOfSecurity) may be helpful and efficient ways to inform parents. It is important to note that telling a parent the child's behavior is "normal" without putting it into a developmental or emotional context may be experienced as rejecting by parents who are worried about their child.

### Encourage Consistency in Child's Caregiving Environment

No matter what the clinical concern, children will benefit from predictable, consistent, and safe responses to both pro-social and negative behaviors. The PCP can encourage the primary caregivers to reflect on and enhance their own consistency. In addition, the PCP can assist the primary caregivers in developing strategies to increase the consistency the child experiences across caregivers, including mother, father, grandparents, babysitters, and child care providers.

### Explore Opportunities for Positive Parent-Child Interactions

Whether a clinical problem seems to be located primarily within the child, the parent, or their relationship, it is likely that all family members are experiencing less joy and fulfillment from their interactions than they would like. Assisting a parent in identifying a child's strengths and positively reinforcing positive behaviors or efforts toward positive behaviors can be a useful first step toward healing. "Time in," as little as 5 minutes a day of interactive play time with the child, can be a way for parents to delight in their child, feel competent, and appreciated, and for the child to enjoy the parent. If a caregiver's own history of problematic relationships or mental health problems is affecting her relationship with the child, it can be useful to explore her readiness to address these problems as part of helping the child.

### Encourage Healthy Habits and Activities

The PCP can encourage healthy child and family habits that will provide a sound foundation for ongoing development. These healthy habits can include opportunities for active play, good nutrition, media-free family meals, regular bedtime routines, and adequate sleep. Discussions of media exposure and the dangers of frightening or violent media can be especially important for parents of children with anxiety, aggressive behaviors, or a history of trauma exposure. Additionally, the AAP media recommended limits to screen time can promote healthy brain development, increase interactive and exploration time, and reduce the potential for exposure to adult content or violence.[18]

The PCP can direct the parent toward high-quality early childhood care and education such as Head Start and programs accredited by the National Association for the Education of Young Children (NAEYC). The PCP can also encourage communication between child care or preschool personnel and home and coach them to praise progress and effort, not just outcomes. The AAP Early Brain and Child Development Resources can be shared with parents to give to child care providers to promote consistency across a child's environments.

### Offer Initial Intervention(s)

Evidence-based psychosocial interventions for social-emotional problems include a number of "common elements" amenable to implementation in the primary care setting. Table 76-3 provides strategies that the physician can suggest to the family.

### Provide Resources

Helpful handouts, fact sheets, and Web sites are included in Tools for Practice at the end of this chapter.

**Table 76-3**
**Strategies for Building Child's Social-Emotional Skills and Resilience and in Addressing Behavior Problems**

| STRATEGY | ADVICE TO CAREGIVERS |
|---|---|
| Promote daily positive joint activities between parent(s) and child. | • Enlist support of extended family, friends, faith group, or involved agency to relieve parent of some stresses and provide emotional support.<br>• Educate about the importance of smiling with and talking and cooing to infants, attending to vocalizations or speech, and reading and playing at all ages.<br>• Assist with recognizing a child's cues by labeling the child's behaviors and needs in the office and support the parent in responding sensitively.<br>• Increase parent's one-on-one time with child (eg, interacting, feeding, reading, playing). Daily routines around mealtime and bedtime, for example, can ensure that these activities are well integrated into family life.<br>• Promote resilience at every visit by using the anticipatory guidance of Bright Futures or the EBCD website and by emphasizing individual strengths. |
| Apply positive parenting principles to toddlers and preschoolers (positive attention for positive behaviors; removing attention for low-level behaviors; and safe, consistent, calm consequences for unacceptable or unsafe behaviors). | • Reinforce desired behaviors using parental attention (eg, "Catch them being good").<br>• Help the child develop vocabulary to describe feelings.<br>• Encourage praise and reinforcement ("rewards") for specific, desired (target) behaviors. The choice of target behaviors and the time intervals for reinforcements should be developmentally appropriate and sustainable.<br>• Teach parents to reduce attention to ("ignore") minor, provocative behaviors. "Pick battles" and focus discipline on priority areas.<br>• Reduce positive reinforcement of disruptive behavior.<br>• Teach parents to recognize the child's anxiety, expose the child only to manageable anxiety-provoking situations, provide support around unavoidable anxiety-provoking situations, and praise the child's management of her feelings.<br>• When possible, reorganize the child's day to avoid trouble by avoiding situations in which the child cannot control himself or herself. Examples include asking a neighbor to look after the child while the parent goes shopping, ensuring that activities are available for long car journeys, and arranging activities in separate rooms for siblings who are prone to fighting.<br>• Talk to the child care center or preschool and suggest that similar principles be applied. |

**Table 76-3**
**Strategies for Building Child's Social-Emotional Skills and Resilience and in Addressing Behavior Problems—cont'd**

| STRATEGY | ADVICE TO CAREGIVERS |
|---|---|
| Encourage parents to be calm and consistent. | Suggest that parents do the following:<br>• Set clear house rules agreed on by the primary caregivers<br>• Give short, specific commands about the desired behavior, not prohibitions about undesired behavior (eg, "Please walk slowly," rather than "Don't run").<br>• Provide consistent and calm consequences for misbehavior. Consequences should not be dangerous, drastic, or of extreme duration.<br>• Use natural consequences, such as the child cleaning up a mess he or she has created.<br>• When enforcing a rule, avoid getting into arguments or explanations, reduce additional attention for the misbehavior, and defer negotiations until periods of calm.<br>• Consider parenting classes or community support. |

## Monitor Progress

Symptoms can be tracked using screening measures described in Table 76-1 or disorder-specific measures. Nonproprietary general measures like the Baby and Preschool Pediatric Symptom Checklists and the Early Childhood Screening Assessment, or the proprietary Strengths and Difficulties Questionnaire, are useful in monitoring symptoms over time. Symptom-specific measures like the Eyberg Child Behavior Inventory (disruptive behaviors), and the Preschool Feelings Checklist (depression) are valuable and validated measures that provide more specific information about a child's course. Child care or preschool reports can be helpful in monitoring progress. Attention-deficit/hyperactivity disorder (ADHD) can be tracked using measures validated on older children, such as the Vanderbilt ADHD Rating Scales and the Conners-3. More extensive measures, such as the Child Behavior Checklist, are validated in children as young as 18 months of age, but are longer than a PCP can use regularly.

## Involve Specialist(s)

Involvement of a specialist may be considered appropriate under the following circumstances:

- A child younger than 5 years has symptoms of social-emotional problems causing functional impairment or distress; for example
  - o The child has symptoms of anxiety, sadness, or irritability that limit participation in family interactions, child care experiences, or other normative experiences.
  - o The child has behaviors that are disruptive in the home or in out-of-home settings, or that limit participation in developmentally appropriate experiences.

- The child does not use the caregiver effectively for emotional support or is indiscriminate in social interactions with strangers.
- The child exhibits sleep or eating problems are not responsive to primary care interventions.

- The parent is very negative toward child, compromised by physical or mental illness, disengaged, inconsistent in providing nurturing, or unresponsive to primary care guidance.
- The parent has difficulty allowing a child to have developmentally appropriate opportunities for exploration.
- The family is not able to maintain a calm, consistent, or safe environment. (In this instance, also consider reporting to child protective services.)

*When specialty care is needed, a PCP should recommend evidence-informed treatment.* A variety of evidence-based and evidence-informed psychosocial interventions are available for the treatment of social-emotional problems in children younger than 5 years of age. See Table 76-4.

No randomized controlled trials of medications have been carried out in young children with disruptive behavior, mood, or anxiety disorders, but ADHD has been studied using 2 different medications (methylphenidate and atomoxetine). Current evidence suggests that these two agents have higher rates of adverse effects in preschoolers than are reported in older children.[13–16]

The PCP and specialist(s) should clarify roles in the child's care. The PCP's role may, for example, include engaging and encouraging the family's positive view of interventions or referral and serving as the care coordination "hub" of the medical home. The specialist may monitor the child and family's progress, observe for and addressing any comorbidities that may develop, and coordinate care provided by parents, child care center, preschool, medical home, early intervention agency, and specialists.

## TOOLS FOR PRACTICE

### Engaging Patient and Family

- *Connected Kids* (fact sheets), American Academy of Pediatrics (shop.aap.org)
- *Everybody Gets Mad: Helping Your Child Cope With Conflict* (Web page), American Academy of Pediatrics (www.healthychildren.org/English/healthy-living/emotional-wellness/Pages/Everybody-Gets-Mad-Helping-Your-Child-Cope-with-Conflict.aspx)
- *Parents' Roles in Teaching Respect* (handout), Bobbi Conner (www.brightfutures.org/mentalhealth/pdf/families/mc/parent_role.pdf)

### Medical Decision Support

- *The Abuse Assessment* (screen), National Institute of Justice (www.crimesolutions.gov/ProgramDetails.aspx?ID=165)
- *Ages & Stages Questionnaires: Social-Emotional (ASQ-SE)* (screen), Brookes Publishing (www.brookespublishing.com/resource-center/screening-and-assessment/asq/asq-se)
- *Edinburgh Postnatal Depression Scale (EPDS)* (screen), Cox JL, Holden JM, and Sagovsky R (www2.aap.org/sections/scan/practicingsafety/toolkit_resources/module2/epds.pdf)
- *M-CHAT* (screen), Diana L. Robbins, PhD (www.mchatscreen.com/Official_M-CHAT_Website.html)
- *The Multidimensional Scale of Perceived Social Support* (article), *Journal of Personality Assessment,* Vol 52, Issue 1, 1988

**Table 76-4**
**Psychosocial and Psychopharmacologic Treatments for Social-Emotional Problems in Young Children**

| EVIDENCE-BASED PARENTING PROGRAMS | |
|---|---|
| **CLUSTER AREA** | **PARENTING PROGRAM** |
| For disruptive behavioral problems | • The Incredible Years (www.incredibleyears.com)<br>• Triple P Positive Parenting Program (www.triplep.net)<br>• Parent-Child Interaction Therapy (http://pcit.phhp.ufl.edu)<br>• "Helping the Noncompliant Child" parent training program (www.strengtheningfamilies.org/html/programs_1999/02_HNCC.html) |
| For first-time, pregnant, low-income women prior to 28 weeks' gestation | • Nurse-Family Partnership (www.nursefamilypartnership.org) |
| For children in foster care | • Attachment and Biobehavioral Catch-up (www.cachildwelfare-clearinghouse.org/program/108/detailed)<br>• Multidimensional Treatment Foster Care Program for Preschoolers (www.uoregon.edu/~snaplab/SNAP/Projects.html)<br>• Parent Child Interaction Therapy[a] |
| For parent-child relationship disturbances and high-risk parenting situations | • Circle of Security (www.circleofsecurity.org)<br>• Promoting First Relationships (www.pfrprogram.org)<br>• Parents as Teachers (www.parentsasteachers.org)<br>• Child Parent Psychotherapy |
| For children exposed to trauma, including sexual abuse or domestic violence | • Child Parent Psychotherapy (www.cachildwelfareclearinghouse.org/program/49/detailed)<br>• Cognitive behavioral therapy[b,c,d] |
| **PSYCHOPHARMACOLOGIC INTERVENTIONS[e]** | |
| There is limited evidence to support psychopharmacologic intervention in this age group. There is a single multisite, placebo-controlled, randomized trial of methylphenidate and another focused on atomoxetine as a treatment for attention-deficit/hyperactivity disorder in preschoolers. Both showed the medication was more effective than placebo, but less effective than in older children and was associated with a higher rate of adverse effects.[f,g] | |

Updates are available at www.aap.org/mentalhealth.

[a]Chaffin M, Funderburk B, Bard D, Valle LA, Gurwitch R. A combined motivation and parent-child interaction therapy package reduces child welfare recidivism in a randomized dismantling field trial. *J Consult Clin Psychol.* 2011;79(1):84.

[b]Cohen JA, Mannarino AP. Factors that mediate treatment outcome of sexually abused preschool children: 6 and 12 month follow-up. *J Am Acad Child Adolesc Psychiatry.* 1998;37(1):44–51.

[c]Cohen JA, Mannarino AP. A treatment study for sexually abuse preschool children: outcome during one year follow-up. *J Am Acad Child Adolesc Psychiatry.* 1997;36(9):1228–1235.

[d]Scheeringa M, Weems CF, Cohen JA, Amaya-Jackson L, Guthrie D. Trauma-focused cognitive-behavioral therapy for posttraumatic stress disorder in three-through six year-old children: a randomized clinical trial *J Child Psychol Psychiatry* 2011;52(8):853–860.

[e]Lahey BB, Pelham WE, Loney J, et al. Three-year predictive validity of DSM-IV attention deficit hyperactivity disorder in children diagnosed at 4–6 years of age. *Am J Psychiatry.* 2004;161(11):2014–2020.

[f]Kratochvil CJ, Vaughan BS, Stoner JA, et al. A double-blind, placebo-controlled study of atomoxetine in young children with ADHD. *Pediatrics.* 2011;127(4):e862–e868.

[g]Greenhill LL, Kollins S, Abikoff H, et al. Efficacy and safety of immediate-release methylphenidate treatment for preschoolers with ADHD. *J Am Acad Child Adolesc Psychiatry.* 2006;45(11):1284–1293.

- *Parent-Child Interaction Therapy* (Web page), University of Florida College of Public Health and Health Professions (pcit.phhp.ufl.edu)
- *Parenting Stress Index* (screen), PAR, Inc (www4.parinc.com/products/Product.aspx?ProductID=PSI-4)

## AAP POLICY STATEMENT

American Academy of Pediatrics Committee on Psychosocial Aspects of Child and Family Health, Committee on Early Childhood, Adoption, and Dependent Care, and Section on Developmental and Behavioral Pediatrics. Early childhood adversity, toxic stress, and the role of the pediatrician: translating developmental science into lifelong health. *Pediatrics.* 2012;129(1):e224–e231 (pediatrics.aappublications.org/content/129/1/e224)

## REFERENCES


1. Knapp P, Mastergeorge AM. Clinical implications of current findings in neurodevelopment. *Psychiatr Clin North Am.* 2009;32:177–197
2. Middlebrooks JS, Audage NC. *The Effects of Childhood Stress on Health Across the Lifespan.* Atlanta, GA: Centers for Disease Control and Prevention, National Center for Injury Prevention and Control. http://www.bvs.is/files/file703.pdf. Published 2008. Accessed February 24, 2010
3. Committee on Integrating the Science of Early Childhood Development, Board on Children, Youth, and Familieis. *From Neurons to Neighborhoods: The Science of Early Childhood Development.* Shonkoff JP, Phillips DA, eds. Washington, DC: National Academy Press; 2000
4. Hagan JF, Shaw JS, Duncan PM, eds. *Bright Futures: Guidelines for Health Supervision of Infants, Children, and Adolescents.* 3rd ed. Elk Grove Village, IL: American Academy of Pediatrics; 2008
5. Transforming Mental Health Care in America: The Federal Action Agenda: "A Living Agenda." Rockville, MD: Substance Abuse and Mental Health Services Administration, US Department of Health and Human Services; 2008. http://store.samhsa.gov/product/Transforming-Mental-Health-Care-in-America/SMA05-4060. Accessed February 8, 2015
6. Ginsburg S, Foster S. *Strategies to Support the Integration of Mental Health into Pediatric Primary Care.* Washington, DC: National Institute for Health Care Management. Published 2009. http://nihcm.org/pdf/PediatricMH-FINAL.pdf. Accessed November 18, 2014
7. Sameroff, AJ, ed. *The Transactional Model of Development: How Children and Contexts Shape Each Other.* Washington, DC: American Psychological Association; 2009
8. Felitti VJ, Anda RF, Nordenberg D, et al. Relationship of childhood abuse and household dysfunction to many of the leading causes of death in adults. The Adverse Childhood Experiences (ACE) Study. *Am J Prev Med.* 1998;14:245–258
9. Anda RF, Felitti VJ, Bremner JD, et al. The enduring effects of abuse and related adverse experiences in childhood. A convergence of evidence from neurobiology and epidemiology. *Eur Arch Psychiatry Clin Neurosci.* 2006;256:174–186
10. Egger HL, Angold A. Common emotional and behavioral disorders in preschool children: presentation, nosology, and epidemiology. *J Child Psychol Psychiatry.* 2006;47:313–337
11. Kim-Cohen J, Arseneault L, Newcombe R, et al. Five-year predictive validity of DSM-IV conduct disorder research diagnosis in 4(1/2)-5-year-old children. *Eur Child Adolesc Psychiatry.* 2009;18:284–291
12. Lahey BB, Pelham WE, Loney J, et al. Three-year predictive validity of DSM-IV attention deficit hyperactivity disorder in children diagnosed at 4-6 years of age. *Am J Psychiatry.* 2004;161:2014–2020
13. Scheeringa MS, Zeanah CH, Myers L, Putnam FW. Predictive validity in a prospective follow-up of PTSD in preschool children. *J Am Acad Child Adolesc Psychiatry.* 2005;44:899–906
14. Briggs-Gowan MJ, Carter AS. Social-emotional screening status in early childhood predicts elementary school outcomes. *Pediatrics.* 2008;121:957–962

15. Nelson CA, Zeanah CH, Fox NA, et al. Cognitive recovery in socially deprived young children: the Bucharest Early Intervention Project. *Science*. 2007;318:1937–1940
16. Dozier M, Manni M, Gordon MK, et al. Foster children's diurnal production of cortisol: an exploratory study. *Child Maltreat*. 2006;11:189–197
17. Kemper KJ, Wissow L, Foy JM, Shore SE. *Core Communication Skills for Primary Clinicians*. Wake Forest School of Medicine. nwahec.org/45737. Accessed January 9, 2015
18. American Academy of Pediatrics Council on Communications and Media. Children, adolescents, and the media. *Pediatrics*. 2013;132(5):958–961

# Chapter 77

# Syncope

*Prema Ramaswamy, MD*

## ▶ DEFINITION

Syncope, defined as a transient sudden loss of consciousness and postural tone, is a fairly common complaint in children, particularly adolescents. Presyncope is the presence of sensory and postural impairment without the actual loss of consciousness. The origin of the word *syncope* is a Greek term meaning *to cut short* or *interrupt*. Regardless of the underlying disorder, syncope is caused by interruption of essential energy substrates to the brain, usually from a transient reduction in cerebral blood flow. In children and adolescents, syncope is most often benign; however, in rare cases, it can be a first signal of potential sudden death, and hence identifying patients at risk is critical. Even when the cause is benign, syncope can result in injury, and it certainly provokes anxiety.

Although the exact incidence of syncope in children is not known, it affects 3.5% of the general adult population. Almost one-third of these adults will have recurrent syncope.[1] The corresponding numbers for children are not known, but recurrence seems to be less common in childhood.

## ▶ CAUSES OF SYNCOPE

The most common cause of benign syncope is neurocardiogenic or vasovagal syncope, also termed the common faint, church faint, reflex syncope, or neurally mediated syncope (NMS). Another common cause of benign syncope is orthostatic hypotension. Together, these 2 causes are even more common in adolescents than in adults, and account for almost 80% of all cases.[2] Both causes are more common during adolescence than at any other time in childhood. Syncope is also common in children from 6 months to 3 years of age, when breath-holding spells are prevalent. In particular, children with the pallid type of breath-holding spell have an increased risk for NMS as adults.[3] Syncope that is not benign can stem from cardiac, neurologic, metabolic, and psychiatric causes. Box 77-1 lists the causes of syncope.

### Neurally Mediated Syncope

Naturally mediated syncope is classified into 3 types[4]

1. *Central syncope* occurs in response to strong emotional stimulation such as pain, anticipated pain, or the sight of blood. In susceptible individuals, emotional stimulation can activate ill-defined areas within the central nervous system that, in turn, trigger sympathetic inhibition and parasympathetic activation.

BOX 77-1

## *Causes of Syncope*

### NEURALLY MEDIATED SYNCOPE

- Emotional
- Postural
- Situational
  - Deglutition syncope
  - Micturition syncope
  - Weight-lifter's syncope
  - Defecation syncope
  - Carotid sinus hypersensitivity
  - Hair-grooming syncope

### ORTHOSTATIC HYPOTENSION

- Primary
- Drugs
- Pregnancy
- Adrenal insufficiency
- Systemic mastocytosis
- Familial dysautonomia
- Postural orthostasis tachycardia syndrome

### BEHAVIORAL OR PSYCHIATRIC

- Hyperventilation
- Hysteria, conversion reaction
- Breath-holding spells
- Cyanotic
- Pallid infantile syncope

### NEUROLOGIC

- Seizure
- Migraine
- Trauma, concussion
- Narcolepsy

### CARDIAC

- Structural abnormalities
  - Aortic stenosis
  - Hypertrophic cardiomyopathy
  - Tetralogy of Fallot
  - Pulmonic stenosis
  - Primary pulmonary hypertension
  - Coronary artery abnormalities
  - Marfan syndrome
- Arrhythmia
  - Bradycardia
  - Sick sinus syndrome
  - Atrioventricular block
  - Supraventricular tachycardia
  - Ventricular tachycardia, fibrillation
    - Myocarditis, pericarditis
    - Postoperative cardiac surgery
    - Prolonged QT syndrome

### METABOLIC

- Hypoglycemia
- Anemia

2. *Postural syncope* is associated with the upright position, typically developing while the person is standing or walking. It is the most common type of NMS, much more frequent than central or situational syncope.
3. *Situational syncope* occurs after the specific stimulation of sensory or visceral afferents, resulting in hypotension and then syncope. Examples include syncope evoked by the hypersensitivity of carotid baroreceptors, micturition syncope, defecation syncope, hair-grooming syncope, swallow syncope, cough syncope, and weight-lifter's syncope, all of which have been described in teenagers but are much less common than in adults.

## Pathophysiologic Features

Although the pathophysiologic mechanism of NMS continues to be debated, investigators think it occurs in persons with a predisposition when they experience peripheral venous pooling and a fall in venous return. An increase in catecholamine release follows as a compensatory mechanism. The primary abnormality in patients who faint is unclear but may include β-adrenergic hypersensitivity, resulting in a relatively empty hypercontractile heart.

Cardiac mechanoreceptors are stimulated, producing the Bezold-Jarisch reflex—a vagal response that includes sinus bradycardia, hypotension, and peripheral vasodilation. The syncope is termed *vasodepressor* if the more prominent element is hypotension, and *cardioinhibitory* if bradycardia is more prominent. In most instances, the syncope is mixed, with both hypotension and bradycardia.

## Clinical Manifestations

In NMS of childhood, loss of consciousness is typically preceded by light-headedness, nausea, yawning, a feeling of being hot, and sounds seeming distant to the ear. Typically brief (from a few seconds to 1 or 2 minutes), the loss of consciousness is most often brought about by pain or by prolonged standing, especially in warm environments such as in a crowded room or in a hot shower. Occasionally, the cause is not identifiable. Symptoms characteristically appear after the person has been upright for at least a few minutes, in contradistinction to the patient with orthostatic hypotension, whose symptoms occur within seconds of standing.

### *Orthostatic Hypotension*

Orthostatic hypotension is the fall in blood pressure after assuming the upright position. The autonomic nervous system provides the principal responses to changes in position.[5] When a person stands, cardiac output and cerebral perfusion are maintained by a combination of pumping action of skeletal muscles, venous valves, and carotid baroreceptor–mediated arterial constriction and cerebral autoregulation. If these mechanisms are unable to maintain the blood pressure, then the decrease in the pressure in the carotid sinus leads to reduced afferent traffic in the carotid sinus and thus to an increase in the heart rate. The compensatory increase in heart rate is inadequate in patients with orthostatic hypotension, and symptoms of weakness and light-headedness develop, typically within seconds of standing. The sinus tachycardia of orthostatic hypotension sets this type of syncope apart from NMS, during which bradycardia is a prominent sign.

Volume depletion from any cause, but in children most often from vomiting and diarrhea, will exacerbate orthostatic hypotension. Drugs that cause vasodilation and diuretics can also stimulate orthostasis.

Pregnancy should always be considered when a woman of childbearing age faints; pregnancy-associated fainting results from increased estrogen and progesterone levels that cause decreased peripheral vascular resistance and hypotension.

In the past few years, an entity called the postural orthostasis tachycardia syndrome (POTS) has been described.[5] The diagnosis of POTS requires orthostatic heart rate acceleration in excess of 120 beats per minute or an absolute increase of 30 beats per minute or greater in the absence of significant orthostatic hypotension. Two forms have been identified. In the more common peripheral variety, persistent tachycardia, associated with fatigue, exercise intolerance, and palpitations, is present while the patient is upright. The onset may occur after a viral illness, trauma, or surgery. The second type of POTS, the β-hypersensitivity (or central) form, is often associated with migraines, tremor, and excessive sweating. Both forms are more common in young women, and treatment can be frustrating.

Familial dysautonomia, an inherited autosomal recessive condition with abnormalities of the autonomic nervous system, is a rare but serious cause of orthostatic syncope, with affected patients at risk for sudden death.

## Behavioral or Psychiatric Causes of Syncope

### Breath-holding Spells

Two types of breath-holding spells typically occur in children between 6 months and 3 years: cyanotic and pallid. In the former, an episode of cyanosis and apnea is precipitated after a child is upset and begins to cry. Stiffening of the body and a loss of consciousness may soon follow. Although the pathophysiologic basis is unclear, crying during expiration may cause increased intrathoracic pressure, which, in turn, leads to low cardiac output. Hypoxia combined with decreased cerebral blood flow leads to the loss of consciousness. The event is brief, and afterward, the child becomes fully conscious. Pallid breath-holding spells (pallid infantile syncope) are less common and usually begin with sudden pain. The mechanism differs in that the child suddenly becomes pale and limp and loses consciousness. The pathophysiologic basis is increased vagal tone, which causes an apparent asystole. The event ordinarily lasts only seconds to minutes, and the child awakens to full consciousness (also see Chapter 78, Temper Tantrums and Breath-holding Spells).

### Hyperventilation

Another benign cause of syncope, hyperventilation is frequent among adolescents, especially in the presence of anxiety. The hyperventilation results in the washing out of carbon dioxide, and the resulting hypocapnia causes reduced cerebral blood flow, dizziness, and syncope. Classically, hypoventilation is also associated with numbness and paresthesia of the hands and feet.

### Psychiatric Syncope

A child with hysterical syncope is likely to be unusually calm. No autonomic effects such as change in heart rate or blood pressure are noted during the episodes, which tend to be recurrent and frequent and to occur in front of an audience. Recovery of consciousness is often prolonged, and no injury is usually sustained.

## Cardiac Syncope

Syncope can result from a low cardiac output secondary to either a structural problem or a dysrhythmia, and the abnormal rhythm underlying the syncope may be either too slow or too fast.

### Bradyarrhythmias

Sick sinus syndrome is extremely rare in a child with a normal heart and is usually seen after extensive surgery in the atria with the Senning and Mustard operations,[6] performed for transposition of the great arteries. Patients who have undergone the Fontan procedure for a single ventricle may also be at risk secondary to atriotomies and dilated atria.

### Atrioventricular Block

Very slow heart rates from atrioventricular (AV) block can lead to syncopal episodes termed *Stokes-Adams attacks.* Congenital AV block in the presence of a structurally normal heart is most commonly associated with a history of systemic lupus erythematosus in the mother. The structural heart disease, which is most commonly associated with congenital AV block and has an ongoing risk for acquired AV block, is corrected transposition of the great arteries. AV block is also occasionally acquired after cardiac surgery or Lyme disease.

### Pacemaker Malfunction

In any child with a pacemaker, syncope should prompt immediate interrogation of the pacemaker for either a malfunction or inappropriate programming.

## *Tachyarrhythmias*

### Supraventricular Tachycardia

Most children with supraventricular tachycardia have a structurally normal heart, and in those children, palpitations and dizziness are more common symptoms of supraventricular tachycardia than syncope. However, with a structural abnormality resulting in reduced hemodynamic reserve, as with a single ventricle, syncope may be a presenting feature. In patients with congenital heart defects, Wolff-Parkinson-White syndrome is most often seen in children with disorders of the AV fibrous valve annuli such as Ebstein disease and corrected transposition of the great arteries.

### Ventricular Tachycardia

Although ventricular tachycardia (VT) is rare in children, it can cause sudden death; early identification of underlying conditions that predispose to VT can be lifesaving. Prolonged QT syndrome is one such condition in which patients are at risk for sudden death secondary to a polymorphic VT termed *torsades de pointes*. The prolongation of the QT interval may be part of a congenital syndrome such as Romano-Ward syndrome, which is autosomal dominant, or Jervell and Lange-Nielsen syndrome, which is autosomal recessive and associated with congenital neural deafness. Both syndromes are caused by mutations in genes encoding cardiac ion channels. Prolonged QT also may be caused by electrolyte imbalances, such as hypokalemia or hypocalcemia, and by a variety of drugs, such as tricyclic antidepressants, certain macrolide antibiotics, and antiarrhythmic medications. VT can also occur in children as a complication of myocarditis or in adolescents with tetralogy of Fallot who have undergone surgical repair in infancy.

## *Structural Heart Disease*

An acute reduction in cardiac output can result in reduced cerebral perfusion and syncope. With certain heart conditions discussed later, patients may be able to maintain an adequate cardiac output at rest but experience syncopal episodes with exercise.

### Aortic Stenosis

An impediment to the forward flow of blood from marked left ventricular hypertrophy, stimulation of the ventricular mechanoreceptors resulting in systemic vasodilation, and subendocardial ischemia causing a ventricular arrhythmia are all mechanisms that may contribute to syncope in children with severe aortic stenosis.

### Hypertrophic Cardiomyopathy

Syncope with exercise may be an important presenting sign of hypertrophic cardiomyopathy. Most affected patients have no left ventricular obstruction at rest; however, with exercise, they can develop a dynamic gradient with an acute reduction in cardiac output. In addition, these patients may develop VT from subendocardial ischemia. The electrocardiogram is frequently abnormal, and an echocardiogram is diagnostic.

### Tetralogy of Fallot

Children with unrepaired tetralogy of Fallot may have syncopal episodes in association with hypercyanotic *tet* spells, often precipitated by crying, straining with a bowel movement, or awakening from sleep.

### Pulmonary Hypertension

With exertion, children with pulmonary hypertension may experience syncope from the inability to maintain transpulmonary flow.

### Coronary Artery Abnormalities

A patient with syncope who is demonstrated to have a coronary artery aberrant either in its origin or course should be presumed at risk for sudden death. Typically, syncope occurs with exercise. Acquired abnormalities of the coronary arteries include coronary artery aneurysms and stenosis caused by Kawasaki disease in early childhood. Cocaine use can cause acute coronary vasoconstriction and ventricular arrhythmias, with consequent syncope.

## *Neurologic Causes of Syncope*

### Seizures

Typically, generalized seizures are preceded by a prodrome and include tonic-clonic activity with loss of consciousness and a period of confusion and lethargy after recovery. However, atypical seizures can occasionally be difficult to differentiate from the benign forms of syncope. Loss of consciousness occurring in the recumbent position is more likely to be from a seizure than from syncope, especially if the heart is normal. Pallor is seen more often in benign syncope, and flushing is more common with seizures. Bowel incontinence points toward a seizure.

### Migraine

The primary care physician should always ask about migraine in a child who has a syncopal episode that does not fit the pattern of typical neurally mediated syncope, particularly if dizziness occurs in the sitting position and no other provoking factors can be elicited. A history of flashing lights, severe headache preceding the episode of syncope, and a family history of migraines usually help clinch the diagnosis.

### Head Trauma

Brief loss of consciousness with head trauma is not uncommon and signals concussion.

## *Metabolic Causes*

Hypoglycemia can cause syncope, most commonly in a child with diabetes on medication. Presyncopal symptoms such as weakness, a feeling of hunger, and confusion may be present, and the syncope is typically not brief. Dehydration and severe anemia also predispose to syncopal episodes.

# EVALUATION

## History

The history is the most important tool in the diagnosis of syncope. It should include a detailed inquiry into the exact circumstances surrounding the event, including the time of the day, presence of an upper respiratory infection, time since last meal, posture during syncope and time spent in this posture before syncope, presence of prodromal symptoms, duration of loss of consciousness, bystander testimony, and any headache or prolonged disorientation after syncope.

Inquiry should also include the circumstances precipitating the event. For example, with vasovagal syncope, the child often is standing in a warm, stuffy room and is hungry, tired, or frightened. The prodrome of a seizure may consist of an aura, whereas a cardiac event often occurs without warning or is induced by exercise. There may also be a history of palpitations just before the episode. The primary care physician should determine whether the child was completely unconscious or whether some degree of responsiveness was present, suggesting hysteria or malingering. A truly unconscious person will not respond if the eyelashes are lightly brushed; a hysterical person will respond, albeit often with just a mild flickering of the lids. Seizure-like movements are important; however, generalized tonic-clonic movements may be seen in any form of syncope. The duration of the episode should be estimated. In general, the conscious state is regained quickly in the case of vasovagal syncope (a few seconds to 1 or 2 minutes), whereas a seizure may last longer, and the postictal state may be characterized by prolonged confusion and fatigue.

A history of congenital heart disease, seizure disorder, or endocrine abnormality such as diabetes would obviously be important. Recurrent syncopal episodes are unusual and may require more extensive testing.

The family history may be helpful. Seizure disorders and cardiac disease leading to syncope (eg, Marfan syndrome, hypertrophic cardiomyopathy, prolonged QT syndrome) may be inherited in an autosomal-dominant fashion. Breath-holding spells can also have a familial pattern.

## Physical Examination

Examination of a patient with a history of syncope should begin with an assessment of the level of consciousness; a child who is not alert and oriented has not had a benign syncopal episode and needs immediate evaluation for potentially life-threatening causes. In most children who are fully alert after a syncopal episode, the findings on physical examination tend to be normal. The presence of a cardiac murmur may point to an obstructive lesion, such as aortic or pulmonic stenosis. Listening to the heart in both the supine and upright positions is important because a mild obstructive gradient in hypertrophic cardiomyopathy may become audible only when the patient is upright. The heart rate and blood pressure should also be obtained in both the supine and upright positions to ascertain the presence of orthostatic intolerance.

## Evaluation

### Electrocardiogram

The only test indicated in most patients with a history typical for benign syncope is an electrocardiogram, which may reveal the presence of AV block or a dysrhythmia. Abnormally large left ventricular forces, especially with left ventricular strain, may be the only evidence of hypertrophic cardiomyopathy in a patient with normal findings on physical examination. The corrected QT interval should be measured in all children with syncope or seizures as an initial screen for prolonged QT syndrome.

### Holter and Event Monitor

A 24-hour electrocardiographic monitoring test is indicated only if a cardiac dysrhythmia is strongly suspected based on either prominent palpitations that occurred before the episode or the presence of cardiac surgical history that may predispose a child to abnormal rhythms. An event recorder is more practical because patients are able to keep the monitor for a month and use it at the time of their symptoms.

### Echocardiogram

When a suspicion exists based either on history (eg, syncope with exercise) or examination of a structural cardiac lesion, an echocardiogram is indicated and can usually adequately demonstrate the origin and course of the coronary arteries.

### Electrophysiologic Testing and Cardiac Catheterization

Electrophysiologic testing and cardiac catheterization must be considered for any patient who has had syncope during active exercise in whom a physical examination, electrocardiogram, and echocardiogram has failed to demonstrate an abnormality.

### Tilt-table Testing

By creating an orthostatic stress, tilt-table testing can provoke symptoms in patients with NMS and orthostatic hypotension. Patients are placed supine on a table that has a foot board. The table is then tilted up between 60 and 80 degrees for 30 to 60 minutes. Patients are monitored closely for a syncopal episode. Some centers use low-dose intravenous isoproterenol infusions to increase the sensitivity of the test, which ranges from 30% to 80%, depending on the laboratory. The specificity of a negative test without isoproterenol ranges from 80% to 100%.[7]

Although the utility of head-upright tilt-table testing in children is still controversial, it has become a means of provoking vasodepressor syncope in susceptible individuals after other more serious causes have been ruled out. Some indications[2] for the use of this test include the following:

1. Three or more syncopal episodes during a 12-month period with no evidence of heart disease
2. Syncope during exertion in which heart disease has been ruled out after an exhaustive workup
3. Recurrent syncopal episodes thought to be hysterical in nature

## ▶ MANAGEMENT

The management of cardiac, neurologic, and psychiatric syncope depends on the cause. The management of NMS includes some of the following approaches.

#### *Reassurance*

The most important interventions for most patients who have NMS or orthostatic hypotension are reassurance and education regarding the cause of the syncope and how to avoid aggravating factors (avoiding extreme heat and standing still for long periods). Patients should be instructed to sit down or lie down at the onset of any prodromal symptoms to avoid injury. Drinking fluids regularly and eating salty foods may be helpful in preventing episodes.

### Isometric Exercises

In a small randomized trial of adults, intense gripping of hands and tensing of the arms for 2 minutes at the onset of the tilt-induced symptoms raised systolic blood pressure. Syncope occurred in 37% of these patients compared with 89% of those who did not perform the maneuver.[8] The value of *tilt training* is still controversial, but it may be helpful to some patients; they are instructed to stand with their backs against a wall, initially for short periods, and slowly increasing the duration to approximately 30 minutes per day.

### Volume Expansion

A reduced frequency of syncope in adolescents with neurocardiogenic syncope was reported after consuming 2 liters of water in the morning.[9]

Fludrocortisone is a synthetic mineralocorticoid that causes salt retention and the expansion of the central blood volume. One randomized trial in adolescents showed similar results to atenolol, but no placebo was studied.[10]

### Beta-blockers

Although beta-blockers have been used for many years as therapy for neurocardiogenic syncope, studies of their effectiveness have at best been equivocal.[10,11]

### Investigational Agents

Midodrine is a direct $\alpha_1$-receptor agonist that has been shown to reduce episodes in adults with severely symptomatic neurocardiogenic syncope.[12] Because serotonin may have a role in regulating the sympathetic nervous system activity, selective serotonin reuptake inhibitors have also been considered for treatment of NMS. In a trial in adults, paroxetine was shown to be superior to placebo.[13]

### Cardiac Pacing

Currently, cardiac pacing has a very limited role in the management of syncope. In pediatrics, cardiac pacing has been used for children in whom asystole is the prominent symptom in recurrent syncope caused by vagal hypertonia, including some patients with deglutition syncope.

## When to Refer

- Patient history of cardiac disease
- Family history of sudden death, cardiac disease, or deafness
- Recurrent episodes
- Recumbent episode
- Exertional syncope
- Prolonged loss of consciousness
- Associated chest pain or palpitations
- Medications that can alter cardiac conduction

## TOOLS FOR PRACTICE

### Medical Decision Support

- *Isometric Arm Counter-Pressure Maneuvers to Abort Impending Vasovagal Syncope* (article), *Journal of the American College of Cardiology*, Vol 40, Issue 11, 2002

## REFERENCES

1. Savage DD, Corwin L, McGee DL, Kannel WB, Wolf PA. Epidemiologic features of isolated syncope: the Framingham Study. *Stroke*. 1985;16:626–629
2. Kanter RJ. *Syncope and Sudden Death. The Science and Practice of Pediatric Cardiology*. 2nd ed. Baltimore, MD: Williams and Wilkins; 1998
3. Prazar GE. Temper tantrums and breath holding spells. In: Hoekelman RA, ed. *Primary Pediatrics*. 3rd ed. Melbourne, Australia: Churchill Livingstone; 1994
4. Mosqueda-Garcia R, Furlan R, Tank J, Fernandez-Violante R. The elusive pathophysiology of neurally mediated syncope. *Circulation*. 2000;102:2898–2906
5. Grubb BP. Neurocardiogenic syncope and related disorders of orthostatic intolerance. *Circulation*. 2005;111:2997–3006
6. Krongrad E. Syncope and sudden death. In: *Moss and Adams' Heart Disease in Infants, Children and Adolescents*. 5th ed. Baltimore, MD: Williams and Wilkins; 1995
7. Fouad FM, Sitthisook S, Vanerio G, et al. Sensitivity and specificity of the tilt table test in young patients with unexplained syncope. *Pacing Clin Electrophysiol*. 1993;16:394–400
8. Brignole M, Croci F, Menozzi C, et al. Isometric arm counter-pressure maneuvers to abort impending vasovagal syncope. *J Am Coll Cardiol*. 2002;40:2053–2059
9. Younoszai AK, Franklin WH, Chan DP, Cassidy SC, Allen HD. Oral fluid therapy. A promising treatment for vasodepressor syncope. *Arch Pediatr Adolesc Med*. 1998;152:165–168
10. Scott WA, Pongiglione G, Bromberg BI, et al. Randomized comparison of atenolol and fludrocortisone acetate in the treatment of pediatric neurally mediated syncope. *Am J Cardiol*. 1995;76:400–402
11. Sheldon R. The Prevention of Syncope Trial (POST) results. Presented at Late-Breaking Clinical Trials, Heart Rhythm 2004: 25th Annual Scientific Sessions, San Francisco, CA, May 19–22, 2004
12. Perez-Lugones A, Schweikert R, Pavia S, et al. Usefulness of midodrine in patients with severely symptomatic neurocardiogenic syncope: a randomized control study. *J Cardiovasc Electrophysiol*. 2001;12:935–938
13. Di Girolamo E, Di Iorio C, Sabatini P, et al. Effects of paroxetine hydrochloride, a selective serotonin reuptake inhibitor, on refractory vasovagal syncope: a randomized, double-blind, placebo-controlled study. *J Am Coll Cardiol*. 1999;33:1227–1230

# Chapter 78

# Temper Tantrums and Breath-holding Spells

*Gregory E. Prazar, MD*

## ▶ TEMPER TANTRUMS

Children exhibit temper tantrums almost inevitably during the second through fourth years of life. Therefore a temper tantrum is generally a *problem behavior* rather than a *behavioral problem*. Helping parents cope with temper tantrums involves providing anticipatory guidance, sharing information on developmental psychology, and offering strategies to deal with tantrums.

Temper tantrums usually become part of the child's emotional repertoire during the second and third years of life. Early signs of the negativism that is part of tantrums can be appreciated as early as 12 months of age. Some children continue to display occasional tantrums until the age of 5 or 6 years. Tantrums typically reappear in a slightly less intense form during adolescence, when independence once more becomes an issue for the developing adolescent.

Several aspects of the toddler's development seem to make tantrums almost inevitable. First, because the 1-year-old can walk and climb, the child begins to achieve physical mastery over the environment. This increased physical independence and an insatiable curiosity frequently place the child in dangerous situations that require parental intervention. Imposition of adult safety limits thwarts and frustrates the child, often precipitating tantrums. Second, the child's increased exploration of the environment immediately creates a conflict because the child must adapt to rules of an adult world. The child enters an environment of adult social values, in which people are expected to use the bathroom appropriately, verbalize dissatisfactions rather than *act* them out physically, sit quietly while eating, and sometimes subjugate their own wants to those of others. This process is too much for the egocentric toddler to bear, and frustration is inevitable. Third, between the ages of 1 and 4 years, the toddler begins to develop an increased awareness of how the child is separate and different from the mother. The child experiences a conflict between desires for autonomy and desires to remain close to the mother. Frustration in dealing with these intense feelings frequently results in tantrums.

Tensions are created in "establishing ego boundaries as separate from those of parents," as Brazelton[1] states, and in coping with physical limitations placed on exploring an adult world. Adults frequently deal with their own tensions and frustrations by verbalizing their feelings; the toddler, however, lacks a sophisticated ability to verbalize. A toddler's frustration with the adult world may be displayed in doing the exact opposite of what the adult requests, by saying "no, no" yet following through with the adult request (what Fraiberg[2] refers to as the "cheerful no"), by dawdling, or by displaying physical behavior outright (eg, kicking, screaming, lying on the floor, hitting, throwing, biting).

Most parents would probably agree that intellectual appreciation of the cause of tantrums does not necessarily aid in coping with a screaming and inconsolable child. Reasons for parental frustration are understandable. Well-meaning relatives and friends (who have likely forgotten their experience as young parents) may propagate myths about tantrums, which intensify parental anxiety and confusion. Myths of causation suggest that children who display tantrums are underdisciplined or parented inadequately. Myths of management suggest that tantrums can be quelled by spanking, dousing with cold water, or threats.

## ▶ ANTICIPATORY GUIDANCE FOR TANTRUMS

The primary care physician should provide anticipatory guidance about temper tantrums. Such guidance may forestall events that precipitate tantrums and prevent future parental confusion in dealing with negative behaviors. The physician has many opportunities during the child's first 2 years to provide behavioral counseling.

Beginning in infancy, parents should be provided with anticipatory guidance regarding opportunities for positive interactions with the child within daily routines and activities such as feeding, pretend play, and reading aloud. Howard and others have recommended "'special time' provided every day as an approach to formalizing time-in."[3]

At the 6-month well-child visit, the importance of parental time away from the infant can be emphasized. Parents who occasionally leave their infants and toddlers with responsible babysitters provide their children with the security that adults can leave and will come back; they also provide themselves with important mental health holidays from the rigors of parenting.

At the 9- or 12-month infant visit, environmental engineering should be discussed.[3] Providing home safety (eg, safety plugs in outlets, safety latches on drawers), removing valuables or breakables from the child's reach, and ensuring a safe place for the child to play (playpen or enclosed area) are examples of such engineering. Therefore this visit not only may reduce chances for childhood accidents but also may forestall potential adult-toddler power struggles over environmental dangers.

The 15- or 18-month visit provides the physician another opportunity to offer the parent alternatives to negative interactions with the toddler. Afternoon naps (to allow for renewal of toddler and parental energy), the importance of praising cooperative toddler efforts, and the concept of limited decision making for the toddler ("Do you want to wear the green or blue shirt today?" versus "Which shirt do you want to wear today?") represent issues that may help parents minimize hostile encounters with their toddler.

The approach here should encourage parents to describe how they think tantrums should be handled, and should not simply display the physician's personal biases about child rearing. Several excellent books describing turbulent toddlerhood can be suggested to parents, including Brazelton's *Toddlers and Parents,*[1] Ilg and Ames' *Child Behavior,* [4] and Schmitt's *Your Child's Health.*[5] Furthermore, general guidelines concerning tantrums can be given. Tantrums are best ignored unless, as Fraiberg[2] states, "they encroach on rights of others or potentially endanger." If safety is the issue, then either environmental engineering should take place or the child should be restricted to the child's bedroom for 2 to 3 minutes (a kitchen timer is helpful to remind both parent and toddler of the time). If the child hits, bites, or throws in anger, then room restriction for 2 to 3 minutes should once again be suggested. Some behavioral psychologists suggest 1 minute of time out for each year of age (so a 5-year-old child would have a 5-minute time-out). Other behaviorists recommend that the time-out not be fixed. Because the goal is to help the child develop self-regulation, the time-out should end when the tantrum subsides.[6] The child should receive a brief hug or be praised and then be allowed to resume previous activity.

Parents may be reluctant to use bedroom restriction because they worry either that the child will associate the bedroom with unpleasant experiences or that the child will not feel adequately remorseful if placed in a room full of toys. Parents should be reassured that room restriction does not cause bedroom fears. Similarly, goals of discipline are to teach rules and to help the child understand which behaviors are acceptable. Discipline does not need to be severe to be effective. The physician should emphasize to parents that once the tantrum is over, the slate is wiped clean and there is no holdover of judgment or anger, even if the child has acted out badly.

Time-outs are an effective method of dealing with temper tantrums. Time-ins represent a method to reward acceptable behavior. Specifically, when a toddler is playing quietly, the parent should pat the child on the shoulder, give a brief hug, or otherwise offer some form of nonverbal affection. Such attention from the parent simply but effectively indicates approval of the current behavior. Some behavioral psychologists consider time-ins to be a more powerful method of encouraging acceptable behavior than time-outs.

Temper tantrums occur much more frequently in the presence of parents; they are much less common in the presence of alternative child care providers. Most experienced child care providers feel comfortable dealing with temper tantrums. If the child care provider expresses concern to a parent about a child's temper tantrums, then several questions should be considered. Does the child care provider have adequate training to deal with such a common behavior? Is this child care setting the most appropriate for the child (in terms of adult-child ratio, philosophy of discipline used by the provider, and realistic developmental expectations for the child's behavior in the child care setting)? Are the child's temper tantrums much more severe or frequent than those of the child's peers? These questions should be addressed with the child care provider. Subsequently, parents and the child care provider should formulate a plan for dealing with the tantrums that is followed consistently at home and at the child care location. If the parent and the child care provider cannot agree on such a plan, then the child's primary care physician should be consulted.

More specific guidelines for managing tantrums may be necessary in other individual situations. Parents should be encouraged by the physician to vent their feelings (to the physician) about tantrums and be reassured that they are doing the best job they can for their toddler.

## ▶ MANAGEMENT OF PROBLEM TANTRUMS

Although tantrums represent a stage of the normal developing toddler's personality, several factors may suggest that further professional intervention is advisable. An important aspect of management is obtaining a detailed history, including the circumstances in which tantrums take place, a specific description of the tantrums, and what happens following the tantrums. This is referred to as antecedent, behavior, and consequence or "A,B,C." Toddlers who display persistent negativism or tantrums may suffer from too restrictive parenting, may receive too little positive reinforcement and affection, or may have parents who place unreasonable behavioral expectations on them. One study of 3-year-olds defined severe temper tantrums as "episodes of shouting, banging, kicking, or screaming occurring 3 or more times a day or lasting more than 15 minutes."[7] Approximately 50% of these children had behavior problems. Furthermore, such severe tantrums were associated with specific psychosocial issues, including maternal depression, use of corporal punishment, marital stress, and low maternal education.

Children who display tantrums regularly beyond 5 or 6 years of age may be displaying signs of depression or poor self-esteem, or they may be children who live in a family in which emotional problems exist. When temper tantrums regularly occur at school, academic problems should be suspected because peer pressure usually inhibits displays of tantrums.

Children exhibiting persistent tantrums along with other associated behaviors (eg, inability to concentrate, stereotypical behaviors, unrealistic fears, inability to display affection) may have more significant underlying problems, such as attention-deficit disorder, oppositional defiant disorder, or autism spectrum disorder. Similarly, parents who verbalize persistent frustration with tantrums or an inability to cope with age-appropriate tantrums may need more comprehensive counseling than the primary care physician can provide.

Many parenting groups are available to help parents cope with negative behaviors. Programs such as Systematic Training for Effective Parenting (STEP) and Parent Effectiveness Training (PET) provide valuable community referral sources for families. If such services are not available, or if more sophisticated professional counseling is obviously warranted, then the family should be referred to a psychiatrically trained counselor.

Referral should be discussed as soon as the physician anticipates its necessity and should stress the involvement of both parents. The physician should maintain contact with the family about the problem after the referral has been made. Such ongoing contact may solidify the family's commitment to obtain and adhere with the counseling.

## ▶ BREATH-HOLDING SPELLS

Breath-holding spells cause particular anxiety for parents. Spells occur between ages 4 months and 5 years, with most occurring between 12 and 36 months of age. According to Menkes,[8] approximately 5% of all children display breath-holding spells. A positive family history of breath-holding spells occurs in approximately 25% of cases.

Such spells are precipitated by anger, frustration, fear, or minor injury (often a very minor head injury) and are categorized as cyanotic or pallid. Both types of spells are unlikely to occur more often than once a day and are not associated with an increased predisposition to epilepsy (although brief seizure-like activity can occur as a terminating event in either form of spell).

Cyanotic breath-holding spells are precipitated more often by anger or frustration than by fear or injury. The child emits a short, loud cry, takes a deep breath, and holds it. Cyanosis occurs after approximately 30 seconds. Either the episode terminates at this point or the child becomes rigid or limp and loses consciousness (loss of consciousness occurs in approximately

50% of all children who have breath-holding spells). In rare situations, mild clonic movements of the extremities follow.

Pallid breath-holding spells are similar to cyanotic spells in most respects but are more often precipitated by fear or minor injury. The initial cry is brief or silent. The spell then proceeds as with a cyanotic spell. Toddlers who suffer from pallid spells are often from families that have a history of syncope, and, in fact, these toddlers have an increased chance (approximately 15%) of syncopal attacks as adults.

Both cyanotic and pallid breath-holding spells are caused by autonomic nervous system dysregulation. Cerebral anoxia is responsible for spells that terminate with loss of consciousness. Furthermore, both forms of spells are involuntary and reflexive, despite spells often being precipitated when the child is angry or frustrated.

Children who display pallid breath-holding spells may, as adults, suffer from neurocardiogenic syncope, a form of vasovagal response to postural changes. Adults who suffer from neurocardiogenic syncope are more likely to faint at the sight of blood or when injured than are adults who do not have this disorder.

Because both forms of breath-holding spells potentially can terminate with seizure-like movements, differentiation between spells and epilepsy is important. The occurrence of a precipitating factor (eg, minor injury, being frustrated) before the onset of the spell indicates that the episode is a breath-holding spell. Patients who have epilepsy display cyanosis during or after the seizures, not before seizure onset. Furthermore, electroencephalograms performed on patients who suffer from breath-holding spells are normal when not holding their breath; patients who have epilepsy often have abnormal electroencephalograms during seizure-free periods.

## ▶ MANAGEMENT OF BREATH-HOLDING SPELLS

No effective medical therapy exists for breath-holding spells, although some toddlers who experience seizure-like activity along with spells are prescribed anticonvulsant therapy. However, the decision to use medication remains controversial among pediatric neurologists.

Iron deficiency anemia has been associated with breath-holding spells. A study involving 67 children who had breath-holding spells revealed that iron therapy reduced spells in the treatment group by 88%. These results suggest that iron may be important in the regulation of the autonomic nervous system.[9]

Coping with breath-holding spells can be extremely difficult for parents. Spells that terminate with loss of consciousness or with seizure-like movements are obviously frightening. Convincing parents that no harm will come to their child is important. Nevertheless, parents of a breath holder will frequently avoid enforcing limits for fear of precipitating the child's anger and a subsequent attack. Such parents need repeated reassurance and encouragement to continue age-appropriate limits on their child's behavior. To do otherwise will create an overindulged child who subsequently may fear loss of parental love because limits have been rescinded.

When to refer a breath-holding patient to a neurologist or a psychiatrically trained professional may not be an easy decision for the physician. If parents request further consultation, then their wish certainly should be respected, even if the physician is confident that further evaluation is unnecessary. If parents indicate agreement with the physician that spells are of no consequence yet continue to withhold appropriate limit setting, then referral to a mental health professional should take place. The physician who is unsure of the diagnosis of breath-holding (especially in situations in which loss of consciousness or seizure-like activity occurs) should always refer the family to a pediatric neurologist. Referral must not end the physician–parent communication concerning the spells: an ongoing dialogue may ensure adherence with the referral.

## ▶ SUMMARY

Temper tantrums and breath-holding spells usually represent benign forms of childhood behavior evolving from the child's preverbal attempts to express feelings of frustration and anger. Unfortunately, parents frequently have difficulty appreciating the benign course of such behaviors when they daily must face a screaming, inconsolable toddler who may even lose consciousness and then display seizure-like movements. Parents can best deal with negative behaviors when they are adequately prepared by the physician before such behaviors occur and when they are offered empathic guidance and positive reinforcement during regular office visits.

### *TOOLS FOR PRACTICE*

#### Engaging Patient and Family

- *Caring for Your Baby and Young Child: Birth to Age 5* (book), American Academy of Pediatrics (shop.aap.org)
- *Temper Tantrums: A Normal Part of Growing Up* (handout), American Academy of Pediatrics (patiented.solutions.aap.org)
- *Top Tips for Surviving Tantrums* (Web page), American Academy of Pediatrics (www.healthychildren.org/English/family-life/family-dynamics/communication-discipline/Pages/Temper-Tantrums.aspx)

### *REFERENCES*

1. Brazelton TB. *Toddlers and Parents*. New York, NY: Dell; 1989
2. Fraiberg S. *The Magic Years*. New York, NY: Charles Scribner's Sons; 1996
3. Hagan JF Jr, Shaw JS, Duncan PM, eds. *Bright Futures: Guidelines for Health Supervision of Infants, Children, and Adolescents*. 3rd ed. Elk Grove Village, IL: American Academy of Pediatrics; 2008
4. Ilg FL, Ames LB. *Child Behavior*. New York, NY: Harper & Row; 1992
5. Schmitt B. *Your Child's Health*. New York, NY: Bantam Books; 2005
6. Carey WB, Crocker AC, Coleman WL, Elias ER, Feldman HM. *Developmental-Behavioral Pediatrics*. 4th ed. Philadelphia, PA: Saunders Elsevier; 2009
7. Needlman R, Stevenson J, Zuckerman B. Psychosocial correlates of severe temper tantrums. *J Dev Behav Pediatr*. 1991;12:77–83
8. Menkes JH. *Textbook of Child Neurology*. 2nd ed. Philadelphia, PA: Lea & Febiger; 1995
9. Daoud AS, Batieha A, al-Sheyyab M, Abuekteish F, Hijazi S. Effectiveness of iron therapy on breath-holding spells. *J Pediatr*. 1997;130:547–550

# Chapter 79

# Tics

*Robert A. King, MD*

*Tics,* which are recurring, nonrhythmic, sudden, rapid, stereotyped, involuntary movements or vocalizations,[1] may be classified as motor or vocal and as simple or complex. The most common *simple motor tics* are eye blinking, neck twisting, shoulder shrugging, and grimacing; the most common *simple vocal tics* are coughing, throat clearing, sniffing, and grunting. *Complex motor tics* include more sustained, orchestrated, or seemingly purposeful gestures, such as touching, stomping on, or sniffing objects; jumping; sustained dystonic movements; copropraxia (obscene gestures); or echokinesis (automatic imitation of another person's movements). *Complex vocal tics* include sudden changes in volume or prosody; syllables, words, or stock phrases spoken out of context; palilalia (repeating one's own words); echolalia (repeating the words of others); and coprolalia (uttering obscenities).

Tic disorders are model neuropsychiatric conditions demonstrating the complex interplay of genetic, neurobiological, environmental, and psychosocial factors. That is, they have a constitutional, probably genetic basis; are influenced by perinatal risk and environmental factors; demonstrate sexual dimorphism; show a changing course over development; and, although neurobiologically determined, can be affected by psychosocial factors, such as stress and cognitive behavioral interventions.

## ▶ CLINICAL MANIFESTATIONS

The most common age at onset for tics is 6 or 7 years. The usual initial motor tics are blinking or facial grimacing, with subsequent rostral-caudal involvement. The most common initial vocal tics are sniffing, coughing, and throat clearing. Not surprisingly, these symptoms are often initially mistaken for allergies or otolaryngologic or respiratory symptoms; but with tics, the other characteristics of such disorders are absent. Characteristically, tics wax and wane in intensity and frequency, with a tic disappearing only to have new ones take its place. Stress or excitement often exacerbates the tics.

Although children are generally unaware of their tics, premonitory urges[2,3] are often reported in more severe cases or in older children. Tics are often transiently suppressible with effort, usually resulting in an increased urge to perform the tic. Many patients describe their tics as neither fully voluntary nor involuntary[3]; some experience the effort to suppress tics in social situations to be as burdensome as are the tics themselves.

## ▶ INCIDENCE

It once was believed that *Tourette syndrome* (TS) was rare, persistent, severe, and disabling. It is now clear that tic disorders, including TS, exist on a clinical spectrum from transient, isolated, inconsequential tics to more persistent multiple motor and vocal tics that interfere with daily functioning. Isolated and transitory tics are common (occurring in as many as 24% of first- and second-graders[4]) and of minimal consequence. Depending on ascertainment methods, childhood prevalence of TS is thought to be 2 to 185 per 10,000—much higher than previously believed, with many milder, uncomplicated cases not coming to clinical attention. Boys are affected more than girls, by a ratio as high as 9:1 to 14:1 in TS.[5]

## ▶ ETIOLOGY

The cause of tics is unknown, but neurobiologic and behavioral research shows the boundaries between psychiatric and neurologic domains to be poorly defined and increasingly obsolete. Most of this research has been on TS rather than on milder forms of tic disorder. Areas of interest have been basal ganglia and cortico-striatal-thalmo-cortical circuitry,[6–8] genetics,[9–11] and immunology.[12–14] A multifactorial etiology for TS, with a convergence of genetic vulnerability, environmental and perinatal risk factors, and disturbances in the prefrontal cortex and basal ganglia, has been proposed.[7,8] Several factors have been shown to be associated with tics and may give clues to their cause.

### *Developmental Stage*

Tics usually have their onset between 5 and 10 years of age, most commonly at 6 or 7 years. Although fluctuating in intensity from hour to hour and day to day, tics are usually at their most severe at around 10 to 13 years of age. Approximately 70% to 80% of the time, tics spontaneously diminish in severity during the course of adolescence and disappear or become minimal by young adulthood. Comorbid conditions, however, such as obsessive compulsive disorder (OCD), attention-deficit/hyperactivity disorder (ADHD), and anxiety disorder, may persist. The factors associated with spontaneous improvement or remission remain unclear and are important areas of research.[15–17]

### *Sex*

Transient tics as well as chronic tic disorders are more common in boys than in girls.[4,5] Androgens are implicated for multiple reasons—postnatal exposure to androgens may elicit TS; antiandrogen therapy may improve tics; and androgen-dependent alterations in prenatal brain development may be associated with TS.[8]

### *Prenatal, Perinatal, and Postnatal Factors*

Factors that have been associated with tic severity also have been associated with other neuropsychiatric symptoms and disorders, such as hyperactivity: in particular, prenatal factors, such as maternal smoking, vomiting, psychosocial stress, drug use, fetal nutrition, and androgen exposure, and perinatal factors, such as low birth weight.[18]

Experts have proposed that, in some cases, the acute onset of tics represents a form of *p*ediatric *a*utoimmune *n*europsychiatric *d*isorder *a*ssociated with *Streptococcus* (PANDAS).[12] This controversial hypothesis posits that group A α-hemolytic streptococcal infection can cause an autoimmune reaction that attacks the basal ganglia, resulting in tics, OCD, or both. Despite much ongoing research, this hypothesized autoimmune condition remains unproven.[13,14,19] In the absence of a biological marker, distinguishing which cases might represent true PANDAS as opposed to the nonspecific coincidental occurrences of 2 common childhood conditions (streptococcal pharyngitis and tics or OCD) is difficult, at least at the onset. In one large study, children subsequently diagnosed with de novo tic disorder were found to have a greatly increased rate of streptococcal infections in the months before diagnosis.[20]

Pending further research to clarify this matter, some primary care physicians have chosen to obtain throat cultures from children with sudden onset or exacerbations of tics and from children with tics or OCD who have pharyngitis or who are exposed to *Streptococcus*. Children with positive throat cultures should receive appropriate antibiotic treatment. There is no established role for repeat posttreatment cultures to prevent streptococcal carrier states, nor does the use of prophylactic antibiotic treatment have any firm basis in evidence. Plasmapheresis or intravenous immunoglobulin therapy are only suitable in intractable cases as part of an approved investigational protocol.[14]

## Psychological Factors

Anxiety, stress, and excitement can all exacerbate tics.[21] Little is known about the psychological status of most children in the general population who have tics, because they are rarely seen in clinics. However, evidence exists for increased autonomic lability in individuals with TS, and children who have anxiety disorders are overrepresented in clinical samples.[22]

## Psychiatric Disorders

Population and clinical studies of tics point to a strong relationship, most marked in TS, between tics and ADHD.[5]

A relationship also exists between tics (especially in TS) and OCD, with symptoms (eg, premonitory urges, intrusive thoughts, compulsive actions), putative anatomic locus (cortical, striatal, or thalamic circuits), hypothesized pathophysiologic features (rogue reverberating microcircuits), and family pedigrees all showing elements in common.[7,23]

Tics should never be assumed to indicate another psychiatric disorder or psychological problem unless they are associated with other signs or symptoms that affect other areas of function beyond the motor system. Although tics can be controlled to some degree in public situations (eg, school or a physician's office), an affected child should not be expected to control them most of the time. Such control requires considerable mental energy and effort and usually cannot be sustained for long. As soon as the child relaxes, is distracted, or lets up concentration, the tics will reappear.

## Genetic Factors

Many cases of tics, especially TS, appear to be genetic in origin. Mild and transient cases of tic disorder may coexist in the same pedigree as cases of TS, suggesting that protective and risk factors also exist. Even with monozygotic twins, the concordance rate is only 77%, which suggests that environmental factors (eg, low birth weight) also play a role. Although specific genes have been identified in a handful of pedigrees, the condition may well be heterogeneous (ie, different specific genes may be responsible in different pedigrees) and perhaps polygenic (ie, reflecting the interaction of multiple vulnerability loci).[9–11] Penetrance increases if OCD is accepted as an alternative expression of the gene.

## Drugs

Amphetamine and other dopaminergic drugs induce stereotypies in rats and occasionally produce or exacerbate tics in children. Cocaine, other stimulants, sympathomimetics, caffeine, serotonin uptake inhibitors and other antidepressants, and anabolic steroids may also produce or exacerbate tics.

## ▶ DIFFERENTIAL DIAGNOSIS

Tics are usually distinguishable from other neurologic disorders by their stereotyped nature, variability over time, transient suppressibility, accompanying premonitory urges, and lack of other neurologic symptoms.[24] The differential diagnosis includes dystonia, myoclonus, chorea, seizures, athetosis, and stereotypies.

Tics are distinguishable from *chorea* (with which they are often confused) by their centripetal location, repetitive form, normal muscle tone, and lack of postural impersistence; and from most other neurologically based abnormal movements by their rapidity and normal muscle tone. Even so, tics rarely reflect or portend a neurologic disorder. Such tics are likely to be much more persistent and accompanied by signs of the disorder that causes them.

A more difficult diagnostic quandary in young children is distinguishing true tics from stereotypies or self-stimulating behaviors, such as rocking, head banging, flapping, or spinning. Tics are characterized by a later onset, lower complexity, fluctuating intensity and locus, and their intrusive, bothersome, disruptive, and involuntary nature. In contrast, stereotypies are most often bothersome to parents but not to the child, who may find them pleasurable and resist adult attempts to interrupt them. Self-stimulating movements mostly occur at times of boredom or excitement, but they rarely disrupt coordinated movements, and they persist without much change in form or anatomical location. Although stereotypies are often associated in many physicians' minds with intellectual disability or autism spectrum disorders, in fact they can also occur in children who are otherwise developmentally normal (see Chapter 69, Self-stimulating Behaviors).

The most recent edition of the American Psychiatric Association's *Diagnostic and Statistical Manual of Mental Disorders*[1] distinguishes 3 arbitrary subtypes of tic disorder: *provisional* (present for less than 1 year since first tic onset); *persistent (chronic)* (motor or vocal tics, but not both, that have persisted longer than 1 year since first tic onset); and *Tourette disorder,* also known as Tourette syndrome (multiple motor and and at least one vocal tic, not necessarily concurrently, persisting at least 1 year from first tic onset). Whether these 3 classifications reflect varying severity of the same disorder is unknown. Most recent research has been restricted to TS but suggests that these subtypes are probably related.

## ▶ COMORBID DISORDERS

Persistent tics, even mild ones, seem to be associated with an increased risk of comorbid ADHD, which predates the tics or any accompanying OCD. This association is not simply the result of the bias toward comorbidity in clinical sample populations because it is also found in community sample populations.[5,25] In addition, many youngsters with TS whose concentration is basically good can become distracted and lose focus when their tics are in a period of exacerbation, presumably because of the tics themselves and the impingement of tic urges and efforts to suppress them.

Individuals with TS are also at risk for other anxiety disorders, depression, fine-motor difficulties, and uneven cognitive profile (performance IQ scores lower than verbal IQ scores).[23] ADHD is common (present in 50% of patients with TS), and children with combined ADHD and tics have the greatest social and academic difficulties. ADHD severity is a better predictor of poor adjustment than tic severity.[26] Although the presence of ADHD with tics increases the likelihood of disruptive behavior and learning problems, chronic tics are often associated with learning impairment independent of ADHD. Investigations of both community and clinical sample populations confirm that the presence of ADHD predicts greater disability than that associated with tic disorders alone.[27]

OCD is found in up to 50% of patients with TS, with compulsions and obsessions most commonly involving symmetry, evening up, *just right* phenomena, sex, and aggression.[23]

## ▶ TREATMENT

Most tics in children are mild and short lived and require no treatment. A careful clinical evaluation is needed to assess not only the current phenomenology, history, and effect of the tics, but also the presence of other symptoms (anxiety, impulsivity, inattention) or adaptive difficulties in the overall context of the child's social, family, and school life.[28]

Once a tic has persisted for several months, treatment may be considered, but only if the tic is conspicuous, disabling, or distressing to the child. No treatment for tics can be said to be simple, entirely effective, or free from side effects. Treatments shown to have some limited efficacy are discussed in the following sections.

### *Behavioral Methods*

Although a variety of behavioral techniques (eg, relaxation, massed practice) have been tried for tic disorders, only comprehensive behavioral intervention for tics (CBIT) seems to have good empirical support.[29] As the name conveys, CBIT is an effective evidenced-based behavioral approach to tics that combines habit reversal and contingency management techniques.[30] Habit-reversal therapy is best carried out by a physician who is experienced in the technique and who is accustomed to working with children. Cognitive behavioral interventions may also be helpful for youngsters whose tic disorder is accompanied by disruptive behavior and explosive outbursts.[31]

### *Anxiety-Reducing and Supportive Procedures*

Relaxation training and biofeedback are not of proven value in treating tics. Psychotherapy (specifically focused on stressful interpersonal difficulties), work with parents, and other means of addressing environmental stresses may be helpful, not because stress causes tics, but rather because stress and high expressed emotion can exacerbate tics. These procedures should not be considered specific; rather, they are ancillary and holistic in meeting therapeutic objectives.

Many youngsters with tic disorders have difficulties at school, either from comorbid ADHD or an uneven neuropsychological profile, or difficulties with peer stigmatization.[26,27] Close collaboration with school staff to ensure appropriate educational programming and accommodations is important.[32]

### *Acceptance*

In most cases, the best management is explaining to parents, teachers, and peers that the tics are a physical disability, that the child cannot help them, and that acceptance of both child and tics is the kindest, safest, and simplest way to deal with them. Criticizing and belittling the child are likely to make tics worse and prolong their course. Peer problems can be a major difficulty for children with tics and TS,[26] and collaboration with school staff to reduce peer teasing and stigmatization is a major therapeutic task.[32] Helping to support and build upon the child's strengths is an important component in bolstering and protecting the child's self-esteem. In emphasizing that children cannot help their tics, the physician and parents should avoid the pitfall of concluding that the child cannot help other problematic behaviors related to impulsivity, for which consistent structure, expectations, and consequences are desirable and beneficial.[31]

### *Pharmacotherapy*

Only physicians thoroughly familiar with the drugs indicated and experienced in their use in children with tics should undertake pharmacotherapy.[33–35] The first consideration is deciding which symptom to target: the tics themselves or 1 of the common comorbid symptoms or conditions, such as OCD or ADHD, which are often a greater source of impairment.[28]

## Pharmacotherapy for Tics

Various medications are effective in partially suppressing tics, but they are not curative in terms of affecting the underlying course or prognosis of tics. Furthermore, because of frequent side effects (especially sedation), medication should be administered only if the tics are significantly bothersome, disruptive, stigmatizing, or painful. The first mandate is to do no harm. In the case of tics, this approach means starting with low doses, titrating the dose upward only gradually, and avoiding sedation, cognitive blunting, or other distressing side effects (eg, acute dystonic reactions) that may be more burdensome than the tics themselves. Setting realistic goals in terms of reducing tics to tolerable levels is important; attempts to suppress tics completely often result in overmedication. Discontinuing anti-tic medications should be done gradually, because even when medications seem ineffective, abrupt discontinuation may produce bothersome acute rebound or withdrawal-related exacerbation of tics that may persist for several weeks.

Many physicians' first choice of anti-tic medication, especially in children with comorbid ADHD, is 1 of the α-adrenergic agonists, clonidine or guanfacine.[36,37] Although these agents are less potent and are effective in fewer patients with severe tics than the neuroleptics, they tend to have fewer and less severe side effects, with the principal dose-related side effects being sedation and hypotension. They are, however, potentially fatal in overdoses. Guanfacine, when available, is the preferred first choice because it is longer acting and less sedating than clonidine, and it seems to be more effective for attentional problems.[38] Although sustained-release forms of both clonidine and guanfacine are available, it is usually preferable with younger children to begin on smaller doses of the short-acting form, titrating slowly with only small-dose increments to avoid sedation.

If the α-adrenergic agents are not effective or if the tics are severe, then the next line of agents is the dopamine-blocking neuroleptics, now known as antipsychotic drugs.[37] These agents seem to be effective because tics, whatever their cause, are executed through the basal ganglia, with an apparent relative overactivity in the dopaminergic nigrostriatal systems that inhibits cholinergic basal ganglia systems. However, the neurochemistry of tic disorder is complex and probably involves several neurotransmitter systems; therefore, inferring underlying deficits from the observed therapeutic effectiveness of various agents is difficult.

Of the traditional *typical* so-called *high-potency* (ie, nonatropinic) neuroleptics, haloperidol, pimozide, or fluphenazine have been shown to be effective,[34,37] but have largely been replaced in clinical practice by the newer, so-called atypical antipsychotics. As with several of the other typical neuroleptics (eg, ziprasidone), caution must be exercised with pimozide in terms of cardiotoxicity and drug interactions, especially with drugs such as erythromycin that are metabolized through the cytochrome P450 3A4 isoenzyme system, because fatal drug interactions can result. Monitoring the QTc interval at baseline and with dose increases is prudent in patients receiving pimozide or ziprasidone. Even at relatively low doses, neuroleptics may produce acute dystonic reactions, sedation, cognitive blunting, medication-induced separation anxiety, parkinsonism, akathisia (restless legs), and, in the longer term, withdrawal or tardive dyskinesias, 1 rare type of which may be a worsening of tics caused by presumed dopamine-2 receptor hypersensitivity. If moderate doses are not effective, then higher doses are not likely to be either, and higher doses almost always increase the risk of side effects and make weaning the patient from the drug difficult without rebound exacerbation.

Although tardive dyskinesias are rare in children who receive modest doses of neuroleptics for tics, the traditional, or typical, antipsychotics are now being replaced by the newer so-called atypical antipsychotics,[34] which seem to have a lower risk of tardive dyskinesia. However, atypical neuroleptics have the same other adverse effects as typical neuroleptics, including acute dystonic or extrapyramidal reactions, sedation, or dysphoria. In addition, risperidone and olanzapine may cause hyperphagia and weight gain, with potentially serious metabolic consequences. Clinical trials have demonstrated the efficacy of risperidone, olanzapine, and ziprasidone for tics, but the lack of efficacy of the paradigmatic atypical neuroleptic clozapine indicates that not all atypical neuroleptics are equally effective.

When neither $\alpha$-adrenergic agents nor neuroleptics are effective, a variety of second-line drugs or augmentation strategies may be tried with caution.[33–35] Although some neurologists use clonazepam to manage tic disorders, it should be used only in rare instances in children. Like the other benzodiazepines, clonazepam can cause cognitive blunting, sedation, irritability, and disinhibition, and its use can lead to dependence and withdrawal symptoms.

Tics should be treated pharmacotherapeutically only if significantly impairing, and only by a physician skilled in the use of the drugs concerned—ordinarily a child or adolescent psychiatrist or a pediatric neurologist. Such treatment should be carefully considered and discussed with parents, closely monitored, and undertaken only with knowledge and consideration of the risks and disadvantages involved.

## Pharmacotherapy for Attention-Deficit/Hyperactivity Disorder, Obsessive-Compulsive Disorder, Anxiety, and Depression

Pharmacotherapy for impairing comorbid ADHD, OCD, anxiety, or depression may be indicated in children with tic disorder, bearing in mind some considerations specific to tic disorder. Because ADHD is often more disabling than the child's tics, a cautious trial of a stimulant may be necessary, beginning with very low doses and increasing only gradually to avoid exacerbating tics. Alternatives to the stimulants are the $\alpha$-adrenergic agents (clonidine or guanfacine), atomoxetine,[39] or 1 of the second-line drugs such as the older tricyclic antidepressants (with appropriate electrocardiogram monitoring).[36] Most children with tics and ADHD are able to tolerate methylphenidate,[36] and the combination of methylphenidate and clonidine seems more effective than either agent alone.[40]

The SSRIs seem to be effective in children with OCD and tics, although evidence suggests that monotherapy with the SSRIs is less effective in the presence of tics. In such cases, augmentation with a low dose of a neuroleptic often boosts the treatment response. In rare cases, SSRIs can exacerbate or even precipitate tics, akathisia, or other movement abnormalities, or can increase suicidal thinking.

## ▶ MANAGEMENT

Most tics last only a few weeks, although they may flit from 1 muscle group to another or change their form at irregular intervals. Even the chronic tics of TS are likely to disappear in later adolescence, with tic severity peaking at age 10 to 12 or so.[17] Although most tics improve by late adolescence, OCD or ADHD symptoms may persist.[15–17] Because the prevalence of tics drops sharply after age 13, tics that persist into later adolescence are more likely to become chronic. Tic severity in adulthood is inversely proportional to caudate volume in childhood and to childhood performance on a dominant hand fine-motor skill test.[15,16]

Children with tics and especially TS can experience related problems of self-image when adult criticism and peer rejection result.[26] Occasionally, severe complex motor tics result in injury or self-mutilation. Finally, OCD may develop during adolescence or late in TS and can be a persistent source of distress despite the improvement in tic severity with age.

Data from community surveys suggest that tic disorders, including TS, exist on a spectrum from transient to persistent multiple motor and vocal tics that in more severe forms interfere with daily living. The presence of isolated and transitory tics is common and seems to be of minimal consequence. On the other hand, persistent tics, even mild ones, seem to be associated with increased prevalence of ADHD, OCD, disruptive behavior, learning problems (although not necessarily a formal learning disability), and vulnerability to anxiety and depression.

Children should be referred to a specialist if the differential diagnosis is unclear, if a psychiatric disorder is present or is a possibility, if psychiatric drugs or treatments are needed, or if an expert opinion is required.

Referral is likely to be influenced as much by associated problems as by the tics themselves. The emphasis of treatment may thus focus less on tics per se than in mapping other areas of dysfunction.

Criteria for referring children to a specialist with expertise in the diagnosis and management of tics are the following: presence of tics associated with additional evidence of psychiatric disorder, such as ADHD, generalized anxiety, or OCD; presence of chronic or recurrent tics that seem to have a clear relationship to stress, particularly if a reason exists to think that psychosocial interventions may be helpful; presence of chronic, disabling, or discomforting tics for which differential diagnosis or treatment is needed; when the primary physician knows little about tics and wants an expert opinion; or when psychoactive drugs such as antipsychotics (neuroleptics) or $\alpha$-adrenergic agents may be indicated, because psychiatrists and developmental-behavioral pediatricians routinely use these medications and are well informed about risks, side effects, dose levels, and newer drugs.

Such referral may be only for consultation, not necessarily for continued management. In general, the preferred mental health specialist is a well-trained child or adolescent psychiatrist, or developmental-behavioral pediatrician—one who has a broad biopsychosocial perspective, including a good grasp of neuropsychiatry and pharmacotherapy but who will not overprescribe and who has a capacity to work closely with behavioral psychologists. This kind of specialist should also be alert to the possibilities of the rare neurologically induced tics and willing to order any appropriate neuroimaging studies and neurologic consultations. When the tic is disabling and no further diagnostic workup is required, or when pharmacotherapy is not an option or is already in place but further relief is necessary, referral should be made to a child psychologist experienced in behavioral types of treatment.[29–31] Consultation from a clinical psychologist is also useful if a child is having difficulties at school that are not simply caused by teasing or the distraction of tics or tic urges.[27] Many children with tic disorders benefit from close collaboration with their school, which may include making the teacher aware of the tics and providing accommodations such as the ability to step out of class briefly when tics especially intrusive or bothersome.[32]

## When to Refer

- Differential diagnosis is unclear
- A psychiatric disorder is present or a possibility
- Psychiatric drugs or treatments are needed
- For expert opinion

## When to Admit

- Never in the first instance (for tics alone)
- Occasionally, for complex assessments to initiate treatments or to taper a child from high doses of multiple medications

## *TOOLS FOR PRACTICE*

### Engaging Patient and Family

- *A Family's Guide to Tourette Syndrome* (book), Walkup JT (store.tsa-usa.org/index.html)
- *Tics, Tourette Syndrome, and OCD* (fact sheet), American Academy of Pediatrics (www.healthychildren.org/English/health-issues/conditions/emotional-problems/Pages/Tics-Tourette-Syndrome-and-OCD.aspx)
- *Tourette Syndrome Association* (Web site), (www.tsa-usa.org)
- *What You Want to Know About TS* (Web page), New Jersey Center for Tourette Syndrome and Associated Disorders, Inc. (www.njcts.org/what-you-want-to-know.php)

## *REFERENCES*


1. American Psychiatric Association. *Diagnostic and Statistical Manual of Mental Disorders.* 5th ed. Washington, DC: American Psychiatric Association; 2013
2. Leckman JF, Walker DE, Cohen DJ. Premonitory urges in Tourette's syndrome. *Am J Psychiatry.* 1993;150:98–102
3. Leckman JF, Bloch MH, Sukhodolsky DG, Scahill L, King RA. Phenomenology of tics and sensory urges: the self under siege. In: Martino D, Leckman JF, eds. *Tourette Syndrome.* New York, NY: Oxford University Press; 2013:1–25
4. Snider LA, Seligman LD, Ketchen BR, et al. Tics and problem behaviors in schoolchildren: prevalence, characterization, and associations. *Pediatrics.* 2002;110:331–336

5. Scahill L, Dalsgaard S, Bradbury K. The prevalence of Tourette syndrome and its relationship to clinical features. In: Martino D, Leckman JF, eds. *Tourette Syndrome.* New York, NY: Oxford University Press; 2013:121–133
6. Leckman JF, Vaccarino FM, Kalanithi PS, Rothenberger A. Annotation: Tourette syndrome: a relentless drumbeat–driven by misguided brain oscillations. *J Child Psychol Psychiatry.* 2006;47:537–550
7. Leckman JF, Bloch MH, Smith ME, Larabi D, Hampson M. Neurobiological substrates of Tourette's disorder. *J Child Adolesc Psychopharmacol.* 2010;20:237–247
8. Spessot AL, Peterson BS. Tourette's syndrome: a multifactorial developmental psychopathology. In: Cicchetti D, Cohen DJ, eds. *Developmental Psychopathology.* 2nd ed. Vol 3. Hoboken, NJ: John Wiley & Sons; 2006
9. Abelson JF, Kwan KY, O'Roak BJ, et al. Sequence variants in SLITRK1 are associated with Tourette's syndrome. *Science.* 2005;310:317–320
10. Fernandez TV, State MW. Genetic susceptibiity in Tourette syndrome. In: Martino D, Leckman JF, eds. *Tourette Syndrome.* New York, NY: Oxford University Press; 2013:137–155
11. Castellan Baldan L, Williams KA, Gallezot JD, et al. Histidine decarboxylase deficiency causes Tourette syndrome: parallel findings in humans and mice. *Neuron.* 2014;81:77–90
12. Swedo SE, Leonard HL, Rapoport JL. The pediatric autoimmune neuropsychiatric disorders associated with streptococcal infection (PANDAS) subgroup: separating fact from fiction. *Pediatrics.* 2004;113:907–911
13. Kurlan R, Kaplan EL. The pediatric autoimmune neuropsychiatric disorders associated with streptococcal infection (PANDAS) etiology for tics and obsessive-compulsive symptoms: hypothesis or entity? Practical considerations for the clinician. *Pediatrics.* 2004;113:883–886
14. Singer HS, Gilbert DL, Wolf DS, Mink JW, Kurlan R. Moving from PANDAS to CANS. *J Pediatr.* 2012;160:725–731
15. Bloch MH, Peterson BS, Scahill L, et al. Adulthood outcome of tic and obsessive-compulsive symptom severity in children with Tourette syndrome. *Arch Pediatr Adolesc Med.* 2006;160:65–69
16. Bloch MH, Sukhodolsky DG, Leckman JF, Schultz RT. Fine-motor skill deficits in childhood predict adulthood tic severity and global psychosocial functioning in Tourette's syndrome. *J Child Psychol Psychiatry.* 2006;47:551–559
17. Leckman JF, Zhang H, Vitale A, et al. Course of tic severity in Tourette syndrome: the first two decades. *Pediatrics.* 1998;102:14–19
18. Mathews CA, Bimson B, Lowe TL, et al. Association between maternal smoking and increased symptom severity in Tourette's syndrome. *Am J Psychiatry.* 2006;163:1066–1073
19. Swedo SE, Schrag A, Gilbert R, et al. Streptococcal infection, Tourette syndrome, and OCD: is there a connection? PANDAS: horse or zebra? *Neurology.* 2010;74:1397–1398; author reply 1398–1399
20. Mell LK, Davis RL, Owens D. Association between streptococcal infection and obsessive-compulsive disorder, Tourette's syndrome, and tic disorder. *Pediatrics.* 2005;116:56–60
21. Lin H, Katsovich L, Ghebremichael M, et al. Psychosocial stress predicts future symptom severities in children and adolescents with Tourette syndrome and/or obsessive-compulsive disorder. *J Child Psychol Psychiatry.* 2007;48:157–166
22. Chappell P, Riddle M, Anderson G, et al. Enhanced stress responsivity of Tourette syndrome patients undergoing lumbar puncture. *Biol Psychiatry.* 1994;36:35–43
23. Martino D, Leckman JF, eds. *Tourette Syndrome.* New York, NY: Oxford University Press; 2013
24. Kurlan, R. The differential diagnosis of tic disorders. In: Martino D, Leckman JF, eds. *Tourette Syndrome.* New York, NY: Oxford University Press; 2013:395–401
25. Peterson BS, Pine DS, Cohen P, Brook JS. Prospective, longitudinal study of tic, obsessive-compulsive, and attention-deficit/hyperactivity disorders in an epidemiological sample. *J Am Acad Child Adolesc Psychiatry.* 2001;40:685–695
26. Bawden HN, Stokes A, Camfield CS, Camfield PR, Salisbury S. Peer relationship problems in children with Tourette's disorder or diabetes mellitus. *J Child Psychol Psychiatry.* 1998;39:663–668

27. Sukhodolsky DG, Landeros-Weisenberger A, Scahill L, Leckman JF, Schultz RT. Neuropsychological functioning in children with Tourette syndrome with and without attention-deficit/hyperactivity disorder. *J Am Acad Child Adolesc Psychiatry*. 2010;49:1155–1164
28. King RA, Landeros-Weisenberger A. Comprehensive assessment strategies. In: Martino D, Leckman JF, eds. *Tourette Syndrome*. New York, NY: Oxford University Press; 2013:402–410
29. Piacentini J, Woods DW, Scahill L, et al. Behavior therapy for children with Tourette disorder: a randomized controlled trial. *JAMA*. 2010;303:1929–1937
30. Woods DW, Piacentini JC, Chang SW, et al. *Managing Tourette Syndrome: A Behavioral Intervention*. Oxford University Press; 2008
31. Sukhodolsky DG, Vitulano LA, Carroll DH, et al. Randomized trial of anger control training for adolescents with Tourette's syndrome and disruptive behavior. *J Am Acad Child Adolesc Psychiatry*. 2009;48:413–421
32. Pruitt SK, Packer LE. Information and support for educators. In: Martino D, Leckman JF, eds. *Tourette Syndrome*. New York, NY: Oxford University Press; 2013:636–655
33. Murphy TK, Lewin AB, Storch EA, Stock S; American Academy of Child and Adolescent Psychiatry Committee on Quality Issues. Practice parameter for the assessment and treatment of children and adolescents with tic disorders. *J Am Acad Child Adolesc Psychiatry*. 2013;52(12):1341–1359
34. Scahill L, King RA, Lombroso P, Sukhodolsky DG, Leckman JF. Assessment and treatment of Tourette's syndrome and other tic disorder. In: Martin A, Scahill L, Kratochvil C, eds. *Pediatric Psychopharmacology: Principles and Practice*. 2nd ed. New York, NY: Oxford University Press; 2011
35. Roessner V, Plessen KJ, Rothenberger A, et al. European clinical guidelines for Tourette syndrome and other tic disorders. Part II: pharmacological treatment. *Eur Child Adolesc Psychiatry*. 2011;20:173–196
36. Bloch MH, Panza KE, Landeros-Weisenberger A, Leckman JF. Meta-analysis: treatment of attention-deficit/hyperactivity disorder in children with comorbid tic disorders. *J Am Acad Child Adolesc Psychiatry*. 2009;48:884–893
37. Weisman H, Qureshi IA, Leckman JF, Scahill L, Bloch MH. Systematic review: pharmacological treatment of tic disorders—efficacy of antipsychotic and alpha-2 adrenergic agonist agents. *Neurosci Biobehav Rev*. 2013;37:1162–1171
38. Arnsten AF, Steere JC, Hunt RD. The contribution of alpha 2-noradrenergic mechanisms of prefrontal cortical cognitive function. Potential significance for attention-deficit hyperactivity disorder. *Arch Gen Psychiatry*. 1996;53:448–455
39. Allen AJ, Kurlan RM, Gilbert DL, et al. Atomoxetine treatment in children and adolescents with ADHD and comorbid tic disorders. *Neurology*. 2005;65:1941–1949
40. Tourette's Syndrome Study Group. Treatment of ADHD in children with tics: a randomized controlled trial. *Neurology*. 2002;58:527–536

involves thickening and tightness of the SCM itself.[2] Finally, *congenital postural torticollis* occurs without the presence of a palpable mass or tightness of the SCM.[3]

The twisted position of the neck can lead to positional plagiocephaly. Skull flattening on the contralateral side may result from sleeping supine.[4] Thus, plagiocephaly can be the presenting sign of mild torticollis.

### Acquired Torticollis

As with congenital torticollis, most cases of torticollis encountered in older children are primarily muscular in origin. Cervical muscle or ligament injury arising from trauma can cause a head tilt and unilateral neck tenderness, a condition that can also occur on awakening, presumably as a result of awkward positioning of the neck during sleep.

*Benign paroxysmal torticollis* is a disease of infancy with an unknown cause, although a familial pattern has been described. Manifestations of the condition begin in the first year of life with recurrent episodes of head tilt that may be associated with emesis, pallor, agitation, ataxia, malaise, and behavioral changes. Attacks may last from several hours to several days. Spontaneous and complete remission usually occurs by 5 years of age. Some patients, however, go on to develop migraines or benign paroxysmal vertigo.

## ▶ DIFFERENTIAL DIAGNOSIS

The differential diagnosis of torticollis is listed in Box 80-1.

### Congenital Torticollis

Several congenital cervical spine anomalies can occur in conjunction with torticollis. Most of these anomalies can be diagnosed by radiographic studies of the cervical spine. *Pterygium colli,* a congenital web of the skin of the neck extending from the acromial process to the mastoid, can be restrictive and result in torticollis. *Congenital remnant cysts* within the body of the SCM are a less common cause of torticollis. Unilateral absence of one SCM results in unopposed action of the other muscle and produces a contralateral torticollis.

### Acquired Torticollis

Conditions that need to be considered in the differential diagnosis of acquired torticollis include cervical spine subluxations, infections of the head and neck (Grisel syndrome), neurologic disorders, and neoplasia. Laxity of the transverse cervical ligaments results in atlantoaxial instability in up to 15% of patients with Down syndrome.[5] Most of these children are asymptomatic, but subluxation of the cervical spine, most commonly a rotational atlantoaxial subluxation, may occur after trauma.[6] Nontraumatic subluxations of the atlantoaxial spine may arise as a result of head and neck infections or juvenile idiopathic arthritis (JIA). Torticollis may be the presenting finding in either the systemic onset or polyarticular forms of JIA, but this is rare. The current theory is that inflammatory reactions around the spine produce hyperemia and edema, which, in turn, lead to laxity of the supporting ligaments and a predisposition to spontaneous subluxations and torticollis.

Torticollis may also arise from acute cervical disk calcification caused by trauma or from an upper respiratory infection. *Ocular torticollis* may be caused by paralysis of the extraocular muscles, strabismus, nystagmus, and refractive errors. *Spasmus nutans,* also known as *nodding spasms* or *salaam spasms,* includes a triad of acquired nystagmus, head nodding,

BOX 80-1

## *Differential Diagnosis of Torticollis*

### CONGENITAL

- Muscular torticollis
- Postural torticollis
- Cervical spine anomalies
- Hemivertebra
- Atlantooccipital fusion
- Klippel-Feil syndrome
- Sprengel deformity
- Pterygium colli (webbed neck)
- Sternocleidomastoid cysts
- Cystic hygroma
- Bronchial cleft cyst
- Unilateral absence of sternocleidomastoid
- Occipital condylar dysplasia

### ACQUIRED

- Muscular
  - Cervical muscle injury
    - Traumatic
    - Awkward positioning during sleep
- Vertebral
  - Atlantoaxial subluxation
    - Laxity of the transverse cervical ligaments results in atlantoaxial instability in up to 15% of patients with Down syndrome.
  - C2–C3 subluxation
  - Rotary subluxation
  - Cervical fractures
  - Cervical vertebral osteomyelitis
  - Juvenile idiopathic arthritis (JIA)
    - Torticollis may rarely be the oresenting finding in either systemic onset or polyarticular JIA.
    - Inflammatory reactions around the spine produce hyperemia and edema, which lead to laxity of the supporting ligaments and a predisposition to spontaneous subluxations and torticollis.
  - Acute cervical disk calcification caused by trauma or respiratory infection
- Infectious
  - Infection of the head and neck (Grisel syndrome)
  - Upper respiratory infection
  - Retropharyngeal abscess
  - Cervical lymphadenitis
  - Cervical vertebral osteomyelitis
  - Dental infection
- Neurologic
  - Ocular torticollis with
    - Strabismus
    - Nystagmus
    - Refractive errors
    - Paralysis of extraocular muscles
  - Spasmus nutans (nystagmus, head nodding, and torticollis)
    - No known cause.
    - Signs and symptoms usually develop within the first 2 years of life.
    - May persist for months to years, but the course is often benign and self-limited.
    - But if accompanied by ataxia, suspect a erebellar tumor.
  - Dystonic torticollis
    - May follow the administration of phenothiazines, carbamazepine, or phenytoin.
    - Presence of other extrapyramidal signs can confirm a dystonic reaction.
  - Syringomyelia
  - Epidural hematoma
  - Labyrinthine torticollis
  - Brachial plexus palsy
  - Arnold-Chiari malformation
  - Accessory nerve palsy
  - Acute disseminated encephalomyelitis
  - Wilson disease
- Neoplastic
  - Cervical cord tumor
  - Posterior fossa tumor
  - Soft tissue tumor
  - Langerhans cell histiocytosis (histiocytosis X)
  - Infantile desmoid fibromatosis
- Other
  - Benign paroxysmal torticollis
  - Psychogenic torticollis
  - Sandifer syndrome
    - An abnormal posturing that includes torticollis and opisthotonos
    - Believed to be a protective mechanism adopted by some patients with gastroesophageal reflux, esophagitis, or hiatal hernia
  - Dermatogenic torticollis
    - A painful, stiff neck resulting from extensive local skin lesions
  - Spurious torticollis
    - Stiffness of the neck from dental malformations or caries

and torticollis, without a known cause. Signs and symptoms usually develop within the first 2 years of life and may persist for months to years. However, the clinical course often is benign and self-limited. A *dystonic torticollis* may follow the administration of several drugs, including phenothiazines, carbamazepine, and phenytoin. The presence of other extrapyramidal signs can often be used to distinguish patients who have dystonic reactions.

Neoplasms associated with torticollis include cervical cord tumors and cerebellar tumors. Posterior fossa masses may manifest similarly to spasmus nutans with nystagmus, head nodding, and torticollis. For patients with cerebellar tumors, however, ataxia is often a cardinal feature. *Sandifer syndrome* is an abnormal posturing that includes torticollis and opisthotonos. This syndrome is believed to be a protective mechanism adopted by some patients with one of several conditions, including gastroesophageal reflux, esophagitis, or hiatal hernia. *Dermatogenic torticollis* is a painful, stiff neck that results from extensive local skin lesions. Stiffness of the neck resulting from dental malformations and caries is called *spurious torticollis.*

## ▶ EVALUATION

### History

The first step in determining the cause of torticollis should be to obtain a thorough and detailed history. Particular attention should be given to duration of symptoms, variation in severity of symptoms at different times of day (morning stiffness), previous trauma, presence of fever, and other systemic manifestations, including other musculoskeletal system symptoms. In younger patients, the birth history is essential.

### Physical Examination

Physical examination should not be limited to the head and neck areas but should include all organ systems. Findings such as craniofacial asymmetry suggest a congenital torticollis of long duration. The presence of webs or cysts in the neck should raise the suspicion of pterygium colli or remnant cysts. Patients with acquired torticollis as a result of trauma often have a tender SCM. Point tenderness over the cervical spine may suggest an underlying fracture or subluxation. Cervical vertebral osteomyelitis should be suspected in patients who have point tenderness in association with an unexplained fever. A thorough examination of the musculoskeletal system is necessary to examine muscle tone, muscle strength, hip positions, and the alignment of the lower extremities and feet. All vertebrae must be examined, with attention paid to the presence of sacral dimples. Examination of peripheral joints should be done to assess for evidence of arthritis in the forms of joint swellings or limitations of movement in association with pain, warmth, or redness. A thorough neurologic exam must be completed, checking cranial nerves and including vision, sensation, reflexes, fine and gross motor skills, and cerebellar testing.

### Laboratory Evaluation

The presence of peripheral leukocytosis and increased sedimentation rate can be helpful adjuncts in diagnosing torticollis caused by infection or inflammation.

### Imaging Studies

Imaging of the cervical spine should be obtained in all neonates with torticollis and in older children who have findings that suggest vertebral involvement or who have persistent torticollis. Ultrasound is the imaging modality of choice for initial evaluation.[7] Patients with neurologic deficits should undergo prompt computed tomography scanning or magnetic resonance imaging of the head and neck.

## ▶ MANAGEMENT

Congenital muscular torticollis responds well to prompt conservative treatment during the first year of life.[8] Medical management includes passive and active stretching of the neck. *Gentle (passive) stretching* can be performed daily by the parents of the child or by a physical therapist. *Active stretching* is achieved by manipulating the infant's environment in such a way that objects of interest are located on the opposite side of the room from the torticollis, inducing the infant to turn the neck in the desired direction.

Surgical correction is essential if the deformity persists beyond the first year of life, if range of motion is restricted more than 30%, or if residual craniofacial deformity exists.[9,10] Craniofacial asymmetry is best reversed at an early age when the child's growth potential is at its maximum. The surgical procedure that has the best results involves a bipolar tenotomy of the affected SCM, followed by casting or bracing to maintain the corrected posture.[11]

Acquired muscular or ligamentous torticollis is managed with local heat, massage, analgesics, muscle relaxants, and a soft cervical collar. Symptoms usually resolve in 7 to 10 days. Notably, however, patients with acquired muscular or ligamentous torticollis experience only mild discomfort. Any child with severe neck pain or tenderness over the vertebra requires immediate cervical immobilization until radiography can be performed to exclude the possibility of vertebral fracture or subluxation.

Drug-induced dystonic reactions are reversed by discontinuing the offending drug and administering intravenous diphenhydramine. The treatment of torticollis arising from other specific diseases should be directed at the cause.

### When to Refer

- Presence of craniofacial asymmetry
- Radiographic evidence of cervical spine abnormality
- More than 30% restriction in range of motion
- Persistence beyond the first year of life

### When to Admit

- Presence of neurologic deficits
- Severe neck pain
- Point tenderness over the vertebrae

### *TOOLS FOR PRACTICE*

#### Engaging Patient and Family

- *Head Tilt* (fact sheet), American Academy of Pediatrics (www.healthychildren.org/English/health-issues/conditions/head-neck-nervous-system/Pages/Head-Tilt.aspx)
- *Positional Skull Deformities and Torticollis* (fact sheet), American Academy of Pediatrics (www.healthychildren.org/English/health-issues/conditions/head-neck-nervous-system/Pages/Positional-Skull-Deformities-and-Torticollis.aspx)

## REFERENCES


1. Davids JR, Wenger DR, Mubarak SJ. Congenital muscular torticollis: sequela of intrauterine or perinatal compartment syndrome. *J Pediatr Orthop*. 1993;13(2):141–147
2. Macdonald D. Sternomastoid tumour and muscular torticollis. *J Bone Joint Surg Br*. 1969;51(3):432–443
3. Hulbert KF. Congenital torticollis. *J Bone Joint Surg Br*. 1950;32:50–59
4. Ta JH, Krishnan M. Management of congenital muscular torticollis in a child: a case report and review. *Int J Pediatr Otorhinolaryngol*. 2012;76(11):1543–1546
5. Pueschel SM, Scola FH, Pezzullo JC. A longitudinal study of atlanto-dens relationships in asymptomatic individuals with Down syndrome. *Pediatrics*. 1992;89(6 Pt 2):1194–1198
6. Msall ME, Reese ME, DiGaudio K, et al. Symptomatic atlantoaxial instability associated with medical and rehabilitative procedures in children with Down syndrome. *Pediatrics*. 1990;85(3 Pt 2):447–449
7. Do TT. Congenital muscular torticollis: current concepts and review of treatment. *Curr Opin Pediatr*. 2006;18(1):26–29
8. Binder H, Eng GD, Gaiser JF, et al. Congenital muscular torticollis: results of conservative management with long-term follow-up in 85 cases. *Arch Phys Med Rehab*. 1987;68(4):222–225
9. Slate RK, Posnick JC, Armstrong DC, Buncic JR. Cervical spine subluxation associated with congenital muscular torticollis and craniofacial asymmetry. *Plast Reconstr Surg*. 1993;91(7):1187–1195
10. Wolfort FG, Kanter MA, Miller LB. Torticollis. *Plast Reconstr Surg*. 1989;84(4):682–692
11. Bharadwaj VK. Sternomastoid myoplasty: surgical correction of congenital torticollis. *J Otolaryngol*. 1997;26(1):44–48

# Chapter 81

# Vaginal Bleeding

*Maria Trent, MD, MPH; Alain Joffe, MD, MPH*

The assessment of vaginal bleeding depends largely on the pubertal status of the patient. In prepubertal girls, vaginal bleeding usually reflects a localized problem in the vagina or uterus. In pubertal girls and young women, the differential diagnosis includes disorders affecting the hypothalamic-pituitary-ovarian (HPO) axis and complications of pregnancy in addition to local causes. In all cases, however, a complete history and thorough physical examination will provide important clues to the diagnosis.

## ▶ PREPUBERTAL GIRLS

In utero, maternal estrogen diffuses across the placenta into the fetal circulation. After birth, estrogen levels in the infant fall, resulting in a physiologic vaginal discharge that can be blood tinged or frankly bloody. No treatment except reassurance is necessary, and the discharge usually disappears within 10 days.

Several conditions can result in vaginal bleeding in the prepubertal child, including vulvovaginal infections, excoriations secondary to pruritus, foreign bodies, sexual abuse, trauma (eg, involving a straddle injury during bike riding), tumors, condylomata, hemangiomas, polyps, and coagulopathies.[1] Any suggestion of sexual abuse, such as bruising, hymenal tears, or other signs of trauma, mandates obtaining a careful, nonthreatening history from the child and caretaker to determine the need for a referral to child protective services for full investigation including forensic interview and subspecialty medical evaluation.

Nighttime pruritus may indicate a pinworm infestation. The Scotch tape slide test, to look for pinworm eggs, can help establish *Enterobius vermicularis* infestation. If petechiae or numerous bruises are noted on physical examination, a platelet count and clotting studies are indicated to screen for a coagulopathy. A foreign body in the vagina should always be considered, even if no history of such exists. Contrary to popular belief, most girls who have bleeding from a foreign body do not have an associated foul-smelling discharge. The physician should also make sure that the bleeding is vaginal in origin, given that a prolapsed urethra can mimic vaginal bleeding.

Excoriation, erythema, or a rash in the perineal area make vaginitis a distinct possibility. If a vaginal discharge is found and microscopic examination demonstrates large numbers of white blood cells, then vaginitis is highly likely. Concern about sexual abuse should prompt cultures for *Neisseria gonorrhoeae* and *Chlamydia trachomatis*. Other bacterial cultures may be necessary. For example, a history of diarrhea in the weeks preceding onset of the bleeding suggests vaginitis caused by *Shigella* organisms. Group A beta-hemolytic streptococcus can also cause vaginitis.

Vaginal bleeding caused by a foreign body or vulvitis will respond to removal of the foreign body and proper perineal hygiene. Occasionally, systemic antibiotics may be necessary. Foreign bodies can often be washed out with a soft, flexible catheter; sharp objects should be removed carefully, under direct visualization. Care should be taken to avoid touching or manipulating the unestrogenized prepubertal hymen as to avoid pain to the child. Referral to a gynecologist may be required if the patient is uncooperative. After removal of a foreign body, bleeding should subside within 10 days. If it does not, then referral to a gynecologist is indicated. The entire foreign body may not have been removed, or a tumor, not readily visualized by the primary care physician, may be the actual cause of the bleeding. Similarly, when treatment of the presumed cause does not end the bleeding, referral for a more thorough examination is indicated.

## ▶ PUBERTAL GIRLS

### Evaluation

Abnormal vaginal bleeding in pubertal girls can indicate a variety of disorders. Evaluation of this symptom depends on the nature of the problem: Is she bleeding between normal periods, or have her previously regular menses become more frequent or heavier? A teenager whose prior menses have been regular might possibly begin to have infrequent but heavy menstrual bleeding. In general, normal periods in adult women (measured from the first day of 1 period to the first day of the next), range from 21 to 35 days with a flow of 3 to 7 days.[2] Flow greater than 1 week is considered excessive. A similar cycle pattern is observed in adolescent girls, but cycle length is more variable, especially in the first few years after menarche. Although the normal blood loss during menses is 30 to 40 mL, with an upper limit of 80 mL,[3,4] the quantity of blood loss is difficult to assess by history unless the patient reports very light flow.[5] History should include an assessment of menstrual pattern and the quantity of pads or tampons used. Although research has demonstrated the value of pictorial assessment to determine menstrual blood loss,[6] laboratory assessment of hemoglobin, hematocrit, or both is useful for determining if significant blood loss resulting in anemia has occurred.

Normal menstrual function requires that the HPO axis function properly. Follicle-stimulating hormone (FSH) causes maturation of ovarian follicles, which produce estrogen. Rising levels of estrogen stimulate the endometrial lining of the uterus to proliferate and, at the same time, induce a midcycle surge of luteinizing hormone (LH) that causes the primary follicle to release an ovum, after which LH and FSH levels fall. The remnants of the follicle (*corpus luteum*) now produce progesterone, which converts the proliferative endometrium to a secretory phase. At the end of a normal cycle, the corpus luteum involutes, and both estrogen and progesterone levels fall. The endometrial lining is shed, and bleeding occurs.[7]

In adolescents, especially young adolescents, the HPO axis is relatively immature and highly sensitive to disturbance by several endogenous and exogenous factors; this perturbation leads to irregular bleeding. Among young adolescents (but in some older adolescents as well), the axis has not yet matured, and most cycles are anovulatory. Thus the endometrium proliferates under estrogen stimulation from the maturing follicle, but the midcycle LH surge is absent, ovulation does not occur, and the progesterone-secreting corpus luteum never forms. Toward the end of the cycle, the follicle involutes, estrogen levels fall, and bleeding occurs.

Influenced by estrogen only, endometrial shedding is incomplete and irregular, accounting for the excessive bleeding of anovulatory cycles. Alternatively, fluctuating estrogen levels during an anovulatory cycle result in estrogen withdrawal bleeding. The occasional ovulatory cycle helps stabilize endometrial growth, and because the corpus luteum produces progesterone, a more organized withdrawal bleed occurs. Hence, any condition that increases the frequency of anovulatory cycles is more likely to produce the kind of uterine bleeding that prompts the teenager to seek medical care.

Most teenagers who seek evaluation for genital bleeding in the first few years after menarche will have abnormal uterine bleeding (AUB) secondary to an immaturity of the HPO axis, with resultant anovulatory cycles.[5] Because this is a diagnosis of exclusion, the primary care physician should search for other causes that affect the integrity of the HPO axis and can mimic AUB from this cause. Anovulatory cycles may also occur in patients with a mature HPO axis who have disorders such as polycystic ovary syndrome,[8] thyroid disease, or conditions resulting in hypothalamic amenorrhea (emotional stress, eating disorders, chronic illness, or intense athleticism). Additional causes of abnormal bleeding in this age group include disorders of pregnancy, other endocrine abnormalities, cervicitis, vaginitis, pelvic inflammatory disease, other sexually transmitted infections, foreign bodies, tumors, coagulopathies, drugs, and systemic disorders (Box 81-1).[3,5,9] Heavy bleeding at menarche, significant anemia, or the need to be hospitalized to control the bleeding all increase the likelihood that a coagulopathy or another pathologic condition is the cause of the bleeding.[7,10] Family history, however, has been shown to be a better predictor of coagulopathy than menstrual history.[11] While the International Federation of Gynecology and Obstetrics [FIGO] and the American College of Obstetrics and Gynecology (ACOG) have disregarded many of the old terms used to describe menstrual abnormalities and developed a new nomenclature for use in adult women termed PALM-COEIN (PALM [structural causes: *p*oly, *a*denomyosis, *l*eiomyoma, *m*alignancy and hyperplasia]; COEIN [nonstructural causes: *c*oagulopathy, *o*vulatory dysfunction, *e*ndometrial, *i*atrogenic, and *n*ot yet classified]),[12,13] it is important to adequately explore the diagnostic entities common in pubertal girls such as anovulatory bleeding, pregnancy, sexually transmitted infections, and von Willebrand disease.

## History

Most causes of vaginal bleeding or abnormal uterine bleeding (see Box 81-1) can be ruled out by history and physical examination. Maternal support during the initial history taking can be useful. Many mothers track the menstrual periods of their adolescent daughters, especially in the first years after menarche, and are keenly aware of the amount of bleeding based on the quantity of feminine products purchased, stained laundry, evidence of fatigue, and general level of their activity and behavior. A mother can often provide detailed family medical histories for first-degree female relatives, as well as that of her daughter.

Certain key aspects of the history may be difficult to obtain. A young woman may hesitate to reveal that she has engaged in sexual intercourse or that she has been sexually abused. The patient should be interviewed alone regarding sexual activity, sexually transmitted infections (including associated symptoms such as cramping, vaginal discharge, and dyspareunia), abuse, stress, weight changes and eating habits, participation in sports and other activities, chronic illnesses, other bleeding problems, medication use (particularly contraceptives), and substance use patterns. If a discharge is foul smelling and bloody, then a foreign body or

BOX 81-1

## *Possible Causes of Abnormal Uterine Bleeding*

### PREGNANCY COMPLICATIONS

- Spontaneous abortion
- Ectopic pregnancy
- Retained gestational products
- Trophoblastic disease

### HEMOSTATIC DISORDERS

- von Willebrand disease
- Idiopathic thrombocytopenia
- Coagulation factor deficiency
- Platelet dysfunction (eg, Glanzmann disease, Bernard-Soulier syndrome)

### THROMBOCYTOPENIA

- Immune thrombocytopenia
- Bone marrow infiltration by malignancy (eg, leukemia)
- Bone marrow failure disease (eg, aplastic anemia)

### SYSTEMIC DISEASE

- Systemic lupus erythematosus
- Renal failure
- Hepatic failure
- Malignancy

### CONDITIONS OF THE REPRODUCTIVE TRACT

#### *Vagina*

- Vaginitis
- Trauma
- Foreign body
- Congenital anomaly (septum)
- Neoplasia

#### *Cervix*

- Cervicitis, erosion
- Cervical polyp
- Neoplasia

#### *Uterus*

- Endometritis
- Endometrial polyp
- Submucosal leiomyoma
- Arteriovenous malformation
- Congenital anomaly
- Neoplasia

#### *Pancreas*

- Diabetes mellitus

#### *Pelvis*

- Endometriosis

### ENDOCRINE DISORDERS

#### *Hypothalamus, Pituitary*

- Immature HPO axis
- Hyperprolactinemia
- Anorexia nervosa, malnutrition
- Excessive exercise

#### *Ovary*

- Polycystic ovary syndrome
- Luteal phase abnormality
- Primary ovarian insufficiency
- Neoplasia (hormone secreting)

#### *Adrenal*

- Congenital adrenal hyperplasia
- Cushing disease
- Adrenal insufficiency
- Neoplasia

#### *Thyroid*

- Hypothyroidism
- Hyperthyroidism

#### *Iatrogenic*

- Hormonal contraceptives
- Anticoagulants
- Neuroleptics
- Intrauterine contraceptive device
- Androgens
- Spironolactone
- Antipsychotic medication
- Platelet inhibitors

retained tampon is likely; however, necrotic tumors can result in similar bleeding patterns. Pruritus or dysuria suggests vaginitis or cervicitis as the cause of the bleeding. Bleeding between periods is common during the first 2 or 3 cycles of oral contraceptive use and generally does not require any additional therapy; however, cervicitis secondary to *N gonorrhoeae* or *C trachomatis* infection or vaginitis secondary to *Trichomonas vaginalis* may also result in intermenstrual spotting. Young women who receive depot medroxyprogesterone acetate (Depo-Provera) injections often have frequent and irregular periods of excess bleeding, particularly in the first months after beginning use of this contraceptive method. Teenagers who forget to take 1 or 2 oral contraceptive pills may also have some bleeding.[3] Occasionally, women may have a small amount of bleeding or spotting after sexual intercourse, and some will have spotting around the time they ovulate. A complete family history is important to determine if other family members have any kind of bleeding problem. Complications of pregnancy (ectopic pregnancy or incomplete abortion) are more likely if a history of 1 or 2 missed periods exists, if the prior menstrual period was lighter than normal, if other symptoms of pregnancy are present (breast tenderness or nausea), or if the bleeding is accompanied by crampy, lower abdominal pain. A history of passing tissue or tissue present in the vaginal canal is also suggestive of complications of pregnancy. Blood dyscrasias, such as thrombocytopenia or von Willebrand disease, can cause heavy vaginal bleeding without other cutaneous manifestations of bleeding. Symptoms of endocrine disorders, such as cold intolerance, polyuria, nipple discharge, headache, acne, and increased facial hair, can be easily assessed using a comprehensive review of systems.

### Physical Examination

The physical examination should include measurement of height, weight, and blood pressure, as well as thorough palpation of the thyroid gland. Visual field and funduscopic examinations are necessary to help rule out a prolactinoma. Increased facial hair is consistent with polycystic ovaries or an adrenal tumor. Striae suggest Cushing disease. An enlarged clitoris is consistent with an androgen-secreting tumor or late-onset 21-hydoxylase deficiency. Normal findings on physical examination, including pelvic examination, help rule out the many causes of vaginal bleeding or abnormal uterine bleeding listed in Box 81-1. Vulvar or vaginal bruising or lacerations suggest the probability of sexual abuse, although the most common finding after sexual abuse is a normal examination without any evidence of trauma.[1] Lack of abdominal pain with adnexal or cervical motion tenderness excludes pelvic inflammatory disease.[14] If the ovaries are of normal size, then ovarian tumors or cysts are unlikely sources of the bleeding. A minimally enlarged uterus, consistent with early pregnancy, may not be noted by an inexperienced examiner. Endometrial polyps or submucous leiomyomas are distinctly unusual in women younger than 20 years, and they cannot be palpated by the examiner on the usual pelvic examination. With a patient who has an intractably heavy flow, these entities should be considered.

### Laboratory Tests

For most cases of vaginal bleeding, relatively few laboratory tests are needed. A complete blood count with indices provides an objective measurement of the amount and duration of bleeding and guides the treatment approach for patients with an otherwise negative evaluation. A urinalysis and urine pregnancy test should also be obtained. Bleeding associated with crampy lower abdominal pain may indicate ectopic pregnancy, and a quantitative serum pregnancy test is indicated. Screening for *N gonorrhoeae, C trachomatis,* trichomonas, and bacterial vaginosis is indicated for sexually active patients or when there is any suspicion of sexual abuse. A pelvic sonogram is indicated if ectopic pregnancy is suspected, if a pelvic mass is found on bimanual examination, or if the pelvic examination is difficult.

Thyroid-stimulating hormone function tests, prolactin, LH and FSH levels, and coagulation tests should be ordered if hormonal therapy is contemplated. Any evidence of hyperandrogenism necessitates measurement of androgens, which may initially include free and total testosterone, and dehydroepiandrosterone sulfate. Coagulation tests such as a prothrombin time, partial thromboplastin time, von Willebrand panel, and platelet aggregation studies are indicated if the patient has profuse hemorrhage, menorrhagia at menarche, a family history of bleeding disorders, or unexplained heavy vaginal bleeding. Measures of iron stores (eg, ferritin, reticulocyte count, hemoglobin content) may also be useful in managing iron deficiency even in the absence of anemia.

## Management

Sexually transmitted infections are easily diagnosed and can usually be treated with antibiotics.[14] The complications of pregnancy, such as threatened or spontaneous abortion, can be managed in the outpatient setting. However, a physician experienced in the management of early pregnancy should be consulted. For patients with bleeding disorders, consultation with a hematologist may be required.

Most cases of vaginal bleeding in adolescent girls are caused by anovulatory cycles. In other instances, the physician must manage the bleeding without knowing the cause. Treatment decisions can be guided using the patient's clinical symptoms and the results of basic laboratory testing. Although some physicians may feel comfortable using hormonal therapy, others may prefer the guidance of a more experienced physician. Because many patients with DUB are early adolescents accompanied by their parents, the primary care physician should include the parents in the decision to begin hormonal treatment in a non–sexually active patient. Assuring the parents that combined oral contraceptives (COCs) are, in this instance, being used as treatment; COCs are the most convenient way to package and deliver hormonal treatment; short-term use of COCs for 3 to 6 months is anticipated; and close follow-up will be provided during the treatment period, will often alleviate concerns about hormonal treatment and prevent rejection of these methods by the family. All patients with abnormal vaginal bleeding should be instructed to maintain a menstrual calendar to facilitate follow-up management.

Mild cases of AUB that do not result in anemia and that do not greatly upset the patient and her parents can be managed expectantly with no immediate, specific therapy. Those who have mild anemia (hemoglobin value 11–12 g/dL) should receive iron supplementation. Some problems will resolve in 3 or 4 cycles. For a sexually active patient, oral contraceptive pills can be prescribed to treat the bleeding, as well as to provide contraception. Nonsteroidal anti-inflammatory drugs (NSAIDs), such as ibuprofen or naproxen, can also be used for their demonstrated antiprostaglandin effects. It should be noted that patients with von Willebrand disease or other hemostatic abnormalities may have increased bleeding if NSAIDs are prescribed. Patients with mild bleeding should be reevaluated in 6 to 8 weeks.

In addition to iron supplementation, hormonal therapy is indicated in teenagers who have moderate AUB (enough to cause a decrease in hemoglobin to less than 11–12 g/dL). Girls who have menses every 1 to 3 weeks also need treatment. Treatment includes COCs or progestin alone. As previously mentioned, COCs are easier to use (1 pill is taken daily every day of the month). If the patient has a condition in which COCs are contraindicated or this method is rejected by the patient or her parents, then medroxyprogesterone 10 mg orally can be given daily for 10 to 14 days, beginning on the first day of each month (calendar method) or on the fourteenth day of the menstrual cycle (day 1 being the first day of bleeding).[2] The patient with moderate bleeding should be reassessed in 4 to 6 weeks.

Patients with severe prolonged heavy AUB accompanied by a drop in hemoglobin to 10 g/dL or less need to be treated more aggressively. In this instance, adolescent medicine or gynecologic consult should be sought, clotting studies obtained, and hospitalization strongly considered.[15] For patients with severe bleeding, COCs (1 tablet taken twice daily for 3 to 4 days) will generally stop the bleeding. However, prescribing a COC such as ethinyl estradiol-norgestrel–28 every 4 hours may be necessary initially until the bleeding stops, then every 6 hours for 24 hours, then every 8 hours for 4 days, and then twice daily to complete 3 weeks of hormonal therapy. Antiemetic medications may be required to counteract the side effects of the high levels of estrogen contained in this regimen. A withdrawal bleed will occur 2 to 4 days after completion of this initial course of therapy. Patients with significant AUB should avoid the placebo pills contained in the COC pill packs and remain on continuous COCs until the hemoglobin and hematocrit begin to normalize. Iron and folic acid supplementation should be included as a part of the therapeutic plan.

The need for blood transfusion will depend on the hemodynamic stability of the patient. Although some physicians prefer to use conjugated estrogens (25 mg intravenously every 4 hours) to stop the bleeding, use of ethinyl estradiol-norgestrel–28 or a similar COC given 6 times a day and then gradually tapered to once a day over the next 7 to 10 days will usually stop the bleeding. Endometrial biopsy or dilation and curettage is rarely indicated. Even when these measures succeed in controlling the vaginal bleeding, affected adolescents require long-term, close follow-up because an appreciable number of them will continue to have menstrual abnormalities.[15]

## When to Refer

- Patient is experiencing severe bleeding or initial attempts to control the bleeding by the primary care physician have failed.
- Vaginal bleeding seems to be secondary to a chronic illness that the primary care physician is unable to manage.
- Primary care physician feels uncomfortable performing a pelvic examination.
- Long-term hormonal therapy is required.
- Evidence of anatomical abnormality exists.
- Evidence of a complicated endocrine disorder exists.
- Evidence of a coagulopathy exists or additional guidance is required for further evaluation of a coagulation or hemostatic disorder.
- Evidence of a malignancy exists.
- Evidence of sexual abuse exists.

## When to Admit

- Patient shows evidence of hemodynamic instability.

### *TOOLS FOR PRACTICE*

#### Engaging Patient and Family

- *All About Menses* (Web page), Nemours Foundation (kidshealth.org/teen/sexual_health/girls/menstruation.html)
- *The Pelvic Exam* (handout), American Academy of Pediatrics (patiented.solutions.aap.org)
- *Puberty—Ready or Not, Expect Some Changes* (handout), American Academy of Pediatrics (patiented.solutions.aap.org)

#### Medical Decision Support

- *American College of Obstetricians and Gynecologists* (ACOG), (www.acog.org)
- *STD Treatment Guidelines* (Web page), Centers for Disease Control and Prevention (www.cdc.gov/std/treatment)
- *Young Women's Health Center* (Web site), Boston Children's Hospital (www.youngwomenshealth.org)

### *AAP POLICY STATEMENTS*

American Academy of Pediatrics Committee on Adolescence, American College of Obstetricians and Gynecologists and Committee on Adolescent Health Care. Menstruation in girls and adolescents: using the menstrual cycle as a vital sign. *Pediatrics.* 2006;118(5):2245–2250 (pediatrics.aappublications.org/content/118/5/2245.full)

American Academy of Pediatrics Committee on Sports Medicine and Fitness. Medical concerns in the female athlete. *Pediatrics.* 2000;106(3):610–613. Reaffirmed May 2008 (pediatrics.aappublications.org/content/106/3/610.full)

Jenny C, Crawford-Jakubiak JE; American Academy of Pediatrics Committee on Child Abuse and Neglect. The evaluation of children in the primary care setting when sexual abuse is suspected. *Pediatrics.* 2013;132(2):e558–e567 (pediatrics.aappublications.org/content/132/2/e558.full)

### *REFERENCES*


1. Adams JA, Knudson S. Genital findings in adolescent girls referred for suspected sexual abuse. *Arch Pediatr Adolesc Med.* 1996;150:850–857
2. Treloar AE, Boynton RE, Behn BG, et al. Variation in the human menstrual cycle through preproductive life. *Int J Fertil.* 1970;12:77–126
3. Emans SJ, Laufer MR, Goldstein DP. *Pediatric and Adolescent Gynecology.* 6th ed. Boston, MA: Lippincott-Raven; 2012
4. Hallberg L, Högdahl AM, Nilsson L, Rybo G. Menstrual blood loss—a population study. Variation at different ages and attempts to define normality. *Acta Obstet Gynecol Scand.* 1966;45:320–351
5. Fraser IS, McCarron G, Markham R. A preliminary study of factors influencing perception of menstrual blood loss volume. *Am J Obstet Gynecol.* 1984;149:788–793
6. Wyatt KM, Dimmock PW, Walker TJ, O'Brien PM. Determination of total menstrual blood loss. *Fertil Steril.* 2001;76:125–131
7. Speroff L, Fritz MA. Dysfunctional uterine bleeding. In: *Clinical Gynecologic Endocrinology and Infertility.* 7th ed. Baltimore, MD: Williams & Wilkins; 2005
8. Franks S. Polycystic ovary syndrome. *N Engl J Med.* 1995;333:853–861

9. Claessens EA, Cowell CA. Dysfunctional uterine bleeding in the adolescent. *Pediatr Clin North Am.* 1981;28:369–378
10. Chi C, Pollard D, Tuddenham EG, Kadir RA. Menorrhagia in adolescents with inherited bleeding disorders. *J Pediatr Adolesc Gynecol.* 2010;23(4):215–222
11. Jayasingehe Y, Moore P, Donath S, et al. Bleeding disorders in teenagers presenting with menorrhagia. *Aust N Z J Obstet Gynaecol.* 2005;45:439–443
12. Committee on Practice Bulletins—Gynecology. Practice bulletin no. 128: diagnosis of abnormal uterine bleeding in reproductive-aged women. *Obstet Gynecol.* 2012;120(1):197–206
13. Committee on Practice Bulletins—Gynecology. Practice bulletin no. 136: management of abnormal uterine bleeding associated with ovulatory dysfunction. *Obstet Gynecol.* 2013;122(1):176–185
14. Division of STD Prevention National Center for HIV/AIDS, Viral Hepatitis, STD, and TB Prevention. Sexually transmitted diseases treatment guidelines, 2010. *MMWR Recomm Rep.* 2010;59:1–110
15. Brawner NA, Koehler CSE. Abnormal uterine bleeding in the adolescent. *Adolesc Med.* 1994;5:157–170

# Chapter 82

# Vaginal Discharge

*Linda M. Dinerman, MD, PC; Alain Joffe, MD, MPH*

Vaginal discharge is a common complaint to pediatricians. However, the presence of discharge is not necessarily abnormal; this symptom may represent the vagina's response to changes in estrogen levels, and the pediatrician need only reassure the patient and her parents. In most circumstances, the age of the patient, her pubertal status, and whether she has ever had sexual intercourse are key elements in sorting out the cause of the discharge.

## ▶ NEWBORN PERIOD

In utero, the vaginal epithelium of the neonate is stimulated by maternal hormones that cross the placenta into the fetal circulation. After delivery, these hormone levels fall rapidly, and the parents may note a thick, grayish-white, mucoid discharge from the neonate's vagina. In many instances, the discharge is blood tinged or even grossly bloody. No treatment is needed, and the discharge usually resolves by 10 days of age.

## ▶ PREPUBERTAL GIRLS

The genital area of prepubertal girls is more susceptible to infection than that of older, pubertal girls. The labial folds are smaller and lack pubic hair, and the distance between the vagina and the rectum is relatively short compared with adolescents and adults.[1] Low levels of circulating estrogen render the vaginal mucosa relatively thin and susceptible to irritation or infection. The alkaline pH (approximately 7.0) of the vaginal secretions affords a hospitable environment to bacteria, which together with poor perineal hygiene, allows fecal flora to establish themselves more easily in the genital area. Box 82-1 lists causes of vaginal discharge in prepubertal girls.

### *Evaluation*

When evaluating a premenarchal girl who has vaginal discharge, the physician should inquire about her hygiene. Wiping from the rectum toward the vagina brings intestinal flora to the vaginal introitus. Use of chemicals such as bubble baths, deodorants, or strong detergents to launder underwear can irritate the vulva and vagina. Occlusive nylon or rayon underwear provides a moist environment for potential pathogens, and the material itself can be an irritant. Although accounting for less than 5% of cases of vaginal discharge, the possibility that the child or an abuser placed a foreign body, such as toilet paper, a coin, a small toy, or other objects, in her vagina should be considered. In such cases, the child has a discharge that can range from scant to abundant; can be white, brown, or bloody; and is frequently malodorous.[2]

BOX 82-1

## *Causes of Vaginal Discharge in Prepubertal Girls*

- Nonspecific vaginitis (the most common cause)
- Irritative (bubble baths, sand); the vulva is often involved as well. Nonabsorbent, occlusive clothing such as nylon undergarments, tights, bathing suits also irritate the vulva, leading to skin breakdown and infection. Although uncommon, *Candida* species infections can arise under these circumstances.
- Poor perineal hygiene
- Foreign body
- Associated systemic illness (group A streptococci, varicella)
- Other respiratory pathogens (eg, *Haemophilus influenzae*) may also cause discharge
- Enteric infections
- *Escherichia coli* with foreign body
- *Shigella* organisms
- *Yersinia* organisms
- *Enterobius vermicularis*
- Sexually transmitted infections (strong presumption of sexual abuse)
- *Neisseria gonorrhoeae*
- *Trichomonas vaginalis*
- *Chlamydia trachomatis* (Whether this organism alone can cause discharge is unclear. *C trachomatis* is often isolated in conjunction with *N gonorrhoeae*.)
- Primary vulvar skin disease
- Tumor, polyps (rare)

The parents should be asked about recent or concomitant illness. For example, vaginal discharge is associated with *Streptococcus pyogenes* infection (with or without scarlet fever) and with *Shigella* infection, occurring coincident with or after an episode of diarrhea. Systemic illnesses such as varicella also may be associated with vaginal discharge. Rectal infestations with *Enterobius vermicularis* (pinworms) can lead to vaginitis if the eggs are deposited around or in the vagina. A history of nocturnal itching accompanying vaginal discharge suggests this diagnosis. *Candida vulvovaginitis* is an uncommon cause of vaginal discharge or vulvovaginitis in prepubertal girls unless the child has recently taken antibiotics, has diabetes mellitus, is still in diapers, or is immunocompromised.[1]

Sexually transmitted organisms, such as *Neisseria gonorrhoeae, Chlamydia trachomatis*, and *Trichomonas vaginalis*, are known to cause vaginal infections in prepubertal girls. Whereas *N gonorrhoeae* clearly causes vaginal discharge, evidence that *C trachomatis* alone does so is limited.[3,4] The possibility of sexual abuse should always be considered in the evaluation of any child with vaginal discharge.

Although these other entities should be considered carefully as the physician evaluates the young patient, nonspecific vaginitis, in which no clear causative agent for the discharge can be established, accounts for 25% to 75% of cases of vulvovaginitis.[1] Rare causes of discharge include polyps or tumors; ectopic ureters, which drain urine into the vagina, resulting in a wetness that is mistaken for discharge; a draining pelvic abscess; or a prolapsed urethra, often associated with a bloody discharge.

The physical examination should include the entire genital and rectal area. The condition of the vulva, urethral meatus, and vaginal introitus should be noted. Infections in prepubertal girls usually involve the vulva as opposed to only the vagina. The presence of bruises, lacerations, or scrapes in the genital area is suggestive of sexual abuse, although it must be remembered that in most cases of child sexual abuse, the examination reveals no evidence of trauma. Excoriations around the rectum or vagina suggest itching caused by pinworms. A rash that spares skin folds is consistent with an irritative cause; one that is predominantly within the skin folds suggests candidiasis.

Having the girl sit on her mother's lap with her legs spread so that they dangle outside her mother's legs will often afford the examiner a clear view of the vulva and vaginal introitus. Alternatively, she may lie on her back in the frog-leg position or face down on the examining table in the knee-chest position. Care should be taken to avoid touching or manipulating the sensitive unestrogenized hymen of a prepubertal child to minimize pain. If a foreign body is thought to be present (because of a thick discharge that is often bloody and sometimes foul smelling) but not visualized, then irrigating the vagina with a soft, flexible catheter and tepid saline solution will often flush out bits of toilet paper or small objects.[1]

If sufficient vaginal discharge is present, then several drops of the secretion should be placed on 2 glass slides. If the discharge is scant, then a saline-moistened cotton swab can be introduced into the vagina to obtain samples for the glass slides. Several drops of normal saline solution should be added to 1 slide to create a wet preparation. Several drops of 10% potassium hydroxide should be added to the second slide, which should then be gently heated to dissolve epithelial cells, allowing visualization of hyphae. Slides should be examined, as indicated in Table 82-1. If indicated, cultures for *N gonorrhoeae* and *C trachomatis* should be performed; alternatively, evaluation with nucleic acid amplification tests may be easier to perform and provide more sensitive testing.[3] A piece of cellophane tape with its sticky side applied to the perianal area and then onto a glass slide for microscopic examination may reveal the typical eggs of *E vermicularis.*

## Management

If the history or physical examination suggests an irritative origin, then parents should discontinue the offending agent and have the child wear cotton underpants. Sitz baths will provide temporary relief until natural healing takes place. Removal of a foreign body will result in rapid improvement and cessation of the discharge. Pinworm infestations should be treated in the usual manner. Infections caused by poor personal hygiene will respond to the general measures just listed, coupled with instructions about proper perineal hygiene. If the discharge is associated with another infection (such as *S pyogenes* or *Shigella* organisms), then it will disappear as the underlying infection is treated.

When the organism causing the vaginal discharge is found to be sexually transmitted, more comprehensive evaluation and treatment are required.[1] Appropriate antibiotic treatment should be prescribed and a report to child protective services made.

Nonspecific vaginitis will usually respond to thorough perineal hygiene, sitz baths, and mild soaps. Patients should be advised to wear white cotton underpants and loose-fitting pants or skirts, to avoid nylon tights and tight pants, to avoid sitting for long periods in nylon bathing suits, and to wipe only from front to back. For persistent cases, the condition can be treated with amoxicillin, amoxicillin clavulanate, a cephalosporin, or clindamycin in standard childhood doses for 10 to 14 days.[1] Alternatively, a 1- to 2-month daily low-dose antibiotic may be helpful. If these approaches are unsuccessful, then antibiotic creams (mupirocin, gentamicin, metronidazole, or clindamycin) or estrogen creams may be used. If symptoms persist, the patient should then be referred to a pediatric gynecologist.

**Table 82-1**
**Major Causes of Vaginal Discharge in Pubertal Girls**

| AGENT | DISCHARGE | ODOR; pH | DYSURIA; PRURITUS | OTHER CLUES | DIAGNOSIS | TREATMENT[a] |
|---|---|---|---|---|---|---|
| *Candida albicans* | Thick, white, curdlike, cheesy | None usually; pH 4.5 (obtained from mid-vagina with nitrazine paper) | Dysuria frequent; pruritus (4+) | Vulva affected; association with use of some oral contraceptives and, in some women, with antibiotic use | Hyphae on potassium hydroxide examination | A variety of effective treatments are available for vaginal candidiasis, including creams, suppositories, and intravaginal tablets. Three-, 5-, and 7-day therapies offer no advantage over single-day treatments. Fluconazole 150 mg orally as a single dose is as effective as other regimens; however, more systemic side effects may occur. Ultimately, the *best* treatment is a combination of patient preference, what treatments are covered by her insurance policy, and whether it is less expensive or more convenient for the patient to obtain a prescription medication or purchase an over-the-counter treatment. |
| *Trichomonas vaginalis* | Frothy; yellow-green or gray | Foul smelling; pH 5.2–5.5 | Dysuria frequent; pruritus | Low abdominal pain; "strawberry" cervix; punctate vaginal hemorrhages | Motile trichomonads on wet preparation; avoid drying specimen; affirm VP III & OSOM tests are commercially available tests when microscopy is not available | Metronidazole 2 g orally in a single dose or tinidazole 2 g orally in a single dose. Alternative regimens include metronidazole 500 mg orally twice daily for 7 days. If failure occurs with either of the indicated regimens (and reinfection is excluded), the patient should be treated with metronidazole 500 mg twice daily for 7 days. Repeated failures should be treated with tinidazole or metronidazole at 2 g orally for 5 days. The patient should be advised to avoid alcohol until 24 hours after completion of therapy with metronidazole or 72 hours after treatment with tinidazole. |
| Bacterial vaginosis[b] | Homogeneous, thin, white discharge that smoothly coats the vaginal walls | A fishy odor of vaginal discharge before or after addition of 10% KOH (ie, the whiff test); pH >4.5 | No dysuria; slight pruritus | Occurs in association with anaerobes and *G vaginalis* | Clue cells on wet preparation (bacteria-coated epithelial cells); affirm VP III & OSOM Blue BV tests are commercially available tests when microscopy is not available | Metronidazole 500 mg orally twice daily for 7 days, metronidazole gel 0.75% 1 full applicator (5 g) intravaginally once daily for 5 days or clindamycin cream 2%, 1 full applicator (5 g) intravaginally every night at bedtime for 7 days. Alternative regimens include tinidazole 2 g orally once daily for 2 days or tinidazole 1 g orally once daily for 5 days or clindamycin 300 mg orally twice daily for 7 days or clindamycin ovules 100 mg intravaginally 1 at bedtime for 3 days. The patient should be advised to avoid alcohol until 24 hours after completion of therapy with metronidazole or 72 hours after treatment with tinidazole. |

[a]Centers for Disease Control and Prevention. Sexually transmitted diseases treatment guidelines. *MMWR Recomm Rep*. 2010;59(RR-12):1–110.
[b]Must have 3 of these 4 criteria to make diagnosis.
Data from Amsel R, et al. *Am J Med*. 1983;74:14; Brunham RC, et al. *N Engl J Med*. 1984;311:1; Rein MF, Chapel TA. *Clin Obstet Gynecol*. 1975;18:73; and Sobel J. *N Engl J Med*. 1997;337:1896.

## ▶ PUBERTAL AND POSTPUBERTAL ADOLESCENTS

With the onset of puberty, circulating estrogen and progesterone levels rise, stimulating vaginal mucus production and an increase in the turnover of vaginal epithelial cells. Bartholin and sebaceous glands are also stimulated. Generally, the clear mucoid discharge that results will not cause problems. The amount of secretion, however, can increase with sexual excitement, as well as midway through a normal menstrual cycle. Discharge is particularly prominent at the onset of puberty (physiologic leukorrhea). Examination of a wet preparation will reveal vaginal epithelial cells only. The high protein content of this discharge, absorbed onto underwear, causes yellow staining. Traditionally, occlusive nylon or rayon underpants have been alleged to cause a nonspecific vaginal discharge; however, that association may be spurious.

A wide variety of organisms are normally found in the vagina. These organisms, especially the lactobacilli, help maintain the normal acidic pH of the vagina, which resists infection. Some of the organisms that cause vaginitis and vaginal discharge in this age group are sexually transmitted or associated with sexual activity.[5] Because many teenagers fear admitting to sexual intercourse, a negative response to queries about sexual activity should not rule out consideration of a sexually transmitted organism as the cause of the discharge. Sexual abuse and the presence of a foreign body (eg, a retained tampon or condom) should also be considered. If a sexually transmitted organism has caused the discharge, then the patient's sexual partner should be notified and treated. Patients should refrain from sexual intercourse until they complete treatment. Otherwise, reinfection from the partner may occur. Use of spermicides or douching can cause vaginitis.[6]

The organisms and conditions commonly responsible for vaginal infections or vaginal discharge in pubertal young women and their treatments are listed in Table 82-1. Although the characteristics of each type of infection are said to be typical, the discharge observed on examination does not always fit these classic presentations.[7,8] The laboratory methods outlined in Table 82-1 therefore are of considerable diagnostic utility. However, they are not 100% sensitive. *T vaginalis* may not be noted during microscopic examination even if the vaginal fluid is examined immediately under the microscope to avoid drying of the organisms. The vaginal wet preparation is 64% to 80% sensitive at identifying trichomonads compared with culture, depending on the presence of symptoms and the experience of the microscopist. Culture is the most sensitive and specific commercially available method of diagnosis for *T vaginalis*. Other, newer tests such as direct fluorescent antibody, polymerase chain reaction, and enzyme immunoassay have higher detection rates but are not yet commonly used in clinical practice.[7,9] Papanicolaou tests also detect the presence of trichomonas, but the sensitivity is less than that of the wet preparation, and false positives can occur.[7,9] Although the Centers for Disease Control and Prevention consider a Gram stain the gold standard for the diagnosis of bacterial vaginosis, it is not widely used in clinical practice. In the absence of a Gram stain, 3 of 4 clinical criteria should be met to make the diagnosis: (1) homogeneous, thin white discharge evenly coating the vaginal walls; (2) clue cells on microscopic examination; (3) vaginal fluid pH higher than 4.5; (4) positive "whiff test"—a fishy odor to the vaginal discharge before or after the addition of 10% KOH. A DNA probe-based test, as well as a card test to detect increased pH and trimethylamine and proline-aminopeptidase, may also be useful in the diagnosis of bacterial vaginosis, but they are not widely used.

The role of *N gonorrhoeae* and *C trachomatis* in causing vaginal discharge has been reassessed recently. The presence of yellow vaginal discharge on speculum examination has been associated with infection by either organism; in contrast, neither profuse vaginal discharge nor a foul or fishy odor predicted infection with either. Nonetheless, because sexually transmitted infections often co-occur, appropriate screening tests for *N gonorrhoeae* and *C trachomatis* should be part of the evaluation of vaginitis if *T vaginalis* is found or if the patient reports a new sexual partner.

Bacterial vaginosis is a complex syndrome characterized by decreased *lactobacilli* and increased concentrations of several anaerobic microorganisms. The pathogenesis of this disorder continues to be poorly understood.[7,9] Bacterial vaginosis is associated with having multiple sex partners, douching, smoking, and the presence of sexually transmitted infections.[8] However, because it sometimes occurs in women who have never had sexual contact, bacterial vaginosis is not considered a sexually transmitted infection. Current evidence indicates that women who have bacterial vaginosis are at increased risk for developing pelvic inflammatory disease after instrumentation of the genital tract and, if pregnant, are more likely to deliver a premature infant or experience postpartum complications. Therefore, prompt treatment is essential. Treatment of sexual partners is not currently recommended because it does not affect the disease process.[7]

Occasionally, herpesvirus infections of the vulvovaginal area or cervix (or both) are associated with vaginal discharge. Typically, pain or a burning sensation is felt in the genital area. The vulva is reddened, and groups of small vesicles are noted on the vulva, in the vagina, or on the cervix. If the vesicles have ruptured, then the examiner sees only small ulcerations. Inguinal adenopathy, fever, and malaise are usually present if this attack is the first one.

A teenager who has a persistent discharge that is unresponsive to therapy may not be complying with treatment or may have become reinfected by an untreated partner. If such is not the case, and if *N gonorrhoeae, C trachomatis*, and *T vaginalis* are excluded, and the discharge does not appear to fit any of the causes described earlier, then a trial of sitz baths, use of cotton as opposed to nylon underwear, and careful attention to perineal hygiene are warranted. If symptoms persist, then the patient should be referred to an adolescent medicine specialist or a gynecologist.

Candidal infections can be especially difficult to treat and may recur. Factors that predispose to candidiasis include oral contraceptive use, broad-spectrum antibiotic use, and diabetes mellitus.[8] In cases of recurrent vulvovaginal candidiasis, either topical therapy for 7 to 14 days or oral fluconazole 150 mg repeated 72 hours after the first dose is recommended as initial treatment. If more intensive treatment is warranted, a recent study of adult women with recurrent vulvovaginal candidiasis demonstrated significant reduction of symptoms among those treated with oral fluconazole 150 mg once weekly for 6 months after initial treatment of 1 dose every 3 days for 3 doses.[10,11] A variety of monthlong antifungal treatments have been successful; however, intravaginal treatment over a long period is inconvenient for most patients. Although long-term ketoconazole has been used to suppress recurrent infection, hepatotoxicity is a concern. Male sexual partners should also be treated if they have any signs or symptoms of penile candidal involvement.

## When to Refer

- Physician is uncomfortable with evaluating genital complaints in prepubertal girls
- Physician lacks experience in performing pelvic examinations
- Evaluation yields evidence of sexual abuse
- Discharge persists despite seemingly appropriate therapy

## TOOLS FOR PRACTICE

### Engaging Patient and Family

- *Center for Young Women's Health* (Web page), Boston Children's Hospital (www.youngwomenshealth.org)
- *Info for Teens* (Web page), Planned Parenthood (www.plannedparenthood.org/info-for-teens)
- *The Pelvic Exam* (handout), American Academy of Pediatrics (patiented.solutions.aap.org)

## AAP POLICY STATEMENTS

American Academy of Pediatrics Committee on Infectious Diseases and Committee on Fetus and Newborn. Recommendations for the prevention of perinatal group B streptococcal (GBS) disease. 2011;128:611–616 (pediatrics.aappublications.org/content/128/3/611)

Kellog N; American Academy of Pediatrics Committee on Child Abuse and Neglect. The evaluation of sexual abuse in children. *Pediatrics*. 2005;116(2):506–512 (pediatrics.aappublications.org/content/116/2/506)

## REFERENCES

1. Emans SJ, Laufer MR, Goldstein DP. *Pediatric and Adolescent Gynecology*. 5th ed. Philadelphia, PA: Lippincott Williams & Wilkins; 2005
2. Smith YR, Berman DR, Quint EH. Premenarchal vaginal discharge: findings of procedures to rule out foreign bodies. *J Pediatr Adolesc Gynecol*. 2002;13:227–230
3. Shapiro RA, Schubert CJ, Siegel RM. Neisseria gonorrhea infections in girls younger than 12 years of age evaluated for vaginitis. *Pediatrics*. 1999;104:e72
4. Stricker T, Navratil F, Sennhauser FH. Vulvovaginitis in prepubertal girls. *Arch Dis Child*. 2003;88:324–326
5. Syed TS, Braverman PK. Vaginitis in adolescents. *Adolesc Med Clin*. 2004;15:235–251
6. Jaquiery A, Stylianopoulos A, Hogg G, Grover S. Vulvovaginitis: clinical features, aetiology, and microbiology of the genital tract. *Arch Dis Child*. 1999;81:64–67
7. Sobel JD. What's new in bacterial vaginosis and trichomoniasis? *Infect Dis Clin North Am*. 2005;19(2):387–406
8. Steele RW. Prevention and management of sexually transmitted diseases in adolescents. *Adolesc Med*. 2000;11:315–326
9. Spigarelli MG, Biro FM. Sexually transmitted disease testing: evaluation of diagnostic tests and methods. *Adolesc Med Clin*. 2004;15:287–299
10. Sobel JD, Wiesenfeld HC, Martens M, et al. Maintenance fluconazole therapy for recurrent vulvovaginal candidiasis. *N Engl J Med*. 2004;351:876–883
11. Centers for Disease Control and Prevention. Sexually transmitted diseases treatment guidelines. *MMWR Recomm Rep*. 2010;59(RR-12):1–110

## ▶ CAUSES AND DIFFERENTIAL DIAGNOSIS

Box 83-1 lists the most frequent causes of vomiting in infants and children. In infancy, regurgitation, or spitting up, is very common and most often a developmental event that has no sequelae and gradually resolves. Pathologic gastroesophageal reflux (ie, gastroesophageal reflux disease) is defined by the association of regurgitation with complications, including esophagitis (sometimes with anemia or stricture), recurrent apnea, aspiration pneumonia, or failure to thrive.[5] Bilious vomiting, especially when associated with the first vomitus, usually occurs only with ileus or intestinal tract obstruction below the ampulla of Vater (second portion of the duodenum). In newborns, bilious vomiting can be associated with necrotizing enterocolitis. In older children who vomit persistently, reflux of bile from the duodenum into the stomach may lead to bilious vomiting without gastrointestinal tract obstruction. Projectile vomiting commonly occurs with pyloric stenosis. When this condition persists, however, gastric atony may eliminate the projectile character. A succussion splash (the splashing sound present when a patient who has fluid in a hollow organ is gently shaken on physical examination) may be present, as in other causes of gastric outlet obstruction. Vomiting associated with increased intracranial pressure may be projectile and may take place in the absence of nausea or retching.

Persistent vomiting in a newborn or young infant who has no evidence of infection usually suggests a congenital gastrointestinal anomaly, inborn error of metabolism, or CNS abnormality such as hydrocephalus or subdural effusion. If the history and physical examination results do not suggest a cause, then evaluating all 3 possibilities simultaneously is best. When the sudden onset of bilious vomiting develops in a previously well newborn, especially within the first few days of life, the physician must consider a malrotation with secondary midgut volvulus. Midgut volvulus is a surgical emergency requiring early diagnosis and surgical intervention. In a sick newborn, the diagnosis of necrotizing enterocolitis must be considered in the event of bilious vomiting, especially with blood in the stool. Beyond the first week of life but within the first 2 months, pyloric stenosis is the most common cause of persistent vomiting in an otherwise well infant. In the older infant or child, the entire spectrum of causes of vomiting listed in Box 83-1 should be considered. Patients who have celiac disease may occasionally have minimal or no diarrhea but prominent vomiting. When an older child exhibits acute vomiting and somnolence, the physician should always consider drug overdose (especially acetaminophen, aspirin, or iron), meningoencephalitis, and inborn errors of metabolism (especially mitochondrial fatty acid oxidation) in the differential diagnosis. Persistent or recurrent vomiting without other symptoms may be the major manifestation of an emotional disorder in childhood. Therefore, a complete psychosocial history is an important part of the evaluation.

Cyclic vomiting is characterized by repeated episodes of intense nausea and vomiting with at least 3 attacks over a 6-month period or 5 attacks in any interval. Episodes last 1 hour to 10 days and are separated by at least a week. In an individual, the attacks are very stereotypic.[6] Uncontrollable vomiting and retching (at least 4 times in an hour for at least 1 hour) are typical of an attack; but between episodes, children act well. Approximately 10% of these children have an identifiable gastrointestinal or extraintestinal (eg, renal, metabolic, or neurologic) disorder as the probable cause.

Abdominal migraine is a common cause of cyclic vomiting and is characterized by the paroxysmal onset of repetitious attacks often relieved with sleep.[7] A strong family history of

**BOX 83-1**

## *Causes of Vomiting (Arranged by Usual Age of Earliest Occurrence)*

### INFANCY/EARLY CHILDHOOD

#### *Gastrointestinal*

Congenital

- Regurgitation—gastroesophageal reflux (developmental or pathologic)
- Atresia—stenosis (tracheoesophageal fistula, antral web, intestinal atresia, annular pancreas)
- Gastrointestinal tract duplication
- Volvulus (secondary to an error in rotation and fixation or to Meckel diverticulum)
- Congenital bands
- Meconium ileus (cystic fibrosis), meconium plug
- Hirschsprung disease

Acquired

- Acute infectious gastroenteritis
- Food allergy, cow milk protein intolerance, eosinophilic gastroenteritis
- Eosinophilic esophagitis
- Pyloric stenosis
- Intussusception
- Celiac disease—risk is inherited, but clinical manifestations occur only after introduction of gluten in diet
- Incarcerated hernia—inguinal, internal secondary to old adhesions
- Postviral gastroparesis[a]
- Adynamic ileus—the mediator for many nongastrointestinal causes of vomiting
- Neonatal necrotizing enterocolitis
- Chronic granulomatous disease with gastric outlet obstruction

#### *Nongastrointestinal*

- Infectious—otitis, urinary tract infection, pneumonia, upper respiratory tract infection, sepsis, meningitis
- Metabolic—aminoaciduria and organic aciduria, galactosemia, fructosemia, adrenogenital syndrome, renal tubular acidosis, hyperammonemia, disorders of fatty acid oxidation (eg, medium-chain acyl-coenzyme A dehydrogenase deficiency), mitochondrial disease
- Central nervous system—trauma, tumor, infection, increased intracranial pressure, ventriculoperitoneal shunt failure, diencephalic syndrome, rumination, autonomic responses (pain, shock), anticipatory nausea and vomiting

### CHILDHOOD/ADOLESCENCE

#### *Gastrointestinal*

- Appendicitis
- Food poisoning (staphylococcal, clostridial)
- Peptic disease—ulcer, gastritis, duodenitis, *Helicobacter pylori* infection
- Trauma—duodenal hematoma, traumatic pancreatitis, perforated bowel
- Pancreatitis—viral, trauma, drug induced, cystic fibrosis, hyperparathyroidism, hyperlipidemia, organic acidemias, hereditary pancreatitis, cystic fibrosis gene mutation
- Gallbladder—cholelithiasis, choledochal cyst
- Crohn disease
- Adhesions—congenital or secondary to previous abdominal surgery
- Visceral neuropathy or myopathy
- Superior mesenteric artery syndrome[b]

#### *Nongastrointestinal*

- Medications—anticholinergics, alcohol, idiosyncratic reaction (eg, codeine), chemotherapy, radiation therapy, overdose (especially aspirin or acetaminophen)
- Central nervous system—cyclic vomiting, migraine, anorexia nervosa, bulimia nervosa
- Motion sickness
- Metabolic—diabetic ketoacidosis, acute intermittent porphyria
- Pregnancy

[a]Sigurdsson L, Flores A, Putnam PE, et al. Postviral gastroparesis: presentation, treatment, and outcome. *J Pediatr.* 1997;131(5):751–754.

[b]Biank V, Werlin S. Superior mesenteric artery syndrome in children: a 20-year experience. *J Pediatr Gastroenterol Nutr.* 2006;42:522.

migraine is common. Headache typical of migraine may rarely occur with episodes; abdominal pain is not unusual. Cyproheptadine, amitriptyline, topiramate, and propranolol are highly effective as prophylactic treatment for abdominal migraine; treatment success helps confirm the diagnosis. Abdominal epilepsy is a much less common cause of cyclic vomiting. A complete history of the sequence of events and electroencephalographic evaluation are useful in the evaluation, and anticonvulsants can be tried when this condition is suspected.

## ▶ EVALUATION

Patient history is often the most helpful in narrowing the wide range of potential causes of vomiting. Evaluation of the gastrointestinal tract usually includes an upper gastrointestinal contrast roentgenographic study. However, in an infant with persistent vomiting between 2 and 12 weeks of age, the first study is often an ultrasound of the abdomen for pyloric stenosis. Food allergy is in the differential diagnosis for gastroesophageal reflux in infants; therefore, with intractable reflux symptoms, it is reasonable to undertake a 2-week feeding trial with hypoallergenic formula. In the older infant or child with intractable reflux symptoms, eosinophilic esophagitis should be a consideration and requires endoscopic evaluation of the esophagus. Endoscopy is feasible in all children, even newborns, if performed by an experienced examiner using an appropriately sized instrument. Esophageal pH monitoring and impedance monitoring, esophageal biopsies, and gastroesophageal scintiscan are all useful in establishing a diagnosis of gastroesophageal reflux. Endoscopically placed wireless esophageal pH capsule monitoring can be performed in children older than 2 to 3 years and is generally well tolerated.

If brain tumor is a consideration, magnetic resonance imaging is more sensitive than a computed tomography scan of the head. Further workup for metabolic or neurologic disease should be considered, as appropriate. With persistent vomiting, the physician should expect to see a metabolic alkalosis; metabolic acidosis raises concerns about an underlying metabolic disorder or drug intoxication. Metabolic workup often includes a urine test for organic acids and amino acids, urinalysis for ketones as well as serum glucose, blood urea nitrogen, electrolytes, lactate, ammonia, and total carnitine and acylcarnitine levels. In a postpubertal girl, pregnancy must always be considered in the differential diagnosis of vomiting.

When a midgut volvulus is suspected in a newborn or older child, a plain radiograph of the abdomen may show a paucity of gas distal to the upper small intestine; however, the radiograph may not be helpful. An upper gastrointestinal contrast radiographic study should be done at once, with the controlled introduction of barium through a nasogastric tube after gastric aspiration. A barium enema investigation of cecal position is a less reliable study when evaluating a patient for malrotation because of the lack of complete correlation of developmental rotation of the cecum with that of the duodenum.

## ▶ COMPLICATIONS

The most significant complications of vomiting include dehydration and electrolyte imbalance, especially when the vomiting is persistent, as well as aspiration pneumonia, hemorrhage from prolapse gastropathy (a hemorrhagic area on the posterior wall of the proximal stomach), or, less commonly, a tear at the gastroesophageal junction (Mallory-Weiss syndrome) and rupture of the esophagus (very uncommon in children). Feeding refusal may follow persistent vomiting, especially in infants.[8]

## ▶ TREATMENT

Acute intercurrent vomiting without serious underlying disease or significant dehydration should be treated by administering clear liquids by mouth (eg, in acute gastroenteritis or otitis media). The usually advisable course is to start with a period of 4 to 6 hours without oral intake and then begin with frequent small quantities of clear liquids (1 teaspoonful every few minutes for infants) and gradually increase the volume and extension of the period between oral fluids. If vomiting is associated with diarrhea and dehydration, then oral rehydration solution is indicated. Carbonated beverages may increase vomiting. Fluids of high osmolality, long-chain triglycerides, and anticholinergic drugs all tend to slow gastric emptying and should be avoided.

The drugs used most commonly, when necessary, for symptomatic improvement of acute or persistent vomiting are ondansetron and promethazine. If emesis interferes with administration, ondansetron is available as an oral disintegrating tablet and promethazine as a suppository. Ondansetron is generally preferred because of fewer side effects. When indicated, ondansetron has been used in children older than 6 months for vomiting associated with gastroenteritis, reducing the frequency of emesis and need for intravenous hydration.[9]

For chemotherapy-induced vomiting, 5-$HT_3$ receptor antagonists (especially ondansetron and granisetron) have been effective. Dexamethasone and $NK_1$ receptor antagonists (aprepitant) can be added when necessary.[2,3] Metoclopramide is added occasionally, but less frequently than in the past. Unfortunately, these treatments are not as effective in controlling nausea as vomiting.

$H_1$ receptor antagonists (including diphenhydramine, dimenhydrinate, meclizine, and promethazine) and muscarinic cholinergic receptor antagonists (eg, scopolamine) prevent motion sickness.[4] Low-dose erythromycin or metoclopramide has been used to treat poor gastric emptying when there is not a mechanical obstruction (eg, postviral gastroparesis).

Patients should be monitored for signs of dehydration. For persistent vomiting with feeding, a nasoduodenal infusion may be useful. Significant vomiting that requires intravenous fluid therapy is usually associated with hypochloremic alkalosis with secondary hypokalemia. Intravenous fluids should repair the deficits.

Management of gastroesophageal reflux must be individualized.[5] The extent of treatment necessary depends on the volume of emesis and the presence of complications of reflux. Medical management for infants includes thickening feedings with cereal (a standard concentration is 1 tablespoonful of cereal for each 1 to 2 ounces of formula) or the use of commercial antiregurgitant formula, which can reduce the amount of overt emesis but not reflux into the esophagus. Although prone positioning of young infants reduces reflux, this should only be done when the infant is observed and awake because the risk for sudden infant death syndrome is increased in this position. Prone positioning may be useful after 1 year of age. Left lateral decubitus positioning is discouraged for sleeping infants as well because these infants may become prone during sleep. Elevating the head of the bed remains standard therapy for older children and adults. Older children may benefit from avoiding snacks or liquids after dinner and agents that exacerbate esophagitis (alcohol, caffeine, and smoking). Medications are commonly used to decrease exposure of the esophageal mucosa to acid (antacids, $H_1$ receptor blockers, or proton pump inhibitors). Attempts to improve lower esophageal function and gastric emptying (eg, metoclopramide) have been less successful because of unacceptable medication side effects. Baclofen has been suggested as an agent to reduce the frequency of inappropriate relaxations of the lower esophageal sphincter, but there is still limited experience in children. A slurry of sucralfate (a cytoprotective agent) is used occasionally for management of acid damage to the esophagus. When a child has severe gastroesophageal reflux, medical management may be unsatisfactory. In this case, antireflux surgery (fundoplication) should be considered. In this group of children, the results of surgery are generally good when performed by an experienced surgeon, and the benefits can be long lasting. In children who have psychomotor retardation and gastroesophageal reflux, antireflux surgery may not eliminate respiratory symptoms because other factors, such as swallowing dysfunction, may contribute to these findings. Among children undergoing a Nissen fundoplication, the risk for postoperative complication may be in the range of 10% to 30% and underscores the need for careful patient selection for this operation.

## When to Refer

- Persistent vomiting
- Recurrent episodes of vomiting
- Vomiting associated with a significant underlying process (eg, surgical abdomen, neurologic problem)

## When to Admit

- Intractable vomiting with dehydration
- Vomiting in association with symptoms or signs of an acute abdominal process (eg, acute appendicitis, pancreatitis, cholecystitis)
- Vomiting in association with symptoms or signs of raised intracranial pressure

## *TOOLS FOR PRACTICE*

### Engaging Patient and Family

- *Caring for Your Baby and Young Child: Birth to Age 5* (book), American Academy of Pediatrics (shop.aap.org)
- *Vomiting* (Web page), American Academy of Pediatrics (www.healthychildren.org/English/tips-tools/Symptom-Checker/Pages/Vomiting.aspx)

### Medical Decision Support

- *Pediatric Gastroesophageal Reflux Clinical Practice Guidelines: Joint Recommendations of the North American Society for Pediatric Gastroenterology, Hepatology, and Nutrition (NASPGHAN) and the European Society for Pediatric Gastroenterology, Hepatology, and Nutrition (ESPGHAN)* (article), *Journal of Pediatric Gastroenterology and Nutrition*, Vol 49, Issue 4, 2009

## *AAP POLICY STATEMENT*

Lightdale JR, Gremse DA; American Academy of Pediatrics Section on Gastroenterology, Hepatology, and Nutrition. Gastroesophageal reflux: management guidance for the pediatrician. *Pediatrics*. 2013;131(5):e1684–e1695 (pediatrics.aappublications.org/content/131/5/e1684.full)

## REFERENCES


1. Grundy D. Nausea and vomiting—an interdisciplinary approach. *Auton Neurosci.* 2006;129:1–2
2. Sanger GJ, Andrews PL. Treatment of nausea and vomiting: gaps in our knowledge. *Auton Neurosci.* 2006;129:3–16
3. Choi MR, Jiles C, Seibel NL. Aprepitant use in children, adolescents, and young adults for the control of chemotherapy-induced nausea and vomiting (CINV). *J Pediatr Hematol Oncol.* 2010;32:e268–e271
4. Golding JF. Motion sickness susceptibility. *Auton Neurosci.* 2006;129:67–76
5. Vandenplas Y, Rudolph CD, Di Lorenzo C, et al. Pediatric gastroesophageal reflux clinical practice guidelines: joint recommendations of the North American Society for Pediatric Gastroenterology, Hepatology, and Nutrition (NASPGHAN) and the European Society for Pediatric Gastroenterology, Hepatology, and Nutrition (ESPGHAN). *J Pediatr Gastroenterol Nutr.* 2009;49:498–547
6. Li BU, Lefevre F, Chelimsky GG, et al. North American Society for Pediatric Gastroenterology, Hepatology, and Nutrition consensus statement on the diagnosis and management of cyclic vomiting syndrome. *J Pediatr Gastroenterol Nutr.* 2008;47:379–393
7. Lewis DW. *Pediatric migraine. Neurol Clin.* 2009;27:481–501
8. Richards CA, Andrews PL. Food refusal: a sign of nausea? *J Pediatr Gastroenterol Nutr.* 2004;38:227–228
9. Freedman SB, Adler M, Seshadri R, Powell EC. Oral ondansetron for gastroenteritis in a pediatric emergency department. *N Engl J Med.* 2006;354:1698–1705

swallowing or occasional choking may be noted at the beginning of the feeding. The mother's motivation to breastfeed and her positive or negative feelings about the experience should be discussed. Encouragement and support should be given for continuation of nursing, including specific suggestions for maternal rest, nutrition, and nursing frequency (every 2–3 hours in the day) to build up the milk supply. Formula or other fluids should not be recommended unless serious concerns exist about the infant's well-being. Recommending discontinuing breastfeeding prematurely is inappropriate for the physician. An appropriate weight gain in the following few days provides evidence that the infant is well and confirms the diagnosis of initial underfeeding. Infants who fail to thrive while breastfeeding require more intensive nutritional rehabilitation while still preserving breastfeeding.

The formula-fed newborn rarely loses more than 5% of birth weight in the first few days, inasmuch as complete nutrition is available beginning a few hours after birth.[6] Weighing less than birth weight at the age of 10 days is unusual for a formula-fed infant, and such an infant should be evaluated thoroughly. An error in feeding caused by maternal inexperience is the usual explanation, with poor caloric intake most often from either inadequate feedings or faulty preparation of formula. If such is not the case, then a thorough search for an organic problem and an evaluation of family dynamics, support mechanisms, and adjustment to the newborn are indicated. In rare instances, a newborn will lose weight as a result of inadequate intake for other reasons, such as infection, congenital heart disease, inborn error of metabolism, somnolence from maternal medications or substance abuse, or poor suck resulting from a craniofacial or central nervous system (CNS) abnormality. Weight loss can also result from excessive fluid loss, such as vomiting associated with congenital gastrointestinal malformations (duodenal atresia, annular pancreas, volvulus), or from diarrhea or polyuria (diabetes insipidus, renal disease) (Box 84-1).

## ▶ OLDER INFANTS, PRESCHOOLERS, AND SCHOOL-AGED CHILDREN

The most common reason for weight loss in older infants and toddlers is fluid loss as a result of fever, vomiting, and diarrhea. The loss of weight typically amounts to less than 10% of premorbid body weight and is usually reversed after a few hours of oral or intravenous fluid replacement.

Infants who lose more than 10% of their body weight from excessive vomiting require further investigation for pyloric stenosis and malrotation as well as for tumors of the CNS, which may cause vomiting, anorexia, and cachexia.

Weight loss may also accompany any severe febrile illness, such as pneumonia, pyelonephritis, septic arthritis, osteomyelitis, or meningitis, as well as less severe illnesses, such as stomatitis and pharyngitis. Resolution of the infection is often followed by a period of catch-up growth and weight gain.

Inefficient use of caloric intake can also result in weight loss. Cystic fibrosis, the most common disease in which malabsorption occurs in childhood, may appear in infancy as poor weight gain or actual weight loss. Intestinal disorders such as celiac disease, Hirschsprung disease, inflammatory bowel disease, and other causes of malabsorption will also lead to weight loss or poor weight gain.

Weight loss from chronic diarrhea may be caused by a variety of infectious diseases, including HIV infection. A diagnosis of tuberculosis should also be considered in every child who has lost weight.

**BOX 84-1**

## *Differential Diagnosis of Weight Loss by Age Group*

**NEWBORNS AND YOUNG INFANTS**

- Difficulties in establishing breastfeeding
- Inappropriate dilution or choice of formula
- Inadequate intake
- Infection
- Metabolic abnormality
- Craniofacial abnormalities
- CNS dysfunction
- Somnolence from maternal medications/substance abuse
- Congenital heart disease
- Maternal depression/inexperience/lack of knowledge
- Excessive losses secondary to vomiting or diarrhea
- Vomiting because of gastrointestinal malformations (duodenal atresia, others)
- Polyuria (diabetes insipidus, renal disease)
- Diarrhea

**OLDER INFANTS, PRESCHOOLERS, AND SCHOOL-AGED CHILDREN**

- Pyloric stenosis
- Gastroesophageal reflux
- CNS tumors
- Vomiting
- Diarrhea
- Fever and infection
- Diabetes mellitus
- Excessive activity
- Inadequate intake
- Fever and infection
- Tuberculosis
- Surgery
- Medication effect (loss of appetite)
- Malignancy
- Congenital heart disease
- Malabsorption syndromes
- Inflammatory bowel disease
- Immunodeficiency disorders, especially HIV infection
- Psychosocial dysfunction
- Poverty
- Neglect; nonorganic failure to thrive
- Parental depression
- Childhood depression
- Rumination
- Childhood eating disorder

**ADOLESCENTS**

- Dieting behavior
- Adolescent eating disorders
- Anorexia nervosa
- Bulimia nervosa
- Other eating disorders
- Psychiatric affective disorders, especially depression
- Malignancy
- Inflammatory bowel disease
- Diabetes mellitus
- Hyperthyroidism
- Tuberculosis

*CNS*, central nervous system; *HIV*, human immunodeficiency virus.

Children with new-onset insulin-dependent diabetes mellitus commonly lose weight (often 10% or more of body weight) despite polyphagia and polydipsia. Hyperthyroidism is another endocrine disorder that may lead to weight loss in childhood.

Malignancies, including leukemia, lymphoma, and neuroblastoma, may have weight loss as part of their presenting picture or even as their initial symptom.

Poverty remains the greatest single risk factor for failure to thrive in the United States; however, other psychosocial factors (poor parent-child interaction, depression, rumination) often underlie an infant's or a child's poor growth and development.[7] Actual weight loss is much less common in this setting than a slowdown or cessation of weight gain and linear growth. Psychosocial dysfunction that results in a child's weight loss requires a prompt and thorough evaluation. Eating disorders have been described in prepubertal children as young as 7 years.[8] In addition, as reported by the Agency for Health Care Research and Quality, the largest increase in the rate of hospitalizations for eating disorders occurred in children younger than 12 years.[9]

## ▶ ADOLESCENTS

Monitoring the adolescent growth curve, including body mass index, is crucial to the recognition of weight loss and should be a part of every encounter. The prevalence of obesity in children and adolescents has increased in the past decade, leading to an unhealthy emphasis on dieting and weight loss among children and adolescents.[10] Planned dieting must be distinguished from an eating disorder such as anorexia nervosa or bulimia nervosa. The 2010 American Academy of Pediatrics policy statement regarding the identification and management of eating disorders estimates that 0.5% of female adolescents have anorexia nervosa, that 1% to 2% meet criteria for bulimia nervosa, and that up to 5% to 10% of all cases of eating disorders occur in boys. The American Psychiatric Association acknowledges that a large number of patients do not meet the strict diagnostic criteria for anorexia nervosa and bulimia nervosa; in the 2013 revision of the *Diagnostic and Statistical Manual of Mental Disorders*, these individuals are labeled OSFED (Other Specified Feeding or Eating Disorder). The prevalence of this diagnosis is estimated to be between 0.8% and 14%; these adolescents remain at risk for both physical and psychological complications from their altered eating habits.

Anorexia nervosa should be suspected when the adolescent is unwilling or unable to maintain body weight over a minimally normal weight for age and height and when attitudes and behaviors about eating or body image are distorted.[11] The anorectic female adolescent may experience amenorrhea associated with emaciation and overactivity. The patient may demonstrate clinical signs of malnutrition such as hypothyroidism, bradycardia, hypothermia, and growth of lanugo-like hair on the body and extremities. Nutritional rehabilitation and psychiatric treatment are indicated. Adolescents who have bulimia indulge in binge eating, followed by self-induced vomiting, self-starvation, overactivity, or the use of cathartics or diuretics to reduce weight. These behaviors are practiced in secret, and the adolescent often denies them. An elevated serum bicarbonate level, hypokalemia, or high urine pH may provide evidence of chronic vomiting. The patient is often depressed and self-deprecating and may seek medical aid when the eating-vomiting pattern becomes compulsive and out of the patient's control. Psychiatric evaluation and intervention are indicated.

Young adults who participate in sports may follow unhealthy weight-control practices to seek advantage in their athletic activities, including food restriction, vomiting, overexercise, diet pills, stimulants, insulin, nicotine, and voluntary dehydration.[12] For adolescents who participate in sports in which weight loss is a goal (eg, wrestling, gymnastics, ice skating, running, swimming, diving, dancing), a thorough dietary and supplement history should be elicited.

Although significant weight loss during adolescence can often be ascribed to eating disorders, other diagnoses must be considered. These conditions include psychiatric disturbances (especially affective disorders), CNS tumors (particularly those of the hypothalamus, sella turcica, or other midline areas), malignancies (especially lymphoma), or gastrointestinal problems such as inflammatory bowel disease or other malabsorption syndromes. Systemic disorders such as diabetes mellitus, hyperthyroidism, autoimmune disease, and renal disease may cause significant weight loss in adolescents. Infectious diseases such as HIV infection and tuberculosis should be considered when an adolescent patient reports weight loss.

## ▶ INITIAL EVALUATION OF A COMPLAINT OF WEIGHT LOSS

The following should be included in the initial evaluation (Table 84-1):

1. A complete history and thorough physical examination, with special attention to dietary intake, family functioning, and the patient's emotional well-being. The growth chart should be reviewed and updated.
2. A complete blood cell count (CBC) and erythrocyte sedimentation rate (ESR). The CBC screens for oncologic factors and provides an overview of the nutritional state. The ESR may be elevated in autoimmune diseases, chronic infections, certain malignancies, and inflammatory bowel disease; it may be abnormally low in anorexia nervosa.

**Table 84-1**
**Laboratory Studies Helpful in Weight Loss**

| SUGGESTED STUDIES | SUGGESTED DIAGNOSES |
|---|---|
| Complete blood cell count, smear | Anemia<br>Infection<br>Nutritional deficiencies<br>Malabsorptive syndromes<br>Malignancy |
| ESR | Autoimmune disease<br>Infection<br>Inflammatory bowel disease<br>Malignancy<br>Anorexia nervosa (very low ESR) |
| Serum electrolytes, kidney function tests | Dehydration<br>Vomiting, self-induced or pernicious<br>Renal dysfunction<br>Adrenal disorders<br>Metabolic disorder (with acidosis)<br>Autoimmune disease |
| Serum protein and albumin levels | Liver dysfunction<br>Malignancy<br>Malnutrition<br>Protein malabsorption<br>Protein-losing enteropathy |
| Tuberculosis skin test | Tuberculosis |
| Stool for occult blood | Gastroenteritis<br>Inflammatory bowel disease<br>Enteropathies |
| Serum carotene; specific tests of malabsorption | Malabsorption syndromes<br>Cystic fibrosis<br>Anorexia nervosa (high carotene) |
| Urinalysis, including specific gravity; urine culture | Diabetes mellitus<br>Diabetes insipidus<br>Dehydration<br>Urinary tract infection<br>Renal disease<br>Adolescent eating disorder (high pH) |

*ESR*, erythrocyte sedimentation rate.

3. Serum electrolyte and kidney function tests should be obtained to evaluate for dehydration, to reveal evidence of pernicious or self-induced vomiting, and to rule out renal or adrenal disease.
4. Serum protein and albumin levels to assess liver function, to determine whether the weight loss represents malnutrition, and to rule out protein malabsorption. Reversal of the albumin-to-globulin ratio is often seen in autoimmune diseases and malignancies.
5. Tuberculosis skin test.
6. Stool for occult blood and tests of malabsorption to diagnose gastroenteritis, inflammatory bowel disease, and the various causes of malabsorption. The serum carotene level may be low in infancy and in malabsorptive conditions but is often elevated in anorexia nervosa.
7. Urinalysis and urine culture to rule out diabetes mellitus, diabetes insipidus, dehydration, urinary tract infection, and renal disease. The urine pH may be high (>8) in adolescents who have eating disorders, particularly when vomiting occurs.

## When to Refer

Evidence or suspicion of

- Malignancy
- Endocrinopathy (thyroid, adrenal, pituitary)
- Gastrointestinal disorder (eg, gastroesophageal reflux; malabsorption, including cystic fibrosis; inflammatory bowel disease)
- Pancreatitis
- Heart disease
- Renal disease
- Pulmonary disease
- Rheumatologic condition
- CNS abnormality
- Metabolic disorder
- Surgical abdominal problem (eg, pyloric stenosis, Hirschsprung disease, volvulus)
- Immunodeficiency
- Unusual infection
- Psychiatric diagnosis in child or caretaker
- Anorexia nervosa or bulimia nervosa in the child or adolescent

## When to Admit

A newborn, when

- Weight loss cannot be managed as outpatient
- Weight loss of more than 12% to 15% of birth weight
- Excessive fluid loss (vomiting, diarrhea, polyuria)
- Evidence of infant hypernatremic dehydration
- Suspicion of infection, metabolic abnormality, congenital heart disease, other conditions requiring evaluation
- Extreme passivity of the infant, which may require tube feeding
- Need for intensive maternal education and support

At any age, when

- Weight loss is excessive (more than 5%–10% of previous weight)
- Excessive fluid loss from vomiting or diarrhea
- New-onset diabetes mellitus (usually)
- Evidence of severe febrile illness (pneumonia, pyelonephritis, osteomyelitis, meningitis, septic arthritis, others)
- Evidence of dehydration
- Physiologic instability
- Severe bradycardia
- Hypotension
- Hypothermia
- Orthostatic changes
- Electrolyte abnormalities (eg, hypernatremia, hypokalemia)
- Evidence of significant psychosocial dysfunction

An adolescent, when

- Eating disorder cannot be managed as outpatient
- Severe malnutrition, with weight
- Evidence of dehydration or electrolyte abnormalities
- Physiologic instability
- Acute food refusal
- Uncontrollable binge eating and purging
- Acute medical complication of malnutrition (syncope, seizures, cardiac failure, pancreatitis)
- Suicidal intent or ideation, or psychosis

## TOOLS FOR PRACTICE

### Engaging Patient and Family

- *About BMI for Children and Teens* (fact sheet), Centers for Disease Control and Prevention (www.cdc.gov/nccdphp/dnpa/bmi/childrens_BMI/about_childrens_BMI.htm)
- *Eating Disorders* (fact sheet), American Academy of Pediatrics (www.healthychildren.org/English/health-issues/conditions/emotional-problems/Pages/Eating-Disorders.aspx)
- *New Mother's Guide to Breastfeeding,* 2nd ed (book), American Academy of Pediatrics (shop.aap.org)

### Medical Decision Support

- *BMI–Body Mass Index: Child and Teen Calculator: English* (interactive tool), Centers for Disease Control and Prevention (apps.nccd.cdc.gov/dnpabmi/Calculator.aspx)
- *Breastfeeding Handbook for Physicians,* 2nd ed (book), American Academy of Pediatrics (shop.aap.org)
- *Eating Behaviors of the Young Child: Prenatal and Postnatal Influences for Healthy Eating* (book), Dietz W, Birch L (shop.aap.org)
- *Growth Charts–tutorials and information* (Web page), Centers for Disease Control and Prevention (www.cdc.gov/growthcharts)
- *Growth Charts* (chart), Centers for Disease Control and Prevention (www.cdc.gov/growthcharts), also available at American Academy of Pediatrics (shop.aap.org)
- *Pediatric Nutrition Handbook,* 7th ed (book), American Academy of Pediatrics (shop.aap.org)

## AAP POLICY STATEMENTS

American Academy of Pediatrics Committee on Sports Medicine and Fitness. Promotion of healthy weight-control practices in young athletes. *Pediatrics.* 2005;116(6):1557–1564 (pediatrics.aappublications.org/content/116/6/1557.full)

American Academy of Pediatrics Section on Breastfeeding. Breastfeeding and the use of human milk. *Pediatrics.* 2012;129(3):e827–e841 (pediatrics.aappublications/org/content/129/3/e827.full)

American Heart Association, Gidding SS, Dennison BA, Birch LL, et al. Dietary recommendations for children and adolescents: a guide for practitioners. *Pediatrics.* 2006;117(2):554–559 (AAP endorsed) (pediatrics.aappublications.org/content/117/2/544.full)

Block RW, Krebs NF; American Academy of Pediatrics Committee on Child Abuse and Neglect, Committee on Nutrition. Failure to thrive as a manifestation of child neglect. *Pediatrics.* 2005;116(5):1234–1237 Reaffirmed May 2009 (pediatrics.aappublications/org/content/116/5/1234.full)

Rosen DS; American Academy of Pediatrics Committee on Adolescence. Identification and management of eating disorders in children and adolescents. *Pediatrics.* 2010;126(6):1240–1253 (pediatrics.aappublications.org/content/early/2010/11/29/peds.2010-2821.abstract)

## REFERENCES

1. Dawson P. Normal growth and revised growth charts. *Pediatr Rev.* 2002;23:255–256
2. National Center for Health Statistics. Clinical Growth Charts. Available at: www.cdc.gov/growthcharts. Accessed November 24, 2014
3. McDonald PD, Ross Sr, Grant L, et al. Neonatal weight loss in breast and formula fed infants. *Arch Dis Child Fetal Neonatal Ed.* 2003;88(6):472–476
4. Stashwick CA. When a breastfed infant isn't gaining weight. *Contemp Pediatr.* 1993;10:116–134
5. Metaj M, Laroia N, Lawrence RA, Ryan RM. Comparison of breast- and formula-fed normal newborns in time to first stool and urine. *J Perinatol.* 2003;23:624–628
6. Lawrence RA, Lawrence RM. *Breastfeeding: A Guide for the Medical Profession.* 7th ed. St Louis, MO: Mosby; 2010
7. Block RW, Krebs NF; American Academy of Pediatrics Committee on Child Abuse and Neglect, Committee on Nutrition. Failure to thrive as a manifestation of child neglect. *Pediatrics.* 2005; 116(5):1234–1237
8. Atkins DM, Silber TJ. Clinical spectrum of anorexia nervosa in children. *J Dev Behav Pediatr.* 1993;14:211–216
9. Agency for Healthcare Research and Quality. Eating disorders sending more Americans to the hospital. AHQR New and Numbers. April 1, 2009. Available at: archive.ahrq.gov/news/newsroom/news-and-numbers/040109.html. Accessed February 26, 2015
10. Rosen DS; American Academy of Pediatrics Committee on Adolescence. Identification and management of eating disorders in children and adolescents. *Pediatrics.* 2010;126(6):1240–1253
11. American Psychiatric Association. *Diagnostic and Statistical Manual of Mental Disorders.* 5th ed. Arlington, VA: American Psychiatric Association; 2013
12. American Academy of Pediatrics Committee on Sports Medicine and Fitness. Promotion of healthy weight-control practices in young athletes. *Pediatrics.* 2005;116(6):1557–1564
13. American Academy of Pediatrics Section on Breastfeeding. Breastfeeding and the use of human milk. *Pediatrics.* 2012;129(3):e827–e841
14. Rosen DS; American Academy of Pediatrics Committee on Adolescence. Identification and management of eating disorders in children and adolescents. *Pediatrics.* 2010;126(6):1240–1253

# Chapter 85

# Wheezing

*Alfin G. Vicencio, MD; Joshua P. Needleman, MD*

## ▶ DEFINITION

Wheezing, a continuous musical sound that represents turbulent intrathoracic airflow, is usually most prominent during expiration, but it may also be present in inspiration. A history of wheezing reported by family members, however, is insensitive and nonspecific because untrained observers without appropriate equipment often mistake many other respiratory sounds for wheezing.

During the normal respiratory cycle, rhythmic expansion and contraction of the thorax lead to dynamic changes in thoracic pressures, allowing air to flow into and out of the lungs (Figure 85-1). On inspiration, the thoracic cavity expands, resulting in negative intrathoracic and airway pressures (relative to atmospheric pressure), allowing air to flow into the lungs. Extrathoracic airway obstruction, signaled by stridor (see Chapter 74, Stridor), is most likely to cause turbulent airflow during this phase of the respiratory cycle (see Figure 85-1, *A*). Expiration is accomplished by contracting the volume of the thoracic cavity, creating positive pressure in the thorax, which is transmitted to the intrathoracic airways. Thus, during expiration, the intrathoracic airways are more prone to obstruction leading to turbulent airflow (see Figure 85-1, *B*). It should be noted that obstruction occurring at the thoracic inlet or severe fixed obstruction at any level of the airway may cause abnormal noises that are not limited to one phase of the respiratory cycle, including biphasic wheezing.

Although wheezing is most commonly associated with the distal airway obstruction seen in viral bronchiolitis or asthma, several other diseases can cause small airway obstruction and can be indistinguishable on physical examination. Similarly, abnormalities causing obstruction of the mid or distal trachea or main-stem bronchi, both of which reside within the thorax, can cause wheezing. Thus, although bronchiolitis and asthma will certainly account for most children who wheeze, the general pediatrician should be prepared to initiate a more extensive evaluation for the wheezing child, particularly for patients with unusual presentations or if conventional treatment yields less than optimal results.

## ▶ DIFFERENTIAL DIAGNOSIS

The differential diagnosis of wheezing is extensive and includes any process that can cause obstruction of intrathoracic airways. Because the intrathoracic airways include large centrally located airways and smaller peripheral bronchioles, determining the level of obstruction is often helpful before generating a list of differential diagnoses (see Evaluation).

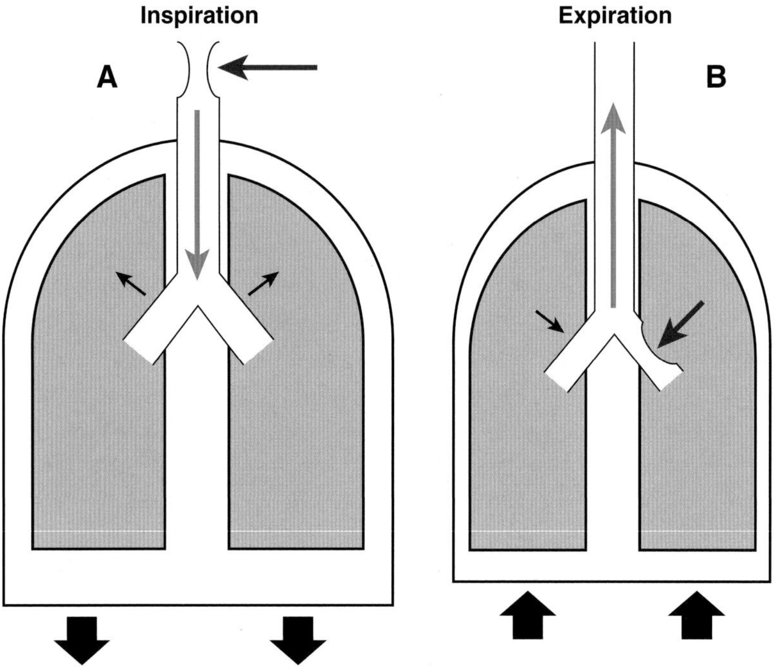


**Figure 85-1**
The respiratory cycle and related airway changes. **A,** During inspiration, negative intrathoracic pressures generated by thoracic expansion are likely to cause obstruction in the extrathoracic airway *(red arrow)* leading to stridor. **B,** During expiration, positive intrathoracic pressures generated by thoracic compression are likely to cause obstruction in the intrathoracic airways, including the mid and distal trachea, main-stem bronchi, and small bronchioles, leading to wheeze.

Viral bronchiolitis and asthma account for most wheezing localized to the small peripheral airways. A major challenge in evaluating the wheezing child is determining when the wheeze is not caused by asthma or bronchiolitis, but rather by a different process requiring different diagnostic approaches and alternate treatment strategies. For example, cystic fibrosis, a severe genetic disease causing progressive small airway obstruction, can be mistaken for poorly controlled asthma. Similarly, early congestive heart failure can produce intractable wheezing from peribronchial edema. Pulmonary hemosiderosis, a rare disorder, can cause anemia and recurrent wheezing because blood irritates the peripheral airways. In a similar manner, gastroesophageal reflux and recurrent aspiration can also result in persistent or recurrent wheezing and may also complicate large airway abnormalities.

Distinguishing large airway obstruction (ie, trachea or main-stem bronchi) from small airway obstruction (ie, asthma) is difficult because both can cause expiratory wheeze. In addition, a variety of abnormalities can cause large airway obstruction, further complicating evaluation and diagnosis. Dynamic lesions of the large airways such as tracheomalacia or bronchomalacia are fairly common causes of congenital wheezing and can also be associated with gastroesophageal reflux, tracheoesophageal fistula, or prolonged mechanical ventilation in premature infants. External compression of large airways can be seen with vascular abnormalities (rings and slings), mediastinal masses, or infectious agents, most notably lymphobronchial tuberculosis or histoplasmosis.

For any child with a sudden onset of wheezing or a history of choking, the possibility of a foreign body should be of particular concern. Importantly, many patients with foreign body aspiration will not have an obvious history of choking, and as such one should always maintain a suspicion for this possibility, even in a child whose wheezing has been present for days or weeks. Finally, intrinsic airway abnormalities, including complete tracheal rings and webs, and acquired obstructions, such as tracheal stenosis or granulation tissue, can cause intractable wheezing.

## ▶ EVALUATION

### *History*

A major challenge in evaluating the wheezing child is to determine when a wheeze is not caused by viral bronchiolitis or asthma. Wheezing caused by viral bronchiolitis is usually preceded by upper respiratory symptoms and fever, often worsens within the first few days of onset, and tends to improve slowly thereafter. Asthma exacerbations are often initiated by vigorous activity, changes in weather, upper respiratory infection, or exposure to a triggering allergen. Such exacerbations typically respond well to inhaled β-agonist therapy with or without systemic corticosteroids. Persistent or recurrent episodes of wheezing that do not fit these profiles and have a family history that supports the diagnosis of asthma should be evaluated more thoroughly.

A detailed and focused history can often provide clues to an accurate diagnosis. Wheezing that appears at birth or soon afterward should prompt an evaluation for congenital airway abnormalities such as tracheomalacia, complete rings, or vascular abnormalities or compression. Wheezing after a recent surgical procedure or intubation suggests acquired obstruction, whereas abrupt onset of wheezing accompanied by a history of choking should prompt an evaluation for aspiration of a foreign body. Other clues that suggest underlying illnesses or abnormalities include constant wheezing, failure to thrive, hemoptysis, difficulty swallowing, frequent vomiting, positional wheezing, worsening with agitation or crying, and poor response to conventional therapy.

### *Physical Examination*

Location of airway obstruction can often be determined by thorough physical examination and can direct the ensuing workup. Unilateral wheezing, most often associated with aspiration of a foreign body, can also accompany unilateral bronchial compression or stenosis and should be evaluated thoroughly. In addition to determining whether the wheezing is bilateral or unilateral, detailed assessment of the auditory characteristics can help determine whether the obstruction is central or peripheral. For example, wheezing that varies in pitch and can be heard throughout the chest (musical, heterophonous) typically represents small airway obstruction. In contrast, central airway obstruction tends to sound more even in pitch (monophonic, homophonous) and can often be heard best in central locations such as the sternal notch, although this may be unreliable in a small infant. In addition, large airway obstruction is more likely than small to be heard throughout the entire expiratory phase.

In addition to the auditory composition of a wheeze, positional characteristics can help determine cause. For example, wheezing caused by a dynamic lesion such as tracheomalacia is often worse when a patient is supine. Mediastinal structures such as the heart and the great vessels, which lie immediately anterior to the trachea, tend to fall posteriorly in the supine position and can be obstructive. In contrast, these structures tend to fall anteriorly when the patient is prone, relieving pressure on the airway and improving the wheeze. Wheezing caused by small airway obstruction or fixed compression of a large airway does not typically change with position.

## *Objective Testing*

Although a detailed history and physical examination can help the physician narrow the list of potential diagnoses, additional testing is often helpful and may guide therapy. Information obtained through the history and physical examination should guide further evaluation. Table 85-1 highlights the features of some common abnormalities that cause wheezing.

**Table 85-1**
**Causes of Recurrent or Persistent Wheeze**

| | FEATURES | OBJECTIVE FINDINGS |
|---|---|---|
| Asthma | Worse with exercise or respiratory infections<br>Responds to bronchodilators<br>Responds to steroids<br>Family history of atopy | Reversible obstruction on PFTs<br>Homophonous wheeze<br>Positive bronchoprovocation |
| Tracheomalacia | Worse with activity or agitation<br>Poor response to bronchodilators<br>Poor response to steroids | Homophonous wheeze<br>Airway collapse on fluoroscopy<br>Collapsible trachea on bronchoscopy |
| Bronchomalacia | Worse with activity or agitation<br>Poor response to bronchodilators<br>Poor response to steroids | Heterophonous wheeze<br>Airway collapse on fluoroscopy<br>Collapsible bronchus on bronchoscopy |
| Foreign body | Sudden onset<br>May have a history of choking | Asymmetrical breath sounds<br>Asymmetrical hyperinflation or collapse on radiograph |
| Heart failure or pulmonary edema | Poor response to bronchodilators<br>Poor growth | Hepatomegaly<br>Radiograph with increased fluid<br>Responds to diuresis |
| Bronchiolitis | Infant: URI symptoms | Positive viral studies |
| Vocal cord dysfunction | Poor response to all therapies<br>Severe distress reported | PFTs: normal or with abnormal inspiratory loop<br>Laryngoscopy: vocal cord adduction during inspiration |
| Cystic fibrosis | Poor growth, GI symptoms<br>Recurrent pneumonia | Positive sweat test |
| Gastroesophageal reflux and aspiration | Variable response to bronchodilators<br>Often worse after meals | Positive reflux evaluation (upper GI, nuclear scan, or pH probe) |
| Vascular compression | Central wheeze<br>No bronchodilator response | Indentation on esophagram<br>Anatomy demonstrated on thoracic MRI |
| Large airway abnormality (stenosis, complete rings, compression) | No response to therapy<br>Worse with activity<br>Stridor noted at times | Flattened or square flow–volume loop<br>Obstruction visible on imaging or bronchoscopy |

*GI*, gastrointestinal; *MRI*, magnetic resonance imaging; *PFT*, pulmonary function test; *URI*, upper respiratory infection.

Laboratory testing may be indicated to diagnose specific clinical entities. For example, a sweat test is required if cystic fibrosis is suspected, and viral studies can identify respiratory syncytial virus or influenza as a cause of small airway wheezing in an infant with upper respiratory symptoms.

Pulmonary function testing can help characterize a wheeze objectively in patients older than 5 or 6 years. The expiratory loop shown in Figure 85-2 demonstrates small airway obstruction that improves after bronchodilator therapy, suggesting asthma as the underlying cause of recurrent wheezing. In contrast, small airway obstruction that does not demonstrate reversibility after bronchodilator therapy may require additional workup; several disease processes, including cystic fibrosis, congestive heart failure, and obliterative bronchiolitis, can cause fixed small airway obstruction. Similarly, expiratory loops suggesting fixed large airway obstruction (Figure 85-3) may require further evaluation for stenosis, rings, or compression.

Radiographic studies can be helpful when evaluating a patient with persistent or recurrent wheeze, particularly when asthma or viral bronchiolitis is not likely the cause. Chest radiography can detect thoracic masses that cause obstruction of airways. In

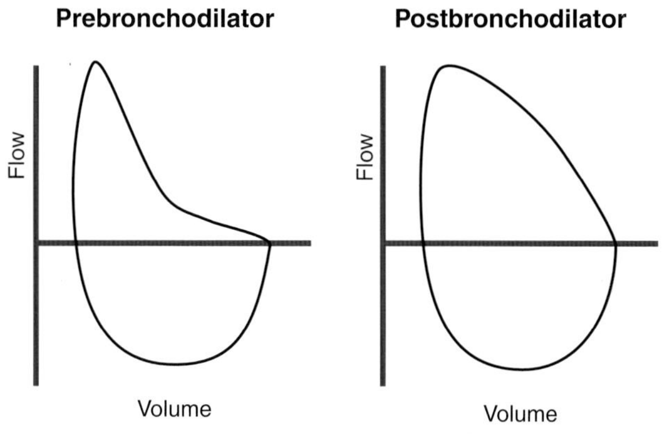


**Figure 85-2**
Pulmonary function test demonstrating small airway obstruction. Small airway obstruction, such as that seen in asthma, has a distinctive scooped appearance on spirometry. Normalization of the flow loop after bronchodilator treatment strongly suggests asthma as the underlying cause of recurrent wheezing.

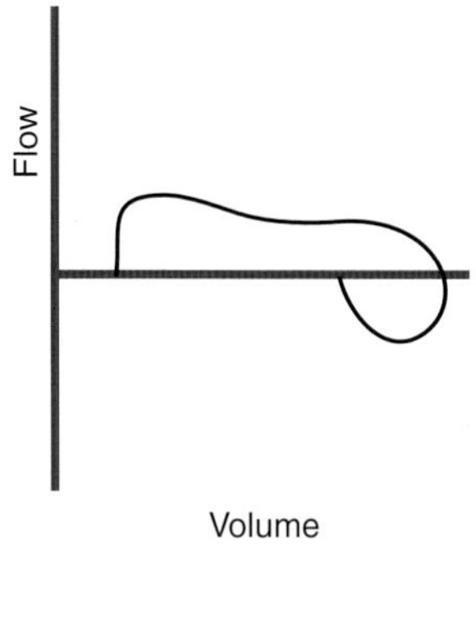


**Figure 85-3**
Pulmonary function test demonstrating large airway fixed obstruction. Fixed obstruction of a large airway by compression or stenosis will result in a characteristic flat expiratory loop on spirometry. No change will occur after administering bronchodilator.

addition, chest radiography with decubitus films or inspiratory and expiratory views can be helpful in diagnosing foreign-body aspiration (Figure 85-4). If history and physical examination suggest tracheobronchomalacia as an underlying diagnosis, then airway fluoroscopy (Figure 85-5) can confirm the diagnosis and help quantify the severity. An esophagram or upper gastrointestinal series is useful if a vascular abnormality is suspected. However, although a vascular abnormality can be easily identified by an esophageal notch in an esophagram, a computed tomographic scan with contrast (Figure 85-6) or magnetic resonance image is ultimately required to determine the exact anatomic variant, which may include a double aortic arch, a right aortic arch with aberrant left subclavian, or a pulmonary artery sling.

Direct visualization of the airway via flexible bronchoscopy is increasingly used to better characterize dynamic lesions such as tracheobronchomalacia (Figure 85-7). Intrinsic airway abnormalities, such as complete cartilaginous rings, often require bronchoscopy to make a diagnosis (Figure 85-8). Improved radiologic techniques, such as 3-dimensional airway reconstruction, may be useful, although the high radiation dose should limit their use (Figure 85-9). Furthermore, rigid bronchoscopy can be useful in both diagnosis and treatment of tracheal stenosis (Figure 85-10). Bronchoscopy can help assess the severity of airway compression by a thoracic mass and confirm patency after resection (Figure 85-11).

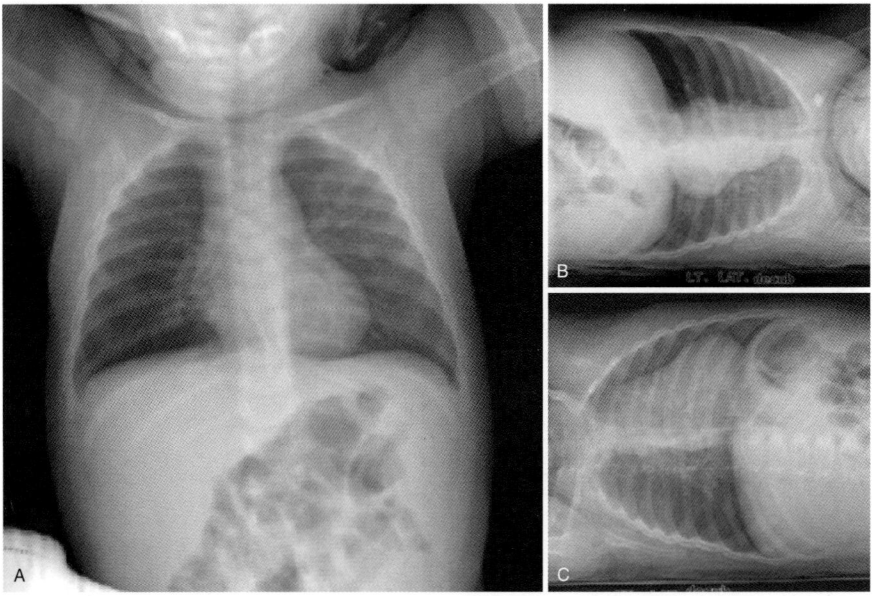


**Figure 85-4**

Foreign-body aspiration. **A,** Chest radiograph demonstrates mild hyperaeration of the right lung and mild flattening of the right hemidiaphragm on anteroposterior view. **B,** On left lateral decubitus view, the hyperaeration of the right lung is accentuated. **C,** On right lateral decubitus view, the heart does not shift with gravity, and the right lung remains well inflated. A peanut was found in the right main-stem bronchus during bronchoscopy.

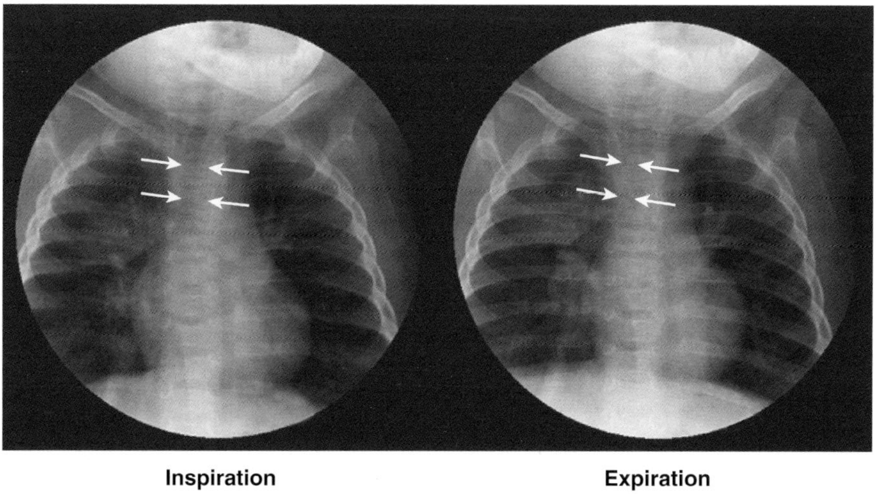


**Figure 85-5**
Airway fluoroscopy. Airway fluoroscopy demonstrates a normal trachea during inspiration *(arrows)*. On expiration, severe collapse of the trachea is demonstrated, indicating tracheomalacia.

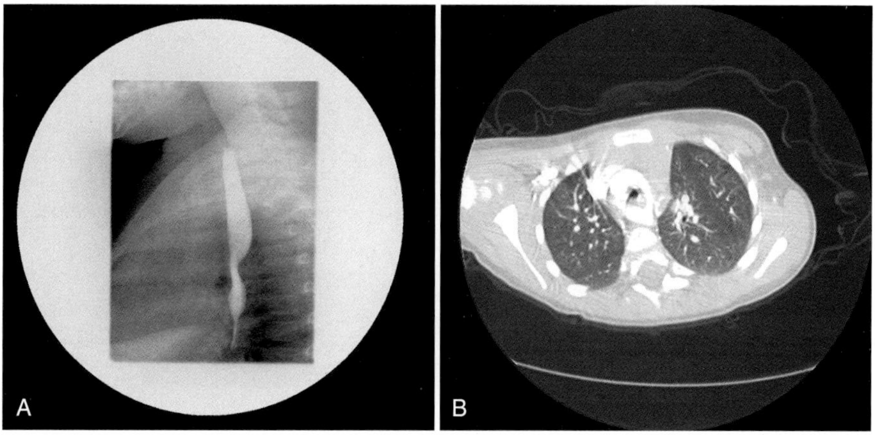


**Figure 85-6**
Esophagram and computed tomographic scan. **A,** Esophagram demonstrates a posterior indentation suggestive of a vascular ring. **B,** Computed tomographic scan of the chest confirms the presence of a double aortic arch

## ▶ MANAGEMENT

Most patients with wheezing have viral bronchiolitis and asthma and should be managed accordingly. Although some children with viral bronchiolitis or asthma require hospitalization for severe respiratory distress, hypoxemia, poor feeding, or dehydration, the general pediatrician can care for most children in an outpatient setting. An important point to note is that, currently, no evidence exists to support the regular use of β-agonist therapy in viral bronchiolitis. Hypertonic 3% saline has recently been used as adjunctive therapy for hospitalized

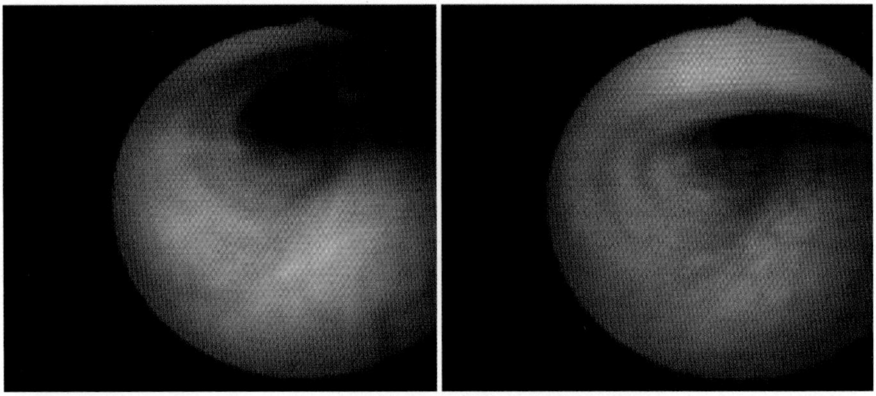

**Figure 85-7**

Images from fiberoptic bronchoscopy. Fiberoptic bronchoscopy demonstrates normal tracheal caliber during inspiration. During expiration, the distal trachea collapses, consistent with tracheomalacia.

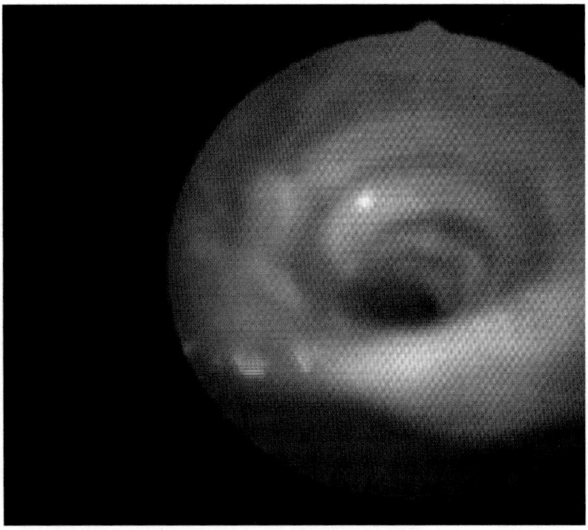

**Figure 85-8**

Image from fiberoptic bronchoscopy. Fiberoptic bronchoscopy demonstrates complete cartilaginous rings causing severe obstruction of the trachea.

patients with bronchiolitis. Hospital admission or referral to a subspecialty physician may be indicated for chronic wheezing associated with failure to thrive, which can be a sign of a significant underlying disease. Similarly, an unusual history or physical examination should prompt more detailed evaluation and may require alternate treatment regimens, depending on the cause. In general, the pediatrician evaluating the child with wheeze should be aware of the various clinical entities that can produce wheezing, be able to recognize by history or physical examination patients who require further workup, initiate simple diagnostic tests, and refer to appropriate subspecialty physicians children with unusual presentations or poor response to conventional therapies.

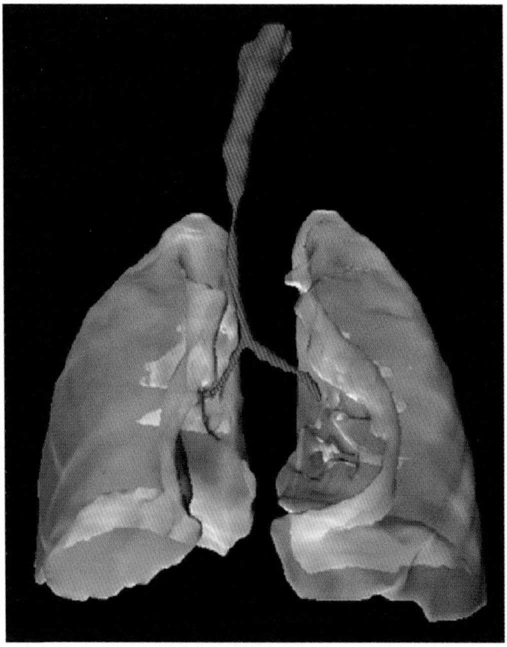

**Figure 85-9**
Three-dimensional reconstruction of computed tomographic image. Severe circumferential narrowing of the trachea starting at the thoracic inlet and extending to the main-stem bronchi.

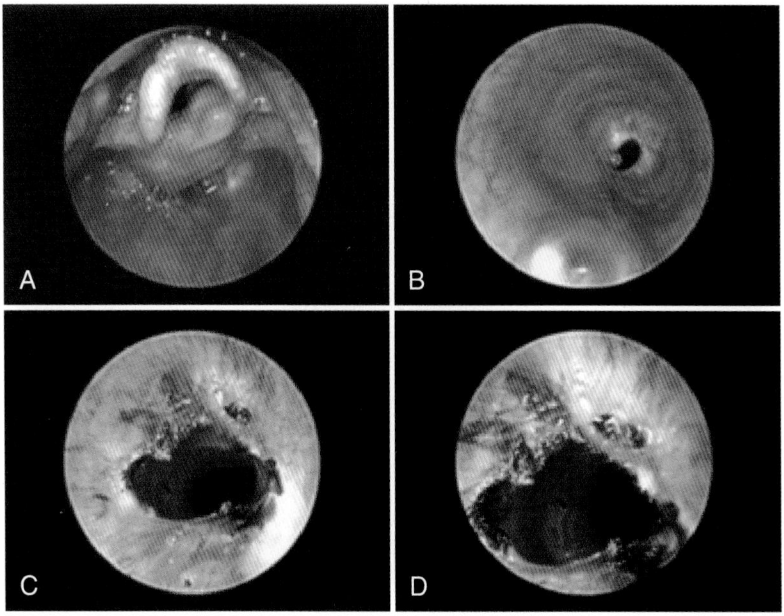


**Figure 85-10**
Images from rigid bronchoscopy. **A,** Epiglottis. **B,** Severe stenosis secondary to a tracheal web. **C** and **D,** After laser resection of the stenosis. *(Courtesy of Sanjay Parikh, MD.)*

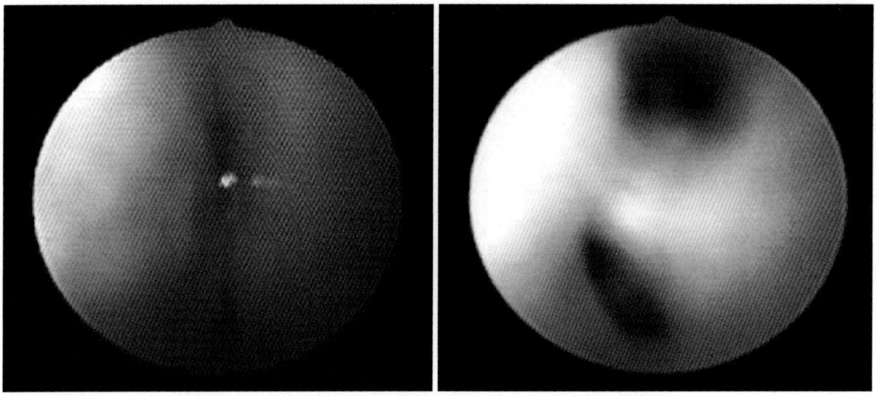

**Figure 85-11**
Images from fiberoptic bronchoscopy. Complete obstruction of the distal left main-stem bronchus secondary to a mediastinal mass. Immediately after resection of the mass, the segmental branch points of the left lung are easily identified.

## When to Refer

- Persistent or recurrent wheezing in an infant younger than 1 year
- Apparent paradoxical response to bronchodilators
- Poor weight gain or growth associated with chronic or recurrent wheezing
- Repeated hospitalization or multiple courses of oral corticosteroids
- Persistent asymmetric wheezing

## When to Admit

- Respiratory distress unresponsive to therapy
- Hypoxemia
- Tachypnea interfering with ability to eat or drink
- Altered mental status or signs of fatigue

### SUGGESTED READINGS

Callahan CW. Primary tracheomalacia and gastroesophageal reflux in infants with cough. *Clin Pediatr.* 1998;37:725–732

Elphick HE, Sherlock P, Foxall G, et al. Survey of respiratory sounds in infants. *Arch Dis Child.* 2001;84:35–39

Finder JD. Primary bronchomalacia in infants and children. *J Pediatr.* 1997;130:59–66

Harty MP, Kramer SS. Recent advances in pediatric pulmonary imaging. *Curr Opin Pediatr.* 1998;10:227–235

Lowe LA, Simpson A, Woodcock A, et al. Wheeze phenotypes and lung function in preschool children. *Am J Respir Crit Care Med.* 2005;171:231–237

Newman KB, Mason UG, Schmaling KB. Clinical features of vocal cord dysfunction. *Am J Respir Crit Care Med.* 1995;152:1382–1386

Schellhase DE, Fawcett DD, Shutze GE, et al. Clinical utility of flexible bronchoscopy and bronchoalveolar lavage in young children with recurrent wheezing. *J Pediatr.* 1998;132:321–328

Taylor WR, Newacheck PW. Impact of childhood asthma on health. *Pediatrics.* 1992;90:657–662

Wood RE. The emerging role of flexible bronchoscopy in pediatrics. *Clin Chest Med.* 2001;22:311–317

# Index

Page numbers followed by "f" denote figures; "t" denote tables; "b" denote boxes.


## A

Abdomen
- tumors of, 8
- tympanitic, 4–6, 6–7

Abdominal distention
- algorithm for, 10f
- causes of, 3b, 5b
- diagnosis of, 4, 5t, 8f
- family history and, 2
- history taking, 1–2
- hospitalization for, 10
- physical examination for, 2–4
- radiographic diagnosis of, 8f, 9, 10f
- symptoms of, 1, 2b

Abdominal masses, 7–8
Abdominal migraine, 972, 974
Abdominal pain
- acute, 13, 15, 16b
- causes of, 17b
- characteristics of, 13, 18–21
- chronic, 18
- diagnosis of, 15b, 16b
- differential diagnosis of, 15–18
- evaluation of, 18–21, 19f
- functional, 14, 19–20
- history taking, 18–20
- hospitalization for, 24
- laboratory evaluation of, 20–21, 21b
- medically unexplained symptoms, 658
- physical examination for, 20
- referral for, 23–24
- treatment for, 21–23

Abdominal sepsis, 489
Abdominal wall hypotonia, 9
Abduction, 373b
Absenteeism, 444, 775–776, 776b
Academic difficulties, 455t
Acanthocytes, 51b
Acetylcholine, 549
Achondroplasia, 652
Acid reflux, 114
Acne, 736f, 739
Acquired autoimmune myasthenia gravis, 555
Acquired hypothyroidism, 821
Acquired immunodeficiency syndrome. *See* AIDS
Acquired torticollis, 948–950
Acrocyanosis, 146, 156
Acrodermatitis enteropathica, 36, 192, 739f
Acute abdomen, 572–573
Acute and recurrent headaches, 443
Acute appendicitis, 13
Acute cerebellar ataxia, 81–82
Acute diarrhea
- causes of, 178b
- description of, 178b, 181b
- evaluation of, 180–181, 181b
- treatment of, 181–185

Acute disseminated encephalomyelitis, 80
Acute phase reactants, 644
Acute stroke, 79–80
Acute surgical abdomen, 15b
Addison disease, 333
Adduction, 373b
Adenomatous polyps, 399
Adenosine, 102
ADHD. *See* Attention-deficit/hyperactivity disorder
Adolescent(s)
- amenorrhea in, 39–45
- anxiety in, 65t, 66
- back pain in, 85–87, 88–92
- bacterial conjunctivitis in, 767
- blood pressure in, 508–509
- brain development in, 887–888
- cardiac arrhythmias in, 98, 104
- exercise guidelines for, 519t
- fatigue in, 333
- gastrointestinal bleeding in, 400
- gonadal hyperandrogenism in, 530–533
- hoarseness in, 541b, 542
- hypertension in, 508b, 519t
- hypothalamic-pituitary-ovarian axis of, 41
- inattention and impulsivity in, 567b
- learning disabilities in, 612
- mortality, cardiac arrhythmias and, 107
- polycystic ovary syndrome in, 530–535
- rashes in, 744b–745b
- substance use by
  - brain development considerations, 887–888
  - screening for, 890t
  - treatment of, 898
- tobacco use by, 888
- transgender, 418–419, 427–429

Adrenal cortex, 527
Adrenal hyperandrogenism, 527–529
Adrenarche
- definition of, 523
- description of, 728
- premature, 527–529
- signs of, 535

Adverse childhood experiences, 68t, 165t, 207t, 562t, 610t, 892t

Aggression. *See* Disruptive behavior and aggression
Agoraphobia, 64t
AIDS, 193, 749
Airway
  compression of, 995f
  fluoroscopy of, 993f
Airway obstruction
  stridor and, 877
  wheezing and, 987–989, 991f
Alagille syndrome, 587
Alanine aminotransferase, 590–591
Albumin-globulin ratio, 367
Alcohol, 891, 891t
Alcoholism, 333
Alkaline phosphatase, 591
Allergic conjunctivitis, 765t, 768–769, 769f
Allergies
  constipation caused by, 124
  diarrhea caused by, 190–191
  red eye caused by, 764, 764f
Almotriptan, 447t
Alopecia
  alopecia areata, 31–33, 32f
  androgenetic, 33
  definition of, 27, 29t
  diagnosis of, 32f
  differential diagnosis of, 28–37
  management of, 37
  prognosis for, 28
  referrals for, 37
  traumatic, 34
Alpha-blockers, 515t
Alpha-thalassemia, 53–54
Ambiguous genitalia, 297
Ambras syndrome, 526
Ambulatory blood pressure monitoring, 510–511
Amenorrhea
  causes of, 40b
  description of, 39–41
  evaluation of, 41–44, 42f
  history taking, 41
  hypoestrogenic, 44
  laboratory testing for, 43–44
  management of, 44–45
  physical examination for, 41–43
  primary, 39, 43
  referrals for, 45
  secondary, 39, 43
  secondary sex characteristics, 42f
  stress and, 41
Amiloride, 706
Amniotic band disruption sequence, 296, 296f
Amphetamines, 938
Anal stenosis, congenital, 123
Androgens, in hair growth, 524
Anemia
  aplastic, 55
  classification of, 47–59, 52t
  definition of, 47
  diagnosis of, 59t
  evaluation of, 56–57, 59–60
  family history of, 59
  fatigue caused by, 332, 338
  hematologic causes of, 55–56
  hemolytic, 56
  iron deficiency, 55
  laboratory findings for, 60
  macrocytic, 52t, 57
  management of, 259
  microcytic. *See* Microcytic anemia
  in newborn, 50f, 57–59
  normocytic, 52t, 54–55, 54–56
  physical examination for, 59–60
  referrals and, 61
  sideroblastic, 54
  treatment of, 60–61
Angiotensin II, 511
Angiotensin-converting enzyme inhibitors, 515t
Angiotensin-receptor blockers, 515t
Ankle, 628–629
Ankylosing spondylitis, 598
Annulus, 741f
Anomalous left coronary artery, 574
Anorectal disorders, 123
Anorexia nervosa
  causes of, 635b
  description of, 982
  differential diagnosis of, 633–634
  evaluation for, 634
  pathophysiologic features, 633
  referral for, 636
  treatment of, 634–636
Antalgic gait, 627t
Anterior horn cell disease, 554–555
Anterior saccular cyst, 884f
Anteversion, 373b
Antibiotic-associated pseudomembranous colitis, 179
Anticipatory guidance
  for family dysfunction, 322
  temper tantrums and, 930–931
Antidepressants, for insomnia, 851
Antiemetics, 975
Antihistamines
  cough treated with, 141
  pruritus and, 721
Anti-inflammatory drugs, nonsteroidal, 222
Antinuclear antibody testing, 629
$\alpha_1$-Antitrypsin deficiency, 586
Anxiety
  in adolescents, 65t, 66
  assessment of, 66–69
  in children, 65t, 66
  chronic medical conditions and, 63
  conditions coexisting with, 68t
  depression and, 68t, 165t
  disruptive behavior and aggression associated with, 207t

findings suggestive of, 63–64, 65t
inattention and impulsivity and, 562t
in infants, 65t, 66
overview of, 64t
in parents, 67, 72
plan of care for, 7–13
symptoms of, 63
tics and, 939
in toddlers, 66
treatment of, 941
Anxiety disorders
assessment of, 66–69
description of, 64t
healthy habits and, 70
identification of, 64–65
interventions for, 71–72
obsessive-compulsive disorder, 64t, 67, 69
overview of, 64t
plan of care for, 7–13
post-traumatic stress disorder, 64t, 67, 69
psychoeducation about, 70
psychopharmacologic treatment of, 74t
psychosocial screening tools for, 64–65, 66t
psychosocial treatment of, 74t
resources for, 73
reward system for, 72, 72t
social-emotional problems versus, 907t
specialist involvement in, 73–74
stress reduction and, 71
substance use and, 892t
tics and, 939
tools for assessing, 64–65, 66t
treatment of, 67, 69
Aortic stenosis
chest pain caused by, 116
syncope and, 923
Aortic valve clicks, 460
Aplastic anemia, 55
Apocrine bromhidrosis, 679
Appendicitis, 13, 573
Appendix testis torsion, 789–790
Appetite, 633
Apraxia, 865
Apt-Downey test, 396
Area postrema, 971
Arnold-Chiari malformation, 878
Arrhythmias
approach to, 97–98
atrial fibrillation, 101f, 104
atrial flutter, 104, 105f
conduction abnormalities, 106–107
normal rhythm variations, 98
premature beats, 98–100
referrals for, 109
sudden cardiac death, 107–109
supraventricular tachycardia, 100–104
ventricular tachycardia, 105–106
Arteriovenous malformation, 79
Arthralgia, 597
Arthritis, 597
juvenile idiopathic, 598, 624
septic, 620, 621t
Arthrogryposis multiplex congenita, 287
Arthropathy, 597
Articulation, 865
Arytenoid dislocation, 546
Ascites, 9, 257
Aspartate aminotransferase, 590–591
Associations, 287, 289
Asthma
chest pain caused by, 115t
dyspnea and, 241
sleep-related, 852t, 853–854
wheezing and, 987–989
Ataxia
acute cerebellar, 81–82
causes of, 78b
definition of, 77
differential diagnosis of, 79–82
episodic, 79b
evaluation of, 77–79
Guillain-Barré syndrome as cause of, 81
history taking for, 77–78
imaging of, 82
intermittent, 79b
laboratory evaluation of, 82
management of, 83
motor, 81
ongoing care for, 83
physical examination of, 78–79
sensory, 81
treatment of, 83
Ataxia-telangiectasia, 752t, 753
Athletes
back pain and, 86–87
extremity pain and, 281–282
Atresia
extrahepatic biliary, 586–587
newborns and, 6f
pulmonary, with ventricular septal defect, 153
tricuspid, 153
Atrial fibrillation, 101f, 104
Atrial flutter, 104, 105f
Atrial premature contractions, 99f, 99–100
Atrial septal defect, 459
Atrioventricular block, 106–107, 107f, 922–923
Atrophy, 742
Attention-deficit/hyperactivity disorder
American Academy of Pediatrics treatment recommendations for, 567b
disruptive behavior and aggression associated with, 207t
inattention and impulsivity in, 559–560, 562t
irritability caused by, 577
learning difficulties and, 610t
pharmacotherapy for, 941
psychoeducation for, 563

Attention-deficit/hyperactivity disorder *(continued)*
psychosocial interventions for, 567
social-emotional problems versus, 907t
substance use and, 892t
tics and, 936, 940–941
Auditory neuropathy/dyssynchrony, 454
Auditory screening, 455
Auscultation, of heart, 462–463
Autism spectrum disorder, 68t, 73, 208t, 577, 611t, 863, 906
Autoimmune diseases
fatigue caused by, 337–338
fever caused by, 364b, 365
hemoptysis and, 482
Autoimmune enteropathy, 193–194
Axillary apocrine bromhidrosis, 681
Axillary hyperhidrosis, 549–550
Axillary odor, 681

## B

Back pain
chronic causes of, 87
diagnosis of, 86–87, 87t
epidemiology of, 85
evaluation of, 88–92
management of, 92–94
psychosocial considerations of, 87–88
referrals for, 94
Bacterial conjunctivitis, 765t, 767f, 767–768
Bacterial infections
fever caused by, 363, 364b
hemoptysis caused by, 480
in infants, 348
joint pain and, 599
lymphadenopathy caused by, 640
in newborn, 350
recurrent, 748
splenomegaly and, 870–871
Bacterial vaginosis, 968
Bad breath, 681–682
Balanitis, 252
Balanoposthitis, 252
Bamboo spine, 598
Banti syndrome, 871
Barium enema, 406
Barky cough, 878
Bartonellosis, 363
Basophilic stippling, 51b
BEARS parent questionnaire, 830
Beckwith-Wiedemann syndrome, 291
Bedtime fears, 839
Behavior
disruptive. *See* Disruptive behavior and aggression
self-injurious. *See* Self-injurious behavior
self-stimulating. *See* Self-stimulating behaviors
Behavioral disorders, 455t
Behavior Analyst Certification Board, 801
Bell clapper deformity, 786
Benign neonatal sleep myoclonus, 675–676
Benign paroxysmal positional vertigo, 217–218
Benign paroxysmal torticollis, 217, 948
Benign paroxysmal vertigo, 674–675
Benign premature adrenarche, 529
Bereavement, 68t, 165t, 207t, 563t, 610t
Bernard-Soulier syndrome, 266
Beta-blockers
hypertension and, 515t
syncope and, 927
Beta-thalassemia, 53
Bezoars, 8
Bezold-Jarisch reflex, 921
Biliary obstruction
hepatomegaly and, 492
jaundice and, 589
Bilious vomiting, 972
Bilirubin
conjugation of, 584
increased production of, 583–584
jaundice and, 581
metabolism, 581–582
Bilirubin UDP-glucuronosyl transferase, 581
Biopsy
liver, 591–592
lymphadenopathy and, 645, 647
renal, 474
Biopsychosocial approaches
abdominal pain and, 22
school refusal and, 779
Bipolar disorder, 166t, 207t, 892t
Bleeding
gastrointestinal
adolescents with, 400, 401b
causes of, 398–400, 401b
diagnostic testing of, 396, 402–403
differential diagnosis of, 396, 398–400
history taking, 401–402
infants and young children with, 398–400, 401b
lower, 395
management of, 403–406
newborns with, 397–398, 401b
nongastrointestinal source of, 396
overview of, 395
physical examination for, 402
terminology associated with, 395–396
vaginal
causes of, 956b
diagnostic testing for, 957–958
evaluation of, 954–958
history taking, 955–957
management of, 958–959
physical examination for, 957
in prepubertal girls, 953–954
in pubertal girls, 954–959
Blepharitis, 765, 769
Blister cells, 51b

Blood cell count
  dyspnea and, 238
  epistaxis and, 267
Blood in diaper or underwear, 476
Blood pressure. *See also* Hypertension
  ambulatory monitoring of, 510–511
  in boys, 498f, 499t–502t
  definition of, 511
  factors influencing, 497, 507
  in girls, 498f, 503t–506t
  measurement of, 509–511
  regulation, 511
Blue-dot sign, 789
Board-certified behavior analyst, 803
Body odor
  causes of, 681–687, 683t–687t
  differential diagnosis of, 681–682
  physical examination of, 680
Body temperature, normal, 343–344
Body twirling, 815
Bone marrow failure, 694–695
Bone scan, 278
Bone scintigraphy, 630
Borderline personality disorder, 800
*Bordetella pertussis,* 150
*Borrelia burgdorferi,* 599–600
Botulism, infantile, 335, 556, 571
Bowed legs, 380–383, 382f
Bowing, 371
Boys
  blood pressure levels, 498f, 499t–502t
  growth patterns in, 819
  puberty in, 723–727
Brachycephaly, 291
Bradyarrhythmias, 922
Bradycardia, 98, 98t
Brain
  development of, in adolescents, 887–888
  injuries to, 569
Breast development
  in boys, 724
  in girls
    delayed, 725–727, 731
    early, 727–730
    normal, 723–724
Breastfeeding
  sleep and, 837, 841
  weight loss in infants and, 979–980
Breath-holding spells
  cyanotic, 156, 673, 932–933
  description of, 673–674, 932–934
  pallid, 933
  syncope and, 919, 922
Breathing disorders
  dyspnea, 235–244
  sleep related, 842–843, 853–854
Bromhidrosis, 550, 679
Bronchiectasis, hemoptysis and, 483, 485–486
Bronchiolitis, 987–988
Bronchitis, 987
Bronchoscopy
  hemoptysis and, 486
  wheezing and, 992, 994f, 995f–996f
Bruit, 463
Bruxism, 847
Budd-Chiari syndrome, 491
Bulimia nervosa, 982
Bullae, 734, 738f
Bullous disease, 738f
Bullying, 209
Bunionette, 390

## C

Café au lait macules, 735f
Calcaneovalgus, 383, 384f
Calcaneus, 373b
Calcium channel blockers, for hypertension, 515t
Canavan disease, 651
Candidal infections, 968
Capillary hemangiomas, 763, 763f
Carbohydrate intolerance, 189
Carbohydrate malabsorption, 187
Carbon monoxide poisoning
  cyanosis caused by, 155
  irritability and, 574
Cardiac arrhythmias
  approach to, 97–98
  atrial fibrillation, 101f, 104
  atrial flutter, 104, 105f
  conduction abnormalities, 106–107
  normal rhythm variations, 98
  premature beats, 98–100
  referrals for, 109
  sudden cardiac death, 107–109
  supraventricular tachycardia, 100–104
  ventricular tachycardia, 105–106
Cardiac catheterization, 926
Cardiac cyanosis, 149–150
Cardiac cycle, 459–460, 460f
Cardiac disease, 462b
Cardiac pacing, 927
Cardiovascular system
  evaluation of, 514
  irritability and, 573–574
  syncope, 922–924
Caregiver Strain Questionnaire, 205
Caroli disease, 492
Cataplexy, 676, 849
Catheterization, cardiac, 926
Cat scratch disease, 356
Cavus, 373b
CBT. *See* Cognitive behavioral treatment
CCAVB. *See* Complete congenital atrioventricular block
Celecoxib, 222
Celiac disease
  description of, 124, 820
  diarrhea associated with, 188

Cellular immunity defects, 752–753
Central alpha-agonist, 515t
Central cyanosis, 146–148, 156
Central diabetes insipidus, 700–702
Central nervous system
abnormalities of, 551
hypotonia, 555
sensation of dyspnea and, 235
Central precocious puberty, 530, 728
Central syncope, 919
Cerebellar hemisphere dysfunction, 79
Cerebellitis, 80
Cerebral palsy
hypotonia and, 551
limp caused by, 625
Cervical adenopathy, 337
Cervicitis, 955
C fibers, 719
CFS. *See* Chronic fatigue syndrome
CGD. *See* Constitutional growth delay
Chalazia, 764
CHARGE association, 289
Chédiak-Higashi syndrome, 753t
Chemical conjunctivitis, 768
Chemoreceptor trigger zone, 971
Chest pain
causes of, 114–117, 115t
diagnosis of, 111
evaluation of, 112–113
exercise-induced, 114, 115t
history and, 112–113
idiopathic causes of, 116–117
laboratory evaluation and, 113
pathophysiologic features of, 111–112
psychogenic, 117
referred, 111
symptoms of, 113b, 115t
Chest radiograph
lymphadenopathy evaluations, 643–644
wheezing evaluations, 992f–993f
Chest wall syndrome, 117
Children. *See also* Infant(s); Neonate; Newborn
hypertension in, athletic participation considerations for, 516
language development in, 860t–861t
mortality of, cardiac arrhythmias and, 107
sexual abuse of, vaginal bleeding and, 953
tobacco use by, 888
*Chlamydia trachomatis,* 968
Choledochal cysts, 587
Cholelithiasis, 589
Cholera, 176
Cholestasis, 591
Cholestatic jaundice, 584
Cholestyramine, 186
Chondromalacia patellae, 284, 601
Chorea, 938
Chromosome analysis, 297
Chronic disease and illness
absenteeism caused by, 776
anemia and, 54–55
constipation, 196
short stature caused by, 820
Chronic edema, 258
Chronic fatigue syndrome
chronic fatigue versus, 334
criteria for, 334
description of, 334–335
diagnosis of, 337
Chronic granulomatous disease, 753t
Chronic inflammation, 54–55
Chronic irritability, 576–578
Chronic nonprogressive headaches, 443–444
Chronic progressive headaches, 443
Chronic tic disorder, 938
Chylous ascites, 9
Circadian rhythms
description of, 829–830
sleep disorder involving, 843
Citalopram, 23
Claudication, 277
Claw toe, 389f, 390
Cleidocranial dysostosis, 652
Clevidipine, 518t
Clitoromegaly, 43
Clonidine, 518t, 940
*Clostridium botulinum,* 335
Clubfoot, 287, 288f, 383–385, 384f
Coarctation of the aorta, 508–509
Cochlear implants, 456
Coefficient of absorption, 173
Cognitive behavioral treatment
abdominal pain and, 22
depression treated with, 170
selective serotonin reuptake inhibitors and, 170
somatic disorders treated with, 662t
Cognitively impaired children, 578
Colic, 572, 577
Colloid osmotic pressure, 255
Colloids, 255
Colon, 119–120
Colonic pain, 13
Columbia Impairment Scale, 560
Combined oral contraceptives, 958–959
Common variable immunodeficiency, 751t
Complementary and alternative medicine, 22
Complement system, 753–754
Complete atrioventricular block, 106
Complete congenital atrioventricular block, 106–107
Complex regional pain syndrome, 602
Complex vocal tics, 935
Concussion, 571
Conduct disorder, 165t, 203, 204b, 209, 212, 563t, 611t
Conduction abnormalities, 106–107, 107f
Confusional arousals, 845–846
Congenital adrenal hyperplasia, 528

Congenital anal stenosis, 123
Congenital aqueductal stenosis, 650
Congenital atrioventricular block, 107f
Congenital chloride-losing diarrhea, 177, 194
Congenital cyanotic heart disease, 151–152, 156–158
Congenital generalized hypertrichosis, 526
Congenital heart defects
  hemoptysis and, 483
  tetralogy of Fallot, 152, 924
Congenital hepatic fibrosis, 492
Congenital hip dysplasia, 623, 623f
Congenital hypertrichosis lanuginosa, 526
Congenital hypotonia, 557
Congenital laryngeal stridor, 882
Congenital laryngeal webs, 539, 541
Congenital muscular dystrophy, 556–557
Congenital myopathies, 556–557
Congenital sodium-secretory diarrhea, 194
Congenital torticollis, 947–950
Congestive splenomegaly, 871
Conjugated bilirubin, 582
Conjugated hyperbilirubinemia, 584–585
Conjunctival abnormalities, 765
Conjunctival papilloma, 770, 770f
Conjunctivitis
  allergic, 765t, 768–769, 769f
  bacterial, 765t, 767f, 767–768
  chemical, 768
  history taking, 759–760
  in Kawasaki disease, 771
  in newborn, 767
  overview of, 759
  physical examination of, 760–761
  types of, 765t
  vernal, 768
  viral, 765t, 766, 766f
Constipation
  causes of, 122–124
  chronic, 196
  complications of, 126
  definition of, 119, 120b
  diagnosis of, 122b, 122–124
  evaluation of, 125–127
  functional, 119–120, 123t, 125–131
  Hirschsprung disease comparison, 123t
  idiopathic, 7
  irritability and, 577
  red flag signs in, 127b
  referrals for, 131
  studies and, 124b
  treatment of, 127–131, 131b
Constitutional growth delay, 819
Contact dermatitis
  illustration of, 740f
  pruritus and, 720
Continuous murmurs, 466–467, 467f
Contraception/contraceptives, 223
Conversion disorder, 660t
Cooley anemia, 53
Coprolalia, 935
Copropraxia, 935
Corneal abrasion, 771, 771f
Corneal and ciliary flash, 772
Corneal ulcer, 771, 772f
Cornelia de Lange syndrome, 815
Coronary arteries, 924
Corticotropin-releasing hormone, 527
Co-sleeping, 834
Costochondritis, 115t
Cough
  classification of, 135–136
  diagnosis of, 136–137
  evaluation of, 137–140
  family and personal history, 137
  laboratory evaluation of, 138–140
  neonatal history, 137
  pathophysiologic features of, 135
  physical examination for, 138
  referrals for, 142
  treatment of, 140–141
Cough suppressants, 141
Coxa vara, 372
Craniosynostosis, 665
C-reactive protein, 367
Crigler-Najjar syndrome, 584
Croup, 150
Curly toe, 389f, 390
Currant-jelly stools, 399
Cushing syndrome, 336, 821
Cuticle biting, 813
Cyanide poisoning, 155
Cyanosis
  acrocyanosis, 146
  cardiac, 149–150
  central, 146–148, 156
  definition of, 145
  dyshemoglobinemias with, 155
  in fetus, 156
  heart disease with
    congenital cyanotic heart disease, 151–152, 156
    description of, 151
    hypoplastic left heart syndrome, 153–154
    right ventricular outflow tract abnormalities, 152–153
    tetralogy of Fallot, 152
    total anomalous pulmonary venous return, 152, 154
    transposition of great arteries, 152–154
    tricuspid valve abnormalities, 153
  hyperoxia test for, 149, 157
  in infant, 156–158
  miscellaneous causes of, 155–156
  in newborn, 156–158
  overview of, 145–146
  peripheral, 146–147
  persistent pulmonary hypertension of the newborn, 157

Cyanosis *(continued)*
pulmonary disease with, 150
pulmonary mechanisms of, 148–149
pulse oximetry evaluations, 149
reverse differential, 152
Cyanotic breath-holding spells, 156, 673, 932–933
Cyberbullying, 778
Cyclic vomiting, 972
Cyst(s)
description of, 734
epithelial, 8
Cystic fibrosis, 188, 852t
description of, 124
hemoptysis and, 482
weight loss and, 980

## D

Dactylitis, 598
Day–night reversal, 836
Deconditioning syndrome, 362
Decongestants, for cough, 141
Defecation, 119
Deformation, 287
Dehydration
in infants, 979
vomiting secondary to, 975
Dehydroepiandrosterone, 527–528
Dehydroepiandrosterone sulfate, 527–528
De Lange syndrome, 667
Delayed puberty
causes of, 726b
description of, 725–727
diagnostic testing for, 727b
referral for, 731
Delayed settling, 836–837
Depot-medroxyprogestone acetate, 223
Depression, 892t, 941. *See also* Major depressive disorder
anxiety and, 68t, 165t
assessment of, 163–164
children and, 850
conditions co-occurring with, 165t–166t
diagnostic criteria for, 164b
disruptive behavior and aggression associated with, 207t
*DSM-5* criteria for, 164b
findings suggestive of, 161–162, 162b, 163t
healthy habits and, 168
identification of, 162–163, 163t
initial interventions for, 169
insomnia caused by, 850
learning difficulties and, 610t
plan of care for, 167–170
prevalence of, 161
psychoeducation for, 167–168
psychopharmacologic treatment of, 171t
psychosocial screening for, 163t
psychosocial treatments for, 171t
resources for, 169
risk factors for, 162b
screening for, 163, 163t
specialist involvement for, 170–171
stress reduction for, 168–169
suicide risk, 166b
symptoms of, 162b
tools for identifying, 162–163, 163t
Dermatitis, contact
illustration of, 740f
pruritus and, 720
Dermatogenic torticollis, 949
Dermatoglyphics, 296
Dermatomal distribution, 741f
Dermatomyositis, 277
Dermatophytes, 682
Desisters, 422
Desmopressin, 706
Developmental delays, 851, 906t
Developmental dysplasia of the hip, 375
Developmental night waking, 842
Diabetes mellitus
fatigue caused by, 331
weight loss and, 981
Diabetic ketoacidosis, 241
Dialectal behavior therapy, for nonsuicidal self-injury, 804
Diamond-Blackfan anemia, 58
Diaphragmatic inflammation, 112
Diarrhea
acute
causes of, 178b
description of, 178, 178b, 181b
evaluation of, 180–181, 181b
treatment of, 181–185
chronic, 186b
differential diagnosis of, 179–180
exudative, 177
factitious, 192
hormone-related, 192–193
in infants
acute, 179–180
chronic, 185–196
description of, 980
medication for, 184
motility, 177–178
osmotic, 175–176
pathophysiologic factors of, 173–178
protracted, 186–188
referrals for, 196–197
secretory, 176–177
Diastolic blood pressure, 510
Diastolic murmurs, 464t, 465, 466f
Diet, hypertension and, 514
Diffuse pulmonary hemorrhage, 481–482
Diffusion block, 149
DiGeorge syndrome, 752t
Dilated cardiomyopathy, 151
Dipstick test, for urine screening, 710

Direct bilirubin, 582
Discoid lupus erythematosus, 36–37
Discoid meniscus, 623
Disimpaction, 128–129, 129t
Diskitis, 86, 89, 93, 599, 621
Disruptive behavior and aggression
  age-based manifestations of, 203–204
  assessment of, 206
  conditions co-occurring with, 206, 207t–208t
  family involvement in care for, 208
  findings suggestive of, 203–204, 204b
  healthy habits for, 209
  identification of, 204–205
  initial interventions for, 209–211
  parents and, 209–210
  plan of care for, 206–213
  prevalence of, 203
  prevention of, 203
  psychoeducation for, 208–209
  psychopharmacologic treatment of, 213t
  psychosocial screening for, 205t
  psychosocial treatment of, 213t
  resources for, 210
  specialist involvement for, 210–213
  stress reduction for, 209
  substance abuse and, 206, 208t
  tools for identifying, 204–205
Disruptive behavior disorders, 907t
Distal airway obstruction, 987
Diuretics, 260, 511, 515t
Dix-Hallpike maneuver, 218
Dizziness
  causes of, 215–216
  definition of, 215
  diagnosis of, 216f, 219t
  evaluation of, 218
  management of, 220
  referrals for, 220
DNA analysis, 297
DNA testing, 555
Dolichocephaly, 291
Dopaminergic drugs, 938
Down syndrome
  description of, 288, 292, 293f, 294, 852t
  hypotonia and, 551
  microcephaly and, 667
Dropping out of school, 781
Drospirenone, 534
Drug(s)
  abdominal pain managed using, 23
  irritability and, 575
  sleep affected by, 851
Drug abuse. *See also* Substance use
  dyspnea caused by, 242
  fatigue caused by, 333
Drug-induced dystonic reactions, 951
Drug-induced liver injury, 589
Dualism, 657
Dubin-Johnson syndrome, 589
Duchenne muscular dystrophy, 556
Dysfluency, 865
Dysfunctional elimination syndrome, 251
Dysfunctional uterine bleeding, 955, 958
Dysfunctional voiding, 251
Dyshemoglobinemias, 155
Dysmenorrhea
  primary, 221–223
  referrals for, 224
  secondary, 223–224
Dysmorphism, facial
  body, 294–297
  causes of, 292t
  craniofacial features, 291–292
  definition of, 287
  description of, 820
  diagnosis of, 290b, 298–299
  growth, 291
  history taking, 289–290
  laboratory evaluation for, 297
  physical examination for, 291–292
  proportions, 291
Dysphagia
  causes of, 228b, 228–229
  clinical manifestation of, 229
  diagnostic studies of, 231–232
  evaluation of, 231–232
  imaging studies for, 230–231
  laboratory studies for, 230
  management of, 232–233
  physical examination for, 229–230
  referrals for, 233
  symptoms of, 230b
Dyspnea
  clinical evaluation of, 236
  clinical presentation of, 237–242
  etiology of, 237–242
  history taking, 236
  hospitalization for, 244
  management of, 242–243
  pathophysiologic features of, 235–236
  psychogenic causes of, 242
  referrals for, 243
Dystonic torticollis, 949
Dysuria
  algorithm for, 249f
  causes of, 249t
  differential diagnosis of, 248–252
  history taking, 247
  hospitalization for, 252
  physical examination of, 248
  prepubertal children with, 250f
  referral for, 252

## E

Early Childhood Screening Assessment, 205t
Eating disorders, 982. *See also* Anorexia nervosa; Bulimia nervosa
Ebstein anomaly, 153

Eccrine bromhidrosis, 679, 682
ECG. *See* Electrocardiogram
Echinocytes, 51b
Echocardiogram, for syncope evaluations, 926
Echokinesis, 935
"E-cigarettes," 888
Edema
  causes of, 256b, 256–257
  evaluation of, 257–258
  history taking, 257–258
  laboratory evaluation of, 258
  management of, 259–260
  pathophysiology of, 255–256
  physical examination for, 258
  referrals for, 260
  test interpretation and, 258
Eflornithine hydrochloride, 534
Ehlers-Danlos syndrome, 277, 552, 601
Eicosapentaenoic acid, 635
Eisenmenger syndrome, 151
Ejection clicks, 460
Ejection murmurs, 464, 465f
Electrocardiogram
  arrhythmia evaluations, 97–98, 101
  chest pain evaluations, 113
  dyspnea evaluations, 240
  syncope evaluations, 925–926
Electroencephalograms, 933
Electrolytes
  absorption of, 176–177, 194–195
  congenital absorption disorders, 194–195
  imbalance of, 974
Electrophysiologic testing, 926
Eletriptan, 447t
Elliptocytes, 51b
Emergency plan, 169
Emotional disorders, 332–333. *See also* Social-emotional problems
Enalaprilat, 518t
Endocrine disorders
  fatigue caused by, 331, 334
  short stature caused by, 821
Endometrial fibrosis, 224
Endometrial polyps, 224
Endometriosis, 223–224
Endoscopic injection sclerotherapy, 405
Endoscopy, 398, 403
Energy
  conditions resulting in deficiency, 306b
  needs in children, 305b
*Entamoeba histolytica,* 180
Enterocolitis, 399
Enterohemorrhagic *E coli,* 180
Enterohepatic circulation, 582
Enterokinase, 189
Enteropathy, 259–260
Environment
  language development and, 860
  school refusal and, 777, 778
Eosinophilic esophagitis, 229
Eosinophilic gastroenteropathy, 191
Epididymal cysts, 795
Epididymitis, 790
Epiglottis, 995f
Epiglottitis, 150
Epilepsy
  electroencephalograms and, 933
  sleep-related, 853
Episcleritis, 774
Episodic ataxia, 79b
Epistaxis
  cause of, 265b
  definitions of, 263
  diagnosis of, 264–266
  epidemiologic factors of, 263
  evaluation of, 266–267, 268t
  management of, 267–272, 269f, 270b
  referrals for, 272–273
  scoring system for, 268t
  treatment of, 269f
Epley maneuver, 217
Epstein-Barr virus, 333
Equinovarus, 383, 384f
Equinus, 373b
Erosions, 734, 739f
Erythema migrans, 599
Erythematous papules, 736f
Erythematous patch, 735f
Erythroblastosis fetalis, 58
Erythrocyte sedimentation rate, 367–368
*Escherichia coli,* 180
Esmolol, 518t
Esophageal manometry, 232
Esophageal pH probe study, 232
Esophagitis, 115t
Esophagogastroduodenoscopy, 232
Esophagram, 993f
Ethnicity
  mean blood pressure and, 507
Event monitors, 926
Eversion, 373b
Evidence-based parenting programs, 212t
Ewing sarcoma, 285
Exclamation-point hairs, 31
Exercise
  dyspnea secondary to, 240
  hypertension and, 514
Exercise-induced chest pain, 114, 115t
Expectorants, 140
Expressive language deficits, 863
External tibial torsion, 377
Extrahepatic biliary atresia, 586–587
Extremity pain
  diagnosis of, 279b–280b, 279–285
  evaluation of, 275–279
  history taking, 275–276
  laboratory examination and, 277–278
  physical examination of, 276–277
  terminology associated with, 275
Eyberg Child Behavior Inventory, 913

Eye, red. *See* Conjunctivitis; Red eye
Eyelid abnormalities, 761–765
Eyelid tumors, 763, 763f

# F

Facial dysmorphism
  body, 294–297
  causes of, 292t
  craniofacial features, 291–292
  definition of, 287
  diagnosis of, 290b, 298–299
  growth, 291
  history taking, 289–290
  laboratory evaluation for, 297
  physical examination for, 291–292
  proportions, 291
Facio-auriculo-vertebral syndrome, 291
Facioscapulohumeral dystrophy, 557
Factitious disorder, 660t
Factitious fever, 356
Factitious hemoptysis, 483
Failure to thrive
  definition of, 301–303
  evaluation of, 306–308
  follow-up for, 309–312, 311–312
  history taking, 307–308
  hospitalization for, 312
  laboratory evaluation of, 309
  pathogenesis of, 304–306
  physical examination for, 308–309
  prognosis for, 312
  referral for, 312
  treatment of, 309–312
  undernutrition as cause of, 310–311, 311b
Familial dysautonomia, 921
Familial short stature, 819, 821–822
Family. *See also* Parent(s)
  blurred boundaries in, 320–321
  characteristics of, 317–318
  divided loyalties in, 320
  functioning of, 317–318
  of gender nonconforming patient, 422
  interpersonal interactions in, 323
  overview of, 317
  parenting styles in, 318–319
  physician's role in, 321–324
  roles in, 322
Family dysfunction
  anticipatory guidance for, 322
  description of, 319
  patterns of, 319–321
  presentation of, in primary care setting, 321
  summary of, 324
Fanconi syndrome, 295
FAS. *See* Fetal alcohol syndrome
Fat excretion, 173
Fatigue
  in adolescents, 333
  definition and etiology of, 329–330
  diagnostic testing of, 336–337
  differential diagnosis of, 330b–331b, 330–335
  in infants, 330
  management of, 338–339
  patient history and, 335–336
  physical examination of, 336
  weakness versus, 329
Favism, 57
Febrile seizures, 345
Fecal impaction, 7f
Feeding
  diarrhea and, 185
  dysphagia caused by, 229
  equipment, 233
  failure to thrive and, 307
  sleep and, 837
Feeding center, 633
Femoral anteversion, 373, 378–380
Femoral retroversion, 378
Femoral torsion deformities, 378–380
Fenoldopam, 518t
Fetal alcohol syndrome
  description of, 292, 293f
  microcephaly and, 667
Fetal hemoglobin, 156
Fever
  algorithms for, 351f–352f, 355f
  behavioral symptoms of, 344
  definition of, 343–344
  differential diagnosis of, 346b, 346–347
  evaluation of, 347–356
  factitious, 356
  in infants, 350, 354
  joint pain and, 599
  laboratory evaluation of, 350–353, 351f
  management of, 349–350
  in newborn, 350
  physical examination of, 344
  presentation of, 345–346
  Rochester criteria for, 353t
  signs and symptoms of, 344–345
  systemic inflammatory response syndrome, 347, 347t
  urinary tract infections as cause of, 354
  weight loss and, 980
Fever of unknown origin
  autoimmune diseases as cause of, 363, 364b
  definition of, 361–363
  diagnostic testing of, 367–368
  differential diagnosis of, 363–366, 364b–365b
  infectious diseases as cause of, 364b, 365
  malignancies as cause of, 364b, 365–366
  patient history and, 366
  periodic fever syndromes as cause of, 363, 364b, 366
  physical examination of, 366–367
  pseudo–fever of unknown origin versus, 362, 362b, 366
Fiber, 130
Fiberoptic endoscopic evaluation of swallowing, 231

Fibrillin, 288
Finasteride, 33
First heart sound, 459
Fitz-Hugh–Curtis syndrome, 17
Flatfoot, 373, 385–387
Flexible flatfoot, 385–386
Flexible laryngoscopy, 883f
Floppy infant, 335
Fluorescent in situ hybridization, 297
Fluphenazine, 941
Focal fat necrosis, 791
Follicle-stimulating hormone, 43–44, 954
Folliculitis, 739f
Food allergy
  description of, 577
  diarrhea caused by, 190–191
Food protein-induced enterocolitis syndrome, 191
Food refusal, 305
Foot disorders
  clubfoot, 383–385
  femoral torsion deformities, 378–380
  forefoot, 374–376
  shoes and, 392
  terminology, 373b
  tibial torsion, 376–378
  toe deformities, 388–390, 389f
  toe-walking, 390–391
Foot odor, 682
Forefoot, 374f–375f, 374–376
Foreign bodies
  aspiration of
    cyanosis caused by, 150
    hemoptysis caused by, 480, 485
    stridor caused by, 879t
    wheezing and, 992f
  in ear, 576
  in eye, 576
  in nose, 576
  odor caused by retention of, 682
  vaginal bleeding caused by, 954
Fourth heart sound, 459–460
FPIES. *See* Food protein-induced enterocolitis syndrome
Fragile X syndrome, 652
Frog-leg position, 335
Frovatriptan, 447t
FTT. *See* Failure to thrive
Functional abdominal pain, 14, 19–20
Fungal infections, 641t, 643
Fungi, splenomegaly and, 871
Fungicidal agents, 35–36
FUO. *See* Fever of unknown origin
Furosemide, 518t
Fusion beats, 100

## G

Gait, 626, 627t
Galactosemia, 585–586
Ganglioneuroblastoma, 193
Ganglioneuroma, 193
Gastrocolic reflex, 173
Gastroduodenoscopy, 404
Gastroenteritis, 184
Gastroesophageal reflux
  chest pain caused by, 115t
  cough caused by aspiration of, 139
  description of, 540, 972, 975
  sleep problems and, 852t, 854
Gastroesophageal varices, 398, 405
Gastrointestinal bleeding
  adolescents with, 400, 401b
  causes of, 49, 398–400, 401b
  diagnostic testing of, 396, 402–403
  differential diagnosis of, 396, 398–400
  history taking, 401–402
  infants and young children with, 398–400, 401b
  lower, 395
  management of, 403–406
  newborns with, 397–398, 401b
  nongastrointestinal source of, 396
  overview of, 395
  physical examination for, 402
  terminology associated with, 395–396
Gastrointestinal obstructions, 4
Gastrointestinal tract, 174f
Gaucher disease, 493
Gender, 409
Gender dysphoria, 410, 433
Gender expression and identity issues
  adverse effects of, 413–416
  advocacy, 437
  coming out, 428
  definitions, 409–412
  developmental well-being, 426
  *DSM-5* inclusion of, 411
  emotional well-being, 426
  etiology of, 412–413
  evaluation of, 416–422
  family considerations, 422
  future of, 429–430
  gender dysphoria, 410
  genetics of, 413
  history taking, 418–420
  isolation concerns, 428
  laboratory evaluation of, 421–422
  management of, 422–430
  overview of, 409
  parents, 435–436, 436b
  physical examination of, 420–421
  physical well-being, 425
  primary care physician considerations, 416–421
  psychosocial theories of, 412
  referral for, 437–438
  relationships, 428–429
  safety considerations, 427–428
  schools and, 415
  self-acceptance, 426–427
  self-disclosure, 428

sexual decision making, 428–429
social well-being, 426
societal stigma associated with, 415
transition care
female-to-male hormone treatment, 434–435
hormone therapy, 433–435
male-to-female hormone treatment, 434
overview of, 430–432
pubertal suppression, 432–433
validation, 426–427
Gender identity, 410
Gender identity disorder, 411
Gender nonconforming, 409, 422
Gender role, 409
Generalized anxiety disorder, 64t
Generalized edema, 258
Generalized lymphadenopathy, 356
Genetic factors
abdominal distention and, 2
epistaxis and, 266
hearing loss and, 453
hepatomegaly and, 492
hypertension and, 507
hypotonia and, 551–552
microcephaly and, 666b, 666–668
tics and, 937
Genital irritation, 814
Genitourinary tract malformation, 4
Genu valgum, 380–381. *See also* Knock-knees
Genu varum, 380
GER. *See* Gastroesophageal reflux
Giant vascular malformations, 696
*Giardia lamblia,* 190
Gilbert syndrome, 584, 587
Girls
blood pressure levels, 498f, 503t–506t
prepubertal
vaginal bleeding in, 953–954
vaginal discharge in, 963–965
puberty in, 723–727
short stature in, 822
Global developmental delay, 551
Glomerular hematuria, 474
Glossoptosis, 230
Glottic web, 884f
Glottis, 882f, 884f
Glucocorticoids, 821
Glucophage, 535
γ-Glutamyltransferase, 591
Gluten-sensitive enteropathy, 173, 820
Glycogen storage diseases, 557
Glycosuria, 703
Glycosylation, 195
Goldenhar syndrome, 291
Gonadarche, 723
Gonorrhea, 767
Goodpasture syndrome, 482
Gottron papules, 277, 625
Gram-positive bacteria, 682
Grief, 168
Griseofulvin, 35–36
Growing pains, 280–281, 601
Growth and development
sleep and, 828t
temper tantrums and, 929
Growth curves, 822
Growth delay, 819
Growth hormone deficiency, 819
Growth patterns, 819
Guaifenesin, 140
Guanfacine, 940
Guillain-Barré syndrome, 179
ataxia caused by, 81
treatment of, 83
weakness caused by, 335
Gynecomastia, 725

## H

Habits, rigid, 904b
*Haemophilus influenzae* type b, 349, 354, 620
Hair
excess. *See* Hirsutism
growth of, 27
loss of, 27. *See also* Alopecia
pulling and twisting of, 815
Hairball, 33, 815
Hair follicle, 523–524
Hair shaft anomalies, 29–30
Hair tourniquet, 576
Halitosis, 679, 681–682
Hallux valgus, 388–389, 389f
Haloperidol, 941
Hammer toe, 389, 389f
Hand flapping, 815
Hartnup syndrome, 176
Headaches
acute and recurrent, 443
algorithm for, 446f
analgesic overuse as cause of, 448
chronic nonprogressive, 443–444
chronic progressive, 443
clinical approach to, 443–449
disability caused by, 444–445
imaging of, 445
migraine
irritability and, 571
principles of, 445–448
prophylaxis for, 447b, 447–448
syncope and, 924
triptans for, 447, 447t
vertigo caused by, 82, 217
physical examination of, 445
principles of, 448–449
prognosis for, 449
referral for, 449
sleep-related, 853
tension type, 443–444, 448

Head banging, 811–812, 815
Head injuries
  irritability and, 569–571
  syncope and, 924
HEADSS assessment, 41, 418, 889
Hearing aids, 455
Hearing loss
  identification of, 454–455
  normal hearing versus, 452f–453f
  parental concerns and, 455t
  signs and symptoms of, 453–454
  speech development affected by, 455t
Heartbeat
  normal rhythm variation, 98
  premature, 98–100
Heart disease
  cyanotic
    congenital cyanotic heart disease, 151–152
    description of, 151
    hypoplastic left heart syndrome, 153–154
    right ventricular outflow tract abnormalities, 152–153
    tetralogy of Fallot, 152
    total anomalous pulmonary venous return, 152, 154
    transposition of the great arteries, 152–154
    tricuspid valve abnormalities, 153
  dyspnea caused by, 240
  hepatomegaly and, 491
  management of, 260
Heart murmurs
  cardiac evaluation and, 461–463, 462b
  evaluation of, 463t, 463–468
  holosystolic, 464
  innocent, 468
  patient evaluation for, 461
  referral for, 468
Heart sounds, 459–460
Height
  hypertension and, 498, 498f, 499t–502t
  short stature, 819–824
Heiner syndrome, 482
Hemangiomas
  gastrointestinal bleeding caused by, 400
  stridor and, 880
  stridor caused by, 879t
Hematemesis, 395, 484t
Hematochezia, 395–396
Hematocrit, 48t
Hematologic diseases and disorders
  dyspnea caused by, 240–241
  edema caused by, 258
  splenomegaly and, 871
Hematuria
  macroscopic, 471f–472f, 471–475
  microscopic, 472b, 475f, 475–476
  referral for, 476
Hemochromatosis, neonatal, 586
Hemoglobin
  deoxygenated, 147
  values for, 48t
Hemoglobin F, 156
Hemoglobin oxygen saturation, 145–146
Hemolysis, 583
Hemolytic anemia, 56
Hemolytic-uremic syndrome, 180, 696
Hemoptysis
  diagnostic testing for, 485–486
  differential diagnosis of, 483, 484t
  etiology of, 480–483, 481t
  history taking for, 483–484
  pathogenesis of, 479–480
  physical examination for, 484–485
  referral for, 487
Hemorrhagic disease of newborn, 397
Hemorrhagic stroke, 79
Henoch-Schönlein purpura, 277
  description of, 696
  joint pain, 599
  scrotal swelling and, 790–791
Hepatitis, 588–589
Hepatoblastoma, 8
Hepatomegaly
  definition of, 489
  diagnostic testing for, 492
  differential diagnosis of, 489–492, 490b
  history taking for, 492
  management of, 492–493
  palpable liver and, 489, 490b
  physical examination for, 492
Hepatorenal tyrosinemia, 586
Hereditary hemorrhagic telangiectasia, 266, 400, 484
Hereditary sensorimotor neuropathies, 555
Hereditary spherocytosis, 57
Hernia, 791–793, 792f
Herpes simplex virus
  conjunctivitis caused by, 766
  description of, 740f
Herpes zoster, 741f
Heterosexual precocious puberty, 728, 729b, 730
Hip dysplasia, congenital, 623, 623f
Hip joint, 627
Hirschsprung disease
  constipation caused by, 122–123, 126
  description of, 123–124
  diarrhea caused by, 179, 187, 190
Hirsutism
  cosmetic removal methods for, 534
  definition of, 523
  electrolysis for, 534
  evaluation of, 525, 525b
  idiopathic, 533
  modified Ferriman-Gallwey scoring system for, 532, 532f
  oral contraceptive pills for, 533–534
  referral for, 535
  treatment of, 533–535

Histiocytic necrotizing lymphadenitis, 363
Histoplasmosis, 871
HIV, 749
Hives, 721
Hoarseness
causes of, 539
definition of, 539
diagnostic testing for, 543–544
differential diagnosis of, 539–543, 540b–541b
history taking, 542–543
management of, 544–546
physical examination for, 543
Holosystolic murmurs, 464, 465f
Holter monitors, 926
Hordeola, 764
Hospitalization
abdominal distention, 10
abdominal pain, 24
anemia, 61
back pain, 94
cardiac arrhythmias, 109
chest pain, 113b, 117
constipation, 131
cough, 142
diarrhea, 197
dizziness, 220
dysmenorrhea, 224
dysphagia, 233–234
edema, 261
epistaxis, 273
failure to thrive, 312
vertigo, 220
HSV. *See* Herpes simplex virus
Human immunodeficiency virus. *See* HIV
Human papillomavirus, 770
Humoral immunodeficiencies, 750–753, 751t
Hurler syndrome, 651
Hydralazine, 518t
Hydrocele, 791–793, 792f
Hydrocephalus
description of, 649–651, 650b
stridor and, 878
Hydrometrocolpos, 7–8
Hydroxyzine, 720
Hyperandrogenism
adrenal, 527–529
definition of, 523
gonadal
in adolescents, 530–533
in children, 530
in infants, 529
precocious puberty, 529
ovarian, 531
Hyperbilirubinemia
conjugated, 581, 583b, 584–585, 588b, 588–589
definition of, 581
unconjugated, 582–584, 583b, 587, 588b
Hypercalciuria
dysuria caused by, 252
microhematuria caused by, 476
Hyperextension test, 90f
Hyperhidrosis, 549–550
Hyper-IgM syndrome, 751t
Hypermobility syndrome, 601
Hyperoxia test, 149, 157
Hypertension. *See also* Blood pressure
antihypertensive drugs and, 514–516, 515t
athletic participation by children with, 516
blood pressure regulation and, 511
body size and, 498, 498f, 499t–502t, 514
causes of, 507–509, 508b
definition of, 497
diagnostic evaluation for, 511–514, 512f, 513b
exercise guidelines for adolescents with, 519t
factors influencing, 497, 507
primary, 507–508
referral for, 518
secondary, 508–509
treatment of, 514–516
Hypertensive emergencies, 516–517, 518t
Hypertensive urgency, 518, 518t
Hypertrichosis
causes of, 526b
classification of, 526
congenital generalized, 526
definition of, 523
lumbosacral, 526
prepubertal, 526
presentation of, 525–526
sexual hair versus, 525–526
treatment of, 527
Hypertrophic cardiomyopathy
chest pain caused by, 115t
syncope and, 923
Hypertrophic pyloric stenosis, 573
Hyperventilation
chest pain caused by, 115t, 117
syncope and, 922
Hyphema, 773, 773f
Hypnagogic hallucinations, 676
Hypoestrogenic amenorrhea, 44
Hypoglycemia
dizziness caused by, 215
irritability and, 574
Hypoplasia, 292
Hypoplastic left heart syndrome, 153–154
Hypospadias, 297
Hypothalamic-pituitary-adrenal axis, 527
Hypothalamic-pituitary-gonadal axis, 530
Hypothalamic-pituitary-ovarian axis, 41, 953–955
Hypothyroidism
description of, 9
fatigue caused by, 331, 336
hypotonia and, 552
short stature and, 821

Hypotonia
causes of, 552–557
definition of, 551
diagnostic testing for, 553–554
history taking, 552–553
physical examination for, 553
referral for, 557
Hypoventilation, 149
Hypoxemia
definition of, 147
hypoventilation-induced, 149
Hypoxia, 147

**I**

Iatrogenic Cushing syndrome, 821
IBD. *See* Inflammatory bowel disease
Ibuprofen, 222
IDEA. *See* Individuals with Disabilities Education Act
Identity issues. *See* Gender expression and identity issues
Idiopathic hirsutism, 533
Idiopathic hypersomnia, 849
Idiopathic intestinal pseudoobstruction, 194
Idiopathic short stature, 821–822
IgA deficiency, 751t
IgG subclass deficiency, 751t
Illness anxiety disorder, 659t
Imiglucerase, 493
Immunodeficiencies
combined, 752t, 752–753
diagnostic testing for, 754–755, 755t
diarrhea and, 193
history taking, 754
physical examination for, 754
primary, 749–754
recurrent infections and, 747
secondary, 748–749, 749t
treatment of, 755–756
Immunoglobulin A nephropathy, 474
Inattention and impulsivity
in adolescents, 567b
anxiety and, 562t
assessment of, 560–561
in attention-deficit/hyperactivity disorder, 559–560, 562t
conditions co-occurring with, 562t–563t
findings suggestive of, 559, 560b
healthy habits and, 564
identification of, 560
initial interventions for, 564–566, 565b
parental involvement, 564
plan of care for, 561–567
psychoeducation for, 563
psychosocial screening of, 561t
resources for, 566
specialist involvement for, 566
stress reduction for, 564
tools for identifying, 560
Inborn errors of metabolism, 575
Indirect laryngoscopy, 543
Individual Education Plan, 614
Individuals with Disabilities Education Act, 614
Indomethacin, 706
Infant(s). *See also* Premature infants
anorexia in, 635b
arrhythmias in, 103
back pain in, 86, 88–89, 93
blood pressure in, 509–511
botulism in, 556, 571
caloric intake in, 979
constipation in, 125–127
cyanosis in, 156–158
development of, 841
diarrhea in
acute, 179–180
chronic, 185–196
description of, 980
diffuse pulmonary hemorrhage in, 486
dysphagia and, 230
fatigue in, 330
fever in, 350, 354
gastrointestinal bleeding in, 398–400, 401b
gonadal hyperandrogenism in, 529
hearing loss in, 451–457
hoarseness in, 539, 541b, 541–542
hypertension in, 508b
hypotonia in, 335, 556
irritability and, 569–571, 576–578
jaundice in, 582–587
language development in, 860t–861t
night feeding of, 841
progressive spinal muscular atrophy, 554, 554t
rashes in, 744b–745b
sleep myoclonus in, 675–676
syncope in, 674
vaginal discharge in, 963
vomiting in, 971, 980
weight gain, 303–304
weight loss, 980
Infantile hypertrophic pyloric stenosis, 767
Infection, recurrent
diagnostic testing for, 754–755
immune disorders and, 747–748
patient history and examination for, 754
primary immunodeficiencies and, 749–754, 750t
referrals for, 756b
secondary immunodeficiencies and, 748–749, 749t
splenomegaly and, 870–871
susceptibility to, 748
treatment of, 755–756
Infiltrative disorders
hepatomegaly and, 491
splenomegaly and, 871
Inflammation
chronic, 54–55
hoarseness and, 545–546

Inflammatory bowel disease
diarrhea caused by, 196
fatigue caused by, 333
gastrointestinal bleeding caused by, 400
short stature caused by, 820
Inflammatory diseases
fatigue caused by, 331–332
hepatomegaly and, 490–491
lymphadenopathy and, 643
splenomegaly and, 871–872
Inguinal hernia
description of, 791–793, 792f
irritability and, 573
Inguinal ring, 794f
Innocent murmurs, 461, 467t, 468
Insomnia, primary, 839–840
Insulin-like growth factor 1, 823
Insulin resistance, 531
Intellectual and developmental disabilities, self-injurious behavior in children with, 799, 804–805
Intermittent ataxia, 79b
Internal tibial torsion, 377, 378f
Interstitial hydrostatic pressure, 257
Intestinal lymphangiectasia, 191–192
Intestinal pseudoobstruction, idiopathic, 194
Intestine(s)
disorders of, 980
malrotation of, irritability and, 573
obstruction of, 4–6
Intra-atrial re-entrant tachycardia, 104
Intracranial pressure, increased
ataxia and, 79
irritability and, 571
Intrathoracic airway obstruction, 987
Intraventricular hemorrhage, 650
Intussusception
gastrointestinal bleeding caused by, 399
irritability and, 572–573
Inversion, 373b
IPEX syndrome, 194
Iritis, 773
Iron deficiency
breath-holding spells and, 933
microcytic anemia caused by, 48–50, 52–53
sleep disturbance and, 847
Iron deficiency anemia, 55
Irritability
acute, 569–575, 570f
causes of, 569–575, 576–578
chronic, 570f, 576–578
Irritable bowel syndrome, 177, 196
Irritants, dysuria caused by, 251
Isoimmune hemolytic anemia, 58
Isometric exercises, 927
Isosexual precocious puberty, 728b, 729–730
Itch, 719–721

## J

Jaundice
bile acid metabolism defects as cause of, 587
bilirubin metabolism and, 581–582
diagnosis of, 590–592
differential diagnosis of, 582, 583b
history taking for, 589–590
management of, 592
metabolic disorders that cause, 585–586
obstructive, 586–587
physical examination for, 590
systemic illnesses that cause, 585
Jervell and Lange-Nielsen syndrome, 108, 923
Job syndrome, 753t
Joint Committee on Infant Hearing, 454
Joint pain
definition of, 597
differential diagnosis of, 597–602
etiology of, 597
evaluation for, 602
referral for, 603–604
treatment of, 602–603
Juvenile dermatomyositis, 598, 625
Juvenile idiopathic arthritis, 624
description of, 598
fatigue caused by, 331
Juvenile nasopharyngeal angiofibroma, 265
Juvenile polyposis coli, 399
Juvenile polyps, 398

## K

Kasabach-Merritt syndrome, 491, 696
Kawasaki disease
conjunctivitis associated with, 771
irritability and, 572
Kidney, multicystic, 7
Kiesselbach plexus, 264
Kikuchi-Fujimoto disease, 363
Kleine-Levin syndrome, 853
Knee joint, 627–628
Knock-knees, 380–383, 382f
Korotkoff sounds, 510
Kussmaul breathing, 241
Kyphosis, 92

## L

Labetalol, 518t
Labial adhesions, 251
Labyrinthitis, 82
Lactic acidosis, 535
Language development
delays in
differential diagnosis of, 866
prognosis for, 867
risk factors for, 859–863, 861t–862t
description of, 859
environmental factors that affect, 860
milestones in, 860t
screening of, 863, 864t

Language disorders
description of, 863, 865
differential diagnosis of, 866
prevalence of, 859
prognosis for, 867
referral for, 866
treatment of, 866–867
Lanugo, 27, 523
Laryngeal clefts, 539, 545
Laryngeal papilloma, 884f
Laryngeal papillomatosis, 879t
Laryngeal saccular cysts, 541, 545
Laryngeal trauma, 546
Laryngeal webs
hoarseness and, 539, 541
stridor caused by, 879t
Laryngitis, 545–546
Laryngomalacia, 878, 879t, 880, 884f
Laryngopharyngeal reflux, 541–542
Laryngoscopy, 544, 882f–883f
Laryngotracheobronchitis, 545–546
Larynx, 882f–883f, 884f
Lateral collateral ligament, 628
Laxatives, 127–128, 129t, 130
Lead poisoning, 54
Learning difficulties
in adolescents, 612
assessment of, 611–613
background on, 607
causes of, 608–611
conditions co-occurring with, 610t–611t
developmental problems as cause of, 609
findings suggestive of, 608t
homework battles, 614b
initial interventions for, 614
lack of school readiness as cause of, 608, 609b
medical problems as cause of, 609
mental health problems as cause of, 609
plan of care for, 613–615
primary care physician's role in, 607
recognition of, 607, 608b
resources for, 614
significance of, 607
specialist involvement in, 614
stress reduction for, 613–614
symptoms of, 608b
Learning disabilities, 68t, 165t, 207t, 562t, 611, 865, 892t
Learning problems, sleep-related symptoms of, 851
Leg disorders
bowed legs, 380–383, 382f
femoral torsion deformities, 378–380
knock-knees, 380–383, 382f
terminology, 373b
tibial torsion, 376–378
Legg-Calvé-Perthes disease, 277, 283, 619, 620f
Leg-length discrepancy, 86–87
Lesch-Nyhan syndrome, 815
Let-down reflex, 979
Leukemia, 622
Leukocyte adhesion defect, 753t
Leydig cell tumors, 794
Lichenification, 742
Limit-setting disorder, 838–839
Limp
antinuclear antibody testing of, 629
bone scintigraphy of, 630
computed tomography of, 630
differential diagnosis of, 619–625
diskitis as cause of, 621
evaluation of, 625–630
gait examination in, 626, 627t
general examination of, 629
history taking for, 625–626
imaging of, 630
infectious causes of, 620–621
inflammatory diseases as cause of, 624–625
joint examination in, 626–629
laboratory testing of, 629–630
Legg-Calvé-Perthes disease as cause of, 619, 620f
magnetic resonance imaging of, 630
malignancies as cause of, 622
musculoskeletal examination in, 626–629
neuromuscular disorders as cause of, 625
osteochondritis dissecans as cause of, 619
osteomyelitis as cause of, 621
physical examination of, 626
radiographs of, 630
referral for, 630–631
skeletal anomalies as cause of, 623–624
trauma as cause of, 619
ultrasound of, 630
vascular causes of, 619
Little League elbow, 281
Liver
bilirubin transport defects, 589
biopsy of, 591–592
enlargement of. *See* Hepatomegaly
palpation of, 489
transplantation of, 592
Liver disease
edema caused by, 259
jaundice and, 588–589
Liver span, 489
Long-chain triglycerides, 175
Long QT syndrome, 108
Loose anagen syndrome, 30
Lower airways diseases, 150
Lower gastrointestinal bleeding, 398–400, 401b, 402, 405–406
Lumbar puncture, for febrile seizure, 345
Lumbosacral hypertrichosis, 526
Lupus erythematosus, 36–37
Luteinizing hormone, 954

Lyme disease, 599
Lymphadenopathy
  age-based incidence of, 639t
  diagnostic testing for, 643–645
  differential diagnosis of, 640–643
  etiology of, 638t–640t
  evaluation of, 646t
  history taking for, 643–644
  infectious, 644–645, 647–648
  physical examination for, 643–644
  referral for, 648
  treatment of, 647–648
Lymphatic system, 637, 640
Lymph nodes
  disease origin in, 638t
  of head and neck, 638f
Lymphonodular hyperplasia, 399

## M

Macrocephaly
  causes of, 650b
  definition of, 649
  diagnostic testing for, 654
  differential diagnosis of, 649–652
  management of, 654
  patient history and examination for, 652–653, 653b
  referral for, 654–655
Macrocytic anemia, 52t, 57
Macroscopic hematuria, 471–475
Macules
  café au lait, 735f
  definition of, 734
Magnesium, 223
Magnetic resonance cholangiopancreatography, 591
Major depressive disorder. *See also* Depression
  diagnostic criteria for, 164b
  *DSM-5* criteria for, 164b
  prevalence of, 161
  psychopharmacologic treatment of, 171t
Malabsorption
  diarrhea and, 176, 184
  syndromes, 173, 188–189
  weight loss caused by, 980
Male-pattern alopecia, 524
Malformations
  definition of, 287–289
  Pierre Robin sequence of, 288
Malignancies. *See also* Neoplasia; Neoplasms; Tumor(s)
  fatigue caused by, 332
  irritability associated with, 575
  limp caused by, 622
  petechiae and purpura caused by, 696
  weight loss and, 981
Mallet toe, 389, 389f
Mallory-Weiss tear, 398
Malnutrition
  protracted diarrhea and, 187
  secondary immunodeficiency and, 749
Malocclusion, 813
Malrotation, with secondary midgut volvulus, 972
Maltreatment, 165t
Marfan syndrome, 92, 114, 288, 295, 601
Masturbation, 813–814
McBurney point, 13
McMurray test, 628
Mean corpuscular hemoglobin, 60
Mean corpuscular volume, 47, 48t, 60
Meatal stenosis, 251
Meckel diverticulum, 399
Meckel scan, 406
Medial collateral ligament, 628
Medial meniscus, 628
Mediastinal masses, 643b
Medically unexplained symptoms
  abdominal pain, 658
  assessment of, 660–661, 661b
  background for, 657
  classification of, 659t–660t, 659–660
  epidemiology of, 658
  etiology of, 658
  interventions for, 662t
  management of, 661–662
  prognosis for, 663
  risk factors for, 658b
Medications. *See also specific medication*
  abdominal pain managed using, 23
  irritability and, 575
  sleep affected by, 851
Medium-chain triglycerides, 175, 592
Mefenamic acid, 222
Megalencephaly, 649, 650b, 651–652
Menarche, 39–40
Ménière disease, 218
Meningitis, 345, 747
Menstrual cycle, 954
Menstruation, 39
Metabolic disorders
  description of, 124, 241, 682, 683t–684t
  hypotonia and, 552
Metabolic syndrome, 507
Metabolism, bilirubin, 581–582
Metatarsus adductus, 371, 374–376
Metatarsus varus, 374, 376, 383
Methemoglobinemia, 155, 574
Methotrexate, 602
Microcephaly
  causes of, 666b
  definition of, 665–666
  description of, 665, 668
  differential diagnosis of, 666–668
  evaluation of, 668–670
  management of, 670
  referral for, 670
Microcytic anemia
  causes of, 52t
  diagnostic approach to, 49f

Microcytic anemia *(continued)*
iron deficiency as cause of, 48–50, 52–53
lead poisoning as cause of, 54
thalassemias as cause of, 53–54
Micrognathia, 230
Microscopic hematuria
causes of, 472b
description of, 471, 475–476
evaluation of, 475f
Microthrombi, 239
Microvillus inclusion disease, 194
Middle-ear disease, 215
Midodrine, 927
Midsystolic apical click, 460
Migraine headaches
irritability and, 571
principles of, 445–448
prophylaxis for, 447b, 447–448
syncope and, 924
triptans for, 447, 447t
vertigo caused by, 82, 217
Milk allergy, 398
Miller-Dieker syndrome, 667
Minoxidil, 518t
Mitochondrial encephalomyopathies, 557
Mitral valve prolapse, 116
Mobitz type I block, 106
Mobitz type II block, 106
Modified Overt Aggression Scale, 204
Monilethrix, 30–31
Mononucleosis, infectious
fatigue caused by, 333
splenomegaly and, 871
Motivational interviewing, 895, 897t
Motor ataxia, 81
Motor tics, 935
Motor unit disorders, 554–557
Mouth odor, 681–682
Mucolytic agents, 141
Multiple suture craniosynostosis, 668
Mumps orchitis, 791
Münchausen syndrome by proxy, 483
Murmurs
cardiac evaluation and, 461–463
evaluation of, 463t, 463–468
holosystolic, 464
innocent, 468
patient evaluation for, 461
referral for, 468
Muscle biopsies, 554
Muscular dystrophy, 625
Duchenne, 556
facioscapulohumeral, 557
hypotonia and, 556
Muscular torticollis, 947, 950–951
Mutational voice disorder, 542
Myasthenia gravis, 335, 555–556
*Mycoplasma* pneumonia, 333
Myocarditis, 115t, 116
Myoclonus, 675–676
Myoneural junction disorders, 555–556
Myopathies, 556–557
Myotonic dystrophy, 556
Myxedema, 260

## N

Nail biting, 812–813
Naratriptan, 447t
Narcolepsy, 676–677, 849
Nasal hemangioma, 265
Nasogastric tubes, 404
Nasolacrimal duct obstruction, 767
Nasopharyngeal carcinoma, 265
National Association for the Education of Young Children, 911
National Center for Health Statistics, 302
National Health and Nutrition Examination Survey, 39
National Health Examination Survey, 39
Necrotizing enterocolitis
gastrointestinal bleeding and, 397
irritability and, 573
*Neisseria gonorrhoeae,* 599, 968
*Neisseria meningitidis,* 599
Neonatal cholestasis, 584
Neonatal drug abstinence syndrome, 195
Neonatal hemochromatosis, 586
Neonate. *See also* Newborn
botulism in, 556, 571
diffuse pulmonary hemorrhage in, 486
gastrointestinal bleeding in, 397, 401b
hemoptysis in, 486–487
hoarseness in, 539, 541b, 541–542
hypertension in, 508b
hypotonia in, 335, 556
irritability in, 569–571
jaundice in, 582–587
measuring blood pressure of, 509–511
rashes in, 742b–743b
sleep myoclonus in, 675–676
testicular torsion in, 789
vaginal discharge in, 963
vomiting in, 971
Neoplasia. *See also* Malignancies
hoarseness and, 545
lymphadenopathy and, 643, 648
Neoplasms. *See also* Malignancies
epistaxis caused by, 265
extremity pain caused by, 285
torticollis and, 949
Nephrogenic diabetes insipidus, 702, 705–706
Neurocardiogenic syncope, 919
Neurocutaneous syndromes, 652
Neurofibromas, 736f
Neurofibromatosis, 735f, 736f
Neurogenic diabetes insipidus, 702
Neuroleptics, 941
Neurologic disorders, sleep-related symptoms of, 851, 853
Neurotransmitters, 971

Newborn. *See also* Infant(s); Neonate
anemia and, 50f, 57–59
bacterial infections in, 350
cardiac arrhythmias and, 99, 105
congenital cyanotic heart disease screening in, 157–158
conjunctivitis in, 767
cyanosis in, 156–158
diarrhea in, 179, 195
dysmorphism and, 289–292
fever in, 350
hemorrhagic disease of, 397
language development in, 860t–861t
persistent pulmonary hypertension of the, 157
tympanitic abdomen in, 4–6
Nicardipine, 518t
Nifedipine, 518t
Nightmare disorder, 846–847
Night terrors, 577, 676
Nighttime pruritus, 953
Night waking, 841–842
Nodding spasms, 948
Nodules, 734
Nonconvulsive periodic disorders, 673–677
Nonconvulsive status epilepticus, 571
Nonpathological proteinuria, 711–712
Nonsteroidal anti-inflammatory drugs, 222
Nonsuicidal self-injury
definition of, 799
diagnostic approach to, 802
dialectal behavior therapy for, 804
epidemiology of, 800
evaluation of, 801
function of, 800–801
gender and, 800
hospitalization for, 806
management of, 804–805
ongoing care for, 805
referral for, 802–803, 805
risk assessment for, 802–803
self-injurious behavior versus, 801
signs and symptoms of, 802
suicide attempts versus, 802
treatment of, 804–805
Noonan syndrome
description of, 292, 294f, 295
short stature and, 820
Normocephaly, 291
Normocytic anemia
causes of, 54–56
characteristics of, 52t
evaluation of, 56–57
Nucleated red blood cells, 52b
Nutrition disorders, short stature caused by, 820
Nylan-Barany test, 218

## O

Obesity
dyspnea caused by, 241
hypertension and, 498, 514
knock-knees and, 381
metabolic syndrome and, 497, 507
Obsessive-compulsive behaviors, 815
Obsessive-compulsive disorder
characteristics of, 64t
description of, 936–937, 941
treatment of, 67, 69
Obstruction
airway
distal, 987
intrathoracic, 987
stridor and, 877
wheezing and, 987–989, 991f
biliary
hepatomegaly and, 492
jaundice and, 589
Obstructive jaundice, 586–587
Obstructive pulmonary disease, 237, 238b
Octreotide, 405
Ocular myositis, 774
Ocular torticollis, 948
ODD. *See* Oppositional defiant disorder
Odor
body
causes of, 681–687, 683t–687t
differential diagnosis of, 681–682
physical examination of, 680
conditions associated with, 686t–687t
foot, 682
infection as cause of, 685t–686t
urine
causes of, 682, 685
differential diagnosis of, 681–682
metabolic abnormalities as cause of, 682, 683t
physical examination of, 682
Oligohydramnios, 2
Oncotic pressure, 255–257
Opitz syndrome, 292
Opportunistic infections, 747–748
Oppositional defiant disorder, 165t, 203, 204b, 209, 212, 563t, 611t
Oral contraceptive pills, 223, 533–534
Oral hygiene, 682
Oral motor therapy, 233
Orbital cellulitis, 761–763, 763f
Orchitis, 790
Ornithine decarboxylase, 534
Orthopedics, 372, 373b
Orthostatic hypotension, 921
Orthostatic proteinuria, 711–712
Osgood-Schlatter disease, 284, 601
Osler-Weber-Rendu disease, 266, 272, 400
Osmidrosis axillae, 681
Osmotic diuresis, 703
Osteochondritis dissecans, 283–284, 619
Osteochondroses, 283–284
Osteoid osteoma, 93, 285, 622, 622f

Osteomyelitis
description of, 86, 93, 572
extremity pain caused by, 284–285
joint pain and, 599
limp caused by, 621
Osteosarcoma, 622
Otitis media
irritability and, 576
recurrent, 748
Ottawa ankle criteria, 278, 278b
Ovarian hyperandrogenism, 531
Overnight sleep study, 836
Overuse syndromes, 281–282
Oxygen delivery, 147–148
Oxygen transport, 147–148
Oxyhemoglobin saturation, 145, 147

## P

Pacemaker malfunction, 923
Pain
abdominal
acute, 13, 15, 16b
causes of, 17b
characteristics of, 13, 18–21
children and, 13, 18–21
chronic, 18
diagnosis of, 15b, 16b
differential diagnosis of, 15–18, 16b
evaluation of, 18–21, 19f
functional, 14, 19–20
history taking, 18–20
hospitalization for, 24
laboratory evaluation of, 20–21, 21b
medically unexplained symptoms, 658
physical examination for, 20
referral for, 23–24
treatment for, 21–23
back
chronic causes of, 87
diagnosis of, 86–87, 87t
epidemiology of, 85
evaluation of, 88–92
management of, 92–94
psychosocial considerations of, 87–88
referrals for, 94
chest
causes of, 114–117, 115t
diagnosis of, 111
evaluation of, 112–113
exercise-induced, 114, 115t
history and, 112–113
idiopathic causes of, 116–117
laboratory evaluation and, 113
pathophysiologic features of, 111–112
psychogenic, 117
referred, 111
symptoms of, 113b, 115t
extremities
diagnosis of, 279b–280b, 279–285
evaluation of, 275–279
history taking, 275–276
laboratory examination and, 277–278
physical examination of, 276–277
terminology associated with, 275
joint
definition of, 597
differential diagnosis of, 597–602
etiology of, 597
evaluation for, 602
referral for, 603–604
treatment of, 602–603
Palilalia, 935
Pallid breath-holding spells, 673, 933
Pallor, 47, 59
Palmoplantar hyperhidrosis, 549–550
PANDAS, 936–937
Panic attacks, 67, 72
Panic disorder, 64t
Pansystolic murmurs, 465f
Papules, 734, 740f
Papulopustules, 736f
Paradoxical vocal fold dysfunction, 542
Paralytic ileus, 6
Parasites, 190
Parasomnias, 843–846
Parenchymal lung disease, 148
Parent(s). *See also* Family
amenorrhea diagnosis and, 41
anxiety in, 67, 72
authoritative role of, 319
breath-holding spells, 932–934
characteristics of, 318–319
constipation and, 121, 127–128
disruptive behavior and aggression management by, 209–210
dysfunction patterns, 319–320
dysmorphism and, 298
of gender nonconforming children, 435–436, 436b
inattention and impulsivity managed by, 564
over-involved, 320
school refusal and, 777–778
sleep disturbance and, 834
temper tantrums and, 930–931
uninvolved, 320
Parenteral diarrhea, 179
Parenteral nutrition, 585
Parenting
evidence-based programs for, 212t
styles of, 318–319
Parietal pain, 13
Patches, 734, 735f
Patellofemoral pain syndrome, 601
Patent ductus arteriosus, 151
Pathological proteinuria, 712–713, 713t
Pathologic gastroesophageal reflux, 972
PCOS. *See* Polycystic ovary syndrome

Pediatric Symptom Checklist, 205t
PEG. *See* Polyethylene glycol
Pelvic examination, 43, 222, 224
Pelvic inflammatory disease
  description of, 223–224
  dysuria caused by, 252
Peppermint oil, 23
Peptic ulcer disease, 400
Pericarditis, 115t, 116
Perihepatitis, 17
Perilymph fistula, 217
Perinatal asphyxia, 668
Period (menstrual), 954
Periodic fever, aphthous stomatitis, pharyngitis, and cervical adenopathy, 363, 366
Periodic fever syndrome, 362
Periodic limb movements, 847
Periorbital edema, 258
Peripheral cyanosis, 146–147
Peripheral nerve disorders, 555
Peripheral puberty, 728
Persistent pulmonary hypertension of the newborn, 157
Pertussis, 150
Pes, 373b
Pes cavus, 387–388
Petechiae
  description of, 691–696
  evaluation of, 691–693, 692f
Phagocytic immunodeficiencies, 753, 753t
Phentolamine, 518t
Phlyctenulosis, 769, 769f
Phobia, school, 776
Phonologic disorders, 866
Phonology, 865
Phonotrauma, 542, 546
Physical abuse, joint pain and, 601
Physiologic anemia of the newborn, 57
Physiologic leukorrhea, 967
Pierre Robin sequence, 230
Pigmented villonodular synovitis, 602
Pili torti, 31
Pimozide, 941
Pink eye. *See* Conjunctivitis
Pinworms, 953
Pitted keratolysis, 682
Plagiocephaly, 291
Plantar hyperhidrosis, 549
Planus, 373b
Plaque
  description of, 734
  scaling, 737f
Plasma volume, 257
Platelet disorders, 691–696
Play, 861t–862t
Pleural effusion, 115t
Pleural pain, 112
Pleurodynia, 112
Pneumococcal vaccine, 349
Pneumonia
  chest pain caused by, 115t
  *Mycoplasma,* 333
  recurrent, 748
Pneumoperitoneum, 6
Pneumothorax
  chest pain caused by, 115t
  spontaneous, 114, 115t
Point of maximal impulse, 462
Poisoning
  carbon monoxide, 574
  lead, 54
Poison ivy, 740f
Polycystic ovary syndrome
  in adolescents, 530–535
  glucophage for, 535
  insulin resistance in, 531
  laboratory evaluation of, 44, 533
  physical examination of, 532
  premature adrenarche risks, 529
  treatment of, 533–535
Polydactyly, 295, 389f, 390
Polydipsia, 699, 705
  psychogenic, 703
Polyethylene glycol, 129–130
Polyhydramnios, 2
Polyps
  description of, 398–399
  gastrointestinal bleeding caused by, 398–399
Polyuria
  definition of, 699
  diagnostic testing for, 703–706, 704t
  differential diagnosis of, 700–703, 701b
  evaluation of, 703–706
  management of, 705–706
  pathophysiologic features of, 699–700, 700f
  referral for, 705, 707
Port wine stain, 735f, 763
Post-concussive syndrome, 571, 577
Posterior drawer test, 628
Postpubertal vaginal secretions, 681
Post-traumatic stress disorder, 64t, 67, 69
Postural hypotension, 674
Postural kyphosis, 92
Postural orthostasis tachycardia syndrome, 921
Postural proteinuria, 711–712
Postural syncope, 920
Posture, 232–233
Poverty, weight loss and, 981
Prader-Willi syndrome
  description of, 815
  hypotonia and, 551
Pragmatic deficits, 865
Precocious puberty
  causes of, 729b
  central, 530, 728
  diagnostic testing for, 730b
  gonadotropin-dependent, 529

Precocious puberty *(continued)*
gonadotropin-independent, 529
referral for, 731
Precocious sexual hair growth, 729
Prednisone, 36
Pregnancy
dysmorphic feature, diagnostic questions about, 289–290
dyspnea caused by, 241–242
Prehn sign, 790
Premature adrenarche, 527–529
Premature infants. *See also* Infant(s)
diffuse pulmonary hemorrhage in, 486
gastrointestinal bleeding in, 397
hemoptysis in, 486–487
necrotizing enterocolitis in, 397
Premature ventricular contractions, 100
Prepubertal girls
vaginal bleeding in, 953–954
vaginal discharge in, 963–965
Prepubertal hypertrichosis, 526
Presenteeism, 444
Preseptal cellulitis, 761–763, 762f
Presyncope, 919
PRICEMMMS mnemonic, 93
Primary amenorrhea, 39, 43
Probiotics, 23
Problem solving, 169
Processus vaginalis, 792
Progressive familial intrahepatic cholestasis, 587
Projectile vomiting, 972
Prostaglandin $E_1$, 152
Prostaglandin $E_2$, 221
Prostaglandin $F_{2\alpha}$, 221
Protein hypersensitivity, 190
Proteinuria
definition of, 709
diagnostic testing for, 709–711, 714, 715f
etiology of, 711–713
history taking for, 713
laboratory evaluation of, 709–711
management of, 714
pathophysiology of, 709
physical examination for, 713
prevalence of, 711
referral for, 716
renal biopsy and, 715b
warning signs of, 714b
Prothrombin time, 591
Pruritus, 719–721
Pseudo–fever of unknown origin, 362, 362b, 366
*Pseudomonas aeruginosa,* 621
Pseudoprecocious puberty, 728
Psoriasis, 598, 737f
Psychiatric syncope, 922
Psychoactive substances, 887
Psychoeducation
for anxiety disorders, 70
for attention-deficit/hyperactivity disorder, 563
for depression, 167–168
description of, 8
for disruptive behavior and aggression, 208–209
for inattention and impulsivity, 563
Psychogenic chest pain, 115t
Psychogenic polydipsia, 703
Psychoneurotic truancy, 776
Psychosis, 68t, 892t
Psychosocial screening
for anxiety disorders, 64–65, 66t
for depression, 163t
for inattention and impulsivity, 561t
Pterygium colli, 948
Pubarche, 523, 527
Puberty
delayed
causes of, 726b
description of, 725–727
diagnostic testing for, 730b
referral for, 731
gynecomastia, 725
onset of, 724t
precocious
causes of, 729b
diagnostic testing for, 730b
referral for, 731
short stature and, 822
suppression of, 432–433
Pulmonary atresia with ventricular septal defect, 153
Pulmonary diseases and disorders
dyspnea caused by, 237–240
fatigue caused by, 332
Pulmonary function tests
cough and, 139
wheezing and, 991f
Pulmonary hemorrhage, 396
Pulmonary hemosiderosis, 482
Pulmonary hypertension, 459, 924
Pulmonary neoplasms, 482
Purpura
description of, 691–696
evaluation of, 691–693, 692f
Henoch-Schönlein
description of, 696
joint pain, 599
scrotal swelling and, 790–791
palpable, 692f
Pustules, 734, 739f
Pyknocytes, 51b

## Q

QRS morphology, 99–100, 105
QT interval, 100, 108
Quickening, 290

## R

Race, hypertension and, 507
Radiographs
abdominal distention evaluations, 9
back pain evaluations, 89

chest pain evaluations, 113
dysmorphism evaluations, 298
dysphagia evaluations, 230
dyspnea evaluations, 237
epistaxis evaluations, 267
extremity pain evaluations, 278, 278b
facial dysmorphism evaluations, 298
limp evaluations, 630
lymphadenopathy evaluations, 643–644
wheezing evaluations, 992f–993f
Radioulnar synostosis, 295
Ramsay-Hunt syndrome, 218
Rash
appearance of, 734–737
color of, 740
crusting of, 741
differential diagnosis of, 742b–743b, 744b–745b, 742–745
distribution of, 737, 739
examples of, 735f–737f
patient history and, 733–734
physical examination of, 734–737
scaling of, 742
secondary changes in, 741–742
types of, 734–737
Reactive arthritis, 600
Receptive language deficits, 863
Recurrent respiratory papillomatosis, 542
Red blood cell(s), 47, 55–56
Red diaper syndrome, 396
Red eye
causes of, 760t
differential diagnosis of
allergic reactions, 764, 764f
blepharitis, 765, 769
capillary hemangiomas, 763, 763f
corneal abnormalities, 771–774
corneal abrasion, 771, 771f
episcleritis, 774
eyelid abnormalities, 761–765
eyelid tumors, 763, 763f
herpetic keratitis, 771
hordeola, 764
hyphema, 773, 773f
iritis, 773
ocular myositis, 774
orbital cellulitis, 761–763, 763f
preseptal cellulitis, 761–763, 762f
scleritis, 774
subconjunctival hemorrhage, 769–770, 770f
trauma, 765
uveitis, 773
varicella-zoster virus, 771, 772f
history taking, 759–760
overview of, 759
physical examination of, 760–761
Referrals
abdominal pain, 23–24
alopecia, 37
amenorrhea, 45
anemia, 61
anorexia nervosa, 636
arrhythmias, 109
back pain, 94
cardiac arrhythmias, 109
constipation, 131
cough, 142
delayed puberty, 731
diarrhea, 196–197
dizziness, 220
dysmenorrhea, 224
dysphagia, 233
dyspnea, 243
dysuria, 252
edema, 260
epistaxis, 272–273
extremity pain, 285
failure to thrive, 312
gender expression and identity issues, 437–438
headaches, 449
heart murmurs, 468
hematuria, 476
hemoptysis, 487
hirsutism, 535
hypertension, 518
hypotonia, 557
joint pain, 603–604
language disorders, 866
limp, 630–631
lymphadenopathy, 648
macrocephaly, 654–655
mental health, 780b
microcephaly, 670
murmurs, 468
nonsuicidal self-injury, 802–803, 805
nosebleeds, 273
polyuria, 705, 707
precocious puberty, 731
proteinuria, 716
recurrent infection, 756b
scrotal swelling, 795
scrotal swelling and pain, 795
self-stimulating behaviors, 812, 816
short stature, 824
sleep disorders, 854
sleep disturbances, 854
speech disorders, 866
splenomegaly, 873
substance use, 897
tics, 942–943
torticollis, 951
vertigo, 220
vomiting, 976
weight loss, 984
wheezing, 996
Referred pain, 17, 111
abdomen and, 17

Reflex, let-down, 979
Reflux
hoarseness and, 541
laryngopharyngeal, 541–542
testing, 544
Refractory shock, 348t
Regulatory difficulties, 904b, 906t
Regurgitation, vomiting versus, 971
Rehydration, 181–184
Reiter syndrome, 276, 600
REM behavior disorder, 847
Renal biopsy, 474
Renal disease
edema caused by, 258–260
proteinuria and, 711
short stature caused by, 820
Renal masses, 7
Renal parenchymal disease, 509
Renin, 511
Renin-angiotensin-aldosterone system, 257
Respiratory cycle, 987, 988f
Respiratory syncytial virus, 150, 345
Restless legs syndrome, 847
Restrictive pulmonary disease, 237–238, 239b
Retching, 971
Reticulocyte count, 56–57
Retropharyngeal abscess, 879t
Retroversion, 373b
Rett syndrome, 666
Reverse differential cyanosis, 152
Rheumatic fever, 600
Rifampin, 584
Right-ventricular hypertrophy, 240
Right ventricular outflow tract abnormalities, 152–153
Rigid flatfoot, 386–387
Rizatriptan, 447t
Rocking, 811–812
Romano-Ward syndrome, 923
Rome I, II, and III criteria, for abdominal pain, 14
Rotavirus, 183
Rotor syndrome, 589
Rubinstein-Taybi syndrome, 667
Russell-Silver syndrome, 820

## S

Sacroiliac joint, 627, 628f
Salaam spasms, 948
*Salmonella* enteritis, 189
Sandifer syndrome, 949
Satiety center, 633
Scheuermann disease, 91–92, 94
Schistocytes, 51b–52b
School health, cardiac arrhythmias and, 109
School phobia, 72, 776
School readiness, 608, 609b
School refusal
child-related factors of, 777
definition of, 775
environmental factors of, 778
family-related factors of, 777
long-term sequelae of, 780t
management of, 778–779
parents and, 778–779, 781
prevalence of, 777
prevention of, 780–781
prognosis for, 779–780
Scintigraphy, 232
Scleritis, 774
Scoliosis, 89, 295, 852t
Scotch tape slide test, 953
"Scotty dog with a collar," 90, 91f
Screen for Child Anxiety Related Disorders 2, 64
Screening
adolescent substance use, 890t
anxiety disorders, 64–65, 66t
auditory, 455
depression, 163, 163t
language development, 863, 864t
for sleep complaints, 831t–833t
substance use, 889–890, 890t
Scrotal skin disease, 791
Scrotum
anatomy of, 787f–788f
swelling of
causes of, 786b
diagnostic testing for, 785–786
evaluation of, 785–786
patient history and examination for, 785, 792–793
referral for, 795
treatment of, 788–790
without pain, 791–795
Seal-like cough, 878
Seckel syndrome, 667
Secondary amenorrhea, 39, 43
Secondary hypertension, 508–509
Second heart sound, 459
Second impact syndrome, 571
Seizure(s)
benign neonatal sleep myoclonus versus, 676
febrile, 345
irritability and, 571
syncope and, 924
Selective mutism, 68t
Selective serotonin reuptake inhibitors, 170, 779, 942
Self-biting, 815
Self-cutting, 802
Self-harm. *See* Self-injurious behavior
Self-injurious behavior. *See also* Nonsuicidal self-injury
analysis of, 803–804
in children with intellectual and development disabilities, 799, 804–805

co-occurring disorders with, 801
definition of, 799
diagnostic approach to, 803
epidemiology of, 800
etiology of, 800–801
functional assessment of, 803–804
nonsuicidal self-injury versus, 801
ongoing care for, 805
signs and symptoms of, 803
similarities and differences, 805
syndromes associated with, 801
types of, 799
Self-mutilation, 815
Self-stimulating behaviors
hair pulling and twisting, 815
head banging and rocking, 811–812
masturbation, 813–814
referral for, 812
thumb sucking and nail biting, 812–813
tics versus, 938
Semont maneuver, 217
Sengstaken-Blakemore tube, 405
Sensory, motor, reflex grid, 88f
Sensory abnormalities, 121
Sensory ataxia, 81
Separation anxiety disorder, 64t
Sepsis
definitions associated with, 348t
jaundice associated with, 585
severe, 348t
Septic arthritis, 620, 621t
Septic shock, 348t
Septo-optic dysplasia, 288
Serum bilirubin, 582
Sever disease, 601
Severe combined immunodeficiency, 752, 752t
Severe sepsis, 348t
Sex hormone binding globulin, 524
Sex-reassignment surgery, 410
Sexual abuse, 953
Sexual hair, 525–526
Sexually transmitted infections
urethritis caused by, 250
vaginal bleeding caused by, 955
vaginal discharge caused by, 964
Sexual orientation, 410, 416
Shin splints, 282
Shivering episodes, 675
Shoes
fitting of, 392
leg problems and, 392
Short bowel syndrome, 191
Short stature
diagnostic testing for, 822–823
differential diagnosis of, 819–822
history taking, 822
management of, 823–824
physical examination for, 822
Shuddering attacks, 675
Sickle cell anemia
irritability and, 574
splenomegaly and, 871
Sickle cell disease, 852t
Sick sinus syndrome, 922
Sideroblastic anemias, 54
Silk stocking sign, 793
Simple vocal tics, 935
Single-photon emission computed tomography, 90
SIRS. *See* Systemic inflammatory response syndrome
Situational syncope, 920
Skin gouging, 815
Skin picking, 815
Skull abnormalities, 649, 650b, 652
SLE. *See* Systemic lupus erythematosus
Sleep
average hours, 829t
awakenings from, 840–841
BEARS parent questionnaire for, 830
developmental milestones of, 828–830, 829t
evaluation of, 830–836
excessive, 848t
hygiene principles and, 835b
inadequate, 839b
violence during, 847
Sleep deprivation, 165t, 207t, 562t, 610t, 906
Sleep disorders
behavioral disorder associations, 850t, 850–851
benign neonatal sleep myoclonus, 675–676
causes of, 838t, 840t
classification of, 836–847
developmental disorder associations, 851
maturational issues and, 836–847
medical problem associations, 851–854, 852t–853t
narcolepsy, 676–677
night terrors, 676
parasomnias, 843–846
questions for evaluation, 831t–833t
referrals and, 854
Sleep log, 833f–834f
Sleep myoclonus, 675–676
Sleep-onset association disorder, 837–838, 841–842
Sleep paralysis, 676
Sleep terrors, 676, 846
Sleep–wake transition disorder, 848
Sleepwalking, 846
Slipped capital femoral epiphysis, 282–283, 601, 623–624
Slow transit, 121
Slump test, 91, 92f
Small-for-gestational-age infants, 820
Smith-Lemli-Opitz syndrome, 296–297
Social-emotional problems
assessment of, 903, 905, 909
background of, 901–903

Social-emotional problems *(continued)*
differential diagnosis of, 906t–908t, 909f
epidemiology of, 901–903
findings suggestive of, 903, 904b
healthy habits and activities, 911
identification of, 903
initial interventions for, 911, 912t–913t
parental considerations, 910
plan of care for, 909–914
positive parent-child interactions, 911
primary care physician's role in, 902
progress monitoring of, 913
reframing of child's behaviors, 910–911
safety considerations, 910
screening for, 905t
specialist involvement for, 913–914
Social phobia, 64t
Social skills, 169
Sodium nitroprusside, 518t
Solvent drag, 174–175
Somatic symptom disorder, 659, 659t
Somnambulism, 846
Sorbitol, 176
Soto syndrome, 291
Soy protein allergy, 398
Space-occupying lesions, 649, 650b, 652
Spasmus nutans, 948
Specialists
for anxiety disorders, 73–74
for depression, 170–171
for disruptive behavior and aggression, 210–213
for inattention and impulsivity, 566
for learning difficulties, 614
for social-emotional problems, 913–914
Specific language impairment, 866
Specific phobia, 64t
Speech and language pathologist, 866–867
Speech disorders
description of, 865
differential diagnosis of, 866
prevalence of, 859
prognosis for, 867
referral for, 866
treatment of, 866–867
Spence Children's Anxiety Scale, 64
Spermatoceles, 795
Spherocytes, 51b
Spina bifida, 853t
Spinal muscular atrophy, 335
Spinning behavior, 815
Spironolactone, 534
Spleen
cysts of, 872
disorders of, 872
dysfunction of, 748
function of, 869
palpation of, 869
Splenomegaly
definition of, 869
differential diagnosis of, 869–872, 870b
imaging for, 872–873
laboratory testing for, 872
patient history and, 872
physical examination for, 872
referral for, 873
treatment of, 873
Splenoptosis, 872
Spondyloarthropathy, 598
Spondylolisthesis, 86, 90
Spondylolysis, 86, 90, 93
Spontaneous pneumothorax, 114, 115t
Sports
classification of, 517f
participation in, by children with hypertension, 516
Sprain, 281
Spurious torticollis, 950
Staphylococcal infection, 93
*Staphylococcus aureus,* 599
Steatorrhea, 173
Steeple sign, 881
Steppage gait, 627t
Stereotypies, 811, 938
Sternocleidomastoid muscle, 947
Still disease, 598
Stimulants
short stature caused by, 820–821
treatment for insomnia, 851
Stokes-Adams attacks, 922
Stomach, distended, 6f
Stomatocyte, 52b
Stool
blood in, 178b, 179, 181
failure to thrive diagnosis and, 307
withholding of, 120–121
Stool-withholding behaviors, 130
Storage disorders, 491
Stork test, 90
Straight-leg raise test, 91
Strengths and Difficulties Questionnaire, 205
Stress reduction, 71, 168–169, 209, 564, 613, 894
Stridor
croup as cause of, 150
definition of, 877
diagnostic testing for, 880–883
differential diagnosis of, 877–878, 879t
history taking for, 878–880
hoarseness and, 543
management of, 883–885
physical examination for, 880
spirometry findings for, 881f
Stroke, 79–80
Students Against Destructive Decisions, 890
Sturge-Weber syndrome, 763
Stuttering, 865

Subconjunctival hemorrhage, 769–770, 770f
Subdural hematomas, 652
Subglottic hemangiomas, 541, 545
Subglottic lesions, 884f
Subglottic obstruction, 881f
Subglottic stenosis, 879t
Subluxation, radial head, 282
Substance use
  in adolescents
    brain development considerations, 887–888
    screening for, 890t
    treatment of, 898
  advice and counseling, 890
  alcohol, 891, 891t
  assessment of, 890–891, 891t
  conditions co-occurring with, 892t
  confidentiality and, 889
  counseling to reduce, 895
  disruptive behavior and aggression, 206, 208t
  dyspnea caused by, 242
  health problems associated with, 888
  interventions based on stage of, 895, 896t
  motivational interviewing for reduction of, 895, 897t
  overview of, 887
  prevalence of, 888
  referral for, 897
  screening tools for, 889–890, 890t
  specialty treatment for, 895, 897–898
Substance use disorders
  assessment of, 890–891, 891t
  classification of, 888–889
  description of, 887
  general care for, 894–898, 896t–897t
  laboratory testing for, 894
  physical examination of, 893
  stress reduction, 894
Sudden cardiac death, 107–109
Sudden death, 116
Suicidal intent, 206
Suicidality, 171t
Suicide attempts, nonsuicidal self-injury versus, 802
Suicide risks, 166b
Sumatriptan, 447t
Supraventricular tachycardia
  definition of, 100–101
  diagnosis of, 101–102, 102f
  in infants, 97
  irritability and, 574
  management of, 102–104
  presentation of, 101–102
  syncope and, 923
Surgery
  abdominal pain treated with, 15, 17
  dysmenorrhea treated with, 224
SVT. *See* Supraventricular tachycardia
Swallowing, 227
Sweating, excessive, 549–550
Symptomatic proteinuria, 713
Syncope
  causes of, 919–924, 920b
  characteristics of, 674
  definition of, 674, 919
  diagnostic testing for, 925–926
  management of, 926–927
  patient history and examination for, 925
Syndactyly, 296, 389f, 390
Synovial fluid, 621t
Systemic inflammatory response syndrome, 347, 347t–348t
Systemic lupus erythematosus
  joint pain and, 598
  limp caused by, 625
Systemic-onset disease, 598
Systolic blood pressure, 510
Systolic murmurs, 464, 464t, 465f

## T

Tachyarrhythmias, 923
Tachycardia
  intra-atrial re-entrant, 104
  supraventricular
    definition of, 100–101
    diagnosis of, 101–102, 102f
    in infants, 97
    irritability and, 574
    management of, 102–104
    presentation of, 101–102
    syncope and, 923
  ventricular
    description of, 105–106, 106f
    syncope and, 923
Tailor bunion, 390
Talc granulomatosis, 242
Taliglucerase alpha, 493
Talipes, 373b
Talipes calcaneovalgus, 383, 384f
Talipes equinovarus, 383, 384f
Talipes varus, 374, 375f, 376
Talocalcaneal coalition, 387
Tardive dyskinesia, 941
Tarsal coalition, 386–387, 623
T cells, 752
Teardrop cells, 51b
Teething, 575
Telogen effluvium, 27
Temper tantrums, 903, 929–932
Tension pneumothorax, 489
Tension type headaches, 443–444, 448
Teratogenic agent, 288
Terbinafine, 35
Terminal hair, 523
Testes
  nonsalvageable, 788f
  tumors of, 793–794
Testicular torsion, 786–789
Testosterone, 524

Tetralogy of Fallot, 152, 924
"Tet spells," 152–153
Thalassemia
  β-, 53
  major, 53
Thelarche, 530, 728
Thigh–foot angle, 377
Thin basement membrane nephropathy, 475
Third heart sound, 116, 459
Three-dimensional airway reconstruction, 995f
Thrombocytopenia
  epistaxis caused by, 266
  petechiae and purpura and, 695–696
Thrombotic thrombocytopenic purpura, 696
Thrush, 747
Thumb sucking, 812–813
Thyroid disease, 338
Tibial torsion, 376–378
Tick bites, 599–600
Tics
  clinical manifestations of, 935
  comorbid disorders, 938–939
  definition of, 935
  differential diagnosis of, 938
  etiology of, 936–938
  incidence of, 935–936
  management of, 942–943
  pharmacotherapy for, 940–942
  referral for, 942–943
  treatment of, 939–943
Tilt-table testing, 926
Timed urine sample, 710
Tinea capitis, 34–36, 35f
Tinea corporis, 741f
To-and-fro murmurs, 466, 467f
Tobacco use, 888
Toddler's diarrhea, 185
Toe deformities, 388–390, 389f
Toe-walking, 390–391
Toilet training, 130
TORCH infections, 585
Torsades de pointes, 923
Torsion, 373b
Torticollis
  clinical manifestations of, 947–948
  congenital, 947–951
  definition of, 947
  differential diagnosis of, 948–950, 949b
  evaluation of, 950
  management of, 950–951
  ocular, 948
  referral for, 951
Total anomalous pulmonary venous return, 152, 154
Tourette syndrome, 935–936, 938, 942. *See also* Tics
Toxic synovitis, 283
Toxins
  ataxia and, 81
  body odor caused by ingestion or inhalation of, 682, 684t, 685
  irritability and, 575
Tracheal stenosis, 994f
Tracheobronchomalacia, 992, 994f
Trained night waking, 841–842
Transactional model, 306
Transgender, 410, 415–417
Transgender adolescents, 418–419, 427–429
Transient hypogammaglobulinemia of infancy, 751t
Transient proteinuria, 712
Transient synovitis, 625
Transposition of the great arteries, 152–154
Trauma
  ataxia and, 80–81
  dysuria caused by, 251
  head, syncope and, 924
  hoarseness and, 542, 546
  irritability and, 569–571, 572
  limp caused by, 619
  red eye caused by, 765
  scrotal pain and swelling caused by, 791
Traumatic brain injuries, 853t
Treacher-Collins syndrome, 293f
Trendelenburg gait, 627t
Trichobezoar, 33, 815
*Trichomonas vaginalis,* 967
Trichorrhexis nodosa, 30
Trichotillomania, 33, 34f, 815
Tricuspid atresia, 153
Tricuspid valve, 153
Triptans, 447, 447t
Truancy, 775, 781
Truncus arteriosus, 154
Trypsinogen, 189
Tufting enteropathy, 194
Tumor(s). *See also* Malignancies; Neoplasms
  abdominal, 8
  ataxia and, 80
  eyelid, 763, 763f
  hoarseness caused by, 542
  testicular, 793–794
  Wilms, 8, 8f
Turner syndrome
  description of, 295, 295f
  short stature in girls and, 820
Tympanitic abdomen
  children and, 6–7
  newborns and, 4–6
Tyrosinemia type 1, 586

## U

Ulcers
  corneal, 771, 772f
  skin, 737
Unconjugated bilirubin, 582

Unconjugated hyperbilirubinemia, 582–584, 583b, 587, 588b
Undernutrition, 310–311, 311b
Unhappy mood, 904b
Upper airway hemorrhage, 484t
Upper airway obstruction, 150
Upper gastrointestinal tract
  barium study of, 231
  bleeding in, 398, 401b
Urethral prolapse, 251
Urethral strictures, 251
Urethritis, 250–251
Urinary tract
  description of, 7
  pain, 247
Urinary tract infections
  dysuria caused by, 248, 250
  fever caused by, 354
Urine
  normal output, 699t
  odor of
    causes of, 682, 685
    differential diagnosis of, 681–682
    metabolic abnormalities as cause of, 682, 683t
    physical examination of, 682
  protein-creatinine ratio, 710
Urticaria
  description of, 737f
  pruritus and, 721
Utah Growth Study, 819, 821
Uterine bleeding, 956b
Uveitis, 773

**V**

Vaccinations, 576
VACTERL, 289
Vaginal bleeding
  causes of, 956b
  diagnostic testing for, 957–958
  evaluation of, 954–958
  history taking, 955–957
  management of, 958–959
  in newborn, 396
  physical examination for, 957
  in prepubertal girls, 953–954
  in pubertal girls, 954–959
Vaginal discharge
  causes of, 964b, 966t
  evaluation of, 963–965
  management of, 965, 967–968
  in newborns, 963
  in prepubertal girls, 963–965, 964b
  in pubertal and postpubertal girls, 966t, 967–968
Vaginal maturation index, 43
Vaginal odor, 681
Vaginitis, 953, 955, 964
Valgus, 373b
Valproic acid, 288
Valsalva maneuver, 120
Variceal bleeding, 405
Varicella zoster
  intraocular manifestations of, 772
  rash, 741f
  recurrent infections and, 747
Varicocele, 795
Varus, 373b
Vascular abnormalities, 993f
Vascular congestion, 491
Vascular lesions, 400
Vascular pulmonary disease, 239–240
Vasculitis, 400
Vasoactive intestinal polypeptide, 177
Vasodilators, 511, 515t
Vaso-occlusive crisis, 86, 93
Vasopressin, 699–700, 704t–705t, 706
Vasovagal syncope, 919
Vaulting gait, 627t
Vein of Galen arteriovenous malformation, 653
Vela-glucerase, 493
Vellus hair, 523, 524f
Venous admixture, 149
Venous hypertension, 257
Venous thromboembolism, 259
Ventilation-perfusion mismatch, 148–149, 151
Ventricular septal defect, 153
Ventricular tachycardia
  description of, 105–106, 106f
  syncope and, 923
Vernal conjunctivitis, 768
Version, 373b
Vertebral osteomyelitis, 86
Vertigo
  benign paroxysmal, 674–675
  causes of, 216–218
  definition of, 216
  diagnosis of, 219t
  evaluation of, 218
  management of, 220
  migraine headache as cause of, 82
  referrals and, 220
Vesicles, 734, 738f, 740f
Videofluorographic swallowing study, 231
Videostroboscopy, 543
Videotaping, 231
Viral conjunctivitis, 765t, 766, 766f
Viral croup, 878, 879t
Viral enteritis, 183
Viral infections
  fever caused by, 363, 364b
  lymphadenopathy caused by, 640t
  splenomegaly and, 870
Viral laryngitis, 545–546
Virilization, 523, 528, 535
Virus
  Epstein-Barr, 333
  herpes simplex, 740f
  respiratory syncytial, 150, 345
  rotavirus, 183

Vitamin $B_{12}$ deficiency, 57
Vocabulary, 863
Vocal cords
  cyst of, 879t
  paralysis of
    hoarseness and, 539, 545
    stridor caused by, 879t
Vocal tics, 935
Volume expansion, 927
Vomiting
  causes of, 972–974, 973b
  complications with, 974
  definition of, 971
  differential diagnosis of, 972–974
  evaluation of, 974
  failure to thrive diagnosis and, 307
  referral for, 976
  treatment of, 975–976
  weight loss and, 980
von Willebrand disease
  description of, 266
  petechiae and purpura caused by, 695
VT. *See* Ventricular tachycardia
Vulnerable child syndrome, 781
Vulvovaginitis, 252

**W**
Wadell test, 88
Wasting, 302
Water deprivation test, 705t
Weakness
  definition of, 329
  diagnostic testing for, 337–338
  differential diagnosis of, 331b
  etiology of, 330
Weight, hypertension and, 498, 498f, 514
Weight gain, healthy, 303–304
Weight loss
  admission for, 984–985
  in adolescents, 982, 985
  diagnostic testing for, 983t, 983–984
  differential diagnosis of, 981b
  in infants, 979–980
  initial evaluation of, 983–984
  in newborns, 979–980
  referral for, 984
Well-child visits
  6-month, 930
  12-month, 930
Wenckebach block, 106
Werdnig-Hoffman disease, 335, 554
Wheals, 734, 737f
Wheezing
  causes of, 990t
  definition of, 987
  diagnostic testing for, 990–992, 991f–996f
  differential diagnosis of, 987–989
  management of, 993–994, 996
  patient history for, 989
  physical examination for, 989
  referral for, 996
Wilms tumor, 8, 8f
Wilson disease, 491, 493, 589
Wiskott-Aldrich syndrome, 752t, 753
Wolff-Parkinson-White syndrome, 101, 923
Woodruff plexus, 264
World Professional Association for Transgender Health, 411, 431

**X**
X-linked agammaglobulinemia, 751, 751t
X-rays. *See* Radiographs

**Y**
*Yersinia* enterocolitis, 179, 190

**Z**
Zinc acetate, 493
Zolmitriptan, 447t